ATLAS OF
Clinical
Neurology

SECOND EDITION

EDITED BY

Roger N. Rosenberg, MD

PROFESSOR OF NEUROLOGY AND PHYSIOLOGY

ZALE DISTINGUISHED CHAIR IN NEUROLOGY

THE UNIVERSITY OF TEXAS SOUTHWESTERN MEDICAL CENTER

SENIOR NEUROLOGIST

ZALE-LIPSHY UNIVERSITY HOSPITAL AND PARKLAND MEMORIAL HOSPITAL

DALLAS, TEXAS, USA

With 56 Contributors

DEVELOPED BY CURRENT MEDICINE, INC.

PHILADELPHIA

Current Medicine, Inc.

400 Market Street, Suite 700
Philadelphia, PA 19106

Developmental Editors
Bill Edelman and Teresa M. Giuliana

Editorial Assistant
Annmarie D'Ortona

Illustrators
Wieslawa Langenfeld, Maureen Looney, Paul Schiffmacher

Cover Design
William Whitman

Interior Design and Layout
John McCullough

Assistant Production Manager
Simon Dickey

Indexing
Susan Thomas

• •

Atlas of clinical neurology / editor-in-chief, Roger N. Rosenberg, with 56 con-
tributors.—2nd ed.
     p. cm.
   Includes bibliographical references and index.
   ISBN 1-57340-175-7 (alk. paper)
   1. Nervous system—Diseases—Atlases. 2. Neurology—Atlases.
   [DNLM: Nervous System Diseases—Atlases. WL 17 A8814 2001]
I. Title: Clinical neurology. II. Rosenberg, Roger N.
RC358.8 .A85 2001
616.8'002'2—dc21

                                            2001017180

• •

Every effort has been made to ensure that the drug dosage schedules within this text are
accurate and conform to standards at the time of publication. However, as treatment recommendations vary in the light of continuing research and clinical experience, the reader
is advised to verify drug dosage schedules herein with information found on product
information sheets. This is especially true in cases of new or infrequently used drugs.

Printed by Jaypee Brothers Medical Publishers (P) Ltd. New Delhi, India

10 9 8 7 6 5 4 3 2 1

Contributors

Hakan Ay, MD
Cayyolu, Ankara, Turkey

Alma R. Bicknese, MD
Assistant Professor
Department of Neurology
St. Louis University
Child Neurologist
Cardinal Glennon Children's Hospital
St. Louis, Missouri

Anish Bhardwaj, MD
Assistant Professor
Department of Neurology, Neurological Surgery,
  Anesthesiology, and Critical Care Medicine
Johns Hopkins University School of Medicine
Associate Director, Neurosciences/Critical Care
  Division
Johns Hopkins Hospital
Baltimore, Maryland

Shawn J. Bird, MD
Associate Professor
Department of Neurology
Director, Electromyography Laboratory
University of Pennsylvania
Philadelphia, Pennsylvania

Thomas D. Bird, MD
Professor
Department of Neurology
University of Washington
Staff Neurologist
VA Medical Center
Seattle, Washington

Susan Bressman, MD
Professor
Department of Neurology
Albert Einstein College of Medicine
Chairman
Department of Neurology
Beth Israel Medical Center
New York, New York

Ufuk Can, MD
Associate Professor
Department of Neurology
Baskent University
Ankara, Turkey

James R. Couch, Jr., MD, PhD
Professor and Chair
Department of Neurology
University of Oklahoma Health Sciences Center
Oklahoma City, Oklahoma

Steven C. Cramer, MD
Assistant Professor
Department of Neurology
University of Washington
Seattle, Washington

Antonio R. Damasio, MD, PhD
M.W. Van Allen Professor and Head
Department of Neurology
University of Iowa College of Medicine
Iowa City, Iowa

Hanna Damasio, MD
Professor
Department of Neurology
University of Iowa College of Medicine
Iowa City, Iowa

Marthand Eswara, MD
Clinical Assistant Professor
Department of Pediatrics
Stanford University
Palo Alto, California
Consultant in Genetics
Santa Clara Valley Medical Center
San Jose, California

Stanley Fahn, MD
Director, Movement Disorder Group
Department of Neurology
Columbia University
H. Houston Merritt Professor of Neurology
New York Presbyterian Hospital
New York, New York

Glen Alan Fenton, MD
Assistant Professor
Department of Neurology
St. Louis University
St. Louis, Missouri

Karen L. Fink, MD, PhD
Assistant Professor
Department of Neurology
University of Texas Medical Center at Dallas
Dallas, Texas

Seth P. Finklestein, MD
Associate Professor
Department of Neurology
Associate Neurologist
Massachusetts General Hospital
Boston, Massachusetts

Blair Ford, MD
Assistant Professor
Department of Neurology
Columbia University
New York, New York

Gary P. Foster, MD, FACC
Director, Echocardiography
Rogue Valley Medical Center and Providence
  Medford Medical Center
Medford, Oregon

Karen Furie, MD, MPH
Instructor
Department of Neurology
Assistant in Neurology
Massachusetts General Hospital
Boston, Massachusetts

Thomas J. Geller, MD
Assistant Professor
Department of Neurology
St. Louis University
Director, Child Neurology Division
Cardinal Glennon Children's Hospital
St. Louis, Missouri

Bruce G. Gold, PhD
Scientist and Associate Professor
Department of Cell and Developmental Biology
Center for Research on Occupational and
  Environmental Toxicology (CROET)
Oregon Health Sciences Center
Portland, Oregon

Thomas J. Grabowski, Jr., MD
Associate Professor
Departments of Neurology and Radiology
University of Iowa College of Medicine
Iowa City, Iowa

Dorothy K. Grange, MD
Associate Professor
Department of Pediatrics
St. Louis University
Director, Division of Medical Genetics
Cardinal Glennon Children's Hospital
St. Louis, Missouri

Steven M. Greenberg, MD, PhD
Assistant Professor
Department of Neurology
Harvard Medical School
Co-Director
Massachusetts General Hospital
Boston, Massachusetts

Paul E. Greene, MD
Associate Professor of Clinical Neurology
Department of Neurology
Columbia University
Associate Attending in Neurology
Columbia-Presbyterian Medical Center
New York, New York

Daniel F. Hanley, MD
Jeffrey and Harriet Legum Professor of Acute Care
  Neurology
Department of Neurology
Cornell University Medical Center
New York, New York
Jeffrey and Harriet Legum Professor of Acute Care
  Neurology
Johns Hopkins Medical Institutions
Baltimore, Maryland

Burk Jubelt, MD
Professor and Chairman
Department of Neurology
SUNY Upstate Medical University
Chief of Neurology
SUNY University Hospital
Syracuse, New York

J. Philip Kistler, MD
Professor
Department of Neurology
Harvard Medical School
Director of Stroke Service
Massachusetts General Hospital
Boston, Massachusetts

Walter J. Koroshetz, MD
Associate Professor
Department of Neurology
Harvard Medical School
Director, NICU
Massachusetts General Hospital
Boston, Massachusetts

Suresh Kotagal, MB, BS
Professor
Department of Neurology
Mayo School of Medicine
Senior Associate Consultant
Mayo Clinic
Rochester, Minnesota

Marc E. Lenaerts, MD
Assistant Professor
Department of Neurology
University of Oklahoma Health Sciences Center
Oklahoma City, Oklahoma

David S. Martin, MD, FACR
Associate Professor
Department of Radiology
St. Louis University
Attending Neuroradiologist
Cardinal Glennon Children's Hospital
St. Louis, Missouri

Marek A. Mirski, MD, PhD
Associate Professor
Departments of Anesthesiology, Neurology, and
  Neurosurgery
Johns Hopkins University School of Medicine
Chief, Neuroanesthesiology
Director, Neuroscience Critical Care Unit
Johns Hopkins Hospital
Baltimore, Maryland

Michael A. Nigro, DO
Professor
Departments of Neurology and Psychiatry
Wayne State University School of Medicine
Detroit, Michigan

Christopher S. Ogilvy, MD
Associate Professor of Surgery
Department of Surgery
Harvard Medical School
Boston, Massachusetts

Thomas Pittman, MD
Associate Professor
Department of Surgery
University of Kentucky
Lexington, Kentucky

David Pleasure, MD
Professor
Departments of Neurology and Pediatrics
University of Pennsylvania
Director, Joseph Stokes, Jr. Research Institute
The Children's Hospital of Philadelphia
Philadelphia, Pennsylvania

Alexander Razumovsky, PhD
Assistant Professor
Departments of Anesthesiology/Critical Care
  Medicine and Neurology
Johns Hopkins University School of Medicine
Baltimore, Maryland

Stacie L. Ropka, PhD
Research Assistant Professor
Department of Neurology
SUNY Upstate Medical University
Syracuse, New York

Guy Rordorf, MD
Assistant Professor
Department of Neurology
Harvard Medical School
Associate Director Neuroscience ICU
Massachusetts General Hospital
Boston, Massachusetts

Elisabeth J. Rushing, MD
Associate Professor
Department of Pathology
University of Texas Southwestern Medical Center
Dallas, Texas

Steven Scherer, MD, PhD
Associate Professor
Department of Neurology
University of Pennsylvania
Philadelphia, Pennsylvania

Jerome V. Schnell, PhD
Research Associate
Center for Research on Occupational and
  Environmental Toxicology
Oregon Health Sciences University
Portland, Oregon

S. Clifford Schold, Jr., MD
Professor
Department of Neurology
University of Pittsburgh Medical Center
Pittsburgh, Pennsylvania

Donald Schotland, MD
Professor Emeritus
Department of Neurology
University of Pennsylvania
Philadelphia, Pennsylvania

John T. Sladky, MD
Professor
Departments of Neurology and Pediatrics
Emory University School of Medicine
Atlanta, Georgia

Martin Smrčka, MD
Research Fellow
Department of Neurosurgery
Massachusetts General Hospital
Boston, Massachusetts

Peter S. Spencer, PhD, FRCPath
Professor
Department of Neurology
Oregon Health Sciences University
Director and Senior Scientist
Center for Research on Occupational and
  Environmental Toxicology
Portland, Oregon

S. Mark Sumi, MD
Professor Emeritus
Departments of Neurology and Pathology
University of Washington
Seattle, Washington

Nijasri C. Suwanwela, MD
Associate Professor
Department of Medicine
Chulalongkorn University
Bangkok, Thailand

Nitaya Suwanwela, MD
Professor
Department of Radiology
Chulalongkorn University
Bangkok, Thailand

Michael R. Swenson, MD, MSc
Professor and Chair
Department of Neurology
University of Louisville
Louisville, Kentucky

Daniel Tranel, PhD
Professor
Department of Neurology
University of Iowa College of Medicine
Iowa City, Iowa

John A. Ulatowski, MD, PhD, MBA
Associate Professor
Department of Anesthesiology
Johns Hopkins University School of Medicine
Vice Chairman for Clinical Affairs
Johns Hopkins Hospital
Baltimore, Maryland

Paul C. Van Ness, MD
Associate Professor
Department of Neurology
University of Texas Southwestern Medical Center
Dallas, Texas

Earl A. Zimmerman, MD
Professor and Bender Endowed Chair
Department of Neurology
Albany Medical School
Albany, New York

Preface

The year 2001 marks the beginning of a new millenium, and the second edition of the *Atlas of Clinical Neurology* highlights and underscores the enormous strides being made in the biologic understanding of neurologic disease. Neurology is a highly visual specialty. The neurologic examination, magnetic resonance imaging, electroencephalography, positron-emission tomographic (PET) and functional magnetic resonance (fMRI) scanning, and light- and electron-microscopy are examples of visual images that define neurologic disease and normal brain functions. This *Atlas of Clinical Neurology* has been designed to provide a pictorial comprehensive visual exposition and integration of all aspects of neurologic disease, including clinical syndromes and related neuropathology, neuroradiology, neurophysiology, neuropharmacology, neurochemistry, and molecular biology. The goal is to provide a holistic visual concept of neurologic disease to allow the clinician an overall image of a specific neurologic disorder. Quality patient management requires the good judgment and factual knowledge of an experienced physician. The *Atlas of Clinical Neurology* is intended to provide essential information about neurologic disease in an immediate and integrated manner to facilitate the neurologist in the primary function of providing excellence in patient care.

There has been great progress in the past decade in our understanding of the cellular and molecular basis of many neurologic diseases. New therapies have been developed as a result of this recent knowledge. Thrombolytic therapy for stroke, pallidotomy for Parkinson's disease, new classes of anti-convulsants, and effective immune therapy for multiple sclerosis represent examples of recent significant therapeutic advances in neurology. A new chapter on headache syndromes and their therapies is included in the second edition because of its clear clinical significance and recent advances in therapy. Of great importance to the understanding of gene structure and function in the nervous system has been the discovery of DNA triplet repeat expansions in autosomal dominant neurogenetic diseases, including Huntington's disease, olivopontocerebellar atrophy (SCA1), Machado-Joseph disease, dentatorubropallidoluysian atrophy, fragile-X disease, myotonic muscular dystrophy, and most recently Friedreich's ataxia. The leading cause of dementia in our society affecting over 4 million Americans and countless millions more around the world, Alzheimer's disease (AD), has been shown to be a clinical syndrome due to specific different genetic mutations in selected families with dominantly inherited disease. Mutations in the amyloid precursor protein gene (chromosome 21), the presenilin 1 gene (chromosome 14), and the presenilin 2 gene (chromosome 1) result in dominantly inherited AD. A major risk factor for AD is the presence of the E4 allele of apolipoprotein E (chromosome 19). Additional detailed images related to the dementias are included in the second edition of the *Atlas*. These clinical-molecular correlations are all very recent and attest to the scientific vigor of current neuroscientific research. It is my view that these new data will lead in the near future to effective new therapy for AD that will slow its rate of progress and reduce significantly the incidence of this major, debilitating disease. Positron-emission tomographic and fMRI brain scanning have effectively defined regional brain areas for behaviors. The clarity of insights into heterogeneous brain functions by PET and fMRI is literally revolutionizing our concepts about how our brain thinks.

The topics covered in this *Atlas* represent the most common and important neurologic diseases authored by authorities in their field. The descriptive text for each disease sets the stage for use of the detailed images both for self-instruction and also for lecture presentations. Several hundred images, algorithms, tables, and schematic drawings have been selected carefully for their clarity in conveying the essence of a particular disorder. The collection of figures for a specific disease is intended to provide a thorough and comprehensive description that enables the clinician to generate a clear concept of current thinking about pathogenesis of that disorder and finally a framework for rational therapy. These images are now available in print in the second edition of the *Atlas* and are also available for convenient use in a CD-ROM format.

I am grateful to my colleagues for conceptualizing the *Atlas* with me initially and for updating the second edition. Our overall educational objectives of integrating illustrated text with well-focused images to provide the final detailed visual imprint of each neurologic disorder have been achieved. We believe our efforts provide highly useful educational material for the student and teacher alike. It is important to recognize those who have assisted in the entire process of formulating and producing this *Atlas*. First to be recognized is Abe Krieger, President of Current Medicine, who conceived the *Atlas* series; and to Bill Edelman, a most efficient and effective Developmental Editor.

It is our hope that the *Atlas of Clinical Neurology* will be of value to neurologists and physicians of all specialties caring for patients with neurologic disorders, as well as neurologic investigators and teachers of neurology, and in the final analysis that it will benefit our patients.

Roger N. Rosenberg, MD

Contents

1

Developmental Diseases of the Nervous System

Suresh Kotagal • Alma R. Bicknese • Marthand Eswara
Glen A. Fenton • Thomas J. Geller • Dorothy K. Grange
David S. Martin • Michael A. Nigro • Thomas Pittman

THIS chapter covers a varied group of disorders of inherited, postinfectious, ischemic, or undetermined etiology. All lead to abnormal development of the nervous system. Some disorders have been selected because of the challenge they pose in diagnosis and management, and others because they illustrate important concepts in neuroembryology or pathophysiology.

Advances in molecular genetics play an ever-increasing role in furthering our understanding of congenital central nervous system malformations; for example, certain cases of schizencephaly have been linked to germline mutations in homeobox genes [1]. Using fluorescent in situ hybridization techniques, most cases of lissencephaly have now been linked to deletions in chromosome 17p13.3 and the *LIS1* gene, located in this region [2]. Prader Willi syndrome, Angelman syndrome, fragile X syndrome, and achondroplasia are some other congenital anomalies with well-established genetic mutations.

A thorough general physical examination provides valuable diagnostic information in infants and children manifesting seizures and developmental delay. Nowhere is this concept more true than with the *phakomatoses*, clues to the specific diagnosis of which become apparent during a careful general physical examination. We now also have a better understanding of the mechanisms underlying abnormal cell proliferation and synaptogenesis in some neurocutaneous syndromes. For example, mutations in the neurofibromatosis type I gene located on chromosome 17 lead to loss of the gene product, neurofibromin, which normally plays a role in down-regulating *ras*, a protooncogene protein [3].

As a general rule, the more severe the disturbance of brain development, the earlier the onset of clinical symptoms. Seizures, microcephaly, macrocephaly, hemiparesis, external defects, and developmental delay therefore regularly accompany developmental disorders presenting in infancy or early childhood.

Myelomeningocele

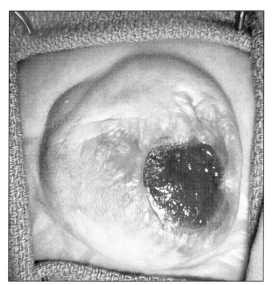

Figure 1-1. A myelomeningocele. About one child in 1000 is born with a myelomeningocele. Symptoms vary depending on the level of the lesion. Bowel and bladder dysfunction are nearly universal, but motor disability is specific to the functional level; that is, children with thoracic lesions have flaccid paraplegia, whereas those with lumbar lesions have various degrees of lower extremity weakness. Almost all affected children have hydrocephalus; many have macrocephaly apparent at birth, but others do not develop signs of intracranial hypertension until the back has been surgically closed. Over 90% of patients with myelomeningocele have asymptomatic type II Chiari malformations that require no treatment. The treatment of children with myelomeningoceles that require intervention involves back closure, usually performed within the first 24 hours of life; delay beyond that time increases the likelihood of infection. A ventriculoperitoneal shunt can be placed at the same time, but many neurosurgeons prefer to perform the two procedures separately. Many children will have problems with bony deformity and contractures, and almost all with higher lesions ultimately develop scoliosis. Recurrent urinary tract infections, ureteral reflux associated with a spastic bladder, and problems with continence and sexual function are also common. Finally, as they grow, some patients with myelomeningocele become symptomatic from tethering of the spinal cord, manifested by back pain, progressive weakness, and changes in bowel and bladder habits. Symptomatic tethering usually requires operative intervention.

The outlook for patients with a myelomeningocele today is much better than in the past. Now a productive life is the norm, and treatment of these children is usually productive. Research on the effect of maternal vitamin supplementation on the incidence of the disease offers hope for prevention, whereas changes in medical management offer better lives for those affected [4,5].

Anencephaly

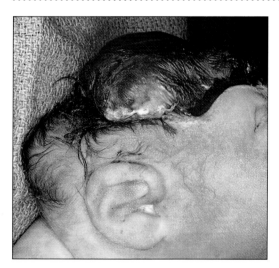

Figure 1-2. Lateral view of an infant with anencephaly showing the lack of normal development of the brain, skull, and scalp. Anencephaly and other neural tube defects can be diagnosed prenatally through maternal serum alpha-fetoprotein screening and fetal ultrasonography. All cases of anencephaly should be detectable by ultrasonography by 14 weeks of gestation with state-of-the-art equipment [6]. After the first affected offspring, the recurrence risk for any neural tube defect in a subsequent pregnancy is approximately 4%. Neural tube defects are thought to result from multifactorial inheritance, in which a group of genes inherited from each parent acts in association with environmental factors to produce the defect [7]. It has been shown that maternal folic acid deficiency can contribute to the incidence of neural tube defects. For women who have had a previous pregnancy with a neural tube defect, the consumption of folic acid, 4 mg/d, can reduce the recurrence risk to 0.5% to 1% [4]. To reduce the overall incidence of neural tube defects, it is now recommended that all women of childbearing age should ingest folic acid, 0.4 mg/d [5]. Since the average intake of dietary folic acid is about 0.2 mg/d, government agencies are recommending peri-conceptional maternal folic acid supplementation [8]. The genes mutated in several mouse models of neural tube defects involve actin regulation, supporting the postulation that actin plays a key role in neurulation [9].

Encephalocele

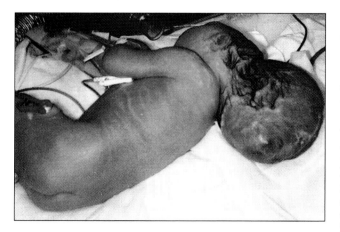

Figure 1-3. Newborn infant with a massive occipital encephalocele. An encephalocele is a neural tube defect that involves extrusion of cranial contents through a bony defect in the skull [10]. The pathogenesis is poorly understood, but

most likely involves defective development of the skull base [11]. Encephaloceles can be located anywhere along the midline of the cranium, although most appear in the occipital (70% to 80%) or frontal locations [7,10]. Parietal, nasal, and nasopharyngeal lesions may occur as well. Temporal lesions are the least common. Most defects are skin covered, although some have only a thin membranous covering that can rupture during delivery or with manipulation. The clinical consequences and prognosis are related directly to the contents of the encephalocele sac rather than the size of the defect. The infant shown had severe microcephaly with a bony defect in the occipital region of the skull; most of the brain tissue was contained within the encephalocele sac. Approximately 20% of affected children are mentally retarded or have neurologic abnormalities [7]. There is a high frequency of associated anomalies of the brain, such as neuronal migrational defects, absent corpus callosum, hydrocephalus, and posterior fossa anomalies, including Dandy-Walker and Arnold-Chiari malformations [7]. Extracranial anomalies occur more often with encephalocele than with other neural tube defects. All infants with encephaloceles should be examined carefully for additional anomalies, because a significant number of recognizable genetic syndromes include encephaloceles. The presence of a specific syndrome would alter the recurrence risk figures for future pregnancies. Encephaloceles occur in 1 in 5000 to 1 in 10,000 births [7]. The recurrence risk for future pregnancies after the first affected child is about 6%. As with other neural tube defects, maternal use of folic acid before and during pregnancy may reduce the risk of recurrence [12].

Caudal Regression Sequence

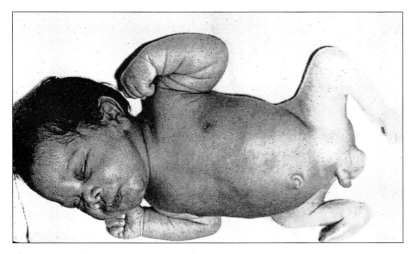

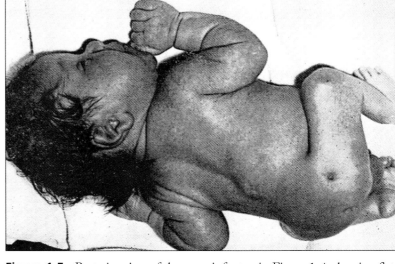

Figure 1-4. Frontal view of an infant with caudal regression sequence showing the "frog leg" appearance of the lower extremities. There are abduction and flexion deformities of the hips as well as popliteal webs, a talipes equinovarus deformity of the left foot, and a calcaneovalgus deformity of the right foot. The upper body appears normal, but there is marked hypoplasia of the lower body. Primary neurulation occurs from embryonic days 18 to 27 and involves the formation of the neural plate, the neural tube and finally, the spinal cord. Secondary neurulation occurs from day 28 to 48 and results in formation of the spinal cord below the lumbosacral junction [13]. The paired somites, derived from mesoderm, develop along the spinal cord. The vertebral segments form from a portion of each somite. The caudal eminence, or tailbud, gives rise to the terminal spinal cord, the caudal notochord, vertebral segments S-2 through the last coccygeal segment and parts of the hindgut and urogenital system. Thus, an insult to the caudal eminence may cause malformations in any of the structures normally derived from it, and might result in agenesis of sacral and coccygeal vertebrae, and lower gastrointestinal and urogenital anomalies [13,14]. (*From* Gellis and colleagues [15]; with permission.)

Figure 1-5. Posterior view of the same infant as in Figure 1-4, showing flat buttocks and sacral dimples, as well as a spinal projection of the lower back. Radiographic examination showed absence of the sacrum and lumbar vertebrae, fused iliac bones, and hypoplastic femurs. Hydronephrosis was present.

Caudal regression sequence is a developmental field defect with absence or defects of structures derived from the embryonic caudal axis [14,16]. Sacral agenesis and variable abnormalities of the lumbar vertebrae are commonly seen. Hypoplasia of the sacrum leads to flattening of the buttocks, shortening of the intergluteal cleft, or dimpling of the buttocks. There is frequently severe lack of growth in the caudal region. Sensory sparing is characteristic and suggests a relative preservation of neural crest cells. There may be abnormalities of the distal spinal cord with neurologic impairment [13]. The occasional association of caudal regression with myelomeningoceles suggests an abnormality of development that arises prior to or during caudal neural tube closure. Other anomalies include imperforate anus or rectal agenesis, hypoplasia of the external genitalia, and renal anomalies or agenesis [17].

Caudal regression has been previously grouped with sirenomelia, or sympodia, in which the lower extremities are fused, with posterior alignment of the knees and feet; these defects are now thought by some investigators to be pathogenetically different, with sirenomelia being caused by vitelline artery steal [17]. Caudal regression sequence should also be distinguished from isolated sacral agenesis with or without spina bifida, which is probably a separate autosomal dominant condition [18]. (*From* Gellis and colleagues [15]; with permission.)

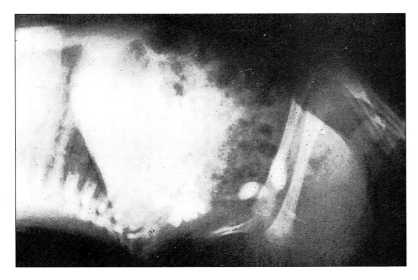

Figure 1-6. Radiograph showing an infant with severe caudal regression sequence. The lumbar spine and sacrum are completely absent, as are several of the lower thoracic vertebrae with associated rib anomalies. The iliac wings are hypoplastic and medially displaced. The infant had hypoplasia of the external genitalia and an imperforate anus. There was severe hypoplasia of the lower extremities with popliteal webbing. The infant was stillborn to a mother with Class B diabetes mellitus. Caudal regression sequence is probably due to a variety of different causes. Most cases are sporadic with an unknown etiology, although there have been reports of mendelian inheritance in some families [18]. Maternal diabetes is thought to be responsible in at least 16% of cases; however, only about 1% of diabetic mothers have offspring with caudal regression [16]. (*From* Gellis and colleagues [15]; with permission.)

Holoprosencephaly Sequence

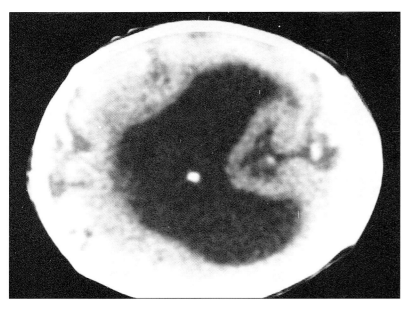

Figure 1-7. Computed tomography (CT) image of the head of an infant who presented with developmental delay, displaying semi-lobar holoprosencephaly. Note the incomplete differentiation of the two lateral ventricles and absence of the septum pellucidum. The interhemispheric fissure is rudimentary in its anterior aspect but better developed in the occipital regions. Holoprosencephaly occurs in approximately 1 in 13,000 live births, but the incidence is 50-fold greater in spontaneously aborted embryos. It lies on the severe end of the spectrum of disorders of prosencephalic development.

Normally, neural tube closure is accomplished by embryonic day 28, followed by its division into three distinct segments: from a rostral to caudal direction, these segments are called the prosencephalon, mesencephalon, and rhombencephalon. The pre-notochordal mesoderm then induces the ventral aspect of the prosencephalon to form the paired cerebral hemispheres, the lateral ventricles, and the diencephalon, as well as the midline

portion of the face. Induction consists of a group of cells secreting chemical signals that cause the surrounding tissue to change. Holoprosencephaly is characterized by noncleavage of the prosencephalon owing to a failure of this normal inductive process. The timing of the insult is invariably prior to the 5th or 6th week of embryonic life. The failure of the telencephalon to cleave into the two cerebral hemispheres may be partial or complete. A single midline ventricle replaces the paired lateral ventricles. The cytoarchitecture of the cerebral cortex surrounding this single ventricle resembles that of the limbic cortex. The extralimbic cortex fails to develop. Neuronal migration abnormalities are also visible. Holoprosencephaly is invariably associated with arhinencephaly (failure of the olfactory bulbs and tracts to develop). The corpus callosum is also usually absent as the presence of an interhemispheric fissure seems essential for the formation of the corpus callosum. Most patients are microcephalic, but patients with macrocephaly from associated hydrocephalus have also been described occasionally. Associated facial anomalies include a single median incisor in the upper jaw, ocular hypotelorism, a single nostril, median cleft lip and palate, and no philtrum. Facial anomalies generally parallel the brain anomalies in severity. When associated with a single median eye, the disorder is termed *cyclopia*. Up to a third of the patients may have normal facial features, however. About three fourths of the patients have additional congenital anomalies involving the cardiovascular, genitourinary, or gastrointestinal systems [19]. Lesser degrees of abnormalities in prosencephalic development may lead to midline disorders like *agenesis* of the corpus callosum (onset no later than 9 to 20 weeks of gestation), absence of the septum pellucidum, and septo-optic dysplasia (unilateral or bilateral optic nerve hypoplasia, absence of the septum pellucidum, hypothalamic dysfunction, and various degrees of cortical dysfunction in the form of seizures or intellectual deficit). Even milder forms of the holoprosencephaly sequence are characterized by subtle midfacial abnormalities such as single midline incisor or arhinencephaly.

Antenatal diagnosis of the more severe forms can be established in the first and second trimesters using cranial ultrasound, which shows fusion of the cerebral hemispheres and thalami, and a single lateral ventricle [20]. Cranial ultrasonography, computed tomography (CT), or magnetic resonance imaging (MRI) can establish the diagnosis after birth, with the MRI being ideal for revealing the associated cortical migration abnormalities.

Etiology of Holoprosencephaly

Chromosomal anomalies
  Chromosome 13: trisomy 13-15, trisomy 13-15 mosaicism, ring 13, deletion 13
  Chromosome 18: trisomy 18, ring 18, deletion 18q
  Chromosome 2, 3, 7 and 21 deletions, trisomies
  Triploidy 69 XX
Familial, without overt chromosomal anomalies
  Autosomal dominant
  Autosomal recessive
  X-linked recessive
In association with normal karyotype and family history

Figure 1-8. Pathogenesis of holoprosencephaly. Using conventional chromosomal studies, approximately half of the patients show normal karyotypes, whereas the remaining have trisomy 13-15, mosaic trisomy 13-15, trisomy 18, or deletion or ring abnormalities of chromosome 18. High-resolution banding and molecular studies may reveal chromosomal abnormalities not otherwise visualized using conventional cytogenetic methods. A mouse model of holoprosencephaly, created by maternal exposure to alcohol during early pregnancy (now considered by many to be a mild form of holoprosencephaly), demonstrates a midline anterior neural plate deficiency that leads to positioning the olfactory placodes too close to the midline and other secondary changes [21]. Retinoic acid administration has also been implicated in the pathogenesis in some animal models of holoprosencephaly [22]. Sporadic and autosomal dominant forms have been associated with mutations of a gene in the 7q36 region, designated *HPE3* [23].

Achondroplasia

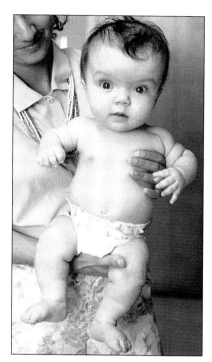

Figure 1-9. Frontal view of a 9-month-old girl with typical achondroplasia. Achondroplasia is the most common skeletal dysplasia and occurs in approximately 1 of 16,000 to 1 of 35,000 newborns [24]. It is characterized by significant macrocephaly, with head circumference well above normal for the age, a relatively normal trunk size, short stature, and rhizomelic shortening of the extremities with redundant folds of skin and soft tissue. Gross motor developmental milestones in infancy and early childhood are delayed because of the large heavy head and short extremities [25]. Individuals with achondroplasia, however, have normal intelligence and can attain normal development within the limits of their short stature.

Potential medical problems include an increased risk for respiratory disturbances, sleep apnea, and even sudden infant death due to upper cervical spinal cord and medullary compression caused by narrowing of the foramen magnum [26,27]. Mild enlargement of the ventricles frequently occurs with true megalencephaly, but frank hydrocephalus requiring treatment occurs only in approximately 5% of patients. Therefore, baseline magnetic resonance imaging with sagittal views through the foramen magnum and serial brain ultrasonography until the patient is 6 months old have been recommended [28]. Fortunately, most cases of cervical spinal cord compression resolve spontaneously by age 2; surgical intervention is rarely required. Kyphosis, lordosis, and gibbus formation may occur. Severe lordosis with spinal stenosis and neurologic symptoms may develop in adults with achondroplasia. Deformities of the lower extremities, such as genu valgum or varus, may require orthopedic intervention.

The phenotype is almost invariable from patient to patient, and the physical features are usually obvious at birth. Some cases can be detected by prenatal ultrasonography in the third trimester of pregnancy. The diagnosis is confirmed by radiographic examination. The interpedicular spaces narrow progressively in the lumbar spine, the sacrum is narrow and oriented horizontally, and the pelvis is short and broad. The vertebral bodies are concave posteriorly, and there may be anterior wedging of some vertebral bodies, especially at the thoracolumbar junction. The long bones show rhizomelic shortening (proximal greater than distal), especially in the upper extremities. The fibula may be longer than normal at the distal end in relationship to the tibia. Achondroplasia is an autosomal dominant disorder with complete penetrance, although at least 80% of cases represent new mutations [24]. The molecular genetic basis was discovered in 1994. Achondroplasia is caused by mutations in the gene for fibroblast growth factor receptor 3 (FGFR3), which is located on chromosome 4 at 4p16.3 [29,30]. Greater than 95% of all patients have either a G-to-A or a G-to-C point mutation in nucleotide 1138 that results in an amino acid change from glycine to arginine in the transmembrane portion of the molecule at position 380. Given that most cases are due to new mutations, nucleotide 1138 is the most highly mutable nucleotide currently known in the human genome. Several atypical cases of achondroplasia, and the related conditions of hypochondroplasia and thanatophoric dysplasia, have different mutations in the FGFR3 gene.

Migrational Defects

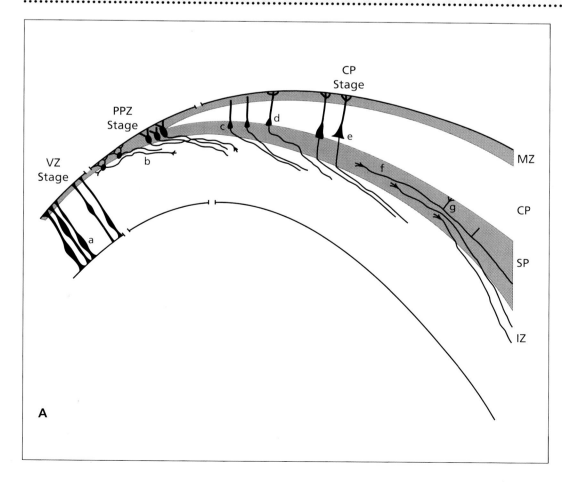

A

Figure 1-10. Formation of early neocortical layering and cortical plate formation. **A,** Schematic representation of the course of early neocortical layering. The preplate zone (PPZ), marginal zone (MZ), and subplate (SP) are highlighted by color. An idealized dorsolateral wall of the telencephalic vesicle is shown, and for convenience, three stages of early cortical development are represented. This compression is indicated by the broken lines at the pial (*upper*) and ventricular (*lower*) borders of the drawing. In the ventricular zone stage (VZ) processes of dividing cells (*a*) and presumptive radial glia extend from pial to ventricular surfaces. In the PPZ stage (*b*), postmitotic neurons collect and extend axons. These cells later form the MZ and the subplate (*c*). The subplate is a precocious neuronal organization, complete with synaptic connections and long axons. The preplate and subplate neurons achieve a high level of morphologic maturity at early cortical stages. Subplate cells form local circuits and interconnections. The subplate receives the earliest afferent connections from outside the cortex, and its axons form the earliest efferent connections from the cortex to subcortical sites. If the subplate is destroyed, normal innervation and patterning of the cortex does not occur.

The cortical plate (CP) cells that are generated later collect between the MZ and SP in an inside-out manner (*d, e*).

(*Continued on next page*)

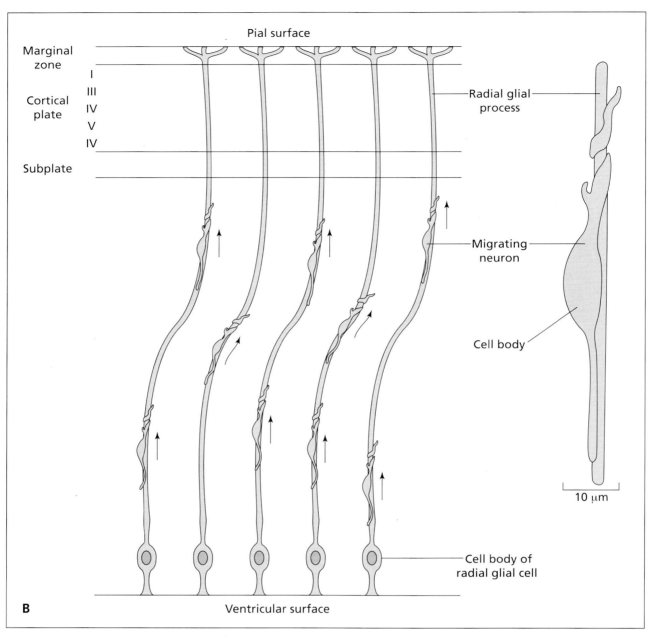

Figure 1-10. (*Continued*) In contrast, neuroblasts of the cortical plate are formed in proliferative regions lining the *lumen* of the neural tube, and post-mitotic cells must migrate over long distances from these regions to the surface of the forebrain. Specialized cells, called radial glial cells, seem essential to this migratory process. Radial glia are elongated glial cells that are anchored on both the pial and the ventricular surfaces. As the cortical wall expands, the radial glia lengthen. These specialized glia provide radial scaffolding for the cortical plate neuroblasts, which appear to climb ameoba-like up the radial glia until reaching their correct position in the cortex. Neuroblasts secrete extracellular proteins like astrotactin and reelin, which provide a receptor system for migration. Later, thalamic axons selectively extend in the SP (*f, g*). **B,** Schematic of cortical plate formation. Radial glia span the cortical wall. Neurons generated in the ventricular zone migrate up radial glia into position in the cortex. The cortical plate is formed in an inside-out manner. Layers IV and V are formed first, and more superficial neurons migrate past these to form the upper layers of the cortex. Cortical plate cells form layers II to VI of the cortex. The radial glia can be considered cells of the original columnar epithelium that became "stretched" as the cortical wall thickened. (Panel A *adapted from* Bicknese and colleagues [31]; Panel B *adapted from* Rakic [32].)

Lissencephaly

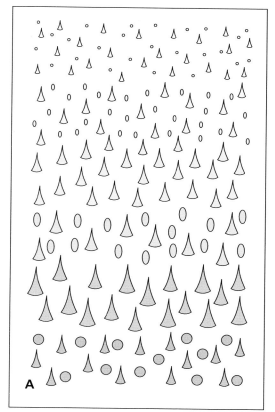 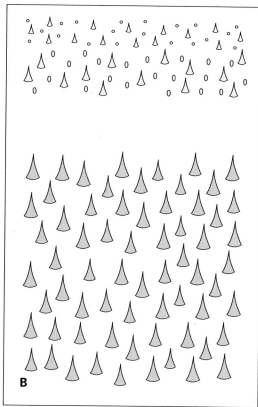 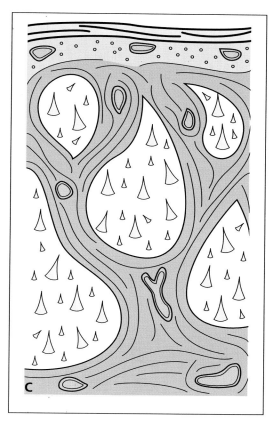

Figure 1-11. A normal cortex compared to a classic lissencephalic cortex. **A,** Schematic representation of normal six-layer cortex. Lissencephaly means smooth brain, and represents a failure to form normal convolutions, resulting in a smooth surface. Cortical development proceeds to cleavage into two hemispheres and the formation of the sylvian fissure, but normal migration fails. **B,** Classic lissencephalic cortex, with four layers: a thick deep layer of cells arrested in migration, a relatively cell-free layer; a layer of disorganized early migrating cells; and a molecular layer. In all forms of lissencephaly, there is an outer layer that may represent the preplate. However, the remaining neurons do not form the normal six-layered cortex and have arrested or stopped during migration. Often the lissencephalic cortex has large, simple gyri called pachygyria; however, the presence of pachygyria does not rule out lissencephaly. Advances in genetics have advanced both the classification and understanding of the etiology of lissencephaly. **C,** Type II lissencephaly thickened meninges obscure the molecular layer in some places. Glio-mesenchymal bundles isolate neuronal heterotopias.

Several classification systems have been used for lissencephaly. In the most commonly used system, lissencephaly was classed as type I, classic or Miller-Dieker lissencephaly, type II, Walker-Warburg syndrome, and sporadic lissencephaly [33]. The different forms of lissencephaly show differences in severity and microscopic anatomy, and they appear to result from defects in separate factors. (*Adapted from* Aicardi [34].)

Miller-Dieker Lissencephaly

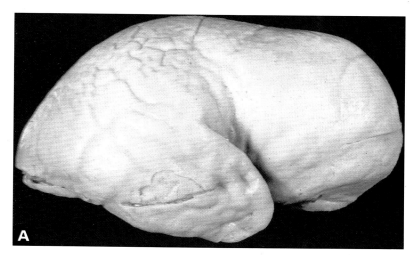 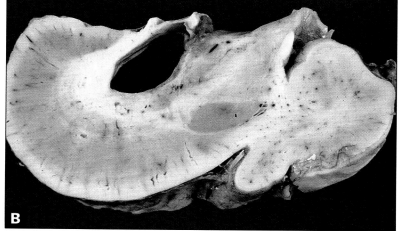

Figure 1-12. A thickened simple cortex showing type I lissencephaly, also called Miller-Dieker lissencephaly or classic lissencephaly [35]. On gross inspection much of the cortical surface is smooth and agyric (**A, B**). The severity of the agyria varies. Many brains have pachygyria, particularly on the inferior and the frontal surfaces of the cortex. Because of the association with pachygyria, some authorities have called type I lissencephaly the agyria-pachygyria complex [34].

(*Continued on next page*)

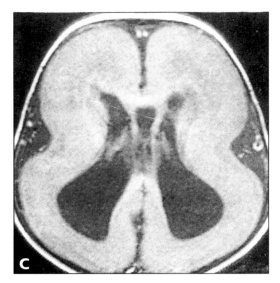

Figure 1-12. (*Continued*) **C,** T1-weighted magnetic resonance image (MRI) of type I lissencephaly. Because the sylvian fissure has formed, transverse sections give a "figure 8" appearance to the cortex. This characteristic shape of the telencephalon is seen on either computed tomography (CT) or magnetic resonance imaging (MRI). The ventricles keep their fetal shape, and thus appear large with occipital dilatation or copolcephaly. The hippocampus is small and may be simple. Often the brain stem is hypoplastic with heterotopia in the olivary nuclei. Usually there is a corpus callosum, although the body may be short or hypoplastic. Myelination of white matter and the corpus callosum occurs at developmentally normal times [36]. Heterotopia may appear along the ventricle within the band of white matter [37].

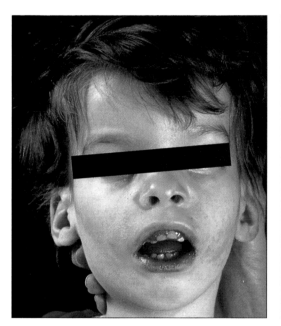

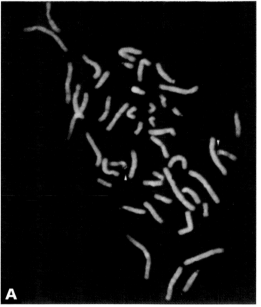

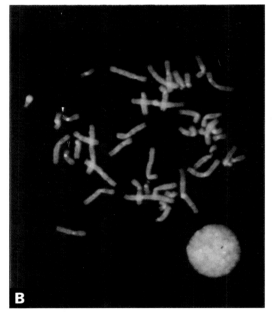

Figure 1-13. The facial features of Miller-Dieker syndrome. Phenotypic features include an upturned nose, micrognathia, and bitemporal hollowing [38]. At birth the head circumference may be normal, but as the growth rate falls off, microcephaly develops. Most affected individuals are hypotonic, severely developmentally delayed, and have intractable epilepsy, including infantile spasms and feeding difficulties. Survival is often short, with many children dying by 5 years of age. Classic lissencephaly occurs in Miller-Dieker syndrome. Because of this association, classic lissencephaly is sometimes called Miller-Dieker lissencephaly. Not all classic lissencephaly patients have Miller-Dieker syndrome, although affected individuals usually have some of the phenotypic features.

Figure 1-14. Fluorescence in-situ hybridization (FISH) probes of chromosomes of a normal and type I lissencephaly patient. Initially described by Miller in 1963 and Dieker in 1969, type I lissencephaly was at first attributed to a familial autosomal recessive disorder with occasional sporadic or isolated cases. High resolution chromosome banding techniques demonstrated deletion of band 17p13 in Miller-Dieker syndrome. Development of FISH probes into the lissencephaly region demonstrated deletions in the 17p13.3 region in the majority of both Miller-Dieker patients and patients with isolated lissencephaly. The *LIS1* gene has been localized to this region [39]. **A,** Chromosomes in metaphase are counterstained with a chromosome-17-specific centromeric α satellite probe (*green*). A cosmid probe from within the smallest deletion interval for lissencephaly is detected with rhodamine (*red*). In a normal individual, the cosmid probe shows two positive signals on each chromosome 17 (*yellow filled arrowheads*). **B,** In a lissencephaly patient with submicroscopic deletion there is one normal chromosome 17 (*filled arrowhead*), and the other homologue shows no hybridization to the cosmid probe (*open arrowhead*). The failure of labelling in the lissencephaly patient indicates a deletion in the 17p13 region. Most, if not all, familial cases are secondary to balanced translocations in one of the parents. Analysis of parental chromosomes is necessary, and will assist in predicting the likelihood of recurrence in a given family. The recent finding of decreased expression of doublecortin in the cerebral cortex of Miller-Dieker syndrome patients also points to the role of doublecortin in neuronal migration [40]. (*Courtesy of* David H. Ledbetter, MD, National Institutes of Health, Bethesda, MD.)

X-linked Lissencephaly and Subcortical Band Heterotopias

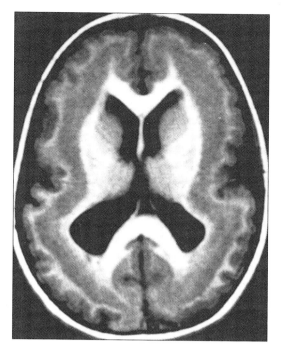

Figure 1-15. T1-weighted magnetic resonance image (MRI) of a double cortex (subcortical band heterotopia). X-linked lissencephaly has been linked to the syndrome of subcortical band heterotopia or double cortex. These syndromes are the sex-dependent expression of the same gene [41]. Hemizygous males have classic lissencephaly, while females express band heterotopia. Females may be asymptomatic, but frequently have severe seizures and may be mentally retarded. MRI scans are recommended in mothers of boys with classic lissencephaly, unless there is documentation of a deletion in the 17p13 region. Recurrence risk in carriers is high, with half of boys having lissencephaly, and half of girls having a double cortex. The gene regulating the expression of doublecortin is localized on chromosome Xq21-24. It contains a tyrosine kinase phosphorylation site, which is important for signal transduction, hence neuronal migration [42]. (*From* Altman and colleagues [43]; with permission.)

Cobblestone Complex

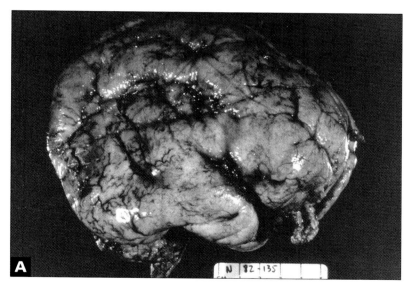

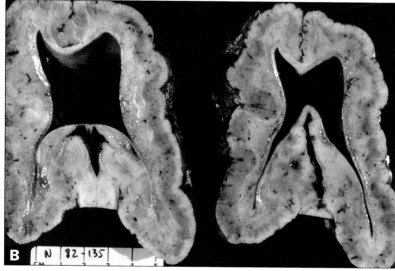

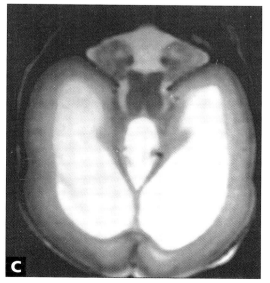

Figure 1-16. Pathologic specimen and magnetic resonance image (MRI) showing lissencephaly type II, now called *cobblestone complex* [33]. **A, B,** The irregular surface of the cortex, with thickened meninges, is from a patient who had cobblestone complex. Cobblestone complex occurs in Walker-Warburg syndrome (WWS). The typical presentation is severe, with macrocephaly secondary to hydrocephalus, weakness, and seizures. Although the cortex has areas of agyria, other pathologic changes clearly separate this from other types of lissencephaly. Four abnormalities are required for the diagnosis of this disorder: lissencephaly, cerebellar malformation, retinal malformation, and congenital muscular dystrophy. WWS is a lethal autosomal recessive disorder with a 25% recurrence risk [44]. The facial appearance varies but usually includes a high forehead and facial weakness. Ocular abnormalities may include microopthalmia, cataracts, congenital glaucoma, coloboma, and optic nerve hypoplasia. Retinal hyperplasia and detachments occur in all patients. Unlike classic lissencephaly, areas of polymicrogyria and pachygyria may "cobblestone" the surface of the brain. The cerebella are small and aplastic, the vermi absent or hypoplastic, and the folia small with microgyria and rosette formations [45]. Agenesis of the corpus callosum is common. **C,** MRI scan of WWS. Neuroimaging of type II lissencephaly demonstrates lissencephaly, a varying degree of hydrocephalus, and a Dandy-Walker malformation. Posterior encephaloceles are common. The meninges are thickened and appear inflamed. Leptomeningeal neuronal and glial heterotopia may partly obstruct the subarachnoid space and cause fusion of the two cerebral hemispheres. Whether ventricular dilatation is secondary to meningeal adhesion, the Dandy-Walker malformation, or aqueductal stenosis is unclear. (*Courtesy of* William Dobyns, MD, University of Chicago, Chicago, IL.)

Pachygyria

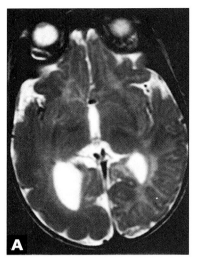
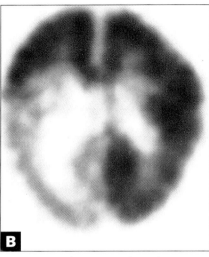

Figure 1-17. Neuroimages and a gross specimen showing pachygyria. **A,** T2-weighted magnetic resonance image (MRI) of left occipital pachygyria. Pachygyria refers to a cerebral cortex developing overly large gyri, instead of the normal development of several smaller gyri. Usually diagnosed on MRI finding, pachygyria may be generalized across the cortex or may be focal or on one hemisphere. Pachygyria are part of type I lissencephaly, and some cases of generalized pachygyria have the lissencephaly deletion on chromosome 17p13 [43]. **B,** A single photon emission computed tomography (SPECT) scan showing decreased perfusion in the area of pachygyria. SPECT scanning may detect subtle areas of cortical malformation, and is performed in many medical centers prior to epilepsy surgery. **C,** Gross specimen of the parieto-occipital region of the brain demonstrating pachygyria (*arrow*). (Panel C *from* Byrd and colleagues [46]; with permission.)

Polymicrogyria

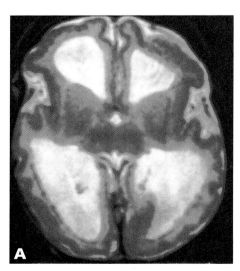
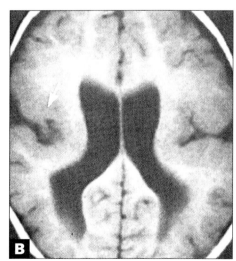
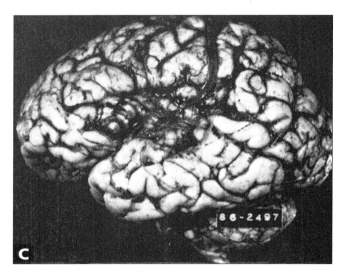

Figure 1-18. Magnetic resonance imaging (MRI) scans showing polymicrogyria. **A,** T2-weighted MRI of polymicrogyria. Polymicrogyria occur in focal areas or are generalized across the cortex. Polymicrogyria is linked to disruptions in cortical genesis after migration has begun. Four-layer polymicrogyria is attributed to laminar necrosis of layer V and VII. One-layer microgyria is generally disorganized and is attributed to cell loss in week 15 to 17 of pregnancy [47].

Superficially, this MRI appears to show pachygyria and ventriculomegaly, but closer inspection of the surface reveals polymicrogyria. The "nubby" surface appearance helps to distinguish polymicrogyria from pachygyria.

Generalized polymicrogyria has been linked to congenital cytomegalovirus infection [48]. **B,** T1-weighted MRI of perisylvian polymicrogyria (*arrow*). **C,** Pathologic specimen of perisylvian polymicrogyria. This disorder was recognized after neuroimaging became a common procedure in cases of epilepsy. Unlike generalized polymicrogyria, symmetric polymicrogyria recurs within families and is believed to have a genetic origin [49]. Symmetric polymicrogyria appears less commonly in the frontal and parietal lobes. (Panels A and B *courtesy of* William Dobyns, MD, University of Chicago, Chicago, IL; Panel C *from* Becker and colleagues [50]; with permission.)

Porencephaly

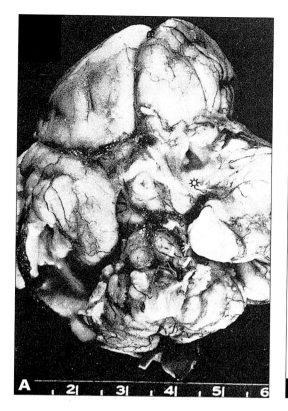

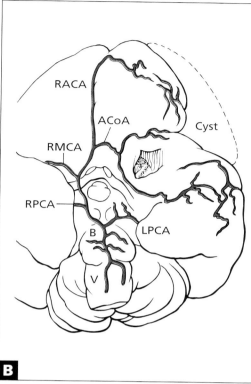

Figure 1-19. Porencephaly. **A,** Ventral surface of the brain of a child who died of multiple congenital defects and porencephaly one hour after birth. Destructive lesions within the vascular distribution of a blood vessel underlie porencephaly. Lesions are more common in twin pregnancies or following maternal hypotension, both of which increase the probability of vascular events occurring in the fetus. The gestational timing of the vascular event determines the appearance of the lesion. Infarction after the period of neuronal migration results in tissue loss and cavitation [51,52] frequently with a membrane, and the cyst may be under tension.

In this specimen, a defect or cleft in the left frontal lobe extends into the ventricular space (*asterisk*). The cystic membrane was destroyed when the brain was removed. **B,** Drawing of the ventral surface of the brain, illustrating the original cystic membrane. The anatomy of the circle of Willis is disrupted, and the left middle cerebral artery is ablated. B—basilar artery; ACoA—anterior communicating artery; LPCA—left posterior cerebral artery; RACA—right anterior cerebral artery; RMCA—right middle cerebral artery; RPCA—right posterior cerebral artery; V—vertebrae. (*From* Stewart [53]; with permission.)

Schizencephaly

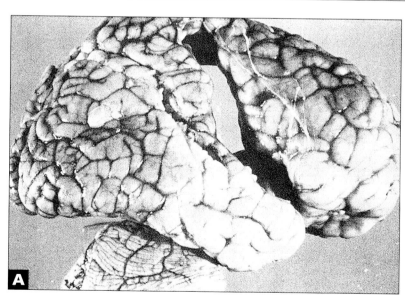

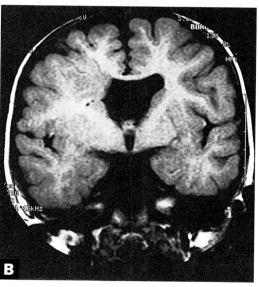

Figure 1-20. Schizencephaly. Destructive events occurring within the period of neuronal migration may cause schizencephaly. Loss of the cortical wall causes a cleft, and if the ependymal lining of the ventricle is damaged, the defect will communicate with the ventricular system. Most clefts occur in the distribution of the middle cerebral artery. However, not all cases of schizencephaly are secondary to vascular events. Germline mutations of the homeobox gene *EMX2* produce a severe form of open lip schizencephaly [54]. There have been several reports of familial schizencephaly, and this lesion may occur in the presence of other congenital defects [55,56]. Schizencephaly is associated with focal or generalized epilepsy. The lesion can be overlooked on computed tomography (CT) and is best seen with magnetic resonance imaging (MRI). **A,** Pathologic specimen showing bilateral large open-lip schizencephaly. Clefts in schizencephaly extend from the cortical surface to the ventricle and are lined with cortex. Mental retardation occurs in 15% of unilateral lesions and approaches 90% in bilateral lesions. **B,** T1-weighted MRI of a unilateral closed-lip schizencephaly in a 5-year-old child. The cleft is lined with polymicrogyria. This child was mildly developmentally delayed and seizure-free. The MRI was obtained following a CT scan for head trauma, which incidentally noted the septal dysplasia. The incidence of septal dysplasia and the association to septo-optic dysplasia sequence is not known, although there is a higher incidence of septal dysplasia. (Panel A *from* Norman [57]; with permission.)

Focal Cortical Dysplasia

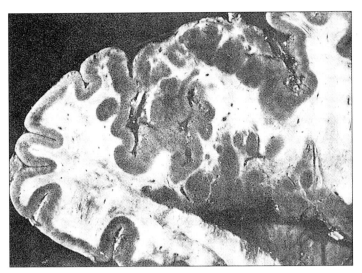

Figure 1-21. Surgical specimen of focal cortical dysplasia. Heterotopia appear between the cortical wall and the pial surface. With the advent of high resolution magnetic resonance imaging, focal cortical defects and dysplasias are being recognized with increasing frequency. These defects occur on a limited portion of the cortical wall, and appear to have a high association with epilepsy. Extratemporal seizure foci are most commonly observed. The seizures are frequently refractory to antiepileptic drug therapy, and can be partial motor, partial complex, or secondarily generalized in type. Histologically there is localized disruption of the cortical laminae, and large, bizarre neurons with astrocytosis. (*From* Layton [54]; with permission.)

Hydranencephaly

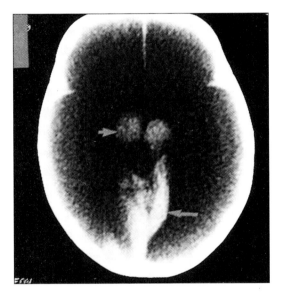

Figure 1-22. Computed tomography (CT) scan of a patient with hydranencephaly. Hydranencephaly is an encephaloclastic disorder in which nearly the entire telencephalon is absent, presumably caused by disruption of bilateral carotid arterial flow. The vertebrobasilar circulation is preserved, which is reflected in the relative preservation of the brain stem and cerebellum, as well as occasional portions of the occipital and inferior temporal cortex. This is a disorder of destruction of previously formed tissue, with onset early enough in gestation to produce cavitation but a minimum of reactive gliosis. The hemispheres are replaced by fluid-filled cavities lined with a thin membrane that abuts the dura mater [59]. The etiology of the vascular disruption varies and includes infections with cytomegalovirus, syphilis, toxoplasmosis, and influenza [60]. Attempted abortions, radiation exposure, and rarely, embryonal tumors of the hemispheres have also been associated with the disorder [61].

Clinically, the child may appear normal if the hypothalamus is intact, and the head size and shape may be normal at birth but grow rapidly thereafter. Lethargy and extreme thermoregulatory instability may be observed in those with impaired diencephalic function. Transillumination of the skull demonstrates the large fluid sacs with small overlying vessels. The patients have a poor prognosis, with anticipated survival of only a few years. They often lack normal diurnal sleep-wake rhythm organization, which also complicates their care [62]. Radiographically, the skull and falx appear normally formed, but the hemispheres are replaced by large cysts. Electrophysiologically, short latency cortical potentials are absent and the electroencephalogram is flat or nearly so. Brain stem responses are generally intact, however. The arrowhead indicates the intact thalamus, and the arrow indicates a segment of the deep venous sinus system.

Williams Syndrome

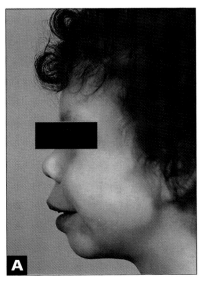

Figure 1-23. Williams syndrome in an 8-year-old child. **A,** Williams syndrome is a relatively common genetic disorder that causes mild to moderate developmental disability. It is easily diagnosed because of characteristic facies and a recognizable behavioral phenotype [63]. **B,** This patient shows the epicanthal folds, flattened bridge of the nose, short nose with upturned nares, relatively long philtrum, and prominent lips that are characteristic of the "elfin" facial features associated with Williams syndrome. Ocular features include epicanthal folds, medial eyebrow flare, strabismus, and periorbital fullness. Individuals with light colored eyes often demonstrate a stellate pattern of the iris. The patient also exemplifies the behavioral phenotype, called "cocktail party manner," characterized by inappropriately friendly and loquacious speech. This feature often persists into adulthood, with many patients describing themselves as too trusting and easily taken advantage of. The relative preservation of verbal skills in the face of impaired reasoning and poor visual motor integration often leads to unrealistic expectations and frustration for the family until the diagnosis has been established.

Medical problems in infancy include irritability, feeding difficulty, failure to thrive, constipation, and hypercalcemia. The hypercalcemia rarely persists beyond infancy, but may occasionally require control measures such as administration of calcitonin or intravenous fluids and diuretics. Cardiovascular anomalies include supravalvular aortic or pulmonic stenosis, but ventricular septal defects and patent ductus arteriosus may also be seen. Hypertension, with or without renal anomalies, may be encountered; indeed some infants with Williams syndrome are diagnosed upon presentation with hypertensive encephalopathy. A history of hyperacusis is often elicited on direct questioning of the parents. (*Continued on next page*)

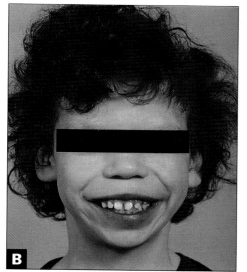

Figure 1-23. (*Continued*) Adults with Williams syndrome are often moderately mentally retarded and found in sheltered work environments. They often have health problems related to hypertension, genitourinary anomalies (multiple urinary tract infections and nephrocalcinosis), or gastrointestinal problems such as ulcer disease or constipation. The facial features change from the elfin appearance during early childhood to a relatively coarse visage. Other problems sometimes encountered include obesity, diabetes, joint contractures, and premature graying [64].

Most instances are sporadic, but there is clear evidence now for autosomal dominant inheritance (the sporadic cases would represent new dominant mutations) [65]. Williams syndrome is an example of a genetic disorder for which a targeted search based on knowledge of the disordered biology led to the discovery of abnormalities in a specific gene. In this case, deletions in the elastin gene on the long arm of chromosome 7 account for at least part of the observed phenotype [66]. Clearly, other genes in the region are implicated in some of the other characteristics, such as the developmental profile and the hypercalcemia; therefore Williams syndrome is best considered a contiguous gene syndrome with many of the other involved genes yet to be isolated. When the diagnosis is suspected, a FISH (fluorescent in situ hybridization) study using a DNA probe derived from the elastin gene is usually diagnostic [66].

Prader-Willi Syndrome

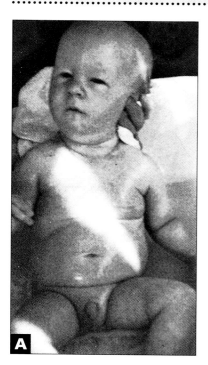

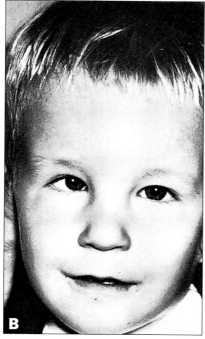

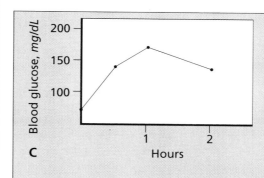

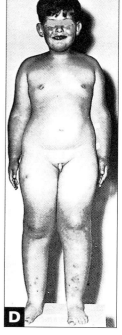

Figure 1-24. Patients with Prader-Willi syndrome (PWS). PWS is characterized by decreased fetal movement, infantile hypotonia, and feeding difficulties. Around ages 12 to 18 months, behavior shifts to marked hyperphagia, resulting in gross obesity as well as major adjustment problems related to food-seeking behavior. In addition, these children have short stature, mental retardation, hypogonadotropic hypogonadism, and a recognizable facial phenotype that includes bifrontal narrowing, slightly upslanting almond-shaped eyes, and full cheeks. Small hands and feet and tapering fingers are seen in most patients. Decreased pigmentation is common, relative to family background, and may sometimes manifest as ocular albinism with the concomitant misrouting of optic ganglion fibers and nystagmus [67].

A patient at 5 months (**A**) and at 4 years and 2 months (**B**), at which time the height age was 3 years and 2 months, developmental quotient was 50, and response to an oral glucose load was abnormal (**C**). A patient at 9 1/2 years old with a height age of 7 1/2 years and a mental age of 5 years (**D**). Beyond midchildhood and adolescence, obesity and behavioral problems may become unmanageable. The patients usually show few or no signs of puberty. During young adulthood, the extreme obesity may bring on cor pulmonale or diabetes mellitus. Sleep disorders include sleep apnea, daytime somnolence, and rapid eye movement-onset sleep periods. Adults with PWS are often emotionally labile, have poor gross motor skills, and significant cognitive impairment. Diagnosis and initiation of an effective program of weight reduction and control often has a salutary effect on many of these long-term clinical problems.

Most PWS cases are sporadic, and occasional familial occurrences were puzzling until the molecular mechanism of the condition became clear. PWS is caused by lack of the paternal segment of chromosome 15q11.2-q12. Imprinting also plays a role in its pathogenesis. Imprinting refers to the phenomenon of suppression of certain genes when they are transmitted through the sperm and their expression when transmitted through the egg, or vice versa. Indeed, PWS was one of the first human genetic disorders recognized as related to imprinting. Interstitial deletions of the paternal chromosome 15q account for about 75% of cases. Unbalanced translocations may also result in PWS when the missing segment on chromosome 15q is paternal; most of these occur *de novo*. The karyotype in the remainder is normal; these cases are caused by maternal uniparental disomy (a phenomenon in which both copies of a chromosome pair, in this case, number 15, are inherited from the mother). The clarification of the genetic mechanisms underlying PWS and its imprinting counterpart, Angelman syndrome, has led to the appreciation of an entirely new mechanism of human disease [68]. (*From* Jones [69]; with permission, *courtesy of* Professor A. Prader.)

Angelman Syndrome

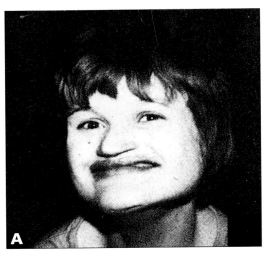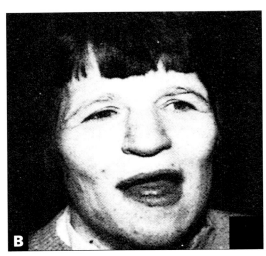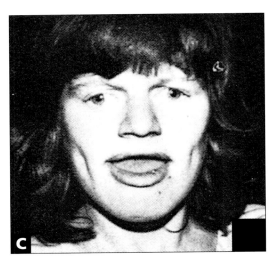

Figure 1-25. An individual with Angelman syndrome (AS) (**A–C**). AS is characterized by severe intellectual and motor deficits, seizures, ataxia, and minimal or no speech. The facial features include a prominent jaw and an open-mouthed expression, repeated tongue thrusting, and a propensity to excessive laughter. The jerky, ataxic movements, along with inappropriate laughter, gave rise to the designation of "happy puppet syndrome," a term that should be avoided due to its derisive nature. Other features include an occipital groove, possibly related to cerebellar atrophy, abnormal choroidal pigmentation, and an electroencephalogram pattern consisting of symmetric, synchronous, high amplitude spike and wave activity. Many patients have hypopigmentation relative to family members, a feature also noted in patients with Prader-Willi syndrome [70].

AS is difficult to diagnose in the first 2 years of life [71], and clinical suspicion is usually delayed until the appearance of the signs described above. Most cases of AS occur sporadically. Multiple instances of recurrence in siblings have been reported, but inheritance of AS is clearly not typically mendelian. The puzzling pattern of inheritance began to yield to molecular genetic understanding after the phenomena of uniparental disomy and imprinting were discovered in the 1980s. Deletions of the long arm of chromosome 15q11.2 have been noted repeatedly in cases of AS. In contrast to Prader-Willi syndrome (PWS), the origin of the deleted chromosome is maternal in AS. An alternative mechanism (in cases with no cytogenetic or molecular deletion detectable) is paternal uniparental disomy. The critical region involved in both AS and PWS has been worked out. One of the candidate genes is an ubiquitin protein ligase; there may also be additional genes [72]. (*From* Williams CA, Frias JL: The Angelman ("Happy Puppet") syndrome. American Journal of Medical Genetics, Copyright © 1982. Reprinted by permission of Wiley-Liss, Inc., a subsidiary of John Wiley & Sons, Inc.)

Arachnoid Cysts

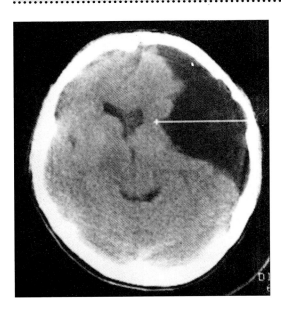

Figure 1-26. An unenhanced computed tomography (CT) scan of an arachnoid cyst of characteristic shape and mass effect, located in the temporal fossa and extending into the sylvian fissure. Arachnoid cysts are congenital lesions that occur intracranially or within the spinal canal. They are cavities filled with cerebrospinal fluid (CSF) and lined by arachnoidal cells and collagen fibers. Some arachnoid cysts may be clinically asymptomatic, being discovered incidentally. Other cysts usually come to attention because of their mass effect; symptoms are related either to local pressure or to hydrocephalus from compression along the CSF pathway [74]. Arachnoid cysts comprise about 1% of all space-occupying intracranial masses. They occur in males slightly more than in females and often present during the first two decades of life. A patient usually has only one arachnoid cyst, and familial occurrence is rare. About two thirds of cysts occur in the supratentorial space; one third are infratentorial. The middle cranial fossa perisylvian region is the most common location for these lesions, but they also occur frequently in the suprasellar region, within the ventricles, between the cerebral hemispheres, and around the cerebral convexities [75].

The most common symptoms are those caused by increased intracranial pressure: headache, macrocephaly, nausea, vomiting, and papilledema. Associated complaints include seizures, developmental delay, and other deficits reflective of local compression. A small group of patients presents with spontaneous hemorrhage into the cyst. Consequently a pre-existing arachnoid cyst should be considered in patients who develop subdural hematomas after minimal trauma.

Magnetic resonance imaging (MRI) is currently the best modality available for imaging these lesions. The cysts appear as CSF density collections without enhancing nodules. Their shapes depend on their locations: middle fossa cysts are frequently trapezoidal and spread the sylvian fissure; suprasellar cysts can bulge into the third ventricle, obstructing both foramina of Monro, giving the appearance of "Mickey Mouse ears." CT scans are useful in the evaluation of these patients if MRI cannot be done [74].

Asymptomatic arachnoid cysts do not require treatment. When associated with mass effect, arachnoid cysts may be decompressed by either a cystoperitoneal shunt or fenestration of the cyst wall. A shunt is a simpler procedure but carries with it the risks of indwelling hardware and shunt failure. Fenestration avoids these problems but requires a craniotomy and is not uniformly successful [76].

Dermal Sinus Tracts, Dermoids, and Epidermoids

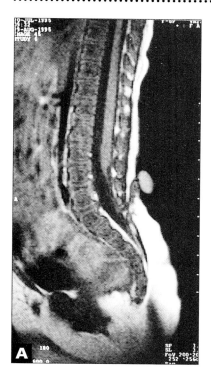 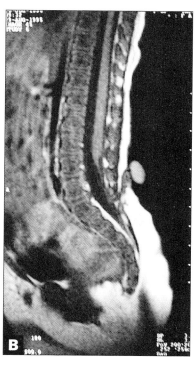

Figure 1-27. Dermal sinus tracts. **A,** A magnetic resonance image (MRI) of a dermal sinus tract with an associated intradural dermoid. Dorsal dermal sinuses are the result of a relatively minor developmental abnormality, but they can have great clinical significance. The lesions appear as small pits or dimples anywhere along the midline from coccyx to nasion, although most occur in either the lumbosacral or occipital areas. The sinus tracts are lined by epithelium and can extend to any depth; about one half enter the subarachnoid space, many of which are attached to neural elements. The significance of these malformations lies in their association with dermoids and epidermoids as well as other tethering lesions and in their role as a conduit for infectious agents. If they are recognized, the evaluation and treatment of these malformations is straightforward, but it is as easy to overlook a sinus tract as it is to underestimate its importance [77].

Dermal sinus tracts are postneurulation defects, arising from incomplete separation or dysjunction of the cutaneous ectoderm from the neural ectoderm. The central nervous system is an ectodermal derivative that begins as a thickening of the ectodermal layer in the area overlying the notochord. Soon a central groove forms and the margins of the neural plate fold in toward the midline, dragging with them the ectoderm attached at their edges. The neural folds meet and fuse. Then the tissue that had been attached to the folds separates from them and joins in the midline over what has become the neural tube. If this separation is incomplete, a potential connection is left between the neural tube and the future skin. The tract may remain patent or part of it may be obliterated, which accounts for the various depths of dermal sinuses. Because cutaneous ectoderm forms the lining of the tract, dermoid and epidermoid tumors may arise at any point along it, which occurs in about half of all cases [78]. Dorsal sinus tracts can be divided into two groups: those that occur within the intergluteal fold and those that occur above it. Sinuses that occur within the fold are common; they can be found in nearly 5% of newborns and are almost uniformly innocuous. If they occur as isolated lesions, neither radiologic nor other evaluation is necessary. Tracts that occur above the intergluteal fold, however, always require investigation whether or not the patient is symptomatic. Common manifestations include: infection, including meningitis or an intraspinal abscess; lower extremity pain or weakness related to root or cord compression from associated tumors; and pain, scoliosis, weakness, and bowel or bladder dysfunction from a tethered cord [79]. Sinus tracts that exit above the gluteal cleft and those that are associated with lipomas or skin markers should be evaluated with MRI, which is the best modality currently available for imaging a dermal sinus. The tract is easily seen and the anatomy of the spinal cord and roots is well defined. Ultrasonography is also useful, especially in young children. Computed tomography myelography gives similar anatomic information, but it should not be performed if active infection is suspected.

B, MRI of a dermal sinus tract that extends into the canal and tethers the spinal cord. Almost all dermal sinuses that occur above the intergluteal fold should be excised. Because of the risk of progressive neurologic dysfunction associated with a tethered cord, lesions that penetrate the dura should be removed soon after diagnosis. If imaging studies do not adequately demonstrate the extent of the lesion, exploration is warranted. The surgery consists of excision of the tract and exploration and removal of any intradural components. A vigorous attempt at complete resection of the tumor should be made, because incompletely removed tumors are likely to recur [79].

Neurenteric Cysts and Diastematomyelia

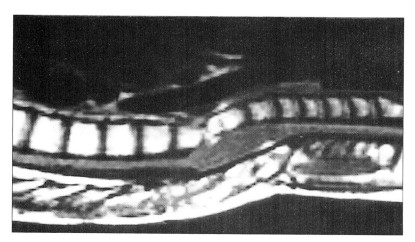

Figure 1-28. Magnetic resonance image (MRI) of a lower thoracic neurenteric cyst. Neurenteric cysts and diastematomyelia belong to a group of postneurulation dysraphic malformations that result from abnormalities in gastrulation. These lesions are usually skin-covered and are often found in patients with good neurologic function. They share a propensity for tethering the spinal cord and are likely to cause progressive disability if left untreated.

Neurenteric cysts are fluid-filled and lined with simple epithelium resembling that seen in the intestines. They can be found anywhere in the midline, but when they occur in the vertebral canal they are usually within the cord or anterior to it. They are most common in the cervical region and are more frequent in males than females. The cysts are often associated with anterior vertebral defects, which are occasionally visible on plain radiographs. Patients usually come to medical attention because of signs and symptoms of myelopathy caused by cord compression or occasionally cord tethering. MRI is the best way to make the diagnosis [80]. Almost all of these lesions require excision, and the prognosis is quite good if the lesions are removed completely.

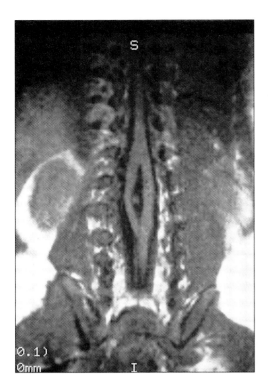

Figure 1-29. Magnetic resonance image of a diastematomyelia with a bony septum. Diastematomyelia describes a malformation characterized by duplication of the spinal cord with varied dural and bony anatomy. Some patients have two hemicords separated by fibrous septae that share the same dural tube. Other patients have two dural tubes with bone or cartilage between. These lesions occur most frequently in the lumbar spine and often have cutaneous markers; a hair-bearing patch is most common. Patients are generally neurologically normal at birth and impairment usually progresses slowly, although several reports of acute decompensation associated with excessive or forced flexion have appeared. Pain and weakness are the most common complaints, but bowel or bladder dysfunction may be the only symptoms of a tethered cord [81]. Magnetic resonance imaging is often sufficient to define the lesion, but bony or cartilaginous septae can be overlooked, and for that reason computed tomography myelography is valuable. Repair is complicated because both cords are usually functional, but owing to the risk of neurologic deterioration associated with tethering lesions, surgery is recommended in all patients with diastematomyelia [81]. (*From* Dias and colleague [81]; with permission.)

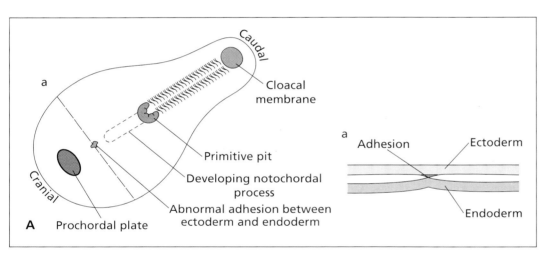

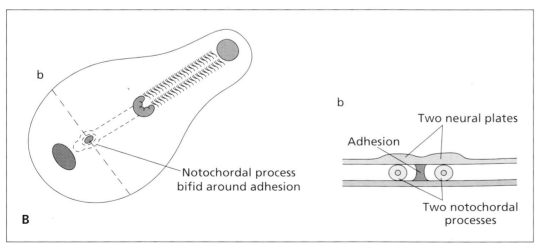

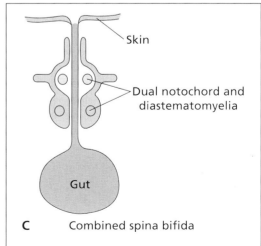

Figure 1-30. Split notochord theory. Although a common defect in embryogenesis is thought to cause both neurenteric cysts and diastematomyelia, the details of the embryopathy are not known. It seems most likely that in these lesions duplication of part of the notochord leads to duplication of various parts of the spinal cord and its surrounding structures. This would potentially allow direct communication between the endoderm and the ectoderm in the area between the split notochords. Notochordal abnormality could have several causes. **A,** An adhesion between the ecdoderm and endoderm of the two-layered embryonic disc may occur, cranial to the developing notochordal process (*cross-sectional view a*). **B,** The notochordal process is forced to divide around the adhesion creating two notochordal processes. Two neural plates may be induced (*cross-sectional view b*), which ultimately could form an area of diastematomyelia. **C,** An enterocutaneous fistula may penetrate through a vertebral body cleft, diastematomyelia, and posterior spina bifida to create a combined anterior-posterior spina bifida. The theories invoking an abnormality of the neurenteric canal are attractive. (*Continued on next page*)

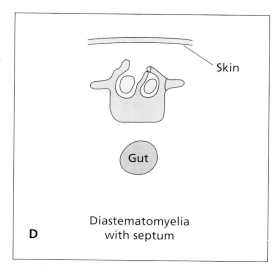

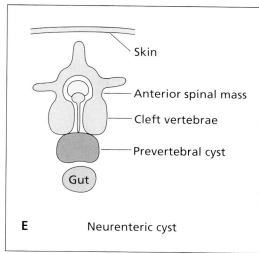

Figure 1-30. (*Continued*) **D,** Healing of the anterior portions of the fistula could lead to diastematomyelia with septum, which is usually accompanied by posterior element and vertebral body abnormalities. **E,** Healing of the posterior and midportions of the fistula could lead to neurenteric cyst, vertebral body anomalies, and various enteric malformations. (*Adapted from* Beardmore and colleague [82].)

Posthemorrhagic Hydrocephalus of the Newborn

Factors Predisposing to Intraventricular Hemorrhage

Fluctuating cerebral blood flow
Increase in cerebral blood flow
Increase in cerebral venous pressure
Decrease in cerebral blood flow
Platelet and coagulation disturbance
Vascular immaturity
Deficient vascular support
Excessive fibrinolytic activity

Figure 1-31. Factors predisposing to intraventricular hemorrhage. Periventricular or intraventricular hemorrhage is a common complication of prematurity, with an incidence of approximately 30% in neonates of birthweight less than 1500 g and a 62% incidence in premature infants with a birthweight of 500 to 700 g [83]. Improved understanding of the factors involved in pathogenesis has resulted in reduced incidence over time [84]. Extensive degrees of hemorrhage are associated with ventricular dilatation, but do not usually progress to require permanent ventriculoperitoneal shunting. Much controversy exists regarding the appropriate management of the ventricular dilatation in these small, fragile babies [85,86]. (*Adapted from* Volpe [84].)

Volpe's Modified Grading of Intraventricular Hemorrhage

Grade I	Germinal matrix hemorrhage with no or minimal intraventricular hemorrhage (<10% of ventricular area on parasagittal view)
Grade II	Intraventricular hemorrhage involving 10%-50% of ventricular area
Grade III	Intraventricular hemorrhage involving >50% of ventricular area, usually with ventricular dilatation
Grade IV	Grade III plus intraparenchymal extension (now felt to be due to periventricular hemorrhagic infarction)

Figure 1-32. Volpe's modified grading of intraventricular hemorrhage. The periventricular germinal matrix in the developing brain is supplied by a vascular rete that is friable, with poorly developed connective tissue support. Fluctuations in the arterial and venous pressure may lead to rupture of these vessels, particularly if they have been previously injured by hypoxia. The germinal matrix involutes after 34 weeks' gestation, and hemorrhage at this site subsequently becomes much less common. Neurosonograms permit serial bedside assessment of the brain anatomy. The most widely used grading system for intraventricular hemorrhage (IVH) is based on that devised by Papile [87] and modified by Volpe [84]. Grade IV hemorrhage actually represents periventricular hemorrhagic infarction consequent to deep vein thrombosis, rather than an "extension" of the intraventricular hemorrhage

due to rupture. Volpe therefore prefers using a separate notation describing the location and extent of the intraparenchymal component [84].

Posthemorrhagic ventriculomegaly is caused by a combination of blockage of resorption of cerebrospinal fluid (CSF) at the arachnoid villi and obliterative arachnoiditis, particularly in the posterior fossa region, impeding flow of CSF through the subarachnoid spaces. Infrequently, the cast of blood may cause obstruction at the cerebral aqueduct, producing noncommunicating hydrocephalus. Elevated intraventricular pressure presents clinically as excessive head growth (more than 2 cm/wk), separation of cranial sutures, and bulging anterior fontanelle, and occasionally with lethargy, respiratory insufficiency, feeding difficulties, and oculomotor disturbances. A lag of 10 to 14 days may occur between the onset of ventricular dilatation and the onset of excessive head growth. Not all cases showing ventriculomegaly progress to the point of requiring ventriculo-peritoneal diversion.

Pharmacologic measures to reduce CSF production (acetazolamide and furosemide) may be helpful in controlling hydrocephalus [85], but frequently cause systemic metabolic derangements. Repeated lumbar punctures have also been used as an interim measure with variable results. A large multicenter European study failed to show its benefit in either arresting hydrocephalus and thus avoiding shunting, or on long-term neurodevelopmental outcome [86]. Placement of a ventriculoperitoneal or ventriculoatrial shunt is fraught with complications (high rates of infection and shunt blockage) when performed early. The temporary use of a subcutaneous ventricular catheter reservoir [88] is safe and effective until the patient's weight reaches 2 kg and CSF protein falls below 1 g/dL (factors associated with better shunt success rate). Ventriculoscopic methods of manipulating the clot and instillation of fibrinolytic agents into the ventricle [89] show promise but require further study before their routine use can be justified. The outcome in patients with intraventricular hemorrhage varies, based on the severity of the hemorrhage. The incidence of major neurologic sequelae is 5% to 15% following low-grade hemorrhage, 35% in grade III hemorrhage, and 90% in those with an intraparenchymal component (100% in those with an extensive intraparenchymal component) [84]. (*Adapted from* Volpe [84].)

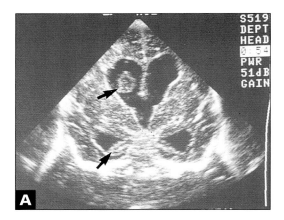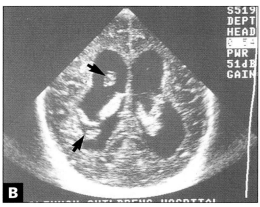

Figure 1-33. Coronal cranial ultrasound images from a 17-day-old premature baby born at 28 weeks' gestation who suffered a grade III intraventricular hemorrhage. **A, B,** They show dilatation of frontal and temporal horns of the lateral ventricles and of the third ventricle with residual blood clots (*arrows*). This patient was treated with serial lumbar punctures to remove cerebrospinal fluid (CSF) until his weight reached 2 kg and CSF protein fell to less than 1 g/dL, at which time a ventriculoperitoneal shunt was placed. Shunt revision was necessary at 17 months. At 30 months of age the patient showed mild global developmental delay.

Dandy-Walker Malformation

Syndromes Associated With Dandy-Walker Malformation

Aase-Smith	Jaeken and Van den Burghe
Aicardi	Joubert
Cerebro-oculo-muscular	Meckel-Gruber
Coffin-Siris	Oro-facio-digital type II
Cornelia de Lange	and III
Dekaban	Ruvalcaba-Myhre-Smith
Ellis-van Creveld	Smith-Lemli-Opitz
Frasier cryptophthalmus	Warburg
Goldenhar	

Figure 1-34. Syndromes associated with Dandy-Walker malformation (DWM). DWM is a developmental disorder characterized by a cystic lesion of the fourth ventricle, partial or complete agenesis of the cerebellar vermis, hydrocephalus (which is usually not present at birth but develops over time), and enlargement of the posterior fossa with elevation of the tentorium and confluence of sinuses (torcular). Several conditions masquerade as DWM (mega cisterna magna, arachnoid cyst, and other "variants" marked by cerebellar vermal agenesis) but can be excluded based on the preceding criteria. DWM accounts for approximately 3% of cases of hydrocephalus and is estimated therefore to occur in 1 per 25,000 to 30,000 births [90]. Although a variable female preponderance has been noted in several reports, it is not statistically significant [91]. Most cases are sporadic. Those with cerebellar vermis agenesis associated with constellations of extraneural anomalies may represent specific syndromes with known inheritance patterns, thus making their distinction important.

Central Nervous System Anomalies Associated With Dandy-Walker Malformation

Anomalies of cerebellar folia
Cerebral and cerebellar hamartomas
Corpus callosum agenesis
Malformation of olivary and dentate nuclei
Microgyria/polymicrogyria
Nonspecific gyral disturbances
Occipital encephalocele
Pachygyria
Uncrossed pyramidal tracts

Figure 1-35. Central nervous system anomalies associated with Dandy-Walker malformation (DWM). With advances in prenatal and neonatal ultrasonography, DWM is being increasingly diagnosed at birth. The diagnosis is made by 1 year of age in approximately 80% of cases [90], the most

common presenting symptom being macrocephaly with a prominent occiput. Hypotonia and signs of hydrocephalus may be present. Associated brain anomalies are present in 68% of cases [91]. Anomalous development of other organ systems (cardiac, genitourinary, skeletal, ocular, facial) frequently coexists.

The etiopathogenesis has been debated widely. DWM is regarded as a developmental disorder of the midline central nervous system with marked genetic and etiologic heterogeneity [92]. A localized defect in differentiation of the roof of the newly closed neural tube in the hindbrain [93] results in absence of the foramen of Magendie, a consistent finding during surgical intervention [90]. Lack of cerebrospinal fluid outflow produces cystic enlargement of the fourth ventricle. Hirsch has estimated that the timing of the development of DWM occurs in the third postovulatory week. This would explain associated cardiovascular and facial anomalies [90]. Hart reviewed pathologic material and believed that the disturbance occurs by the end of the second month [91].

The management of DWM has changed and is still controversial. Initially, excision of the cyst membrane was proposed, but showed a high failure rate. Currently favored options include shunting the ventricular system, the cyst, or both. The outcome depends on the presence of coexistent neural and extraneural malformations, in addition to the timing and effectiveness of the surgical intervention. The percentage of patients with DWM who possess an intelligence quotient of 80 or above varies from 29% to 67% [90].

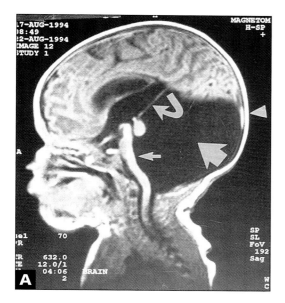
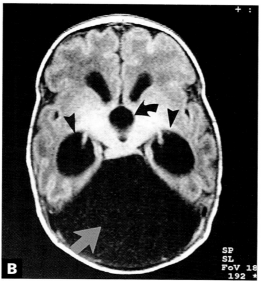

Figure 1-36. T1-weighted magnetic resonance image in the midline sagittal (**A**) and transaxial section at the level of the third ventricle (**B**) from a 7-day-old baby with Dandy-Walker malformation. The sagittal view shows the typical cystic enlargement of the fourth ventricle (*large arrow*), with anterior displacement of the brain stem (*small arrow*), aplasia of the cerebellar vermis, and elevation of the tentorium (*curved arrow*), as well as the confluence of sinuses (*arrowhead*). The transaxial view shows the fourth ventricular cyst (*large arrow*) with cerebellar aplasia and dilatation of the temporal horns of the lateral ventricles (*arrowheads*) and third ventricle (*curved arrow*). This patient was treated with a diversion procedure in which both the fourth ventricular cyst and the hydrocephalus were decompressed using a single catheter. Postoperatively, the patient is stable but development is significantly delayed.

Chiari Malformations

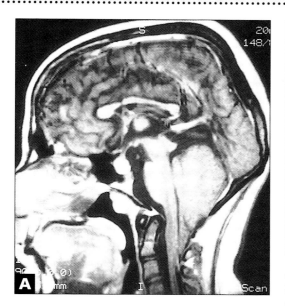
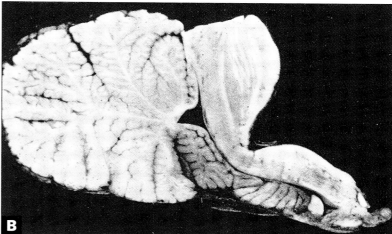

Figure 1-37. Type II Chiari malformations. **A,** Magnetic resonance image (MRI) of a type II Chiari malformation, the lesion most commonly associated with a myelomeningocele. **B,** Pathologic specimen of the same lesion. The extent of the cerebellar displacement is easily seen. The medulla is elongated and kinked and the fourth ventricle can be seen to extend well into the cervical spine. In patients with a type I Chiari malformation, the cerebellar tonsils extend below the level of the foramen magnum but the position of the brain stem and midline cerebellar structures is normal. Syringomyelia occurs frequently, but not universally, among these patients [94]. Most patients with type I malformations come to medical attention in adulthood, complaining of headaches, neck pain, upper extremity weakness, and unsteady gait. Only occasionally do children have symptomatic lesions; those who do often present with scoliosis, a complication of the malformation that rarely occurs in adults [95]. Diagnosis is made most easily with MRI, although computed tomography myelography can be used if MRI is not available. Treatment is surgical decompression of the lesion. The best way to treat patients with associated syringomyelia is still uncertain. Some favor decompression alone, whereas others recommend more extensive procedures [96]. Interestingly, iatrogenic symptomatic Chiari I malfunctions have been reported as a result of lumboperitoneal shunts [97].

In type II Chiari malformations, both the cerebellar vermis and the tonsils are displaced into the cervical canal. In addition, the brain stem and fourth ventricle are elongated and displaced. These lesions appear almost exclusively in children with myelomeningoceles, in whom they are often associated with a constellation of other anomalies, most notably hydrocephalus, cortical heterotopia, and a small posterior fossa. Chiari malformations may be symptomatic at birth, with stridor, respiratory abnormalities, and feeding difficulties being the most common signs. The problems usually resolve with placement of a ventriculoperitoneal shunt. Most patients with Chiari II malformations who do develop symptoms do so during childhood. Many have upper extremity pain, incoordination, or weakness with or without myelopathy. Cranial neuropathies are also common, as is headache. Diagnosis is made by MRI and the treatment is surgical decompression. Because the site of compression generally lies within the cervical canal, the bony decompression is performed primarily at that level. Shunt malfunction may mimic symptomatic Chiari malformation and should be excluded prior to surgery.

The cause of Chiari malformation is not known, but there is general agreement that the pathogenesis of the two types of malformation is different. Evidence is growing that many cases of type I anomaly are acquired rather than congenital. In those born with the lesion, the developmental abnormality most likely occurs late in embryogenesis, because the cerebellar hemisphere and the deep nuclei are normal. The pathogenic mechanism of the type II malformation probably operates earlier in development. Current theories focus on mechanical or hydrodynamic effects of the accompanying myelomeningocele or primary dysgenetic mechanisms as the cause of the lesion [98]. Research is ongoing, and mouse models of abnormal neurulation offer hope of advances in this area.

Choroid Plexus Papilloma

Microscopic Features of Malignant Choroid Plexus Tumors

Invasion

Loss of differentiation

Nuclear pleomorphism

Increased mitoses

Necrosis

Figure 1-38. Microscopic features of malignant choroid plexus tumors. Choroid plexus neoplasms are essentially the only cause of hydrocephalus resulting from cerebrospinal fluid (CSF) overproduction. Choroid plexus neoplasms account for up to 6% of childhood intracranial neoplasms [99]. They can present at any age, 40% being in children less than 15 years old [99]. Most childhood series have noted a tendency in children under 2 years. Cases presenting in adulthood tend to favor the fourth ventricular location, whereas in the pediatric population, 80% are located in the lateral ventricle, 16% in the fourth ventricle, and 4% in the third ventricle [99]. The most common presenting symptoms are increased intracranial pressure (irritability, lethargy, vomiting), intellectual dysfunction, and seizures. Examination reveals an enlarged head size, and computed tomography or magnetic resonance imaging reveal an enhancing mass lesion within the enlarged ventricular system. Uniform enhancement of a lobulated mass that does not invade the parenchyma favors diagnosis of choroid plexus papilloma (CPP), whereas a variegated appearance with local invasion suggests malignancy (carcinoma). The cytologic features of CPP are similar to those of normal choroid plexus. The papillae are composed usually of a single layer of columnar or cuboidal epithelium supported by a stroma of vascularized connective tissue [100]. Although histologic examination distinguishes papilloma from carcinoma [101], not all papillomas behave in a benign fashion [99]. Ploidy analysis seems to allow greater prediction of neoplastic behavior, because aneuploid choroid plexus neoplasms (whether papilloma or carcinoma) have a significantly increased mortality rate (67%) compared with diploid papillomas (9%) [102]. In addition to choroid plexus carcinoma, the differential diagnosis of CPP includes medulloepithelioma, teratoma belonging to the embryonal carcinoma or endodermal sinus tumor group, metastatic adenocarcinoma from elsewhere in the body, and villous hypertrophy of the choroid plexus [100].

The treatment typically consists of alleviation of hydrocephalus with either external temporary or internal permanent CSF shunting, followed by removal of the tumor. Not all patients require permanent ventricular diversion once the tumor has been removed completely [103]. Removal of these highly vascularized tumors is frequently complicated by bleeding. The optimal method of tumor removal entails reaching the arterial feeder(s) first, although this is not always possible [103]. Carcinomas require additional therapy. Complete resection of the carcinoma may be curative but is not always possible. Irradiation of the neuraxis is recommended owing to the high rate of leptomeningeal metastases. Unfortunately, irradiation in the developing infant may cause intellectual deterioration, endocrinopathies, and spinal growth failure. Postoperative chemotherapy, using vincristine, cyclophosphamide, cisplatinum, and etoposide, has shown promise in stabilizing the disease and delaying the need for irradiation [104]. (*From* Ho and colleagues [101].)

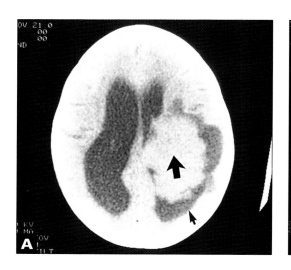
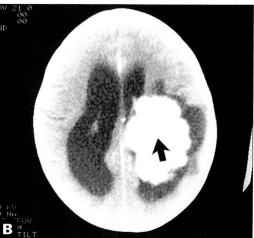

Figure 1-39. Computed tomography scans from a 10-month-old baby who presented with enlarging head size and symptoms of increasing intracranial pressure. The noncontrast scan (**A**) shows a mass in the left lateral ventricle (*large arrow*) causing localized enlargement of the left lateral ventricle (*small arrow*) and diffuse hydrocephalus. Following contrast infusion (**B**), the typical lobulated appearance becomes more obvious and uniform enhancement (*arrow*) suggests choroid plexus papilloma, which in this case was proven histologically following removal of the tumor.

Klippel-Feil Anomaly

Classification of Klippel-Feil Anomaly

Type I   Complete fusion of cervical vertebrae into blocks; may include upper thoracic vertebrae

Type II   Involvement at a few cervical levels with hemivertebrae and atlanto-occipital fusion

Type III   Cervical fusions plus lower thoracic or lumbar fusions

Figure 1-40. Classification of Klippel-Feil anomaly. The Klippel-Feil anomaly consists of a congenital fusion of the cervical vertebrae. It occurs between the 21st and 37th day of gestation through failure of segmentation of adjacent sclerotomes in the fetus [105]. The genetic basis of the defect is not yet known, but the processes of appropriate segmentation and somite differentiation appear to be under the control of a group of paired homeobox or "Hox" genes that have been conserved through the genomes of many vertebrate species and are normally expressed in a specific anteroposterior sequence. At present no specific Hox defects have been detected in patients with the Klippel-Feil syndrome, but it is likely that such a relationship eventually will be found [106,107]. The anatomic feature that defines Klippel-Feil syndrome is fusion of vertebral bodies, laminae, pedicles, and posterior spinous processes. The classification system developed by Gunderson [108] divides the syndrome into three types. Type I anomalies include those with massive fusion of multiple cervical and high thoracic vertebrae into solid blocks of bone. Despite the fusion, intervertebral foramina remain patent and the brachial plexus formation is preserved. Clinically, the head is typically retroflexed or tilted and appears to sit on the shoulders. In type II Klippel-Feil anomaly, only one or two cervical vertebrae are fused, although hemivertebrae and fusion of the atlas and occipital bone often occur. Patients with this most common form of the anomaly have less restriction of motion but may develop complications such as scoliosis, spinal stenosis, and subluxation as they grow older. They frequently have other musculoskeletal anomalies, such as absent ribs, Sprengel's deformity (congenital raised scapula), kyphosis, torticollis, microtia, or conductive hearing deficits. Diplomyelia and hydromyelia have also been described. Associated malformations of the urinary tract and other organs have been reported [109,110]. The type III anomaly includes patients with fusions lower in the thoracic spine or lumbar spine with associated type I or type II anomalies in the cervical region.

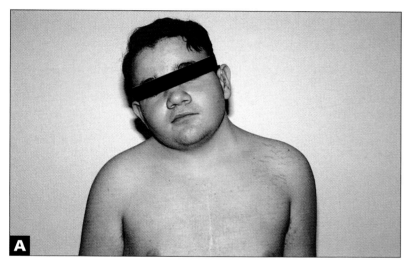 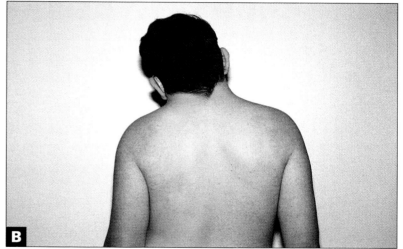

Figure 1-41. A 15-year-old patient with type II Klippel-Feil anomaly who has a short neck, low hairline, and conductive deafness (**A**). The patient's neck mobility is impaired, especially in lateral rotation and tilt (**B**). These clinical findings are characteristic of the Klippel-Feil anomaly. Neurologic findings include radicular pain and paresthesias, particularly about the roots that are not involved in fusion, where open disc spaces allow excessive compensatory mobility and eventual osteoarthritic spurring. Vertebral artery compression may develop in older patients via a similar mechanism and cause posterior circulation symptoms [106,107]. Cervical instability can precipitate symptoms and signs of cord compression, including transient quadriparesis, spastic gait, reflex asymmetry, and Lhermitte's paresthesia. The association of synkinesia or mirror movements with the Klippel-Feil syndrome is ascribed to inadequate decussation of the pyramidal tracts. Special consideration and precautions should be taken to prevent traction on the neck during anesthesia and intubation in Klippel-Feil patients. Participation in gymnastic activities such as tumbling should be avoided.

Neurofibromatosis

Two or More Criteria Necessary for Diagnosis of Neurofibromatosis Type 1

1. Five or more café-au-lait macules over 5 mm in diameter in a prepubertal child or 15 mm in a postpubertal child

2. Two or more cutaneous neurofibromas or one plexiform neurofibroma

3. Axillary or inguinal freckles

4. Two or more iris (Lisch) nodules

5. Osseous lesions—sphenoid wing hypoplasia, thinning of long bone cortex, or pseudoarthrosis

6. Bilateral optic pathway glioma

7. First degree relative with neurofibromatosis type 1

Figure 1-42. Criteria for the diagnosis of neurofibromatosis type 1 (NF1). NF1 (von Recklinghausen's disease) is the most common nervous system disorder, with an incidence of about 1 in 3000 [113]. Although the nervous system, bone, and skin are most prominently affected, other organ systems might also be involved. Clinical diagnosis is established when an individual expresses at least two of the classic features of NF1.

Café-au-lait spots are often present at birth and increase in pigmentation, size, and number with age. Axillary freckles have identical colors and are an important diagnostic sign specific for NF1. Sessile, pedunculated, and flat cutaneous neurofibromas range in size from several millimeters to centimeters. Less often seen are hypopigmented macules. Lisch nodules are an important diagnostic sign of NF1 and appear over the iris with increasing frequency from 10% in the first decade to 100% after the sixth decade. They are hyperpigmented melanotic hamartomas of the iris and are usually bilateral.

Skull abnormalities include absence of the sphenoid wing (empty orbit), enlarged sella turcica and middle cranial fossa arachnoid cysts. Spinal involvement includes scoliosis, enlarged vertebral foraminae, and a widened spinal canal due to anterior meningocele [114]. Tumors are relatively nonprogressive benign astrocytomas [115]. The optic nerve chiasm and optic radiations may also be affected by hamartomas. Astrocytomas are pilocytic, usually benign with rare grade IV tumors, and are found in the hypothalamus, brain stem, and cerebellum [116]. Ependymomas and medulloblastoma are also more frequent. Intracranial schwannomas of cranial nerve V is rare, whereas extracranial plexiform neurofibromas are more common. Unlike its occurrence in NF2, acoustic neuroma is rare in NF1. Ventricular dilatation is usually asymptomatic, although acute hydrocephalus associated with aqueductal stenosis has been reported. Cerebral vascular dysplasia is associated with acute and progressive cerebrovascular accidents.

Most often spinal cord compression results from adjacent nerve neurofibromas (dumbbell lesions) or vertebral compression. Short stature occurred in 27% of North's series [117]. Neurofibromas can affect nerves at any level—small distal radicles, larger nerves, trunks, and plexuses. Plexiform neurofibromas may be massive and are more prone to undergo malignant transformation to neurofibrosarcomas. Orbital and periorbital plexiform neurofibromas may be particularly deforming. Pheochromocytoma occurs in less than 1% of NF1 patients. Hypertension unrelated to pheochromocytoma may be secondary to renal artery stenosis associated with fibromuscular disease. Rhabdomyosarcoma may occur in preexisting plexiform neurofibromas. Gastrointestinal involvement was estimated at 10% by Hochberg and colleagues, and included neurofibromas, leiomyomas, and sarcomas predominantly affecting the serosa and extending from stomach to colon [118].

The diagnosis is made by clinical examination. Molecular analysis provides confirmation in questionable cases, defines sporadic and familial forms, and allows prenatal screening if desired. Clinical monitoring is needed for signs of insidious neurologic involvement, such as spinal cord compression and visual loss. Cranial magnetic resonance imaging (MRI) studies are helpful in explaining obvious problems such as megalencephaly, and also in defining asymptomatic lesions that warrant close clinical assessment, such as optic pathway tumors. Conventional radiographic studies are warranted in the presence of obvious skeletal and cranial involvement. Body MRI scans of plexiform lesions may define the size and complexity of the lesions and may be useful for comparative studies. Visual and auditory evoked responses are valuable in defining the significance of neuroimaging abnormalities and in detecting functional impairment in asymptomatic patients. Somatosensory evoked responses have questionable benefit in asymptomatic patients with negative scan studies.

Genetic counseling is a valuable service to families and should be initiated when the diagnosis is made and mode of inheritance determined. Parents should be aware that cutaneous neurofibromas can enlarge in adolescence, may be uncomfortable, and require removal. No therapy is currently available to prevent or reduce neurofibroma growth. Ultimately, therapy will need to be aimed at somehow minimizing the effects of neurofibromin loss. In children with symptomatic or suspected neurologic involvement, psychometric testing is helpful in determining the extent of cognitive impairment, central processing dysfunction, and behavioral problems that might affect learning and social adjustment. Families should be referred to the National Neurofibromatosis Foundation for information about the disease and available resources [119].

Genetically, this autosomal dominant disorder exhibits complete penetrance and variable expressivity and has an approximate 50% mutation rate. The NF1 gene resides on the long arm of chromosome 17q11.2 [120]. This defective gene, a truncated polypeptide, can be used in the molecular detection of approximately 70% of mutations responsible for NF1. The gene spans 350 kb of genomic DNA, encodes an mRNA of 11–13 kb, and is organized into 50 exons. The gene product, neurofibromin, is ubiquitous, with its greatest levels occurring in the brain. One role of neurofibromin appears to be inactivation of *ras*, a protooncogene protein. Guttman and Collins postulated that a mutational loss of neurofibromin could result in a loss of down regulation of *ras* leading to cell proliferation and transformation [121]. A portion of neurofibromin accelerates the hydrolysis of *ras*-guanidine triphosphate (GTP) to *ras*-guanidine diphosphate (GDP) and converts *ras* from the inactive to active forms. Further proof was suggested by increased *ras*-GTP levels with reduced neurofibromin levels in neurofibrosarcoma cell lines [121]. Mutations affecting mRNA splicing appear to be the most common molecular defect in NF1 [122].

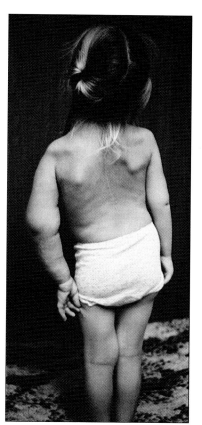

Figure 1-43. Patient with neurofibromatosis. The patient's right arm plexiform neurofibroma extends from the deltoid proximal humerus to the hand. Her humerus is affected by multiple midshaft fractures associated with thinning of bone cortex and pseudoarthrosis. She also has scoliosis, short stature, and enlargement of the lumbar intraspinal canal due to anterior meningocele.

Café-au-lait spots may be seen within a few weeks of life and typically increase in pigmentation, number, and size through early childhood. Dermal fibromas are rarely seen prior to puberty. Plexiform neurofibromas may be present at birth. They typically occur along nerve roots and may produce large and disfiguring masses. Developmental delay, learning disabilities, frank mental retardation, and attention deficit disorder with hyperactivity are nonprogressive manifestations of NF1 that should be identifiable at an early age [112,117,123]. Macrocephaly also occurs in 8% to 27% of patients and is often asymptomatic. Learning disability may be the only manifestation of central nervous system involvement. Symptoms from progressive tumor growth, for example, spinal cord compression, seizures, and hemiparesis due to malignant cerebral or cerebellar tumor, and optic glioma are typically insidious until significant compromise occurs. Cerebrovascular complications of NF1 from moyamoya syndrome or fibromuscular vascular dysplasia are usually acute in onset and may be progressive. Seizure frequency is uncommon in our experience and is reported at 3.5% to 30%. Wong's study indicates the lack of significant variation in ethnic expression of NF1 [123]. Recurrent migraine and tension headaches are also extremely common [124].

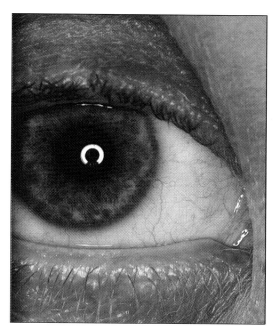

Figure 1-44. Iris (Lisch) nodule. Lisch nodules of the iris are present in most adults with neurofibromatosis type 1 (NF1) and are seen with increasing size, number, and pigmentation. They are hyperpigmented melanotic hamartomas.

Optic pathway lesions may involve the optic nerves, chiasm, or retrochiasmal pathways. These lesions might not be gliomas but rather hamartomas, which may become less evident over time or remain stable. Acoustic neuromas, optic gliomas, astrocytomas, and meningiomas have a collective incidence of 7% to 8%. In NF1, sarcomatous degeneration of pre-existing neurofibromas is uncommon, although in the Mount Sinai study, a 3.6% incidence was reported [125]. In Listernick's study, optic pathway tumors were found in 19% of available NF1 patients [115]. Of this population, 88% had optic nerve tumor (one half intraorbital alone, and one half orbital and chiasmal); 12% had isolated chiasmal lesions; and 42% had clinically evident tumors at the time of diagnosis, exhibiting either proptosis, diminished visual acuity, or precocious puberty. Lack of progression in tumor growth and visual loss was characteristic (only three patients exhibited progression). Symptomatic patients with proptosis and glaucoma had a median age of 1.9 years versus 5.3 years for asymptomatic NF1 patients with optic pathway tumors. Chiasmal lesions were more likely to be associated with visual loss and precocious puberty. In the study by North, cognitive impairment was seen most often in children with abnormal cerebral magnetic resonance imaging (MRI) signals [126].

Tuberous Sclerosis

Diagnostic Criteria for Tuberous Sclerosis

Primary features
  Facial angiofibromas*
  Multiple ungual fibromas*
  Cortical tuber (histologically confirmed)
  Subependymal nodule or giant cell astrocytoma (histologically confirmed)
  Multiple calcified subependymal nodules protruding into the ventricle
    (radiographic evidence)
  Multiple retinal astrocytomas
Secondary features
  Affected first-degree relative
  Cardiac rhabdomyoma (histologic or radiographic confirmation)
  Other retinal hamartoma or achromic patch*
  Cerebral tubers (radiographic confirmation)
  Noncalcified subependymal nodules (radiographic confirmation)
  Shagreen patch*
  Forehead plaque*
  Pulmonary lymphangiomyomatosis (histologic confirmation)
  Renal angiomyolipoma (radiographic or histologic confirmation)
  Renal cysts (histologic confirmation)
Tertiary features
  Hypomelanotic macules*
  "Confetti" skin lesions*
  Renal cysts (radiographic evidence)
  Randomly distributed enamel pits in deciduous and/or permanent teeth
  Hamartomatous rectal polyps (histologic confirmation)
  Bone cysts (radiographic evidence)
  Pulmonary lymphangiomyomatosis (radiographic evidence)
  Cerebral white-matter "migration tracts" or heterotopias (radiographic evidence)
  Gingival fibroma*
  Hamartoma of other organs (histologic confirmation)
  Infantile spasms
Definite tuberous sclerosis
  Either one primary feature, two secondary features, or one secondary plus two
    tertiary features
Probable tuberous sclerosis
  Either one secondary plus one tertiary feature, or three tertiary features
Suspect tuberous sclerosis
  Either one secondary feature or two tertiary features

Histologic confirmation is not required if the lesion is clinically obvious.

Figure 1-45. Diagnostic criteria for tuberous sclerosis. Tuberous sclerosis complex (TSC) is an autosomal dominant neurocutaneous hamartomatous disease exhibiting variable expression in multiple organs. The incidence of TSC is variably reported at 1 in 12,000 to 1 in 6000. In 1880, Bourneville described the relationship of cerebral cortical tubers, epilepsy, and hemiplegia. Subsequently, numerous authors described involvement of skin, retina, lung, heart, kidney, and other organs along with variable degrees of mental and behavioral involvement. The term *phakoma* was coined for TSC because of the lentil-shaped retinal lesions and then applied to other neurocutaneous diseases as the *phakomatoses*. Clinical diagnostic criteria were established by a consensus of the Diagnostic Criteria Committee of the National Tuberous Sclerosis Association [127]. Clinical heterogeneity is common within the same pedigree. Clinical manifestation of TSC may be present at birth with cardiac and neurologic involvement. Perinatologists are able to identify cardiac rhabdomyomas prenatally, thus allowing for neurologic diagnosis at birth. Rhabdomyomas of spontaneous mutational origin are also commonly seen in symptomatic newborns and are usually the first clue in the diagnosis of TSC. The lesions usually are not significant clinically and decrease in relative size as the child grows and the heart enlarges normally.

All of the infants that we have evaluated for TSC at birth exhibited seizures and electroencephalographic abnormalities within one week of birth. Magnetic resonance imaging (MRI) is the preferred study, because it reveals changes in tissue and hydration of cerebral lesions in both the gray matter and the hypomyelinated subcortical white matter. The advantage of computed tomography (CT) imaging is the identification of calcified lesions. Shepherd and colleagues described sulcal islands, gyral cores, radial migration lines, wedges, and subependymal nodules as MRI imaging abnormalities of tuberous sclerosis [128]. On rare occasions the diagnosis is made during the evaluation of learning disability or polycystic kidney disease. Angiomyolipomas increase in number and size with age. In childhood they are usually asymptomatic except for microscopic hematuria. Renal cysts are also usually asymptomatic. Both renal lesions are readily identified by ultrasonography. Polycystic kidneys may be associated with progressive renal disease that may require transplantation.

Pulmonary lymphangiomyomatosis may result in adult-onset pulmonary disease in women. Gastrointestinal hamartomas may produce recurring pain and bleeding but are usually asymptomatic. Dental enamel pitting is a common finding in 90% of patients and is more apparent in adults. Hepatic hamartomas occur in 25% of children and are clinically insignificant. Bone cysts are small and clinically insignificant. TSC most often presents as seizures. Gomez found that seizures were the initial presenting sign in 92% of TSC patients and occurred in 84% of all affected individuals.

effect could be associated with lack of cell surface markers [129].

In the majority of children seizures are present from infancy and occur in 84% of all TSC patients. Although these seizures may initially be responsive to conventional antiepileptic drugs such as phenobarbital, phenytoin, or carbamazepine, the emergence of infantile spasms at 2 to 11 months of age is common, with the greatest incidence occurring between 4 and 5 months. Atypical features of infantile spasm of TSC include the appearance of lateralizing features, such as asymmetric tonic and atonic components, unilateral grimacing, head turning, eye deviation, and unequal limb movements. Multifocal electroencephalographic epileptiform abnormalities usually arise from more abnormal or dominant structural foci (cortical tuber). Progression from multifocal to generalized spike and wave discharges on electroencephalograms, with sudden voltage attenuation is as prevalent as hypsarrhythmia. Earlier onset infantile spasm is associated with posterior temporal and occipital tuber foci. The emergence in time of infantile spasms in TSC relates to the development of dysplastic neuronal populations and expanded dendritic arborization, providing an enhanced connective pathway to propagate epileptiform abnormalities from focal and multifocal to generalized. Although an infant with TSC and partial epilepsy may appear to be developing normally, regression of cognitive, behavioral, and motor skills commonly accompanies the onset of infantile spasms, and reversibility and severity parallel the location and number of cortical tubers. Children with multiple tubers and spasms resistant to antiepileptic drugs are more likely to be permanently impaired. The reported excellent response of TSC infantile spasms to vigabatrin is probably related to their focal origin. When seizures are intractable, despite aggressive antiepileptic drug therapy, surgery for epilepsy must be considered [130]. Even in the presence of multiple cortical tubers or astrocytic hamartomas, if the seizure focus can be consistently localized to a dominant cerebral lesion, after resection of the primary focus the less prominent or secondary foci may gradually diminish [131]. Mental subnormality occurs in approximately 38% to 68% of TSC patients and is evident in early childhood [131]. More intractable seizures and multiple bilateral tubers are more commonly associated with mental retardation [132].

Although a high incidence of autism has been described in TSC studies [133], a prospective comprehensive behavioral analysis of a large unselected TSC population is warranted [133]. Developmental evaluation and psychometric studies are warranted in all patients with TSC to define learning disabilities, mental impairment, and behavioral disorders.

TSC is an autosomal dominant condition with variable expression, and two thirds of cases are new mutations. Linkage studies have identified loci on chromosome 9q34 (*TSC1*) [134] and 16p13 (*TSC2*) [135]. Locus heterogenity may also explain the clinical heterogenity. The gene on chromosome 16 (*TSC2*) has been identified and mutational analysis is available. Linkage analysis may determine whether the TSC patient's genetic abnormality is linked to chromosome 9 or 16. In a new mutation, the risk of another sibling being affected is 2% to 5%. Mutations in either the *TSC1* or the *TSC2* gene may lead to decreased expression of the gene products, tuberin and hamartin [136]. To identify an asymptomatic TSC parent, examination should include careful cutaneous examination, neuroimaging, and ophthalmologic and renal evaluations. Rarely, an asymptomatic parent can be identified, redefining the genetic risk at 50%. Coexistence of NF1 and TSC in a patient has also been reported [137].

Genetic counseling and, when applicable, linkage analysis are necessary after evaluation of family members. In the case of a new mutation, the risk for another affected sibling is 2% to 5%. The National Tuberous Sclerosis Association is a valuable resource for patients, families, and professionals [138].

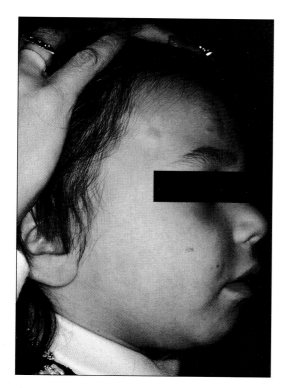

Figure 1-46. Patient with tuberous sclerosis complex (TSC). In this patient, a large forehead plaque was present at birth. She also exhibited asymptomatic rhabdomyoma and at 3 years of age had microscopic hematuria and renal angioleiomyoma determined by ultrasound. The facial sebaceous adenomata were just developing at 3 years and were actually angiofibromas. Although initially responsive to adenocorticotropic hormone (ACTH), she ultimately had maximum seizure control with vigabatrin and carbamazepine. Similar pathologic phenomena could result from different mutations; for example, altered chromosome 11 function could result in abnormal neuronal cell adhesion molecule function, thus affecting neuronal migration. A similar

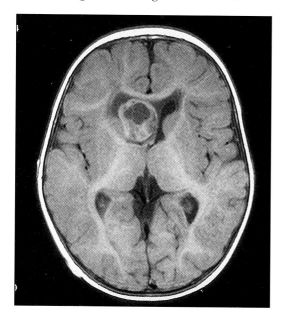

Figure 1-47. T1-weighted transaxial magnetic resonance image of a large right foramen of Monro astrocytic hamartoma with a central cystic component. This lesion was enlarging and causing progressive ventriculomegaly. Right frontal cortical and left parietal cortical tubers with gyral cores were associated with multifocal epileptiform activity. Partial seizures followed infantile spasms. The ventricular mass was resected without incident. Expressive language was delayed and affect was appropriate.

Cortical tubers occur most often in the cerebrum and to a lesser extent in the cerebellum. The tubers are present at birth and vary in number, size, and location. The frontal and parietal lobes are involved most often. Macroscopically, the tubers are firm, flat, or slightly elevated and paler than the surrounding cortex. Normal cytoarchitecture is lost, with enlarged multinucleate glial cells and enlarged neurons irregularly distributed. The cortical gray-white interface shows hypomyelination. Rarely, the cortical tubers undergo necrosis. Subependymal nodules typically occur in the body of the lateral ventricles and are composed of large multinucleated astrocytes and large spindle cells. Microscopic mineralization is seen in at least 50% of cases. Nodules in the region of foramen of Monro may grow to greater than 3 cm and cause hydrocephalus. While approximately 6% of patients may experience malignant tranformation of lesions, the actual frequency of this neoplastic change is poorly defined. DiMario recently reported brain stem tubers and cerebellar dysgenesis with calcification in a patient with central apnea [128].

Hypomelanosis of Ito

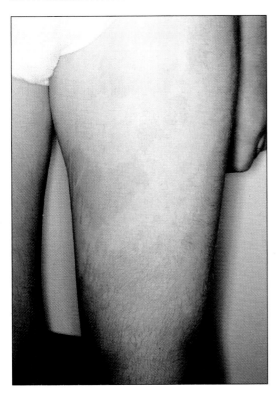

Figure 1-48. A patient with hypomelanosis of Ito. Hypomelanosis of Ito (HOI), or incontinentia pigmenti achromians, was described by Minor Ito in 1952 and is characterized by variable cutaneous macular hypopigmented whorls, streaks, and patches that usually occur on the trunk and the limbs, and to a lesser extent, on the face [139]. Neurologic involvement is reported at 40% to 100%, and the degree of severity and type and extent of neuropathologic involvement varies. Hypopigmentation may be apparent at birth, but as in tuberous sclerosis, the lesions may become obvious only with increasing skin pigmentation after several months of age. Ocular abnormalities include choroidal atrophy and corneal opacities. Anomalies of teeth, facial bones, scoliosis, limb length irregularities, strabismus, macrocephaly, craniofacial dysmorphism, and syndactyly have been described. In this patient a large hypopigmented patch became evident after 12 months of age. The hypomelanotic lesions are wide with irregular borders, and the biopsy specimen revealed decreased melanocytes and melanin deposition. Wood's lamp (ultraviolet) examination can be helpful in identifying the hypopigmented whorls in the younger, fair-skinned infant. This patient also had macrocephaly and learning disabilities with no focal deficit or epilepsy.

Familial case reports make it likely that HOI is a dominantly inherited disorder with variable expression and a high mutation rate, which would explain the frequency of sporadic cases.

Chromosomal abnormalities described include balanced translocations of chromosomes 2 and 8 and mosaicisms in cultured fibroblast [140]. Trisomy 14 mosaicism seen in cultured fibroblasts may underlie the pigmentation abnormalities [141]. The significance of the different chromosomal abnormalities remains ill-defined, however.

Wyburn-Mason Syndrome

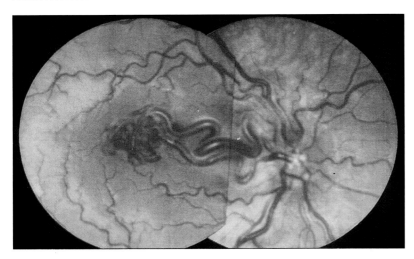

Figure 1-49. Patient with Wyburn-Mason syndrome (WBS). WBS, neuroretinal angiomatosis (retinocephalic vascular malformation), is a spontaneous nonfamilial neurocutaneous disorder characterized by the coexistence of ocular and intracranial arteriovenous malformations (AVMs). Although described by others earlier, Wyburn-Mason in 1943 reviewed the available literature on retinal AVMs and pointed out the association in 22 of 27 patients of associated intracranial vascular malformations, particularly in the midbrain [142]. Subsequent reports of WBS have included patients with optic atrophy without retinal vascular malformation but exhibiting intraorbital or chiasmal AVMs and associated cerebral AVMs [143,144]. Additionally, vascular malformations of the face and mandible have been associated with WBS. From these descriptions, it is apparent that facial, ocular, and intracranial arteriovenous malformations may be heterogeneous in their clinical presentation. This is a spontaneous nonfamilial disorder. The cerebral and ocular malformation has its origin in the first trimester of fetal development. WBS and Sturge-Weber syndrome have been reported in the same patient [145].

Retinal lesions are macroscopic and visualized by funduscopy. Vessels are tortuous, dilated, and arteriovenous shunts can be identified. The retinal lesions are unilateral. Intracranial AVMs are typically ipsilateral to the retinal lesion and lie deep within cerebral parenchyma, including mesencephalon, diencephalon, optic chiasm, and basal ganglia. Patel and Gupta described a child with bilateral neuroretinal involvement [146]. Nonneural involvement is also frequent, and includes facial angioma and palatal, oral mucosal, mandibular, and maxillary vascular malformations in up to 50% of patients. Vision is usually impaired, but it may be difficult to define in the young child. Proptosis, nystagmus, impaired pupillary reaction, conjunctival hyperemia, and variable degrees of visual loss are common. Central nervous system involvement varies depending on the location and size of the intracranial AVM. Intraorbital and midbrain cranial nerves may be affected (III, IV, VI, VII, and VIII). Upper motor neuron and cerebellar dysfunction may be unilateral or bilateral or asymmetrically bilateral.

WBS should be considered when retinal, facial, mandibular, or maxillary vascular malformations are present. Retinal examination reveals AVMs or optic atrophy. Also, the examiner should auscultate for cranial or orbital bruits. Contrast-enhanced cerebral and orbital computed tomography or magnetic resonance imaging scans or angiography generally reveal the extent of intraocular and intracranial involvement. Selective angiography is necessary to delineate the origin and extent of the arteriovenous malformation. Definitive treatment is determined by the extent and location of the AVMs. Depending on the individual circumstances, intravascular occlusive therapy, gamma irradiation, direct surgical intervention, or no treatment may be to the patient's advantage.

Sturge-Weber Syndrome

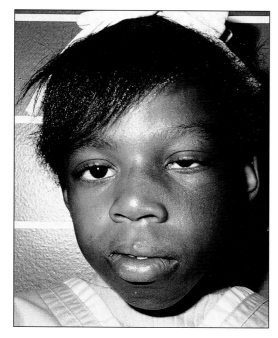

Figure 1-50. Patient with Sturge-Weber syndrome (SWS). SWS is a nonfamilial spontaneous neurocutaneous disease affecting all ethnic groups. This disorder has its onset in infancy in most patients, with a high frequency of seizures, developmental delay, and mental impairment. Sujansky and Courodi analyzed data on 171 patients with SWS and provided valuable information on clinical expression of the disease [147]. Glaucoma is a common feature and is usually ipsilateral to the nevus. Because of variable clinical expression, Roach described three forms of SWS: type I has associated facial and leptomeningeal angiomas, often accompanied by glaucoma; type II has facial angioma

without cerebral leptomeningeal angioma and may have accompanying glaucoma; type III has cerebral leptomeningeal angioma without facial nevus. An extensive capillary venous angioma overlies the affected cerebral tissue; typically it affects the occipital region but can involve the entire hemisphere. The leptomeninges are thickened, containing extensive thin-walled capillaries and veins that often exhibit hyaline thickening of their walls. Cerebral cortical vascular changes are similar, and in time, calcification of the gyral angiomas produce railroad-track calcifications. Progressive cerebral atrophy and external hydrocephalus are long-term effects of SWS. The cerebral lesions are unilateral in 85% of patients.

Facial nevi, present at birth, may involve the oral and nasopharyngeal mucosa. Port wine stains appear on the trunk and limbs of 44% of SWS patients. Facial port wine stains occur along the distribution of the fifth cranial nerve (V) as follows: 16% in V_1 (ophthalmic) alone; 18% in V_1 plus V_2 (maxillary); 38% in V_1, V_2, and V_3 (mandibular); and the remainder exhibiting various degrees of bilateral involvement. The port wine nevus is present at birth, and the extent of involvement impacts the degree of neurologic involvement. Seizures occur in 80% of patients with 75% experiencing onset in the first year of life and 95% by 5 years [148]. Partial, complex partial, and secondarily generalized seizures are typical, and initially may be less responsive to aggressive antiepileptic drug (AED) therapy than in the chronic epileptic disorder of SWS. This may partly be caused by relatively acute neuropathologic changes such as cerebral cortical microinfarction owing to progressive venous occlusive phenomena. Ocular choroid membrane angioma is the cause of glaucoma, with 48% of patients affected; two thirds unilateral and one third bilateral. Approximately 60% of patients exhibit glaucoma by one year of age [147]. It is more common when the port wine stain involves both the upper and lower eyelids [149].

Developmental delay and subsequent mental impairment occur in approximately 50% of SWS patients. The greatest risk for retardation occurs in children with bilateral cerebral abnormalities and those with seizure onset in the first year of life, especially if the epilepsy remains poorly responsive even to aggressive anticonvulsant therapy. Progressive intellectual decline with motor impairment in the presence of widespread hemispheric angioma and intractable seizures is considered to be a potentially preventable condition responsive to epilepsy surgery [150]. Progressive hemiplegia with accompanying hemianopia and specifically localized impairments can be attributed to occlusive venous infarction and cerebral atrophy. Symptomatic external hydrocephalus with macrocephaly may further complicate the condition. If seizures begin after 4 years of age, intellectual impairment is generally infrequent, although seizures may be less responsive to antiepileptic drug (AED) therapy.

Cerebral involvement is best defined by gadolinium-enhanced MRI and magnetic resonance angiography. Electroencephalographic (EEG) findings are representative of focal structural abnormalities and epileptiform potentials, and may extend beyond the extent of angiomatosis, calcification, and atrophy. This patient showed facial angioma port wine nevus involving V_1, V_2, and V_3 distribution with conjunctival and choroidal angioma and ipsilateral glaucoma. The child experienced complex partial seizures and had ipsilateral focal occipital cortical venous angioma. Skull radiography revealed "railroad tracks" in the affected occipital region, and the EEG was abnormal due to frequent epileptiform discharges in the left occipital and parietal regions.

Incontinentia Pigmenti

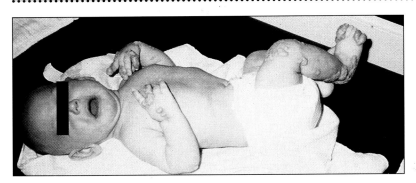

Figure 1-51. A patient with incontinentia pigmenti. Multiple verrucous lesions are present on her upper and lower limbs. They consist of papules and hyperkeratotic streaks and thick crusts. They were preceded by bullae that began 2 weeks after the onset of partial seizures at 6 weeks of age. During the verrucous stage, the patient exhibited recurrent complex partial seizures and regression in milestones.

Incontinentia pigmenti (IP) is a unique progressive genodermatosis that occurs almost exclusively in females, with one third exhibiting neurologic complications [151]. Most patients develop evolving cutaneous lesions (stage 1, bullae; stage 2, verrucae) in the first year of life, although the cutaneous manifestations may appear at single or multiple stages at birth with accompanying neurologic symptoms. Overall systemic involvement occurs in 80% of patients who manifest cutaneous lesions. The female to male ratio is 35 to 1. X-linked dominant inheritance is the likely basis for the predominance of affected females and presumed lethality in affected males. In our own experience, fathers with cutaneous lesions of IP had no neurologic symptoms, and the literature indicates that surviving affected males have no greater degree of neurologic involvement. Curtis and colleagues showed probable linkage to the DXS52 and F8C loci in Xq28 and confirmed inactivation of the maternally inherited X chromosome in affected females [152]. Traupe and Vehring

attribute mosaic disease expression of IP in males to an unstable premutation, which ordinarily remains silent in males during embryogenesis. Surviving affected infant males have a mosaic state of full and premutation alleles [153].

Acute neurologic manifestations may be present at birth when stages 1 and 2 (skin bullae and verrucae) are also present [153,154]. Seizures may precede the skin lesions by days or weeks. Significant neurologic impairment occurs more often with neonatal or infantile onset of symptoms. Mental retardation occurs in approximately 12%, epilepsy in 13%, and spastic cerebral palsy in 11%. Behavioral problems and learning disabilities are also seen in children with less severe neurologic involvement. Neuropathologic features include acute hemorrhagic encephalopathy of white matter with associated edema and chronic effects similar to residua of encephalitis, including neuronal loss, gliosis, ventriculomegaly, and cortical atrophy [153–155]. Acute hemiplegia due to middle cerebral artery occlusive disease affecting both a mother and child was reported by Pellegrino [156]. Lee and colleagues described magnetic resonance imaging (MRI) and magnetic resonance spectroscopy findings indicative of small and large vessel cerebrovascular occlusive disease with probably shared common pathophysiologic mechanisms of retinal vasculopathy of IP [157]. Neuroimaging abnormalities are determined by the acute or chronic phase of the disease. At the onset of central nervous system (CNS) symptoms, cerebral edema is suggested by loss of gray-white interface, effacement of lateral ventricles, and increased MRI signal in the affected areas [154]. Acute cerebrovascular abnormalities appear as focal ischemic lesions. Chronic effects include focal and diffuse cortical atrophy, ventriculomegaly, and microcephaly.

Dental abnormalities include adontia, late dentition, hypodentia, and abnormal (notched and conical) tooth formation [151]. Ocular abnormalities occur in up to 35% of IP cases. Seen in decreasing frequency are strabismus, blindness, congenital cataracts, micropthalmia, nystagmus, iris pigmentation, uveitis, chorioretinitis, and papillitis. Wald and colleagues reported four patients with traction retinal detachments [158]. Retinal vascular abnormalities suggest retinal arteriolar occlusion with ischemic infarction. Eosinophilia occurs during the acute phase in two thirds of patients; it ranges from 5% to 65% and subsides with resolution of the CNS symptoms and cutaneous lesions [151].

Four Stages in the Evolution of the Cutaneous Lesions in Incontinentia Pigmenti

Stage 1   Vesicular lesions occur initially and may be present at birth in 50% of patients. They are usually erythematous and occur on the extremities and trunk and usually resolve over 1 to 2 weeks, although rarely they recur over several months. Ninety percent of patients manifest vesicles by 1 year of age. Microscopically, the vesicles contain and are surrounded by numerous eosinophils with extensive intercellular edema.

Stage 2   Verrucae usually follow vesicles and rarely occur simultaneously with them. The lesions are wart-like and have papular hyperkeratotic formation. These occur in 70% of patients and only on the extremities. Dyskeratosis is prominent; basal cells exhibit vacuolization with loss of pigment.

Stage 3   This is the pigmentary phase. Lesions present over the trunk or limbs and are irregular, whorling, marbled, or reticulated. Although the hyperpigmented stage may occur at birth, it is usually evident at 3 to 6 months of age. There is a subtle fading of the pigmented streaks in the late teens. Microscopically, melanin is heavily deposited in melanophages in the upper dermis.

Stage 4   Atrophic scars occur in one third of cases and follow the fading hyperpigmented lesions. Ultimately, the scars flatten. Although the cutaneous lesions of IP appear to evolve from one stage to the next, different stages may appear simultaneously, and in time the following stage may appear at a different site.

Figure 1-52. Four stages in the evolution of the cutaneous lesions in incontinentia pigmenti. They usually occur in sequence, although two stages may be present simultaneously. The stages are vesicular lesions, verrucae, a pigmentary phase, and atrophic scars.

Secondary Microcephaly

Characteristics of Primary and Secondary Microcephaly

	Primary Microcephaly	Secondary Microcephaly
Etiology	Gene loci on 8p22/19q13/9q34	Environmental, toxic, or infectious cause
Pathology	Abnormally shaped skull; primary migrational disturbances of microgyria, heterotopias	Destructive lesions; cortical atrophy, focal necrosis, mineralizing angiopathy
Neuroimaging	Heterotopias, hypoplasia or aplasia of cerebellar vermis and corpus callosum, periventricular T2 hyperintense lesions	Calcifications, cystic encephalomalacia, relative ventriculomegaly, thinned cortex

Figure 1-53. Characteristics of primary and secondary microcephaly. Microcephaly with a nongenetic basis is frequently encountered. It may be associated with a number of environmental insults to the developing brain, including malnutrition, exposure to toxins such as alcohol, exposure to radiation, and exposure to congenital viral infections. Infectious agents that produce intrauterine microcephaly include toxoplasmosis, cytomegalovirus, rubella, herpes simplex type II (when infection occurs early in pregnancy), lymphocytic choriomeningitis virus, and infrequently, the influenza virus and human immunodeficiency viruses [159,160]. The cortex demonstrates diffuse atrophy, focal necrosis, or gliosis. Deeper structures are frequently affected by degeneration of blood vessel walls, resulting in mineralizing microangiopathy and calcification that is detectable on neuroimaging studies [108]. The mechanism by which viral infections affect specific immature cell populations leading to microcephaly with disordered cell migration, microgyria, and changes of encephalomalacia is not absolutely clear. However, one theory relates to the role of vasoactive intestinal peptide (VIP) in neurodifferentiation in cell cultures [161]. VIP causes glia to release molecules that promote mitosis of astrocytes and neuroblasts. All of the neuropathologic features of microcephaly can be induced in mice following prenatal administration of a specific VIP antagonist (neurotensin-VIP 7-28) intraperitoneally between the 9th and 12th gestational days.

Clinically, patients with secondary microcephaly tend to have more neurologic handicaps and intellectual dysfunction compared with those with primary microcephaly, who present more commonly with mental retardation with or without seizures [162]. Because congenital infections can involve the developing optic nerve and auditory system, patients should be evaluated thoroughly for deafness and optic atrophy.

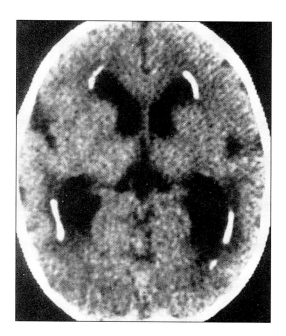

Figure 1-54. Computed tomography (CT) scan of microcephaly due to cytomegalovirus infection, demonstrating periventricular mineralizing angiopathy as well as diffuse atrophy. Maternal viremia allows transplacental passage of the virus into the most vascularized tissues of the fetus. This allows rapid proliferation of the virus in the subependymal germinal matrix, resulting in the periventricular distribution of calcification that is evident on this scan. CT is helpful in detecting gross brain abnormalities. A magnetic resonance imaging (MRI) scan, however, enables better visualization of associated gyral malformations, the corpus callosum, and neuronal heterotopias. If a suspicion of calcific lesions is present on the MRI scan based on low T1 and T2 signal from specific regions, spin-echo sequences can be used to confirm calcification. Alternatively, an unenhanced CT scan can be performed.

Down Syndrome With Atlanto-Axial Subluxation

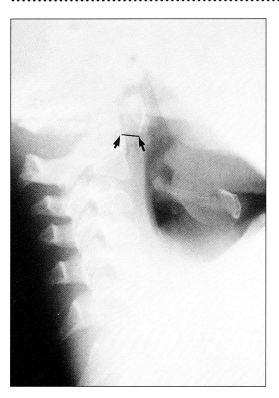

Figure 1-55. Lateral radiograph of the cervical spine in flexion in a 10-year-old boy with Down syndrome, which is the most common chromosomal anomaly, affecting 1.5 of 1000 live births. Over 90% of patients with Down syndrome have trisomy of chromosome 21, whereas a minority have translocations [163]. Atlantoaxial instability (AAI), with an incidence of 9.5% to 27% [164], is a common reason for referral of the patients to neurologists and neurosurgeons. Extreme cases may develop spinal cord compression. The instability of the upper cervical spine is due to laxity of the transverse atlanto-axial ligaments, but hypoplasia or aplasia of the dens may also play a role [164]. The arrows indicate the distance between the posterior aspect of the arch of the C1 vertebra and the anterior aspect of the odontoid process.

Most patients are neurologically asymptomatic. Asymptomatic AAI is not a risk factor for developing subsequent symptomatic AAI [164]. In the symptomatic patient, the disturbance evolves gradually over years. In rare instances, however, abrupt onset may follow otologic or adenotonsillar surgical procedures that predispose to linear and rotational stresses on the cervical spine [165]. Gait abnormalities with a tendency to fall, urinary incontinence in a previously toilet-trained child, neck pain, and head tilt are the most common symptoms [166]. The neurologic examination may be unremarkable. Alternatively, it may show loss of the normal cervical lordosis, altitudinal changes in reflexes (normal jaw jerk with exaggerated upper and lower extremity tendon reflexes), impaired proprioception in the upper and lower extremities, or bilateral extensor plantar responses. Quadriplegia has also been reported in rare instances.

This patient developed progressive clumsiness of gait and a stooped posture over an 18-month period. The neurologic examination disclosed a normal jaw jerk but symmetrically exaggerated upper and lower extremity tendon reflexes, and bilateral extensor plantar responses. The distance from the anterior aspect of the odontoid process to the posteroinferior aspect of the arch of the first cervical vertebra was 3 mm in the neutral position, 2 mm during neck extension, and 6 mm upon neck flexion. AAI is diagnosed when the distance between the posteroinferior aspect of the arch of the atlas and the anterior surface of the odontoid process exceeds 4.5 mm [164].

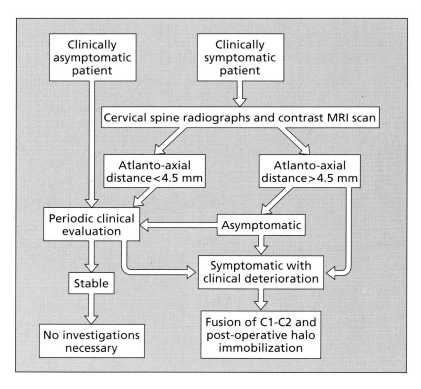

Figure 1-56. Algorithm for evaluation of the cervical spine in Down syndrome. Lateral spine radiographs should be obtained in the neutral, neck flexion, and neck extension positions to detect the abnormality; it is usually apparent on the flexion views. Radiographic reproducibility of the subluxation may be questionable in some patients [167]. Clinical assessment for cervical spinal cord compression therefore assumes greater importance. Translational instability of 10 mm or more on radiographs or neurologic findings on examination that suggest spinal cord compression are indications for operative fusion of C1 to C2 [168]. Postoperative halo immobilization may be necessary for 10 to 12 weeks. All patients with Down syndrome should have periodic clinical neurologic examinations that focus on detecting cervical spinal cord compression. The predictive value of spinal radiographs for evidence of subluxation is uncertain [164]. Parents should be counseled against allowing the child to participate in vigorous physical activities that could predispose to cervical spine dislocation, for example, tumbling, trampoline jumping, diving, high jump, and gymnastics.

Dysostosis Multiplex Secondary to Lysosomal Storage Disease

Syndromes With Dysostosis Multiplex

Disorder	Deficient enzyme	Elevated urinary mucopolysaccharide	Inheritance	Severity of skeletal changes
Hurler (MPS I)	α-Iduronidase	Yes	AR	Severe
Hunter (MPS II)	Iduronate sulfatase	Yes	X-linked	Severe
Sanfilippo (MPS III)				
Type A	Heparan-*N*-sulfatase	Yes/no	AR	Mild
Type B	α-*N*-acetylglucosaminidase	Yes/no	AR	Mild
Type C	Acetyl CoA: α-glucosaminide acetyltransferase	Yes/no	AR	Mild
Type D	*N*-acetylglucosamine-6-sulfatase	Yes/no	AR	Mild
Morquio (MPS IV)				
Type A	Galactosamine-6-sulfatase	Yes	AR	Severe, plus additional
Type B	β-Galactosidase	Yes	AR	changes from other MPS
Maroteaux-Lamy (MPS VI)	Arylsulfatase B	Yes	AR	Severe
Sly (MPS VII)	β-Glucuronidase	Yes	AR	Severe
I Cell Disease (ML II)	*N*-acetylglucosamine phospho-transferase	No	AR	Severe
Pseudo-Hurler Polydystophy (ML III)	*N*-acetylglucosamine phospho-transferase	No	AR	Moderate
α-Mannosidosis	α-Mannosidase	No	AR	Severe
β-Mannosidosis	β-Mannosidase	No	AR	Mild/absent
Sialidosis type II	Sialidase	No	AR	Severe
Aspartylglucosaminuria	Aspartylglucosaminidase	No	AR	Mild
Fucosidosis	α-Fucosidase	No	AR	Moderate
Carbohydrate-defiacient glycoprotein syndrome type Ia	Phosphomannomutase	No	AR	Moderate to severe

Figure 1-57. Storage disorders in which dysostosis multiplex can be seen [159–161]. *Dysostosis multiplex* is a term used to describe skeletal abnormalities seen in lysosomal storage diseases, particularly the mucopolysaccharidoses and mucolipidoses [169]. These bony changes typically are not present at birth, but develop over the first 6 to 12 months of life and may constitute the first sign of the disease. The ribs become thickened anteriorly. The long tubular bones become broad and irregular, especially at the metaphyses [172,173]. The long bones have multiple linear streaks in the trabecular pattern and loss of normal tubulation. The skull becomes enlarged and thickened; frequently, dolichocephalic scaphocephaly might also occur. The sella turcica may be J-shaped. The vertebral bodies develop anterior beaking and wedge deformities, leading to gibbus formation of the back. The metacarpals become broad and irregular, with conical deformities of the proximal metaphyses. Accumulation of storage material in the flexor tendons and sheaths leads to the claw-like deformity of the hands. AR—autosmal recessive; ML II—mucolipidosis type II; ML IV—mucolipidosis type IV; MPS I—mucopolysaccharidosis type I; MPS II—mucopolysaccharidosis type II; MPS III—mucopolysaccharidosis type III; MPS IV—mucopolysaccharidosis type IV; MPS VI—mucopolysaccharidosis type VI.

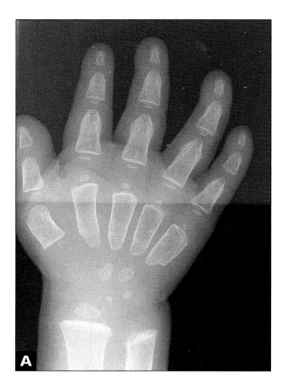
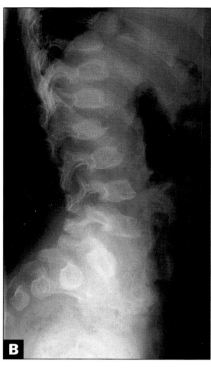

Figure 1-58. Radiographs of a boy with Hurler syndrome. **A,** The hand shows bony changes of dysostosis multiplex. The second through fourth metacarpals are broad and irregular, with cone-shaped and pinched proximal epiphyses. The phalanges are short, thickened, and irregular with a bullet-like configuration. The distal radius and ulna tilt toward each other. **B,** Lateral spine radiograph showing anterior beaking and hook-like projections of the vertebral bodies. This patient has retrolisthesis of T12 on L1 and focal kyphosis of T12–L1. Many patients with dysostosis multiplex develop a gibbus of the lumbar spine.

References

1. Burnelli S, Faiella A, Capra V, *et al.*: Germline mutations in the homeobox gene EMX2 in patients with severe schizencephaly. *Nat Genet* 1996, 12:94–96.

2. Dobyns W, Reiner O, Carrozzo R, Ledbetter D: Lissencephaly: a human brain malformation associated with deletion of the LIS-1 gene located on chromosome 17p13. *JAMA* 1993, 270:2838–2842.

3. Guttman RH, Collins FS: Recent progress toward understanding the molecular biology of von Recklinghausen's neurofibromatosis. *Ann Neurol* 1992, 31:555–561.

4. Use of folic acid for prevention of spina bifida and other neural tube defects—1983–1991. *MMWR* 1991, 40(30):513–516.

5. Recommendations for the use of folic acid to reduce the number of cases of spina bifida and other neural tube defects. *MMWR* 1992, 41(RR-14):1–7.

6. Watson WJ, Chescheir NC, Katz VL, Seeds JW: The role of ultrasound in evaluation of patients with elevated maternal serum α-fetoprotein: a review. *Obstet Gynecol* 1991, 78(1):123–128.

7. Hunter AGW: Brain and Spinal Cord. In *Human Malformations and Related Anomalies*, vol 2. Edited by Stevenson RE, Hall JG, Goodman RM. New York: Oxford University Press; 1993:109–137.

8. Romano PS, Waitzman NJ, Scheffler RM, Randy D: Folic acid fortification of grain: an economic analysis. *Am J Public Health* 1995, 85(5):667–676.

9. Juriloff DM, Harris MJ: Mouse models for neural tube closure defects. *Hum Mol Genet* 2000, 9(6):993–1000.

10. Shapiro K: Encephalocele. In *Birth Defects Encyclopedia*. Edited by Buyse ML. Dover, MA: Center for Birth Defects Information Services in association with Blackwell Scientific Publications; 1990:614–615.

11. Marin-Padilla M. Cephalic axial skeletal-neural dysraphic disorders: embryology and pathology. *Can J Neurol Sci* 1991, 18(2):153–169.

12. Daly LE, Kirke PN, Molloy A, Weir DG, Scott JM: Folate levels and neural tube defects: implications for prevention. *JAMA* 1995, 274(21):1698–1702.

13. Estin D, Cohen AR: Caudal agenesis and associated caudal spinal cord malformations. *Neurosurgery Clinics of North America* 1995, 6(2):377–391.

14. Johnston MC: Understanding human embryonic development. In *Human Malformations and Related Anomalies*, vol 1. Edited by Stevenson RE, Hall JG, Goodman RM. New York: Oxford University Press; 1993:31–63.

15. Gellis SS, Feingold M, Tunnessen WW Jr, Raettig JA: Caudal regression syndrome: picture of the month. *Am J Diseases Childhood* 1968, 116:407–408.

16. Escobar LF, Weaver DD: Caudal regression syndrome. In *Birth Defects Encyclopedia*. Edited by Buyse L. Dover, MA: Center for Birth Defects Information Services in association with Blackwell Scientific Publications; 1990:296–297.

17. Jones KL: *Smith's Recognizable Patterns of Human Malformation*, edn 4. Philadelphia: WB Saunders; 1988.

18. Welch JP, Aterman K: The syndrome of caudal dysplasia: a review, including etiologic considerations and evidence of heterogeneity. *Pediatr Pathol* 1984, 2:313–327.

19. Volpe JJ, ed: *Neurology of the Newborn* edn 3. Philadelphia: WB Saunders; 1994.

20. Hamada H, Oki A, Tsunoda H, Kubo T: Prenatal diagnosis of holoprosencephaly by transvaginal ultrasonography in the first trimester. *Asia Oceania J Obstet Gynaecol* 1992, 18:125–129.

21. Johnston MC, Bronsky PT: Prenatal cranio-facial development: new insights on normal and abnormal mechanisms. *Crit Rev Oral Biol Med* 1995, 6:25–79.

22. Johnston MC, Bronksy PT: Animal models of human cranio-facial malformations. *J Craniofac Genet Dev Biol* 1991, 11:277–291.

23. Muenke M, Gurrieri F, Bay C, Yi DH, *et al.*: Linkage of a human brain malformation, familial holoprosencephaly, to chromosome 7, and evidence for genetic heterogeneity. *Pro Natl Acad Sci USA* 1994, 91:8102–8106.

24. Gorlin RJ, Cohen MM Jr, Levin LS: *Syndromes of the Head and Neck*. New York: Oxford University Press; 1990.

25. Todorov AB, Scott CI Jr, Warren AE, Leeper JD: Developmental screening tests in achondroplasia. *Am J Med Genet* 1981, 9:19–23.

26. Pauli RM, Scott CI, Wassman ER, *et al.*: Apnea and sudden unexpected death in infants with achondroplasia. *J Ped* 1984, 104(3):342–348.

27. Reid CS, Pyeritz RE, Kopits SE, *et al.*: Cervicomedullary compression in young patients with achondroplasia: value of comprehensive neurologic and respiratory evaluation. *J Ped* 1987, 110(4):522–530.

28. Seashore MR, Cho S, Desposito F, *et al.*: Health supervision for children with achondroplasia. *Pediatrics* 1995, 95(3):443–451.

29. Bellus GA, Hefferon TW, Ortiz de Luna RI, *et al.*: Achondroplasia is defined by recurrent G380R mutations of FGFR3. *Am J Hum Genet* 1995, 56:368–373.

30. Shiang R, Thompson LN, Zhu Y-Z, *et al.*: Mutations in the transmembrane domain of FGFR3 cause the most common genetic form of dwarfism, achondroplasia. *Cell* 1994, 78:335–342.

31. Bicknese AR, Sheppard AM, O'Leary DDM, Pearlman AL: Thalamocortical afferents extend along a chondroitin sulfate proteoglycan-enriched pathway coincident with the neocortical subplate and distinct from the efferent pathway. *J Neurosci* 1994, 14(6):3500–3510.

32. Rakic P: Mode of cell migration to the superficial layers of fetal monkey neocortex. *J Comp Neurol* 1972, 145:61–83.

33. Dobyns WB, Gilbert EF, Opitz JM: Further comments on the lissencephaly syndromes. *Am J Med Genet* 1985, 22:197–211.

34. Aicardi J: The agyria-pachygyria complex: a spectrum of cortical malformations. *Brain Devel* 1991, 13(1):1–8.

35. Dobyns W, Truwit C: Lissencephaly and other malformations of cortical development: 1995 update. *Neuropediatr* 1995, 26:132–147.

36. Barkovich A, Koch T, Carrol C: The spectrum of lissencephaly: report of ten patients analysed by magnetic resonance imaging. *Ann Neurol* 1991, 30(2):139–146.

37. Dieker H, Edwards R, ZuRhein G, *et al.*: The lissencephaly syndrome. *Birth Defects* 1969, 5(2):53–64.

38. Dobyns W, Reiner O, Carrozzo R, Ledbetter D: Lissencephaly: a human brain malformation associated with deletion of the LIS1 gene located at chromosome 17p13. *JAMA* 1993, 270(23):2838–2842.

39. Reiner O, Albrecht U, Gordon M, *et al.*: Lissencephaly gene (LIS1) expression in the CNS suggests a role in neuronal migration. *J Neurosci* 1995, 15(5):3730–3738.

40. Qin J, Mizuguchi M, Itoh M: Immunohistochemical expression of doublecortin in the human cerebrum: comparison of normal development and neuronal migration disorders. *Brain Res* 2000, 863(1-2);225–232.

41. Pinard J, Motte J, Chiron C, *et al.*: Subcortical laminar heterotopia and lissencephaly in two families: a single X linked dominant gene. *J Neurol Neurosurg Psychiat* 1994, 57:914–920.

42. Gleeson JG, Allen KM, Fox JW, Lamperti ED, *et al.*: Doublecortin, a brain-specific gene mutated in human X-linked lissencephaly and double cortex syndrome, encodes a putative signaling protein. *Cell* 1998, 92(1):63–72.

43. Altman N, Palasis S, Pacheco-Jacome E: Advanced magnetic resonance imaging of disorders of neuronal migration and sulcation. *Internat Pediat* 1995, 10(suppl 1):16–25.

44. Dobyns W: The neurogenetics of lissencephaly. *Neurol Clin* 1989, 7(1):89–105.

45. Gelot A, Billette de Villemeur T, Bordarier C, *et al.*: Developmental aspects of type II lissencephaly: comparative study of dysplastic lesions in fetal and postnatal brains. *Acta Neuropathol* 1995, 89:72–84.

46. Byrd S, Osborn R, Radkowski M: The MR evaluation of pachygyria and associated syndromes. *Eur J Radiol* 1991, 12:53–59.

47. Barkovich A, Rowley H, Bollen A: Correlation of prenatal events with the development of polymicrogyria. *Am J Neuroradiol* 1995, 16:822–827.

48. Hayward JC, Titelbaum DS, Clancy RR, Zimmerman RA: Lissencephaly-pachygyria associated with congenital cytomegalovirus infection. *J Child Neurol* 1991, 6(4):109–114.

49. Kuzniecky R, Andermann F, Guerrino R: Infantile spasms: an early epileptic manifestation in some patients with the congenital bilateral perisylvian syndrome. *J Child Neurol* 1994, 9:420–423.

50. Becker P, Dixon A, Troncoso J: Bilateral opercular polymicrogyria. *Ann Neurol* 1989, 25(1):90–92.

51. Myers R: Cerebral ischemia in the developing primate fetus. *Biomed Biochim Acta* 1989, 48(2/3):S137–142.

52. Dominguez R, Aguirre Vila-Coro A, Slopis J, Bohan T: Brain and ocular abnormalities in infants with in utero exposure to cocaine and other street drugs. *Am J Dis Child* 1991, 145(6):688–695.

53. Stewart R: Ventral porencephaly: a posterior cerebral defect associated with multiple congenital anomalies. *Acta Neuropathol* 1978, 42:231–235.

54. Brunelli S, Faiella A, Capra V, *et al.*: Germline mutating in the homebox gene EMX2 in patients with severe schizencephaly. *Nat Genet* 1996, 12:94–96.

55. Robinson R: Familial schizencephaly. *Devel Med Child Neurol* 1991, 33:1010–1012.

56. Barkovich A, Chuang S, Norman D: MR of Neuronal Migration Anomalies. *Am J Roentgen* 1988, 150(1):179–187.

57. Norman M, Ludwin S: Congenital Malformations of the Nervous System. In *Textbook of Neuropathology* edn 2. Edited by Davis R, Robertson D. Baltimore: Williams and Wilkins; 1991:207–280.

58. Layton DD: Heterotopic cerebral gray matter as an epileptogenic focus. *J Neuropathol Exp Neurol* 1962, 21:244–249.

59. Lemire RJ, Loeser JD, Leech RW, Alvord EC: Forebrain Cortex. In *Normal and Abnormal Development of the Nervous System*. New York: Harper & Row; 1975:251–253.

60. Kubo S, Kishino T, Sutuke N, *et al.*: A neonatal case of hydranencephaly caused by obstruction of the aortic arch. *J Perinatol* 1994, 14:483–486.

61. Velasco ME, Brown JA, Kini J, Ruppert ES: Primary congenital rhabdoid tumor of the brain with neoplastic hydranencephaly. *Child's Nerv Syst* 1993, 9:185–190.

62. Hashimoto T, Fukuda K, Endo S, Miyazaki M, *et al.*: Circadian rhythm in patients with hydranencephaly. *J Child Neurol* 1992, 7:188–194.

63. Williams JC, Barratt-Boyes BG, Lowe JB: Supravalvular aortic stenosis. *Circulation* 1961, 24:1311–1318.

64. Morris CA, Demsey SA, Leonard CO, *et al.*: Natural history of Williams syndrome: physical characteristics. *J Pediat* 1988, 113:318–326.

65. Sadler LS, Robinson LK, Verdaasdonk KR, Gingell R: The Williams syndrome: evidence for possible autosomal dominant inheritance. *Am J Med Genet* 1993, 47:468–470.

66. Ewart AK, Morris CA, Atkinson D, *et al.*: Hemizygosity at the elastin locus in a developmental disorder, Williams syndrome. *Nature Genet* 1993, 5:11–16.

67. Holm VA, Cassidy SB, Butler MG, *et al.*: Prader-Willi syndrome: consensus diagnostic criteria. *Pediatrics* 1993, 91:398–402.

68. Nicholls RD, Knoll JHM, Butler MG, *et al.*: Genetic imprinting suggested by maternal heterodisomy in non-deletion Prader-Willi syndrome. *Nature* 1989, 342:281–285.

69. Jones KL: *Smith's Recognizable Patterns of Human Malformation*, edn 4. Philadelphia: WB Saunders; 1988:170–173.

70. Clayton-Smith J: Clinical research on Angelman syndrome in the United Kingdom: observations on 82 affected individuals. *Am J Med Genet* 1993, 46:12–15.

71. Fryburg JS, Breg WR, Lindgren V: Diagnosis of Angelman syndrome in infants. *Am J Med Genet* 1991, 38:58–64.

72. Rougeulle C: Angelman syndrome: how many genes to remain silent? *Neurogenet* 1998, 1(4):229–237.

73. Williams CA, Frias JL: The Angelman ("Happy Puppet") syndrome. *Am J Med Genet* 1982, 11:453–460.

74. Raffel C, McComb JG: Arachnoid Cysts. In *Pediatric Neurosurgery Surgery of the Developing Nervous System*. edn 3. Philadelphia: WB Saunders; 1994:104–110.

75. Oberbauer RW, Haase J, Pucher R: Arachnoid cysts in children: a European co-operative study. *Childs Nerv Sys* 1992, 8(5):281–286.

76. Ciricillo SF, Cogen PH, Harsh GR, Edwards MSB: Intracranial arachnoid cysts in children: a comparison of the effects of fenestration and shunting. *J Neurosurg* 1991, 74:230–235.

77. McLone DG, Naidich TP: The Tethered Spinal Cord. In *Disorders of the Developing Nervous System: Diagnosis and Treatment*. Boston: Blackwell Scientific Publications; 1986:71–96.

78. Lemire RJ, Loeser JD, Leech RW, *et al.*: *Normal and Abnormal Development of the Human Nervous System*. New York: Harper & Row; 1975:71–83.

79. Kanev PM, Park TS: Dermoids and dermal sinus tracts of the spine. *Neurosurg Clin North Am* 1995, 6(2):359–366.

80. Steinbok P: Dysraphic lesions of the cervical spinal cord. *Neurosurg Clin North Am* 1995, 6(2):367–376.

81. Dias MS, Pang D: Split cord malformations. *Neurosurg Clin North Am*. 1995, 6(2):339–358.

82. Beardmore HE, Wiggelsworth FW: Vertebral anomalies and alimentary duplications. *Pediatr Clin North Am* 1958, 5:457–474.

83. Perlman JM, Volpe JJ: Intraventricular hemorrhage in extremely small premature infants. *AJDC* 1986, 140:1122–1124.

84. Volpe JJ: *Neurology of the Newborn*. Philadelphia: WB Saunders; 1995:403–463.

85. Shinnar S, Gammon K, Bergman EW, *et al*.: Management of hydrocephalus in infancy: use of acetazolamide and furosemide to avoid cerebrospinal fluid shunts. *J Pediatr* 1985, 107:31–37.

86. Ventriculomegaly Trial Group: Randomised trial of early tapping in neonatal posthaemorrhagic ventricular dilatation: results at 30 months. *Arch Dis Child* 1994, 70:F129–F136.

87. Papile L, Burstein J, Burstein R, Koffler H: Incidence and evolution of subependymal and intraventricular hemorrhage: a study of infants with birth weights less than 1500 gm. *J Pediatr* 1978, 92:529–534.

88. Anwar M, Doyle AJ, Kadam S, *et al*.: Management of posthemorrhagic hydrocephalus in the preterm infant. *J Ped Surg* 1986, 21:334–337.

89. Whitelaw A, Rivers RPA, Creighton L, Gaffney P: Low dose intraventricular fibrinolytic treatment to prevent posthaemorrhagic hydrocephalus. *Arch Dis Child* 1992, 67:12–14.

90. Hirsch JF, Pierre-Kahn A, Renier D, *et al*.: The Dandy-Walker malformation: a review of 40 cases. *J Neurosurg* 1984, 61:515–522.

91. Hart MN, Malamud N, and Ellis WG: The Dandy-Walker syndrome: a clinicopathological study based on 28 cases. *Neurology* 1972, 22:771–780.

92. Pascual-Castroviejo I, Velez A, Pascual-Pascual SI, *et al*.: Dandy-Walker malformation: analysis of 38 cases. *Child's Nerv Syst* 1991, 7:88–97.

93. Volpe JJ: Neural Tube Formation and Prosencephalic Development. In Volpe JJ, ed. *Neurology of the Newborn*. Philadelphia: WB Saunders; 1995:34–36.

94. Carmel P: The Chiari Malformation and Syringomyelia. In *Disorders of the Developing Nervous System: Diagnosis and Treatment*. Boston: Blackwell Scientific Publications; 1986:133–151.

95. Dauser RC, DiPietro MA, Venes JL: Symptomatic Chiari I malformation in childhood: a report of 7 Cases. *Pediatr Neurosci* 1988, 14:184–190.

96. Levy WJ, Mason L, Hahn JF: Chiari malformation presenting in adults: a surgical experience in 127 cases. *Neurosurgery* 1983, 12(4):377–390.

97. Sullivan LP, Stears JC, Ringel SP: Resolution of Syringomyelia and Chiari malformation by ventriculoatrial shunting in a patient with pseudotumor cerebri and a lumboperitoneal shunt. *Neurosurgery* 1991, 22(4):744–747.

98. McClone DG, Knepper PA: The cause of Chiari II malformation: a unified theory. *Pediatr Neurosci* 1989, 15:1–12.

99. Pascual-Castroviejo I, Villarejo F, Perez-Higueras A, *et al*.: Childhood choroid plexus neoplasms: a study of 14 cases less than 2 years old. *Eur J Pediatr* 1983, 140:51–56.

100. Russell DS, Rubinstein LJ: *Pathology of Tumors of the Nervous System*. Baltimore: Williams & Wilkins; 1989:394–404.

101. Ho DM, Wong TT, Liu HC: Choroid plexus tumors in childhood: histopathologic study and clinico-pathological correlation. *Child's Nerv Syst*, 1991, 7:437–441.

102. Qualman SJ, Shannon BT, Boesel CP, *et al*.: Ploidy analysis and cerebrospinal fluid nephelometry as measures of clinical outcome in childhood choroid plexus neoplasia. *Pathol Annual* 1992, 27(pt1):305–320.

103. Yettou H, Marchal JC, Vinikoff L, *et al*.: Choroid plexus papillomas in childhood. Report of 11 cases. *Neurochirurgie* 1994, 40:227–232.

104. Duffner PK, Kun LE, Burger PC, *et al*.: Postoperative chemotherapy and delayed radiation in infants and very young children with choroid plexus carcinomas. *Pediatr Neurosurg* 1995, 22:189–196.

105. Greipp M: Klippel-Feil syndrome. *Orthoped Nurs* 1992, 11:13–18.

106. Burke A, Nelson C, Morgan B, Tabin C: Hox genes and the evolution of vertebrate axial morphology. *Development* 1995, 121(2):333–346.

107. Smith C, Tuan R: Human PAX gene expression and development of the vertebral column. *Clin Orthop* 1994, 302:241–250.

108. Lemire R, Loeser J, Leach R, Alvord E: Suprasegmental structures, CNS associated structures and related considerations. In *Normal and Abnormal Development of the Human Nervous System*. Hagerstown, MD: Harper & Row; 1975: 239–392.

109. da Silva E: Preaxial polydactyly and other defects associated with Klippel-Feil anomaly. *Hum Hered* 1993, 43:371–374.

110. Dubey S, Ghosh L: Klippel-Feil syndrome with congenital conductive deafness: report of a case and review of literature. *Int J Pediatr Otorhinolaryn* 1993, 25:201–208.

111. Erbengi A, Oge H: Congenital malformations of the craniovertebral junction: classification and surgical treatment. *Acta Neurochir* 1994, 127:180–185.

112. Ritterbusch J, McGinty L, Spar J, Orrison W: Magnetic resonance imaging for stenosis and subluxation in Klippel-Feil syndrome. *Spine* 1991, 16:S539–S541.

113. Rubenstein AH: Neurofibromatosis. A review of the clinical problem in neurofibromatosis. *Ann New York Acad Sci*. 1986, 486:1–13.

114. Crawford AH: Neurofibromatosis in children. *Acta Orthoped Scand* 1986, 57(suppl 218): 9–60.

115. Listernick P, Chauren J, Greenwald M, Mets M: Natural history of optic pathway tumors in children with neurofibromatosis type I: a longitudinal study. *J Pediatr* 1994, 125(VI):63–66.

116. Nelson JS: The neuropathology of selected neurocutaneous diseases in seminars in pediatric neurology. *Pediat Neuropathol* 1995, 2:192–199.

117. North K: Neurofibromatosis type I: review of the first 200 patients in an Australian clinic. *J Child Neurol* 1993, 8:395–402.

118. Hochberg FH, DaSilva AB, Galbadini J, et al. Gastrointestinal involvement in von Recklinghausen's neurofibromatosis. *Neurology* 1974, 24:1144–1151.

119. National Neurofibromatosis Foundation, 95 Pine Street, 16th Floor, New York, NY 10005; 212-344-6633, 212-747-0004, 800-323-7938; e-mail NNFF@aol.com; web page HTTP:\\www.nf.org.

120. Heim RA, Silverman LM, Farber RA, *et al*.: Screening for truncated NF-1 proteins. *Nat Genet* 1994, 8:218–219.

121. Guttman RH, Collins FS: Recent progress toward understanding the molecular biology of von Recklinghausen's neurofibromatosis. *Ann Neurol* 1992, 31:555–561.

122. Ars E, Serra E, Garcia J, *et al*.: Mutations affecting mRNA splicing are the most common molecular defects in patients with neurofibromatosis type 1 [published correction appears in *Hum Mol Genet* 2000, 9(4):659]. *Hum Mol Genet* 2000, 9(2):237–247.

123. Wong VC: Clinical manifestations of neurofibromatosis-1 in Chinese children. *Pediat Neurol* 1994, 11:301–307.

124. DiMario FJ Jr, Langshur S: Headaches in patients with neurofibromatosis-1. *J Child Neurol* 2000, 15(4):235–238.

125. Riccardi VM: Neurofibromatosis in neurologic clinics. 1987, 5:341–349.

126. North K, Joy P, Yuille D, *et al*.: Specific learning disabilities in children with neurofibromatosis type I: significance of MRI abnormalities. *Neurology* 1994, 44:878–883.

127. Roach ES, Smith M, Huttenlocher P, *et al*.: Diagnostic criteria: tuberous sclerosis complex. Diagnostic criteria committee of the national tuberous sclerosis association. *J Child Neurol* 1992, 7:221–224.

128. Di Mario FT: Brainstem tubers presenting as disordered breathing in tuberous sclerosis complex. *J Child Neurol* 1995, 10:407–409.

129. Roach ES: International tuberous sclerosis conference. *J Child Neurol* 1990, 5:269–272.

130. Bebin EM, Kelly PJ, Gomez MR: Surgical treatment for epilepsy in cerebral tuberous sclerosis. *Epilepsia* 1993, 4:651–657.

131. Webb SW, Osborne JP, Fryer AE: On the incidence of fits and mental retardation in tuberous sclerosis. *J Med Genet* 1991, 28:385–388.

132. Shepherd CW, Houser OW, Gomez MR: MR findings in tuberous sclerosis complex and correlation with seizure development and mental impairment. *AJNR* 1995, 16:149–155.

133. Hunt A, Shephard C: A prevalence study of autism in tuberous sclerosis. *J Autism Dev Disord* 1993, 23:323–329.

134. Janssen B, Sampson J, Vander Est M, *et al*.: Refined localization of TSC by combined analysis of 9q34 and 16p13 in 14 tuberous sclerosis families. *Hum Genet* 1994, 887:1–4.

135. The European chromosome 16 tuberous sclerosis consortium: Identification and characterization of the tuberous sclerosis gene on chromosome 16. *Cell* 1993, (7):1305–1315.

136. Mizuguchi M, Ikeda K, Takashima S: Simultaneous loss of hamartin and tuberin from the cerebrum, kidney and heart with tuberous sclerosis. *Acta Neuropathol (Berl)* 2000, 99(5):503–510.

137. Lee TC, Sung ML, Chen JS: Tuberous sclerosis associated with neurofibromatosis: report of a case. *J Formosa Med Assoc* 1994, (9):797–801.

138. National Tuberous Sclerosis Association, 8181 Professional Place, Suite 110, Landover, MD 20785; 800-225-NTSA; e-mail NTSA@aol.com; website HTTP://www.sky.net/adamse/TS.HTM.

139. Ito M: Studies of melanin XI. Incontinentia pigmenti achromians, a singular case of nevus depigmentosus systematicus bilateralis. *J Exp Med* 1972, 55:57.

140. Lenzini E, Bertoli P, Artifoni L, *et al.*: Hypomelanosis of Ito: involvement of the chromosome aberrations in this syndrome. *Ann Genet* 1991, 34(1):30–32.

141. Tunca Y, Wilroy RS, Kadandale JS, *et al.*: Hypomelanosis of ito and a 'mirror image' whole chromosome duplication resulting in trisomy 14 mosaicism. *Ann Genet* 2000, 43(1):39–43.

142. Wyburn-Mason R: Arteriovenous aneurysm of midbrain, retina, facial naevi and mental changes. *Brain* 1943, 66:163.

143. Davis R, Appen RE: Optic atrophy and the Wyburn-Mason syndrome. *J Clin Neuro-Ophthalmol* 1984, 4(2):91–95.

144. Brom DG, Hilal SK, Tenner MS: Wyburn-Mason syndrome. Report of two cases without retinal involvement. *Arch Neurol* 1973, 28:67–68.

145. Ward JB, Katz NN: Combined phakomatoses: A case report of Sturge-Weber and Wyburn-Mason syndrome occurring in the same individual. *Ann Ophthal* 1983, 15(12):1112–1116.

146. Patel U, Gupta SC: Wyburn-Mason syndrome—a case report and review of the literature. *Neuroradiol* 1990, 31(6):544–546.

147. Sujansky E, Couradi S: Sturge-Weber syndrome: age of onset of seizures and glaucoma and the prognosis for affected children. *J Child Neurol* 1995, 10:49–58.

148. Arzimanoglou A, Aicardi J: The epilepsy of Sturge-Weber syndrome: clinical features and treatment in 23 patients. *Acta Neurol Scan* (suppl) 1992, 140:18–22.

149. van Emelen C, Goethals M, Dralands L, Casteels I: Treatment of glaucoma in children with Sturge-Weber syndrome. *J Pediatr Ophthalmol Strabismus* 2000, 37(1):29–34.

150 Roach ES, Riela AR, Chugani HT, *et al.*: Sturge-Weber syndrome: recommendations for surgery. *J Child Neurol* 1994, 9:190–192.

151. Cohen BA: Incontinentia pigmenti. *Neurol Clin North Am* 1987, 5:361–377.

152. Curtis ARJ, Lindsay S, Boye E, *et al.*: A study of X chromosome activity in two incontinentia pigmenti families with probably linkage to Xq28. *Eur J Hum Genet* 1994, 2:51–58.

153. Traupe H, Vehring KH: Unstable premutation may explain mosaic disease expression of incontinentia pigmenti in males. *Am J Med Genet* 1994, 49:397–398.

154. Chatkupt S, Gozo AO, Wolansky LJ, Sun S: Characteristic MR findings in a neonate with incontinentia pigmenti. *AJR* 1993, 372–374.

155. Yang JH, Ma SY, Tsai CH: Destructive encephalopathy in incontinentia pigmenti: a case report. *J Dermatol* 1995, 22:340–343.

156. Pellegrino RJ, Shah AJ: Vascular occlusion associated with incontinentia pigmenti. *Pediatr Neurol* 1994, 10:73–74.

157. Lee AG, Goldberg MF, Gillard JH: Intracranial assessment of incontinentia pigmenti using magnetic resonance imaging angiography and spectroscopic imaging. *Arch Pediatr Adolesc Med* 1995, 149:573–580.

158. Wald KJ, Mehta MC, Katsumi O, *et al.*: Retinal detachments in incontinentia pigmenti. *Arch Opthalmol* 1993, 111:614–617.

159. Barton L, Budd S, Morfitt W, *et al.*: Congenital lymphocytic choriomeningitis virus infection in twins. *Pediatr Infect Dis J* 1993, 12:942–946.

160. Perlman J, Argyle C: Lethal cytomegalovirus infection in preterm infants: clinical, radiological and neuropathological findings. *Ann Neurol* 1992, 31:64–68.

161. Gressens P, Hill J, Paindaveine B, *et al.*: Severe microcephaly induced by blockade of vasoactive intestinal peptide function in the primitive neuroepithelium of the mouse. *J Clin Invest* 1994, 94:2020–2027.

162. Sugimoto T, Yashuhara A, Nishida N, *et al.*: MRI of the head in the evaluation of microcephaly. *Neuropediatrics* 1993, 24:4–7.

163. Jones KL, ed: *Smith's Recognizable Patterns of Human Malformations.* Philadelphia: WB Saunders; 1988:10–15.

164. Committee on Sports Medicine & Fitness, American Academy of Pediatrics: Atlantoaxial instability in Down syndrome: subject review. *Pediatrics* 1995, 96:151–154.

165. Harley EH, Collins MD: Neurologic sequelae secondary to atlanto-axial instability in Down syndrome. *Arch Otolaryngol Head Neck Surg* 1994, 120:159–165.

166. Chaudhry V, Sturgeon C, Gates AJ, Myers G: Symptomatic atlanto-axial dislocation in Down syndrome. *Ann Neurol* 1987, 21:606–609.

167. Selby KA, Newton RW, Gupta S, Hunt L: Clinical predictors and radiological reliability in atlanto-axial subluxation in Down syndrome. *Arch Dis Child* 1991, 66:876–878.

168. Smith MD, Phillips WA, Hensinger RN: Fusion of the upper cervical spine in children and adolescents. An analysis of 17 patients. *Spine* 1991, 16:695–701.

169. Neufeld EF, Muenzer J: The Mucopolysaccharidoses. In *The Metabolic and Molecular Bases of Inherited Disease.* Edited by Scriver CR, Beaudet AL, Sly WS, Valle D: New York: McGraw-Hill, 1995, 2465–2494.

170. Kornfeld S, Sly WS: I-Cell Disease and Pseudo-Hurler Polydystrophy: Disorders of Lysosomal Enzyme Phosphorylation and Localization. In *The Metabolic and Molecular Bases of Inherited Disease.* Edited by Scriver CR, Beaudet AL, Sly WS, Valle D. New York: McGraw-Hill, 1995:2495–2508.

171. Thomas GH, Beaudet AL: Disorders of Glycoprotein Degradation and Structure: α-Mannosidosis, β-Mannosidosis, Fucosidosis, Sialidosis, Aspartylglucosaminuria, and Carbohydrate-deficient Glycoprotein Syndrome. In *The Metabolic and Molecular Bases of Inherited Disease.* Edited by Scriver CR, Beaudet AL, Sly WS, Valle D. New York: McGraw-Hill, 1995:2529–2561.

2

Genetic Diseases of the Nervous System

Thomas D. Bird • S. Mark Sumi

ALL human diseases, including those of the nervous system, are the result of interactions between genetic factors and the environment. In some diseases the genetic factors are relatively minor and of little importance. Other disorders are strictly inherited conditions, and genetic factors are paramount. The major categories of genetic influence are single gene (mendelian), gross chromosomal aberration, mitochondrial, and multifactorial/polygenic. Examples of neurologic diseases representing each of these categories are illustrated in this chapter.

Autosomal dominant disorders affect multiple generations, both males and females; there is male-to-male transmission; and each child of an affected person is at 50% risk for inheriting the mutated gene. In autosomal recessive inheritance, carriers of a single copy of the mutation (heterozygotes) are clinically normal. The offspring of carrier parents are at 25% risk of inheriting the mutation from each parent and thus carry two copies of the mutation (homozygote). Such homozygous individuals demonstrate the full manifestations of the disease. Autosomal recessive disorders are usually seen in only a single sibship unless there is intermarriage (consanguinity) within other generations of the family.

X-linked inheritance is a special situation in which the gene locus is on the X chromosome. In X-linked recessive inheritance females with a single mutation on one X chromosome generally show no signs of the disease. However, each of their sons is at 50% risk for inheriting the mutation, and those sons show signs of the disorder. Daughters of carrier females are at 50% risk for also being carriers. Men with X-linked mutations cannot pass them on to their sons (because sons receive only the Y sex chromosome from their father), but daughters of men with X-linked mutations are at 100% risk for being carriers (because fathers always pass on their single X chromosome to their daughters). Occasionally, female carriers of X-linked recessive diseases will show mild or moderate signs of the disorder because of random X inactivation. Also, a few conditions are X-linked dominant, in which case female carriers of the mutation also frequently show signs of the disease, albeit generally milder than affected males in the family.

Mitochondrial inheritance is a special case in which mutations in mitochondrial DNA produce neurologic diseases. Mitochondrial DNA is found in the cytoplasm of cells, not in the nucleus. Sperm do not contain mitochondria, so all mitochondrial DNA is inherited from the cytoplasm of the mother's egg. Therefore, mitochondrial disorders are only transmitted by females. All children of mothers with a mitochondrial mutation inherit some variable proportion of mitochondria containing the mutation. It is the relative proportion of these mitochondria with mutations that determines the expression and severity of the disease in the mother's offspring.

The diseases illustrated in this chapter are presented in anatomic order, that is, from cortex through white matter, basal ganglia, and cerebellum into spinal cord and out to peripheral nerve, muscle, and skin. Examples of neurogenetic diseases of the vasculature and multifactorial conditions are illustrated at the end.

Dementia, Mental Retardation, and Epilepsy

Alzheimer's Disease

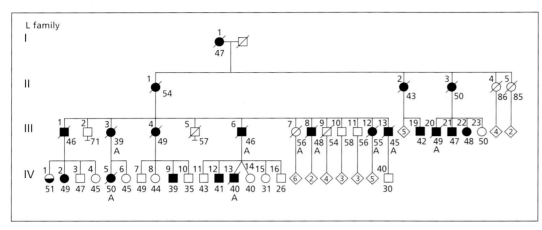

Figure 2-1. The pedigree of a kindred with early-onset familial Alzheimer's disease (FAD) [1]. The disorder has affected male and female family members over four generations in an autosomal dominant pattern. The mean age of onset of dementia in this family is 41 years and the typical duration of disease is approximately 8 years. The numbers beneath each symbol indicate the present age or age at death. The letter *A* indicates those persons who have had an autopsy. The closed symbols represent persons who are affected with dementia, open symbols are persons without dementia, and half-closed symbols are persons with probable dementia. The circles represent females, and the squares represent males; a slash through a symbol indicates death, a number above a symbol is the position in that generation of pedigree, and numbers within a symbol indicate the number of children. The neuropathology in this family demonstrates the typical findings of Alzheimer's, including neuritic amyloid plaques, neurofibrillary tangles, and amyloid angiopathy. This family contains a mutation in the Alzheimer's disease gene on the long arm of chromosome 14 (presenilin 1).

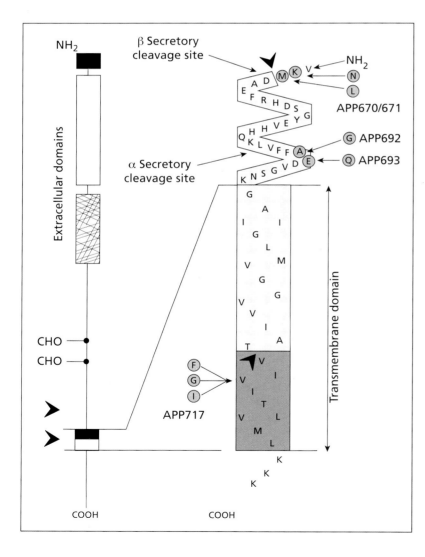

Figure 2-2. The amyloid precursor protein (APP) coded for by a gene on chromosome 21. The region between the black arrowheads indicates where the APP protein is clipped to produce the Aβ amyloid that is deposited in the brains of individuals with Alzheimer's disease. The right side of the diagram shows the location of various mutations that have been discovered in cerebral amyloid disorders. For example, most families with early-onset familial Alzheimer's disease (FAD) and APP mutations have substitution of some other amino acid (usually isoleucine) for valine at position 717. Mutations at positions 692 and 693 result in hereditary cerebral amyloidosis of the Dutch type [2]. The double amino acid substitutions at positions APP 670/671 have caused early onset FAD in a Swedish kindred. A closed box represents signal sequence; an open box represents cysteine-rich domain; a hatched box represents highly negatively charged domain (45% aspartic acid and glutamic acid residues). (*From* Van Broeckhoven [2]; with permission.)

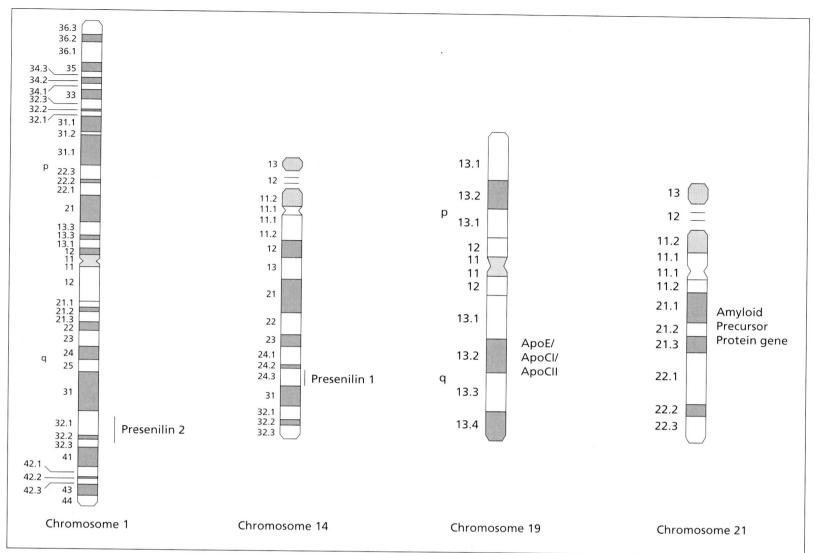

Chromosome 1

Chromosome 14

Presenilin 2

Presenilin 1

Chromosome 19

ApoE/
ApoCI/
ApoCII

Chromosome 21

Amyloid
Precursor
Protein gene

Figure 2-3. Four different chromosomes that contain genes influencing the development of Alzheimer's disease. The amyloid precursor protein (APP) gene is on chromosome 21. Several mutations in this gene result in a form of early-onset, familial Alzheimer's disease (FAD). The presence of the APP gene in triplicate is responsible for the frequent occurrence of Alzheimer's disease in individuals with Down syndrome (trisomy 21). Mutations in a gene called *S182* or presenilin 1 are responsible for early-onset FAD in families showing linkage to chromosome 14, such as the kindred in Figure 2-1 [3]. A gene on chromosome 1 called *STM2* or presenilin 2 is responsible for FAD in Volga German kindreds as well as families of other ethnic backgrounds [4]. Finally, the apolipoprotein E (APO E) gene is on chromosome 19. The ε4 allele of APO E shows a strong association with late-onset (FAD) and sporadic cases of Alzheimer's disease. The ε4 allele of APO E apparently promotes earlier onset of the disease, which is especially true in individuals who are homozygous ε4/4 [5].

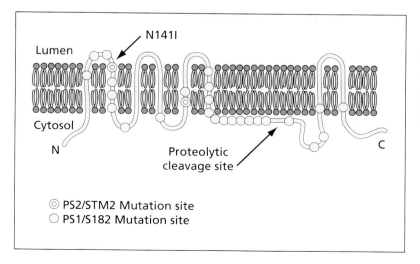

Lumen

N141I

Cytosol

N

Proteolytic
cleavage site

C

⊚ PS2/STM2 Mutation site
◯ PS1/S182 Mutation site

Figure 2-4. The most commonly accepted structure for the presenelin 1 (*S182*) and presenelin 2 (*STM2*) proteins. They are highly homologous and presumably have eight transmembrane domains. The normal function of these two proteins is unknown and it is not yet understood how mutations in them cause Alzheimer's disease. It is possible that the presenilins cleave the amyloid precursor protein at the gamma secretase site. The N141I site is the location of the mutation found in several Volga German kindreds with early onset of Alzheimer's disease [6,7]. C—C terminal; N—N terminal.

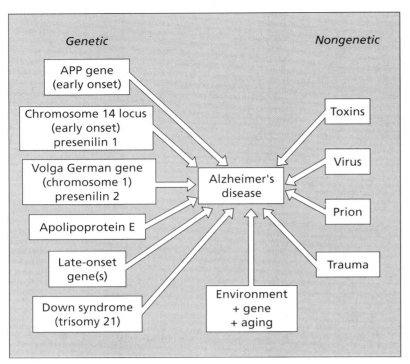

Figure 2-5. The pathogenesis of Alzheimer's disease (AD) as presently understood [6]. Presumably there are nongenetic influences such as toxins, trauma, prions (small proteinaceous infectious particles that resist inactivation), and viruses, but none of these have been identified for certain as causes of AD. As shown in Figure 2-3, there are at least four different genes involved in the pathogenesis of some forms of Alzheimer's disease. However, the most common form of Alzheimer's disease in the general population may be caused by the interaction between as yet unidentified genetic factors and unidentified environmental influences as indicated at the bottom of the diagram. The chromosome 14 gene is called presenilin 1 and the chromsome 1 gene is called presenilin 2. APP—amyloid precursor protein.

Down Syndrome (trisomy 21)

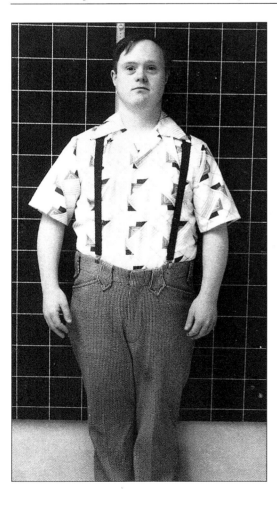

Figure 2-6. Many typical physical features of Down syndrome. These features include short stature, frontal balding, thin hair, epicanthal folds, thick neck, and mild truncal obesity. This young man is moderately mentally retarded but able to perform in a sheltered workshop.

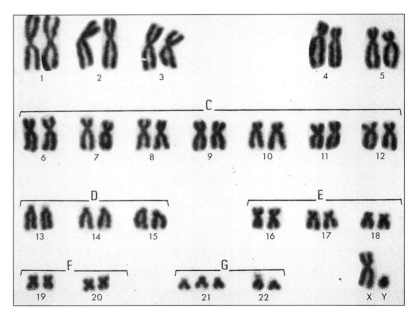

Figure 2-7. Chromosomal karyotype showing typical trisomy 21. Except for chromosome 21, all the other chromosomes occur in pairs, one inherited from the father and the other inherited from the mother. Owing to the phenomenon of nondisjunction, this male child has inherited an extra chromosome 21 (trisomy) and has the phenotypic characteristics of Down syndrome.

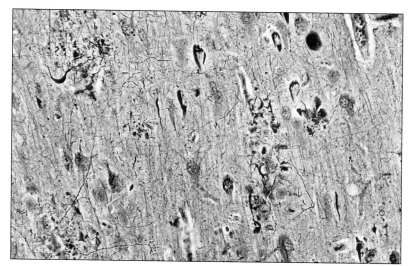

Figure 2-8. Micrograph of cerebral cortex in a woman with Down syndrome who died at age 49 following 2 years of a progressive dementing illness that included incontinence, myoclonic seizures, and mutism. Essentially all individuals with trisomy 21 show neuropathologic hallmarks of Alzheimer's disease if they survive beyond age 40. Neuropathologically the brain met all the criteria for Alzheimer's disease, as shown by the neuritic plaques and neurofibrillary tangles in the hippocampus (Holmes' stain, magnification × 20). This condition is presumably caused by an extra copy of the APP gene on chromosome 21.

Prion Disorders

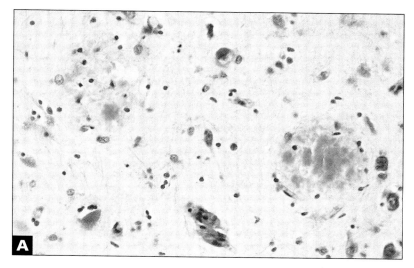

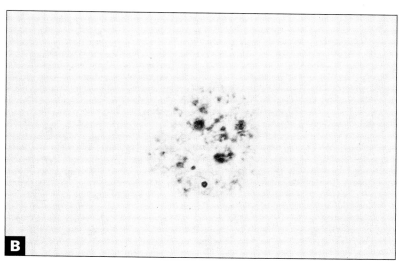

Figure 2-9. Two examples of prion disorders. Prions (small proteinaceous infectious particles that resist inactivation) contain an abnormal isoform of a cellular protein that is a major and necessary component for transmission of disease. The four major prion diseases of humans are kuru, Creutzfeldt-Jakob disease, Gerstmann-Straussler-Scheinker disease (GSS), and fatal familial insomnia [8]. These diseases often produce some combination of progressive dementia, ataxia, myoclonus, and seizures. Usually the diseases are sporadic, but occasionally mutations in the prion gene produce autosomal dominant varieties. **A**, Periodic acid–Schiff (PAS)-positive plaques found in the amygdala of a demented 61-year-old man who died with an inherited form of GSS having an arginine substituted for valine at position 117 of the prion gene (PAS stain, magnification × 25) [9]. **B**, PrP prion antibody–positive plaques in amygdala (magnification × 25). (*Courtesy of* D. Nochlin, MD, University of Washington, Seattle, WA.)

Frontotemporal Disorders

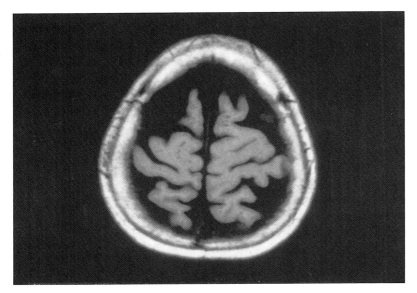

Figure 2-10. A magnetic resonance imaging scan of a 60-year-old woman with familial frontotemporal dementia (FTD) showing severe atrophy of frontal cortex. FTD refers to a group of disorders typically having two major characteristics: lobar atrophy of the frontal and/or temporal lobes and a progressive dementing disorder characterized by behavioral and personality changes (typically disinhibition) and relatively intact memory. FTD may also be associated with cytoplasmic neuronal inclusions representing aggregates of *tau* protein. Various mutations in the *tau* gene have been identified in kindreds with FTD; these mutations disturb the microtubule binding function of *tau*. Pick's disease is considered a subcategory of FTD [10].

Tay-Sachs Disease

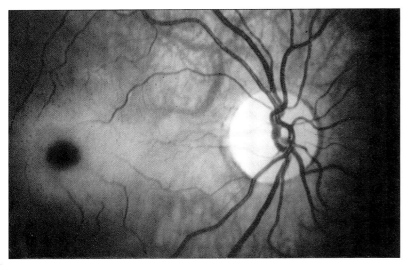

Figure 2-11. The classic cherry red spot macula of Tay-Sachs disease. Tay-Sachs disease is an autosomal recessive lipid storage disorder resulting from a deficiency of the lysosomal hydrolase β hexosaminidase A (Hex A). Accumulation of GM_2 ganglioside in neuronal lysosomes results in a clinical syndrome of progressive hypotonia, blindness, dementia, seizures, and death. The most common form of the disease occurs in infants of Eastern European Jewish ancestry and results in death by 3 to 5 years of age. The bright red color is caused by accumulation of lipid in ganglion cells and visible exaggeration of the normal vascular red appearance of the macular choroid. (*Courtesy of* D.F. Farrell, MD, University of Washington, Seattle, WA.)

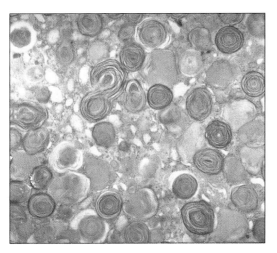

Figure 2-12. Adult Tay-Sachs disease. The adult form of Tay-Sachs disease begins in the second or third decade of life and is often associated with depression or other psychotic features, lower motor neuron signs, cerebellar ataxia, and involvement of the long motor pyramidal tracts [11]. The disease shows more clinical variability and a much longer duration than the infantile form. This electron micrograph is from a rectal biopsy of a 36-year-old man with adult Tay-Sachs disease. Lamellar lipid inclusions in rectal ganglion cells are demonstrated. The patient's symptoms began with depression and cognitive decline in late adolescence followed by slowly progressive ataxia and lower motor neuron disease. He is still alive in a wheelchair at age 52.

Nieman-Pick Type C Disease

Figure 2-13. Cholesterol storage in Nieman-Pick type C disease shown by excessive staining of skin fibroblasts with fillipin. Niemann-Pick type C disease is an autosomal recessive disease associated with progressive ataxia, dystonia, dementia, and supranuclear gaze palsy. It is a disorder of lipid metabolism in which there is decreased esterification of cholesterol and intracellular accumulation of cholesterol. The onset is usually in childhood and lifespan is shortened. The affected gene (*NPC1*) may be important in intracellular cholesterol trafficking [12]. (*Courtesy of* John O'Brien, PhD, Mayo Clinic, Rochester, MN.)

Fragile X Mental Retardation

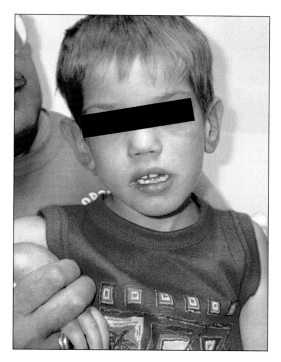

Figure 2-14. The fragile X mental retardation syndrome. This is the most common inherited form of mental retardation [13]. It is characterized by an X-linked inheritance pattern in which affected males show moderate-to-severe mental retardation and occasional carrier females demonstrate mild mental retardation. Affected patients such as this 2-year-old boy often show relatively elongated faces with large jaws and ears, which may be subtle in early childhood. Testicular enlargement also commonly occurs. (*Courtesy of* L. Hudgins, MD, Children's Hospital, Seattle, WA.)

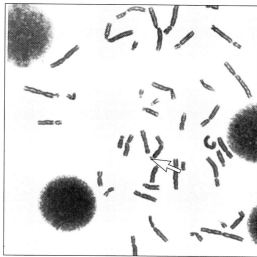

Figure 2-15. Karyotype of fragile X. Fragile X mental retardation is associated with a fragile site at Xq27.3, as shown by the arrow. (*Courtesy of* K. Leppig, MD, University of Washington, Seattle, WA.)

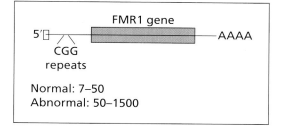

Normal: 7–50
Abnormal: 50–1500

Figure 2-16. Fragile X mental retardation gene. At the molecular level, fragile X mental retardation is characterized by an unstable CGG repeat at the 5′ end of the FMR1 gene. Normally there are seven to 50 CGG repeats in this region. The mechanism of mutation is expansion of the CGG repeat to greater than 50 (sometimes more than 1000) with subsequent hypermethylation of the adjacent CPG island, resulting in silencing of the FMR1 gene. The fragile X syndrome diagnosis can now be confirmed by obtaining a blood sample and identifying an increased CGG repeat expansion in the FMR1 gene. Expansions in the 52- to 200-repeat range are considered premutations, and usually are not associated with mental retardation. Expansions of greater than 200 repeats are always associated with mental retardation in males and in approximately 40% to 50% of females. AAAA show a polyadenine tail.

Familial Epilepsy

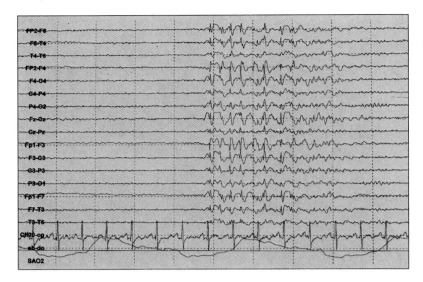

Figure 2-17. Spike and wave electroencephalogram characteristics of a generalized seizure disorder. Numerous forms of inherited epilepsy have been reported.

Figure 2-18. Chromosomal locations of primary epilepsy syndromes. Several genetic forms of epilepsy have been identified by genetic linkage and gene cloning studies [14]. Baltic myoclonic epilepsy is also known as progressive myoclonic epilepsy of Unverricht-Lundborg. AD—autosomal dominant; AR—autosomal recessive.

Chromosomal Locations of Primary Epilepsy Syndromes

Epilepsy syndrome	Inheritance	Localization	Gene
Generalized			
Benign familial neonatal convulsions	AD	20q	KCNQ2
		8q24	KCNQ3
Benign familial infantile convulsions	AD	19q	—
		16 pericen-tromeric	
Febrile seizures	AD	8q	FEB1
		19p	FEB2
		2q23-q24	FEB3
Generalized epilepsy with febrile seizures +	AD	19q	SCN1B
		2q21-q33	
Childhood absence epilepsy	AD	8q24	—
Juvenile myoclonic epilepsy	AD, AR?	6p	EJM1
		15q	
Adult myoclonic epilepsy	AD	8q24	—
Baltic myoclonic epilepsy	AR	21q22	Cystatin B
Generalized tonic-clonic seizures upon awakening	AD	6p	EJM1
Partial			
Nocturnal frontal lobe epilepsy	AD	20q	CHRNA4
		15q	
Partial epilepsy with auditory features	AD	10q	—
Familial temporal lobe epilepsy	AD	10q	—
Rolandic epilepsy	?AR	15q	—
Partial epilepsy with variable foci	AD	2q	—

Leukodystrophies

Metachromatic Leukodystrophy

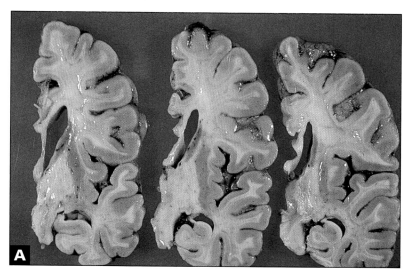

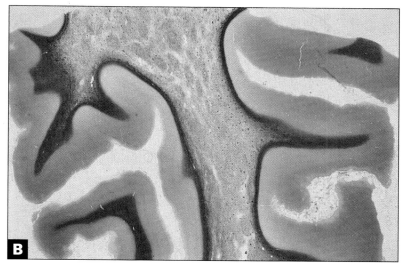

Figure 2-19. Metachromatic leukodystrophy (MLD). This autosomal recessive lysosomal storage disorder is characterized by demyelination in the central and peripheral nervous systems. The disease is caused by deficiency of the enzyme aryl sulfatase A (ASA), which hydrolyzes various sulfatides. The gene coding for ASA is on chromosome 22q13. Deficiency of ASA results in accumulation of sulfatides in numerous tissues including kidneys, brain, and peripheral nerve. There are late infantile, juvenile, and adult forms of the disease. Affected individuals typically have gait disturbance, behavioral problems, and peripheral neuropathy. The late infantile form is rapidly progressive and fatal. The adult form may produce primarily a dementing illness. **A** and **B** demonstrate severe demyelination of cerebral white matter with preservation of subcortical U fibers in a 5-year-old boy (toluidine blue).

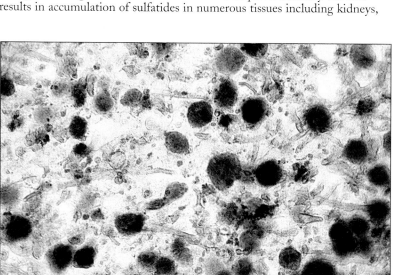

Figure 2-20. Metachromatic staining granules in cerebral macrophages in a case of metachromatic leukodystrophy (toluidine blue, magnification × 20).

Adrenoleukodystrophy

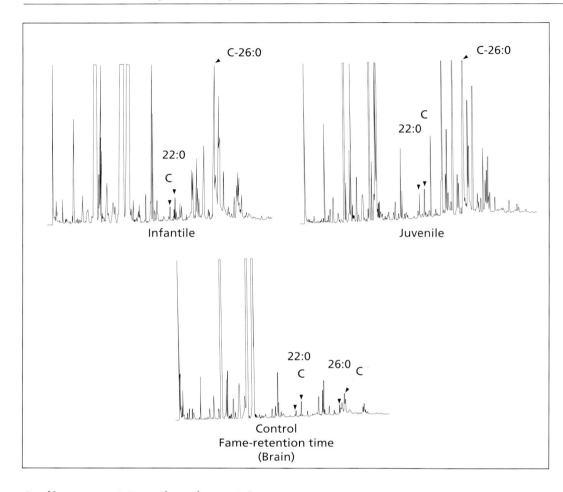

Figure 2-21. Gas chromatograph showing brain lipid profiles from a control individual compared with a juvenile X-linked adrenoleukodystrophy (ALD) patient and a rare form of infantile autosomal recessive ALD. Adrenoleukodystrophy is an X-linked demyelinating disorder of the central and peripheral nervous systems associated with elevated plasma and tissue levels of very long chain fatty acids. The gene for the most common form of the disorder maps to the long arm of the X chromosome (Xq28) and codes for a peroxisomal membrane protein [15]. Boys with the disease may manifest a severe and progressive disorder associated with mental deterioration, spasticity, and seizures. A more indolent form of the disease is called *adrenomyeloneuropathy*, which manifests in early adulthood and primarily involves the spinal cord and peripheral nerves. A few patients present with Addison's disease from adrenal involvement. About 20% of carrier females have neurologic signs or symptoms. A tremendous increase in the relative amount of C26:0 very long chain fatty acids is shown. Fame—fatty acid methyl esters. (*Courtesy of* D.F. Farrell, MD, University of Washington, Seattle, WA.)

Pelizaeus-Merzbacher Disease

Figure 2-22. Pathology sample from the brain of a 10-year-old boy who has Pelizaeus-Merzbacher disease (luxol fast blue and periodic acid–Schiff stain), showing severe demyelination of central white matter. Although not seen here, there are often preserved islands of myelin giving a "tigroid" appearance. Pelizaeus-Merzbacher disease is an X-linked recessive leukodystrophy characterized by infantile or early childhood onset of transient nystagmus, failure to attain motor developmental milestones, and progressive spasticity and ataxia. The disease results from mutations in the proteolipid protein gene on the long arm of the X chromosome [16]. (*Courtesy of* C.M. Shaw, MD, University of Washington, Seattle, WA.)

Genetic Diseases of the Basal Ganglia

Huntington's Disease

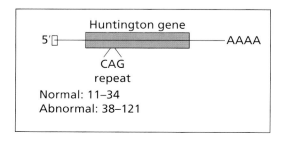

Figure 2-23. The Huntington's disease gene. The gene is located on chromosome 4 at 4p16.3. The gene codes for a protein termed *huntingtin*, whose function is presently unknown. The gene contains a CAG trinucleotide repeat that is expanded to more than 38 repeats in affected persons. There is a rough correlation of larger repeats with earlier onset of disease, and this repeat forms the basis of a diagnostic DNA blood test [17].

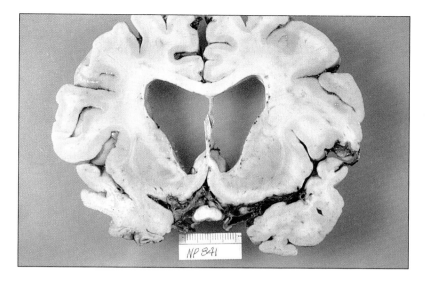

Figure 2-24. Coronal section from the brain of a 67-year-old woman with Huntington's disease (HD) demonstrating the severe bilateral caudate atrophy and enlargement of the lateral ventricles. Huntington's disease (HD) is an autosomal dominant disorder that manifests clinically as slowly progressive chorea and variable cognitive and behavioral deficits. The onset is usually in the fourth or fifth decades, but the range of onset is very broad—it can occur as early as before the age of 10 and as late as after the age of 70. The disease process is especially severe in the striatum.

Wilson's Disease

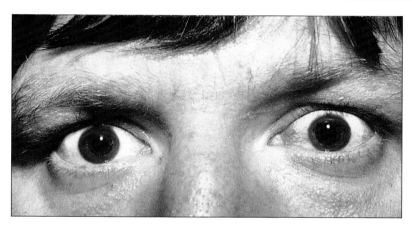

Figure 2-25. Kayser-Fleischer ring. Wilson's disease is an autosomal recessive disorder of copper metabolism that can present with hepatic failure, psychiatric or personality disorder, or neurologic signs, including dysarthria, dystonia, rigidity, and tremor. Serum ceruloplasmin and urinary copper levels are elevated, and hepatic copper level is increased. The abnormality is the golden brown ring contrasted against the blue-gray iris bilaterally. (*From* Finelli [18]; with permission.)

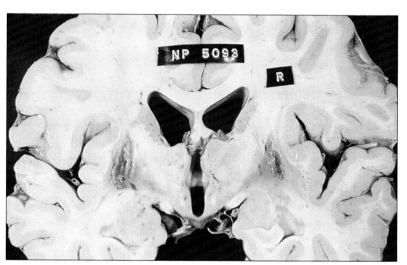

Figure 2-26. The brain of a 35-year-old patient with Wilson's disease demonstrating severe bilateral cystic degeneration of the putamen. Combined with the liver disease, this condition is referred to as *hepatolenticular degeneration*. The Wilson's disease gene is on chromosome 13 and codes for a copper-transporting ATPase. The disease can be treated with copper-chelating agents such as penicillamine.

Chorea-Acanthocytosis Syndrome

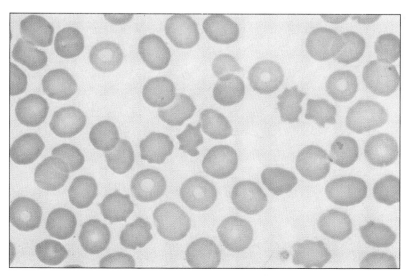

Figure 2-27. Acanthocytes. Some individuals with slowly progressive chorea have associated acanthocytes in their peripheral erythrocytes. Note the spiny appearance of the erythrocytes. Oromandibular dyskinesias, peripheral neuropathy, and caudate atrophy are common. The gene(s) has not been identified.

Familial Parkinson's Disease

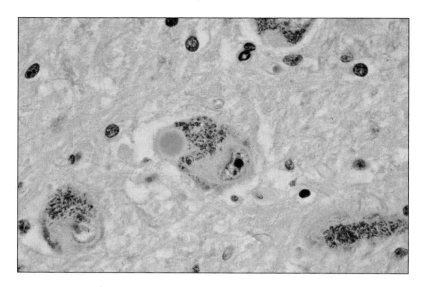

Figure 2-28. Lewy body in a pigmented neuron of the substantia nigra. This cytoplasmic inclusion stains with periodic acid–Schiff, ubiquitin, and α-synuclein antibody and is surrounded by a clear halo. It is considered a hallmark of classic Parkinson's disease.

Familial Parkinson's Disease

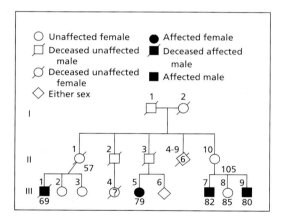

Figure 2-29. Pedigree of a family with familial Parkinson's disease (PD). PD usually occurs as a sporadic condition. Because it is relatively common, it is not unusual to have two cases in a family. Several cases in a single kindred may represent multifactorial inheritance, that is, an unknown genetic predisposition to an unknown environmental agent. Presumably that explains the four affected cousins in this pedigree. Family member III-1 had early onset of PD symptoms at age 36, died at age 69, and had Lewy bodies in both substantia nigra and cerebral cortex. His cousins have had later onset of PD. Other families have been described in which PD is inherited as a single-gene autosomal dominant disease linked to the α-synuclein locus on chromosome 4 [40]. A number above a symbol is the position in that generation of pedigree; numbers within a symbol indicate the number of children.

Genes Causing Parkinsonism

Disorder	Inheritance pattern	Gene
Familial PD (adult onset)	AD	α-Synuclein
Early onset PD (juvenile)	AR	Parkin
	AD (reduced penetrance)	
Dopa-responsive dystonia	AD (reduced penetrance)	GTP cyclohydrolase I
FTDP-17	AD	Tau

Figure 2-30. Four different genes implicated in hereditary causes of the parkinsonian syndrome [20]. Autosomal dominant familial Parkinson's disease caused by mutations in the *alpha*-synuclein gene is associated with Lewy bodies in the substantia nigra. The other three disorders are not associated with Lewy bodies. *Parkin* mutations are associated with early onset of Parkinson's disease, often before age 30. Mutations in GTP cyclohydrolase I cause a childhood-onset dystonia that often has a diurnal variation (worse in the afternoon) and is very responsive to L-dopa. Although autosomal dominant, this condition is more common in women. FTDP-17—frontotemporal dementia with parkinsonism-chromosome 17; PD—Parkinson's disease.

Familial Calcification of the Basal Ganglia

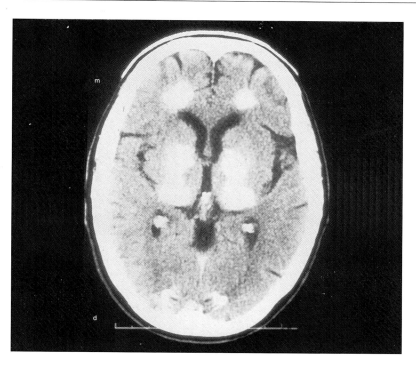

Figure 2-31. Computed tomography scan demonstrating prominent bilateral calcification of the basal ganglia and deep nuclei of the cerebellum. There are many causes of basal ganglia calcification, including pseudohyperparathyroidism. Mild calcification of the basal ganglia can occur normally with aging. Familial idiopathic basal ganglia calcification (Fahr's disease) can be associated with dystonia or parkinsonian features and can be inherited in an autosomal dominant. One family with Fahr's disease has shown genetic linkage to chromosome 14q [21].

Hereditary Ataxias

Dominant Ataxias

Figure 2-32. Various autosomal dominant ataxias defined by genetic linkage. Several are associated with trinucleotide repeat expansions for which there are commercially available DNA tests.

Autosomal Dominant Ataxias Defined by Genetic Linkage Studies

Type	Chromosome location
SCA1	6p (CAG repeat)
SCA2	12q (CAG repeat)
SCA3/MJD	14q (CAG repeat)
SCA4	16q (Neuropathy)
SCA5	11 (Lincoln family)
SCA6	19p (CAG repeat)
SCA7	3p (CAG repeat, retinopathy)
SCA8	13q (CTG repeat, reduced penetrance)
SCA9	22q (Seizures, ATTCT repeat)
SCA10	15q
SCA11	5q (Tremor, dementia)
SCA12	19q (Mild MR)
SCA13	6q
SCA14	
EA-1	12p (Episodic ataxia, myokymia)
EA-2	19p (Episodic ataxia, migraine)
DRPLA	12p (Seizures, chorea)

DRPLA—Dentatorubropallidoluysian atrophy.
MJD—Machado-Joseph disease.
SCA—Spinocerebellar ataxia.

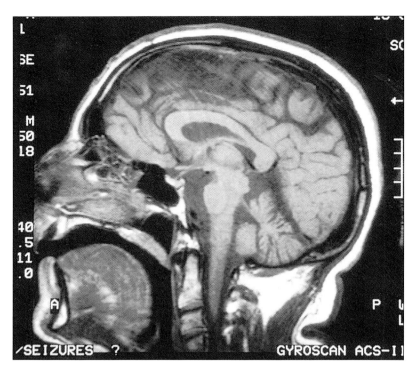

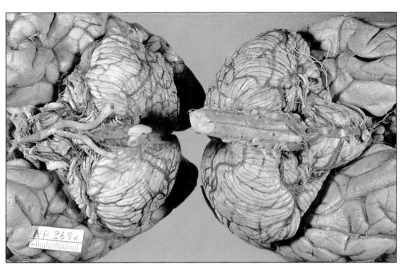

Figure 2-34. The ventral surface of the brain from a 58-year-old man with many years of progressive ataxia, dysarthria, and nystagmus (*left*). A control brain is on the right. Note that the patient with ataxia has a smaller cerebellum and considerable atrophy of the pons, which is almost obscured by the basilar artery.

Figure 2-33. A midline sagittal magnetic resonance imaging scan of a 61-year-old man with slowly progressive ataxia and dysarthria demonstrating atrophy of the cerebellum and pons. His clinical diagnosis is probable olivo-pontocerebellar atrophy (OPCA). Some cases of OPCA are sporadic and of unknown cause; others are clearly genetic.

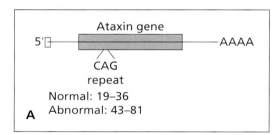

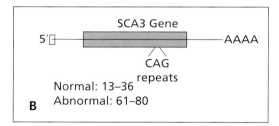

Figure 2-35. Schematic representation of two autosomal dominant hereditary ataxia genes. **A**, SCA1 (hereditary ataxia gene; located on chromosome 6p24). **B**, SCA3 (Machado-Joseph disease gene; located on chromosome 14q 24-32). Both genes contain a CAG repeat, which is expanded in affected individuals and forms the basis for a diagnostic DNA blood test [22,23,24].

Autosomal Recessive Ataxias

Type	Chromosome location
Friedreich's ataxia	9q (GAA repeat)
Ataxia telangiectasia	11q (Immune deficiency)
Vitamin E deficiency ataxia	8q (Mimics Friedrich's ataxia)
Infantile onset ataxia	10q (Neuropathy, deafness)
ARSACS	13q (Neuropathy)
Marinesco-Sjögren syndrome	? (Cataracts, weakness)
Ataxia/oculomotor apraxia	9q

Figure 2-36. Seven different causes of autosomal recessive hereditary ataxia. Most have childhood onset and relatively distinct clinical characteristics. ARSACS—autosomal recessive spastic ataxia of Charlevoix-Saguenay.

Autosomal Recessive Ataxias

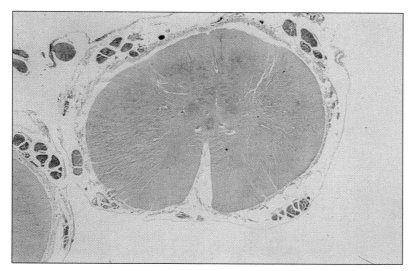

Figure 2-37. Transverse section of thoracic spinal cord from a 20-year-old man with Friedreich's ataxia who developed cardiomyopathy and diabetes. Friedreich's ataxia is an autosomal recessive disorder usually beginning in childhood and presenting with slowly progressive gait ataxia associated with depressed tendon reflexes, bilateral Babinski's reflexes, position and vibration sensory deficits, dysarthria, and nystagmus. Decreased lifespan is primarily because of an associated cardiomyopathy. There is loss of myelin staining in the posterior columns and the lateral cortical spinal tracts (luxol fast blue, periodic acid–Schiff stain, hematoxylin). Of interest is the fact that Friedreich's ataxia is not associated with significant cerebellar atrophy. The gene for Friedreich's ataxia is on chromosome 9 and contains a GAA repeat in an intron [25]. In addition, there are other autosomal causes of ataxia, one of which maps to chromosome 8 and is associated with mutations in the α-tocopherol–transfer protein and is an important condition in the differential diagnosis [24].

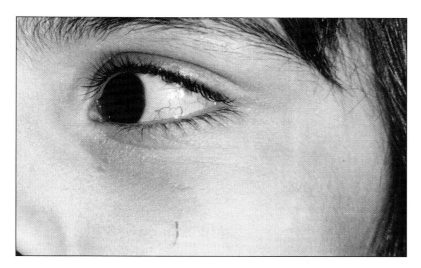

Figure 2-38. The conjunctival telangiectasia. Ataxia telangiectasia is an autosomal recessive disorder beginning in childhood and characterized by progressive cerebellar ataxia and telangiectasias of the conjunctiva and skin. Deficiencies of the immune system commonly associated with recurrent sinopulmonary infections may occur. Growth retardation and an increased frequency of lymphoreticular malignancies may also occur. There is sensitivity to ionizing radiation and a propensity for chromosomal instability and breakage. Serum α-fetoprotein is almost always elevated and is useful as a diagnostic test. Adventitious movements such as chorea may also occur. The neuropathology includes degeneration of the cerebellum associated with loss of Purkinje's cells. Asymptomatic carriers of the ataxia telangiectasia gene have an increased frequency of malignancy, including breast cancer. The ataxia telangiectasia gene is on chromosome 11 and has been identified and cloned [26].

Genetic Disorders of Brain Stem and Spinal Cord

Familial Amyotrophic Lateral Sclerosis

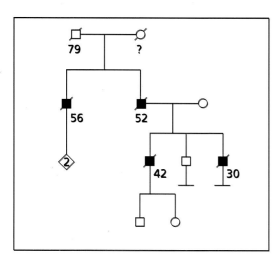

Figure 2-39. Pedigree of a family with early-onset rapidly progressive amyotrophic lateral sclerosis (ALS). ALS is usually a sporadic disease without an obvious hereditary component. However, 5% to 10% of patients with ALS have a similarly affected relative. The inheritance is typical of an autosomal dominant disease, with male-to-male transmission. Affected members of the family have had a combination of both upper and lower motor neuron signs, including weakness, muscle atrophy, fasciculations, and hyperactive tendon reflexes. This family has been found to have a point mutation in exon 1 of the superoxide dismutase (SOD) gene on chromosome 21. Mutations in exon 1 have been associated with an especially aggressive, rapidly progressive form of ALS. Affected members of this family usually survive less than 2 years. Some but not all kindreds with familial ALS have been discovered to have mutations in the SOD gene [27]. The closed symbols represent persons who are affected with ALS, open symbols are persons without ALS. The circles represent females, and the squares represent males; a slash through a symbol indicates death, a number above a symbol is the position in that generation of pedigree, and numbers within a symbol indicate the number of children. (DNA finding *Courtesy of* R.H. Brown, Jr, MD, Massachusetts General Hospital, Boston, MA.)

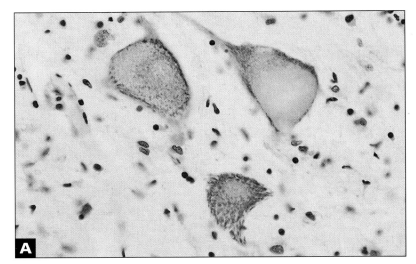

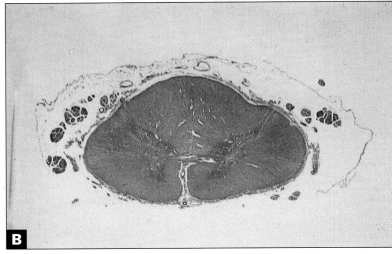

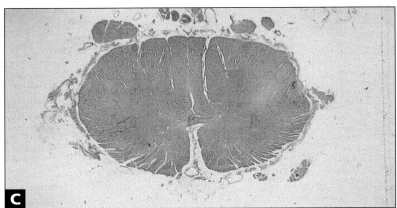

Figure 2-40. Histologic slides from patients with early-onset rapidly progressive amyotrophic lateral sclerosis (ALS). **A**, Anterior horn cells in lumbar spinal cord of a 56-year-old man from the pedigree shown in Figure 2-39 showing chromatolysis of the neuron on the right (Nissl stain, magnification × 40). **B**, Transverse section of cervical spinal cord from a 60-year-old woman from another kindred with familial ALS and **C**, her 57-year-old son showing loss of myelin in lateral corticospinal tracts as well as posterior columns (luxol fast blue, periodic acid–Schiff, hematoxylin). (Panel A *courtesy of* D. Nochlin, MD, University of Washington, Seattle, WA.)

Kennedy's Spinobulbar Muscular Atrophy

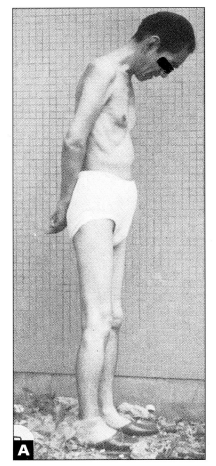

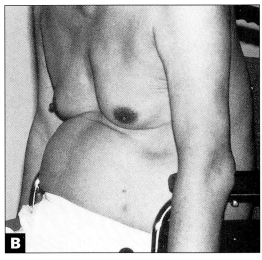

Figure 2-41. Appearance of two brothers with Kennedy's spinobulbar muscular atrophy (SBMA). This X-linked recessive disorder affects lower motor neurons in the brain stem and spinal cord. Affected males have onset of weakness and atrophy beginning in adulthood, which is usually slowly progressive and compatible with several decades of life (**A**). Fasciculations of tongue and perioral muscles are common. Upper motor neuron signs are absent. Gynecomastia is a frequent feature (**B**). Carrier females are asymptomatic and there is no male-to-male transmission of the disease. (Reprinted *from* J Neurol Sci, volume 87, Nagashima T, Seko K, Hirose K, et al., Familial bulbo-spinal atrophy associated with testicular atrophy and sensory neuropathy (Kennedy-Alter-Sung syndrome); autopsy case reports of two brothers, pages 141–152, Copyright 1988, with permission from Elsevier Science [28].)

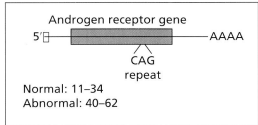

Figure 2-42. Kennedy's spinobulbar muscular atrophy (SBMA) gene. The gene for Kennedy's SBMA is the androgen receptor gene on chromosome Xq21.3. This gene contains a CAG repeat that is expanded in affected men and carrier women and represents a basis for a diagnostic DNA blood test. Dysfunction of the androgen receptor causes the gynecomastia as well as the SBMA.

Childhood Spinal Muscular Atrophy

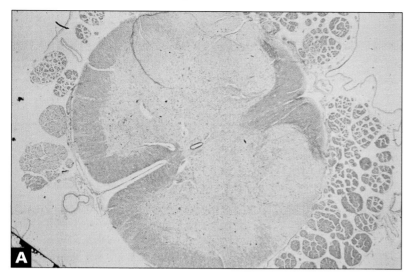

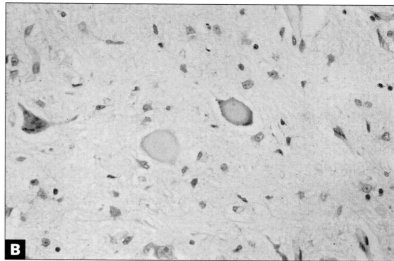

Figure 2-43. Spinal muscular atrophy. Most forms of spinal muscular atrophy (SMA) occurring in childhood are autosomal recessive. Infantile onset is referred to as Werdnig-Hoffman disease and childhood onset is referred to as Kugelberg-Welander disease. The condition is associated with progressive hypotonia, weakness, fasciculations, and loss of reflexes. **A,** Lumbar spinal cord from a 6-month-old child who died with spinal muscular atrophy. It demonstrates loss of neurons in the anterior horns and decreased myelin in the ventral roots (luxol fast blue and Nissl stain). **B,** Chromatolysis of motor neurons in the 12th cranial nerve nucleus of a 4-month-old child who died with SMA (hematoxylin and eosin stain, magnification × 40). The most common form of infantile—SMA has been associated with deletions in the survival motor neuron gene at chromosome 5q13 [29].

Hereditary Spastic Paraplegias

Figure 2-44. Genetic classification of hereditary spastic paraplegias. Hereditary spastic paraplegia refers to several genetic disorders in which the major clinical phenomenon is slowly progressive spasticity in the lower limbs characterized by hyperreactive tendon reflexes, Babinski responses, and increased muscle tone. They may be autosomal dominant, autosomal recessive, or X-linked and complicated or uncomplicated [30]. Genes have been identified for one dominant type (spastin in SPG 4), one recessive type (paraplegin in SPG 7), and two X-linked types (L1CAM in SPG 1 and PLP in SPG 2). ARSACS—autosomal recessive spastic ataxia of Charlevoix-Saguenay; GI—gastrointestinal.

Hereditary Spastic Paraplegias

Type	Chromosome locus
Autosomal dominant forms	
SPG 4	2p (Spastin gene
SPG 13	2q (Uncomplicated)
SPG 8	8q (Uncomplicated)
SPG 10	12q (Uncomplicated)
SPG 3	14q (Early onset)
SPG 6	15q (Uncomplicated)
SPG 12	19q (Early onset)
SPG 9	10q (Cataracts, GI reflux)
Autosomal recessive forms	
SPG 5	8p (Uncomplicated)
SPG 11	15q (Uncomplicated)
SPG 7	16q (Paraplegin gene)
ARSACS	13q (Spastic ataxia with neuropathy)
X-linked forms	
SPG 1	Xq28 (L1 cell-adhesion molecule, hydrocephalus)
SPG 2	Xq28 (Proteolipid protein gene, leukodystrophy)

Hereditary Neuropathies and Charcot-Marie-Tooth Syndrome

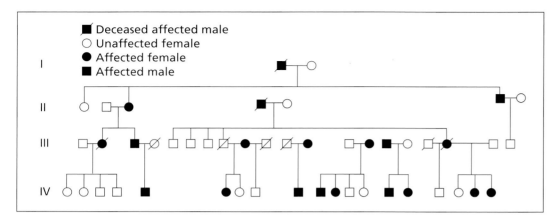

■ Deceased affected male
○ Unaffected female
● Affected female
■ Affected male

Figure 2-45. The pedigree of a family with autosomal dominant Charcot-Marie-Tooth (CMT) disease. CMT is one of a large number of hereditary neuropathies that are described by various terminologies, including peroneal muscular atrophy and hereditary motor and sensory neuropathies. The most common form is CMT type 1 with slow nerve conductions.

Genetic Classification of Charcot-Marie-Tooth Syndrome

Type	Nerve conduction	Inheritance pattern	Chromosome or gene
CMT 1A	Slow	AD	17p11.2 duplication (PMP22)*
HNPP	Normal or mildly slow	AD	17p11.2 deletion
CMT 1B	Slow	AD	1q (P_0 protein)
CMT 1C	Slow	AD	Unknown
CMT 2A	Normal or mildly slow	AD	1p
CMT 2B	Normal or mildly slow	AD	3q
CMT 2C	Normal or mildly slow	AD	Unknown
CMT 2D	Normal	AD	7p
CMT 4†	Slow	AR	8q, 11q, 11p, 5q
CMT X	Variable	X-linked	Xq (Connexin 32)
EGR 2	Slow	AD or AR	10q

Rare forms of CMT 1A have point mutations in the PMP22 gene.

†There are many types of autosomal recessive (AR) CMT.

Figure 2-46. Classification of the Charcot-Marie-Tooth (CMT) hereditary neuropathy syndrome based primarily on genetic characteristics [31]. Commercial DNA diagnostic tests are available for CMT 1A, CMT 1B, CMT X, and hereditary lability for pressure palsies (HNPP). [22]. AD—autosomal dominant; EGR 2—early growth response 2; PMP22—peripheral myelin protein 22kD.

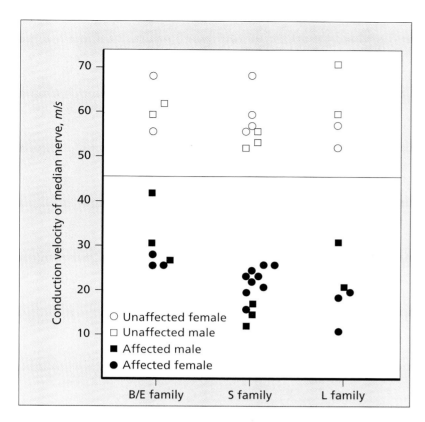

Figure 2-47. The median nerve conduction velocities in affected and unaffected individuals from three separate families with Charcot-Marie-Tooth (CMT) syndrome. CMT type 1 is associated with slow motor nerve conduction velocities. The affected persons all have slow nerve conduction velocities that are frequently less than half the velocity of their unaffected relatives.

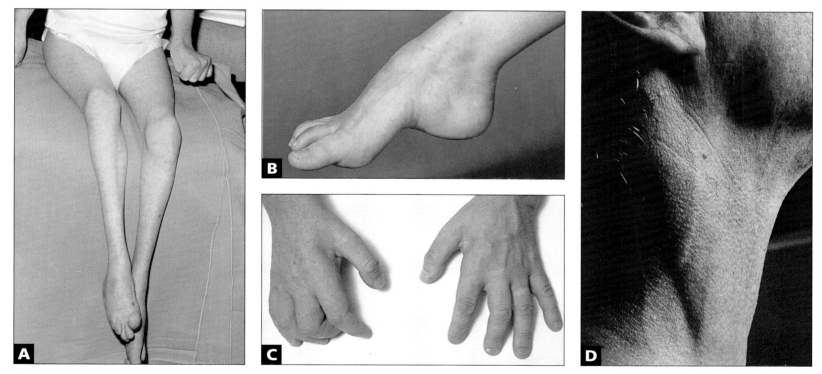

Figure 2-48. Physical manifestations of Charcot-Marie-Tooth 1 (CMT 1) disease. **A**, The marked distal atrophy of leg muscles in an unusually severe case of CMT. **B**, The typical high arch, contracted heel cord, and foot drop posture of CMT. **C**, Clawing of the fingers and interosseous muscle atrophy of the hands. **D**, Hypertrophy of the greater auricular nerve running vertically between the base of the neck and the mastoid in a man with CMT 1A. CMT 1A is associated with a DNA duplication at chromosome 17p11.2, which includes the PMP22 (peripheral myelin protein) gene.

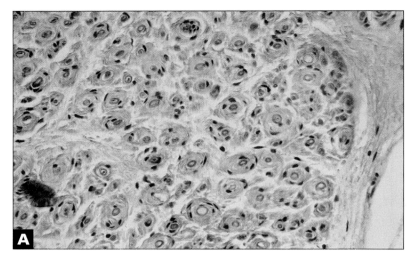

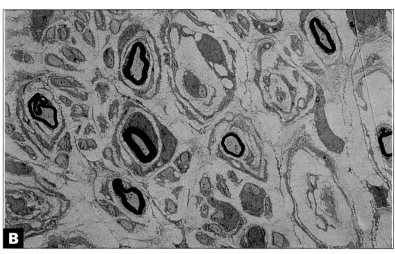

Figure 2-49. Sural nerve biopsy specimens of Charcot-Marie-Tooth (CMT) disease. **A,** Sural nerve biopsy specimen from a 58-year-old man with CMT type 1, demonstrating hypertrophy of tissue surrounding individual nerves

(Gomori-Wheatley stain, magnification × 20). **B,** Electron micrograph of a sural nerve biopsy specimen from a 33-year-old man with CMT demonstrating the excessive Schwann cell wrappings around individual axons.

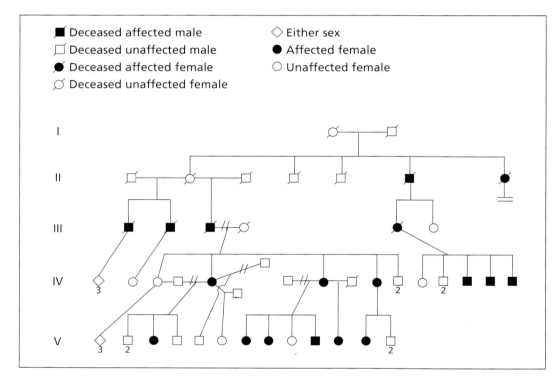

■ Deceased affected male
□ Deceased unaffected male
● Deceased affected female
⊘ Deceased unaffected female
◇ Either sex
● Affected female
○ Unaffected female

Figure 2-50. The pedigree of a family with the Charcot-Marie-Tooth (CMT) syndrome having X-linked dominant inheritance. Male and female members are both affected. However, female members tend to be less severely affected and there has never been male-to-male transmission of disease. X-linked dominant CMT is often the result of mutations in the connexin 32 gene on the long arm of the X chromosome. Isolated ("sporadic") males with the CMT syndrome should have DNA testing to determine if they have the X-linked type of disease. Each number in the figure represents the position in that generation of pedigree.

Genetic Diseases of Muscle

Duchenne-Becker Muscular Dystrophy

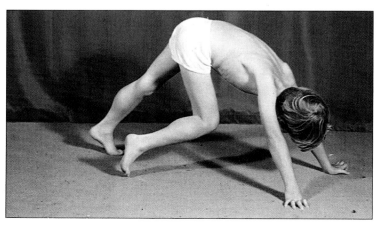

Figure 2-51. A boy with Duchenne muscular dystrophy (DMD) demonstrating pseudohypertrophy of his calves and a positive Gower's maneuver ("climbing" from a sitting position because of proximal muscle weakness). DMD is the most common inherited form of muscle disease. It is transmitted in an X-linked recessive fashion. The disease presents as a slowly progressive weakness of the proximal lower extremities typically beginning between ages 3 and 5. The disease is associated with highly elevated serum creatine kinase levels, wheelchair dependence by age 12, and death usually in the third decade from pneumonia or cardiomyopathy. Female carriers of the gene rarely have symptoms of muscle disease. However, because of random inactivation of the X chromosome, female carriers often have an elevated serum creatine kinase level (about 70% of carriers) and occasionally have enlarged calves and mild muscle weakness. Many patients also develop a cardio myopathy.

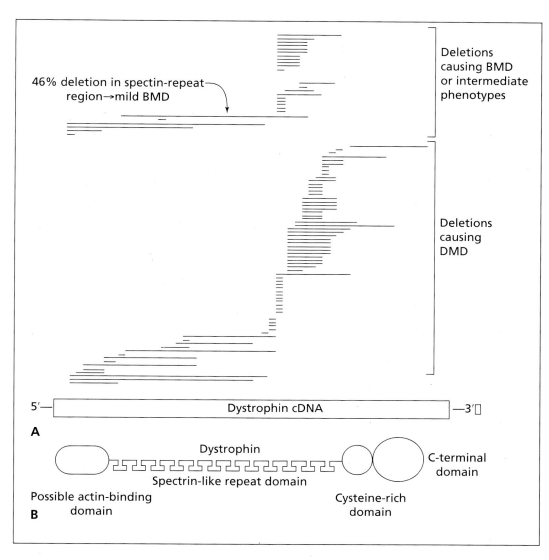

46% deletion in spectin-repeat region→mild BMD

Deletions causing BMD or intermediate phenotypes

Deletions causing DMD

5'— Dystrophin cDNA —3'

A

Dystrophin

Spectrin-like repeat domain

Possible actin-binding domain

Cysteine-rich domain

C-terminal domain

B

Figure 2-52. The Duchenne muscular dystrophy (DMD) gene on the short arm of the X chromosome at Xp21. **A,** The DMD gene, which contains approximately 2000 kb of DNA (more than 2 million base pairs). The gene codes for a muscle protein called dystrophin. The position of various deletions of the DMD gene, resulting in muscle disease. Deletions causing elimination of dystrophin production result in the classic DMD phenotype. Deletions associated with some production of dystrophin are associated with a less-severe phenotype called Becker muscular dystrophy (BMD). The BMD phenotype also shows X-linked recessive inheritance with elevated creatine kinase level and progressive muscle weakness with calf enlargement but a later age of onset, less severe course, and longer life span. **B,** Simplified structure of dystrophin protein. (*Adapted from* Thompson and colleagues [32]; with permission.)

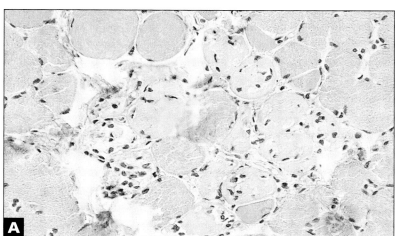

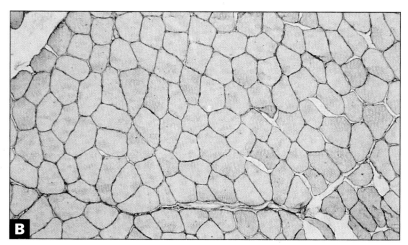

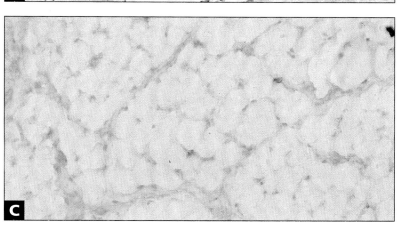

Figure 2-53. Dystrophin staining of muscle biopsy specimens. **A,** Typical light microscopic findings in the muscle biopsy specimen of an 8-year-old boy with Duchenne muscular dystrophy (DMD). There is degeneration of some muscle fibers with round cell infiltration, and "ballooning" with loss of angulation of other fibers (hematoxylin-eosin stain, magnification × 20). **B,** Normal dystrophin antibody immunostaining of a normal control muscle biopsy specimen. The dystrophin is represented by the dark enhancement around the periphery of each muscle fiber (magnification × 10). **C,** The dystrophin immunostaining of a muscle biopsy specimen from a patient with DMD showing a lack of dystrophin. Dystrophin staining of muscle biopsy specimens is very useful in the diagnosis of Duchenne and Becker muscular dystrophy [53,54].

Myotonic Dystrophy

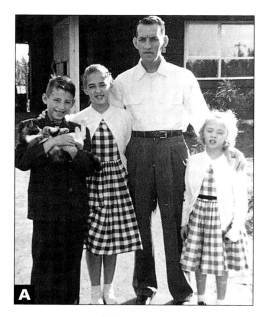 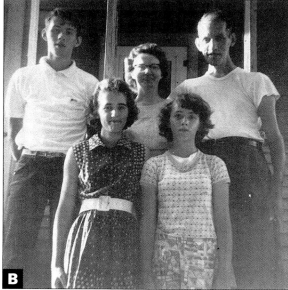 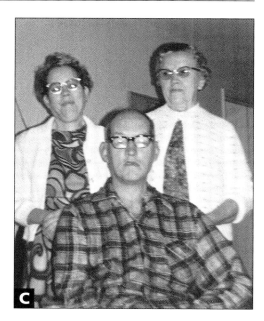

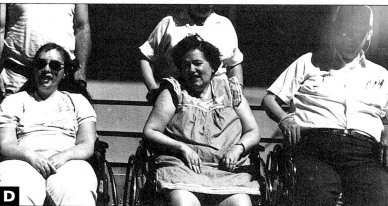

Figure 2-54. The progression of myotonic dystrophy in a single family over a 35-year period. Myotonic muscular dystrophy is an autosomal dominant disorder with highly variable expression. Myotonia refers to a delay in relaxation of muscle contraction and can be found in several different muscle disorders. **A,** A 37-year-old man with his three juvenile children. Temporalis muscle wasting can be seen in the father and possible facial weakness in the youngest daughter. **B,** The father is 41 years old and his facial weakness is more apparent. The adolescent children appear normal. **C,** The father is now 50 years old and in a wheelchair with severe diffuse muscle weakness and cataracts that required surgery. He died at age 57. **D,** All three children have developed the disease and are in wheelchairs in their 40s.

Variable Expression of Myotonic Dystrophy

Common findings	Other occurrences
Myotonia	Mental retardation
Muscle weakness	Infantile hypotonia
Cataract	Clubfoot
Testicular atrophy	Cardiomyopathy
Frontal balding	Gastrointestinal tract dysmotility
Facial diplegia	Diabetes mellitus
Electrocardiographic abnormality	Gallbladder sphincter dysfunction
	Polyhydraminos and prolonged labor
	Thickened skull with large sinuses

Figure 2-55. The variability in expression of myotonic dystrophy. The typical patient has the onset of grip myotonia or muscle weakness, noted in adolescence or adulthood, which slowly progresses to moderate disability later in life. Cataracts in middle age are common. The disease demonstrates genetic anticipation, which means increasing severity of disability with each subsequent generation. The severest manifestation of myotonic dystrophy is infantile disease characterized by marked neonatal hypotonia and respiratory distress, sometimes resulting in death. Infants that survive are frequently mentally retarded.

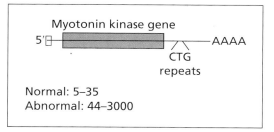

Normal: 5–35
Abnormal: 44–3000

Figure 2-56. The myotonic dystrophy gene on the long arm of chromosome 19 (19q16.3). It codes for a muscle kinase called myotonin. The 3′ noncoding portion of the gene contains a CTG repeat that is abnormally expanded in persons with myotonic dystrophy. Individuals with relatively small expansions may be asymptomatic. Longer expansions are associated with symptoms and signs of the disease and there is a correlation between expansion length and severity of the disease. This triplet repeat forms the basis for a diagnostic DNA blood test for myotonic dystrophy. The longest expansions (greater than 1000) are often associated with severe congenital disease.

Muscle Ion Channel Disorders

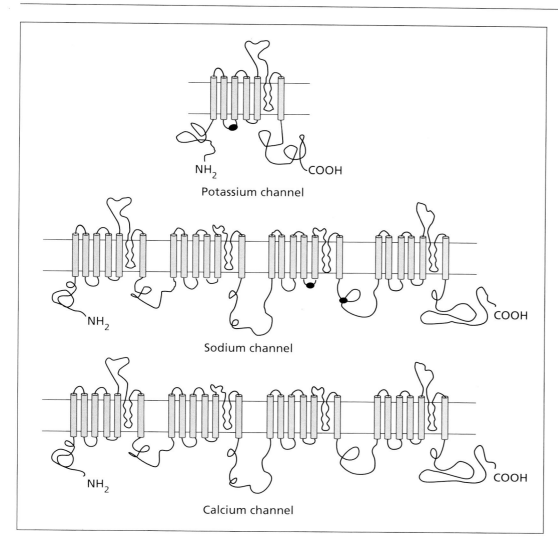

Potassium channel

Sodium channel

Calcium channel

Figure 2-57. The proposed structure of three voltage-gated cation channels and the location of known mutations in these proteins. Several neurologic disorders have been discovered to be the result of mutations in genes coding for ion channels. The potassium channel has six transmembrane segments; the red dots indicate the site of a mutation that clinically produces a syndrome of autosomal dominant periodic ataxia with myokymia. The sodium and calcium channels consist of four transmembrane domains arranged in tandem. Mutations in various sites of the sodium channel have been associated with hyperkalemic periodic paralysis and paramyotonia congenita. Mutations in the calcium channel are associated with autosomal dominant hypokalemic periodic paralysis. Finally, mutations in a chloride channel (not shown) are associated with autosomal dominant myotonia congenita. (*Adated from* Ptaáek [35].)

Nemaline Rod Myopathy

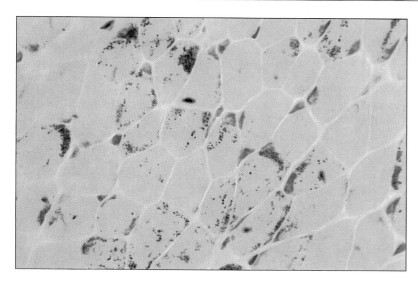

Figure 2-58. Muscle biopsy specimen of nemaline rod myopathy. There are several forms of congenital myopathy, including nemaline rod, central core, and myotubular. Muscle biopsy specimen from a 6-week-old baby girl with muscle weakness caused by nemaline rod myopathy (modified Gomori-Wheatley stain, magnification × 40). The abnormal patchy dark staining material represents the nemaline rods, which appear as dark, elongated material under electron microscopy. The disease is most often an autosomal dominant condition with considerable variability of muscle weakness. Typically there is mild hypotonia in infancy associated with mild-to-moderate weakness. The condition may be nonprogressive or there may be slow deterioration and death from respiratory muscle involvement. The nemaline rods are composed, in part, of α actinin. The disease has been found to be a result of a mutation in the α tropomyosin gene on the short arm of chromosome 1 [36].

Fascioscapulohumeral Muscular Dystrophy

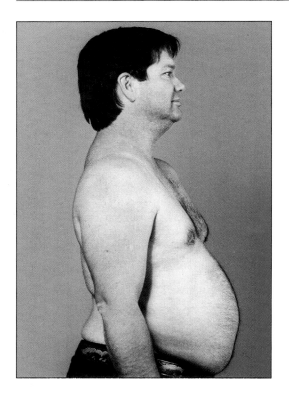

Figure 2-59. Pectoral muscle atrophy and lax abdominal muscles in a man with fascioscapulo-humeral muscular dystrophy. The condition is autosomal dominant with highly variable severity [37]. Some patients are quite compromised by facial diplegia and prominent atrophy and weakness of the serratus anterior (causing scapular winging) and pectoralis muscles. Other individuals have only minor findings and are asymptomatic. The condition is associated with DNA deletions in the telomeric region of the long arm of chromosome 4.

Mitochondrial Diseases

Myoclonic Epilepsy With Ragged Red Fibers

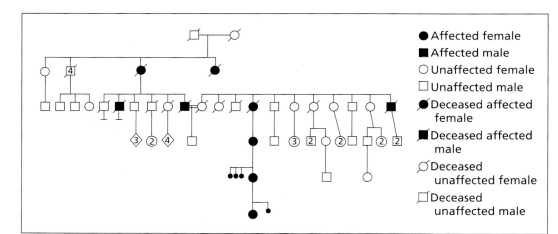

● Affected female
■ Affected male
○ Unaffected female
□ Unaffected male
◕ Deceased affected female
◪ Deceased affected male
⦸ Deceased unaffected female
⬚ Deceased unaffected male

Figure 2-60. Pedigree of a kindred transmitting a mitochondrial mutation causing the syndrome of myoclonic epilepsy with ragged red fibers (MERRF). Mitochondrial DNA codes for 13 proteins involved in oxidative phosphorylation and ribosomal and transfer RNA. Mitochondrial DNA is contained in the cytoplasm (not the nucleus) of cells, thus mitochondrial DNA is inherited in the cytoplasm of a mother's egg but not from the sperm of a father. Therefore, mitochondrial disorders are transmitted only by mothers and never by fathers (cytoplasmic inheritance). Male and female children can both be affected and the disease may appear in all children of an affected mother. Transmission never occurs through an affected male. Each child of an affected mother may inherit a variable number of mitochondria that contain the DNA mutation. The proportion of mutant mitochondria can vary considerably from cell to cell in any affected person (heteroplasmy). Mitochondrial disorders, therefore, often show remarkable variability in clinical expression both within and between families. Individuals affected with MERRF may have any combination of myoclonus, myopathy, ataxia, or seizures. Occasionally, cognitive decline, neuropathy, or hearing loss also occur. The most common mutation is an A to G substitution at nucleotide 8344 of mitochondrial DNA [38]. Numbers within a symbol indicate the number of children.

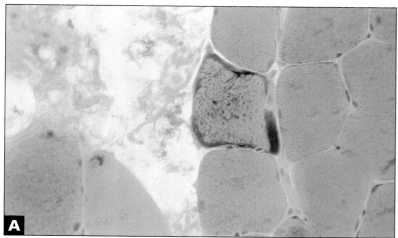

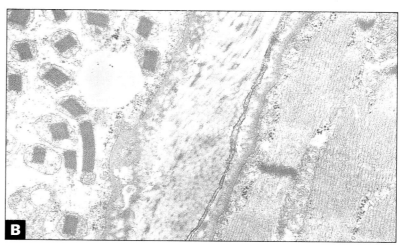

Figure 2-61. Myoclonic epilepsy with ragged red fibers. **A,** Muscle biopsy specimen from a person with myoclonic epilepsy with ragged red fibers (modified Gomori-Wheatley stain, magnification × 40). **B,** Electron microscopic image of ragged red fibers. The ragged red fibers are shown to be crystalline-like inclusions in the mitochondria.

Mitochondrial Myopathy, Encephalopathy, Lactic Acidosis, and Stroke-like Episodes

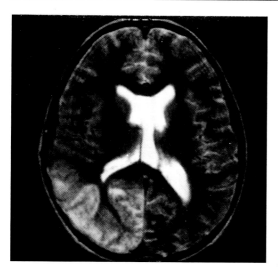

Figure 2-62. Magnetic resonance imaging scan of a 13-year-old boy with MELAS (mitochondrial myopathy, encephalopathy, lactic acidosis, and stroke-like episodes). Shown with the MELAS syndrome is a right occipital stroke, producing a left visual field defect. Mitochondrial mutations may cause MELAS, with the most common being an A to G point mutation at base pair 3243.

Leber's Optic Neuropathy

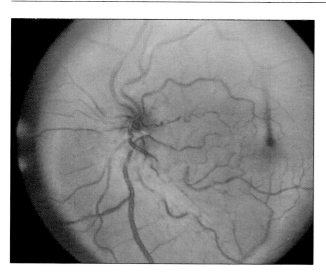

Figure 2-63. Retinal photograph of Leber's hereditary optic neuropathy (LHON). LHON presents with acute or subacute painless loss of central vision typically occurring between age 12 and 30. Males and females may both be affected, but the condition is much more frequent in males for unknown reasons. There may be swelling of the nerve fiber layer around the optic disc, as shown in this photograph. The most common mutation underlying LHON is a change from G to A at base pair 11,778. Some affected individuals may have electrocardiographic abnormalities, and a few cases have been reported with other neurologic signs, including findings typical of multiple sclerosis (*Courtesy of* R. Kalina, MD, University of Washington, Seattle, WA.)

Leigh Encephalopathy

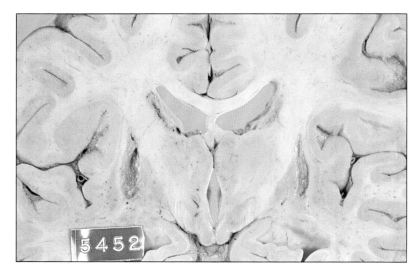

Figure 2-64. Computed tomographic image of the brain of a 15-year-old girl who died of Leigh encephalopathy. Severe bilateral cystic degeneration of the caudate and putamen can be seen. This condition typically begins in the first 2 or 3 years of life, with a downhill course resulting in death within 5 years. Juvenile and adult cases have also been described. Clinical manifestations may include optic atrophy, ophthalmoplegia, nystagmus, ataxia, hypotonia, and spasticity. The neuropathologic lesions are primarily demyelination and gliosis involving the basal ganglia, brain stem, and cerebellum. There are several different causes of the Leigh encephalopathy syndrome. One fairly common cause is point mutations at position 8993 of mitochondrial DNA [39].

Neurocutaneous Disorders

Neurofibromatosis 1

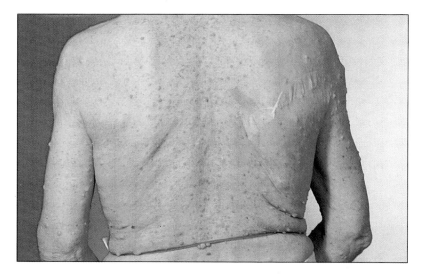

Figure 2-65. The physical manifestations of neurofibromatosis (NF1). NF1 is an autosomal dominant disorder of highly variable expression primarily affecting the skin and nervous system. The hallmarks of the disease are multiple café-au-lait spots and neurofibromas of peripheral nerves. The back and arms of this 69-year-old man are covered with small neurofibromas and there is a café-au-lait spot just medial to his right scapula.

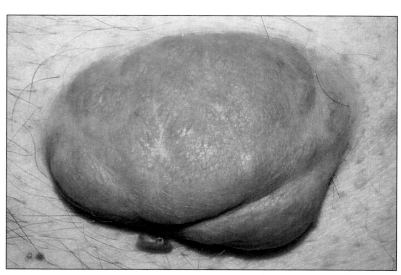

Figure 2-66. A closeup of a 3-cm diameter neurofibroma that is soft, violaceous, and nontender (same patient as in Figure 2-65).

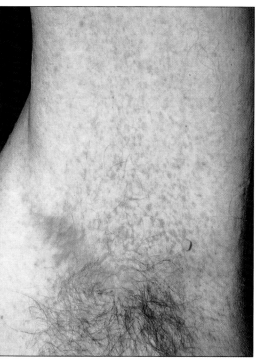

Figure 2-67. Axillary freckling in neurofibromatosis (NF1). The freckling shown here (same patient as in Figure 2-65) is common in NF1. Other characteristics include Lisch nodules of the iris and central nervous system tumors, including astrocytomas, meningiomas, and optic nerve gliomas. The gene for NF1 is on the long arm of chromosome 17 and codes for a protein called neurofibromin, which has tumor suppression properties [40].

Hereditary Bilateral Acoustic Neuroma (Neurofibromatosis 2)

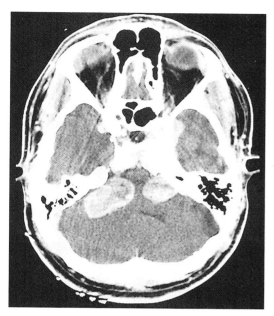

Figure 2-68. Computed tomography (CT) scan of a 40-year-old man with neurofibromatosis 2 (NF2). The hallmark of NF2 is bilateral acoustic neuromas, as dramatically shown in this CT scan. The tumors are schwannomas of the eighth cranial nerve and can be seen indenting the cerebellum and compressing the brain stem. This autosomal dominant disease can also manifest with café-au-lait spots and peripheral neurofibromas, but these are less frequent than in NF1. Initially, NF1 and NF2 were thought to be variants of the same disorder, but it is now clear that they are distinct diseases with different genes. Multiple other nervous system tumors have been associated with NF2 as well as lens opacities. The gene for NF2 lies on chromosome 22 and codes for a tumor-suppressor protein termed *merlin* [41]. (*Courtesy of* M. Mayberg, MD, University of Washington, Seattle, WA.)

Tuberous Sclerosis

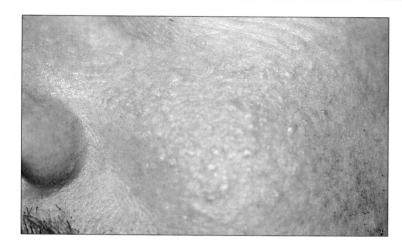

Figure 2-69. Prominent facial angiofibromas ("adenoma sebaceum") that are typical of tuberous sclerosis. These multiple, small, raised, red papules are actually vascular hamartomas. They are commonly mistaken for acne. Tuberous sclerosis is an autosomal dominant disorder primarily characterized by hamartomas of the skin, brain, heart, kidney, and other organs. The prevalence of the disease is approximately one in 10,000 population, and approximately 60% of cases seem to represent sporadic new dominant mutations. The most common neurologic problems are mental retardation and seizures, which occur in approximately half the patients. There are several cutaneous manifestations that are important diagnostic clues to the disease [42]. (*Courtesy of* V. Sybert, MD, Children's Hospital, Seattle, WA.)

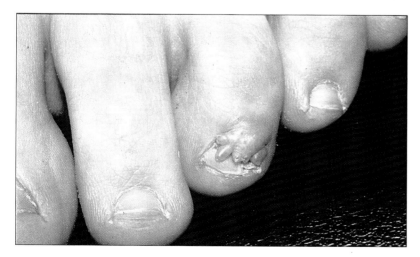

Figure 2-70. Typical periungual fibromas in the toes of a patient with tuberous sclerosis. These small wartlike tumors develop under or around finger- and toenails. (*Courtesy of* V. Sybert, MD, Children's Hospital, Seattle, WA.)

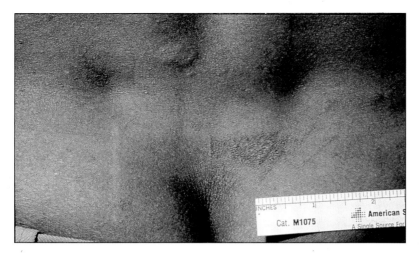

Figure 2-71. The back of a patient with tuberous sclerosis that has two shagreen patches. These elevated and thickened areas of skin have a pebbly texture like that of orange peel and are frequently found over the lumbar area. Another common skin lesion in tuberous sclerosis (not shown) is the depigmented or achromic patch, also called *hypomelonatic macule.* These lesions often have an oval shape resembling the leaf of an ash tree and may best be seen under ultraviolet light using Wood's light. (*Courtesy of* V. Sybert, MD, Children's Hospital, Seattle, WA.)

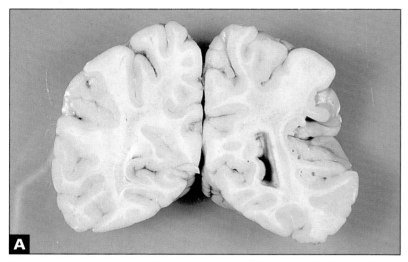

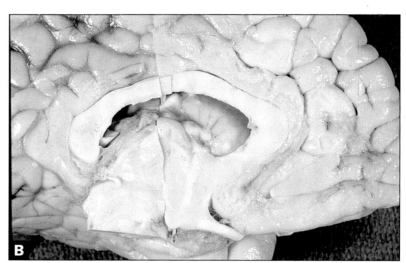

Figure 2-72. The brain from a 25-year-old woman with tuberous sclerosis. **A,** A cortical tuber in the right frontal region appears as a white, smooth, slightly raised area in the gyrus. **B,** A midline sagittal section of the brain shows numerous subependymal nodules projecting into the lateral ventricle. Other relatively common tumors include cardiac rhabdomyomas, retinal hamartomas, renal cysts, and renal angiomyolipomas. Tuberous sclerosis represents an example of genetic heterogeneity [43]. One gene associated with the disease has been located on chromosome 16p and codes for a protein called tuberin, which has similarities to a GTPase-activating protein. Other families with tuberous sclerosis have shown genetic linkage to markers on chromosome 9q encoding another tumor suppressor called <I> hamartin <I>.

Fabry's Disease

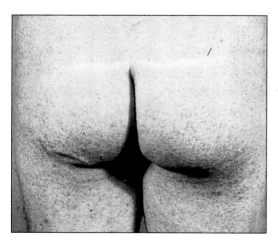

Figure 2-73. Characteristic clinical feature of Fabry's disease. Fabry's disease is also known as diffuse angiokerotoma or Anderson-Fabry's disease. This X-linked recessive disorder is associated with a deficiency of α-galactosidase associated with storage of ceramide primarily in blood vessels. The most characteristic clinical feature is the presence of angiokeratoma on the skin, especially over the buttocks (as shown) and around the navel. These small, red, raised, vascular lesions are easily overlooked when occurring in small numbers. Accumulation of lipid in the vasculature of the kidneys commonly results in hypertension, and renal failure is a frequent cause of death. Lipid accumulation in the cerebral blood vessels produces a multiple recurrent stroke syndrome. Association with a peripheral neuropathy including the autonomic nervous system may produce childhood or adolescent attacks of fever, arthralgia, and abdominal pain. Carrier females may have mild symptoms and signs of the disorder, including characteristic tortuous retinal vessels. The disease results from a deficiency of α-galactosidase and accumulation of trihexosides.

Sjögren-Larsson Syndrome

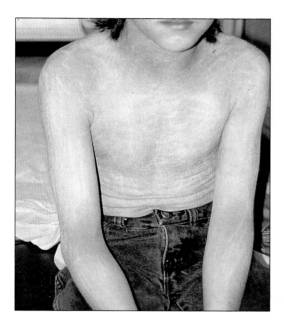

Figure 2-74. The raised, dry, somewhat rough and lightly brownish skin lesions seen on the chest, neck, and cheek of this 12-year-old boy with Sjögren-Larsson syndrome. Sjögren-Larsson syndrome is an autosomal recessive disorder causing congenital ichthyosis and spastic quadriplegia. It is most common in northern Sweden. Approximately half of the patients have pigmentary degeneration of the retina. Short stature, mental retardation, and seizures are common. The gene maps to the long arm of chromosome 17. (*Courtesy of* V. Sybert, MD, Children's Hospital, Seattle, WA.)

Cerebrotendinous Xanthomatosis

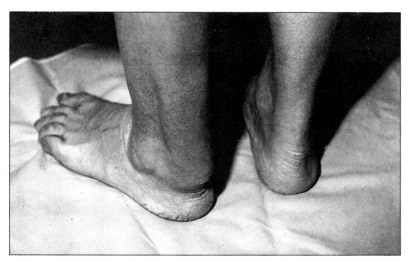

Figure 2-75. Clinical features of cerebrotendinous xanthomatosis (CTX). CTX is an autosomal recessive disorder characterized by lipid deposits in large tendons and lungs as well as cataracts, progressive ataxia, and dementia. The photo shows the enlarged, firm, lipid-impacted deposits in the Achilles tendon. (*From* Schimschock and colleagues [44]; with permission.)

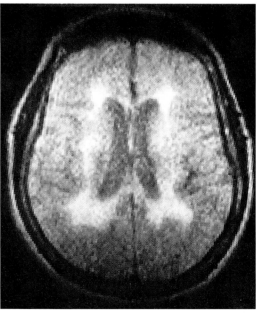

Figure 2-76. A magnetic resonance imaging scan of a 48-year-old woman with cerebrotendinous xanthomatosis (CTX), demonstrating areas of diffuse demyelination in the cerebral white matter. She presented with progressive confusion and had large, thick Achilles tendons. Her speech was slow and unsteady, but there were no focal or reflex abnormalities. CTX is caused by mutations in the sterol 27 hydroxylase gene, resulting in high tissue and plasma levels of dihydrocholesterol (cholestanol). The gene is on the long arm of chromosome 2. Early treatment with chenodeoxycholic acid may be beneficial. (*From* Swanson and colleague [45]; with permission.)

Blue Rubber Bleb Nevus Syndrome

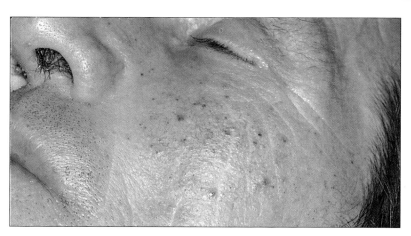

Figure 2-77. The cheek of a 60-year-old man who presented with a small pontine hemorrhage. His brother had a similar facial appearance. The family is presumed to have the blue rubber bleb nevus syndrome. Multiple dark blue hemangiomas of variable size may appear in the skin, the gastrointestinal tract, or the central nervous system. They refill after being compressed. Gastrointestinal tract bleeding frequently occurs. Central nervous system hemorrhage is uncommon but has been reported [46]. The disorder is autosomal dominant with variable expression.

Genetic Neurovascular Diseases

von Hippel-Lindau Disease

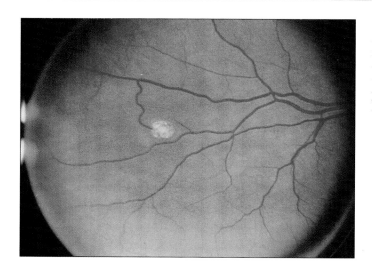

Figure 2-78. The raised, yellow, lumpy-appearing angiomata of the retina, characteristic of von Hippel-Lindau (VHL) disease. VHL disease is an autosomal dominant familial cancer syndrome characterized by a variable number of tumors at different organ sites, including renal cell carcinoma, cerebellar hemangioblastoma, retinal angiomata, and pheochromocytoma. Pancreatic tumors and cysts of the kidneys, pancreas, and epididymis may also occur. (*Courtesy of* R. Pagon, MD, Children's Hospital, Seattle, WA.)

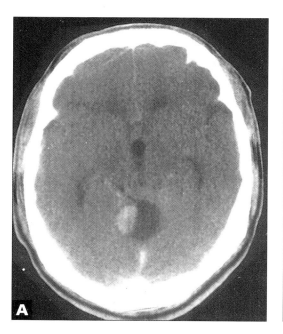

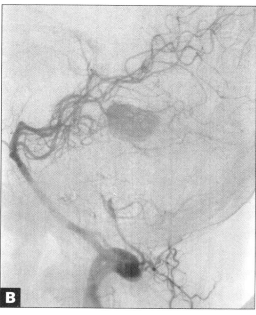

Figure 2-79. Effects of von Hippel-Liandau (VHL) disease on the brain. Neurologists most commonly see VHL patients because of hemorrhage or pressure from hemangioblastomas of the cerebellum, brain stem, or spinal cord. **A,** CT scan showing an enhancing tumor nidus surrounded by a cyst in the cerebellum. **B,** The angiographic blush during vertebral artery injection of this cerebellar hemangioblastoma. (*Continued on next page*)

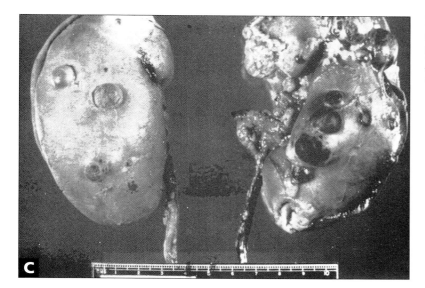

Figure 2-79. (*Continued*) **C**, Bilateral renal cysts and multicentric renal adenocarcinoma. VHL is caused by a tumor suppressor gene on chromosome 3p that has been identified and cloned [47]. (Panel B *courtesy of* J. Eskridge, MD, University of Washington, Seattle, WA; Panel C *from* Lamiell and colleagues [48]; with permission.)

Familial Cavernous Angioma

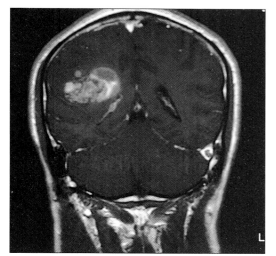

Figure 2-80. Magnetic resonance imaging (MRI) scan of a 31-year-old man who presented with a focal seizure disorder. Multiple small and large intracerebral lesions typical of cavernous angiomas are shown. These congenital blood vessel hamartomas are composed of dense, irregular, venous channels separated by fibrous septi without intervening nervous or glial tissue. Hemosiderin deposition and calcification are common. The disease may occur as an autosomal dominant disorder linked to markers on chromosome 7q [99]. The gene encodes a member of the RAS family of GTPases [50]. The clinical expression is quite variable, and although many carriers of the gene may have no symptoms, MRI scans may reveal the typical asymptomatic lesions. The disorder appears to have an increased frequency in the Hispanic population.

Multifactorial Disorders

Familial Multiple Sclerosis

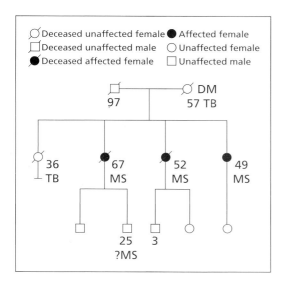

○ Deceased unaffected female ● Affected female
□ Deceased unaffected male ○ Unaffected female
● Deceased affected female □ Unaffected male

Figure 2-81. Pedigree of familial multiple sclerosis (MS). MS is a remitting and relapsing demyelinating disorder that is relatively common in the northern latitudes of the western hemisphere. Its cause is unknown and cases are usually sporadic, without a positive family history. Approximately 10% to 20% of MS patients will have another affected family member. Less commonly, there may be three or more family members with MS, as demonstrated in this kindred. It is assumed that this phenomenon of multiplex MS families represents multifactorial inheritance. That is, some unknown environmental agent (such as a virus) is provoking the disease in a genetically predisposed host (such as an individual with a certain vulnerable HLA type). In persons with MS, the risks for developing the disease in first-degree relatives is approximately 2% to 3% [57]. Although this is a relatively small risk, it should be noted that the lifetime age-corrected risk for the sibling of a patient with MS to develop MS represents more than a 25-fold increase over the lifetime risk for the general population. DM—diabetes mellitus; TB—tuberculosis.

References

1. Lampe T, Bird TD, Nochlin D, *et al.*: Phenotype of chromosome 14-linked familial Alzheimer's disease in a large kindred. *Ann Neurol* 1994, 36:368–378.

2. Van Broeckhoven CL: Molecular genetics of Alzheimer disease: identification of genes and gene mutations. *Eur Neurol* 1995, 35:8–19.

3. Sherrington R, Rogaev EI, Liang Y, *et al.*: Cloning of a gene bearing missense mutations in early-onset familial Alzheimer's disease. *Nature* 1995, 375:754–760.

4. Levy-Lahad E, Wasco W, Poorkaj P, *et al.*: Candidate gene for the chromosome 1 familial Alzheimer's disease locus. *Science* 1995, 269:973–977.

5. Roses AD: Apolipoprotein E genotyping in the differential diagnosis, not prediction, of Alzheimer's disease. *Ann Neurol* 1995, 18:6–14.

6. Levy-Lahad E, Bird TD: Alzheimer's Disease: Genetic Factors. In *Neurogenetics*. Edited by Pulst SM. New York: Oxford University Press, 1999:317–333.

7. Rosenberg RN: The molecular and genetic basis of AD: the end of the beginning: the 2000 Wartenberg lecture. *Neurology* 2000, 54:2045–2054.

8. Nochlin D, Sumi SM, Bird TD, *et al.*: Familial dementia with PrP-positive amyloid plaques: a variant of Gerstmann-Straussler syndrome. *Neurol* 1989, 39:910–918.

9. Mastrianni JA: The prion diseases: Creutzfeldt-Jakob, Gerstmann-Straussler-Scheinker, and related disorders. *J Geriatr Psychiatry Neurol* 1998, 11:78–97.

10. Wilhelmsen KC: Frontotemporal dementia genetics. *J Geriatr Psychiatry Neurol* 1998, 11:55–60.

11. Navon R, Argov Z, Frisch A: Hexosaminidase A deficiency in adults. *Am J Med Genet* 1986, 24:179–196.

12. Millat G, Marcais C, Rafi M, *et al.*: Niemann-Pick C1 disease: the I1061T substitution is a frequent mutant allele of Western European descent and correlates with a classic juvenile phenotype. *J Hum Genet* 1999, 65:1321–1329.

13. Rousseau F, Heitz D, Tarleton J, *et al.*: A multicenter study on genotype-phenotype correlations in the fragile X syndrome, using direct diagnosis with probe StB 12.3: the first 2,253 cases. *Am J Hum Genet* 1994, 55:225–237.

14. Fernandez M, Bird TD: Epilepsy. *The Genetic Basis of Common Diseases*. Edited by King R, Rotter J, Motulsky A.. New York, Oxford University Press; 2001, in press.

15. Watkins PA, Gould SJ, Smith MA, *et al.*: Altered expression of ALDP in X-linked adrenoleukodystrophy. *Am J Hum Genet* 1995, 576:292–301.

16. Garben J, Cambi F, Shy M, *et al.*: The molecular pathogenesis of Pelizaeus-Merzbacher disease. *Arch Neurol* 1999, 56:1210–1214.

17. Nance MA: Huntington disease: clinical, genetic, and social aspects. *J Geriatr Psychiatry Neurol* 1998, 11:61–70.

18. Finelli PF: Kayser-Fleischer ring: hepatolenticular degeneration (Wilson's disease). *Neurology* 1995, 45:1261–1262.

19. Vieregge P: Genetic factors in the etiology of idiopathic Parkinson's disease. *J Neural Transm Dement Sect* 1994, 8:1–37.

20. Payami H, Zareparsi MS: Genetic epidemiology of Parkinson's disease. *J Geriatr Psychiatry Neurol* 1998, 11:98–106.

21. Geschwind DH, Loginov M, Stern JM: Identification of a locus on chromosome 14q for idiopathic basal ganglia calcification (Fahr disease). *Am J Hum Genet* 1999, 65:764–772.

22. Genis D, Matilla T, Volpini V, *et al.*: Clinical, neuropathologic, and genetic studies of a large spinocerebellar ataxia type 1 (SCA1) kindred: (CAG)$_n$ expansion and early premonitory signs and symptoms. *Neurology* 1995, 45:24–30.

23. Matilla T, McCall A, Subramony SH, *et al.*: Molecular and clinical correlations in spinocerebellar ataxia type 3 and Machado-Joseph disease. *Ann Neurol* 1995, 38:68–72.

24. Pulst SM, Perlman S: Hereditary Ataxias. In *Neurogenetics*. Edited by Pulst SM. New York: Oxford University Press, 1999:231–263.

25. Martin JJ, Martin L, Lofgren A, *et al*: Classical Friedreich's ataxia and its genotype. *Eur Neurol* 1999, 42:109–115.

26. Savitsky K, Bar-Shira A, Gilad S, *et al.*: A single ataxia telangiectasia gene with a product similar to PI-3 kinase. *Science* 1995, 268:1749–1753.

27. Rosen DR, Siddique T, Patterson D, *et al.*: Mutations in Cu/Zn superoxide dismutase gene are associated with familial amyotrophic lateral sclerosis. *Nature* 1993, 362:59–62.

28. Nagashima T, Seko K, Hirose K, *et al.*: Familial bulbo-spinal muscular atrophy associated with testicular atrophy and sensory neuropathy (Kennedy-Alter-Sung syndrome): autopsy case report of two brothers. *J Neurol Sci* 1988, 87:141–152.

29. Lefebvre S, Burglen L, Reboullet S, *et al.*: Identification and characterization of a spinal muscular atrophy-determining gene. *Cell* 1995, 80:155–165.

30. Fink JK, Hedera P: Hereditary spastic paraplegia: genetic heterogeneity and genotype-phenotype correlation. *Semin Neurol* 1999, 19:301–10.

31. Nelis E, Timmerman V, De Jonghe P, *et al.*: Molecular genetics and biology of inherited peripheral neuropathies: a fast-moving field. *Neurogenetics* 1999, 2:137–148.

32. Thompson MW, McInnes RR, Willard HF, eds: The Molecular and Biochemical Basis of Genetic Disease. In *Genetics in Medicine*, edn 5. Philadelphia: WB Saunders; 1991:289–293.

33. Witkowski JA: Dystrophin-related muscular dystrophies. *J Child Neurol* 1989, 4:251–271.

34. Arikawa E, Hoffman EP, Kaido M, *et al.*: The frequency of patients with dystrophin abnormalities in a limb-girdle patient population. *Neurology* 1991, 41:1491–1496.

35. Ptaáek L: Ion channel shake-down. *Nature Genet* 1994, 8:111–112.

36. Laing NG, Wilton SD, Akkari PA, *et al.*: A mutation in the alpha tropomyosin gene TPM3 associated with autosomal dominant nemaline myopathy. *Nature Genet* 1995:75–79.

37. Kissel JT: Facioscapulohumeral dystrophy. *Semin Neurol* 1999, 19:35–45.

38. Silvestri G, Ciagaloni E, Santorelli FM, *et al.*: Clinical features associated with the A → G transition at nucleotide 8344 of mtDNA ("MERRF mutation"). *Neurology* 1993, 43:1200–1206.

39. Santorelli FM, Shanske S, Macaya A, *et al.*: The mutation at nt 8993 of mitochondrial DNA is a common cause of Leigh's syndrome. *Ann Neurol* 1993, 34:827–834.

40. Gutmann DH, Collins FS: Recent progress toward understanding the molecular biology of Von Recklinghausen neurofibromatosis. *Ann Neurol* 1992, 31:555–561.

41. Parry DM, Eldridge R, Kaiser-Kupfer MI, *et al.*: Neurofibromatosis 2 (NF2) clinical characteristics of 63 affected individuals and clinical evidence for heterogeneity. *Am J Med Genet* 1994, 52:450–461.

42. Crino PB, Henske EP: New developments in the neurobiology of the tuberous sclerosis complex. *Neurology* 1999, 53:1384–1390.

43. Jones AC, Shyamsundar MM, Thomas MW, et al: Comprehensive mutation analysis of TSC1 and TSC2- and phenotypic correlations in 150 families with tuberous sclerosis. *Am J Hum Genet* 1999, 64:1305–1315.

44. Schimschock JR, Alvord E Jr, Swanson PD: Cerebrotendinous xanthomatosis: clinical and pathological studies. *Arch Neurol* 1968, 18:688–698.

45. Swanson PD, Cromwell LD: Magnetic resonance imaging in cerebrotendinous xanthomatosis. *Neurology* 1986, 36:124–126.

46. Satya-Murti S, Navada S, Eames F: Central nervous system involvement in blue-rubber-bleb-nevus syndrome. *Arch Neurol* 1986, 43:1184–1186.

47. Duan DR, Pause A, Burgess WH, *et al.*: Inhibition of transcription elongation by the VHL tumor suppressor protein. *Science* 1995, 269:1402–1406.

48. Lamiell JM, Salazar FG, Hsia YE: Von Hippel-Lindau disease affecting 43 members of a single kindred. *Medicine* 1989, 68:1–29.

49. Rigamonti D, Hadley MN, Drayer P, *et al.*: Cerebral cavernous malformations: incidence and familial occurrence. *N Engl J Med* 1988, 319:343–347.

50. Sahoo T, Johnson EW, Thomas JW, *et al.*: Mutations in the gene encoding KRIT1, a Krev-1/rap1a binding protein, cause cerebral cavernous malformations (CCM1). *Hum Molec Genet* 1999, 12:2325–2333.

51. Chataway J, Feakes R, Coraddu F, *et al.*: The genetics of multiple sclerosis: principles, background and updated results of the United Kingdom systematic genome screen. *Brain* 1998, 121:1869–1887.

3

Neuroendocrine Disorders

Earl A. Zimmerman

THE brain participates in the endocrine system through the hypothalamus, which contains the neurosecretory system that produces releasing hormones. Some of these hormones are secreted into the hypothalamohypophysial portal system to regulate anterior pituitary hormones and others into the general circulation in the posterior pituitary to control water conservation and breast milk ejection. The hypothalamus and its connections with the anterior and posterior pituitary gland comprise the hypothalamic-pituitary unit [1,2] (Fig. 3-2). The hypothalamus regulates additional vegetative and autonomic functions, including eating, drinking, and temperature. Lesions in or around the hypothalamic-pituitary unit cause various clinical syndromes in the endocrine system associated with decreased or increased hormonal secretions. Tumors in or around the hypothalamus also produce other vegetative symptoms and involve other neural structures nearby; the optic nerves and chiasm are particularly vulnerable. At times extension into the cavernous sinus causes eye movement difficulties. Occasionally obstruction of the third ventricle and its outflow result in hydrocephalus. Headache can be caused by traction on the pain-sensitive dura of the diaphragm of the sella.

Lesions affecting the hypothalamus or pituitary stalk directly (parapituitary) vary with the age of the patient; craniopharyngioma is more common at younger ages and meningioma occurs later in life [1,3]. Many of these tumors are congenital. Involvement of the vasopressin system at this level frequently causes diabetes insipidus, which is much less common with pituitary tumors. Prolactin may also be elevated in hypothalamic hypopituitarism when all other anterior pituitary secretions are diminished (growth hormone [GH], thyroid-stimulating hormone [TSH], adrenocorticotropic hormone [ACTH], luteinizing hormone [LH], follicle-stimulating hormone [FSH]). Prolactin (PRL) secretion is mainly under inhibitory control by dopamine, which originates in the hypothalamus [1,2,4].

A diagnostic work-up includes measurements of the pituitary hormones and their target glands. In addition to an endocrine and neurologic history and examination, screening should begin with assessment of the most critical endocrine functions, especially thyroid (thyroxine, [T4]) and adrenal function (cortisol, intravenous ACTH test) and a blood PRL determination. Visual field and acuity assessments are always important. Imaging, usually by magnetic resonance imaging (MRI) with gadolinium for contrast, is important to localize the lesion. Treatment is total surgical removal of the lesion if possible. Microsurgical techniques have significantly improved the cure rate and reduced morbidity in craniopharyngioma in the last decade. Progress in the postoperative management of diabetes insipidus (DI) with short-acting vasopressin (dDAVP) and control of syndrome of inappropriate secretion of vasopressin (SIADH) and adrenal hypofunction has improved therapy. Similar progress has been made for other lesions. Others, such as infiltrating optic or hypothalamic glioma, require radiotherapy.

Pituitary tumors are either hyposecretory or hypersecretory and associated with specific endocrine syndromes. Some hypersecretory tumors are associated with diminished secretion or reduced glandular function in other systems. For example, hyperprolactinemia due to oversecretion by a pituitary prolactinoma is associated with hypogonadism, commonly seen in the amenorrhea-galactorrhea syndrome. Thyroid and adrenal deficiency—other aspects of hypopituitarism—may be seen in prolactinoma or somatotropic adenoma owing to destruction by compression of normal pituitary tissue. Pituitary hypopituitarism due to pituitary compression or infarction is associated with loss of all the anterior pituitary hormones including PRL (except in prolactinoma). Diabetes insipidus, which usually does not occur, responds nicely to the administration of intranasal dDAVP. Treatment of hypopituitarism is the replacement of the most necessary hormones in adults: thyroid, adrenal glucocorticoid, estrogen, and androgen. GH replacement is important in children, although the importance of its role in adults is still debated.

The hypersecretory pituitary syndromes include SIADH, caused by oversecretion of vasopressin, and the three most common secreting pituitary adenomas: prolactinoma, somatotropinoma, and basophilic adenoma, which causes Cushing's disease [1,4]. SIADH is uncommon and transient and readily managed if recognized or even anticipated. SIADH is very dangerous, causing seizures and coma in the face of rapidly diminished serum sodium levels and osmolality; it occasionally occurs in an inpatient setting when intravenous solutions are given to an obtunded patient.

Prolactinoma is the most common secretory adenoma, producing the amenorrhea-galactorrhea syndrome. In younger patients, most often infertile women, it is often associated with microadenoma. These small tumors may be visualized on MRI or computed tomography (CT). Patients have galactorrhea, hyperprolactinemia, and otherwise normal anterior pituitary function [1,4]. Some prolactinomas resolve over the years and no treatment is given. If fertility and pregnancy are important to the patient, treatment with bromocriptine or removal of the adenoma by transsphenoidal surgery provides excellent results. Larger prolactinomas tend to be associated with hypopituitarism and visual disturbance.

The second most common secretory tumor produces GH and gigantism in children and acromegaly in adults. It is a life-threatening and debilitating condition, which fortunately is often associated with adenomas that can be surgically removed, most often by the transsphenoidal route, resulting in a cure. Larger tumors associated with hypopituitarism are more difficult to cure by surgery; they tend to recur but may be controlled with the administration of bromocriptine, somatostatin analogues, and radiotherapy [1,4]. Control of the GH secretion—as in prolactoma—can be followed by measuring the hormone in blood by radioimmunoassay. Half of the patients with acromegaly oversecrete PRL as well as GH.

The other hypersecretory pituitary syndrome causes Cushing's syndrome from basophilic cells that form ACTH. These are often chromophobic adenomas, as demonstrated by histochemistry. Cushing's disease (caused by a pituitary tumor) is a common cause of Cushing's syndrome, but other causes, such as ectopic ACTH-secreting lung tumor or an ACTH-independent adrenal tumor, need to be considered [1,4,5]. Many Cushing's tumors are pituitary microadenomas too small or diffuse to be visualized on MRI, and require inferior petrosal sinus measurements of ACTH [5] to determine which side of the pituitary to operate on by the transsphenoidal approach, which often results in a cure. Fortunately, aggressive adenomas secreting ACTH and melanocyte-stimulating hormone (MSH) (with hyperpigmentation) were more common in the past after bilateral adrenalectomy (Nelson's syndrome). Some tumors recur after surgery, requiring reoperation, drugs to suppress the adrenal gland, or radiotherapy. This serious hypersecretory state causes medical deterioration in a few years if untreated. Some tumors secrete more than one of the hormones mentioned, on occasion all, and at times others, such as TSH, LH, or FSH.

Normal Functional Anatomy

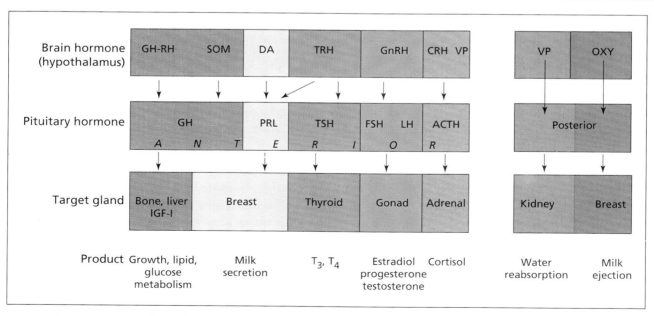

Figure 3-1. The endocrine system. The brain participates in the endocrine system by secreting hormones known as releasing factors, which act in the anterior pituitary gland to regulate the production of specific trophic hormones. These act on other glands and control functions in the body: growth and metabolism, milk secretion, and thyroidal, gonadal, and adrenal functions. The target glands and their hormonal products in turn influence the brain, as feedback systems generally operate between endocrine organs. Thyroid hormones and adrenocortical steroids have significant feedback effects on the brain and pituitary gland. The hypothalamus region of the brain also secretes vasopressin and oxytocin into the general circulation through the posterior pituitary gland; these serve as an antidiuretic hormone (regulating water reabsorption by the kidney) and as a hormone regulating breast milk ejection.

ACTH—adrenocorticotropic hormone; DA—dopamine; CRH—corticotropin releasing hormone; FSH—follicle-stimulating hormone; GH—growth hormone; GH-RH—growth hormone releasing factor; GnRH—gonadotropin releasing factor; IGF-I—insulin-like growth factor; LH—luteinizing hormone; OXY—oxytocin; PRL—prolactin; SOM—somatotrophic hormone; T_3—triiodothyronine; T_4—thyroxine; TRH—thyrotropin-releasing hormone; TSH—thyroid-stimulating hormone; VP—vasopressin.

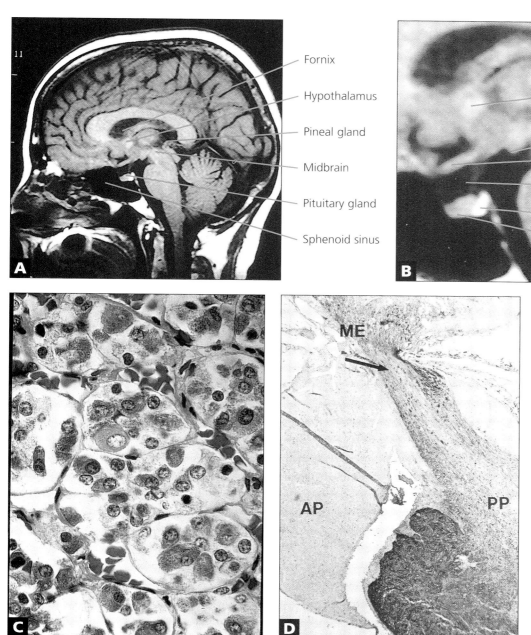

imity to the pituitary stalk and hypothalamus. The thin pituitary stalk, an extension of the hypothalamus, connects with the posterior pituitary, which appears as a bright spot on this MRI scan, compared to the anterior pituitary gland. The anterior commissure, thalamus, and mammillary body are readily apparent.

C, This specimen of the anterior pituitary gland, with trichrome stain under light microscopy, appears generally similar to other glands of the body, such as the pancreas, and dissimilar to the posterior pituitary. Red or reddish-brown cells, which take up acidic stains, are the most numerous cells of the pituitary, producing either growth hormone (GH) or prolactin (PRL). Cells that appear green here, or blue with basic stains, produce thyroid-stimulating hormone (TSH), luteinizing hormone (LH), follicle-stimulating hormone (FSH), or adrenocorticotropic hormone (ACTH). Cells that react with neither acidic nor basic stains are called chromophobes.

D, A sagittal low-power light microscopic image of a monkey pituitary gland specimen prepared with immunohistochemical methods. The posterior pituitary gland (PP) is composed primarily of nerve fibers that descend from the hypothalamus through the internal median eminence (ME). AP—anterior pituitary. (Panel C *courtesy of* Richard Defendini, MD, College of Physicians and Surgeons, Columbia University, New York, NY; panel D *from* Antunes and Zimmerman: The hypothalamic magnocellular system of the Rhesus monkey: an immunocytochemical study. *J Comp Neurol,* Copyright @ 1978. Reprinted by permission of Wiley-Liss, Inc., a subsidiary of John Wiley & Sons, Inc.

Figure 3-2. The hypothalamic-pituitary unit, in which the endocrine system and the brain interact. **A,** Midsagittal view of a magnetic resonance image (MRI) scan of a normal human brain. This "cut" goes right through the third ventricle, which forms the midline of the paired hypothalami. The rostral border is the anterior commissure and inferior to it, the lamina terminalis (not shown). The lateral border is formed by the columns of the fornix, a major hippocampal output. The pineal gland, posterior hypothalamus, and mammillary body form the posterior region, and the thalamus forms the dorsal limit. The sphenoid sinus is separated from the pituitary gland by a thin layer of the sella turcica bone, not visualized by MRI.

B, A higher magnification of the same MRI reveals the optic nerve and chiasm in close prox-

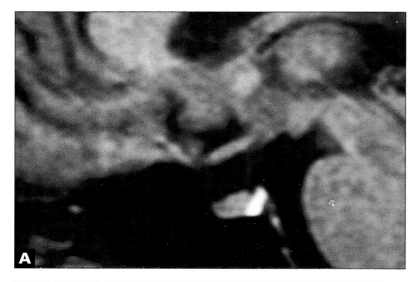

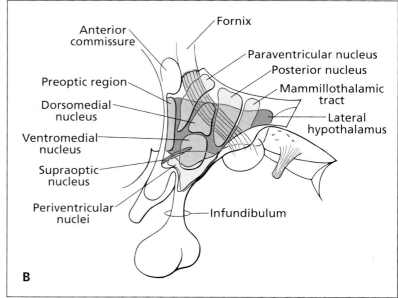

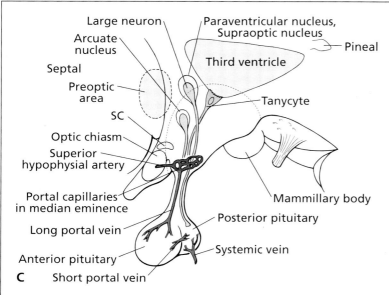

D. Hypothalamic Hormones' Nuclear Group of Origin

Hypothalamic hormone	Nuclear group of origin
CRH/VP TRH	Paraventricular (parvocellular)
Dopamine (DA) GH-RH	Infundibular (arcuate)
GnRH	Preoptic-infundibular
SOM	Periventricular
VP (to posterior pituitary) OXY	Magnocellular paraventricular and supraoptic

Figure 3-3. Anatomic organization of the hypothalamus. **A,** Sagittal magnetic resonance image (MRI) scan showing the hypothalamus has been further detailed by microscopic studies. **B,** Nuclear groups reflecting the cellular organization; some of these contain known releasing secretory systems (*D*). **C,** Large neurons (magnocellular) that form posterior pituitary hormones are concentrated in the supraoptic and paraventricular nuclei. Smaller cells (parvocellular), located in the arcuate nucleus (infundibular), paraventricular nucleus, periventricular region and preoptic areas, secrete hypothalamic releasing hormones into the hypophysial portal capillaries

in the external zone of the median eminence in the lower infundibulum-upper pituitary stalk. Tanycytes are specialized ependyma typically seen in the infundibular region lining the third ventricle; they send long processes to the portal capillary bed and are thought to regulate secretory terminals.

D, Hypothalamic hormones' nuclear group of origin. CRH/VP—corticotropin releasing hormone; GH-RH—growth hormone releasing factor; GnRH—gonadotropin releasing factor; OXY—oxytocin; SC—suprachiasmatic nucleus; SOM—somatotrophic hormone; TRH—thyrotropin-releasing hormone; VP—vasopressin. (Panel B *adapted from* Nauta [7].)

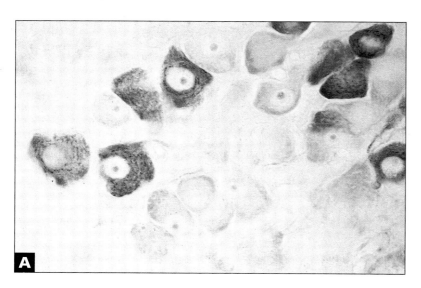

Figure 3-4. Neurosecretory neurons identified by light and electron microscopy using immunoperoxidase technique. **A,** Cell bodies secreting oxytocin (*brown*) and vasopressin (*blue*) in rat supraoptic nucleus.

(*Continued on next page*)

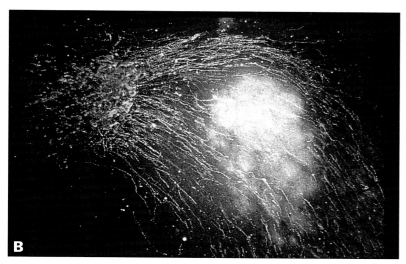

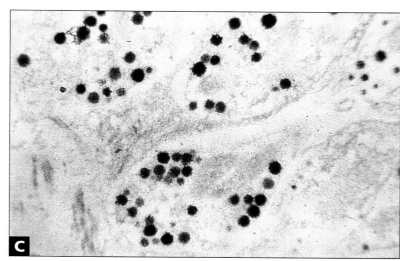

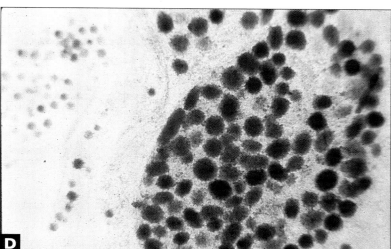

Figure 3-4. (*Continued*) **B,** Dark field photomicrograph of vasopressin-containing axons leaving paraventricular magnocellular neurons laterally and coursing through and around the fornix on their ventral pathway to the pituitary stalk. Massive numbers of fibers provide the hormone to the posterior pituitary gland for the minute-to-minute regulation of tightly controlled osmolality. **C,** Vasopressin-containing granules in nerve terminals in the zona externa of the median eminence co-exist with corticotropin releasing hormone–containing granules and serve to stimulate adrenocorticotropic hormone secretion. **D,** These granules and others containing releasing hormones for the anterior pituitary targets are smaller than the vasopressin granules in the posterior pituitary gland. (Panel A *courtesy of* E.A. Zimmerman, MD and H. Sokol, MD; Panel B *from* Zimmerman and colleagues [8]; with permission; Panels C, D *courtesy of* A.J. Silverman, MD, College of Physicians and Surgeons, Columbia University, New York, NY and E.A. Zimmerman, MD, Albany Medical College, Albany, NY.)

Pathophysiologic States

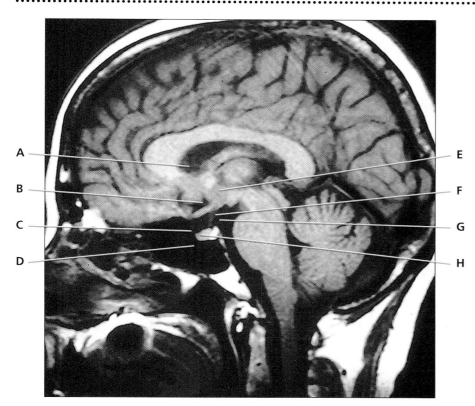

Figure 3-5. Clinical presentations of pituitary and parapituitary lesions. **A,** Hydrocephalus is caused by the tumor blocking the foramen of Monro. **B,** There is a loss of visual acuity due to the optic nerve being affected or a visual field defect due to a disturbance of the optic chiasm. **C,** Cavernous sinus syndrome affecting cranial nerves V_1, III, IV, and VI due to bleeding into the adenoma (pituitary apoplexy). **D,** Cerebrospinal fluid rhinorrhea and possibly the tumor extending into the nose due to erosion of the floor of the sella into the sphenoidal sinus. **E,** Hypothalamic symptoms: hypopituitarism, hyperprolactinemia, and diabetes insipidus. **F,** Hypopituitarism due to disruption of the pituitary stalk by trauma, surgery, or tumor. **G,** Retro-orbital headache due to pressure on the diaphragm sella. **H,** Anterior pituitary failure.

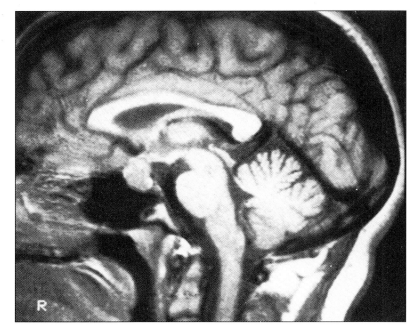

Figure 3-6. Midsagittal magnetic resonance image (MRI) showing a large pituitary adenoma extending upward to involve the pituitary stalk, optic chiasm, and inferior hypothalamus. (*From* Abrams and colleague [4]; with permission.)

Hypothalamic Lesions and Symptoms

Lesions	Symptoms
VMN, Medial hypothalamus	Obesity, excitability
Lateral hypothalamus	Aphagia, placidity
Anterior hypothalamus	Hyperthermia
Posterior hypothalamus	Hypothermia in cold
Preoptic area, OVLT, SFO	Abnormal thirst (adipsia)
PVN, SON, tract	DI or SIADH if stimulated
MBH	Hypopituitarism

Figure 3-7. Hypothalamic lesions and symptoms. DI—diabetes insipidus; MBH—medial basal hypothalamus; OVLT—organum vasculosum of the lamina terminalis; PVN—paraventricular nucleus; SFO—subformical organ; SIADH—syndrome of inappropriate secretion of vasopressin; SON—supraoptic nucleus; VMN—ventromedial nucleus.

Some Lesions Affecting the Hypothalamus

Craniopharyngioma—arises from the pituitary stalk, most commonly presents in childhood with visual changes, diabetes insipidus

Optic glioma—begins in optic nerve or chiasm, causing visual loss
Occurs in neurofibromatosis type 1

Dermoid, teratoma, colloid cyst of the third ventricle—congenital tumors

Pinealoma—choriocarcinoma and germ cell type may secrete B-human chorionic gonadotropin causing precocious pseudopuberty in male boys

Meningioma in adults

Pituitary adenoma by upward extension, causing bitemporal hemianopia

Granulomatous lesions—sarcoidosis, histiocytosis X

Metastatic—lung, breast, most often to the pituitary gland

Figure 3-8. Some lesions affecting the hypothalamus. Craniopharyngioma and optic glioma are more common in children, and pituitary adenoma and meningioma are more often seen in adults.

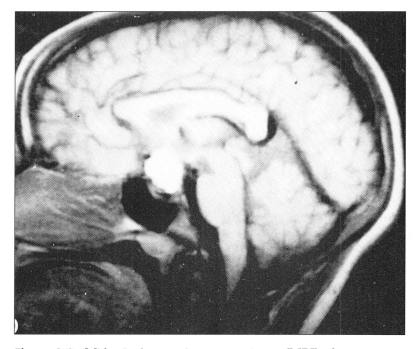

Figure 3-9. Midsagittal magnetic resonance image (MRI) of a craniopharyngioma involving the pituitary stalk and hypothalamus. Hyperintensity of the lesion is due to cyst contents. (*From* Zimmerman and colleague [3]; with permission.)

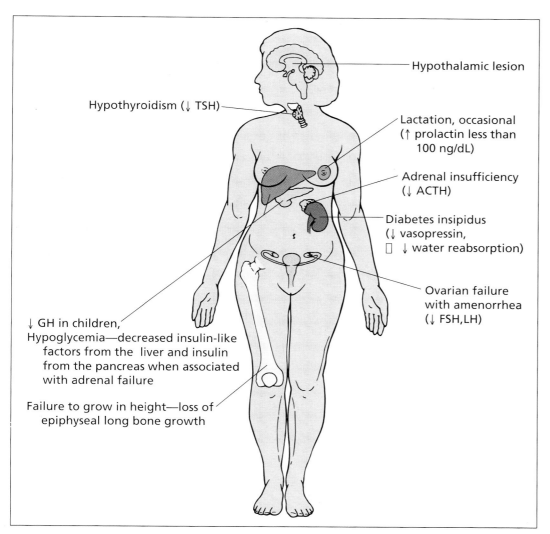

Hypothalamic lesion

Hypothyroidism (↓ TSH)

Lactation, occasional
(↑ prolactin less than
100 ng/dL)

Adrenal insufficiency
(↓ ACTH)

Diabetes insipidus
(↓ vasopressin,
☐ ↓ water reabsorption)

Ovarian failure
with amenorrhea
(↓ FSH,LH)

↓ GH in children,
Hypoglycemia—decreased insulin-like
factors from the liver and insulin
from the pancreas when associated
with adrenal failure

Failure to grow in height—loss of
epiphyseal long bone growth

Figure 3-10. Clinical manifestations of hypothalamic hypopituitarism. ACTH—adrenocorticotropic hormone; FSH—follicle-stimulating hormone; GH—growth hormone; LH—luteinizing hormone; TSH—thyroid-stimulating hormone.

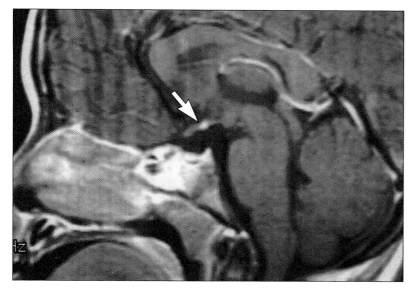

Figure 3-11. Magnetic resonance imaging changes in hypothalamic hypopituitarism. The "bright spot" (*arrow*) appearance of the posterior pituitary gland is missing from its normal location in the sella turcica. Instead it is located in the lower hypothalamus and upper pituitary stalk in this child with congenital growth hormone and thyroid-stimulating hormone deficiency. Damage to the stalk interrupts the hypophysial portal system and vasopressin fibers. These fibers regenerate forming a new, usually smaller, posterior pituitary in this location (ectopic). Such patients may recover from or have partial diabetes insipidus. More proximal lesions in the hypothalamic nuclei and tracts to the vasopressin system do not regenerate. Interruption of the releasing factor pathways and the portal system results in anterior pituitary deficiencies.

Causes of Diabetes Insipidus

Primary: hereditary, idiopathic
Secondary
  Trauma: accident, surgery
  Neoplasm
    Large pituitary adenoma with upward growth to involve
      hypothalamus
    Craniopharyngioma
    Meningioma
    Epidermoid
    Dermoid
    Teratoma
    Chordoma
    Optic glioma
    Metastatic carcinoma
  Infection: meningitis, encephalitis
  Systemic: sarcoidosis, lymphoma, histiocytosis X

Figure 3-12. Causes of diabetes insipidus. The appearance of diabetes insipidus is important to investigate, as it suggests a brain lesion [9].

Clinical Features of Diabetes Insipidus

Polyuria—volumes, often 5–8 quarts when severe

Polydypsia—often a craving for cold water

Hypernatremia and dehydration

Dilute urine (low specific gravity, low osmolality)

Rapid response to intranasal or subcutaneous administration of vasopressin

Figure 3-13. Clinical features of diabetes insipidus. When fully developed, no disease other than hypothalamic diabetes insipidus causes such a large need for drinking very large volumes in 24 hours (*eg*, kidney disease and psychogenic water drinking usually do not exceed a quart or two at most).

Syndrome of Inappropriate Secretion of Vasopressin

Causes

Iatrogenic
  Parenteral administration of fluids in patients not regulating their own fluid intake, in a clinical setting in which vasopressin is oversecreted (*eg*, postoperative patients, especially following thoracic or neurologic surgery)
Central nervous system (overstimulation of vasopressin secretion)
  Head trauma
    Basilar skull fracture
    Damage to hypothalamus and pituitary stalk
  Neurosurgery
    Craniopharyngioma
  Subarachnoid hemorrhage
  Meningitis
  Suprahypothalamic lesions
      Stroke
      Subdural hematoma
Pulmonary disease (lung afferents stimulate the central nervous system)
  Pneumonia
  Pulmonary tuberculosis

Ectopic hormone production
  Carcinoma of the lung
  Other cancers
Metabolic conditions
  Acute intermittent porphyria
  Myxedema
Drugs
  Carbamazepine
  Chlorpropamide
  Clofibrate
  Cyclophosphamide
  Vincristine
  Chlorthiazide
  Cyclophosphamide

Clinical manifestations

Hyponatremia and low serum osmolality due to excessive vasopressin secretion
  Slow lowering of sodium (*eg*, ectopic vasopressin secretion by lung carcinoma)
    May have no clinical signs
  Rapid lowering of sodium (*eg*, obtunded postoperative patient receiving intravenous fluids)
    Seizures
    Obtundation
    Coma
    Death (very low sodium levels, *eg*, 110 mEq/dL)
High urine osmolality, inappropriate with low serum osmolality

Diagnostic procedures

Rule out thyroid, kidney, and adrenal failure

Management

Eliminate the cause

Restrict fluid intake

Replace sodium chloride (carefully—too rapidly may cause central demyelination)

Prescribe diuretics (furosemide)

Figure 3-14. Causes, clinical manifestations, diagnostic procedures, and management of syndrome of inappropriate secretion of vasopressin (SIADH).

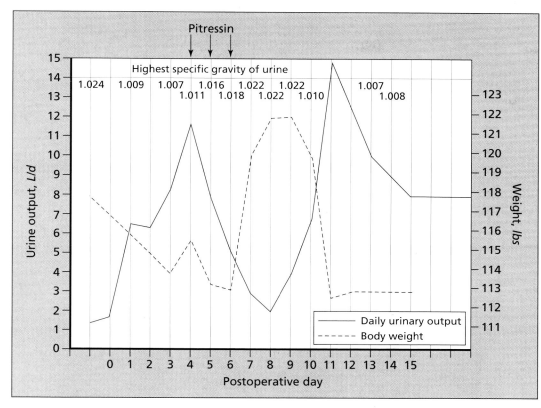

Figure 3-15. Diabetes insipidus alternating with syndrome of inappropriate secretion of antidiuretic hormone—triphasic diabetes insipidus (DI). Triphasic DI was first demonstrated in experimental animals with lesions in the pituitary stalk; it is now anticipated in patients following surgery in the region of the pituitary stalk. It is especially seen in relation to surgery for craniopharyngioma, which often arises from and is attached to the pituitary stalk as in this graph. In this patient the daily urinary output (*dark line*) rose significantly to 10 to 12 L and body weight (*dashed line*) fell by the 4th postoperative day, indicating diabetes insipidus and failure of secretion of vasopressin (antidiuretic hormone) by damaged nerve fibers in the pituitary stalk. This was treated by a long-acting (24-hour) preparation

of vasopressin such as pitressin (Parke-Davis, Morris Plains, NJ) administered by injection. While the patient was receiving intravenous fluids, on day 6 the situation reversed with marked weight gain and a great decrease in urinary output, which hit its lowest point on day 8. Pitressin was discontinued by day 7, but urinary specific gravity continued to rise due to excessive secretion of vasopressin by degenerating nerve terminals in the posterior pituitary gland distal to the damage to the pituitary stalk; this second phase was due to SIADH. By day 10 the situation again reversed, with marked diuresis of 15 L per 24 h and a 10-lb weight loss by postoperative day 11. Urinary specific gravity fell and remained low. This phase of DI was due to elimination of the vasopressin released from degenerating nerve terminals. Partial DI appeared to persist. Regeneration of the proximal vasopressin-secreting nerve terminals, beginning about 2 weeks postoperatively, may result in partial or complete recovery from DI. Interruption of the hypophysial portal system is likely to cause failure of anterior pituitary function (Fig. 3-11).

The phenomenon of triphasic DI still occurs in patients, but the risk of major swings in water and electrolyte balance have been eliminated from practice by anticipating it; administrating short-acting preparations of vasopressin for DI, including the intranasal form when appropriate; and especially monitoring intravenous (IV) fluid intake and urinary output when patients are not regulating their own fluid intake by their own thirst mechanisms. Removing patients earlier from IV fluids permits them to regulate their own fluid intake needs sooner and makes management easier.

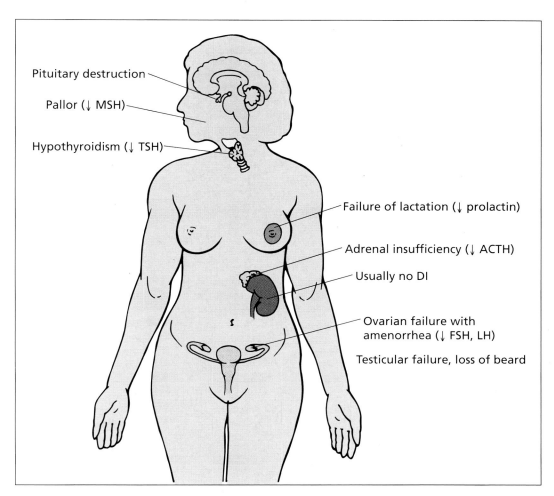

Figure 3-16. Clinical manifestations of pituitary hypopituitarism. The causes of pituitary hypopituitarism include pituitary adenoma, metastatic carcinoma, postpartum pituitary necrosis (which is sometimes called Sheehan's syndrome), and hemorrhage into an adenoma, pituitary apoplexy. ACTH—adenocorticotropic hormone; DI—diabetes insipidus; FSH—follicle-stimulating hormone; LH—luteinizing hormone; MSH—melanocyte-stimulating hormone; TSH—thyroid-stimulating hormone.

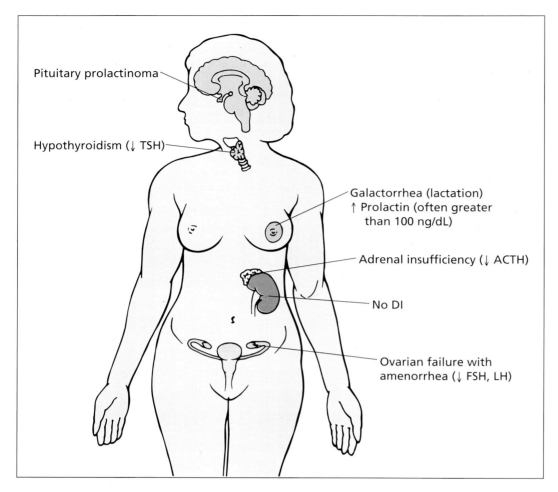

Figure 3-17. Clinical features of a prolactin secreting pituitary adenoma. A prolactin micro-adenoma is less than 1 cm in diameter. The only presenting symptoms may be an amenorrhea-galactorrhea syndrome. A larger tumor may have intracranial symptoms such as bitemporal hemianopia and retro-orbital headaches and possible pituitary failure with thyroid, gonadal, and adrenal insufficiency. ACTH—adenocorticotropic hormone; DI—diabetes insipidus; FSH—follicle-stimulating hormone; LH—luteinizing hormone; TSH—thyroid-stimulating hormone.

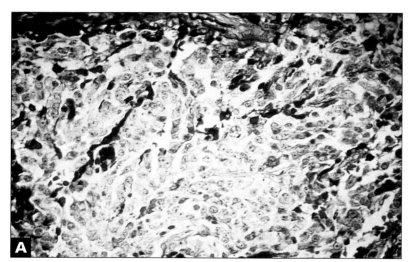
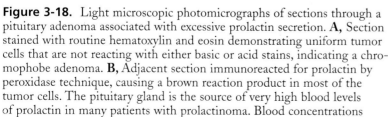
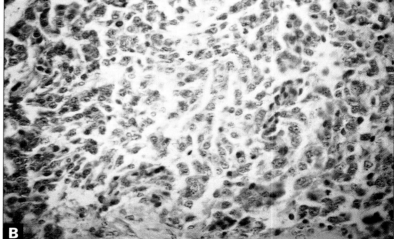

Figure 3-18. Light microscopic photomicrographs of sections through a pituitary adenoma associated with excessive prolactin secretion. **A,** Section stained with routine hematoxylin and eosin demonstrating uniform tumor cells that are not reacting with either basic or acid stains, indicating a chromophobe adenoma. **B,** Adjacent section immunoreacted for prolactin by peroxidase technique, causing a brown reaction product in most of the tumor cells. The pituitary gland is the source of very high blood levels of prolactin in many patients with prolactinoma. Blood concentrations over 100 or 200 ng/dL are nearly diagnostic of prolactinoma. Levels can be as high as several thousand. However, patients with proven prolactinoma and amenorrhea-galactorrhea syndrome may only have slightly elevated concentrations, often less than 100 ng/dL. These tend to be microadenomas. (*Courtesy of* R.F. Defendini, MD, A.G. Frantz, MD, College of Physicians and Surgeons, Columbia University, New York, NY; E.A. Zimmerman, MD, Albany Medical College, Albany, NY.)

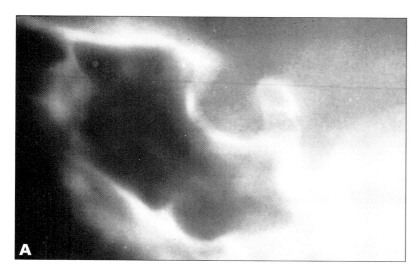

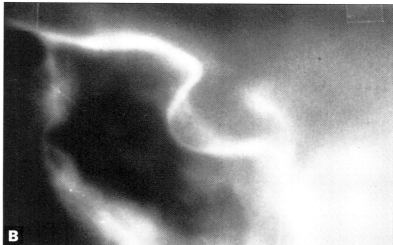

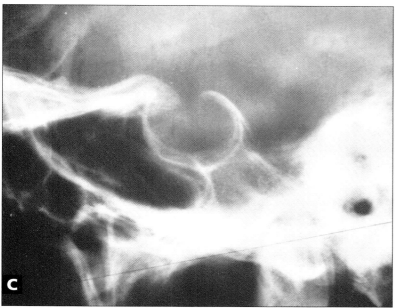

Figure 3-19. Radiographic tomograms showing changes in the sella that indicate skull changes in pituitary adenoma. Prior to advanced computed tomography (CT) and magnetic resonance imaging (MRI), radiographic

tomography was an important tool for detecting pituitary adenoma by showing changes in the sella.

A, Sagittal tomographic view of a small prolactinoma in a 35-year-old woman with amenorrhea-galactorrhea syndrome which demonstrates the normal right side of the sella. **B,** A depression of the floor on the left side by the tumor into the sphenoid sinus in the same patient. More aggressive tumors can erode through the floor, causing cerebrospinal fluid (CSF) to leak into the sphenoid sinus and rarely forming a portal for sinus infection to enter the brain to cause meningitis or brain abscess. These tumors can also grow into the nasal cavity, so the patient presents with epistaxis. Aggressive adenomas, prolactin-secreting or not, may also grow upward, affecting the visual apparatus and eventually blocking the third ventricle and its outflow, causing hydrocephalus.

C, Midsagittal tomogram showing a generally enlarged sella ("ballooned sella") characteristic of a large pituitary adenoma expanding the sella. This particular tomogram was taken from a patient with "empty sella syndrome" (ESS): a large sella with a small amount of pituitary tissue usually plastered on the floor, with most of the intrasellar space filled with CSF. Pituitary function was normal in this patient, but some patients with ESS have pituitary insufficiency and, on rare occasions, visual field abnormalities. In these cases, it is suspected that a pituitary adenoma had been present but shrank due to spontaneous small hemorrhage and infarction that went unrecognized. Larger hemorrhages result in the syndrome of pituitary apoplexy with acute pituitary failure and a neurologic syndrome: headache, cavernous sinus syndrome. Radiotherapy could also shrink a pituitary adenoma, as could bromocriptine therapy administered for prolactinoma.

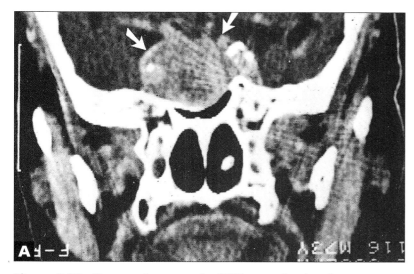

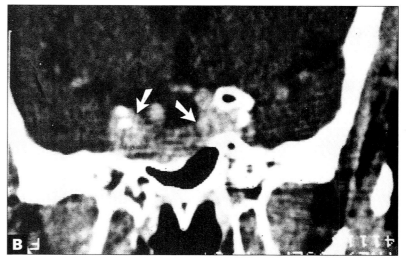

Figure 3-20. Computed tomography (CT) scans showing the treatment of prolactinoma with bromocriptine. **A,** Frontal view of the brain and sella turcica with a prolactinoma before treatment. Arrows point to the top of the adenoma extending above the sella. **B,** Frontal view 1 year after treatment of the prolactinoma with bromocriptine showing shrinkage of the tumor into the sella (*arrows*). Dopamine agonists such as bromocriptine have been the preferred therapy for many patients with prolactin

microadenomas; menses and fertility are restored in most. Prolactin microadenomas frequently shrink significantly in response to the drug [10], but they often recur after discontinuing its use. Tumor response may be partial, requiring additional therapy such as surgical debulking or radiotherapy. Transsphenoidal surgery is usually safe and successful for patients who plan a pregnancy but do not tolerate bromocriptine. (*From* Molitch and colleagues [10]; with permission.)

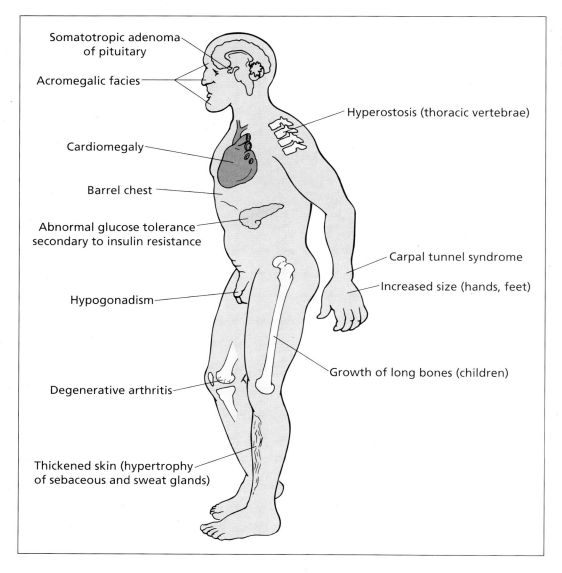

Figure 3-21. Clinical features of growth hormone-secreting adenoma. Growth hormone-secreting adenoma causes acromegaly in adults and gigantism in children.

Somatotropic adenoma of pituitary

Acromegalic facies

Hyperostosis (thoracic vertebrae)

Cardiomegaly

Barrel chest

Abnormal glucose tolerance secondary to insulin resistance

Carpal tunnel syndrome

Increased size (hands, feet)

Hypogonadism

Growth of long bones (children)

Degenerative arthritis

Thickened skin (hypertrophy of sebaceous and sweat glands)

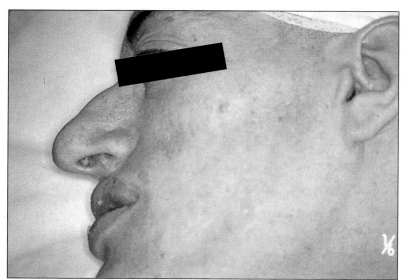

Figure 3-22. Facial features of a woman with acromegaly. Note the thickened skin and large nose and lips. Serial photographs over several years can be very helpful in appreciating these changes.

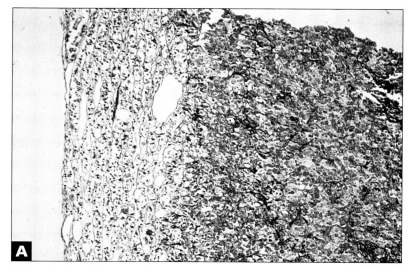

Figure 3-23. Histologic features of growth hormone-secreting tumors. **A,** Light photomicrograph of a routine histologic specimen stained with hematoxylin and eosin, from a section through a pituitary adenoma from a patient with acromegaly. The specimen demonstrates eosinophilia (acid stain) in many cells concentrated in the adenoma; normal compressed tissue on the left margin also contains normal eosinophils. Classic eosinophilic adenoma is associated with growth hormone hypersecretion.

(Continued on next page)

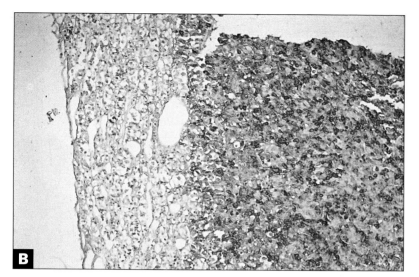

Figure 3-23. (*Continued*) **B,** Another section from the same patient. This specimen was prepared with an immunoperoxidase technique using antiserum to growth hormone (GH). The brown reaction product demonstrated even more GH concentrated in the tumor. Immunologic stains are more sensitive than histologic stains. About 50% of these tumors produce prolactin, which is also normally located in eosinophils, but most prolactinomas are not eosinophilic (Fig. 3-18). Many GH-secreting tumors appear chromophobic on tinctorial staining. (*Courtesy of* R. Defendini, MD, College of Physicians and Surgeons, Columbia University, New York, NY, and E.A. Zimmerman, MD, Albany Medical College, Albany, NY.)

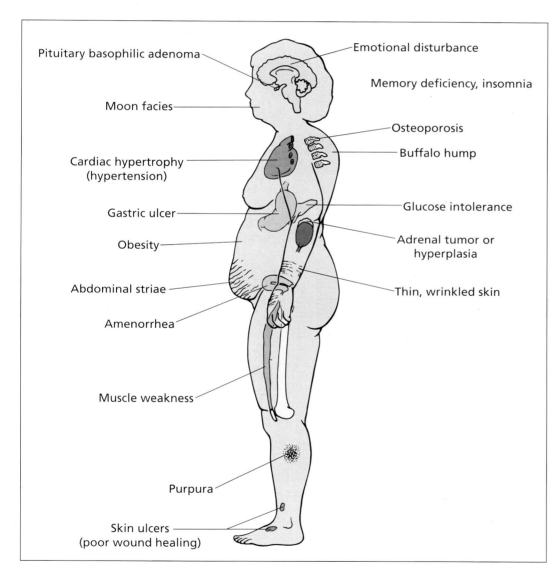

Figure 3-24. Clinical aspects of Cushing's syndrome. The causes of Cushing's syndrome include pituitary adenomas that secrete adenocorticotropic hormone (ACTH), adrenal tumors that secrete cortisol, ectopic tumors (*eg*, lung tumors) that secrete ACTH, and the administration of glucocorticoids (iatrogenic).

Etiology of Spontaneous Cushing's Syndrome

	Proportion of all causes, %
ACTH-Dependent	83
Pituitary Cushing's syndrome (79%)	66
Ectopic ACTH (14%)	12
ACTH source unknown (6%)	4
Macronodular hyperplasia (1%)	1
ACTH-Independent	17
Adrenal adenoma (58%)	10
Adrenal carcinoma (42%)	7

Figure 3-25. The etiology of spontaneous Cushing's syndrome in 225 patients seen at St. Bartholomew's Hospital, London, England, 1969 to 1991. ACTH—adrenocorticotropic hormone. (*Adapted from* Trainer and colleague [5].)

Work-up for Differential Diagnosis of Cushing's Syndrome

	Clinical features	Cortisol suppression with high-dose dexamethasone	ACTH blood levels	Imaging
ACTH-Dependent tumors				
Pituitary Cushing's syndrome	Headache (large tumor) Pigmentation (Nelson's syndrome)	Partial response	Some elevation; ↑ to CRH	MRI—small adenomas present, but few visualized*
Ectopic ACTH-producing tumors	Wasting Clinical diabetes mellitus Pigmentation Marked hypokalemia	No suppression	Often very high; no ↑ to CRH	CT and MRI of lung and thymus
ACTH-Independent tumors				
Adrenal tumor	Carcinoma in children	No suppression	Very low	CT and MRI of adrenal gland

See Figure 3-27.

Figure 3-26. Work-up for differential diagnosis of Cushing's syndrome, after initial screening with a dexamethasone suppression test: urinary free cortisol levels were not suppressed, following the administration of 1 mg of dexamethasone at midnight. ACTH—adrenocorticotropic hormone; CRH—corticotropin-releasing hormone; CT—computed tomography; MRI—magnetic resonance imaging.

Inferior Petrosal Sinus Sampling for ACTH

	Plasma ACTH (ng/L) after IV CRH 100 mg			
	0 Min	5 Min	10 Min	15 Min
Left inferior petrosal sinus	14	477	280	123
Right inferior petrosal sinus	16	23	28	54
Simultaneous peripheral vein	17	19	25	32

Figure 3-27. Inferior petrosal sinus venous sampling for adrenocorticotropic hormone (ACTH) on both sides of the pituitary gland, compared with peripheral venous sampling, both before and after stimulation with corticotropin-releasing hormone (CRH). Many pituitary adenomas cannot presently be visualized with imaging methods, including magnetic resonance imaging with gadolinium enhancement. This procedure may indicate on which side of the gland the microadenoma is located in preparation for transsphenoidal surgery, which is the definitive treatment for Cushing's disease. IV—intravenous. (*Adapted from* Trainer and colleague [5].)

References

1. Biller BMK, Daniels GH: Neuroendocrine Regulation and Diseases of the Anterior Pituitary and Hypothalamus. In *Harrison's Principles of Internal Medicine.* Edited by Fauci AS, Braunwald E, Martin JB. New York: McGraw-Hill; 1998:1972–1999.

2. Reichlin S: Neuroendocrine Control of Pituitary Function. In *Clinical Endocrinology.* Edited by Besser GM, Thorner MO. London: Mosby-Wolfe; 1994:1.2–1.16.

3. Zimmerman EA, Cohen BH: Congenital Tumors. In *Merritt's Textbook of Neurology.* Edited by Rowland LP. Baltimore: Williams & Wilkins; 1995:375–384.

4. Abrams GM, Zimmerman EA: Endocrine Diseases. In *Merritt's Neurology.* Edited by Rowland LP. Philadelphia: Lippincott Williams & Wilkins; 2000:849–864.

5. Trainer PJ, Besser GM: Cushing's Syndrome. In *Clinical Endocrinology.* Edited by Besser GM, Thorner MO. London: Mosby-Wolfe; 1994:8.2–8.10

6. Antunes JL, Zimmerman EA: The hypothalamic magnocellular system of the Rhesus monkey: an immunocytochemical study. *J Comp Neurol* 1978, 181:539–566.

7. Nauta WJH, Haymaker W: Hypothalamic Nuclei and Fiber Connections. In *The Hypothalamus.* Edited by Haymaker W, Anderson E, Nauta WJH. Springfield IL: Charles C. Thomas; 1969:136–209.

8. Zimmerman EA, Hou-Yu A, Nilaver G, Silverman A-J: Anatomy of Pituitary and Extrapituitary Vasopressin Neurosecretory Systems. In *The Neurohypophysis.* Edited by Reichlin S. New York: Plenum; 1984:5–33.

9. Maghnic M, Cosi G, Genovese E, *et al.*: Central diabetes insipidus in children and young adults. *N Engl J Med* 2000, 343:998–1007.

10. Molitch ME, Elton RL, Blackwell RE, *et al.*: Bromocriptine as primary therapy for prolactin-secreting macroadenomas: results of a prospective multicenter study. *J Clin Endocrinol Metab* 1985, 60:698–705.

4

Coma and Intensive Care Neurology

Daniel F. Hanley • Anish Bhardwaj
John A. Ulatowski • Alex Razumovsky
Marek A. Mirski

NEUROCRITICAL care is a subspecialty that has grown during the past 15 years. Critical care is care that is rendered in an acute and emergent setting in which the absence of care is associated with severe disability or death. The critical care concept evolved out of the need to render time-dependent emergent therapies in acute respiratory failure during the polio epidemics and for arrhythmia experienced by heart attack victims. Critical care grew rapidly in the 1970s to provide supportive care for the sickest patients with cardiologic, pulmonologic, and gastrointestinal disorders. In the 1980s the analogous subsets of neurologic and neurosurgical patients began to be identified. Neurocritical Care Units are now populated with head trauma victims, subarachnoid hemorrhage patients, the small numbers of patients who have treatable stroke, and patients with infectious disorders, including meningitis, encephalitis, and the parainfectious diseases, such as Guillain-Barré syndrome and myasthenia gravis. This chapter illustrates the time dependence and therapeutic complexities associated with these patients.

Altered Consciousness and Sedation

Sedation

Modified Ramsey Sedation Scale

Scale	Level criteria
1	Patient anxious, agitated, and restless
2	Patient cooperative, oriented, and tranquil
3	Patient drowsy but responds to commands
4	Patient asleep and exhibits a brisk response to light glabellar tap or loud auditory stimulus
5	Patient asleep and exhibits a sluggish response to light glabellar tap or loud auditory stimulus
6	Patient asleep; no response

Figure 4-1. Modified Ramsey sedation scale. Patients with critical illness often benefit from the use of sedation to optimize their management in an intensive care unit (ICU) environment. Preservation of the neurologic examination is paramount in documenting clinical improvement or deterioration in the critically ill neurologic patient. Pharmacologic sedation in this unique population of acute care patients requires careful consideration of the underlying neurophysiologic disturbances and potential adverse effects introduced by sedative drugs. To maintain patients at an ideal level of sedation, careful monitoring is required. One of the most widely used sedation scales was developed by Ramsey and colleagues and includes six levels of cognitive neurologic functioning. (*Adapted from* Ramsay and colleagues [1].)

Neurologic Effects of Common Sedative Drugs

Agent	Advantages	Disadvantages
Benzodiazepines	Anxiolysis and amnesia Anticonvulsant action Hemodynamic stability Decreased cerebral metabolism Decreased intracranial pressure Effects reversible	Respiratory depression Tachyphylaxis Antagonism decreases seizure threshold
Opioids	Analgesia Effects reversible Minimal alteration of intracranial dynamics	Respiratory depression Addictive Antagonism increases pain
Barbiturates	Sedation and hypnosis Decreased cerebral metabolism Decreased intracranial pressure Anticonvulsant effect	Cardiovascular depression Respiratory depression Alters hepatic drug metabolism Withdrawal phenomenon
Neuroleptics	Antipsychotic action Antiemetic effect	Cardiovascular depression Decreased seizure threshold Neuroleptic malignant syndrome Endocrine changes Anticholinergic effects Hypothermia Extrapyramidal symptoms
Ketamine	Sedation and analgesia Lack of respiratory and cardiovascular depression Amnesia	Increased cerebral metabolism Increased intracranial pressure Proconvulsant Hallucinations and delusions Dissociative state
Propofol	Sedation and hypnosis Ultrashort duration of action Decreased cerebral metabolism Decreased intracranial pressure No drug accumulation	Hypotension Respiratory depression Infection
Clonidine	Sedation and analgesia Blunt sympathetic response	Hypotension Withdrawal hypertension

Figure 4-2. Neurologic effects of common sedative drugs. Each class of sedative drugs has distinct mechanisms of action and a spectrum of physiologic effects that may be advantageous or deleterious to the neurologically ill patient. (*Adapted from* Mirski and colleagues [2].)

Pharmacokinetics and Dosage Ranges for Selective Sedative Drugs

Sedative class agent	$T_{1/2}\alpha$* (min)	$T_{1/2}\beta$† (h)	Clearance (mL/kg/min)	Dosage range	
				Bolus dose (IV)	Infusion (IV)
Benzodiazepines					
Diazepam	50–120	20–40	0.2–0.5	0.03–0.1 mg/kg	
Lorazepam	3–10	10–20	0.8–1.0	0.02–0.05 mg/kg	
Midazolam	7–10	2.0–2.5	4.0–8.0	0.02–0.08 mg/kg	0.05–0.1 mg/kg/h
Opioids					
Morphine	4–11	2–4	12–15	0.03–0.1 mg/kg	
Meperidine	9–15	3–5	12–22	0.5–1.0 mg/kg	
Fentanyl	10	3–4	11–15	0.25–1.5 µg/kg	0.3–1.5 µg/kg/h
Alfentanil	4–10	1–2	2–4	0.25–0.75 µg/kg	10–100 µg/kg/h
Barbiturates					
Thiopental	2–4	7–10	3–4	0.25–0.75 mg/kg	2–3 mg/kg/h
Pentobarbital	22–26	18.2	0.3–0.4	0.5–1.0 mg/kg	0.2–0.4 mg/kg/h
Secobarbital		19	0.7	0.5–1.0 mg/kg	
Phenobarbital	1–2	48–144	3.7	0.5–1.0 mg/kg	
Neuroleptics					
Chlorpromazine	95	30	8.6	0.25–0.50 mg/kg (infused at <1 mg/min)	
Haloperidol	5–17	10–19	9–14	0.01–0.05 mg/kg	
Droperidol	8–21	1–2	10–18	0.01–0.1 mg/kg	
Other sedatives					
Propofol	2–4	40–50	22–32	0.1–0.3 mg/kg	0.6–6.0 mg/kg/h
Ketamine	2–14	2–4	10–30	0.2–0.5 mg/kg	
Clonidine	6–14	7–10	2–4	0.1–0.2 mg (po)	

$T_{1/2}\alpha$—plasma elimination half-life of the distribution phase. †$T_{1/2}\beta$—plasma elimination half-life during the elimination phase.

Figure 4-3. Pharmacokinetic and dosage ranges for selective sedative drugs. A knowledge of the onset and duration of action of common sedative drugs, as well as the dosage range, is important in choosing the agent. IV—intravenous; po—per os (by mouth).

Neurophysiologic Effects of Sedative Drugs

Figure 4-4. Neurophysiologic effects of sedative drugs. CBF—cerebral blood flow; CMRO$_2$—cerebral metabolic rate of oxygen utilization; CPP—cerebral perfusion pressure; ICP—intracranial pressure; MAP—mean arterial pressure. (*Adapted from* Mirski and colleagues [2].)

Sedative agent	CBF	MAP	ICP	CPP	CMRO$_2$
Benzodiazepines	↑	↓	↓	⟷	↓
Opioids	⟷	↓	⟷	⟷	↓
Barbiturates	↓↓	↓↓	↓↓	↓	↓↓
Neuroleptics	↓	↓	↑	↓	⟷
Propofol	↓↓	↓↓	↓↓	↓	↓↓
Ketamine	↑↑	↑	↑	⟷	⟷
Clonidine	↓	↓		↓	⟷

Key: ↑—modest increase; ↓—modest decrease; ⟷—no clear effect; ↓↓—pronounced decrease; ↑↑—pronounced increase

Coma

Glasgow Coma Scale

Eye opening:

Spontaneous	4
To speech	3
To pain	2
Nothing	1

Best *motor* response:

Obeys	6
Localizes	5
Withdraws	4
Abnormal flexion	3
Extensor response	2
Flaccid	1

Best *verbal* response:

Oriented	5
Confused conversation	4
Inappropriate words	3
Incomprehensible sounds	2
Nothing	1
Total (E + M + V)	3–15

Figure 4-5. Glasgow coma scale. The value of routine and standardized evaluation of all patients with any diminution in level of consciousness after head injury is paramount. The Glasgow coma scale (GCS) was developed as a semiquantitative method of measuring head injury, taking into account three reliable indicators of post-traumatic dysfunction (eye opening, language capability, and movement). The examination is invalid in children and intoxicated patients, or when concomitant orbital or spinal cord injury is present. (*Adapted from* Teasdale and colleague [3].)

Correlation Between Levels of Brain Function and Clinical Signs

Structure	Function	Clinical sign
Cerebral cortex	Conscious behavior	Speech (including any sounds) Purposeful movement Spontaneous To command To pain
Brain stem sensory pathways (reticular activating system)	Sleep-wake cycle	Eye opening Spontaneous To command To pain
Brain stem motor pathways	Reflex limb movements	Flexor posturing (decorticate) Extensor posturing (decerebrate)
Midbrain CN III	Innervation of ciliary muscle and certain extraocular muscles	Pupillary reactivity
Upper pons CN V	Facial and corneal sensation	Corneal reflex–sensory
CN VII	Facial muscle innervation	Corneal reflex–motor response Blink Grimace
Lower pons CN VII (vestibular portion) connects by brain stem pathways with CN III, IV, VI	Reflex eye movements	Doll-like eyes Caloric responses
Medulla	Spontaneous breathing Maintained blood pressure	Breathing and blood pressure do not require mechanical or chemical support
Spinal cord	Primitive protective responses	Deep tendon reflexes Babinski's response

Figure 4-6. Correlation between levels of brain function and clinical signs. Neurologic signs can be correlated with specific anatomic sites to establish the severity and extent of central nervous system dysfunction. (*Adapted from* Ropper [4].)

Neurologic Conditions That Produce Unresponsiveness

Condition	Self-awareness	Sleep-wake cycles	Motor function	Experiences suffering	Respiratory function	Electroen-cephalogram	Prognosis for neuro-logic recovery
Persistent vegetative state*	Absent	Intact	No purposeful movement; no visual tracking	No	Normal	Polymorphic delta and theta; some-times slow alpha	Traumatic PVS (1-y outcome): PVS, 15% of patients; dead, 33%; GR, 7%; MD, 17%; SD, 28%
							Nontraumatic PVS (1-y outcome): PVS, 32% of patients; dead, 53%; GR, 1%; MD, 3%; SD, 11%
Brain death	Absent	Absent	None or only reflex spinal movements	No	Absent	Electrocerebral silence	None
Locked-in syndrome	Present	Intact	Quadriplegia; pseudobulbar palsy; preserved vertical eye movements	Yes	Normal	Normal or mildly abnormal	Recovery unlikely; patients remain quadriplegic; prolonged survival possible
Akinetic mutism	Present	Intact	Paucity of movement	Yes	Normal	Nonspecific slowing	Recovery very unlikely and depends on cause

*Adults only.

Figure 4-7. Neurologic conditions that produce unresponsiveness. Due to the overlap of clinical and laboratory findings, these generalizations do not apply to every patient. Magnetic resonance imaging or computed tomography may be able to further differentiate the above conditions. GR—good recovery; MD—moderately disabled; PVS—persistent vegetative state; SD—severely disabled. (*Adapted from* Wijdicks [5].)

Metabolic Coma

Etiology	Specific neurologic signs	Diagnostic steps
Hypoxia	Flaccid muscle tone, myoclonus	Preceding cardiac disease, polytrauma, resuscitation, attempted suicide
Hyperosmolar diabetic coma	Frequently: coma, seizures (20%–25%), focal signs	Blood glucose >1100 mg %, high serum osmolarity
Diabetic ketoacidosis	Clouding of consciousness but rarely coma	Ketonuria, blood glucose >400 mg %
Hypoglycemia	High variability, including coma, seizures, focal signs	Blood glucose <30 mg %
Hepatic encephalopathy	Tremor, asterixis (wing beating); final stage: severe clouding of consciousness	Ammonia
Uremia	Delirium, seizures, myoclonus, asterixis; final stage: clouding of consciousness	Serum creatinine, urea, potassium
Dysequilibrium syndrome	Muscle cramps, seizures, coma	Postdialysis, urea, sodium, osmolarity
Hyponatremia	Clouding of consciousness; seizures and coma only in case of rapid change of serum sodium level	Serum sodium <126 mmol
Hypernatremia	Delirium, "muscle weakness"; coma only in case of rapid change	Serum sodium >156 mmol, reduced urinary sodium excretion
Hypercalcemia	Delirium, headache, "muscle weakness"	Calcium and phosphate in serum and urine, parathormone
Hypocalcemia	Tetanic syndrome, delirium, pseudopsychotic behavior, seizures	Calcium and phosphate in serum and urine, parathormone
Thiamine deficiency	Wernicke encephalopathy; rarely coma	Vitamin B_1 level, 100 mg vitamin B_1 IV

Figure 4-8. Causes, specific neurologic signs, and diagnostic tests in metabolic coma. Specific neurologic signs may be indicative of an etiologic cause of metabolic coma and diagnostic steps should be undertaken to confirm the diagnosis. IV—intravenous. (*Adapted from* Hacke [6].)

Clinical Features and Diagnostic Steps in Patients in Coma After a Drug Overdose

Drug	Main clinical features*	Main diagnostic steps
Alcohol (ethanol)	Hypothermia, average to wide pupil size, tachycardia, vomiting, typical smell	Blood level of alcohol
Antidepressants (tricyclic)	Myoclonus, epileptic seizures	Urine level of drug
		ECG: sinus tachycardia, arrhythmia, conduction defects
Atropine-scopolamine	Raised body temperature, flush, dry skin, dilated pupils	ECG: tachycardia
Arsenic	Diarrhea, seizures, hemolysis	Arsenic at hair roots
		ECG: arrhythmia
Barbiturates	Flaccidity, apnea, blisters, hypothermia, hypotension	EEG: burst-suppression
		Urine/serum level of drug
Benzodiazepines	Usually stupor, no severe cardiac or respiratory alteration	Urine/serum level of drug
Biologic toxins		
Plants containing atropine	See atropine-scopolamine	Investigate for ingestion of plants
Poisonous mussels (containing domoic acid)	Within 1.5–48 h after ingestion: myoclonus, seizures	Investigate for exposure to or ingestion of contaminated seafood, domoic acid levels in feces
Mushrooms, *eg*, *Amanita* spp.	Nausea, vomiting, diarrhea, jaundice, seizures	Investigate for ingestion of mushrooms
Carbon monoxide	Hypoxia	CO hemoglobin
		CT scan: hypodensities in basal ganglia
Cocaine	Seizures, cerebrovascular ischemia	Serum level of drug
Cyclosporine	Status post kidney transplantation, flaccid tetraparesis, seizures	CT (MRI) scan: white matter changes
		Serum level of drug
Ethanol	See alcohol	
Glycol	Myocloni	Renal failure (oxalate in urine), acidosis
		CT scan: hypodensities in basal ganglia
Heroin (opiates)	Seizures, pulmonary edema, rhabdomyolysis, needle marks, extreme miosis	Opiate in urine creatine kinase, myoglobin in urine
Lead	Seizures, anemia, neuropathy, lead line in gingiva	Anemia, basophilic stippling, lead levels in blood and tissue
Lithium	Preceding abdominal pains, vomiting, exsiccosis, myocloni, seizures	Renal failure
		Lithium levels in serum
Methanol	Blindness	Blood level of methanol, acidosis
Opiates: see heroin		
Pesticides (organophosphates)	Agricultural background, abdominal pains, profuse sweating, miosis, paraparesis, seizures	Low cholinesterase in serum, tachycardia, tachyarrhythmia
Phenytoin	Nystagmus	Serum level of phenytoin
Salicylate	Seizures, hyperventilation, hyperthermia	Acidosis, CT scan: brain swelling, salicylate level
Tricyclic antidepressants	See antidepressants	
Thallium	Neuralgia, seizures, loss of hair, constipation	Coagulation disturbance, thallium at hair roots
		Raised blood pressure

*In addition to coma.

Figure 4-9. Clinical features and diagnostic steps in patients in coma after drug overdose. CO—carbon monoxide; CT—computed tomography; ECG—electrocardiography; EEG—electroencephalography; MRI—magnetic resonance imaging. (*Adapted from* Hacke [6].)

Clues Suggesting Possible Intracranial Mass

History: trauma, focal neurologic symptoms (*eg*, arm or leg weakness), known cancer, alcoholism, bleeding disorder, anticoagulant treatment, recent sinusitis

General examination: hypertension (suggests increased intracranial pressure), bradycardia, signs of trauma, bleeding, cancer, or infection

Neurologic examination: papilledema, asymmetric pupils, eye movement, limb movement, limb posture or tendon reflexes, unilateral Babinski's sign, diffusely hyperactive tendon reflexes

Figure 4-10. Clues suggesting possible intracranial mass. Defining the cause of coma demands a thorough history, detailed medical and neurologic examinations, and thoughtful use of laboratory tests. A guiding principle in early management is to search for clues from the history and examination suggesting an intracranial mass lesion. If the clues are present, an emergency computed tomography scan of the head is required to diagnose the lesion and guide immediate decisions about surgery, treatment of intracranial pressure, and management of blood pressure and fluids. (*Adapted from* Grotta [7].)

Causes of Alteration in Consciousness and Coma in Critically Ill Patients With Normal Initial Computed Tomography Scan

Drug overdose
Anoxic-ischemic encephalopathy
Diffuse axonal brain injury
Bilateral isodense subdural hematomas*
Fat embolization
Cholesterol embolization
Diffuse intravascular coagulation†
Thrombotic thrombocytopenic purpura
Connective tissue disease with vasculitis
Prolonged hypoglycemia
Acute severe hyponatremia
Acute severe hypercalcemia
Acute nonketotic hyperglycemia
Metabolic alkalosis
Acute hypercapnia with hypoxemia
Adrenal crisis
Myxomatous coma
Thyrotoxic coma‡
Acute uremia
Acute increase in arterial ammonia
Hypothermia
Acute bacterial, viral, or fungal meningitis
Nonconvulsive status epilepticus
Central pontine myelinolysis
Acute brain stem stroke§
Hyperpyretic-hyperkinetic syndromes¶
Wernicke's encephalopathy

More often in patients with multitrauma who have low hematocrit measurements.

†*Occasionally multiple intracerebral hemorrhages.*

‡*Elderly patients.*

§*May be locked-in syndrome.*

¶*Catatonia more prominent.*

Figure 4-11. Causes of alteration in consciousness and coma in critically ill patients with normal initial computed tomography (CT) scan. The reason for unresponsiveness is often clear by focal neurologic signs and abnormal CT scan findings, but in some patients, the cause of bilateral hemispheric dysfunction remains challenging, particularly when results of the initial CT scan are normal. (*Adapted from* Wijdicks [5].)

Neurologic Syndromes After Cardiac Arrest

Transient CNS deficits after brief coma (<12 h)
  Pathology: No damage or scattered ischemic neurons
  Clinical: Transient confusion often followed by antegrade amnesia
  Outcome: Rapid, complete recovery; delayed deterioration (rare)
Persistent focal CNS deficits after coma (>12 h)
Cerebral syndrome
  Pathology: Focal or multifocal infarcts of cortex, especially in boundary zones
  Clinical: Amnesia
                 Dementia
                 Bibrachial or quadriparesis
                 Cortical blindness, visual agnosia
                 Also may occur: seizures, myoclonus (acute state); ataxia, intention myoclonus, parkinsonism (chronic stage)
  Outcome: Slow, often incomplete, recovery
Spinal cord syndrome (may occur in isolation or accompany cerebral syndrome)
  Pathology: Focal or multifocal infarcts of spinal cord, especially in the lower thoracic boundary zone
  Clinical: Flaccid paralysis of lower limbs
                 Urinary retention
                 Loss of pain and temperature sense
                 Preserved touch and position sense
  Outcome: No or incomplete recovery
Global CNS damage (no recovery of consciousness)
Destruction of hemispheres alone
  Pathology: Laminar necrosis of cortex
  Clinical: Vegetative state (awake but unaware)
  Outcome: Prolonged survival in vegetative state
Brain death
  Pathology: Necrosis of cortex + brain stem ± spinal cord
  Clinical: No evidence of cortical activity, no brain stem reflexes; reflexes of purely spinal origin may persist
  Outcome: Systemic death within days

Figure 4-12. Neurologic syndromes after cardiac arrest. Generalized brain anoxia is most commonly a consequence of systemic circulatory arrest caused by cardiac arrhythmias or arrest. A spectrum of clinical disorders can result, depending on the severity of cerebral anoxia. CNS—central nervous system. (*Adapted from* Ropper [4].)

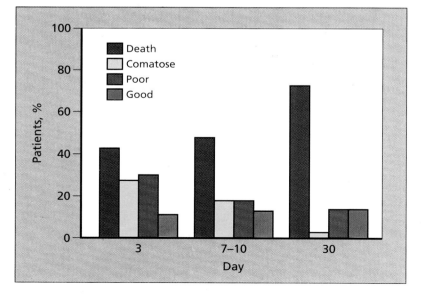

Figure 4-13. Neurologic outcome in postanoxic coma. Patients who remain comatose after resuscitation have a high mortality rate during hospitalization from withdrawal of support or recurrent arrhythmias. There are several clinical and laboratory prognosticators of a poor outcome in postanoxic coma after cardiac arrest when present more than 6 hours after cardiopulmonary resuscitation. Clinical prognosticators include: fixed pupils, myoclonus status, and a sustained upward gaze. Laboratory prognosticators are the absence of bilateral cortical response on somatosensory evoked potentials and a burst–suppression pattern on electroencephalogram. (*Adapted from* Wijdicks [5].)

Horizontal Displacement of Midline Structures on Computed Tomography Scans and Level of Consciousness

Level of consciousness	True dimension from midline (mm)	
	Pineal	Septum pellucidum
Awake	0–3	2–7
Drowsy	3–6	2–10
Stupor	6–9	7–14
Coma	9–15	12–18

Figure 4-14. Horizontal displacement of midline structures on computed tomography scans and the level of consciousness. A correlation has been made between lateral deep brain structures in altering levels of consciousness and unilateral space-occupying lesions. There is general correspondence between pineal displacement and the level of consciousness. Shift of other midline structures, such as the septum pellucidum, is less closely related to the level of consciousness. (*Adapted from* Ropper [4].)

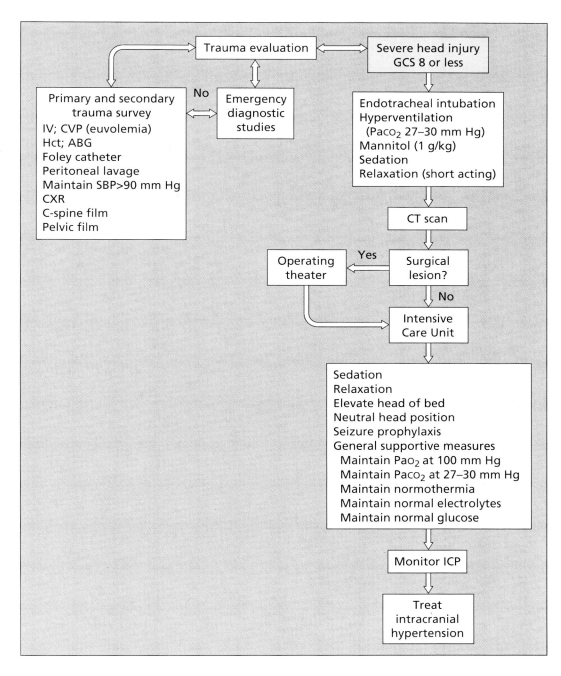

Figure 4-15. Algorithm for the initial resuscitation and treatment of the severely head-injured patient. The fundamental concepts of management of the severely head-injured patient are the early recognition of the existence or potential existence of the severe head injury, avoidance of secondary insults during the early postinjury course, rapid transport of the patient to a center with resuscitation, computed tomography imaging, neurosurgical support, and rapid therapeutic response based on the patient's condition and on the specific intracranial diagnosis. A useful operational definition for severe head injury is any patient with a Glasgow coma score (GCS) of 8 or less (Fig. 4-5). ABG—arterial blood gas; CT—computed tomography; CVP—central venous pressure; CXR—chest roentgenogram; GSC—Glasgow coma score; Hct—hematocrit; ICP—intracranial pressure; IV—intravenous; $PaCO_2$—arterial carbon dioxide pressure; PaO_2—arterial oxygen pressure; SBP—systolic blood pressure. (*Adapted from* Ropper [4].)

**Proposed Head Injury Diagnostic Categories Based on Abnormalities
Visualized on CT Scan Based on Data from the Traumatic Coma Data Bank**

Diffuse injury I	No visible pathology seen on CT
Diffuse injury II	Cisterns are present with shift 0–5 mm. No high or mixed density lesion >25 mL. May include bone fragments and foreign bodies
Diffuse injury III (swelling)	Cisterns compressed or absent. Shift 0–5 mm. No high or mixed density lesion >25 mL
Diffuse injury IV (shift)	Shift >5 mm. No high or mixed density lesion >25 mL
Evacuated mass lesion	Any lesion surgically evacuated
Nonevacuated mass lesion	High or mixed density lesion >25 mL not surgically evacuated
Brain dead	No brain stem reflexes. Flaccid. Fixed, nonreactive pupils. No spontaneous respirations with normal $PaCO_2$. Spinal reflexes are permitted

Figure 4-16. Proposed head injury diagnostic categories based on abnormalities on computed tomography (CT) scan based on data from the Traumatic Coma Data Bank (TCDB). Absence or compression of the basilar cisterns as seen on the cerebral CT scan is associated with a significant risk of intracranial hypertension. Analysis of data from the TCDB has suggested that the division of head injury into groups based on CT imaging can be useful in predicting a patient's course, particularly the probability of developing intracranial hypertension. $PaCO_2$—arterial carbon dioxide pressure. (*Adapted from* Ropper [4].)

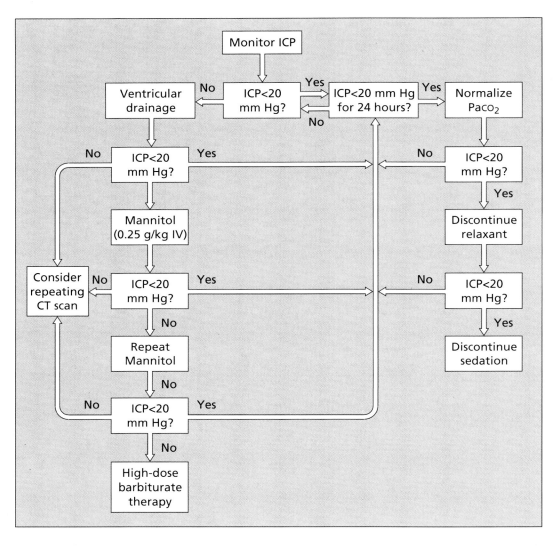

Figure 4-17. Suggested algorithm for managing the severely head-injured patient with elevated intracranial pressure (ICP) with an ICP monitor in place. CT—computed tomography; IV—intravenous. (*Adapted from* Ropper [4].)

Prognosticators of Poor Outcome in Closed Head Injury

Postresuscitation Glasgow coma score of 3

Age older than 65 years

Abnormal pupil or pupils for at least one observation

Shock on admission (blood pressure <80 mm Hg) and during hospital stay

Persistent increased intracranial pressure (>20 mm Hg)

Hypoxia on admission (Po$_2$ <60 mm Hg)

Computed tomography scan abnormalities (absent cisterns, intraventricular hemorrhage, midline shift, shearing in corpus callosum, bilateral epidural hematomas)

Figure 4-18. Prognosticators of poor outcome in closed head injury. Although numerous clinical variables determine the outcome in head injuries, trauma data banks have consistently identified factors with high predictive power. The Glasgow coma scale remains a strong clinical predictor. Poor outcome can be expected in patients who have these clinical features and computed tomography scan abnormalities. Po$_2$—oxygen pressure. (*Adapted from* Wijdicks [5].)

Acute Cerebrovascular Disorders

Stroke

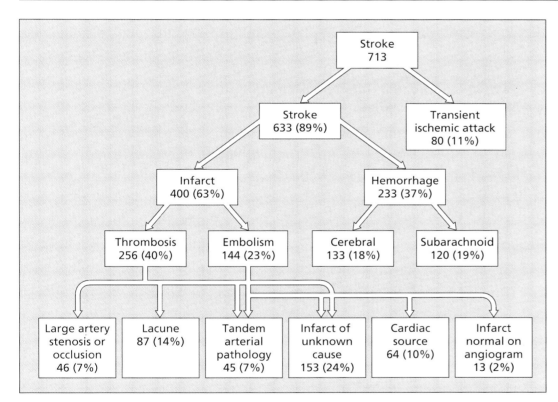

hemorrhage can be subdivided into either subarachnoid or intracerebral, depending on the site and origin of the blood.

The term *stable stroke* refers to a patient with stroke who has shown little change in deficit over a specified period of time (*eg*, a new measurable neurologic deficit within the previous 24 hours that persisted for at least 24 hours) [8]. Anything less is considered a transient ischemic attack (TIA). Many TIA patients are actually found to have a stroke if a brain image is performed at an appropriate time. Therefore, shorter duration of symptoms (*eg*, 1 hour or 15 minutes) may be more pertinent for distinguishing between TIA and stroke.

With cerebral infarction, the differentiation of several clinical, pathophysiologic, and etiologic subtypes may be crucial to rational treatment and prediction of outcome. With the use of computed tomography, magnetic resonance imaging, and lumbar puncture, bleeding into and around the brain can be diagnosed, and these types of strokes can be separated from the more common ischemic stroke. The classification of ischemic stroke is difficult. Ischemic strokes classically are divided into thrombotic (two thirds) and embolic (one third) [9]. Ischemic infarction can be classified by the mechanism of ischemia (hemodynamic or thromboembolic) and the pathology of the vascular lesion: atherosclerotic, lacunar, cardioembolic, or indeterminate. Although the two subtypes can present in the same way, thrombotic infarcts more frequently have progressive onset, as opposed to the sudden onset of embolic strokes. (*Adapted from* Mohr and colleague [9].)

Figure 4-19. Subtypes of ischemic stroke. Stroke is the leading cause of life-threatening neurologic disease and the third leading cause of death in the United States, with an incidence of 500,000 cases per year.

Stroke is a generic term for a clinical syndrome that includes infarction and hemorrhage (intracerebral, intraventricular, and subarachnoid). This term usually applies to any sort of cerebrovascular disease, either ischemic or hemorrhagic, with either permanent or transient symptoms. Intracranial

Percent Distribution of Neurologic Examination Features of Stroke in Relation to Cardiac Source Risk Groups

Examination feature		Cardiac source risk groups			
		Low ($n = 873$)	Medium ($n = 167$)	High ($n = 250$)	$P*$
Diminished LOC	Yes	17.0	23.4	36.0	<0.001
	No	83.0	76.6	64.0	
Multifocal deficits	Yes	8.4	9.6	11.6	NS
	No	91.6	90.4	88.4	
Visual field deficit	Yes	15.2	27.5	30.0	<0.001
	No	84.8	72.5	70.0	
Neglect	Yes	9.2	13.8	20.8	<0.001
	No	90.8	86.2	79.2	
Aphasia	Yes	23.4	22.8	32.8	0.006
	No	76.6	77.2	67.2	
Nonlanguage cognitive deficit	Yes	29.2	35.3	34.0	NS
	No	70.8	64.7	66.0	
Bruit	Yes	6.3	13.2	5.6	NS
	No	93.7	86.8	94.4	
Brain stem signs	Yes	34.5	27.5	36.0	NS
	No	65.5	72.5	64.0	
Noncortical hemiparesis	Yes	29.6	21.0	13.2	<0.001
	No	70.4	79.0	86.8	
Noncortical sensorimotor stroke	Yes	14.0	13.2	8.0	0.017
	No	86.0	86.8	92.0	
Noncortical hemisensory deficit	Yes	1.7	1.8	2.8	NS
	No	98.3	98.2	97.2	

Mantel-Haenszel chi-squared test for trend.

Figure 4-20. Percentage of distribution of neurologic examination features of stroke in relation to cardiac source risk groups. In a National Institute of Neurological Disorders and Stroke Data Bank study, 1290 patients with cerebral infarcts were divided into groups of high, medium, and low risk of a cardiogenic mechanism for their strokes [10]. Diminished level of consciousness, visual field deficit, neglect, and aphasia were significantly related to an increasing risk of having a cardiac source of embolism. In contrast, noncortical hemiparesis and, more weakly, noncortical sensorimotor stroke were inversely associated with a cardiac source of emboli. LOC—level of consciousness; NS—not significant. (*Adapted from* Kittner and colleagues [10].)

Conditions Associated With Cerebral Ischemia Due to Cerebral Embolism

Cardiogenic (cardiac source)
  Atrial fibrillation in all forms of cardiac disease
  Sick sinus syndrome
  Rheumatic heart disease without arrhythmia (mitral stenosis, aortic stenosis)
  Acute myocardial infarction
  Acute and subacute bacterial endocarditis
  Mitral valve prolapse
  Ventricular aneurysm with mural thrombus
  Cardiac valve prosthesis
  Nonbacterial thrombotic endocarditis (marantic)
  Libman-Sacks endocarditis
  Cardiomyopathy (several types)
  Patent foramen ovale, septal defect
  Pulmonary arteriovenous malformation
  Atrial myxoma
  Chagas' disease
  Trichinosis

Figure 4-21. Conditions associated with cerebral ischemia due to cerebral embolism. Arterial embolism from the heart or a carotid artery to the brain represents a major mechanism for stroke. As a cause of stroke, embolism accounts for between 15% and 30% of cases [11,12]. Atherosclerotic plaque in the carotid arteries can produce emboli by two mechanisms: the rupture of its contents into the bloodstream or the breaking off of a thrombus formed on an ulcerated surface or in the bloodstream when flow distal to the plaque is slowed. Intracardiac pathology is the other well-recognized cause of cerebral ischemia and infarction. Factors predisposing to cardiac embolism include left atrial enlargement, spontaneous left atrial fibrillation, atrial septal aneurysm, interatrial shunts, atrial fibrillation, and valvular disease (including rheumatic, endocarditis, mitral valve prolapse, mitral valve calcification, and prosthetic valves). Additionally, abnormal ventricular wall motion (including aneurysm and globally reduced left ventricular function resulting from myocardial infarction or cardiomyopathy) can produce emboli. (*Adapted from* Fisher [13].) (*Continued on next page*)

(*Table continued on next page*)

Conditions Associated With Cerebral Ischemia Due to Cerebral Embolism (*Continued*)

Arteriogenic embolism (artery-to-artery embolism)
  Atheroma thrombosis in aorta, innominate, subclavian, cervicocerebral, internal carotid, vertebral, or basilar artery (platelet, fibrin–platelet, atheroma, cholesterol crystals), from sites of dissection
  Complications of neck and thoracic surgery
Idiopathic carotid mural thrombosis
Miscellaneous
  Arteriographic complications
  Cardiopulmonary mycosis (aspergillosis, candidiasis, etc.)
  Disseminated intravascular coagulation
  Thrombosis in pulmonary veins
  Transfusion of incompatible blood
  Fat
  Air
  Tumor
  Reflux from a radial monitoring catheter
Embolism from undetermined site
Suspected embolism

Figure 4-21. (*Continued*)

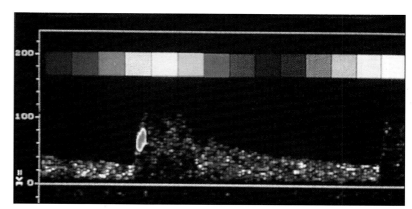

Figure 4-22. The middle cerebral artery embolus detection (*orange*) in a patient who had a cardiac embolic source. Time base is 1.25 seconds. Color scale for signal intensity is at the top. The emboli caused Doppler signals (*orange*) of a much greater intensity compared with those reflected from erythrocytes (*blue*). Although cerebral embolism is one of the major causes of stroke, until recently, we did not have methods that could routinely be used to detect emboli. The development of a transcranial Doppler ultrasound (TCD), therefore, represents a real gold standard for emboli detection and a significant advance in the initiation of appropriate treatment to prevent further emboli from entering the cerebral circulation. Noninvasive, long-term monitoring of intracranial arterial blood flow velocity spectra can reveal abnormal, high-pitched intensity signals indicating emboli. (*Adapted from* Brucher and colleague [14].)

Conditions Associated With Nonembolic Cerebral Ischemia

Atherosclerosis
Dissection (spontaneous and traumatic)
Vasospasm of subarachnoid hemorrhage
Procoagulant states—antiphospholipid antibody, disseminated intravascular thrombosis, intravascular thrombosis with carcinoma, protein C or S deficiency
Thrombosis of undetermined origin
  Associated with estrogen therapy (contraceptive medication), pregnancy, or puerperium
  In young adults, male and female
  Terminal internal carotid arterial occlusion with moyamoya syndrome
  Idiopathic carotid mural thrombus
Crack cocaine
Migrainous accompaniments
Systemic hypotension—syncope, acute blood loss, myocardial infarction, Stokes-Adams syndrome, carotid sinus sensitivity, shock, postural hypotension, antihypertensive medication, insufficiency during open cardiac surgery, cough syncope

Arteritis
  Primary—periarteritis nodosa, granulomatous angiitis (Churg-Strauss syndrome), Wegener's granulomatosis, primary cerebral granulomatous angiitis (intraparenchymal and subarachnoid), temporal arteritis, Takayashu's syndrome, postzoster angiitis, AIDS-associated cerebral arteritis
  Secondary (to meningitis)—pyogenic, tuberculous, syphilitic, or fungal arteritis
Lipohyalinosis
Acute hypertensive encephalopathy
Hematologic disorders—thrombotic thrombocytopenic purpura, polycythemia, thrombocythemia, macroglobulinemia, hemoglobinopathy, cryoglobulinemia
Miscellaneous—reversible cerebral segmental vasoconstriction, dolichoectasia, fibromuscular dysplasia, carotid kinking, intravascular lymphoma, subclavian steal, regional enteritis, radiation angiopathy, homocystinuria, thrombus in saccular and fusiform aneurysms, Behçet's syndrome, Fabry's disease, MELAS, delayed anoxic demyelination, Binswanger's disease (chronic progressive subcortical encephalopathy)
Thrombosis of dural sinuses and cerebral veins

Figure 4-23. Conditions associated with nonembolic cerebral ischemia. Besides atheroembolism from a carotid plaque and cardioembolism, other causes of ischemic stroke have been recognized. Occasionally, hematologic abnormalities, nonatherosclerotic arteriopathies, illicit drug use, oral contraceptive, migraine, or cerebral venous thrombosis are presumed causes of infarction, particularly when the patient is younger than 50 years of age. MELAS—mitochondrial myopathy, encephalopathy, lactic acidosis, and stroke-like episodes. (*Adapted from* Fisher [13].)

Diagnostic Studies for Stroke

Studies	Variables investigated
Laboratory investigation	Hemogram
	Platelet count
	Sedimentation rate
	Electrocardiogram
	Chest radiograph
	Conventional and transesophageal echocardiography
	Blood urea nitrogen, creatinine, and electrolytes
CT scan	Hemorrhage or any unsuspected condition
MRI	The presence and extent of ischemic damage
Ultrasound evaluation	The dynamics of blood flow in and the patency of the cervical and intracranial segments of the internal carotid and vertebral arteries, the proximal parts of the middle and anterior cerebral arteries, and the basilar artery (proximal, middle, and distal)
Magnetic resonance angiography	Clinical diagnosis of large artery disease
Digital subtraction angiography	Clinical diagnosis of large and small artery disease

Figure 4-24. Diagnostic studies for stroke. Every patient with stroke should have these diagnostic investigations. Acute cerebral infarction is presumed when a patient presents with an acute neurologic deficit and when other diagnostic possibilities are excluded by computed tomography (CT) or magnetic resonance imaging (MRI) and laboratory tests. CT scan immediately on arrival in the emergency department is the most reliable way to distinguish between infarct and hemorrhage and should be done in any patient suspected of having a stroke. However, in the first 24 to 48 hours following stroke, the CT scan often fails to reveal any detectable abnormality—it is negative in 25% to 50% of cases [15]. Angiography during this period carries risks and may be of limited availability. MRI has been shown to be more sensitive in the imaging of acute stroke—up to 82% of MRI studies are abnormal on admission, compared with 58% of CT scans during the first 24 hours [15]. Magnetic resonance angiography (MRA) is a noninvasive method of visualizing the cerebrovascular anatomy, and preliminary studies of patients with cerebrovascular disease have been performed [16,17]. Transcranial Doppler ultrasonography (TCD) is another noninvasive, nonionizing, and inexpensive method of assessing cerebral blood flow velocities. The TCD technique has been used in the diagnosis of intracranial and extracranial disease and for the sequential monitoring of patency of cerebral arteries in stroke [18–20]. Both techniques (MRA and TCD) allow noninvasive detection of intracranial vascular stenosis or occlusion with considerable accuracy, but each of these techniques has specific and different limitations [16–20]. The limitations of both methods can produce mistakes or misinterpretations in the acute period of cerebral ischemia because of possible early spontaneous revascularization, development of collateral pathways, evolution of infarction, time of scanning, and so forth.

Evolution of Cerebral Infarction With Time

Time	CT scan appearance
First few hours	Normal
12–36 hours	Decreased radiodensity (darker)
1 week to 1 month	Patchy contrast enhancement (breakdown of blood-brain barrier)
1 month	Area of infarct approaches attenuation of cerebrospinal fluid

Figure 4-25. Evolution of cerebral infarction with time. Cerebral infarction occurs after a sustained deficiency of cerebral profusion, from either an ulcerated thrombus or embolic event. The initial computed tomography (CT) scan is usually negative, but later scans show the localization and size of the infarct. The appearance of cerebral infarction varies with time.

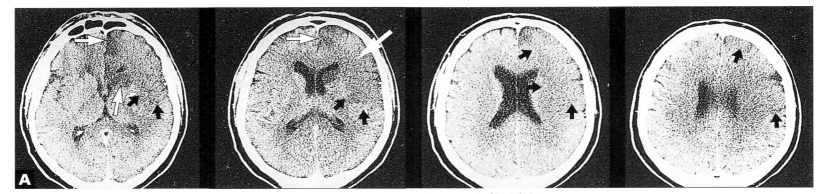

Figure 4-26. Computed tomography (CT) scans of a patient taken after a stroke. **A,** CT scans of a patient taken within the first 6 hours after a stroke. The sharp margins between normal and hypodense gray matter are an unusual finding during the first hours after the ictus. Neuroradiologic findings show a well-defined hypodensity of the left head of the caudate nucleus, the anterior part of the putamen, and the superior frontal gyrus. The open arrows show old infarctions in the territory of the anterior cerebral artery.

(Continued on next page)

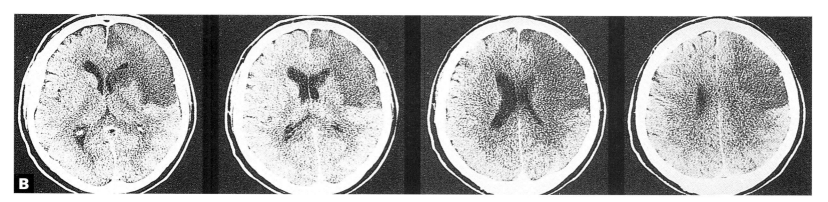

Figure 4-26. (*Continued*) The short arrows indicate less distinct, but already well-demarcated, hypodensity of the lateral left frontal lobe; the long arrow indicates effacement of the left frontal sulci.

Parenchymal hypodensity as shown by CT scan within the first 6 hours after symptom onset, and variably accompanied by focal brain swelling, represents ischemic brain edema. CT scan signs of brain edema in stroke patients do not directly indicate viable brain at risk for ischemia, but they do indicate tissue volume that will invariably undergo irreversible brain damage [21].

B, A second CT scan of the same patient obtained 35 hours after the onset of symptoms, following treatment with recombinant tissue-plasminogen activator (rt-PA). Now a marked hypodensity of precisely that area that was slightly hypodense on the first CT scan is seen. There is lateral compression of the left frontal horn and a slight midline shift. Making a differentiation between areas of old and new recent infarction is now barely possible. (*From* Von Kummer and colleagues [21] of the European Cooperative Acute Stroke Study; with permission.)

Comparison of Five Series of Intraarterial Thrombolysis for Vertebrobasilar Occlusion

	Brandt series [24]	Hacke series [25]	Zeumer series [26]	Bockenheimer series [27]	Becker series [28]
Patients, *n*	51	43	28	13	13
Average time to therapy	≤48 h	≤24 h	8 h	≥12 h	≤24 h
Overall mortality rate	69%	67%	46%	54%	75%
Recanalization rate	51%	44%	75%	54%*	75%
Recanalized mortality rate	46%	26%	NR	71%*	60%
Intracerebral hemorrhage	12%	9%	7%	0%	15%
Rethrombosis	NR	NR	10%	NR	30%

*Bockenheimer reported four patients with partial recanalization, seven patients with complete recanalization, and two who were not recanalized. The mortality rate in the partially recanalized group was 50%, but survivors were severely impaired. The mortality rate with complete recanalization was 57%, with one of the survivors being locked in. The numbers reported in the table reflect a combination of the data from the recanalized and partially recanalized groups.

Figure 4-27. Comparison of five series of intraarterial thrombolysis for vertebrobasilar occlusion. Antithrombotic therapy, with antiplatelet drugs or anticoagulants (heparin or warfarin), is commonly used but remains unproven therapy for acute stroke.

Reperfusion therapies are aimed at improving cerebral blood flow (CBF). Initially, vasodilators were tried, but they have generally been ineffective because blood vessels in ischemic regions are already maximally dilated. Other methods to improve regional CBF under the setting of acute stroke may include angioplasty, emergency thromboendarterectomy of the extracranial internal carotid artery, and embolectomy of the middle cerebral artery.

Neuronal protection is based on the effort to block calcium entry into neurons and prevent the production of free radicals. The dihydropyridine calcium antagonists nimodipine and nicardipine dilate cerebral vessels and also block calcium entry into neurons. Antagonists of the excitatory neurotransmitter glutamate are more potent blockers of calcium entry into neu-

rons but may have behavioral side effects. Free radical scavengers (lazaroids) have shown dramatic results in experimental studies and are also under clinical investigation.

Intraarterial thrombolysis has emerged as a promising treatment for strokes. Thrombolysis with fibrinolytic agents, streptokinase, recombinant tissue plasminogen activator (rt-PA), urokinase, or acetylated plasminogen streptokinase activator complex (APSAC) may proceed with reconstitution of cerebral blood flow (CBF) to ischemic tissue [22,23]. The treatment of vertebrobasilar thrombosis differs from that of carotid or middle cerebral artery thrombosis because of the vital brain stem structures involved. To justify the routine clinical use of thrombolytics in stroke, it must be shown that the benefits outweigh the risks. Given the very poor prognosis in vertebrobasilar thrombosis, realization of even small improvement in outcome would satisfy such a criterion. Further studies will be needed to prove whether this is an effective treatment. NR—not reported. (*Adapted from* Becker and colleagues [28].)

Hemorrhage

Brain Hemorrhages: Common and Clinical Syndromes

Location	Syndrome
Putaminal	Hemiparesis (smooth and steady onset); may progress to involve hemisensory loss, hemianopia, and aphasia (dominant hemisphere) or neglect (nondominant hemisphere); often associated with gaze deviation. Syndrome may progress to coma and death
Lobar	
Occipital	Pain around eye and dense hemianopsia
Temporal	Mild pain anterior to ear, aphasia (posterior), partial field defect
Frontal	Begins with severe arm weakness, minimal leg and face weakness, and frontal headache. Behavior changes, including abulia, are often seen
Parietal	Anterior temporal headache, hemisensory deficit; may also see cognitive and behavioral abnormalities along with visual neglect
Thalamic	Initial deficit of hemisensory loss, later hemiparesis. With enlarging size, there may be vertical gaze palsy, retraction nystagmus, skew deviation, loss of convergence, ptosis and miosis, anisocoria, or unreactive pupils. If the hematoma is large, coma may be present from the onset. Compression of cerebrospinal fluid pathways may lead to hydrocephalus
Cerebellar	Sudden onset of nausea, vomiting, and inability to walk. Also present may be headache, dizziness, impaired consciousness, appendicular ataxia, facial palsy, and ipsilateral gaze palsy
Pontine	Rapid onset of quadriplegia, decerebrate posturing, pinpoint pupils, oculomotor disturbances (bilateral horizontal gaze palsy), fever, and coma
Caudate	Headache, vomiting, decreased alertness, and stiff neck, because of their common association with intraventricular extension

Figure 4-28. Common and clinical syndromes associated with brain hemorrhages. Intracerebral hemorrhage (ICH) usually originates from a single artery or arterialized vein. It may continue for many hours or days. Hypertensive cerebrovascular disease accounts for 70% to 90% of cases of spontaneous ICH. The most common sources of hemorrhage are small penetrating arteries, including the thalamoperforating and lenticulostriate arteries, and paramedian branches of the basilar artery. There appears to be hypertension-induced degeneration of the media of the arterial wall, or fibrinoid necrosis, resulting in progressive weakening or development of microaneurysms. What precipitates the actual hemorrhage is unclear, although sudden elevation in blood pressure coincident with exertion or activity is common. There are core nonfocal features common to all ICHs, which include the sudden onset of headache, vomiting, nausea, and stiff neck; seizures, drowsiness, or loss of consciousness (within 24 hours); high diastolic blood pressure after 24 hours; and bilateral extensor plantar responses. (*Adapted from* Brass [29].)

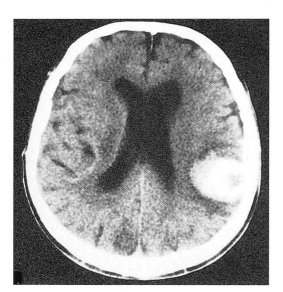

Figure 4-29. A computed tomography (CT) scan showing intracerebral hemorrhage within the left parietal lobe. Cerebral hemorrhage can be caused by (in decreasing order) aneurysm, arteriovenous malformation, trauma, tumor, abnormal coagulation, amyloid angiopathy, sympathomimetic drugs, arteritis, and hemorrhagic infarction (especially from venous occlusion). Hypertensive bleeds occur most frequently in the thalamus, basal ganglia, pons, and cerebellum. Intraventricular blood usually begins as a parenchymal bleed breaking through the ependymal layer of the ventricular system. CT scan should be performed promptly and the acuity of the cerebral hemorrhage classified. At the acute stage, less than 24 hours after the onset of a cerebral hemorrhage, the CT scan shows a high-density lesion surrounded by low density; at the subacute stage, days to a month after the cerebral hemorrhage, a gradual decrease in density from the periphery appears; at the chronic stage, 1 month to years after the cerebral hemorrhage, there is hypodensity. Additionally, CT scan permits determination of hematoma size and location, ventricular extension, and edema. The CT scan may suggest tumor, aneurysm, or vascular malformation as the cause. (*From* Kelly [30]; with permission.)

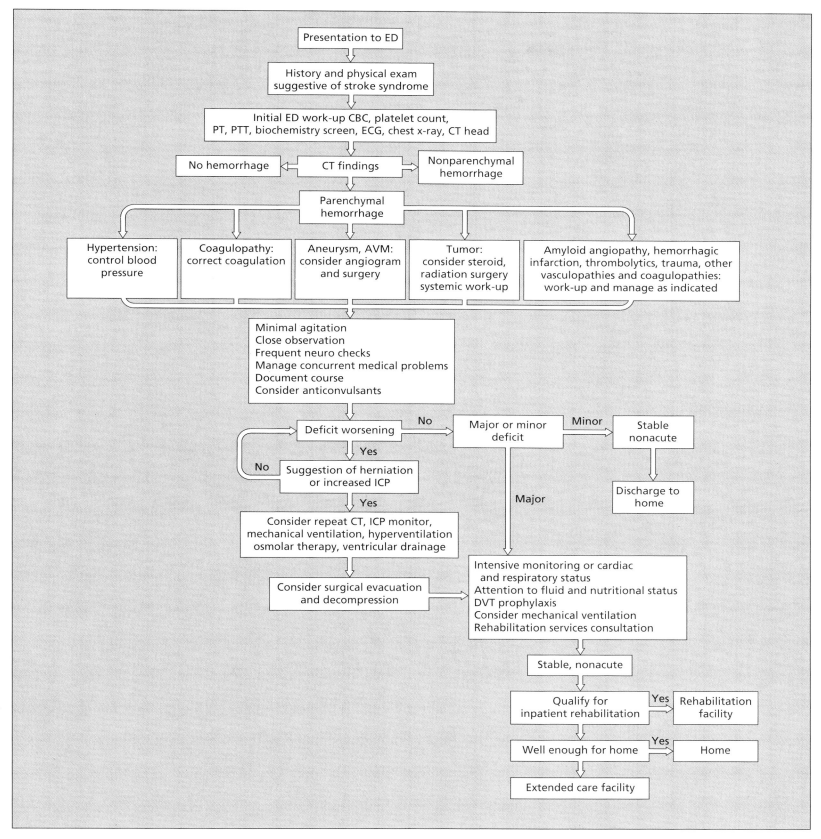

Figure 4-30. A treatment algorithm for management of intraparenchymal hemorrhage. This algorithm demonstrates the sequence of events that follow initial diagnosis. AVM—arteriovenous malformation; CBC—complete blood count; CT—computed tomography; DVT—deep vein thrombosis; ECG—electrocardiogram; ED—emergency department; ICP—intracranial pressure; PT—prothrombin time; PTT—partial thromboplastin time. (*Adapted from* Kelly [30].)

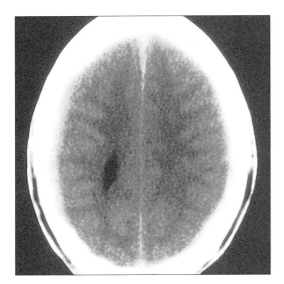

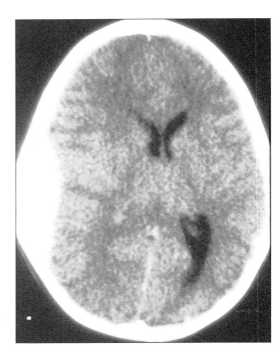

Figure 4-32. Computed tomography scan of an epidural hematoma. An epidural hematoma occurs primarily from an arterial bleed, the middle meningeal artery. The vessel is disrupted following a temporal bone of the skull. The blood fills and occupies the space between the dura and inner table of the skull. The blood conforms to a lenticular shape (biconvex) just beneath the skull. Because these are arterial bleeds, blood may accumulate quickly. A third nerve palsy is a sign of cerebral herniation, and thus a medical emergency.

Figure 4-31. Computed tomography (CT) scan of a subdural hematoma. A subdural hematoma usually appears due to the venous bleeding from bridging veins (subdural veins). The blood occupies space between the dura and the leptomeninges, which conforms to a crescent shape. Subdural hematoma is usually divided into acute and chronic types. This classification can usually be determined by the history and the signal of the blood on the CT scan. In the acute stage, less than 1 week after onset, the CT scan appears hyperdense (white); in the subacute stage, 1 to 3 weeks after onset, the CT scan is isodense (gray); and in the chronic stage, 3 to 4 weeks after onset, the CT scan is hypodense (black).

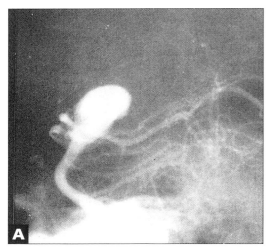

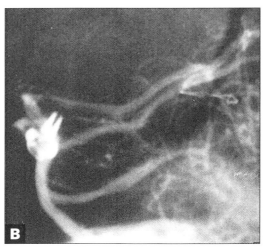

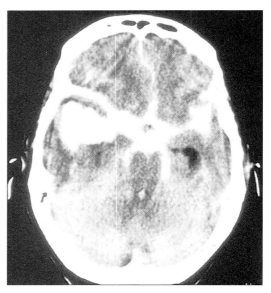

Figure 4-33. Computed tomography scans of a subarachnoid hemorrhage (SAH). **A,** Giant aneurysm at the top of the basilar artery. **B,** Postsurgical obliteration of the same aneurysm. Subarachnoid hemorrhage (SAH) most often presents with an acute onset and a dramatic clinical picture, often striking a patient who has been previously in good condition. The etiology can be divided into three major groups: aneurysmal rupture (75%), arteriovenous malformation (AVM) (5%), and unknown causes (20%). The first and second groups are defined as SAH with an aneurysm or AVM present on angiograms. The third group includes aneurysms not discovered on angiograms and other rare causes. Arterial hypertension is the most widely accepted risk factor for the development and rupture of aneurysm.

Aneurysmal SAH is known to result in both generalized and focal disturbances of the brain function. A combination of different factors of similar pathogenic importance is thought to lead eventually to these alterations. First, the normal brain metabolism is disrupted by direct exposure of the brain tissue to blood. Second, the raised intracranial pressure resulting from the sudden entry of blood into the subarachnoid space may injure the brain tissue. Third, the brain tissue may be rendered ischemic by the reduced arterial perfusion pressure and spasms of the cerebral vessels that frequently accompany SAH. (*From* Kistler and colleagues [31]; with permission.)

Figure 4-34. Computed tomography (CT) scan of subarachnoid hemorrhage (SAH). The clinical diagnosis is based on the classic picture with an acute onset of headache, often starting in the neck and spreading to a diffuse headache. Within minutes, nausea and vomiting may follow. One third of patients remain conscious, while one third are unconscious for more than 1 hour. A few experience an atypical history; this figure would probably increase if more cases with minimal SAH were included. Confirmation may require a lumbar puncture in up to 10% of cases because of a negative CT scan.

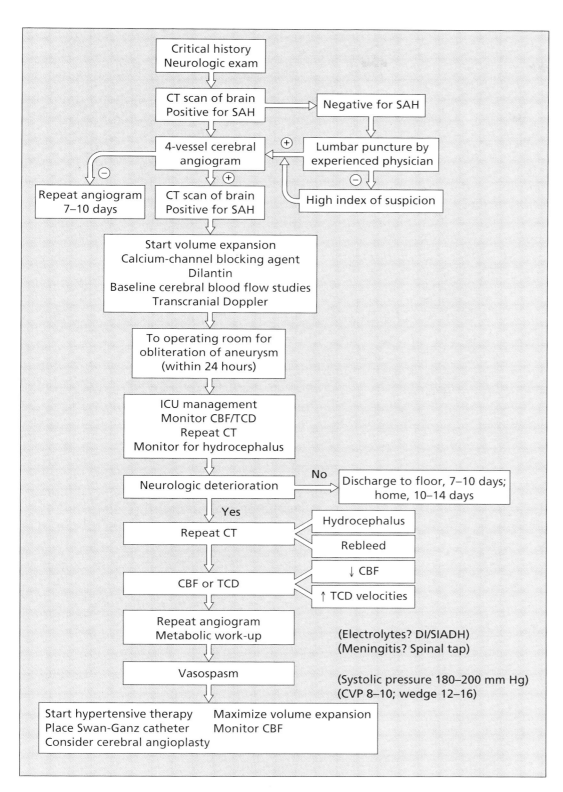

Figure 4-35. Management of patients with subarachnoid hemorrhage (SAH). The management of SAH requires the integration of clinical diagnosis in the emergency room, urgent neuroimaging evaluation, special operative and anesthetic considerations, conventional intensive care and unit-based critical care. The rational and intelligent approach to intensive care, therefore, requires an appreciation of the overall management protocol. CBF—cerebral blood flow; CT—computed tomography; CVP—central venous pressure; DI—diabetes insipidus; ICU—intensive care unit; SIADH—syndrome of inappropriate antidiuretic hormone; TCD—transcranial Doppler. (*Adapted from* Origitano [32].)

Vasospasm Management Protocol Without TCD or CBF Monitoring

Ischemic deficit	Treatment
All SAH patients	Nimodipine 60 mg by mouth or nasogastric tube every 4 h
	5% albumin 250 mL intravenously every 6 h
Deficit present	ICU admission
	Volume expansion (to PCWP 15 mm Hg)
	HCT 33%–37% hypertension (to 170–220 mm Hg systolic blood pressure)
Deficit refractory to medical treatment	Transluminal angioplasty
Deficit resolved	Gradual withdrawal of hypervolemia, hypertension

Figure 4-36. Vasospasm management protocol without transcranial Doppler (TCD) or cerebral blood flow (CBF) monitoring. Delayed ischemia due to cerebral vasospasm after subarachnoid hemorrhage (SAH) is a significant cause of morbidity and mortality after aneurysmal hemorrhage. In a literature review, more than 30,000 cases were found in which vasospasm after SAH was discussed. The incidence of angiographic vasospasm was 43.3% overall, and 67.3% when angiography was done at a time of maximum expected spasm. Symptomatic vasospasm or delayed ischemic deficit (DID) occurred in 32.5% [33]. Several therapeutic protocols have been employed for the management of vasospasm following aneurysmal rupture. The classic strategy, which is the standard at most medical centers, involves prophylactic management with nimodipine and maintenance of normovolemia or moderate hypervolemia, augmented by aggressive hypervolemic hemodilution and systemic arterial hypertension only when patients develop clinical signs of ischemic neurologic deficit. HCT—hematocrit; ICV—intensive care unit; PCWP—pulmonary capillary wedge pressure. (*Adapted from* Martin and colleagues [34].)

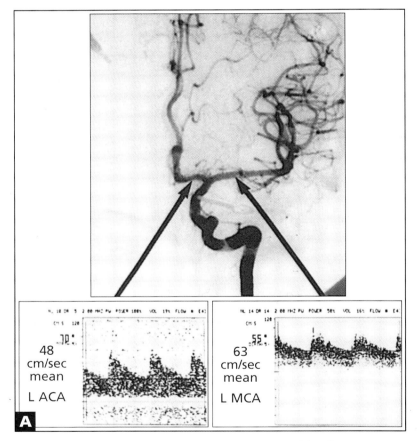

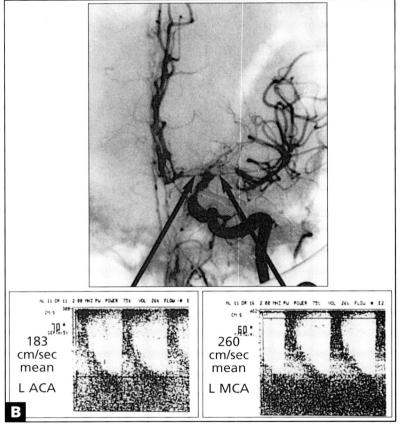

Figure 4-37. Angiographic and transcranial Doppler (TCD) findings in a patient shortly after undergoing early surgery for a ruptured posterior communicating artery aneurysm. For the evaluation of any treatment, the development and evolution of the arterial narrowing should be monitored. Angiography, the standard method of assessing cerebral vasospasm, is an invasive and risky procedure that cannot be repeated at frequent intervals. With the TCD technique, it is possible to register the increased blood flow velocity in the spastic arterial segment. Because the blood flow velocity is inversely related to the lumen area, the arterial narrowing can be evaluated by this method. **A,** Angiogram and normal blood flow velocities in a left anterior cerebral artery (LACA) segment (48 cm/sec) and a left middle cerebral artery (LMCA) segment (63 cm/sec). **B,** Angiogram and abnormally increased blood flow velocities in an LACA segment (183 cm/sec) and an LMCA segment (260 cm/sec) in the same vessels in the same patient after developing symptoms of delayed ischemia. (*From* Seiler and colleague [35]; with permission.)

Encephalitis

Viral Causes of Encephalitis

Togaviridae: alphaviruses	Rhabdoviridae: rabies
Eastern equine	Reoviridae: Colorado tick fever
Western equine	Orthomyxoviridae
Venezuelan equine	Mumps
Flaviviridae	Measles
St. Louis	Picornaviridae: enteroviruses
Japanese	Poliovirus
Murray Valley	Coxsackievirus
West Nile	Echovirus
Tick-borne complex	Herpesviridae
Bunyaviridae	Herpes simplex 1 and 2
California/La Crosse	Epstein-Barr
Rift Valley	Varicella-zoster
Adenovirus	Cytomegalovirus
Arenavirus	Retroviridae: HIV

Figure 4-38. Viral causes of encephalitis. A wide variety of viruses may cause encephalitis, but four families contain most of these: Flaviviridae, Togaviridae, Bunyaviridae, and Herpesviridae. The illnesses caused by these various agents may be clinically indistinguishable without laboratory testing, although epidemiologic features of the illnesses, including seasonality, geographic occurrence (or travel), patient age, and recent animal or insect bites, may aid in the diagnosis.

In temperate climates of the northern hemisphere, the viral encephalitides have distinct seasonal occurrences that may be helpful in the differential diagnosis. Encephalitis caused by the mosquito-borne and tick-borne arboviruses peaks in the spring and summer, paralleling the periods of activity for their insect vectors. Others, such as the herpesvirus infections, may occur year-round. (*Adapted from* Griffin [36].)

Postinfectious Viral Encephalitis

Varicella-zoster
Mumps
Measles
Rubella
Influenza A and B

Figure 4-39. Postinfectious viral encephalitides. Postinfectious encephalitides typically develop 2 to 12 days after the onset of the primary illness and are characterized by a sudden recrudescence of fever and obtundation, with a perivascular demyelination of the brains of patients. Virus is rarely isolated from the brain, and the condition may represent an autoimmune or allergic response. Mumps can cause both primary and postinfectious central nervous system involvement. (*Adapted from* Hanley and colleagues [37].)

Nonviral Conditions Causing or Simulating Encephalitis

Infectious causes

Bacterial	Brain abscess
	Subacute bacterial endocarditis
	Tuberculosis, *Mycoplasma* pneumonia, brucellosis, listeriosis, cat scratch fever
	Syphilis, relapsing fever, Lyme disease, leptospirosis
Fungal	Cryptococcosis, coccidioidomycosis, histoplasmosis, candidiasis, nocardiosis, blastomycosis, actinomycosis
Rickettsial	Rocky Mountain spotted fever, typhus, *Ehrlichia canis*, Q fever
Parasitic	Amebic meningoencephalitis, malaria, toxoplasmosis, cysticercosis, trichinosis, trypanosomiasis

Noninfectious causes

Toxins, drugs	Heavy metals, salicylates, barbiturates, phencyclidine
Metabolic diseases	Electrolyte imbalances, hyperglycemia, hypoglycemia, acute porphyria, pheochromocytoma
Systemic diseases	Sarcoidosis, collagen disease, neoplasms, vasculitis, Whipple's disease, Behçet's disease
Others	Subdural empyema, subdural hematoma, cerebral infarction, demyelinating diseases, acute psychosis

Figure 4-40. Nonviral conditions causing or simulating encephalitis. Most nonviral causes of encephalitis are treatable and should be ruled out when evaluating a patient. Infectious causes of encephalitis include bacterial, rickettsial, fungal, and parasitic diseases. Many noninfectious conditions may have clinical presentations that mimic viral encephalitis. (*Adapted from* Mateos-Mora and colleague [38].)

Causes of Encephalopathy in Immunodeficient Patients

Viral	Other
HIV	*Acanthamoeba*
CMV	*Toxoplasma*
HSV	*Cryptococcus*
Enteroviruses	*Nocardia*
Adenoviruses	*Histoplasma*
Measles	Primary CNS lymphoma
Papovavirus (PML)	

Figure 4-41. Causes of encephalopathy in immunodeficient patients. The causes of encephalitis are different in immunodeficient patients. In those with AIDS, various unusual agents may cause central nervous system disease, either singly or in combination. For further discussion of encephalopathy, see Figures 12-57–12-59 and 12-66. CNS—central nervous system; CMV—cytomegalovirus; HSV—herpes simplex virus; PML—progressive multifocal leukoencephalopathy. (*Adapted from* Hanley and colleagues [37].)

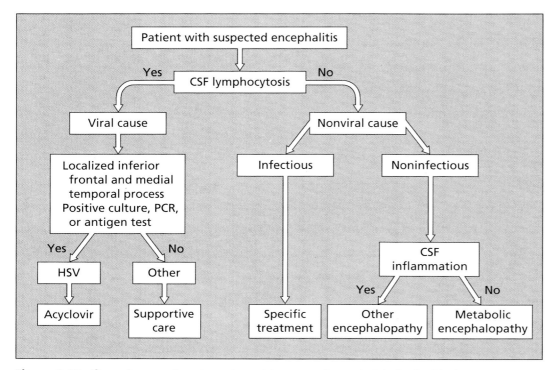

Figure 4-42. General approach to the patient with suspected encephalitis. In the febrile patient with depressed mental status, nonviral causes of encephalitis must first be considered and excluded because treatment is available for many. Epidemiologic, clinical, and laboratory data are important in the differential diagnosis. If a viral encephalitis is suspected, a diagnosis of herpes simplex virus (HSV) encephalitis should next be considered. For HSV encephalitis, early treatment with acyclovir may be beneficial, whereas for most other viral encephalitides, treatment is supportive. Laboratory diagnosis of viral encephalitis. A range of diagnostic tests is available to help in the evaluation of the patient with suspected encephalitis, and their use is guided by the clinical situation. Cerebrospinal fluid (CSF) examination is a key part of the evaluation of every patient, and assays for CSF virus–specific IgM (enzyme-linked immunosorbent assay) can aid in the rapid diagnosis of arbovirus infection. CSF cultures usually are negative for viruses but may be positive in bacterial infection. Serologic studies are useful in selected infections. Brain biopsy is usually necessary to diagnose herpes simplex virus encephalitis definitively, although polymerase chain reaction holds promise as a substitute for biopsy. Computed tomography, magnetic resonance imaging, and electroencephalography are used to identify or help exclude alternative diagnoses and to help establish the presence of a focal encephalitic process. For further discussion of cerebrospinal fluid evaluation in viral encephalitis, see Figure 12-51. PCR—polymerase chain reaction. (*Adapted from* Hanley and colleagues [37].)

Herpes Simplex Virus Encephalitis

Clinical and Neurologic Signs in Herpes Simplex Encephalitis

Signs	%
Altered consciousness	97
CSF pleocytosis	93
Fever	85–87
Headache	79
Personality changes	70–80
Dysphasia	71
Autonomic dysfunction	58
Seizures (focal and generalized)	42–64
Vomiting	51
Ataxia	40
Hemiparesis	30–41
Cranial nerve defects	33
Memory loss	22
Visual field loss	13
Papilledema	13

Figure 4-43. Clinical and neurologic signs in herpes simplex virus (HSV) encephalitis. A history of personality changes, bizarre behavior, hallucinations, focal seizures, or focal signs suggesting a temporal lobe lesion are common in HSV encephalitis because this viral encephalitis usually is localized to the medial temporal and orbitofrontal areas and is often unilateral or asymmetric. Signs do not differ significantly between patients with positive or negative cultures of brain biopsy material. CSF—cerebrospinal fluid. (*Adapted from* Whitley and colleagues [39].)

Diseases That Mimic Herpes Simplex Encephalitis

Treatable (*n* = 38)		Nontreatable (*n* = 57)	
Infection		Nonviral (*n* = 17)	
Abscess/subdural empyema		Vascular disease	11
Bacterial	5	Toxic encephalopathy	5
Listerial	1	Reye's syndrome	1
Fungal	2	Viral (*n* = 40)	
Mycoplasmal	2	St. Louis encephalitis	7
Tuberculosis	6	Western equine encephalitis	3
Cryptococcal	3	California encephalitis	4
Rickettsial	2	Eastern equine encephalitis	2
Toxoplasmosis	1	Epstein-Barr virus	8
Mucormycosis	1	Cytomegalovirus	1
Meningococcal meningitis	1	Echovirus	3
Tumor	5	Influenza A	4
Subdural hematoma	2	Mumps	3
Systemic lupus erythematosus	1	Adenovirus	1
Adrenal leukodystrophy	6	PML	1
		Lymphocytic choriomeningitis	2
		SSPE	2

Figure 4-44. Diseases that mimic herpes simplex encephalitis. PML—progressive multifocal leukoencephalopathy; SSPE—subacute sclerosing panencephalitis. (*Adapted from* Whitney and colleague [40].)

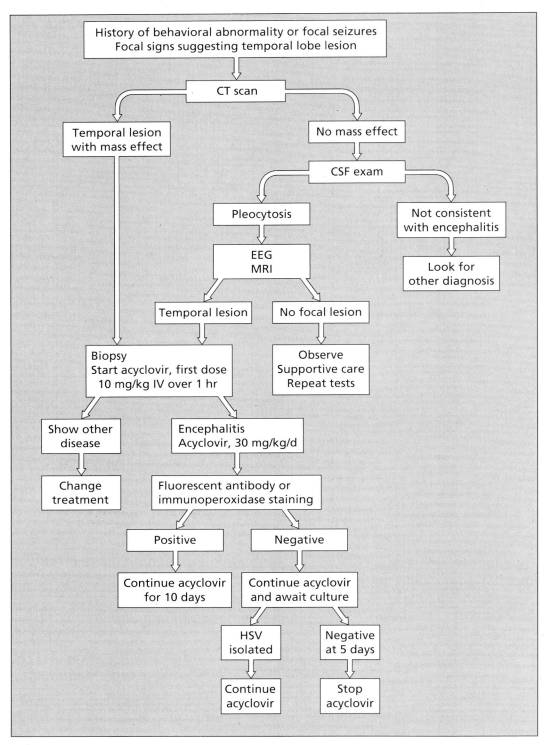

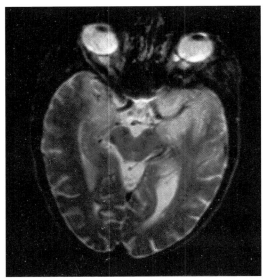

Figure 4-46. Brain edema in herpes simplex virus encephalitis. A magnetic resonance image shows signal intensity in the bilateral anterior temporal lobes, consistent with brain edema. This finding is commonly seen after 5 to 10 days of symptoms. Note the absence of compartment shift. (*From* Hanley and colleagues [37].)

Figure 4-45. Steps in the management of suspected herpes simplex virus encephalitis. CSF—cerebrospinal fluid; CT—computed tomography; EEG—electroencephalogram; HSV—herpes simplex virus; IV—intravenous; MRI—magnetic resonance imaging. (*Adapted from* Johnson [41].)

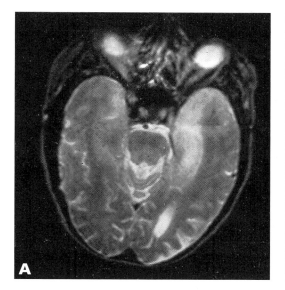
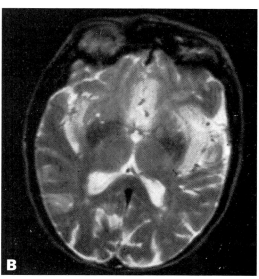
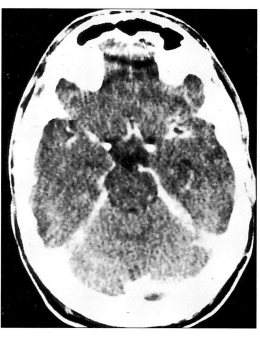

Figure 4-47. Brain edema in herpes simplex virus encephalitis. **A,** A rostral magnetic resonance image (MRI) section demonstrates contiguous medial and temporal extension of brain edema. The presence of medial and temporal findings suggests contiguous spread from the trigeminal ganglia, across the meningeal space to the inferior space of the temporal lobe, and then direct rostral extension. **B,** The most rostral MRI section demonstrates direct extension to the insular cortex from the medial aspect of the temporal lobe. (*From* Hanley and colleagues [37].)

Figure 4-48. Temporal lucency and surface vessels on computed tomography (CT) scan. A contrast-enhanced CT scan shows a medial temporal lucency and small linear enhancement suggestive of a cortical surface vessel. Dilation of surface vessels, increased number of surface vessels, and small areas of lucent tissue are early positive CT findings. However, the most common early CT picture in the first week of symptoms of herpes simplex virus encephalitis is that of a normal CT. (*From* Hanley and colleagues [37].)

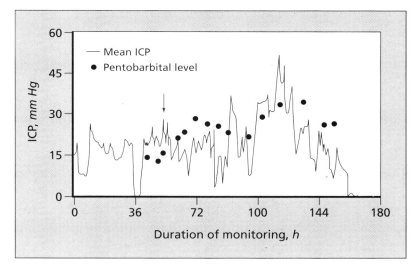

Figure 4-49. Time course of intracranial hypertension in herpes simplex encephalitis. Time course of intracranial hypertension is seen in a patient who underwent an unsuccessful attempt at high-dose barbiturate treatment of brain swelling. The arrow designates the time at which the patient experienced uncal herniation; the herniation appeared to occur without a severe alteration of intracranial pressure (ICP). (*Adapted from* Hanley and colleagues [37].)

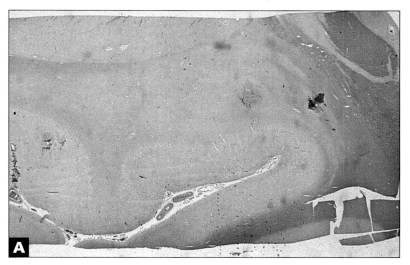

Figure 4-50. Temporal cortex from a patient with herpes simplex virus encephalitis. **A,** A low-power photomicrograph shows white matter and cortical involvement with hemorrhage. This bleeding is frequently punctate and can involve superficial cortex, white matter, or meningeal spaces.

(*Continued on next page*)

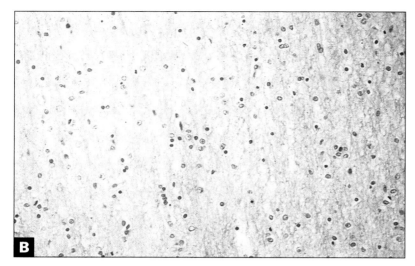

Figure 4-50. (*Continued*) **B**, A high-power photomicrograph of this specimen shows inclusion bodies in both neurons and glia. Herpes simplex inclusion bodies can occur in vascular tissue as well. (*From* Hanley and colleagues [37].)

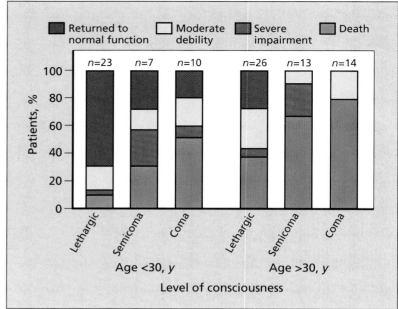

Figure 4-51. Prognostic factors in herpes simplex virus (HSV) encephalitis. The level of consciousness and age are proven major determinants of clinical outcome in HSV encephalitis. Patients younger than 30 years of age and with a more normal level of consciousness (lethargic vs comatose) are more likely to return to normal functioning after HSV encephalitis than older patients, especially those who are semicomatose or comatose. Mortality rates approach 70% in patients older than 30 years of age, whether comatose or semicomatose, but are 25% in those younger than 30 years of age. (*Adapted from* Whitney and colleague [40].)

Status Epilepticus

Classification of Status Epilepticus

Generalized status epilepticus
  Convulsive status epilepticus
    Myoclonic
    Tonic-clonic
    Tonic
    Clonic
  Nonconvulsive status epilepticus
    Absence
Partial status epilepticus
  Convulsive status epilepticus
    Tonic-clonic
    Simple partial (somatomotor)
  Nonconvulsive status epilepticus
    Complex partial

Figure 4-52. Classification of status epilepticus (SE). SE is a relatively common neurologic emergency that is associated with a high degree of morbidity and mortality. There is general agreement that a state of continuous seizures persisting beyond 30 minutes represents SE, although episodes lasting as little as 10 minutes should be considered as SE, and treatment should be initiated to prevent irreversible brain injury. There are several subtypes of SE, and the major classification depends on whether the seizures are generalized or partial, convulsive (motor) or nonconvulsive. Convulsive SE is usually easily identified, whereas nonconvulsive SE may be subtle in its clinical presentation, and diagnosis can only be confirmed by electroencephalography. (*Adapted from* Cascino [42].)

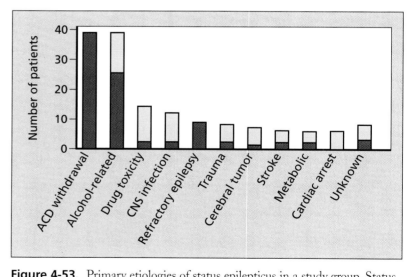

Figure 4-53. Primary etiologies of status epilepticus in a study group. Status epilepticus (SE) has many etiologies. By far the most common, however, are acute withdrawal of anticonvulsant drugs (ACD) and alcohol-related seizures. Acute alcohol withdrawal seizures typically present with generalized convulsive SE, whereas ACD withdrawal–related SE is dependent on the underlying seizure disorder. Other relatively common causes of SE include infection, metabolic disturbances, brain tumors, and ischemic or hypoxic brain injury. CNS—central nervous system. (*Adapted from* Lowenstein and colleague [43].)

Progressive Sequence of Electroencephalographic Patterns in Generalized Convulsive Status Epilepticus

Discrete seizures with interictal slowing
Waxing and waning of ictal discharges
Continuous ictal discharges
Continuous ictal discharges punctuated by flat periods
Periodic epileptiform discharges on a flat background

Figure 4-54. Progressive sequence of electroencephalographic patterns in generalized convulsive status epilepticus (SE). Initially, discrete periods of ictal seizure activity are well defined between periods of postictal depression. As SE continues, a waxing and waning ictal pattern emerges that soon becomes a continuous pattern of epileptiform activity. Thereafter, the continuous seizure pattern breaks up, with longer and longer periods of relative flattening. Finally, the record becomes one of brief periodic epileptiform discharges against a flat background. (*Adapted from* Treiman [44].)

Differential Diagnosis of Complex Partial Status Epilepticus

Epilepsy-related
  Absence status
  Postictal states
Neurologic
  Transient ischemic attacks
  Toxic-metabolic encephalopathy
  Transient global amnesia
  Stroke with delirium
  PLEDs
  Migraine
Psychiatric
  Somatiform disorder
  Psychosis

Figure 4-55. Differential diagnosis of complex partial status epilepticus (SE). Complex partial SE may frequently present with subtle clinical manifestations. Characteristically, there is an alteration of mental status with variable responsiveness. Automatisms and bizarre behavior may be present, and the seizures may be accompanied by lateralizing neurologic deficits. The differential diagnosis of complex partial SE includes a wide variety of neurologic and psychiatric disorders. A high degree of suspicion must be present, and the diagnosis is confirmed by electroencephalogram. PLEDs—periodic lateralized epileptiform discharges. (*Adapted from* Cascino [42].)

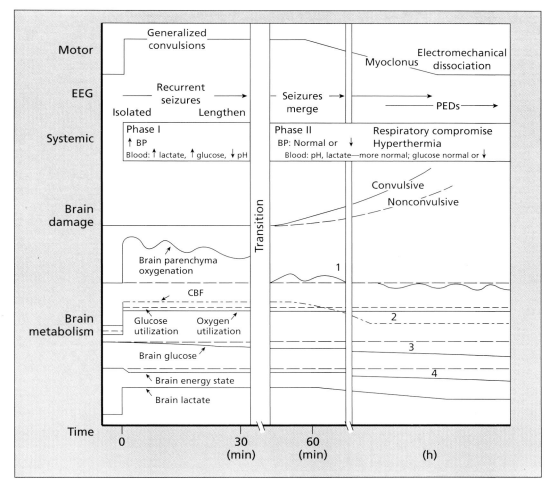

Figure 4-56. Summary of systemic alterations and brain metabolism in status epilepticus (SE). There is general agreement between the clinical progression of SE and experimental models of convulsive SE insofar that two distinct pathophysiologic periods during the evolution of seizures have been identified. In the first phase, typically lasting about 30 minutes, motor seizures steadily intensify and lengthen in duration, with shorter and shorter interictal periods. A rise in both cerebral blood flow and systemic hemodynamic parameters, such as blood pressure (BP) and tachycardia, reflects the high energy demand by the cerebral cortex. Systemic and cerebral lactate production are observed with a fall in blood pH. As the seizures merge and become continuous, the second phase begins, marked by a normalization or fall in hemodynamic indices. Tissue lactate normalizes, and there is a general fall in cerebral metabolism. Initial studies investigating SE-induced brain injury suggested that a mismatch between cerebral metabolism and blood flow resulted in ischemia. Further elaborate experiments controlling for systemic hemodynamics and oxygenation demonstrated only modest declines in cerebral glucose concentrations and normal cerebral blood flow, supporting the hypothesis that a lack of energy substrate is not the etiology of subsequent brain injury. Recent work has identified the excitatory amino acids such as glutamate as probable prime culprits in SE-induced neuronal injury. CBF—cerebral blood flow; EEG—electroencephalogram; PED—periodic epilepiform discharges. (*Adapted from* Lothman [45].)

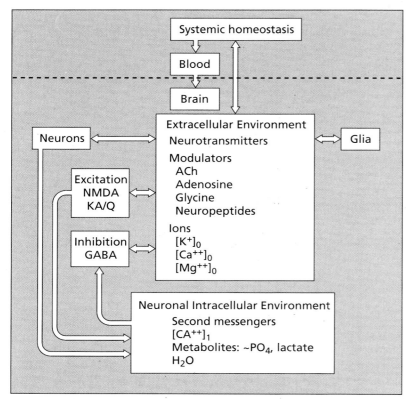

Figure 4-57. Pathophysiologic mechanisms for status epilepticus (SE). Experimental models of SE have elegantly demonstrated that during the course of SE, there is a gradual loss of gamma aminobutyric acid (GABA) inhibition within the brain that usually would assist in the termination of seizure activity. Such dysfunction of GABAergic transmission appears surprisingly early, within 30 to 60 minutes and may in part explain the clinical observations that SE lasting longer than this period is more difficult to terminate than that which lasts for only 10 to 20 minutes. Enhancement of excitatory neurotransmission also occurs, leading to a pronounced increase in toxic intracellular calcium ion by activation of glutaminergic receptors, especially the *N*-methyl-D-aspartate (NMDA) receptor–channel complex. This scenario explains why regions high in glutamate receptors, such as the hippocampus and the middle layers of cerebral cortex, are particularly vulnerable to damage during SE. ACh—acetylcholine; Ca^{++}—calcium; H_2O—water; K^+—potassium; KA/Q—kainate/quisqualate receptor; Mg^{++}—magnesium; PO_4—phosphate. (*Adapted from* Lothman [45].)

Treatment Protocol for Generalized Convulsive Status Epilepticus

Make diagnosis by observing one additional seizure in a patient with a history of recent seizures or impaired consciousness or by observing continuous seizure activity for >30 minutes. Call technician and start EEG recording as soon as possible, but do not delay treatment unless EEG is needed to verify the diagnosis.

Establish IV catheter with normal saline.

Draw blood for serum chemistries, hematologic studies, and antiepileptic drug concentrations.

Administer 100 mg thiamine followed by 50 mL 50% glucose by direct push into the IV line.

Administer lorazepam, 0.1 mg/kg, by IV push (<2 mg/min).

If SE does not stop, start phenytoin, 20 mg/kg by slow IV push (<50 mg/min) directly into IV port closest to patient. Monitor blood pressure and ECG closely during infusion. If SE does not stop after 20 mg/kg of phenytoin, give an additional 5 mg/kg and if necessary another 5 mg/kg until a maximum dose of 30 mg/kg is administered.

If SE persists, intubate patient and give phenobarbital, 20 mg/kg, by IV push (<100 mg/min).

If SE still persists, induce coma with barbiturate. Give pentobarbital, 5 mg/kg, slowly, as initial IV dose to induce an EEG burst-suppression pattern. Continue 0.5 to 2 mg/kg/h to maintain burst-suppression pattern. Slow the rate of infusion every 2 to 4 h to determine whether seizures have stopped. Monitor blood pressure, ECG, and respiratory function closely.

Figure 4-58. Treatment protocol for generalized convulsive status epilepticus. Optimal treatment of status epilepticus (SE) is dependent on a rapid diagnostic and therapeutic algorithm that provides appropriate medical intervention to stop the seizures before permanent neurologic injury occurs. The protocol provided for here illustrates a general guideline toward evaluation and therapy. Pharmacologic anticonvulsant treatment begins with a benzodiazepine because of rapid onset of action and intravenous push capability with this class of drug. Three common agents, midazolam, diazepam, and lorazepam, differ in their pharmacokinetics, but none has been demonstrated to be more efficacious than the others. Phenytoin is typically the second agent used to treat SE. In the near future, fosphenytoin may become a first-line agent because it can be administered rapidly. For SE unresponsive to benzodiazepines, phenytoin, and phenobarbital, general anesthesia should be administered promptly. A number of agents can be selected to induce electrocerebral suppression, including the short-acting barbiturates, such as thiopental or pentobarbital, propofol, or even the volatile anesthetic gases if readily available. Electroencephalograph monitoring should be used in concert to titrate the drugs to cessation of electrical seizure activity. Invasive hemodynamic monitoring is frequently required during administration of these agents. Intubation and intensive care unit management are, of course, mandatory. The key to good recoveries are the prompt termination of seizure activity. Treatment must be instituted aggressively and quickly if seizures persist, ideally within 30 to 45 minutes after onset of SE. ECG—electrocardiogram; EEG—electroencephalogram; IV—intravenous. (*Adapted from* Treiman [46].)

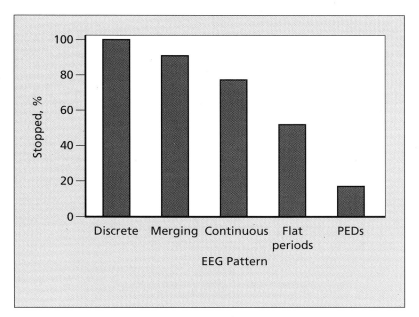

Figure 4-59. Response to treatment of status epilepticus (SE). The higher success rate of treating status epilepticus (SE) early is supported by clinical electroencephalogram (EEG) evidence demonstrating that therapeutic success is maximal when the EEG pattern consists of discrete seizure episodes, moderate with merging or continuous seizure patterns, and poor when the EEG shows periodic epileptiform discharges (PEDs). (*Adapted from* Treiman [47].)

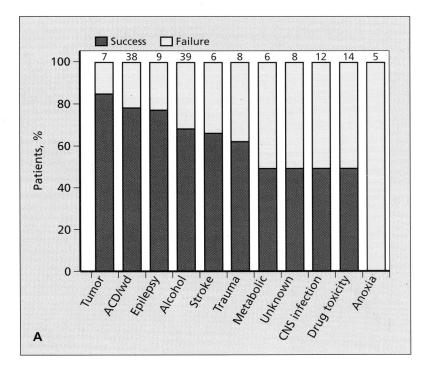

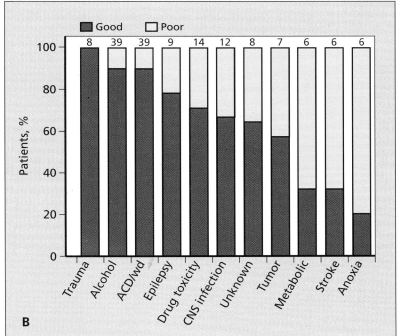

Figure 4-60. Relationship between the primary etiology of status epilepticus and response to first-line therapy and short-term outcome. In addition to the time dependency for successful termination of status epilepticus (SE), the etiology of the seizures also is important in determining the likelihood of stopping SE using first-line therapy. **A,** Patients suffering from SE as a result of common etiologies such as acute anticonvulsant withdrawal (ACD/wd), alcohol abuse, or mass lesions have a relatively high response rate to intravenous benzodiazepine therapy. In contrast, patients with anoxic brain injury have an almost uniformly poor response to pharmacologic therapy. **B,** Correlating with their good response to first-line drug therapy, patients with SE secondary to alcohol use or acute anticonvulsant drug withdrawal generally have a good outcome. Patients with mass lesions, however, do less well owing to underlying brain pathology. Anoxic brain injury has the least favorable outcome, consistent with near-total lack of response to anticonvulsant medication. Numbers along the right side of the graphs represent the total number of patients in each etiologic group. CNS—central nervous system. (*Adapted from* Lowenstein [43].)

Published Studies of Barbiturate Coma Therapy for Refractory Status Epilepticus

Study	Patients, n	Ages, y	Type SE	Drug	Mortality, %	Time of followup
Young *et al.*, 1980	5	19–62	GSE	PB	0	Discharge
Partinen *et al.*, 1981	5	19–57	GSE	TP	0	Discharge
Rashkin *et al.*, 1987	9	15–82	GSE?	PB	77	Discharge
Lowenstein *et al.*, 1988	14	14–79	GSE	TP, MH, PB	43	Discharge
Osorio and Reed, 1989	12	18–67	GSE	PB	17	≥6 mo
Van Ness, 1990	7	17–79	Mixed	PB	43	Discharge
Yaffe and Lowenstein, 1993	17	25–84	GSE	PB	53	>1 1/2 y

Figure 4-61. Published studies of barbiturate coma therapy for refractory status epilepticus (SE). In situations in which status epilepticus (SE) is refractory to initial anticonvulsant drug options, pharmacologic therapy to terminate the seizures by reducing or completely inhibiting cortical brain electrical activity is advocated. Drugs, such as the barbiturates, have been the mainstay of this type of therapy, although general anesthesia using the volatile inhalational agents, such as insoflurane, or newer intravenous anesthetics such as midazolam and propofol, have been considered appropriate alternatives. As these data describe, patients requiring pharmacologic coma to terminate SE have a relatively poor ultimate outcome with a high mortality rate. These patients typically begin with a poor prognosis, suffering from etiologies of SE that do not respond well to first-line anticonvulsant therapy. In addition, by the time coma is induced, SE has likely persisted for such a duration as to result in considerable brain injury. GSE—generalized status epilepticus; MH—methohexital; PB—pentobarbital; TP—thiopental. (*Adapted from* Yaffe and colleague [48]; Kumar and colleague [49].)

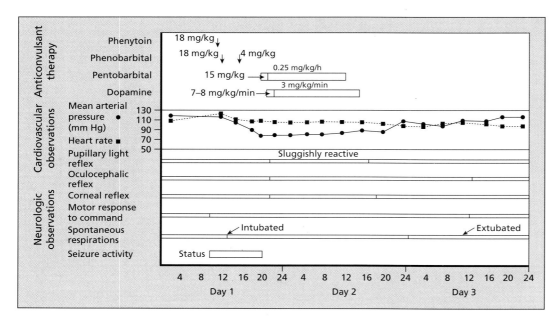

Figure 4-62. Response to barbiturate anesthesia in a patient with status epilepticus (SE). Induction of barbiturate coma for treatment of refractory SE results in significant hemodynamic derangement as well as loss of the neurologic examination. Invasive cardiovascular monitoring is mandatory, and inotropic and vasopressor support is frequently required. The neurologic examination is often limited to pupil reactivity during the drug-induced coma. (*Adapted from* Lowenstein and colleagues [50].)

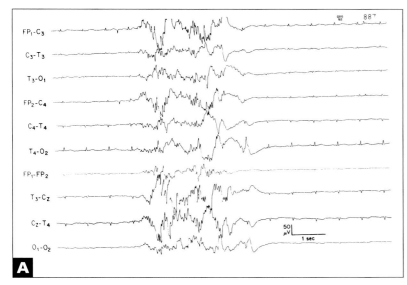

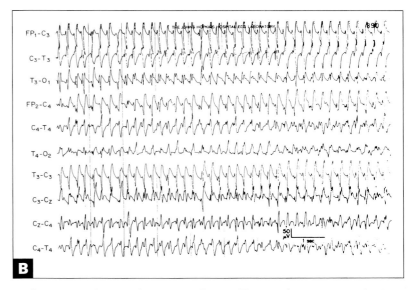

Figure 4-63. Electroencephalograms (EEGs) in status epilepticus (SE) assessment. **A,** The objective of pharmacologic coma is to terminate status epilepticus (SE), as shown here in an 18-year-old man with encephalitis of unclear etiology. This does not usually require electrocerebral silence, as may be the goal when treating intractable elevated intracranial pressure. The therapeutic endpoint is to arrive at an EEG pattern demonstrating no overt epileptiform activity, or to establish a burst suppression pattern as shown in **B**. This EEG pattern is maintained for several hours before attempts are made to wean pharmacologic coma therapy. During this time, optimization of serum levels of selected anticonvulsant agents, such as phenytoin, is performed to provide chronic seizure protection. In unusual cases, it may be necessary to extend the barbiturate coma for several or more days before weaning from the barbiturate infusion. In this case, pharmacologic coma was maintained for 53 days before successful withdrawal was accomplished, with no return of SE. (*From* Mirski and colleagues [51]; with permission.)

Relationship Between Total Duration of Status Epilepticus and Patient Outcome

	Good outcome		Poor outcome		P value
Group	N	Duration*	N	Duration	
All patients	115	2.4 (6.9)	34	11.2 (18.2)	0.0001
Anticonvulsant withdrawal	35	1.7 (2.1)	4	4.6 (6.9)	0.059
Alcohol related	35	1.5 (1.2)	4	4.1 (2.9)	0.001
Drug toxicity	10	1.9 (1.7)	4	32.5 (58.4)	0.102
CNS infection	8	1.7 (1.5)	4	18.5 (22.5)	0.050

*Average hours (SD).

Figure 4-64. Relationship between total duration of status epilepticus (SE) and patient outcome. In keeping with the fact that SE lasting more than 30 to 60 minutes is well associated with irreversible neuronal pathology, there is a clear relation between duration of SE and outcome. Regardless of etiology, SE that persists for more than 3 to 4 hours is likely to be associated with a poor neurologic outcome. These data highlight the therapeutic approach to treatment of SE: aggressive use of the therapeutic algorithm for treatment, with utmost attention paid to minimizing seizure duration. Defaulting to pharmacologic coma if SE has persisted beyond 30 to 60 minutes can only be encouraged to terminate ictal activity while other long-term management strategies are employed. CNS—central nervous system. (*Adapted from* Lowenstein and colleague [43].)

References

1. Ramsay MAE, Savege TA, Simpson BRJ, Goodwin R: Controlled sedation with alphaxalone-alphadolone. *BMJ* 1974, 2:656–659.

2. Mirski MA, Muffelman B, Ulatowski JA, *et al.*: Sedation for the critically ill neurologic patient. *Crit Care Med* 1995, 23:2038–2053.

3. Teasdale G, Jennett B: Assessment of coma and impaired consciousness. *Lancet* 1974, 1:878–881.

4. Ropper AH: *Neurological and Neurosurgical Intensive Care*, edn 3. New York: Raven Press; 1993.

5. Wijdicks EFM: *Neurology of Critical Illness*. Philadelphia: FA Davis, 1995.

6. Hacke W, ed: *Neurocritical Care*. Berlin: Springer-Verlag, 1994.

7. Grotta JC: *Management of the Acutely Ill Neurological Patient*. New York: Churchill Livingstone, 1993.

8. Classification of cerebrovascular disease III. Special report from the National Institute of Neurological Disorders and Stroke. *Stroke* 1990, 21:637–676.

9. Mohr JP, Barnett HJM: Classification of Ischemic Strokes. In *Stroke: Pathophysiology, Diagnosis and Management*. Edited by Barnett HJM, Mohr JP, Stein BM, Yatsu FM. New York: Churchill Livingstone; 1986:281–292.

10. Kittner SJ, Sharkness CM, Sloan MA, *et al.*: Infarcts with a cardiac source of embolism in the NINDS Stroke Data Bank. *Neurology* 1992, 42:299–302.

11. Mohr JP, Caplan LR, Melski JW, *et al.*: The Harvard registry of cases hospitalized with stroke. *Neurology* 1978, 28:754–762.

12. Kunitz S, Gross CR, Heyman A, *et al.*: The pilot stroke data bank: definition, design, data. *Stroke* 1984, 15:740–746.

13. Fisher MC: Principles of Diagnosis and Management of Occlusive Cerebrovascular Disease. In *Neurological and Neurosurgical Intensive Care*, edn 3. Edited by Ropper HH. New York: Raven Press; 1993.

14. Brucher R, Russell D: Methods and Clinical Potential. *Neurosonology*. Edited by Tegeler CH, Babikian VL, Gomez CR. St. Louis: Mosby–Year Book; 1995:231–234.

15. Bryan RN, Levy LM, Whitlow WD, *et al.*: Diagnosis of acute cerebral infarction: comparison of CT and MR imaging. *AJNR* 1992, 8:245–263.

16. Yuh WT, Crain MR, Loes DJ, *et al.*: MR imaging of cerebral ischemia: findings in the first 24 hours. *AJNR* 1991, 12:621–629.

17. Mathews VP, Barker PB, Bryan RN: Magnetic resonance evaluation of stroke. *Magnetic Resonance Quarterly* 1992, 4:245–263.

18. Aaslid R, ed: *Transcranial Doppler Sonography*. New York: Springer-Verlag; 1986.

19. Hereda P, Traubner P, Bujdakova J: Short-term prognosis of stroke due to occlusion of internal carotid artery based on transcranial Doppler ultrasonography. *Stroke* 1992, 23:1069–1072.

20. Halsey JH Jr: Prognosis of acute hemiplegia estimated by transcranial Doppler ultrasonography. *Stroke* 1988, 19:648–649.

21. Von Kummer R, Bozzao L, Manelfe C: Early CT diagnosis of hemispheric brain infarction. Berlin: Springer-Verlag; 1995.

22. Del Zoppo GJ: Thrombolytic therapy in acute stroke: recent experience. *Cerebrovasc Dis* 1993, 3:256–263.

23. Brott TL: Thrombolytic therapy. *Neurol Clin North Am* 1992, 10:219–232.

24. Brandt T, Muller-Kuppers M, von Kummer R, *et al.*: Thrombolytic therapy for acute basilar artery occlusion: predictors for recanalization and outcome. *Stroke* 1996, 27:875–881.

25. Hacke W, Zeumer H, Ferbert A, *et al.*: Intra-arterial thrombolytic therapy improves outcome in patients with acute vertebrobasilar occlusive disease. *Stroke* 1988, 19:1216–1222.

26. Zeumer H, Freitag H-J, Zanella F, *et al.*: Local intra-arterial fibrinolytic therapy in patients with stroke: urokinase versus recombinant tissue plasminogen activator (r-TPA) *Neuroradiology* 1993, 35:159–162.

27. Bockenheimer St, Reinhuber F, Mohs C: Intraarterielle thrombolyse himversorgender Gefäße. *Radiologe* 1991, 31:210–215.

28. Becker KJ, Monsein LH, Ulatowski JA, *et al.*: Intraarterial thrombolysis in vertebrobasilar occlusion. *AJNR* 1996, 17:1–8.

29. Brass LM: Clinical Syndromes of Intracerebral Hemorrhage. In *Intracerebral Hemorrhage*. Edited by Feldmann E. Armonk, NY: Futura Publishing; 1994:223–255.

30. Kelly MA: Management of Intracerebral Hemorrhage. In *Atlas of Cerebrovascular Disease*. Edited by Gorelick PB. Philadelphia: Current Medicine; 1996:20.1–20.10.

31. Kistler JP, Gress DR, Crowell RM: Subarachnoid Hemorrhage Due to a Ruptured Saccular Aneurysm. In *Clinical Atlas of Cerebrovascular Disorders*. Edited by Fisher M. London: Mosby-Wolfe; 1994:12.1–12.14.

32. Origitano TC: Treatment of Aneurysmal Subarachnoid Hemorrhage. In *Atlas of Cerebrovascular Disease*. Edited by Gorelick PB. Philadelphia: Current Medicine; 1996:19.1–19.11.

33. Dorsch NW, King MT: A review of cerebral vasospasm in aneurysmal subarachnoid hemorrhage. Part I: Incidence and effects. *J Clin Neurosci* 1994, 1:19–26.

34. Martin N, Khanna R, Rodts G: The Intensive Care Management of Patients with Subarachnoid Hemorrhage. In *Neurocritical Intensive Care*. Edited by Andrew BT. New York: McGraw-Hill; 1993:291–310.

35. Seiler R, Newell DW: Subarachnoid hemorrhage and vasospasm. In *Transcranial Doppler*. Edited by Newell DW, Aaslid R. New York: Raven Press; 1992:101–107.

36. Griffin DE: Encephalitis, Myelitis, and Neuritis. In *Principles and Practice of Infectious Diseases*, edn 4. Edited by Mandell GL, Bennett JE. New York: Churchill Livingstone; 1995:874–881.

37. Hanley DF, Glass JD, McArthur JC, Johnson RT: Viral Encephalitis and Related Conditions. In *Atlas of Infectious Diseases*, vol 3. Edited by Mandell GL, Bleck TP. Philadelphia: Current Medicine; 1995:3.1–3.36.

38. Mateos-Mora M, Ratzan KR: Acute Viral Encephalitis. In *Infectious of the Nervous System*. Edited by Schlossberg D. New York: Springer-Verlag; 1990:105–134.

39. Whitley RJ, *et al.*: Herpes simplex encephalitis: Clinical assessment. *JAMA* 1982, 247:317–320.

40. Whitney RJ, Schlitt M: Encephalitis Caused by Herpesviruses, Including B Viruses. In *Infections of the Central Nervous System*. Edited by Scheld RJ, Whitley RJ, Durack DT. New York: Raven Press; 1991:53–55.

41. Johnson RT: *Current Therapy in Neurologic Disease*, edn 2. Philadelphia: BC Decker; 1987.

42. Cascino GD: Nonconvulsive status epilepticus in adults and children. *Epilepsia* 1993, 34(suppl 1):S21–S28.

43. Lowenstein DH, Alldredge BK: Status epilepticus at an urban public hospital in the 1980s. *Neurology* 1993, 43:(3 Pt 1):483–488.

44. Treiman DM: The role of benzodiazepines in the management of status epilepticus. *Neurology* 1990, 40:32–42.

45. Lothman E: The biochemical basis and pathophysiology of status epilepticus. *Neurology* 1990, 40(suppl 2):13–23.

46. Treiman DM: Status Epilepticus. In *Current Therapy in Neurological Diseases*, edn 2. Edited by Johnson RT. Philadelphia: BC Decker; 1987:38–42.

47. Treiman DM: Generalized convulsive status epilepticus in the adult. *Epilepsia* 1993, 34:S2–S11.

48. Yaffe K, Lowenstein DH: Prognostic factors of pentobarbital therapy for refractory generalized status epilepticus. *Neurology* 1993, 43:895–900.

49. Kumar A, Bleck TP: Intravenous midazolam for the treatment of refractory status epilepticus. *Crit Care Med* 1992, 20:483–488.

50. Lowenstein DH, Aminoff MJ, Simon RP: Barbiturate anesthesia in the treatment of status epilepticus: clinical experience with 14 patients. *Neurology* 1988, 38:395–400.

51. Mirski MA, Williams MA, Hanley DF: Prolonged pentobarbital and phenobarbital coma for refractory generalized status epilepticus. *Crit Care Med* 1995, 23:400–403.

5

Cerebrovascular Disease

Karen L. Furie • Christopher S. Ogilvy • Martin Smrčka
Nijasri C. Suwanwela • Ufuk Can • Hakan Ay
Steven C. Cramer • Steven M. Greenberg
Guy Rordorf • Seth P. Finklestein
Gary P. Foster • Walter J. Koroshetz
Nitaya Suwanwela • J. Philip Kistler

CEREBROVASCULAR disease, the third leading cause of death after heart disease and cancer in developed countries, has an overall prevalence of 794 per 100,000. In the United States, more than 400,000 patients are discharged each year from hospitals after stroke. The loss of these patients from the work force and the extended hospitalization they require during recovery make the economic impact of the disease one of the most devastating in medicine.

Cerebrovascular disease is caused by one of several pathologic processes involving the blood vessels of the brain. The process may be intrinsic to the vessel, as in atherosclerosis, lipohyalinosis, inflammation, amyloid deposition, arterial dissection, developmental malformation, aneurysmal dilation, or venous thrombosis; originate remotely, as occurs when an embolus from the heart or extracranial circulation lodges in an intracranial vessel; result from decreased perfusion pressure or increased blood viscosity with inadequate cerebral blood flow; or result from rupture of a vessel in the subarachnoid space or intracerebral tissue.

A *stroke* is the acute neurologic injury that occurs as a result of one of these pathologic processes, manifesting either as brain infarction or hemorrhage. About 80% of strokes are due to ischemic cerebral infarction and 20% to brain hemorrhage.

For both *ischemic stroke* and *primary hemorrhagic stroke*, the prelude to proper therapy is precise diagnosis that includes not only the extent and location of the infarcted brain, but knowledge of the arterial pathology and the extent of the spared collateral circulation. This is essential to try to devise therapy to prevent further cerebral damage and recurrence of the stroke. The clinical syndrome characterized by the history and physical examination, including a clear account of the temporal course before the stroke, remains the hallmark of the diagnostic approach. Refinements in laboratory and neuroradiologic diagnostic methods allow confirmation of the suspected clinical syndrome. We approach both ischemic and hemorrhagic stroke, with emphasis on prompt arrival at the precise pathophysiologic diagnosis. Although they carry risk, modern medical and surgical therapeutic options offer significant benefit not only for the management of acute stroke but also for prevention of primary and secondary stroke. This is true, however, only if a precise pathophysiologic diagnosis of the stroke or stroke-producing vascular lesion can be made. In this chapter, cerebrovascular disease is divided into the main primary ischemic and hemorrhagic stroke pathophysiologies.

Ischemic cerebrovascular disease is divided into two broad categories: thrombotic and embolic. Cerebral embolic strokes usually occur abruptly but may present with stuttering, fluctuating symptoms. Thrombotic strokes are heralded in 50% to 75% of patients by transient symptoms, transient ischemic attacks (TIAs), or a minor stroke leading to a more devastating event.

The clinical characteristics and temporal course of ischemic stroke are produced by the same pathophysiologic mechanism responsible for TIAs: large vessel thrombosis low flow, artery-to-artery, cardiogenic, or unknown source embolism, or small intracerebral penetrating vessel occlusion producing a lacuna. Of the many causes of primary thrombotic and embolic stroke, thrombosis complicating atherosclerosis accounts for most cases of thrombotic stroke, and embolus of an unknown or cardiac source accounts for most cases of embolic stroke. The symptoms and signs resulting from an ischemic stroke depend on the precise location of the occlusion and the extent of the spared collateral flow. The following descriptions apply to infarction and ischemia in specific arteries due to atherothrombosis, although similar syndromes may occur with other types of arterial pathology, after primary embolic stroke, and occasionally after primary intracerebral hemorrhage.

Primary hemorrhagic cerebrovascular disease requires the same precise pathophysiologic diagnostic rigor as ischemic cerebrovascular disease. Although the temporal course of the onset is abrupt, the potential posthemorrhagic course requires anticipatory clinical, laboratory, and neuroradiologic diagnostic assessments that often dictate further interventional treatment. Because neurosurgical intervention is often the treatment of choice, close collaboration between neurology and neurosurgery is required.

Large Vessel Atherothrombotic Cerebrovascular Disease

Risk Factors for Ischemic Stroke

Modifiable	Treatment options
Hypertension	Diet, exercise, medication
Hyperlipidemic states	Diet, exercise, medication
Diabetes	Diet, exercise, medication
Smoking	Cessation
Nonmodifiable	
Family history	

Figure 5-1. Risk factors for large vessel atherosclerosis. With the exception of smoking, the exact relation of the modifiable risk factors to the development of extracranial and intracranial atheromatous disease is uncertain. The control of weight through diet and exercise is essential when considering all the risk factors. Treatment options for specific risk factors are outlined elsewhere in this and other texts. Specific algorithms for the management of hypertension and hyperlipidemia exist and are reasonably effective [1].

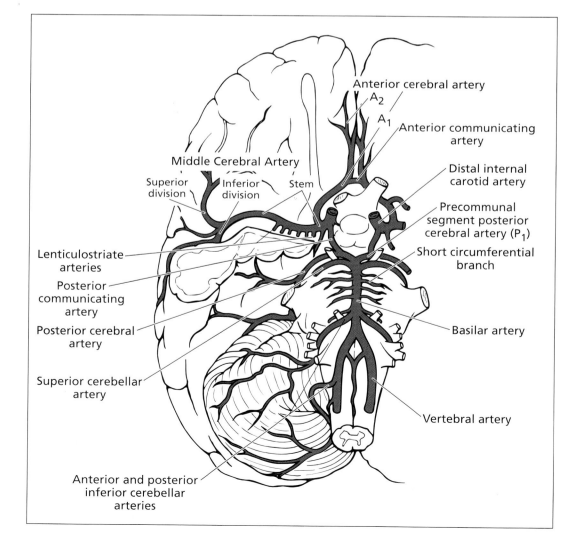

Middle Cerebral Artery
- Superior division
- Inferior division
- Stem

Anterior cerebral artery
- A2
- A1

Anterior communicating artery

Distal internal carotid artery

Precommunal segment posterior cerebral artery (P1)

Short circumferential branch

Lenticulostriate arteries

Posterior communicating artery

Posterior cerebral artery

Superior cerebellar artery

Anterior and posterior inferior cerebellar arteries

Basilar artery

Vertebral artery

Figure 5-2. Circle of Willis. When flow is reduced in an extracranial or intracranial large artery, the availability of collateral flow determines whether low-flow transient cerebral ischemia or infarction will ensue. The circle of Willis [2] is the main source of collateral flow when atheromatous lesions reduce flow in the internal carotid artery or in the basilar arteries. The circle of Willis is incomplete, with one or more atretic segments, in about 20% to 30% of the population.

Large vessel atherothrombotic cerebrovascular disease accounts for 15% of all ischemic strokes [3]. It conveniently divides into that which occurs in the internal carotid artery and its branches and that which occurs in the vertebrobasilar posterior cerebral artery system. Atherothrombotic stroke from these large vessels occurs when the atheromatous process forms thrombus and either occludes or hemodynamically significantly narrows the lumen of the vessel to produce the setting for low-flow stroke. In either case, available collateral circulation determines the final extent and location of the infarction. Both embolic and low-flow transient cerebral ischemic attacks can precede the development of infarction.

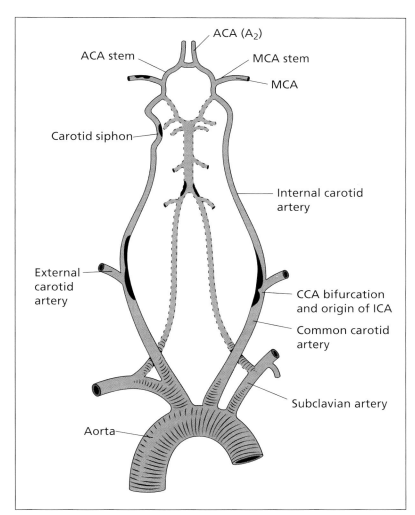

Figure 5-3. Common locations of atherosclerotic plaques in the anterior circulation. Although atherosclerosis is a generalized disease, atherosclerotic plaque deposition tends to be a strategically focal process. Plaques are predominantly located at arterial branch points and bifurcations. Furthermore, certain arteries, such as carotid and coronary arteries and those of the lower extremities, are particularly susceptible to plaque formation, while others, such as those of the upper extremities, are rarely affected. The reasons for the focal location and selective distribution of atheroma formation is uncertain. Many believe that it is related to local hemodynamic conditions. Atherothrombotic disease of the internal carotid system that most often leads to stroke tends to occur at four specific sites, listed in order of frequency: 1) the bifurcation of the common carotid artery (CCA) and the origin of the internal carotid artery (ICA) [4]; 2) the distal internal carotid artery (siphon or petrous portion); 3) the middle cerebral artery (MCA) stem; 4) the proximal anterior cerebral artery (ACA) stem and the origin of the proximal branches of the middle and anterior cerebral arteries. Atheroma of the bifurcation of more distal branches of the middle and anterior cerebral arteries are rare.

At the bifurcation of the common carotid artery–internal carotid artery origin, atherothrombotic occlusion is by far the most common cause of occlusion. Embolic occlusion is rare, as is primary thrombosis in the absence of atheromatous disease. In the distal portion of the internal carotid artery, however, embolic occlusion is more common, although less so than atherothrombotic cause. By contrast, in the middle cerebral artery (MCA) and anterior cerebral artery stems (M_1 and A_1 segments), primary embolic occlusion is the most common mechanism. When arterial occlusion occurs proximal to an adequate circle of Willis, the most common pathophysiologic mechanism of stroke is embolism rather than low flow. Only when collateral flow is limited do low-flow ischemia and infarction ensue. (*Adapted from* Kistler [1].)

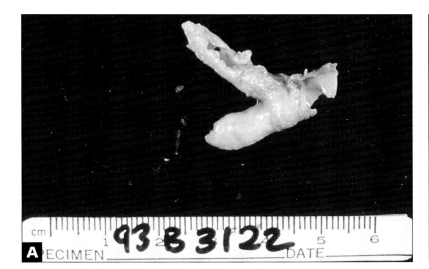

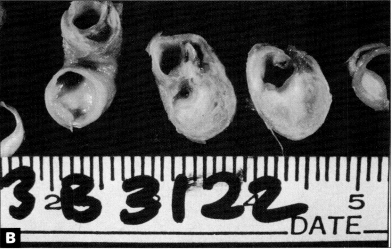

Figure 5-4. Pathologic specimen showing carotid atherosclerosis. **A,** Intact endarterectomy specimen. Note the bifurcation of the common carotid artery into the internal carotid artery below and the external carotid artery above. **B,** The same specimen as in *A,* cross-sectioned at 2-mm intervals and magnified. Note the 1-mm residual lumen diameter at the origin of the internal carotid artery. Most of the atheroma builds up on the internal carotid side (posterior portion of the bifurcation).

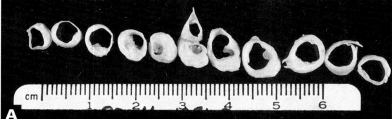

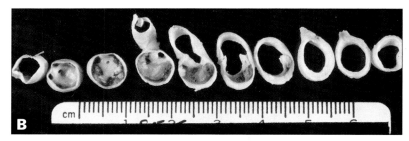

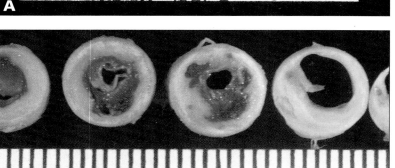

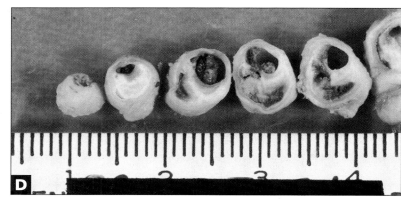

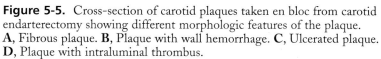

Figure 5-5. Cross-section of carotid plaques taken en bloc from carotid endarterectomy showing different morphologic features of the plaque. **A**, Fibrous plaque. **B**, Plaque with wall hemorrhage. **C**, Ulcerated plaque. **D**, Plaque with intraluminal thrombus.

The medical management of patients with acute ischemic stroke due to large vessel atherothrombotic disease consists of rapidly establishing the precise pathophysiologic arterial lesion responsible for the ischemia and the extent and location of the ischemia or infarct, as described in the previous section on laboratory investigation. After this is accomplished, urgent consideration of thrombolytic and antithrombotic therapy to help prevent clot propagation and to promote clot lysis should be considered.

It is also appropriate to consider strategies to protect ischemic brain from infarction. These therapeutic strategies are discussed in Figures 5-119–5-123. In all patients, with or without symptoms, when an extracranial or intracranial large vessel atherothrombotic lesion is discovered, therapy to prevent further progression of that lesion and possibly regression is paramount. Such therapy consists of standard treatment of risk factors as well as consideration of long-term antithrombotic or antiplatelet therapy, and in the case of carotid artery disease, acute or elective endarterectomy. Consideration of angioplasty for extracranial and intracranial arterial disease is under investigation but not considered standard practice except as innovative care.

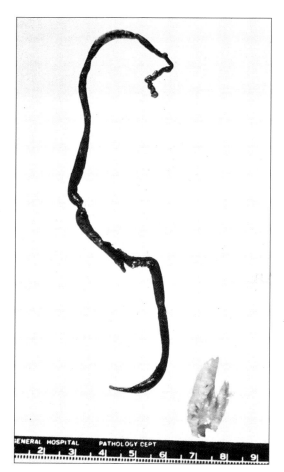

Figure 5-6. Pathologic specimen of endarterectomy with propagating thrombus. The endarterectomy specimen and propagating thrombus removed at the time of endarterectomy may have been long enough to extend into the middle cerebral artery origin. The patient had sudden onset of global aphasia and hemiplegia at angiography and was taken directly to the operating room. She was greatly improved after surgery. Thrombus propagation from the internal carotid artery origin to the middle cerebral artery stem is a less common cause of stroke in carotid occlusion than artery-to-artery embolism.

Pathophysiology and Clinical Syndromes of Carotid Stroke and Transient Ischemic Attacks

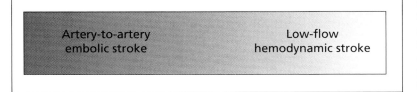

may occur together but usually occur separately. Low-flow stroke usually results from inadequate perfusion distal to a hemodynamically significant stenosis or occlusion of the internal carotid artery. It implies an inadequate collateral circulation from either the external carotid–ophthalmic artery anastomotic system or the circle of Willis. Embolic stroke occurs when a portion of the thrombus (platelet–fibrin complex) that accumulates in the area of the carotid stenosis or ulcerated plaque dislodges and travels into intracranial arteries. Clinical experience and pathologic examination suggest that in carotid disease, emboli, rather than low flow, cause most strokes. Embolism from atherosclerotic plaques may also cause TIAs, but when the events are short-lived, repetitive, and stereotypical, a low-flow cause is more likely.

Figure 5-7. Pathophysiology of carotid stroke and transient ischemic attacks (TIAs). Except for carotid occlusion and clot propagation into the middle cerebral artery stem, the two basic mechanisms of carotid artery stroke are low-flow hemodynamic and artery-to-artery embolism. They

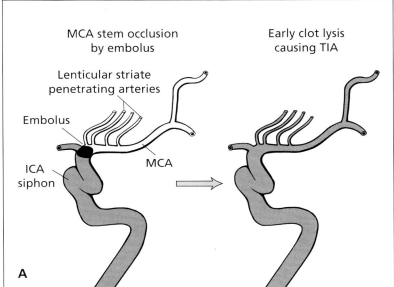

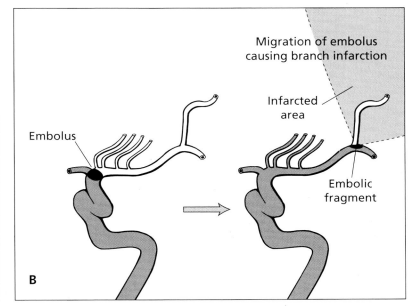

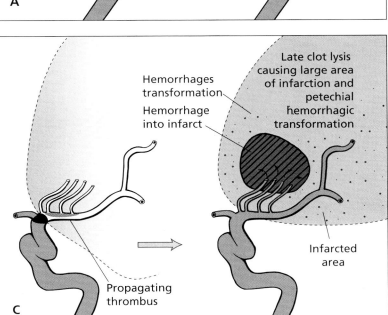

Figure 5-8. Carotid artery-to-artery embolic stroke. An embolus arising from a thrombus formed at the site of an atheromatous lesion may occlude the middle cerebral artery (MCA) stem or a more distal branch. Migration and lysis occur spontaneously. Reperfusion into an infarcted territory due to embolus lysis is thought to be the cause of hemorrhagic conversion of a blind infarct [5]. Migration, lysis, and dispersion of emboli as part of their natural evolution may result in fluctuating symptoms and signs. **A,** Clot lysis, if it occurs early enough, can lead to reversible ischemia. The deficit may resolve completely or in part. When emboli lyse and the symptoms resolve within 24 hours, a clinical diagnosis of transient ischemic attack (TIA) is customary. If the symptoms last only a few hours, however, an area of clinically silent infarction often is present and can be demonstrated by imaging studies. Thus, a better term, as proposed by Fisher, might be an *acceptable minor embolism.* Therefore, we generally refer to transient cerebral ischemia in the territory of the large vessel as either embolic or low flow. **B,** In some cases of proximal MCA stem embolism, the embolus may not completely block flow, allowing some distal MCA territory antegrade flow. If this embolus then migrates and lyses, it may block a distal branch, causing a distal branch territory infarct. **C,** On occasion, however, it may not lyse and becomes the nidus for further thrombus formation, Often the embolic MCA occlusion with propagated thrombi will eventually lyse, leading to recirculation in the infarcted brain. Petechial hemorrhagic transformation will likely ensue. Hemorrhage into infarct occurs less often. This is usually located in the territory supplied by the lenticular striate penetrating arteries. When this occurs, a complete MCA territory stroke that involves not only the deep white matter but also the cortical surface territory can ensue.

Factors Determining Clinical Findings of Carotid Artery-to-Artery Embolic Stroke

Size of the embolus and location of the arterial occlusion

Migration, lysis, and dispersion of the emboli and its timing

Presence or absence of cortical surface collateral circulation distal to the circle of Willis

Figure 5-9. Three main factors determining clinical findings of embolic stroke originating in the extracranial carotid artery. A small embolus that travels to a distal branch of the parent vessel usually causes a wedge-shaped ischemic infarct at the cortical surface. Conversely, a larger embolus that typically lodges in the middle cerebral artery stem generally results in cortical surface and deep white and gray matter infarcts. Rarely, cortical surface pial collateral flow is adequate enough so that the resulting infarct is mainly deep. (*Adapted from* Kistler and colleagues [2].)

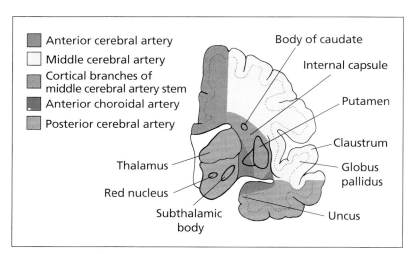

- Anterior cerebral artery
- Middle cerebral artery
- Cortical branches of middle cerebral artery stem
- Anterior choroidal artery
- Posterior cerebral artery

Body of caudate
Internal capsule
Putamen
Claustrum
Globus pallidus
Uncus
Subthalamic body
Red nucleus
Thalamus

Figure 5-10. Internal carotid artery embolic stroke in the distal main branch territory. The anterior cerebral artery is involved less often than the middle cerebral artery. Clinical manifestations include leg and foot weakness (cortical surface), a quiet state with delayed response, abulia (inferior frontal), and incontinence (cingulate gyrus). The middle cerebral artery stem is in the lenticulostriate artery territory. Hemiplegia (internal capsule) is a clinical manifestation. The anterior choroidal artery involves the branch of the distal internal carotid artery. Clinical manifestations include hemiplegia (internal capsule), hemisensory symptoms (thalamus and its cortical projections), and hemianopsia (geniculocalcarine optic radiation)—partial syndromes exist. In some patients, the postcommunal segment of the posterior cerebral artery (P_2) is an extension of the posterior communicating artery arising from the distal internal carotid artery. Hemianopic defects and memory loss may occur (calcarine medial temporal lobe). (*Adapted from* Kistler and colleagues [2].)

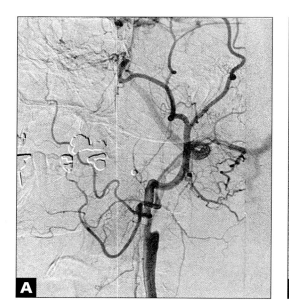

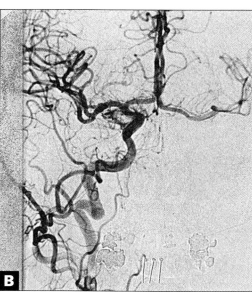

Figure 5-11. Internal carotid artery (ICA) occlusion with collateral flow across the circle of Willis (**A, B**). Asymptomatic occlusion of the ICA. Anterior (*A*) ICA origin occlusion. Collateral flow across the circle of Willis in a patient with transient symptoms in the nonoccluded carotid territory. Low-flow stroke and embolic stroke did not occur in the carotid territory of the occluded side.

Atherothrombotic Disease of the Siphon Portion of the Internal Carotid Artery

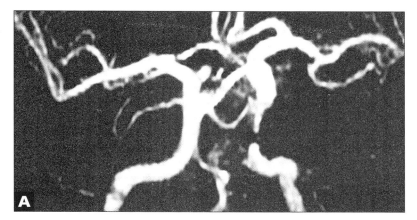

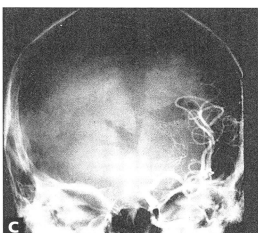

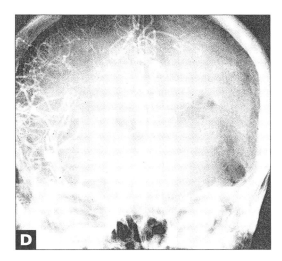

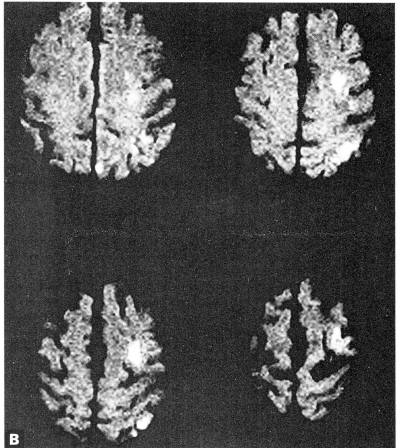

wide open carotid bifurcation, but Doppler examination identified low diastolic flow velocity and a sharp blunted systolic upstroke. A significant stenosis of the petrous part of the left carotid artery is seen on MRI angiography. **B**, Diffusion-weighted MRI of the brain between attacks showed a clinically relevant lesion in the right frontal cortex. Atherosclerosis of the carotid siphon is not as common as proximal internal carotid artery disease. Increased incidence of stroke is found when the lesions become large enough to produce a stenosis of more than 50% [8]. Clinically, stroke or TIA secondary to intracranial carotid stenosis is indistinguishable from the bifurcation stenosis. Noninvasive carotid examination and transcranial Doppler may help in diagnosis. High-resistance flow at the origin of the internal carotid artery, indicated by a very low diastolic velocity and sharp systolic upstroke, may suggest distal stenosis. Ophthalmic artery flow may be reduced or reversed if the siphon stenosis is proximal to its origin; but in contrast to common carotid bifurcation stenosis, it is usually normal. **C**, **D**, Angiogram (*C*) demonstrating a stenotic lesion in the siphon portion of the left internal carotid artery (*left side* of angiogram) in a 74-year-old diabetic woman with recurrent 10- to 20-minute episodes of difficulty with speech without arm, hand, or face weakness. The left internal carotid artery supplies the left middle cerebral artery stem (M_1 segment) but not the left anterior cerebral artery stem (A_1 segment). The angiogram (*D*) of the right carotid artery demonstrates that it fills the distal (A_2) segments of both anterior cerebral arteries by the anterior communicating artery. It does not fill the left A_1 anterior cerebral artery, suggesting that it is atretic. The distal left anterior cerebral artery (A_2) branches fill out the cortical surface border zone. We interpret the symptoms of difficulty forming words as recurrent stereotyped transient ischemia in the cortical surface motor–speech area. Even though the patient had recurrent episodes for several weeks, she became symptom free shortly after aspirin was started. She died 3 years later of acute myocardial infarction.

Figure 5-12. Atherothrombotic disease of the siphon portion of the internal carotid artery. Distal (postophthalmic) internal carotid artery stenosis presents as an embolic stroke or transient ischemic attack (TIA), with the circle of Willis intact, or as a low-flow stroke or TIA, with the circle of Willis incomplete [6,7]. We subscribe to the theory of a low-flow, as opposed to an embolic, cause of the ipsilateral hemispheric symptoms, that is, the availability of adequate collateral flow through the circle of Willis [6]. **A**, Magnetic resonance image (MRI) of a patient who presented with recurrent stereotypic episodes of right hand weakness associated with aphasia. Each episode lasted about 1 to 2 minutes, and the patient reported up to 20 spells per day for at least 1 week. Carotid duplex ultrasonography showed a

Atherosclerotic Disease of the Middle Cerebral Artery

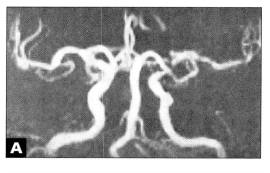

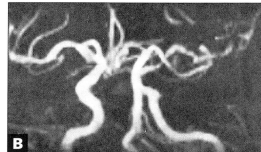

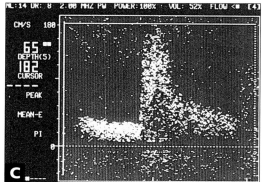

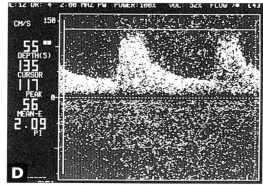

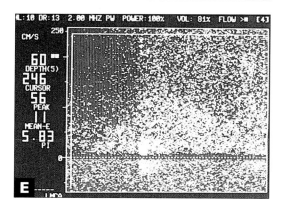

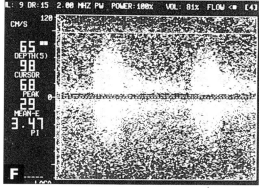

Figure 5-13. Middle cerebral artery (MCA) (M_1) origin stenosis with recurrent focal low-flow transient ischemic attacks (TIAs). In relation to internal carotid artery (ICA) origin or siphon stenosis, atheromatous lesions of the MCA stem are relatively rare. Patients with MCA stenosis tend to be female, young, and black or Asian. They have relatively less ischemic heart disease and hypercholesterolemia [9]. When the MCA stem is stenosed, collateral circulation comes from the anterior cerebral artery and the posterior cerebral artery through the cortical surface pial–pial anastomotic branches. Warning low-flow, recurrent, short-lived stereotypical TIAs usually occur before the stroke develops. Symptoms of MCA stem stenosis occur as a result of ischemia either in the distal field lenticulostriate territory or in the cortical surface distal field of the upper and lower divisions of the MCA stem. They may resemble those of low-flow hemodynamic TIAs and stroke associated with a tight carotid stenosis. **A, B,** Magnetic resonance angiogram of an 85-year-old man with 5- to 20-minute episodes of right arm numbness and heaviness without speech difficulty. Note the very proximal left MCA stem stenosis and the widely patent right MCA stem as well as both distal internal carotid arteries and the basilar artery. **C–F,** Transcranial Doppler depiction of flow in both the MCA (M_1) and the anterior cerebral artery (ACA) (A_1) stems. Note the high-peak systolic flow velocities in the right ACA stem (*C*), compared with the left ACA stem (*D*). Does this suggest collateral flow across the anterior communicating artery and up the A_2 anterior communicating segment of the left ACA to the left ACA–MCA border zone? The high-peak systolic velocity and high end-diastolic velocity with spectral broadening noted in the left MCA stem (*E*) indicates the presence of proximal MCA severe stenosis as compared to the normal (*F*).

Atherothrombotic Disease of the Vertebral Artery

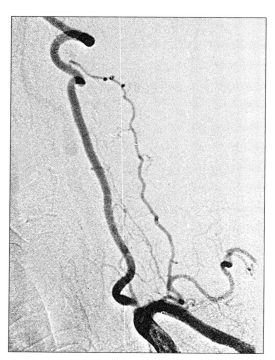

Figure 5-14. Atheromatous lesions of the proximal vertebral artery. Angiogram showing an atherosclerotic lesion of vertebral artery origin in a patient without symptoms. Atherothrombotic lesions in the vertebral artery have a predilection for the first and fourth segments [1,2]. In patients with proximal stenosis, a bruit may be heard over the supraclavicular region. Although the atheromatous narrowing at the origin (first segment) may be significant, it seldom causes low-flow brain stem stroke. Collateral flow from the contralateral vertebral artery, the ascending cervical and ascending thyrocervical arteries, or the occipital branch of the external carotid artery is usually sufficient to prevent ischemia from a low-flow state [1,2]. Artery-to-artery embolic stroke may also arise from these proximal lesions. In 10% to 20% of patients, one of the two vertebral arteries is too small (atretic vertebral artery) to contribute significant blood to the brain stem. In this case, if there is an atherothrombotic lesion, particularly in the distal segment of the larger vertebral artery, low-flow transient ischemic attacks (TIAs) or stroke in posterior circulation may occur. Symptoms of the TIAs are dizziness or vertigo, numbness of the ipsilateral face and contralateral limbs, diplopia, hoarseness, dysarthria, and dysphagia. Dislodging of part of the atherothrombotic lesion from the proximal vertebral artery can also cause embolic stroke in the distal vertebral or basilar artery. Lesions in the fourth segment of the vertebral artery proximal to the origin of the posteroinferior cerebellar artery can cause stroke or TIA in the lateral medulla (Wallenberg's syndrome) and in the posterior surface of the cerebellum [1,2]. (*From* Kistler and colleagues [2]; with permission.)

A. Sites of Arterial Occlusion in Patients With Medullary Infarction

Sites of arterial occlusion	Patients, *n*	Total, %
Vertebral artery	16	38
Vertebral artery and PICA	11	26
PICA alone	6	14
Artery of lateral medullary fossa	1	2
None found	8	19
Total	42	

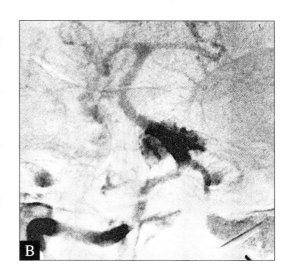

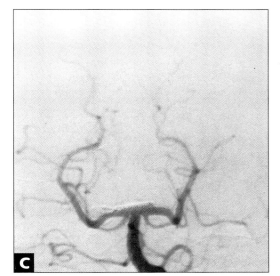

Figure 5-15. Sites of arterial occlusion in patients with lateral medullary infarction. **A**, The common arteriopathologic etiologies of lateral medullary infarction [10]. In patients with lateral medullary infarction, the most common vascular lesion is the occlusion of the intracranial vertebral artery proximal to the posterior inferior cerebellar artery (PICA) origin. Less often, lateral

medullary stroke is caused by occlusion of the PICA alone. The clinical syndrome of the lateral medullary infarction is distinct because of its anatomic location in the medulla.

Distal vertebral disease leading to recurrent stereotyped transient ischemic attack (TIA). **B**, The angiogram demonstrates a right vertebral pre-PICA stenotic lesion with flow distally that refluxes down the left vertebral artery, which is occluded more proximally at its pre-PICA segment. **C**, Bilateral carotid angiogram demonstrated that there was no collateral supply through the posterior communicating arteries to the posterior cerebral arteries and top of the basilar artery. Thus, there was no chance for reversed flow down the basilar artery to supply the collateral. The patient, a 65-year-old man with coronary disease, experienced many episodes of being pulled to the left and a general feeling of profound fatigue, sometimes associated with focal left face, arm, and leg weakness. Episodes lasted no longer than 10 to 20 minutes. He was placed on heparin and then converted to warfarin. The symptoms cleared but returned a year later. The patient was again placed on heparin for 2 weeks and then warfarin. Thereafter, symptoms subsided. The patient has subsequently undergone a successful coronary artery bypass graft procedure. These episodes represented a transient ischemia of the distal left vertebral artery territory in the medial and lateral left medulla. The generalized fatigue for 10 to 20 minutes is more difficult to localize but occurs often in patients with basilar territory ischemia.

Medial medullary infarction is rare. It occurs with distal vertebral occlusion or occlusion of a penetrating branch of the distal vertebral artery. Presumably, atheromatous occlusion rather than embolism is the main cause. Rarely, both medial and lateral medullary infarctions are combined. Lateral medullary infarction alone, however, is by far the most common result of vertebral occlusion and posterior inferior cerebellar artery occlusion. Partial lateral medullary syndromes are more common than the complete syndrome. Explanations of this variation are based on whether the vertebral artery or the PICA is occluded, whether the occlusion is atherothrombotic or embolic with lysis, the availability of collateral flow, and whether only a vertebral or proximal PICA penetrator is involved. Vertebral artery or PICA occlusion, which may be extensive, can lead to extensive posterior inferior cerebellar surface infarction with edema. Surgical decompression can be life-saving, with excellent recovery. It should be considered when the patient becomes stuporous or has bilateral upgoing toes, worsening dysarthria, or diplopia.

Atherothrombotic Disease of the Basilar Artery

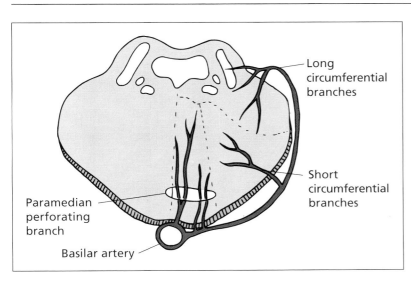

Figure 5-16. Anatomy of the basilar artery. The normal anatomy of the basilar artery and its branches can be divided into three groups: 1) Seven to ten paramedian branches, which supply the ventral side of pons (basis pontis) on either side of the midline. 2) Five to seven short circumferential artery (SCA) branches, which supply the lateral two thirds of the pons and middle and superior cerebellar peduncles. 3) Two pairs of long circumferential arteries (superior cerebellar and anterior inferior cerebellar arteries), which course around the pons to supply the cerebellar hemispheres and cranial nerves.

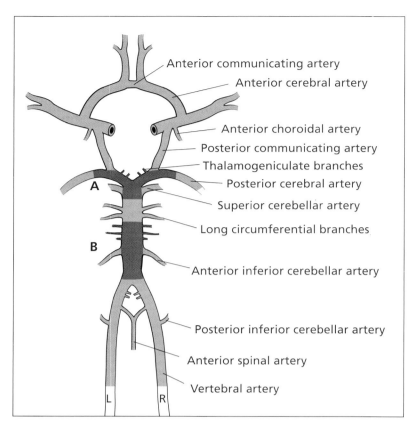

tends to localize in the most distal part, where the basilar artery bifurcates into two posterior cerebral arteries. The resulting so-called top of basilar syndrome begins with loss of consciousness and quadriparesis. As it evolves, the patient often develops hypersomnia, bilateral ptosis, and impaired vertical gaze. When both distal posterior cerebral artery (PCA) territories are involved, cortical blindness may ensue. **B**, Atherothrombotic disease, on the other hand, commonly affects the proximal part of the artery, although it can affect any part of the vessel [11]. The clinical picture varies depending on the availability of retrograde collateral flow from the posterior communicating arteries. Among 18 cases of basilar artery occlusion studied by Kubik and Adams [11], 11 were atherothrombotic. The other eight were embolic. The locations of the arterial occlusion are shown.

In general, atherothrombotic occlusion of a branch of the basilar artery affects one side of the brain stem, causing unilateral symptoms and signs of motor, sensory, and cranial nerve dysfunction. Occlusion of a perforating branch that supplies the basis pontis causes unilateral weakness. Perforating branch infarction never crosses the midline except at the top of the basilar artery. There, the penetrating branches arising from the very top of the basilar artery as it bifurcates to each posterior cerebral artery stem may supply both sides of the brain stem. When the basilar artery is occluded, the infarction usually causes bilateral brain stem symptoms and signs. Basilar occlusion is often heralded by transient cerebral ischemia also involving both sides of the brain stem. The clinical findings of basilar artery occlusion may be progressive or may fluctuate for days before the fixed deficit occurs. When the basis pontis is involved bilaterally, a "locked-in" state may occur. In the complete locked-in syndrome, the midbrain is also involved, and the patient is quadriplegic with bilateral facial weakness and severe eye movement abnormality. Although consciousness is preserved owing to the sparing of the midbrain and pontine tegmentum, the patient is not able to respond owing to the lack of motor control of the eyes, face, mouth, tongue, or extremities. Some patients have been able to respond by blinking. When the particular activating system is involved in the midbrain tegmentum, stupor and coma ensue.

Figure 5-17. Top of basilar syndrome and atherothrombotic disease. **A**, Stroke in the basilar artery territory may occur as a result of local thrombosis or secondary to an embolism. Embolic occlusion of the basilar artery

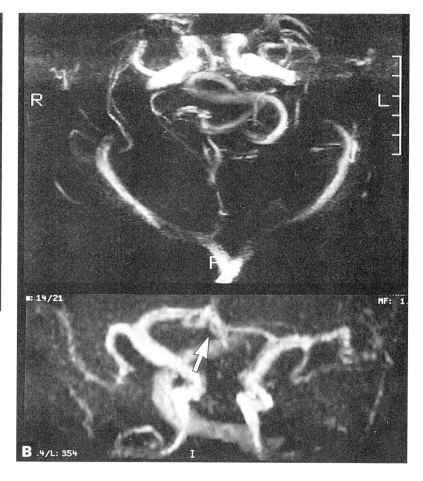

Figure 5-18. Dolichoectasia of the basilar artery. A 51-year-old man presented with recurrent episodes of ataxia, diplopia, and vertigo. **A**, Magnetic resonance image of the patient's brain shows an ectatic basilar artery with significant mass effect on the brain stem and kinking at the pontomedullary junction as well as a bilateral paramedian pontine tegmental infarction. The absence of a signal void area in the basilar artery may represent intraluminal thrombus or slow flow. The dolichoectatic basilar artery (*arrow*) and distorted brain stem (*arrowhead*) are also seen. **B**, Magnetic resonance angiogram with slow-flow susceptibility demonstrates an S-shaped basilar artery. The basilar artery (*arrow*) is seen.

(*Continued on next page*)

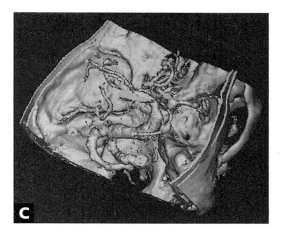
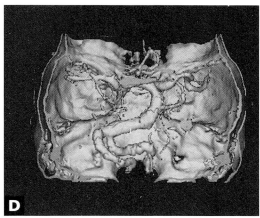

Figure 5-18. (*Continued*) **C, D,** Three-dimensional reconstruction of the computed tomographic angiography of the dolichoectatic basilar artery. Dolichoectasia of the basilar artery is sometimes referred to as a *fusiform aneurysm.* Symptoms and signs may be caused by pressure from the dilated artery on nearby cranial nerves and on the brain stem. Occasionally, ischemic strokes occur, which are thought to result from three mechanisms: occlusion of the basilar artery by intraluminal thrombus, blockade of the orifice of the penetrators by intraluminal thrombus, and distal embolization [12–14].

Investigation of Large Vessel Atherothrombotic Disease

A. Extracranial and Intracranial Arterial Investigation

Arterial test	Methods	Purpose
Carotid ultrasonographic studies Direct tests	Range-gated pulsed Doppler flow analysis and B-mode imaging	To visualize (by B-mode image) and assess the velocity and pattern of blood flow (by Doppler) at the bifurcation of the common carotid artery
Duplex ultrasound study		To look for evidence of a more distal stenotic lesion that might affect the flow in the proximal internal carotid artery
Indirect tests		To assess flow in the proximal to midvertebral artery
Oculoplethysmography	Oculosystolic pressure measurement	To assess whether a proximal ICA lesion is hemodynamically significant
Ophthalmic artery transcranial Doppler	Range-gated pulsed Doppler measurement of ophthalmic artery flow velocity, pattern, and direction	To assess whether a proximal ICA lesion is hemodynamically significant
Transcranial Doppler (anterior)	Range-gated pulsed Doppler measurement of ophthalmic, distal ICA, anterior, middle, and posterior cerebral artery flow velocity and spectral configuration, in both vertebral arteries	To identify a hemodynamically significant stenotic lesion at the ICA origin or in the siphon portion of the ICA, the posterior, middle, and anterior cerebral artery stems
		To identify the availability of collaterals and, the presence of a flow-reducing lesion in both vertebral arteries and in the basilar artery
Transcranial Doppler (posterior)	Range-gated pulsed Doppler measurement of flow velocity and spectral configuration in both distal vertebral arteries and in the basilar artery	To identify the presence of a flow-reducing lesion in both vertebral arteries and in the basilar artery
MRA	MRI of the brain and the extracranial and intracranial arterial system	To detect the location and severity of atherosclerotic lesions at the origin of the ICA, the vertebrobasilar junction, and the posterior, middle, and anterior cerebral artery stems
		To determine the availability of collateral flow
Spiral CT angiography	CT imaging of the extracranial and intracranial arterial system enhanced by intravenous contrast agents	To detect the location and severity of atherosclerotic lesions at the origin of the ICA, the vertebrobasilar junction, and the posterior, middle, and anterior cerebral artery stems
		To determine the availability of collateral flow
Conventional cerebral angiography*	Selective cerebral arterial angiography	To detect the location and severity of atherosclerotic lesions at the origin of the ICA, the vertebrobasilar junction, and the posterior, middle, and anterior cerebral artery stems
		To determine the availability of collateral flow

*Used only when the above methods do not clarify the pathophysiologic arterial lesion and proper therapy depends on that clarification.

Figure 5-19. Diagnosis of cerebral ischemia [1,15]. (*Continued on next page*)

B. Imaging Techniques for Evaluation of Acute Ischemic Stroke

Cerebral imaging technique	Methods	Purpose
CT	X-ray CT	To rule out intracerebral hemisphere delayed detection and resolution at the cortical surface and in the posterior fossa make it less sensitive than MRI in detecting infarcts
MRI		
MRI standard T1, T2 proton density	Nuclear magnetic resonance CT	Reliably detects cerebral infarction within the first 24 hours with adequate resolution of the cortical surface and posterior fossa
Diffusion MRI	Diffusion pulse sequence	Reliably detects cerebral infarction down to 3 mm within minutes; resolution not as good as with standard MRI
Perfusion MRI	Perfusion pulse sequence	Detects areas of decreased perfusion that can be compared to areas of actual infarction determined by diffusion techniques, thereby identifying presumed areas of ischemia that have not yet infarcted
Susceptibility MRI	Susceptibility pulse sequence	Detects areas of recent and prior intracerebral hemorrhage
PET scanning	PET using radionucleotides and CT techniques to look at oxygen and glucose metabolism in an effort to distinguish ischemic viable tissue from infarcted tissue	Largely research

Figure 5-19. (*Continued*) When a patient presents with transient or sustained symptoms that suggest cerebral ischemia, the neurologic history and physical examination should suggest á possible presumed pathophysiologic diagnosis that includes the area of ischemia or infarction and the nature of the arterial pathology. The laboratory assessment is meant to confirm that presumed diagnosis. New developments and refinements in older diagnostic techniques allow the diagnosis to be made noninvasively in most cases. In the case of large vessel atherothrombotic disease, the precise location, suggested pathology (atheromatous, dissection, or other), and severity of the lesion can be identified. If infarction has set in, the precise area of infarction can be localized. The evaluation of the patient with suspected stroke, therefore, should be complete enough to rule in or out large vessel atherothrombotic disease or dissection as a cause of the cerebral ischemia and infarction; that is, it should rule out embolism (from a cardiac, aortic, or uncertain source) (Figs. 5-42–5-64) or lacunar (small vessel) infarction (Figs. 5-35–5-41) and other causes of extracranial and intracranial arterial disease, including dissection, vasculitis, and so forth. Thus, the immediate goal of the evaluation of a patient with suspected stroke is to rule in or out large vessel atherothrombotic disease or dissection and to decide whether the suspected stroke is small vessel lacunar, embolic, or of another cause. If, for example, non–artery-to-artery embolus is suspected because large vessel disease is excluded, then further evaluation of the embolic source should be undertaken, usually after preventive therapy is instituted. The first line of laboratory investigation for any stroke patient, after an electrocardiogram and blood work have been obtained, includes investigation of possible large vessel extracranial and intracranial pathology and investigation of the intracranial territory suspected of undergoing infarction (*ie*, brain imaging) (pathology in the parent vessel).

A, Arterial techniques should be used in a focused manner depending on the nature of the problem and on the individual institution's standard of practice. For example, to evaluate a patient with a suspected internal carotid artery (ICA) origin stenotic lesion that is asymptomatic and detected by the presence of a bruit, we use duplex Doppler and transcranial Doppler tests initially. If these tests provide clear indication that a hemodynamically significant stenosis is present with a residual lumen diameter of 1.5 mm or less, we then consider endarterectomy [6,7,16–18]. If this consideration suggests that the patient represents an appropriate medical or cardiac risk, and surgery is suggested, we then proceed to a magnetic resonance angiogram for confirmation of the lesion and identification of distal intracranial arterial stenoses missed by transcranial Doppler. If that is nonconfirmatory, then spiral computed tomographic angiography is considered. Conventional angiography is considered only after these studies are equivocal or cannot be done and the risk of angiography is deemed appropriate [1,15].

B, Magnetic resonance imaging (MRI) techniques are now in standard use for evaluation of patients with acute ischemic stroke. Computed tomography (CT) scanning is reserved for ruling out hemorrhage as a cause of the acute symptoms and signs. The value of MRI over CT is reduced after the first 24 hours unless the stroke consists of subtle cortical surface areas of infarct or small areas of infarct in the posterior fossa. It is most important to identify not only the extent and location of the infarct but also the presence or absence of the offending arterial lesion. Depending on the pathophysiology and timing of the stroke, this may require only a CT scan combined with carotid duplex and transcranial Doppler extracranial and intracranial arterial flow. Within 24 hours of an acute stroke, diffusion-weighted MRI imaging and MRI angiography are generally required. MRA—magnetic resonance angiography; PET—positron-emission tomography.

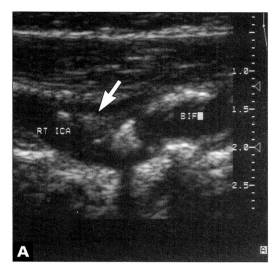

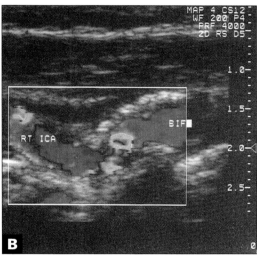

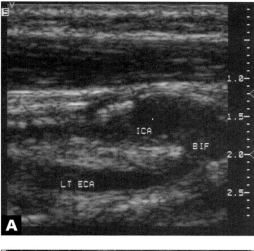

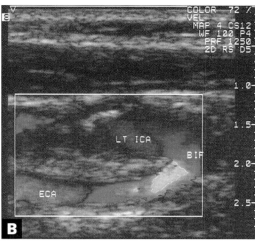

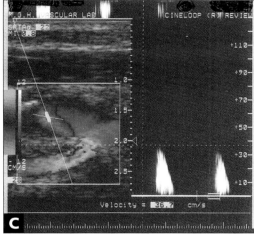

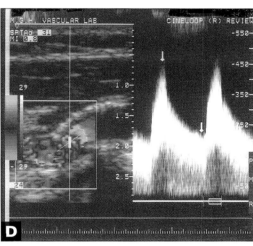

Figure 5-20. Duplex (triplex) scan of the bifurcation of the common carotid artery combined with color-coded real-time assessment of flow. **A**, Dense plaque with calcification (*arrow*) at the anterior portion of the internal carotid artery (ICA). **B**, Color-coded Doppler flow data that present an almost real-time picture of flowing blood. Data can be converted back to frequency intensity depiction of the Doppler shift frequency of flowing blood. Thus, they can provide information about the peak systolic and end-diastolic flow velocities in an artery. The B-mode imaging of the arterial wall provides information about atheromatous plaque location and morphology. Areas of calcification in the atherosclerotic plaque appear as an echolucent acoustic shadow on the B-mode imaging. Dense fibrous plaque appears bright (white) and homogeneous, whereas hypodense fatty plaque appears dull and gray. Ulcer craters appear as an irregular surface between the B-mode static image and the color-coded image of flowing blood in the lumen of the vessel.

Figure 5-21. Carotid duplex (triplex) Doppler scan of a tightly stenotic lesion at the origin of the internal carotid artery. **A**, Carotid duplex examination of the extracranial carotid artery of a patient with severe internal carotid artery (ICA) stenosis. The B-mode ultrasound image shows dense fibrous plaque in the ICA distal to the bifurcation. **B**, The color-coded B-mode image shows sluggish flow in the area of stenosis. **C**, The range-gated pulsed-wave Doppler image of the area proximal to the stenosis shows no flow in the diastolic phase, a finding consistent with a high-resistance Doppler flow pattern of a distal occlusion. **D**, At the level of stenosis, markedly increased peak systolic and end-diastolic flow velocities and a low pulsatility index are demonstrated. Turbulent flow is also demonstrated by the mixed color in the color-coded B-mode image and by the loss of acoustic window in the Doppler waveform. The range-gated pulsed-wave Doppler samples a small volume of flowing blood inside the vessel at specific points seen on B-mode pictures. This method analyzes the frequency and intensity components of flow. The higher the velocity of the flow, the higher is the frequency in both peak systole and in diastole, and the tighter is the stenosis. Turbulent flow is detected by spectral broadening. The narrower the residual diameter, the more spectral broadening is detected.

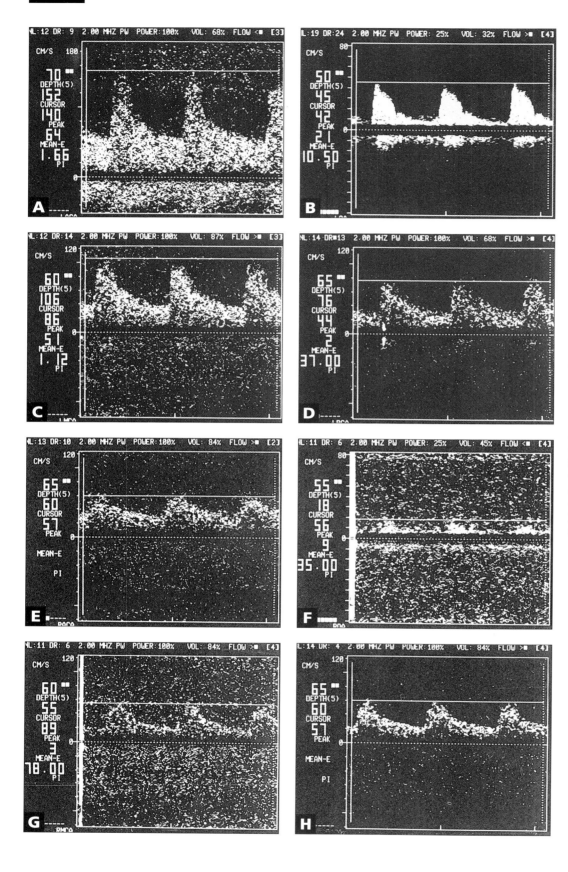

Figure 5-22. Transcranial Doppler examination. Transcranial Doppler is used for assessment of blood flow velocity and direction in the distal internal carotid artery (ICA), middle cerebral artery (MCA), anterior cerebral artery (ACA), and posterior cerebral artery (PCA) stems, the ophthalmic arteries, and the distal vertebral and basilar arteries. Transcranial Doppler is useful for evaluating and understanding the collateral flow above a stenotic lesion at the origin of the ICA [1,16,17]. In addition, it can detect the presence of significant stenosis in the ipsilateral MCA stem and determine if the flow is reduced in the MCA stem owing to a hemodynamically significant ICA lesion [1]. Transcranial Doppler signs of hemodynamically significant stenosis in the proximal ICA include the following [16,17]: 1) reversal of ophthalmic artery (OA) flow or attenuation of flow velocity compared with the contralateral side; 2) attenuation of ipsilateral MCA flow velocity suggesting inadequate collateral circulation; 3) reversed direction of flow in ipsilateral ACA; 4) increased flow velocity in the contralateral A_1 segment of ACA; 5) increased velocity in the ipsilateral PCA, usually occurring in the case of an atretic or absent anterior communicating artery.

This is an example of a transcranial Doppler study of a patient with hemodynamically significant right ICA stenosis with a residual lumen diameter of 1 mm. Note the low peak systolic flow velocity in the right MCA compared with the left side. The right ACA and ophthalmic artery flow are reversed to serve as collateral vessels. **A,** Left ACA; **B,** left OA; **C,** left MCA; **D,** left PCA; **E,** right ACA; **F,** right OA; **G,** right MCA; **H,** right PCA.

Common Carotid Duplex Doppler and Transcranial Doppler Criteria for a Hemodynamically Significant Stenotic Lesion

ICA duplex Doppler

Peak systolic velocity (PSV) >440 cm/s

End-diastolic velocity (EDR) >155 cm/s

Carotid index (PSV/EDR) >10

Transcranial Doppler

Transorbital approach

Reversed flow in the ophthalmic artery

≥50% Peak systolic velocity difference between the distal ICAs (contralateral > unilateral) in patients with only unilateral stenosis*

Transtemporal approach

≥35% Reduction in ipsilateral middle cerebral artery (MCA) peak systolic velocity relative to the contralateral MCA*

≥50% Increase in the contralateral anterior cerebral artery (ACA) peak systolic velocity relative to the ipsilateral ACA*

≥35% Decrement in ipsilateral MCA peak systolic velocity relative to the ipsilateral posterior cerebral artery (PCA)*

Criteria requiring that the contralateral carotid artery does not have a significant stenosis.

Figure 5-23. Common carotid duplex Doppler and transcranial Doppler criteria for a hemodynamically significant stenotic lesion (pressure drop across it) at the origin of the internal carotid artery (residual lumen diameter 1.5 mm or less). These Doppler criteria have been developed by examining the residual lumen diameter of the intact endarterectomy specimen. The goal is to identify more accurately carotid stenosis that, by conventional angiographic criteria (North American Symptomatic Carotid Endarterectomy Trial [NASCET]), are 70% or more stenotic [16,17]. Because, in our practice, angiography is largely avoided in favor of these Doppler techniques combined with magnetic resonance angiography when assessing patients with symptomatic and asymptomatic internal carotid artery (ICA) origin stenosis, the percentage of stenosis is not applicable. In our experience, a residual lumen diameter of 1.5 mm or less, of ICA origin, usually reflects the degree of narrowing associated with a pressure drop across it, and peak systolic flow velocity changes distally. Given a distal ICA diameter of 5 to 6 mm, this is a 70% to 75% stenosis by NASCET criteria. Each of the five Doppler criteria noted in this table have a 100% specificity but a low sensitivity in identifying such a lesion. When they are taken together with carotid duplex ultrasound, the sensitivity increases [16,17].

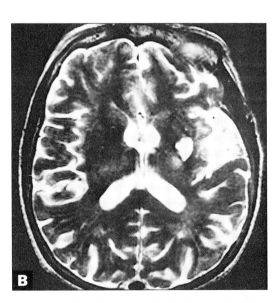

Figure 5-24. T2-weighted magnetic resonance imaging (MRI) scans of a middle cerebral artery (MCA) territory ischemic stroke in a patient with a tightly stenotic interior carotid artery origin atherothrombotic lesion (**A–D**). Note the area of infarction in the corona radiata and also at the cortical surface gray-matter–white-matter junction. MRI is superior to computed tomographic scanning in detecting small areas of cortical surface infarction. The corona radiata infarct is too large to be a lacunar infarction, and the cortical surface involvement virtually excludes occlusion of a single lenticulostriate penetrating artery arising from the MCA stem as a cause. We suspect the cause was a single artery-to-artery embolus.

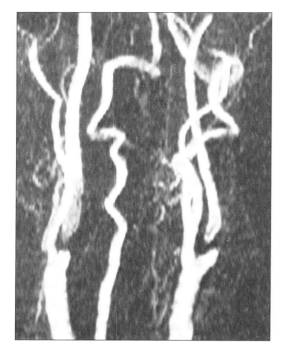

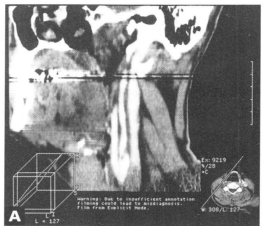

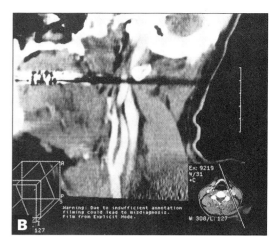

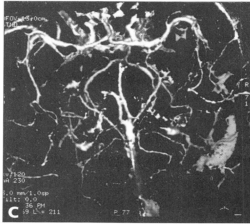

Figure 5-25. Two-dimensional time-of-flight magnetic resonance angiography (MRA) of a patient with severe bilateral internal carotid artery (ICA) stenosis. The signal dropout (an area where the column of flowing blood is interrupted on the image) at the origin of the ICA usually signifies stenosis of 70% or greater. The signal loss is attributed to disturbed or turbulent flow immediately distal to the severe stenosis. The signal dropout is due to phase dispersion as a result of turbulence. Signal loss may also occur as a result of magnetic susceptibility effects of bone–air interfaces, for example, at the carotid siphon. MRA cannot reliably detect the difference between near occlusion and complete occlusion, nor can it detect ulcers. Furthermore, a gap is not always present at the site of an ICA origin stenotic lesion with a residual lumen diameter of 1.5 mm [18].

Figure 5-26. Computed tomographic angiography (CTA) images of the neck. **A**, CTA images of the neck showing a tightly stenotic lesion of the proximal internal carotid artery (ICA). **B**, Normal common carotid bifurcation. **C**, Three-dimensional reconstruction CTA of the arteries at the base of

the brain showing a right middle cerebral artery stem stenosis. CTA uses rapid-sequence computed tomography (CT) scanning during intravenous bolus injection of contrast media. Using computerized reconstruction of the images, the vascular structure can be visualized. The images can be viewed in three dimensions. Because the CT scan visualizes bone, the relations of the vessels to the bony structure can be determined. Moreover, for the bifurcation of the common carotid artery, calcific components of the carotid plaque can sometimes be detected. Computed tomographic angiography can also visualize the vertebrobasilar junction, the stem of the middle cerebral artery, and the siphon portion of the carotid artery, which are the four most common sites of symptomatic atheromatous disease of the extracranial and intracranial arterial system. We use CTA when noninvasive Doppler techniques and magnetic resonance angiography suggest but do not confirm the presence of a stenotic lesion at these sites. Conventional angiography is used if its risks outweigh its benefits for establishing a diagnosis with a therapeutic implication.

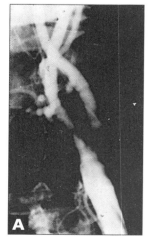

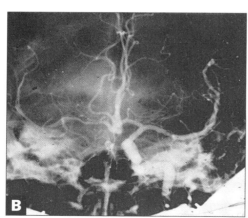

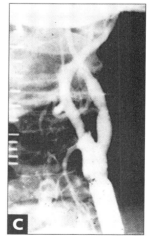

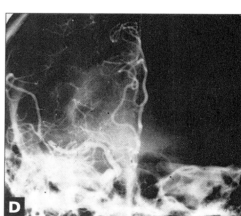

Figure 5-27. Angiogram showing a tightly stenotic lesion at the origin of the right internal carotid artery (ICA) (**A**). A normal left ICA filling both anterior cerebral arteries and the right middle cerebral artery stem across the anterior circle of Willis (**B**). The left ICA opened 6 days after endarterectomy, after the lesion had given rise to an artery-to-artery embolic stroke, noted in the lower right (**C**). The right ICA supplies both the right middle cerebral artery stem and the right anterior cerebral artery since it is open. The cross-flow across the circle of Willis is now not necessary. Unfortunately, the middle cerebral stem was occluded distally by the artery-to-artery embolus (**D**).

The patient was a 71-year-old man with an asymptomatic stenosis of right ICA origin who developed an artery-to-artery embolic stroke 6 days after the angiogram while he was waiting for an endarterectomy. The stenotic lesion of the right ICA origin was hemodynamically significant enough to reduce distal ICA pressure and flow and to allow the anterior circle of Willis collateral to take over, in part, the blood supply to the right hemisphere. It is our view that this circumstance is a precursor to thrombus formation and subsequent embolism in patients with stenotic lesions at the origin of the internal carotid artery [1,2,6].

Management of Atherothrombotic Cerebrovascular Disease

Therapy for Atherothrombotic Cerebral Vascular Disease

Risk factor management

Surgical management

  Carotid endarterectomy

    In patients with symptoms

    In patients without symptoms

  Angioplasty

    Of the internal carotid artery origin

    Of intracranial atherothrombotic lesions

  Extracranial–intracranial bypass grafting

Medical management

  Antiplatelet therapy

  Antithrombotic

  Thrombolitic therapy

  Neuroprotective therapy

Figure 5-28. Therapy for atherothrombotic cerebral vascular disease. The three main aspects of management of patients with atherothrombotic stroke to limit further progression of the arterial lesion, cerebral infarct, or recurrent infarction are risk factor management, surgical management, and medical management (Figs. 5-29–5-34.) Hypertension, hyperlipidemia, diabetes, and smoking are known to be major modifiable risk factors of atherosclerosis and stroke [1,2,6]. The control of blood pressure not only prevents large vessel atherosclerosis but also reduces the risk of stroke caused by small vessel disease (lacunar stroke). Hyperlipidemic states are also known to have correlations with atherosclerosis and stroke. Apolipoprotein E phenotypes and an elevated lipoprotein A are reported to be predictors of atherosclerotic stroke [19]. Evidence in the cardiac literature suggests that strict control of blood lipid by a combination of diet and drug therapy can reduce lesion progression; this has been associated with regression of the atherosclerotic lesion [1]. Our treatment goal for patients with serious extracranial and intracranial disease is to reduce the triglycerides to less than 200 mg/dL (150 mg/dL for diabetic patients), to restrict the total cholesterol to less than 150 mg/dL, and to raise the high-density lipoprotein level (HDL) to more than 40 mg/dL. As with coronary disease, 3-hydroxy-3-methylglutaryl coenzyme A reductase (HMG coA reductase) and niacin are the mainstays of pharmacologic therapy. Their use depends on the type of hyperlipidemia. Evidence is emerging that antioxidants, particularly vitamin E, can reduce the risk of coronary artery disease; these are believed to prevent formation and progression of atherosclerotic plaque by blocking the oxidative modification of low-density lipoprotein (LDL) [1].

Surgical Management of Symptomatic Carotid Stenosis

	NASCET				ECST				VA			
Patients, *n*	659				778				189			
Medical group	331				323				98			
Surgical group	328				455				91			
Followup	2 y				Average, 2.7 y				Average, 11.9 mo			
Angiographic measurement	70%–99% stenosis				70%–99% stenosis				Men, >50% stenosis			
	% Stenosis = [(1-a)/b] x 100				% Stenosis = [(1-a)/b] x 100				% Stenosis = [(1-a)/b] x 100			
Medical treatment	Aspirin, 1300 mg/d								Aspirin, 325 mg/d			
	Med Rx	Surg Rx	Abs RR	Rel RR	Med Rx	Surg Rx	Abs RR	Rel RR	Med Rx	Surg Rx	Abs RR	Rel RR
Stroke	64(28)	34(13)	15	54	58(18)	48(11)	8	42	8(8)	4(4)	NS	NS
Ispilateral stroke	61(26)	26(9)	17	65	44(14)				7(7)	4(4)	NS	NS
Death	21(6)	15(5)	NS	NS	41(13)	45(10)	NS	NS	2(2)	7(8)	NS	NS
Stroke and death	73(32)	41(16)	17	51	89(28)	88(19)	9	32	10(10)	11(12)	NS	NS

Figure 5-29. Surgical management of symptomatic carotid stenosis. Three prospectively randomized, controlled trials have reported the benefit of carotid endarterectomy over medical treatment in symptomatic patients who were found to have a significantly stenotic lesion at the common carotid bifurcation [20–23]. The North American Symptomatic Carotid Endarterectomy Trial (NASCET) concluded that endarterectomy is highly effective in preventing ipsilateral stroke when the stenosis is 70% to 99% [20]. In addition, the efficacy increased when the stenosis was tighter. The European Carotid Surgery Trial (ECST), although using different methods of measurement, found similar results for lesions causing 70% to 99% stenosis [22]. The third trial, the Veterans Administration (VA) trial, had similar findings and stopped early because of the strongly significant results of the other two trials [23]. Although there is strong evidence that carotid endarterectomy is the most appropriate treatment for patients with high-grade carotid stenosis, some patients' lesions are inoperable, or the risk of surgery is too high. Medical management using antiplatelet or anticoagulant therapies may be the treatment of choice in these patients [24]. No data comparing the use of antiplatelet and anticoagulant therapy in this situation are available. Given the high rate of strokes among patients treated with aspirin in the NASCET study, it is possible that anticoagulants such as warfarin may be more effective than aspirin in patients who are not operative candidates. NASCET II has recently demonstrated efficacy for carotid endarterectomy in patients with 50% to 70% internal carotid artery stenosis and symptoms above it [21]. However, this is not as statistically robust as 70% to 99% stenosis found in NASCET I. Abs RR—absolute risk reduction; Med Rx—medical treatment; NS—not significant; Rel RR—relative risk reduction; Surg Rx—surgical treatment.

Most Significant Endarterectomy Trials for Asymptomatic Stenosis

	ACAS	CASANOVA	VA	Mayo Clinic
Patients, *n*	1662	410	441	158
Follow up	Median, 2.7 y	>3 y	Mean, 4 y	Early termination
Medical treatment	"Best medical treatment"	ASA, 990 mg plus dipyridamole, 225 mg/d	ASA, 1300 mg/d	ASA, 80 mg/d
Carotid stenosis, %	>60	50–99	>50	>50 linear stenosis >75% cross-sectional area stenosis

Figure 5-30. The most significant randomized endarterectomy trials for asymptomatic stenosis. The Veterans Administration (VA) trial [25] stopped early because the North American Symptomatic Carotid Endarterectomy Trial (NASCET) suggested the benefit of surgery for patients with a transient ischemic attack (TIA) or stroke who had a 70% or less stenosis. The latter study found significant efficacy when the combined endpoints of stroke, TIA and death, were used. For ipsilateral stroke, there was a nonsignificant trend in favor of surgery in the VA study, but the study was stopped early because the combined endpoints of stroke and TIA were significant. Had the study been allowed to continue, it might have proved efficacious for stroke alone. In the Asymptomatic Carotid Atherosclerosis Study (ACAS) [26], the relative risk reduction of surgery was high, but there were a small number of total strokes. The absolute risk reduction was only 1.2% per year. At 2 and 5 years of follow up, the numbers of endarterectomies per stroke prevented were 67 and 17, respectively. For the NASCET study, the numbers were 10 and 6, respectively. Fortunately, ACAS had a lower surgical morbidity than the national average (2.2% versus 4.5%); it demonstrated a benefit to surgery with so few strokes so late in the trial. If the surgical morbidity were the same (5.4%) as that of the NASCET trial, then there would have been no benefit to surgery. Although ACAS found no correlation with degree of stenosis and surgical efficacy, the total number of strokes was too small, and over 80% of the patients had a 75% or less stenosis. NASCET only found greater benefit to surgery with stenosis from 75% to 99%. ACAS simply did not evaluate that question. CASANOVA—Carotid Artery Stenosis with Asymptomatic Narrowing: Operation versus Aspirin.

Massachusetts General Hospital Stroke Service Algorithms for Managing Asymptomatic Carotid Stenosis

Carotid noninvasive test	Degree of internal carotid stenosis
CDUS criteria or TCD criteria	Negative for residual lumen diameter of 1.5 mm Follow every 4 to 6 to 12 to 24 mo, depending on lesion severity

CDUS criteria or TD criteria	Positive for residual lumen diameter of 1.5 mm
	 Consider surgery
	 Magnetic resonance imaging or angiography
	 Cardiac evaluation
	 Appropriate surgical candidate
	   Endarterectomy
	 Inappropriate surgical candidate
	   Medical therapy

Figure 5-31. Massachusetts General Hospital stroke service algorithms for managing asymptomatic carotid stenosis. Carotid duplex ultrasound (CDUS) and transcranial Doppler (TCD) criteria for diagnosing a stenotic lesion at the origin of the internal carotid artery with a residual lumen diameter of 1.5 mm or less (laboratory tests) [7,21]. These criteria are based on pathologic examination of the residual lumen diameter of the intact endarterectomy specimens. At 1.5-mm residual lumen diameter, a pressure drop across the stenosis begins to occur. This is reflected intracranially by changes in peak systolic velocity and flow direction in the carotid territory arteries and the arteries of the circle of Willis. Because we and others use CDUS and magnetic resonance angiography (MRA) in place of angiography in many patients, the percentage of stenosis is not relevant. The actual residual lumen diameter becomes the most important indicator of severity of stenosis.

MRA provides a picture of flowing blood at the bifurcation of the common carotid artery, confirming the severity of stenosis at that site; however, MRA is not as specific as CDUS and TCD criteria. When MRA, CDUS, and TCD criteria are equivocal, computed tomographic angiography and finally conventional angiography are considered. The latter is considered only if the benefit of endarterectomy is expected to be significant. Thus, we rarely use conventional angiography in the evaluation of patients with asymptomatic carotid stenosis.

Algorithms for combining clinical cardiac findings with stress thallium scanning are widely used [27]. Avoidance of surgery in patients at high risk of myocardial infarction is essential if asymptomatic endarterectomy is to be effective. Endarterectomy should carry a risk of no greater than 3% to have some effect on primary stroke prevention in patients with hemodynamically significant carotid stenosis (a residual lumen diameter of 1.5 mm or less). Medical therapy in addition to controlling the risk factors may include aspirin (antiplatelet therapy) or warfarin (antithrombotic therapy). Neither of these agents has been subjected to clinical trial in patients with asymptomatic carotid stenosis.

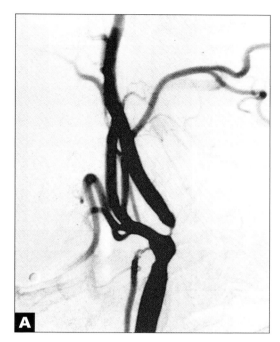 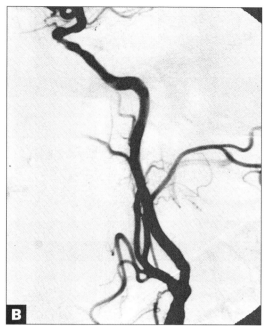

arm weakness lasting 20 minutes or less. He was medically unable to have an endarterectomy. **B,** Angiogram done after the angioplasty of the left ICA stenotic lesion shown in *A.* Transarterial angioplasty at the origin of the ICA and intracranially in the arteries at the base of the brain is now possible. The risk-to-benefit ratio of this procedure, however, has not been established, although several uncontrolled series have shown that, for the ICA origin, transarterial angioplasty is possible at low risk [28]. The benefits and potential long-term complications are unknown. Does rapid restenosis occur at the edge of the sheaths? What is the risk of endarterectomy after angioplasty, and can it even be done? At the least, because of the low risk of endarterectomy, a carefully controlled randomized trial is essential before this technique can be substituted for endarterectomy. We reserve angioplasty for the patient with symptoms in whom endarterectomy is medically contraindicated. Angioplasty of atheromatous lesions in the intracranial ICA, in the middle cerebral artery stem, and at the vertebrobasilar junction is possible as well. At these sites, however, safety data are lacking, and as at the ICA origin, the procedure must be considered innovative therapy.

Figure 5-32. Internal carotid artery (ICA) origin angioplasty. **A,** Angiogram showing the left ICA origin stenotic lesion in a 65-year-old man. The patient had recurrent episodes of speech difficulty and right

Management for Stroke Prevention in Patients With Symptomatic and Asymptomatic Large Vessel Atherothrombotic Disease

Artery	Therapeutic options
Atherothrombotic disease in the carotid circulation	
Internal carotid origin stenosis	
>70% symptomatic or asymptomatic*	Endarterectomy if surgery in contraindicated, then antithrombotic vs antiplatelet therapy
<70% symptomatic*	Antiplatelet vs antithrombotic therapy vs endarterectomy (50% to 70% stenosis)
60%–70% asymptomatic	
<60% asymptomatic	Endarterectomy? (need more data)
Internal carotid siphon stenosis	Antiplatelet therapy
Asymptomatic	
Symptomatic >70%	Antiplatelet therapy
Middle anterior or posterior cerebral artery stem stenosis	Antithrombotic vs antiplatelet therapy
Asymptomatic	
Symptomatic	Antiplatelet vs antithrombotic therapy
Atherothrombotic disease of the vertebrobasilar system	Antithrombotic vs antiplatelet therapy
Distal vertebral stenosis	
Asymptomatic	
Symptomatic	Antiplatelet vs antithrombotic therapy
Basilar artery stenosis	Antithrombotic vs antiplatelet therapy
Asymptomatic	
Symptomatic	Antiplatelet vs antithrombotic therapy
	Antithrombotic vs antiplatelet therapy

*We substituted our Doppler criteria for a residual lumen diameter of 1.5 mm instead of 70% stenosis.

Figure 5-33. Suggested therapeutic options for long-term management of large vessel atherosclerosis. The therapeutic options mentioned are specific for the artery suspected of giving rise to stroke and are used by our Stroke Service. Surgical treatment is considered in all patients with severe (greater than 70%) proximal internal carotid artery stenosis (symptomatic or asymptomatic). Medical contraindication and local surgical morbidity must be thoroughly considered before surgery can be recommended as beneficial management. Medical management is suggested for patients if endarterectomy is contraindicated and for patients with intracranial atherothrombotic disease. The table underlines our preferred therapeutic options. There is no proven difference in efficacy between antithrombotic and antiplatelet therapy in these settings, but antithrombotic therapy is preferred for symptomatic patients. The ongoing National Institutes of Health–sponsored Warfarin Aspirin Recurrent Stroke Study [29] includes patients with primary stroke as a result of intracranial lesions or as a result of small vessel disease or cerebral embolism of unknown source. The anticipated goal is to provide better guidelines for deciding whether thrombolytic or antiplatelet therapy is more efficacious and safer in each of these settings. In all cases, efforts to normalize the serum lipid values, homocystine levels, blood sugar, and blood pressure are considered. (*Adapted from* Kistler [1].)

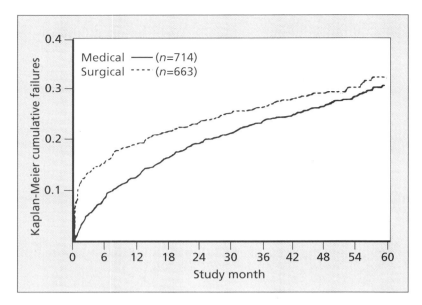

Figure 5-34. Extracranial–intracranial (EC–IC) Bypass Graft Study evaluating the efficacy of surgery that joined a branch of the superficial temporal artery (extracranial) with a cortical surface branch of the middle cerebral artery. This procedure was performed in patients with recurrent symptoms of internal carotid artery (ICA) origin occlusion or primary symptoms of distal ICA or middle cerebral artery stem atherothrombotic stenotic lesions [30]. No statistically significant benefit of EC–IC bypass grafting over medical therapy (aspirin or warfarin per local standard of practice) could be found. The uncertainty of antiplatelet (aspirin) versus antithrombotic (warfarin) therapy in this setting has, in part, prompted the National Institutes of Health–sponsored Warfarin Aspirin Recurrent Stroke Study [29] (Fig. 5-33).

Lacunar Disease

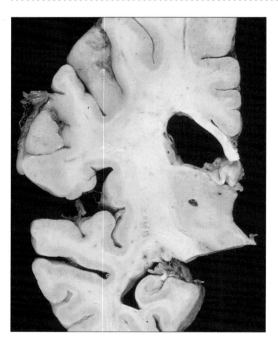

Figure 5-35. Lacunar infarction. Lacunar strokes represent about 25% of all strokes [30,31]. This pathologic specimen shows a lacunar infarction in the basal ganglia, which is seen as a small fluid-filled cavity. This cavity formed after the infarcted tissue was removed by phagocytes. By definition, lacunar infarcts are caused by occlusion of a single penetrating vessel that has a diameter of 200 to 600 μm, resulting in a small infarct with a diameter ranging from 0.3 to 2.0 mm [32]. The medial lenticulostriate branches have lumen diameters ranging from 100 to 200 μm, whereas the more lateral lenticulostriate arteries have larger lumen diameters (200 to 400 μm) [33]. The diameters of paramedian penetrating arteries that arise from the basilar artery vary from 40 to 500 μm [34]. (*Courtesy of* Jean-Paul Vonsattel, MD, C.S. Kubik Laboratory for Neuropathology, Massachusetts General Hospital, Boston, MA.)

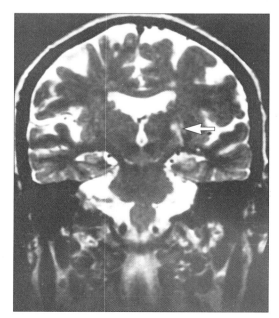

Figure 5-36. Location of the lacunar infarct. Coronal magnetic resonance image showing a lacunar infarction (*arrow*) at the left basal ganglia. The common sites of lacunar infarct are at the basal ganglia (especially the putamen), the internal capsule, the thalamus, the pons, and the subcortical white matter [32]. Most lacunar infarcts occur in the territories of the lenticulostriate branches of the middle cerebral arteries, the thalamoperforators of the posterior cerebral arteries, and the paramedian branches of the basilar artery. Because of the lack of collateral blood supply for the penetrating arteries, the lacunar infarct usually spreads all the way from the point of occlusion through the entire territory of the vessel. Thus, the infarct is often longer in images in the coronal plane than in the axial plane [35].

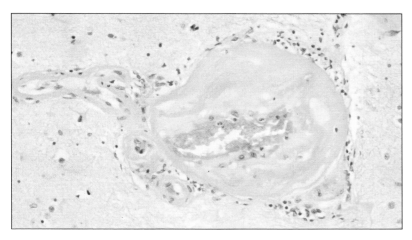

Figure 5-37. Histologic slide of lipohyalinosis of a penetrating artery showing a putaminal vessel with a thickened hyaline wall and optically empty spaces that once contained lipids (lipohyalinosis). This local pathology in the vascular wall of the penetrating artery is the most common cause of lacunar infarction. The other cause is microatheroma of the

proximal penetrating artery, lipohyalinosis, and atherosclerosis of the parent vessel that occludes the origin of the penetrating artery. Microatheroma usually causes a stenosis or occlusion in the first half of the course of the penetrating artery. Lipohyalinosis usually occurs after the origin of the penetrating artery. In some reported cases, pathologic sections of the arteries have been normal, and microembolism was thought to be the cause [33,36]. In addition, polycythemia, chronic meningitis, and neurosyphilis have been associated with lacunar infarct [34,37,38], but serial section data was missing from these studies. The pathologic process could have involved more than one penetrating vessel, thereby excluding the classic definition of a lacunar infarction, *ie*, an infarct due to occlusion of a single penetrating vessel. Note here the relative preservation of adjacent vessels. Pathologically, lipohyalinosis of a penetrating artery is characterized by thickening of the arterial wall, fibrinoid necrosis, hyalinosis, and angionecrosis. It usually affects the penetrating arteries in a segmental fashion. Lipohyalinosis often occurs in the smaller penetrating arteries, especially those with less than a 200-μm diameter. Therefore, it accounts for smaller lacunar infarctions, which are usually asymptomatic [32]. Hypertension is the principal risk factor of this pathologic condition [35]. (*Courtesy of* Jean Paul Vonsattel, MD, C.S. Kubik Laboratory for Neuropathology, Massachusetts General Hospital, Boston, MA.)

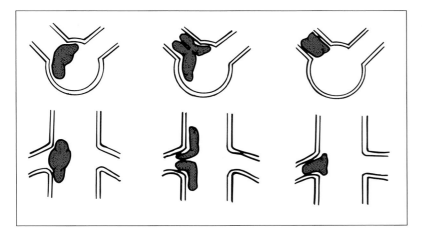

Figure 5-38. Atheromatous disease of a penetrating artery and parent artery. Microatheroma of the vessel is a common mechanism of arterial stenosis underlying lacune. It is found most often at the origin of the penetrating arteries arising from the basilar artery and less often in the posterior cerebral artery and the middle cerebral artery stem [33,39,40]. Microatheroma usually involves penetrating arteries that range in size from 400 to 900 μm, thereby accounting for larger lacunes, which are usually symptomatic [32].

Fisher [36] has demonstrated that the atheromatous lesion may arise in the parent artery and also block the orifices of the penetrating arteries or can extend into the penetrating artery and block it there. This is common in the basilar artery with regard to penetrating branches that supply the pons [40,41]. Different types of basilar artery branch occlusion by atherosclerotic plaque are shown here. Middle cerebral artery atheromatous disease can also cause infarction in the lenticulostriate territory by blocking the orifices of these small vessels [34], but this has never been documented by pathologic study but only by inference based on infarct topology. (*Adapted from* Fisher and colleague [40].)

Lacunar Syndromes

Pure sensory stroke or transient ischemic attacks

Pure motor hemiparesis (PMH)

Ataxic hemiparesis

Dysarthria–clumsy hand syndrome

Modified PMH with motor aphasia

PMH sparing the face

Mesencephalothalamic syndrome

Thalamic dementia

PMH with horizontal gaze palsy

PMH with crossed third nerve palsy (Weber's syndrome)

PMH with crossed nerve palsy

PMH with confusion

Cerebellar ataxia with crossed third nerve palsy (Claude's syndrome)

Sensorimotor stroke (thalamocapsular)

Hemiballism

Lower basilar branch syndrome, with dizziness, diplopia, gaze palsy, dysarthria, cerebellar ataxia, and trigeminal numbness

Lateral medullary syndrome

Lateral pontomedullary syndrome

Loss of memory (?)

Locked-in syndrome (bilateral PMH)

Miscellaneous

  Weakness of one leg with ease of falling

  Pure dysarthria

  Acute dystonia of thalamic origin

Figure 5-39. List of lacunar syndromes described by Fisher [32].

Lacunar Syndromes, Infarct Locations, and Clinical Findings

Lacunar syndrome	Infarct location	Clinical findings
Pure sensory stroke	Thalamus (ventral posterior) Pons Deep white matter (Cerebral cortex)	Sensory loss on one side of the body
Pure motor stroke	Posterior limb of the internal capsule Basis pontis Cerebral peduncle Medullary pyramid	Severe motor weakness of the face, arm, and leg (weakness may be incomplete, affecting only the proximal part of the limbs) Transient hypesthesia and paresthesia are compatible with the syndrome Dysarthria is common
Ataxic hemiparesis	Upper pons Posterior limb of the internal capsule Thalamus Middle and lower pons	Weakness and cerebellar sign on the same side Slight hypesthesia may be found
Dysarthria–clumsy hand syndrome	Basis pontis Genu of the internal capsule Corona radiata, cortical lesion	Dysarthria and clumsiness of one hand Often associated with ipsilateral lower facial paralysis, Babinski's sign (brisk deep tendon reflexes), deviation of the tongue, and dysphagia
Sensorimotor stroke	Thalamocapsular lacunes	Motor and sensory involvement The motor or sensory deficit may be incomplete

Figure 5-40. Lacunar syndromes, infarct locations, and clinical findings. *Pure sensory stroke.* Pure sensory stroke syndrome was initially described by Fisher [42] in 1965. It is characterized by subjective numbness involving the face, arm, and leg without evidence of motor weakness, dysarthria, visual field defect, or neuropsychologic disturbances. Sensory symptoms are generally described as numbness, tingling, or being "asleep." Unpleasant and painful dysesthesia has also been reported. The neurologic examination may demonstrate a decrease in pain and cold sensation, but often joint position sensation and vibration are preserved. The sensory loss may be subtle and difficult to demonstrate by neurologic examination. The sensory symptoms may progress within seconds to hours [42]. They may start in the hand or foot and spread to the whole side of the body. In general, pure sensory lacunar syndrome is associated with infarction at the ventral posterior nuclei of the thalamus [39]. Rarely, cortical surface and deep white matter infarction or a pontine lesion may be responsible for pure sensory symptoms. According to Fisher's observation [43], when the abdomen is involved, thalamic lesion is much more likely. The prognosis of this syndrome is favorable. Marked improvement within weeks is common [34].

Pure motor hemiplegia and pure motor hemiparesis. Pure hemiplegia is one of the most common lacunar syndromes, accounting for 46% to 50% of the cases [44]. It is characterized by weakness of the face, arm, and leg on one side without sensory signs or visual field defect. Prodromal transient ischemic attacks were recorded in 16.1% to 57% of patients, usually within 48 hours [45]. We have seen cases with transient symptoms up to 10 days before developing the fixed deficits. The motor deficit is usually incomplete and often affects the proximal part of the extremity. In our experience, fine motor movement of the fingers and toes is usually present as well. There may be transient hypesthesia or paresthesia [33], and occasionally, the patient may refer to the onset of symptoms as a numbness. Dysarthria is also found. Lacunar infarction associated with pure motor hemiparesis has been reported in the posterior limb of the internal capsule, basis pontis, cerebral peduncle, and medulla [46]. An embolic infarct in an upper division of middle cerebral artery territory can sometimes mimic this type of lacunar syndrome. The deficit in the face, arm, and leg due to cortical infarction, however, is usually disproportional. Moreover, in pure motor lacunar infarction, the tendon reflexes of the affected limbs often become brisker within the few hours of onset, which is faster than in most cases with similar deficit due to cortical infarction [45].

Ataxic hemiparesis. Ataxic hemiparesis is a syndrome in which pyramidal and cerebellar signs occur on the same side of the body. The weakness is mild, and the cerebellar ataxia is apparent in the least affected limb. Motor weakness is usually proportional in the face, arm, and leg, but it may be more severe in the leg or the arm. This syndrome was originally described by Fisher in 1965 [47] as "homolateral ataxia with crural paresis." The description was based on 14 patients who had weakness of the lower limb and Babinski's sign associated with dysmetria. In the ataxic hemiparesis syndrome, transient mild sensory symptoms, dysarthria, and nystagmus have been reported. Ataxic hemiparesis usually results from infarction at the junction of the upper third and inferior two thirds of the basis pontis [45]. Other locations, including internal capsule, thalamus, and lower pons, however, have been shown on imaging studies to cause hemiparesis and ataxia [45].

Dysarthria–clumsy hand syndrome. Dysarthria–clumsy hand syndrome is characterized by dysarthria, dysphagia, and slight weakness and clumsiness of the hand [48,49]. Several additional signs, including lower facial paralysis, ipsilateral brisk tendon reflexes, Babinski's sign, and deviation of the protruded tongue may be present. Fisher [45] stated that writing impairment is common when the dominant hand is affected. Sensory deficit is not a part of the syndrome. Fisher's pathologic study [45] suggests that dysarthria–clumsy hand syndrome is associated with a lacunar infarct at the genu of the internal capsule or at the junction of the upper one third and lower two thirds of the basis pontis. Occasionally, small cortical infarction can mimic this syndrome, but with cortical lesions, sensory deficit on the affected lips is usually present [32].

Sensorimotor stroke. Sensorimotor lacunar stroke syndrome is characterized by sensory loss and motor weakness on one side of the body without evidence of cortical involvement. Pathologically, it has been associated with an infarction in the posterolateral thalamus with extension into the adjacent posterior limb of the internal capsule [50].

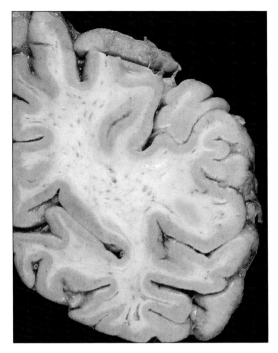

Figure 5-41. Pathologic specimen showing multiple lacunar infarction in the basal ganglia and subcortical white matter. It was initially described as l' État lacunare by Marie in 1901 [51]. Clinically, patients with multiple lacunar infarction may have a history of recurrent slight weakness associated with progressive subcortical dementia, dysarthria, and pseudobulbar palsy. Short-step gait, imbalance, and incontinence are also common.

Cerebral Embolism

Clinical Manifestations of Embolic Stroke

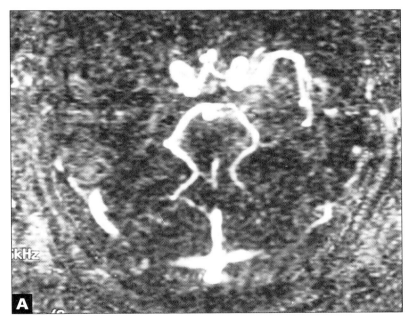

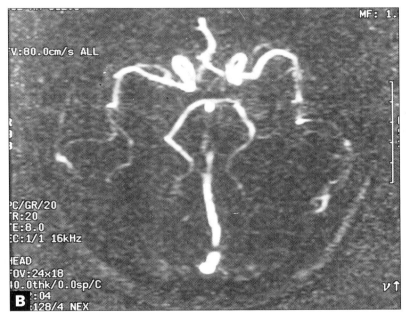

Figure 5-42. Spontaneous recanalization. Once an embolus occludes a vessel, it usually lyses and migrates. The frequency of spontaneous recanalization in acute carotid artery territory thromoembolism has been reported to be 30% to 69% in several studies that used serial angiography [52–54]. Embolic fragments tend to lodge at the bifurcations of the arteries because the diameters of the branches are considerably smaller than the diameter of the parent artery. The tip of the internal carotid artery, the top of the basilar artery, and the middle cerebral artery (MCA) trifurcation are the most common sites of embolic occlusion. **A,** Magnetic resonance angiogram (MRA) done 2 hours after the onset of symptoms showing no flow in the right MCA stem and its main branches. Usually, embolic fragments are lysed and further fragmented by intrinsic thrombolytic mechanisms leading to symptomatic or asymptomatic occlusion of smaller arteries. Depending on the timing of this spontaneous recanalization, the deficits may shrink or disappear. **B,** MRA of the same patient taken 5 days later, showing flow in the right MCA. The timing of recanalization and the quality of leptomeningeal anastomoses are important factors that determine the size and location of the infarction and the patient's clinical outcome. In the case of an MCA stem embolus, the embolus may block some of the origins of the lenticulostriate arteries, which do not have a collateral supply. Even in the event of spontaneous recanalization, if the delay has taken more than a couple of hours, a deep infarction may occur only in the territory of these penetrating arteries. A computed tomography scan taken 5 days later showed an infarction in the lenticulostriate territory in the same patient whose symptoms gradually resolved in 24 hours after the first MRA shown in *A*. The patient had a complete clinical recovery.

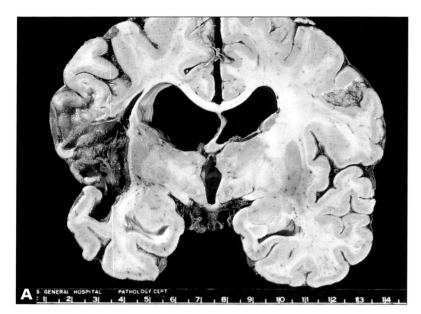
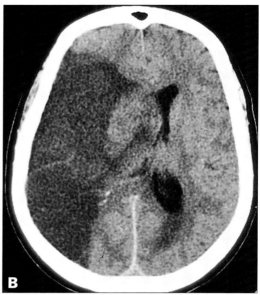

C. Classic Findings in Dominant and Nondominant Middle Cerebral Artery Occlusion

Dominant stem occlusion	Nondominant stem occlusion
Paralysis of contralateral face, arm, leg	Paralysis of contralateral face, arm, leg
Contralateral sensory impairment of face, arm, leg	Contralateral sensory impairment of face, arm, leg
Global aphasia	Contralateral neglect, anosognosia
Contralateral homonymous hemianopia	Contralateral homonymous hemianopia
Paralysis of conjugate gaze to the opposite side	Paralysis of conjugate gaze to the opposite side
Loss or impairment of optokinetic nystagmus	Loss or impairment of optokinetic nystagmus
Superior division occlusion	
Paralysis of contralateral face, arm, leg	Paralysis of contralateral face, arm, leg
Contralateral sensory impairment of face, arm, leg	Contralateral sensory impairment of face, arm, leg
Expressive aphasia, neglect	Neglect
Paralysis of conjugate gaze to the opposite side	Paralysis of conjugate gaze to the opposite side
Inferior division occlusion	
Minimal paralysis of contralateral face, arm, leg	Minimal paralysis of contralateral face, arm, leg
Receptive aphasia	Constructional apraxia
Minimal contralateral sensory impairment of face, arm, leg	Minimal contralateral sensory impairment of face, arm, leg
Homonymous hemianopia or upper quadrantopia	Homonymous hemianopia or upper quadrantopia

Figure 5-43. Middle cerebral artery infarction. Cerebral embolism is the most common pathophysiologic cause of ischemic stroke, occurring in up to 60% of patients [55–57]. The refinement of extracranial and intracranial arterial ultrasound flow analysis, magnetic resonance imaging (MRI) of the brain, and magnetic resonance angiography (MRA) of the extracranial and intracranial circulation allow the physician to exclude reliably large vessel atherothrombotic stroke, lacunar stroke, or even dissection as a cause of cerebral infarction and thus to diagnose embolic stroke. **A,** Gross pathologic sample of the brain showing an old left middle cerebral artery (MCA) territory infarction. **B,** Computed tomography scan showing a large right MCA territory infarction. Occlusion of the MCA or one of its branches is usually due to embolus (artery-to-artery, known cardiac, aortic atheroma, or unknown source) rather than atherothrombosis. A complete MCA syndrome occurs most often when an embolus occludes the stem of the artery. **C,** Clinical findings classically found in dominant and nondominant MCA stem or main branch occlusions. Cortical collateral flow from anastomotic vessels of the anterior and posterior cerebral arteries is responsible for the development of partial MCA syndromes. Partial MCA syndrome may also be due to an embolus that enters the MCA stem and moves distally, causing the recovery of ischemic noninfarcted tissue and its deficits. Partial syndromes resulting from embolic occlusion of the branches of MCA include hand weakness or arm and hand weakness (brachial syndrome) [58]. (Panel C *adapted from* Adams and colleague [59].)

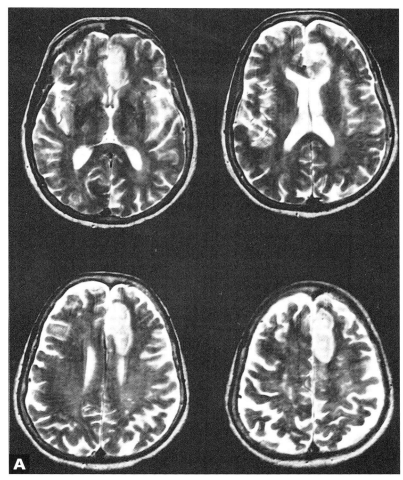

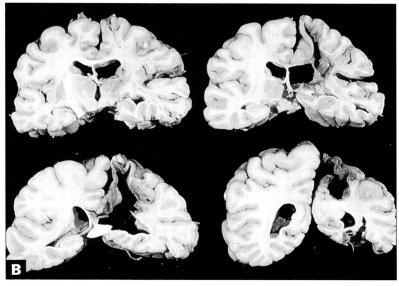

cally found in unilateral ACA occlusions include distal to proximal paralysis of the opposite leg, foot, hip, and arm; cortical sensory loss of the opposite leg; urinary incontinence; abulia; contralateral grasp reflex, sucking reflex, gegenhalten, "frontal tremor"; and left limb apraxia. Clinical findings in bilateral ACA occlusions include paraplegia; profound abulia; cortical sensory loss of both legs; urinary incontinence; contralateral grasp reflex, sucking reflex, gegenhalten, and frontal tremor. Infarction in the ACA territory is uncommon and is most often due to embolism rather than atherothrombosis. Occlusion of the A_1 segment of the ACA is usually well tolerated because of collateral flow from the anterior communicating artery. If both A_2 segments rise from the same ACA stem (contralateral A_1 segment atresia), the occlusion of one A_1 segment affects both ACA territories. The recurrent artery of Heubner usually arises either at the level of the anterior communicating artery or just proximal to it. Pronounced weakness of the arm and face in the presence of ACA occlusion has been attributed to the involvement of this artery because its territory includes the anterior limb and genu of the internal capsule.

Figure 5-44. Clinical finding of anterior cerebral artery (ACA) infarction. **A,** T2-weighted magnetic resonance images (MRIs) showing a left anterior cerebral artery territory infarction. **B,** Gross pathologic picture of the brain showing an old right ACA territory infarct. Clinical findings that are classi-

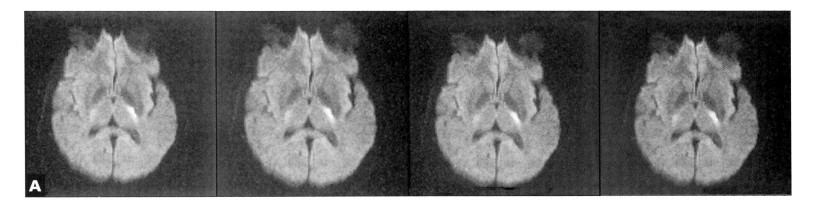

B. Clinical Findings in Anterior Choroidal Artery Occlusions

Right	Left
Contralateral hemiplegia, hemihypesthesia, homonymous hemianopia	Contralateral hemiplegia, hemihypesthesia, homonymous hemianopia
Possibly, left spatial neglect and constructional apraxia	Possibly, slight disorders of speech and language

Figure 5-45. Clinical findings in anterior choroidal artery occlusions. A, A magnetic resonance image–diffusion-weighted image of an anterior choroidal artery territory infarct. **B,** The most consistent syndrome seen in anterior choroidal artery territory infarction includes hemiparesis, hemisensory loss, and hemianopia [60]. Hemiataxia may accompany the sensory symptoms. Anterior choroidal artery territory infarctions may result from a variety of mechanisms, such as cardiac or artery-to-artery embolism or low flow. The anterior choroidal artery may supply as much as the posterior two thirds of the posterior limb of the internal capsule, including its retrolenticular portion, the medial aspect of the globus pallidus, the posterior portion of the optic tract, the uncus of the temporal lobe, the tail of the caudate nucleus, the lateral choroid plexus, and superficial areas of the thalamus [61]. Its territory in an individual patient varies according to its relation to other adjacent arterial territories.

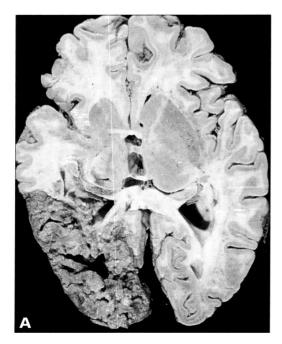

Figure 5-46. Posterior cerebral artery (PCA). **A**, Pathologic sample of the brain showing a left PCA territory infarct. **B**, Clinical findings classically seen in unilateral dominant, nondominant, and bilateral PCA occlusions. Embolic occlusions affecting the PCA or its branches are less common than those affecting the middle cerebral artery. A cardiac or an artery-to-artery source can be the cause. In the latter, embolic material usually arises from plaque in the distal vertebral artery or from the proximal basilar artery. Occlusion of the proximal PCAs can produce a wide variety of symptoms because these arteries supply the upper brain stem, the medial occipital lobes, and the medial and inferior portions of the temporal lobes. The site of the ACA occlusion and the

B. Clinical Findings in Unilateral and Bilateral PCA Occlusions

Unilateral

Dominant	Nondominant
Homonymous hemianopia or homonymous upper quadrantanopia usually sparing macular region	Homonymous hemianopia or homonymous upper quadrantanopia usually sparing macular region
Alexia without agraphia, color anomia	Contralateral sensory impairment of the face, arm, leg
Memory defect	
Contralateral sensory impairment of the face, arm, leg	Visual hallucinations (metamorphopsia, teleopsia, illusory visual spread, palinopsia, distortion of outlines, photophobia)
Visual hallucinations (metamorphopsia, teleopsia, illusory visual spread, palinopsia, distortion of outlines, photophobia)	Topographic disorientation and prosopagnosia
Simultagnosia	

Bilateral

Bilateral homonymous hemianopia, cortical blindness
Unawareness or denial of blindness
Achromatopsia, apraxia of ocular movements
Topographic disorientation and prosopagnosia
Simultagnosia
Memory defect

anatomic variations of the circle of Willis determine the extent of the infarction.

There are variations in the circle of Willis [59]. In about 70% of patients, both PCAs arise from the basilar artery. The posterior communicating arteries may be available for collateral flow or one or both may be atretic. In 20% to 25% of patients, one PCA comes from the basilar artery and the other comes from the internal carotid artery through a large posterior communicating artery. In the remaining cases, both originate from the internal carotids [62]. (Panel B *adapted from* Adams and colleague [59].)

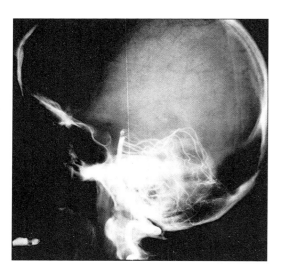

Figure 5-47. Selective vertebral angiogram (lateral view) showing an embolus at the top of the basilar artery causing a filling defect. Neither posterior cerebral artery is filling from vertebral injection. The symptoms caused by cerebral embolism are obviously directly related to the cerebral territory that artery supplies [63]. The size of the embolus and the presence and quality of collateral flow determine the size of the infarction. Clinical findings of the top of the basilar artery syndrome include paralysis of conjugate lateral or vertical gaze, internuclear ophthalmoplegia, horizontal or vertical nystagmus; various visual field defects; bilateral ptosis and third nerve palsy; stupor or hypersomnia; bilateral cerebellar ataxia; quadriparesis or plegia and paralysis of bulbar muscles; various sensory deficits; locked-in syndrome; and memory deficit. If the embolus is small enough to pass through the vertebral artery, it easily passes through the length of the basilar artery, which is of greater diameter than either vertebral artery. If neither proximal nor mid-basilar atherosclerotic lesion is present, the embolic fragment lodges at the tip of the basilar artery, where it bifurcates into one of the posterior cerebral arteries. The size of the embolus, the length of time it obstructs the basilar artery, and the adequacy of collateral flow determine the extent of the infarction and the clinical picture of the patient. Patients may present with a variety of symptoms. T2-weighted magnetic resonance images in this patient showed multiple areas of infarction due to a single basilar tip embolus. The infarct was in the cerebellum, lower and upper pons, midbrain, and thalamus. The left posterior cerebral artery territory was spared.

Evaluation of Embolic Stroke

Diagnostic Tests Used in the Evaluation of Embolic Stroke

Test	Reason
Cardiac	
Electrocardiogram	To diagnose atrial fibrillation and myocardial infarction
Transthoracic echocardiography	For visualization of left ventricular apex, left ventricular thrombus, and some aspects of prosthetic valves
Transesophageal echocardiography	More sensitive in detecting left atrial thrombus and smoke, interatrial septum, atrial aspect of mitral and tricuspid valves, vegetations less than 5 mm in size, endomyocardial abscess, ascending aortic atheromatous disease, and spontaneous echo contrast
Holter monitoring	To detect paroxysmal atrial fibrillation or sick sinus syndrome
Cerebral (brain and arteries)	
Carotid duplex ultrasound	To rule out carotid bifurcation atherosclerotic disease
Transcranial Doppler ultrasound	To rule out evidence of middle cerebral artery stem stenosis or siphon disease, to show if there is an occlusion of intracranial vessels or if they are open (embolus lysed)
MRI or MRA of the head and neck	To rule out lacunar stroke and atherosclerosis of large vessels and to evaluate intracranial collateral flow
Cerebral angiography	In the acute phase, to evaluate for intraarterial thrombolysis
Coagulation	
Hypercoagulable state evaluation, proteins C and S, fibrinogen, D-dimer, anticardiolipin Ab, F_{1+2}	To identify hypercoagulable conditions as a source of thromboembolism

Figure 5-48. Diagnostic tests used in the evaluation of embolic stroke. These diagnostic tests are used to establish that embolism is the underlying pathophysiology of the ischemic stroke and to determine the precise source of the embolism for preventive therapy. The indications for transesophageal echocardiography (TEE) in the evaluation of a stroke and transient ischemic attacks depends on the severity of the stroke and the need to document all suspected sources of emboli precisely. The decision to order a transesophageal study should be based on the therapeutic implications of the information that might be gained. TEE is superior to transthoracic echocardiography in identifying left atrial thrombi, spontaneous left atrial contrast, aortic debris, intracardiac tumors, atrial septal aneurysms, patent foramen ovale or atrial septal defects, native or infective valve vegetations or strands, and prosthetic valves except for infective vegetation [64]. Many physicians favor antithrombotic therapy when these entities are noted in a patient with embolic stroke. The National Institutes of Health–sponsored Warfarin Aspirin Recurrent Stroke Study (WARSS) [27] and a substudy of it using TEE to identify potential cardioaortic sources may provide some valuable information regarding the efficacy of antithrombotic versus antiplatelet therapy. The cerebral tests are needed to document the extent and location of the infarct and to rule out large artery atherothrombotic disease as the cause. The coagulation evaluation may identify a coagulation defect that leads to an overly active hemostatic system. In that case, anticoagulation may be an effective therapeutic strategy for stroke prevention. The Hemostatic System Activation Substudy of WARSS is examining the level of activity of the hemostatic system in WARSS patients and may find an association with increased clotting in a particular cardioembolic stroke–prone group of patients. MRA—magnetic resonance angiogram; MRI—magnetic resonance imaging.

Embolic Sources

Embolic Stroke (Classification by Source)

Definite sources (clinical diagnosis)	Possible sources (diagnosed by echocardiogram)
Prophylactic antithrombotic therapy generally accepted	Chronic left ventricular thrombus
Atrial fibrillation age >65	Left atrial thrombus (or atrial appendage thrombus documented by TEE)
Prosthetic heart valve	Mitral annular calcification
Status post-left ventricular myocardial infarction <3 months	Patent foramen ovale (bubble study) with or without septal aneurysm
Rheumatic valvular heart disease	Valve strands
Marantic (noninfective) endocarditis	Left ventricular dysfunction
	Ascending aortic atheromatous disease documented by TEE >4 mm in diameter

Unknown source (definite clinical and possible echocardiographic sources excluded)

Figure 5-49. Suspected definite and possible cardiac sources for embolic stroke. Cardiac emboli are usually fresh and have a high fibrin content and a high plasminogen count. Atherothrombotic emboli are usually old, have a low fibrin content, are platelet rich, contain cholesterol, and include atheromatous material. Differences in thrombus composition between cardiac source emboli and emboli from atherothrombotic disease at the cervical level may be important for recanalization. Cardiac source emboli from relatively fresh thrombi may be associated with high recanalization rates. Some cardiac emboli, however, may be from old, well-organized thrombus or calcific valve debris, which resist clot lysis. We speculate that emboli from aortic or carotid atherothrombotic disease may also not be associated with rapid lysis. Hacke hypothesizes that at least for thrombolytic therapy, three aspects of embolus subtypes affect the prospect of clot lyses and recanalization: size, origin, and composition [65]. Antithrombotic therapy efficacy has been proven by randomized trial. TEE–transesophageal echocardiography.

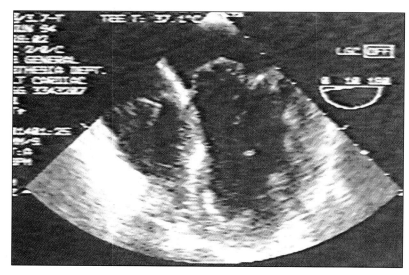

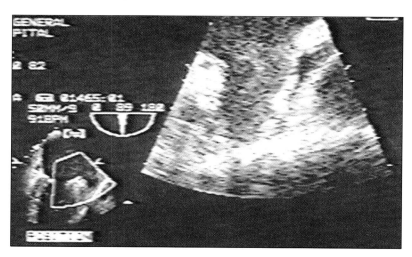

Figure 5-50. Transesophageal echocardiogram (TEE) showing the posterior leaflet prolapse of the mitral valve. A high frequency of association between acute ischemic stroke and mitral valve prolapse has been reported, especially in patients younger than 45 years [66]. This study, primarily based on M-mode echocardiography, found mitral valve prolapse in up to 40% of young patients with stroke or transient ischemic attack, but also in 7% to 21% of otherwise healthy patients. Another recent study using more specific echocardiographic criteria based on three-dimensional analysis of the valve shape showed that patients with uncomplicated mitral valve prolapse did not have an increased risk of stroke [67]. Other recent studies found that age, valve thickness, redundant leaflets, and annular abnormalities in association with mitral valve prolapse resulted in a higher incidence of embolism [68,69], but the power in these studies was not great.

Figure 5-51. Transesophageal echocardiogram of the left atrium showing a spontaneous echo contrast. Spontaneous echo contrast has been seen in patients with mitral stenosis and atrial fibrillation. It usually occurs in association with an obstruction of the atrial outflow. It is almost never found independent of other pathologic conditions in the heart. Laboratory studies suggest that the echo visualization of contrast material represents reversible microaggregation of red blood cells and has been associated with blood stasis, elevated serum fibrinogen level, and elevated blood viscosity [70–72]. Studies have associated spontaneous echo contrast with embolic stroke and previous peripheral embolism, and with an increased rate of stroke among patients with mitral stenosis and atrial fibrillation [73]. Because patients with atrial fibrillation and mitral stenosis have embolic strokes independent of spontaneous echo contrast [74], however, the presence of spontaneous echo contrast cannot be an absolute predictor of cerebral embolism. If atrial fibrillation or mitral stenosis is present, anticoagulation (international normalized ratio [INR] of 2 to 3) is recommended whether or not a spontaneous echo contrast has appeared.

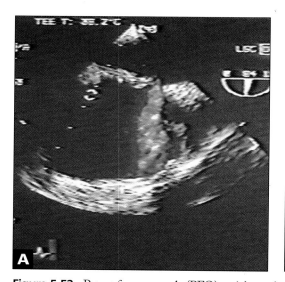

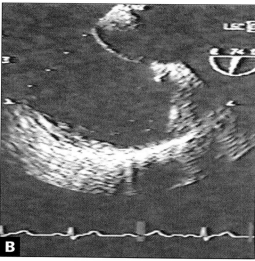

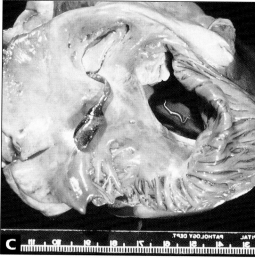

Figure 5-52. Patent foramen ovale (PFO), atrial septal aneurysm. **A,** Transesophageal echocardiogram (TEE) of a PFO with left-to-right shunt. **B,** TEE of a PFO without a left-to-right shunt. **C,** Pathologic specimen showing opened left atrium with the embolus protruding from a PFO in a patient with stroke who had not had any other identifiable risk factors for stroke. PFO has been well recognized as a cause of paradoxical embolism [75,76]. The exact natural history in terms of stroke risk, however, has remained obscure. TEE has been demonstrated to be superior to transthoracic echocardiograms in identifying PFO, particularly when right-to-left shunt is not observed [77]. The significance of these small PFOs is not clear. Two studies suggest that the size of the PFO and the amount of right-to-left shunt is greater in patients with cryptogenic stroke than in patients with an identifiable cause of embolic stroke [78,79]. Other studies conclude that a right-to-left shunt associated with an atrial septal aneurysm carries a higher incidence of stroke in patients with PFOs [80–82]. TEE using a multiplanar 5 MHz probe has demonstrated a dramatic increase in the odds ratio for embolic stroke in patients with PFO greater than 4 mm in diameter (82). Conflicting reports from Europe suggest that PFO may have little relation to embolic stroke [83]. The relative risk of embolic stroke in patients with PFO is uncertain. In our view, quantification of the entire cardiopathologic process, along with the level of activity of the hemostatic system, will be important in establishing the relative risk. Patients with PFOs and embolic strokes have been recommended for primary closure of the defect, either by open heart surgery or by transcatheter closure using a prosthetic double-umbrella device [84,85]. The efficacy and risks of these procedures have not been tested in a randomized controlled trial. The efficacy of either antithrombotic or antiplatelet therapy in preventing secondary stroke when a PFO is suspected as the cause of the primary stroke has also not been tested. The TEE substudy of the National Institutes of Health–sponsored Warfarin Aspirin Recurrent Stroke Study may establish some guidelines. Embolic strokes associated with PFO, however, often occur in young patients for whom long-term anticoagulation is a definite disadvantage. Therefore, transcatheter percutaneous closure has been suggested as an alternative to direct surgical closure [84,85]. We suggest prospectively following a cohort of patients with and without primary stroke who have a PFO gap greater than 4 mm in diameter, assessing their hemostatic system and fibrinolytic system activity. Based on that research, a stroke rate high enough to allow a randomized clinical trial with an acceptable number of patients could be developed comparing the therapeutic efficacy of mechanical closure versus medical therapy. We suggest that the volume or diameter of the PFO together with the level of activity of the hemostatic system may determine the stroke rate over time (85).

Major Features of Dilated Cardiomyopathy

Ventricular dilation
Left ventricular dysfunction
Moderate to severe cardiac enlargement
Intracavity thrombus formation
Systemic and pulmonary embolism
Atrial and ventricular arrhythmias

Figure 5-53. Major features of dilated cardiomyopathy (DCM). DCM is believed to be a predisposing factor to stroke [86,87]. Mural endocardial plaque, recognized as mural thrombi in an autopsy series, occurred in 75% of the cases of dilated cardiomyopathy [88]. Clinically apparent embolism occurs with an annual incidence of 3.5% in patients with DCM [87]. The embolic events are usually related to an intracardiac, ventricular, or atrial thrombus as a result of intracavitary stasis of blood. In contrast to myocardial infarction, which carries a high risk of embolization in early weeks that declines rapidly after 3 months, a thrombus in DCM has a fairly constant risk of embolization over time [89]. Atrial fibrillation, the most common cardiac disorder predisposing patients to embolization, afflicts about 20% of DCM patients [90]. Patients with DCM who have nonvalvular atrial fibrillation or previous systemic embolization should receive anticoagulation to an international normalized ratio of 2 to 3 unless contraindicated. Recommendations for patients with DCM in normal sinus rhythm without previous thromboembolism cannot be made with certainty. Many physicians recommend antithrombotic therapy for patients with DCM and evidence of congestive heart failure or a reduced left ventricular ejection fraction. A prospective, controlled randomized trial evaluating the risk-to-benefit ratio of antithrombotic therapy in prevention of systemic thromboembolism has been suggested [86,89].

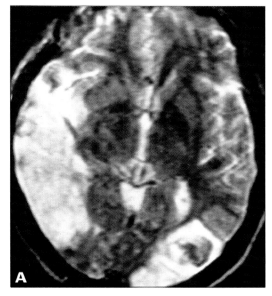 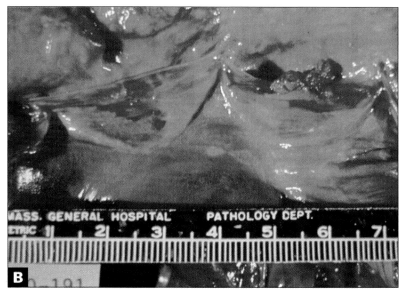

Figure 5-54. Nonbacterial thrombotic endocarditis (NBTE). NBTE causes verrucous valvular heart lesions, which form in association with a wide spectrum of diseases, including malignancies, with their concomitant hypercoagulable states [91,92]. An association with lung, gastrointestinal, and pancreatic adenocarcinomas is especially common. NBTE also occurs in patients with disseminated intravascular coagulation [91,92]. Systemic emboli occur in nearly half of patients with NBTE, most frequently involving the cerebral (**A**), coronary, renal, and mesenteric circulations [93]. The diagnosis of NBTE is usually made at autopsy, but NBTE is being diagnosed clinically more frequently owing to increased awareness and the use of two-dimensional echocardiography (**B**). NBTE is found in 0.3% to 9.3% of autopsy cases, most of which are associated with malignancy [91]. Cerebral infarction occurs in 33% to 53% of patients with NBTE, making neurologic events the most common manifestation [91]. Cerebral infarction is generally noted in the territory of large or medium-sized branches of the middle cerebral artery, the posterior cerebral artery, or the basilar artery. The pathophysiologic mechanism of these malignancy-associated thrombotic vegetations is not clear [94].

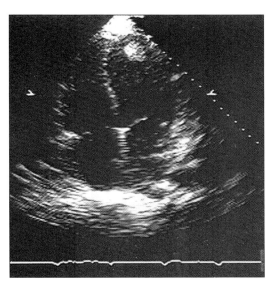

Figure 5-55. Transthoracic echocardiogram showing a thrombus in the left ventricular apex. Myocardial infarction that produces left ventricular (LV) aneurysm and thrombi carries a high risk for systemic embolization [95]. LV thrombi are thought to form in three clinical settings: acute myocardial infarction, chronic left ventricular aneurysm secondary to myocardial infarction, and dilated cardiomyopathy. Endocardial injury, regional circulatory stasis, and activation of the intrinsic coagulation are all factors that favor thrombus formation and systemic embolization. Several studies suggest that the risk is higher during the first 1 to 3 months after infarction. The risk of embolism is highest during the first 10 days for patients with large anterior infarcts. To prevent LV thrombosis and systemic embolism, full-dose heparinization followed by warfarin therapy is suggested for patients with large anterior infarctions and for those with heart failure [96–98]. One prospective nonrandomized trial demonstrated that warfarin is superior to no warfarin in preventing recurrent myocardial infarction, death, or stroke after myocardial infarction [98]. Two studies of patients with thrombus after acute myocardial infarction have demonstrated that antithrombotic therapy with warfarin was associated with the disappearance of ventricular thrombus in 88% of treated patients, compared with 24% of untreated patients [99,100]. The use of thrombolytic therapy, however, has not been shown to reduce the risk of LV thrombus formation [101].

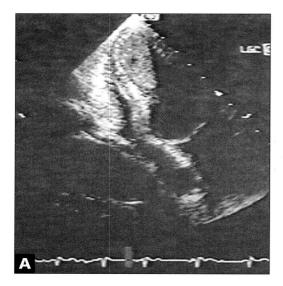

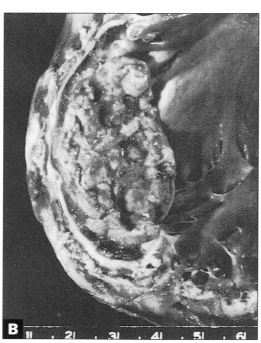

Figure 5-56. Ventricular septal aneurysm. **A,** Echocardiogram showing a ventricular septal aneurysm with thrombus formation after myocardial infarction. **B,** Pathologic specimen of the heart showing a mural thrombus overlying an old myocardial infarction of the left ventricle. Left ventricular (LV) aneurysm, another sequel to myocardial infarction, occurs 3 months or more after acute myocardial infarction [95]. The incidence of mural thrombi in patients with LV aneurysm ranges from 39% to 66% in autopsy and surgical series [95,102]. In contrast to newly formed LV thrombus, chronic organized laminated thrombi rarely embolize, and chronic anticoagulation therapy is not routinely indicated. Thrombus mobility occurs in about one quarter of patients who develop ventricular thrombus acutely after myocardial infarct. About 35% to 83% of these patients have systemic embolization [101]. Thus, current practice is not to treat patients who have chronic LV thrombi with antithrombotic therapy unless they have had a previous embolus or echocardiography has shown a protruding and mobile thrombus [101]. (Panel B *from* the case records of the Massachusetts General Hospital [103]; with permission. Copyright © 1970 Massachusetts Medical Society. All rights reserved.)

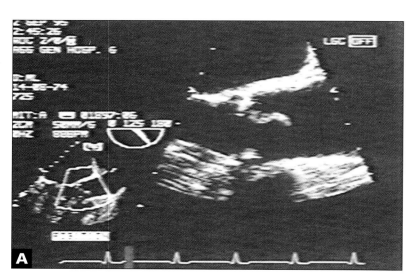

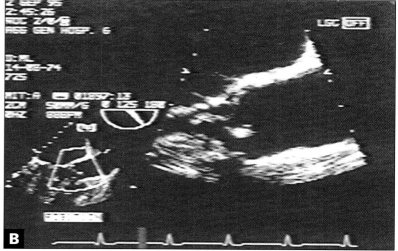

Figure 5-57. Rheumatic valvular disease. **A, B,** Transesophogeal echocardiogram showing a vegetation on the aortic valve moving in and out of the aorta during systole and diastole. Cerebral embolism is a common complication of rheumatic valvular disease. Sources of embolic material from rheumatic valves include vegetations on the valve surface, roughened endocardium, and thrombi on the wall of the atrium and the appendage, which usually coexist with atrial fibrillation. Rheumatic valve disease may be asymptomatic at the time of systemic embolization, but atrial fibrillation is a common complication that often occurs with mitral stenosis. If valvular heart disease is associated with atrial fibrillation, anticoagulation is recommended with an international normalized ratio of 2 to 3 [104]. In 1964 Szekely [105] demonstrated that anticoagulation in the setting of rheumatic mitral valvular disease was associated with fewer strokes. Although this study was not randomized, it established anticoagulation as standard therapy in these patients.

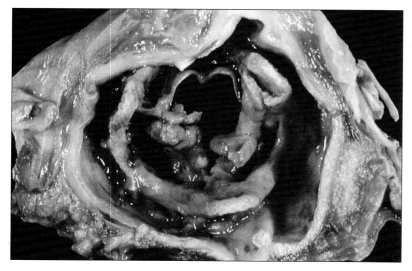

Figure 5-58. Pathologic slide of an aortic bioprosthetic valve containing vegetations and bridging across the cusps. The cardiac valve prostheses currently used are either mechanical or tissue valves (homografts or porcine valves). Cerebral embolism associated with prosthetic heart valves is usually associated with mechanical prosthetic devices rather than bioprosthetic valves. For bioprosthetic valves, anticoagulation (international normalized ratio [INR] of 2 to 3) is recommended in the first 3 months after valve replacement [104,106]. Long-term anticoagulation is recommended only if patients had myocardial infarction, stroke, atrial fibrillation, or left atrial thrombus noted at the time of surgery. If none of these complicating factors exists at the end of 3 months, replacing anticoagulant therapy with antiplatelet therapy (aspirin 325 mg/d) is recommended [104,106]. If vegetations are noted on bioprosthetic valves, infection should be ruled out before considering antithrombotic therapy. The current guidelines strongly recommend anticoagulation with an INR of 2.5 to 3.5 in patients with mechanical prosthetic valves [104,106].

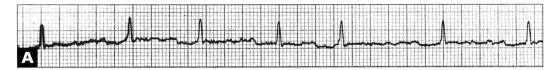

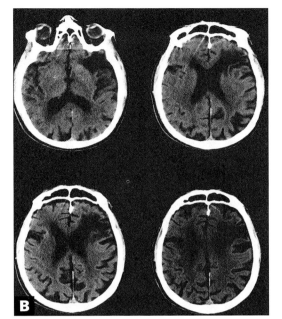

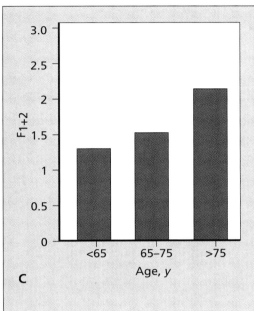

anticoagulation was low, prothrombin time ratio of 1.2 to 1.5, corresponding to an International Normalized Ratio (INR) of 1.5 to 2.7, and use of warfarin was safe. INRs above 3 have been associated with an increased risk of intracranial hemorrhage, especially in elderly patients [115]. Guidelines recommend a target INR of 2 to 3 in the treatment of patients with chronic atrial fibrillation [116,117]. **C**, Age-related increase in the rate of thrombin generation (the plasma level of F_{1+2}) among control patients in the Boston Area Anticoagulation Trial for Atrial Fibrillation [118]. Half of the patients in the control group were taking aspirin, and their mean F_{1+2} was the same as those not taking aspirin [118]. The age-related increase in the level of activity of the hemostatic system may suggest a mechanism to explain the age-related increase in stroke rate among patients with atrial fibrillation [118,119]. Similarly, the lack of effect of aspirin in reducing the level of activity of the hemostatic system may explain its relative lack of stroke-protective effect compared with warfarin in the atrial fibrillation trials [114,119]. The concept of vascular bed-specific hemostasis to explain thrombosis in specific vascular beds in different disease states, *eg*, acute myocardial infarction, thrombotic thrombocytopenic purpura, and deep vein phlebothrombosis, has been suggested (119). We hypothesize that the level of activity of the hemostatic system in the left atrial appendage in patients with atrial fibrillation determines their rate of embolism (120). Our F_{1+2} data suggest that some patients with atrial fibrillation and an adequate INR (2 to 3) still have a heightened level of thrombin generation (118). We anticipate that their vascular bed-specific increased hemostasis can be detected by refined analysis of the hemostatic and fibrinolytic systems combined with genetic markers (85). If so, instead of treating 100 patients with atrial fibrillation per year to prevent four to eight strokes as the atrial fibrillation investigators' collaborative working group suggests (114), only those truly at risk for stroke could be treated.

Figure 5-59. Atrial fibrillation (AF). **A**, Electrocardiogram of a patient with AF. **B**, Computed tomography scans of an 89-year-old man who had chronic AF for 15 years and was on no medication. This scan was done in the first hour after the patient presented with a right middle cerebral artery territory stroke. The new infarct is not yet visible but an old infarct in the territory of the left middle cerebral artery is noted. The Framingham study showed that, after the age of 50 years, AF is the strongest independent risk factor for stroke. The overall attributable risk for stroke in patients with atrial fibrillation who are 50 to 59 years of age (1.5%) increased to 23% for those older than 80 years of age [107,108]. Five randomized trials studying the safety and efficacy of warfarin in the prevention of primary ischemic stroke among patients with AF have demonstrated that warfarin dramatically reduced the rate of stroke in patients 65 years and older [109–114]. Patients younger than 65 years also had significant benefit if they had diabetes, hypertension, or previous stroke as risk factors. The risk of intracranial hemorrhage was less than 0.25% per year. The highest rate of intracranial hemorrhage among the five trials was 0.89% per year [110]. In the two largest trials [111,113], the intensity of

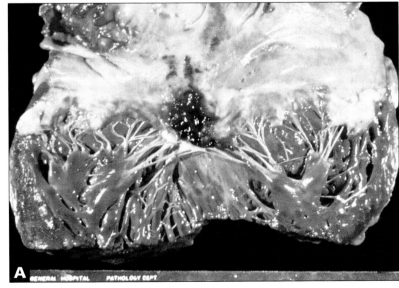

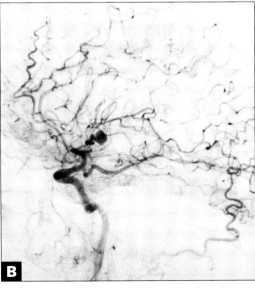

Figure 5-60. Infective endocarditis (IE). **A**, Pathologic specimen of the mitral valve showing a large hemorrhagic bacterial vegetation. Stroke is one of the most common presentations in patients with IE, accounting for one half to two thirds of the neurologic manifestations [121,122]. Up to 30% of these strokes occur within the first 2 weeks after diagnosis and the initiation of the antibiotic therapy [122]. Most emboli related to IE are the result of disrupted fragments from cardiac vegetations. IE due to virulent microorganisms, particularly *Staphylococcus aureus*, is associated with friable vegetations and an increased frequency of embolization. IE due to *Haemophilus* sp. or fungi tends to produce large, mobile vegetations with the risk of large vessel emboli [123]. Emboli occurring before the initiation or the completion of successful antibiotic therapy may contain microorganisms capable of producing secondary infectious complications. These include cerebral microabscesses, meningitis, arteritis, and mycotic aneurysms. **B**, Left common carotid angiogram showing an aneurysm of a proximal branch of the left middle cerebral artery.

(*Continued on next page*)

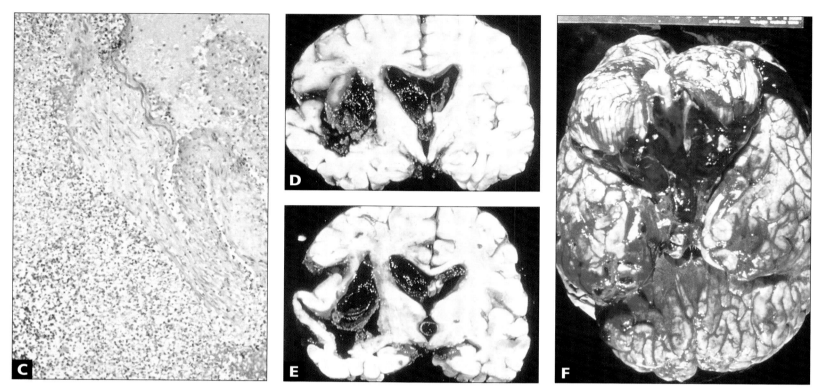

Figure 5-60. (*Continued*) **C,** Microscopic examination of the middle cerebral artery showing acute inflammation and destruction of the wall.

Two types of emboli may occur during IE. First, microemboli result in punctate cerebral infarctions, which may cause fluctuating neurologic deficits or may be asymptomatic. The second, major arterial emboli, is seen in 17% of IE patients [121]. Hemorrhagic transformation frequently occurs in cases of large embolic infarction. The intracerebral hemorrhage noted in 7% to 25% of IE patients (**D, E,** coronal sections of the brain showing a large intracerebral hemorrhage) may be due to ruptured mycotic aneurysms, (**F,** massive subarachnoid hemorrhage at the base of the brain due to a ruptured mycotic aneurysm). Usually, however, subarachnoid hemorrhage from a ruptured mycotic aneurysm occurs on the cortical surface rather than in the basal cisterns. In contrast to berry aneurysms, mycotic aneurysms occur after the first bifurcation of the arteries at the base of the brain or after the first bifurcation of their major branches.

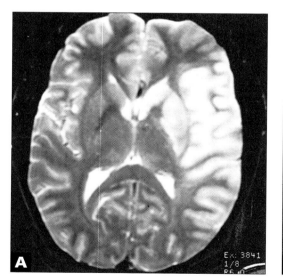
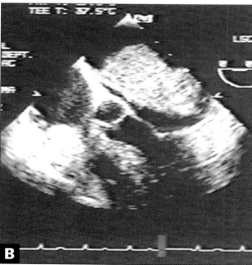
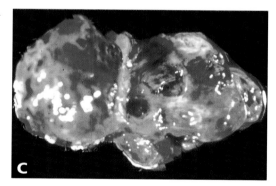

Figure 5-61. Atrial myxoma. Previous studies report that 18% to 67% of patients with left atrial myxoma have neurologic complications, including embolic cerebral infarction and transient cerebral ischemic attacks [124]. **A,** T2-weighted magnetic resonance image of the brain of a patient who presented with global aphasia and right hemiplegia as the result of atrial myxoma embolization. The image shows evolving infarction in the left middle cerebral artery territory. Although atrial myxomas are rare, failure to recognize them may deprive patients of potentially life-saving tumor resection. The prognosis for patients treated early is good, but the prognosis for patients who have developed neurologic complications is much poorer [124]. Half or more of patients with atrial myxoma have systemic symptoms, including fever, weight loss, and generalized aching. Laboratory assessment may show increased gamma-globulin ratio, increased erythrocyte sedimentation rate, and anemia. Atrial myxoma can be diagnosed with a high sensitivity by two-dimensional echocardiography. **B,** Echocardiogram showing a large atrial myxoma floating above the mitral valve during systole. **C,** Pathologic specimen showing bisected gelatinous atrial myxoma with numerous cysts.

(*Continued on next page*)

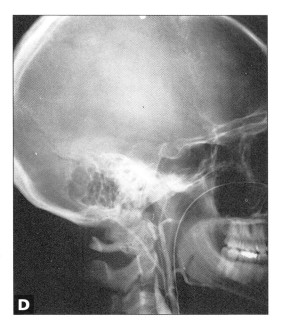
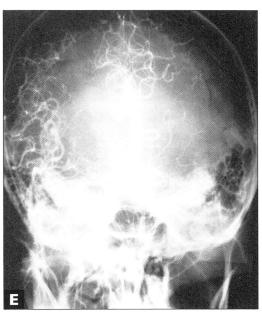

Figure 5-61. (*Continued*) Microscopically, the tumor consists of an amorphous matrix of interstitial ground substance, predominantly an acid mucopolysaccharide [124]. Myxomas may be sessile or pedunculated; however, friable, pedunculated tumors are more likely to embolize [125,126]. Embolic myxoma has been described as invading, displacing, and destroying normal elements of arterial walls, usually in the distal branches of the cerebral arteries. The associated connective tissue proliferation and a mild inflammatory reaction provide the substrate for aneurysm or pseudoaneurysm formation [127]. **D,** Left carotid angiogram showing an occluded left internal carotid artery and **E,** a right carotid angiogram showing cross-filling of the left anterior cerebral artery and an occluded left middle cerebral artery. The right carotid angiogram shows myxomatous aneurysms in the distal branches. Generally, mycotic aneurysms occur after the first major branch of the arteries at the base of the brain, while sterile berry aneurysms occur only at the first branch points of the arteries at the base of the brain. Aneurysm formation and rupture after surgical resection of primary myxoma was an infrequent complication in two recent series [128,129].

Ascending Aortic Atheroma

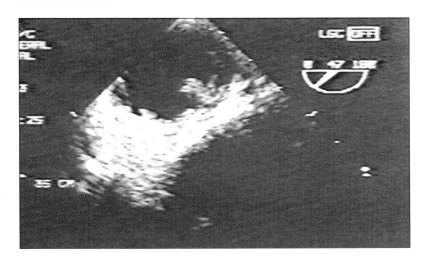

Figure 5-62. Transesophageal echocardiogram that confirms the diagnosis of ascending aortic atheromatous disease [130–134]. Ulcerated atheromatous plaque and lesions 4 mm or more in thickness have been associated with embolic stroke [132]. Aggressive blood pressure and lipid management are important therapeutic goals in attempting to stabilize atheromatous lesions. The efficacy of antithrombotic versus antiplatelet therapy in this setting is uncertain [134]. Patients with primary embolic stroke and an associated aortic atheromatous lesion larger than 4 mm are at especially increased risk for recurrent stroke [135]. A randomized trial studying the stroke prevention efficacy of warfarin versus aspirin in these patients is needed [134,135]. Because of the high recurrence rate, this is a plausible study. Not only would its results help guide the decision to antithrombotic therapy, they also would likely answer whether warfarin therapy is associated with cholesterol crystal embolism [58,134].

Preventive Therapy for Ascending Aortic Atheroma

	Antithrombotic (warfarin, INR 2–3)	Antiplatelet
Known cardioembolic*	++	+, if antithrombotic therapy contraindicated
Possible cardioembolic		+
Ascending aortic atheroma		+

Figure 5-63. Preventive therapy for ascending aortic atheroma. The National Institutes of Health–sponsored Warfarin Aspirin Recurrent Stroke Study is addressing the efficacy question. The number of cases of each entity will probably be too small to answer the question with statistical confidence. (*) Myoma and bacterial endocarditis are exceptions to the recommendation of antithrombotic therapy because they are associated with myxomatous and mycotic intracranial arterial aneurysm formation and subsequent hemorrhage. Antithrombotic therapy is considered only in special circumstances. INR—international normalized ratio.

$$\text{Relative risk of embolism} = \text{presence and severity of cardiac or aortic pathophysiologic process} + \text{the level of activity of the hemostatic system}$$

Figure 5-64. Hypothesis for risk of cerebral embolism. The level of activity of the hemostatic system is, in some measure, related to the ease with which clot formation can occur. It is best measured by the radioimmune assay of the peptide fragment F_{1+2} that splits off prothrombin when it is converted to thrombin. This step is the final common step combining the intrinsic and extrinsic clotting systems before thrombin triggers the conversion of fibrinogen to fibrin. Therefore, it represents a summation of all the procoagulant and anticoagulant factors involved in hemostasis. The hypothesis was conceived because of the age-related increase in stroke risk in patients with atrial fibrillation and our demonstration of the age-related increase in the level of activity of the hemostatic system in patients with atrial fibrillation [111,120]. Warfarin reduced this age-dependent effect in the population of patients studied in the Boston Area Anticoagulation Trial in Atrial Fibrillation [58,111,120,134].

Vasculitis of the Central Nervous System

Types of Vasculitis

Infectious	Noninfectious
Bacterial	Systemic vasculitides that often affect the CNS
Fungal	Vasculitis associated with collagen vascular disease
Rickettsial	Primary CNS vasculitis
Parasitic	Miscellaneous
Viral	

Figure 5-65. Types of vasculitis. Infectious vasculitis of the central nervous system usually occurs as a complication of central nervous system (CNS) infections, such as meningitis or paracranial infection. Systemic infections, however, especially bacterial endocarditis, can also cause severe and diffuse CNS vascular complications. The details about infective endocarditis and its CNS complications are discussed in Fig. 5-60. Noninfectious vasculitis can be part of a systemic illness, such as collagen vascular disease. In this case, CNS complications usually occur late in the course of disease. When vasculitis is the main feature of the illness, as in polyarteritis nodosa or Wegener's granulomatosis, the frequency and distribution of neurologic complications vary with the underlying disorder. In some cases, however, a neurologic manifestation is the only presenting symptom. In granulomatous angiitis of the CNS, the vasculitic process is almost always restricted to the CNS. Most of the noninfectious vasculitides are related either directly or indirectly to immunopathologic mechanisms. In humans, immune complex deposition may be the main pathologic process in hypersensitivity vasculitis and polyarteritis nodosa, whereas cell-mediated immune mechanism may play an important role in vasculitis with granuloma.

It is always prudent to look for infectious causes of vasculitis because most infectious causes need specific treatment, and prompt definitive management may improve the clinical outcome. Treatment of noninfectious vasculitis is based on the immunopathologic mechanisms. Immunosuppressive agents and steroids are the most commonly used medications.

Infectious Vasculitis of the Nervous System

Bacterial
  Bacterial meningitis
  Infective endocarditis
  Cavernous sinus thrombophlebitis
  Syphilitic arteritis
  Lyme disease
  Tuberculous meningitis
Fungal
  Aspergillosis
  Mucormycosis
  Cryptococcosis

Rickettsial
  Rocky Mountain spotted fever
Parasitic
  Cysticercosis
  Malaria
Viral
  Herpes zoster
  Cytomegalovirus
  HIV

Figure 5-66. Infectious vasculitis of the nervous system. Infectious vasculitis affecting cerebral vessels can cause ischemic or hemorrhagic complications. In most cases, the principal mechanism is a direct invasion of organisms into the vascular wall, leading to an inflammatory reaction [135–137]. Occasionally, immune complex–mediated vasculopathy is the primary pathophysiologic mechanism. Various types of organisms have been shown to be associated with cerebral vasculitis, including bacteria, fungi, viruses, protozoa, and parasites [138–140]. Stroke is a common complication of severe bacterial and tuberculous meningitis. Cavernous sinus thrombophlebitis and bacterial meningitis may result in mycotic aneurysm formation [141]. Vasculopathy can also be found in CNS fungal infections, such as aspergillosis, mucormycosis, and cryptococcosis. In the past, syphilitic arteritis (meningovascular syphilis) was a common cause of stroke, but as a result of effective antibiotic treatment, it is now less prevalent. For viral infection, herpes zoster of the fifth cranial nerve and upper cervical roots can be followed by cerebral infarction. This is thought to be caused by direct invasion of the virus into the blood vessel wall. The common clinical finding is contralateral hemiplegia from middle cerebral artery infarction [142].

Noninfectious Vasculitis of the Nervous System

Systemic vasculitides that often affect the CNS
  Systemic necrotizing vasculitis
    Classic polyarteritis nodosa
    Allergic angiitis and granulomatosis (Churg-Strauss syndrome)
  Wegener's granulomatosis
  Giant cell arteritis
    Temporal arteritis
    Takayasu's arteritis
  Hypersensitivity vasculitis
    Henoch-Schönlein purpura
    Serum sickness
    Drug-induced vasculitis: LSD, amphetamine, ephedrine, cocaine, etc.
  Cryoglobulinemia (essential mixed cryoglobulinemia)

Vasculitis associated with collagen vascular disease and other systemic disease
  Systemic lupus erythematosus
  Rheumatoid arthritis
  Scleroderma
  Sjögren's syndrome
  Behçet's disease
  Sarcoidosis
Primary CNS vasculitis
  Granulomatous angiitis of the nervous system
Miscellaneous
  Cogan's syndrome
  Thromboangiitis obliterans
  Kawasaki syndrome
  Eale disease

Figure 5-67. Noninfectious vasculitis of the nervous system. Noninfectious causes of nervous system vasculitis fall into four categories. Classic polyarteritis nodosa and allergic angiitis and granulomatosis (Churg-Strauss syndrome) are prototypes of systemic necrotizing vasculitis. Classic polyarteritis nodosa is a multisystem disease that involves every organ except lung and spleen. Pathologically, it usually affects small and medium-sized arteries at their bifurcations and branching points [143]. The giant cell arteritides consist of two main diseases: temporal arteritis and Takayasu's arteritis. The characteristic pathologic feature of the giant cell arteritides is granulomatous vasculitis of medium-sized and large arteries. Hypersensitivity vasculitides are a group of disorders that include Henoch-Schönlein purpura, drug-induced vasculitis, serum sickness, and sometimes cryoglobulinemia. Neurologic complication in this group of vasculitis is uncommon. Vasculitis can be associated with collagen vascular disease, such as systemic lupus erythematosus, rheumatoid arthritis, or scleroderma. In granulomatous angiitis of the nervous system, the vasculitis is strictly limited to the central nervous system (CNS) [144–146].

Mechanisms of Vascular Inflammation in Vasculitis

Direct infection of vessels
  Bacterial vasculitis (*eg*, neisserial)
  Mycobacterial vasculitis (*eg*, tuberculous)
  Spirochetal vasculitis (*eg*, syphilitic)
  Rickettsial vasculitis (*eg*, Rocky Mountain spotted fever)
  Fungal vasculitis (*eg*, aspergillosis)
  Viral vasculitis (*eg*, herpes zoster)
Immunologic injury
  Immune complex–mediated vasculitis
    Cryoglobulinemic vasculitis
    Henoch-Schönlein purpura
    Lupus vasculitis
    Rheumatoid vasculitis
    Serum sickness vasculitis
    Infection-induced immune complex vasculitis
     Viral (*eg*, hepatitis B and C virus)
     Bacterial (*eg*, group A streptococcal)
    Some paraneoplastic vasculitis
    Some drug-induced vasculitis (*eg*, sulfonamide-induced vasculitis)
    Behçet's disease

Direct antibody attack–mediated vasculitis
  Goodpasture's syndrome (mediated by anti–basement membrane antibodies)
  Kawasaki disease (possibly mediated by antiendothelial antibodies)
ANCA–mediated vasculitis
  Wegener's granulomatosis
  Microscopic polyangiitis (microscopic polyarteritis)
  Churg-Strauss syndrome
  Some drug-induced vasculitis (*eg*, thiouracil-induced vasculitis)
Cell-mediated vasculitis
  Allograft cellular vascular rejection
  Giant cell (temporal) arteritis
  Takayasu's arteritis
  Isolated (granulomatous) CNS vasculitis

Figure 5-68. Mechanisms of vascular inflammation in vasculitis. This is the putative pathogenesis of vasculitides that induces a final pathway of vascular inflammation. The inflammatory process is characterized by the adhesion and penetration of leukocytes into the vascular endothelial surface and the release of mediators. In infectious vasculitis, direct invasion of the vessels may trigger a common inflammatory process, which leads to similar pathologic findings. Some infectious diseases, such as viral hepatitis, may cause immune complex formation and deposition resulting in inflammation. Noninfectious vasculitis is generally related to an immunologic injury to the vessel wall caused by immune complex, direct antibody attack, antineutrophil cytoplasmic antibody (ANCA), or cell mediation. Immune complex–mediated vasculitis is typically found in vasculitis associated with collagen vascular disease and serum sickness. ANCA-mediated diseases usually present as a pure vasculitic syndrome, such as Wegener's granulomatosis, periarteritis nodosa, and Churg-Strauss syndrome. Granulomatous inflammation found in temporal arteritis, Takayasu's arteritis, and isolated granulomatous angiitis of the nervous system are generally cell mediated. CNS—central nervous system. (*Adapted from* Jennette and colleagues [147].)

Bacterial Meningitis

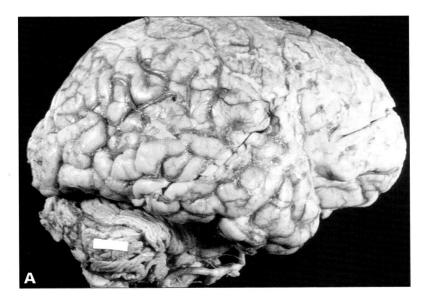

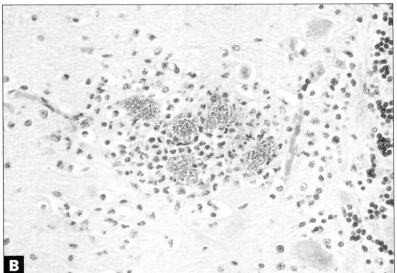

Figure 5-69. Bacterial meningitis. Bacterial meningitis usually causes an acute inflammatory lesion in the leptomeninges at the convexity. In severe cases, the inflammation may involve the meningeal vessels, resulting in vasculitis and stroke. Venous sinus involvement, especially of the superior sagittal sinus and cortical veins, occasionally leads to cerebral venous infarction [148,149]. **A,** Pathologic specimen showing thick exudate from bacterial meningitis covering the convexity of the brain. **B,** Microscopic picture of cerebral cortical arterioles in a patient who presented with bacterial meningitis. The lumen is occupied by clumps of bacteria. Polymorphonuclear infiltration is seen in the vascular adventitia. (*Courtesy of* Jean Paul G. Vonsattel, MD, C.S. Kubik Laboratory for Neuropathology, Massachusetts General Hospital.)

Syphilitic Arteritis

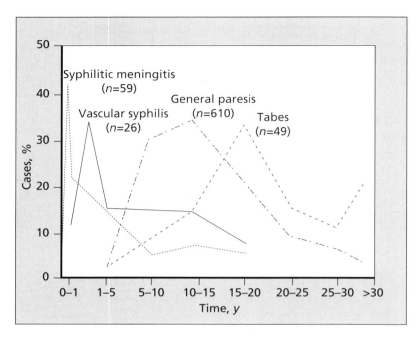

Figure 5-70. Interval between primary infection and symptomatic neurosyphilis. In immunocompetent hosts, the onset of meningovascular complications ranges from a few months to 12 years, with an average latency of 7 years after primary infection [150]. In patients infected with HIV, vascular complications occur earlier in the course (often within 1 year after primary infection). Vasculitis is one of the known complications of syphilis. Progressive neurologic deficit in the distribution of the middle cerebral artery is common. Half of the patients present with insidious prodromal symptoms, such as headache, vertigo, insomnia, or personality changes, several weeks to months before the onset of a focal neurologic deficit. (*Adapted from* Simon [150].)

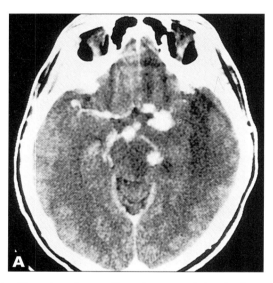
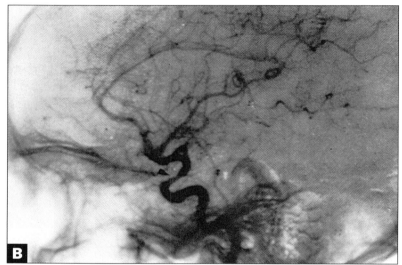

Figure 5-71. Neuroimaging studies of neurosyphilis. **A,** Contrast computed tomography scan of a brain that shows multiple basal–meningeal enhancement around the circle of Willis. It is caused by an inflammatory process and gummatous reaction around the vessels of the circle of Willis. **B,** Cerebral angiogram of another patient showing multifocal concentric narrowing of the intracranial carotid artery and proximal part of the middle cerebral and anterior cerebral arteries. In patients with meningovascular syphilis, vertebrobasilar involvement has also been reported. Aneurysmal dilation is occasionally found on angiography as a result of thinning of the tunica media. (*Panel A from* the case records of Massachusetts General Hospital [151]; with permission. Copyright © 1991 Massachusetts Medical Society. All rights reserved.)

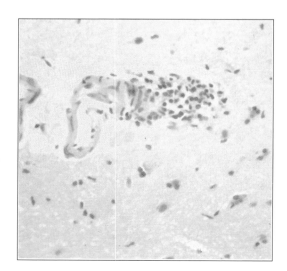

Figure 5-72. Pathologic findings in neurosyphilis. Microscopic brain biopsy specimen of a patient with neurosyphilis demonstrates a lymphoplasmocytic infiltration involving a cerebral blood vessel. The characteristic panarteritis, consisting of lymphocytes and plasma cells, that involves the intima, media, and adventitia is generally referred to as Heubner's arteritis. (*From* the case records of Massachusetts General Hospital [151]; with permission. Copyright © 1991 Massachusetts Medical Society. All rights reserved.)

Tuberculous Arteritis

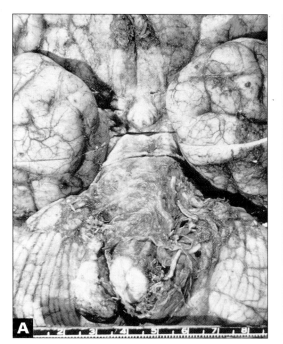
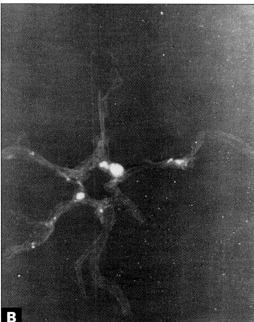
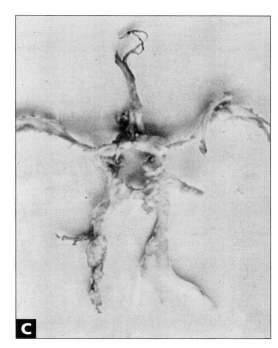

Figure 5-73. Tuberculous arteritis. **A,** Basal exudate at the base of the brain in a patient with tuberculous meningitis. The most common locations of tuberculous arteritis are at the basal arteries of the circle of Willis, especially middle cerebral arteries. The inflammatory exudate can produce inflammation and occlusion of small penetrating vessels. Inflammation in this area can also cause major narrowing, occlusion, and calcification of the main arteries of the circle of Willis and may sometimes lead to a moyamoya type of collateral circulation. **B,** Radiographic findings of **C,** a pathologic specimen of circle of Willis in a patient who had severe vasculopathy from tuberculous meningitis. Note the calcification of the arteries demonstrated by white areas in the radiograph picture. Tuberculous meningitis usually presents as a subacute illness. Patients with tuberculous meningitis generally have fever, malaise, and headache for about 1 week, followed by symptoms and signs of meningeal irritation, deteriorating mental status, cranial nerve palsies, and vasculopathy [152]. Stroke has been reported in up to 20% of patients. (Panel A *courtesy of* Jean Paul G. Vonsattel, MD, C.S. Kubik Laboratory for Neuropathology, Massachusetts General Hospital.)

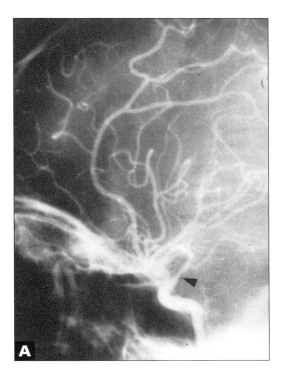
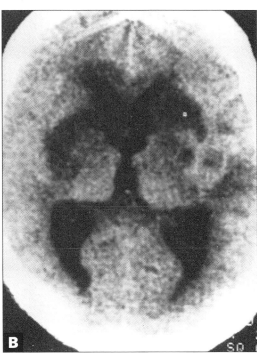

Figure 5-74. Neurologic imagings of stroke secondary to tuberculous meningitis (TBM). **A,** Angiogram demonstrating bilateral infarction at the corona radiata in the distribution of deep branches of the middle cerebral artery (*arrowhead*). Cerebral infarction typically occurs in the deep territory of the middle cerebral artery, leading to sensorimotor hemiplegia [153]. **B,** Computed tomography (CT) scan showing narrowing of the distal part of the internal carotid artery and middle cerebral artery secondary to tuberculous meningitis. Angiographic signs of tuberculous arteritis consist of segmental narrowing of major arteries at the base of the brain and occlusion of smaller vessels. The treatment of stroke syndromes associated with TBM is the same as for acute TBM. Once the diagnosis is established, antituberculous drugs should be administered because the prognosis depends significantly on prompt treatment. Delayed treatment leads to an increase in both morbidity and mortality. Concurrent steroid therapy in severe cases has been reported to reduce morbidity; therefore, short-term use of oral steroids is recommended in patients with evidence of tuberculous vasculitis secondary to meningitis [152].

Central Nervous System Aspergillosis

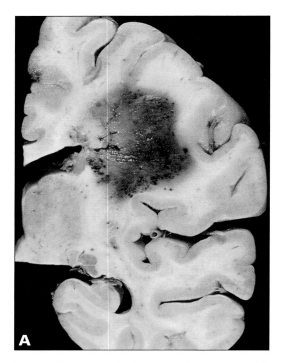

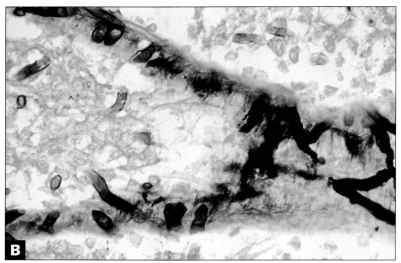

Figure 5-75. Pathologic findings in a patient with central nervous system (CNS) aspergillosis. **A,** Coronal section of a cerebral hemisphere showing hemorrhagic area at centrum semiovale due to vascular involvement of aspergillosis. **B,** Microscopic slide (silver stain) demonstrating invasion of the fungus, seen as uniform 3 to 6 microns, regularly septated branching hyphae, distributed throughout the blood vessel wall. Aspergillosis in humans occurs in two phases. Primary aspergillosis, which is usually asymptomatic, occurs in patients without underlying pulmonary disease or immune defect. Secondary aspergillosis is a reactivation of a primary infection and is generally encountered in an immunocompromised host. Predisposing conditions include malignancy, previous organ transplantation, prolonged antibiotic therapy, immunosuppressive treatment, and intravenous drug addiction. In general, CNS aspergillosis results from a direct extension of a paranasal sinus or orbital infection, or from hematogenous dissemination from lung or endocarditis. The forms of CNS aspergillosis include meningitis, meningoencephalitis, brain abscess, and vasculopathy. The most common vascular complication of aspergillosis is intracranial bleeding. Intracerebral or subarachnoid hemorrhage can occur as a result of either direct invasion by the fungus of a vessel wall or rupture of a mycotic aneurysm [154,155]. (*Courtesy of* Jean Paul G. Vonsattel, MD, C.S. Kubik Laboratory for Neuropathology, Massachusetts General Hospital.)

Central Nervous System Cysticercosis

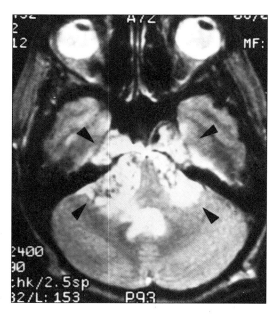

Figure 5-76. Magnetic resonance image showing a subarachnoidal form of cysticercosis at the base of the brain in a patient who presented with progressive ataxia with multiple cranial nerve dysfunction followed by brain stem ischemic stroke. A biopsy confirmed the presence of cysticercosis. The brain stem and the basilar artery are severely compressed and distorted by the clump of cysts (*arrowheads*). Cysticercosis is an infective process caused by pig tapeworm, *taenia solium*. A human becomes an incidental intermediate host when ingested eggs hatch and the parasites penetrate the host's intestinal mucosa to form cysts in various organs. Skin, muscles, and the central nervous system are the most common sites that harbor the cysts. The four forms of cysticercosis in the nervous system are the parenchymal, subarachnoidal, intraventricular, and spinal forms [156]. Cysts in the brain parenchyma may cause focal deficit and seizure and sometimes manifest as transient neurologic deficits mimicking stroke or transient ischemic attacks. The subarachnoidal form is usually located at the basal cistern around the brain stem and may cause chronic inflammation and basal meningitis. Vascular complications may occur as a result of inflammation around the circle of Willis. Occasionally, cysts at the basal cistern obstruct the cerebrospinal fluid pathway and lead to hydrocephalus. Moreover, a large clump of cysts may compress the brain stem or vascular structures. The intraventricular form of cysticercosis is usually asymptomatic unless the cyst obstructs the cerebrospinal fluid pathway. This may result in intermittent hydrocephalic attack and headache [157].

Noninfectious Cerebral Vasculitis

Type of vasculitis	Pathology	Clinical features	CNS involvement	Stroke syndrome
Systemic vasculitides often affecting the CNS				
Polyarteritis nodosa	Necrotizing vasculitis of small and medium-sized arteries	Renal, hepatic, and visceral vessel involvement with aneurysmal dilation, hypertension, anemia, PNS involvement (75%), and HBsAG positive (30%)	20%–40%; usually diffuse or multifocal; headache, confusion, psychosis, seizures, papilledema	Uncommon (13%); saccular aneurysms may be found
Wegener's granulomatosis	Necrotizing granulomatous vasculitis of small and medium-sized vessels	Upper and lower respiratory tract, glomerulonephritis; antineutrophil cytoplasmic antibody positive	23%–50%; peripheral and cranial neuropathy	Very rare
Lymphomatoid granulomatosis	Polymorphonuclear leukocyte infiltration and angiodestruction	Nodular infiltration in the lung and kidney, fever, malaise, weight loss, rapid, progressive	20%–35%; multifocal process; aphasia, frontal lobe signs, confusion, cranial neuropathy	Rare
Temporal arteritis	Granulomatous vasculitis predominantly in the media of medium-sized and large elastic arteries: superficial temporal, occipital, and vertebral arteries	Headache, fever, jaw claudication, polymyalgia, rheumatica, anemia, elevated ESR	Blindness (ischemic optic neuropathy), syncope, confusion, ataxia	Uncommon (10%)
Takayasu's arteritis	Granulomatous vasculitis of large arteries: aorta and its branches	Prodromal systemic illness, absent radial pulse, hypertension	Visual symptoms, syncope, and dizziness related to cerebral hypoperfusion	Rare; secondary to extracranial artery involvement
Hypersensitivity vasculitis	Leukocytoclastic vasculitis of small vessels: capillaries and postcapillary venules	Palpable purpura; possible antigen exposure; may associate with serum sickness, essential mixed cryglobulinemia, connective tissue disease, and malignancies	Uncommon; encephalopathy, seizures, coma, and peripheral neuropathy are found in serum sickness	Very rare
Churg-Strauss syndrome	Necrotizing vasculitis of arterioles, capillaries, and venules	Asthma, eosinophilia, systemic vasculitis, PNS involvement (60%)	Very rare but encephalopathy and focal CNS dysfunction have been reported	Very rare
Vasculitis associated with collagen vascular disease and other systemic disease				
Systemic lupus erythematosus	Vasculopathy (endothelial swelling and proliferation); true vasculitis is unusual	Multiorgan involvement	Encephalopathy, psychosis common	Uncommon (5%–15%), often related to Libman-Sacks endocarditis; TTP and antiphospholipid antibody
Rheumatoid arthritis	Leukocytoclastic vasculitis of the small venules; fulminant disseminated vasculitis is also seen	Arthritis, systemic symptoms, elevated ESR, rheumatoid factor	Compressive myelopathy from C1–C2 subluxation	Rare, may associate with thrombocytosis or hyperviscosity syndrome secondary to polyclonal gammopathy
Scleroderma	CNS vasculitis is very rare	Skin involvement	Rare; trigeminal neuropathy	Rare, hemorrhage from renal hypertension
Sneddon's disease	Mainly occlusive noninflammatory vasculopathy; true vasculitis is very rare	Livedo reticularis, recurrent cerebral infarction; may associate with antiphospholipid syndrome	Transient ischemic attacks or stroke with prominent cortical sign; unknown mechanism; may associate with antiphospholipid antibody and noninfective endocarditis	Common
Behçet's disease	Small vessel vasculitis, especially venules	Oral ulcers, genital ulcers, uveitis, thrombophlebitis	6%–28%, headache, meningoencephalitis, corticospinal tract involvement, pseudotumor cerebri, brain stem dysfunction, encephalopathy	Uncommon; dural venous sinus thrombosis
Primary CNS vasculitis	Segmental granulomatous arteritis of small arteries and veins of the CNS, predilection for the small leptomeningeal vessels	No systemic symptoms	CNS involvement 100%; headache, nausea, dementia, confusion, amnestic state, stepwise progression of multifocal neurologic symptoms and seizures; ESR may be normal; elevated cerebrospinal fluid protein	Common

Figure 5-77. Pathologic and clinical findings of common types of noninfectious vasculitis [136–139,143–147]. CNS—central nervous system; ESR— erythrocyte sedimentation rate; HBsAg—hepatits B surface antigen; PNS— peripheral nervous system; TTP—thrombotic thrombocytopenic purpura.

Screening Tests for Noninfectious CNS Vasculitic Disease

History and physical examination
  Evidence of multiple organ involvement
  Past medical history of connective tissue disease or vasculitis
  Family history
Laboratory tests
  Complete blood count
  Urinalysis
  Blood urea nitrogen and creatinine
  Plasma glucose
  Erythrocyte sedimentation rate, C-reactive protein
  Liver function tests
  Serum Venereal Disease Research Laboratory (VDRL)
  Prothrombin time, partial thromboplastin time,
    coagulation studies
  Antinuclear antibodies (ANA)
  Anticardiolipin antibody
  Antineutrophil cytoplasmic antibody (ANCA)
  Hepatitis B surface antigen
  Serum immunoelectrophoresis
  Coombs' test
  Cryoglobulin
  Cerebrospinal fluid analysis
  Chest radiograph
Imaging studies
  Computed tomography scan of the brain
  Magnetic resonance imaging of the CNS
  Cranial angiography
  Visceral angiography
  Ultrasonography
Tissue diagnosis
  Temporal artery biopsy
  Leptomeningeal and brain biopsy
  Skin biopsy

Figure 5-78. Screening tests for patients with suspected noninfectious central nervous system (CNS) vasculitic disease. A correct diagnosis of noninfectious vasculitic disease depends equally on detailed clinical information and laboratory tests. The patient's history may reveal evidence of connective tissue disease or systemic vasculitis. Skin rashes, unexplained prolonged fever, headache, spontaneous abortion, multiorgan disease, or a family history of connective tissue disease or vasculitis are all helpful clues. Routine laboratory tests, including complete blood count, urinalysis, prothrombin time, partial thromboplastin time, chest radiograph, liver function tests, blood urea nitrogen, creatinine, and plasma glucose, may suggest specific organ involvement and lead to further studies. For example, anemia is common in patients with temporal arteritis, and hypereosinophilia may suggest hypersensitivity vasculitis. Erythrocyte sedimentation rate and C-reactive protein are also helpful, although not specific, in detecting an acute inflammatory process. Several primary vasculitic syndromes, such as Wegener's granulomatosis, Churg-Strauss syndrome, and polyarteritis nodosa have an association with antineutrophil cytoplasmic antibody. The perinuclear antinuclear cytoplasmic antibody is very specific for Wegener's granulomatosis, whereas the cytoplasmic type is specific for Churg-Strauss syndrome. These are not very sensitive, however, and are absent in most patients [147]. Histologic evaluation of the biopsied specimen may be needed as a gold standard for diagnosis of some specific diseases, such as leptomeningeal biopsy for granulomatous angiitis of the CNS, temporal artery biopsy for temporal arteritis, and skin biopsy for systemic vasculitic disease [139].

Takayasu's Arteritis

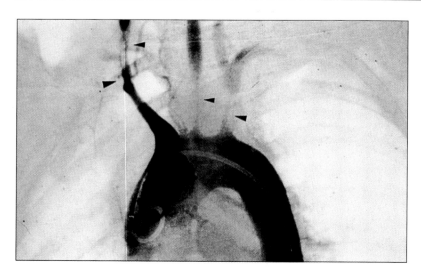

Figure 5-79. The classic angiographic findings in Takayasu's arteritis, as characterized by narrowing or occlusion of the origin of the branch vessels of the aortic arch (*arrowheads*). Takayasu's arteritis is a primary, nonspecific, inflammatory disease that involves the aorta and its main branches. Occasionally, coronary and pulmonary arteries are affected. The disease has a predilection for young Asian women, with a female to male ratio of 2.4:1 to 9.4:1. The age prevalence is greatest in the second and third decades. The cause of this disease is still unclear, but much evidence suggests an autoimmune mechanism. Hereditary factors may also play an important role [158].

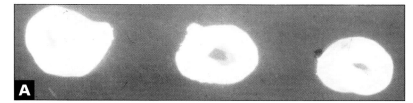

Figure 5-80. Pathologic specimen of the common carotid artery of a young female patient with Takayasu's arteritis who presented with an ischemic stroke. **A**, Cross-section of the artery shows thickening of the wall with a narrow lumen. **B**, Microscopic image of a carotid artery showing the destruction of elastic fibers associated with atrophy and replacement of smooth muscle cells by fibrosis in the tunica media, which is characteristic of Takayasu's arteritis. The cell infiltrations are composed of lymphocytes and multinucleated giant cells. Thickening of the intima occurs secondary to impairment of blood supply within the arterial wall, leading to segmental narrowing of the lumen. Occasionally, the vessel wall becomes thin, and an aneurysm may develop [159,160].

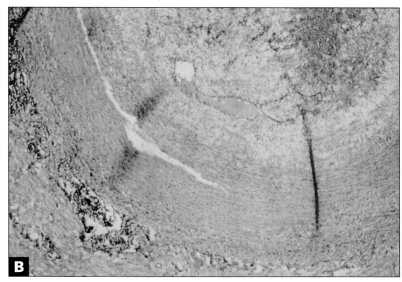

Areas of Involvement and Angiographic Findings in Takayasu's Arteritis

Arterial involvement of Takayasu's arteritis	%
Aorta	38.2
Abdominal aorta	20.2
Renal artery	18.7
Subclavian artery	14.3
Common carotid artery	7.3
Mesenteric artery	6.7
Vertebral artery	5.3
Angiographic findings	
Stenosis	29
Dilation	26
Occlusion	19
Irregular contour	17
Aneurysm formation	9

Figure 5-81. Common areas of involvement and angiographic findings of Takayasu's arteritis in 63 patients. Characteristic lesions of Takayasu's arteritis occur in elastic arteries and often spread to the origins of muscular arteries, which branch off directly from the aorta. The most common location is the aorta, with a predilection for the abdominal part. The second most common site of involvement is the renal artery, followed by the subclavian artery. Lesions of the neck vessels, the carotid and vertebral arteries, are frequently seen. Among the angiographic and pathologic findings, stenosis and irregular contours of the vessels are found in most cases. Aneurysmal formation and dilation of the vessel, secondary to the weakness of the vessel wall, are also seen [158].

Symptoms and signs of Takayasu's arteritis are variable. Hypertension, generalized malaise, fever, arthralgia, and symptoms of low cerebral perfusion and vertebrobasilar insufficiency, such as dizziness, vertigo, fainting spells, and visual disturbances, are common. Hypertension is found in 75% of cases. Absence or diminution of radial pulse as a result of subclavian stenosis or occlusion is an important sign; this disease is also known as the "pulseless" disease. A vascular murmur resulting from a narrowing of the vessels in the neck, back, and abdomen may be heard. Stroke occurs in 22% of patients. Ischemic stroke is not common but has been reported in patients with severe carotid disease. Intracranial hemorrhage is usually related to hypertension [158]. Congestive heart failure and aortic regurgitation are other clinical manifestations.

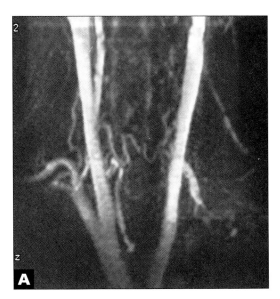
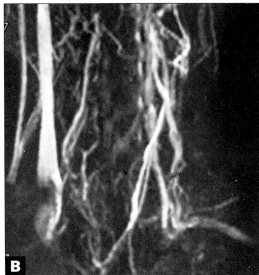
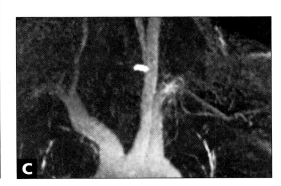

Figure 5-82. Neuroimages of a patient with Takayasu's arteritis. This patient presented with subclavian steal syndrome. **A**, The left vertebral and the left subclavian arteries are not seen on superior saturation pulse magnetic resonance angiogram (MRA). **B**, An inferior saturation pulse MRA, however, shows these arteries, indicating reversal of flow. **C**, Three-dimensional time-of-flight magnetic resonance angiogram (MRA) of the aortic arch showing occlusion of the left subclavian artery with collateral vessels and occlusion of the right common carotid artery.

Clinical and Laboratory Findings in 64 Patients With Giant Cell Arteritis

	%
Abnormal temporal artery	66
Headache	65
Myalgia or arthralgia	46
Visual symptoms	37
Fever	35
Weight loss	28
Anorexia	23
Malaise	23
Jaw claudication	23
Anemia	13
ESR >50 mm/h	91

Figure 5-83. Clinical and laboratory findings in 64 patients with biopsy-proven giant cell arteritis. Giant cell arteritis, or temporal arteritis, is characterized by systemic granulomatous inflammation of large and medium-sized arteries. Usually, it affects people older than 50 years of age [160–163]. The symptoms and signs are most commonly referable to the affected temporal artery. Tender and nodular temporal arteries were found in 66% of patients. A unilateral headache at the temporal region is also common. It is usually worse at night and is sometimes associated with scalp tenderness. Systemic symptoms and signs of polymyalgia rheumatica are found in half the cases. Constitutional symptoms, such as fever, malaise, anorexia, and weight loss, are common. Visual symptoms were found in 37% of patients. Ischemic optic neuropathy is a serious complication of temporal arteritis and can lead to permanent blindness. Jaw claudication is found in 23%. Ischemic stroke can occur, usually because of narrowing of the carotid arteries at the siphon or of the vertebral arteries before they pierce the dura mater. Erythrocyte sedimentation rate (ESR) is a helpful test. Ninety-one percent of patients have an ESR of greater than 50 mm/h. A normal ESR, however, does not exclude the diagnosis [162]. (*Adapted from* Procter and colleagues [164].)

Temporal Arteritis

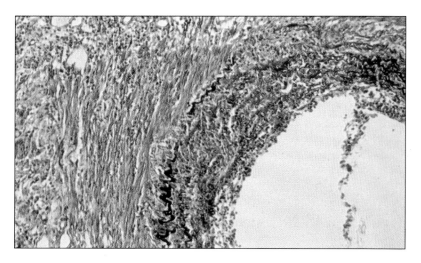

Figure 5-84. Pathologic specimen from a temporal artery biopsy showing thickening of the intimal layer of the blood vessel in a patient with temporal arteritis. Lymphocytic infiltration is found throughout the intima, media, and adventitia of the artery. The most striking appearance in this disease is an irregular destruction of the elastic lamina in the wall of the artery (seen as areas blackened by elastin stain) with granulomatous reaction. A circumscribed granuloma is present in the adventitia. (*From* the case record at Massachusetts General Hospital [165]; with permission. Copyright © 1986 Massachusetts Medical Society. All rights reserved.)

Granulomatous Angiitis

Clinical and Laboratory Findings of Granulomatous Angiitis

Clinical findings	Patients, %	Laboratory findings	Patients, %
Diffuse cortical dysfunction	95	Cerebrospinal fluid findings at the time of diagnosis	
Headache	68	Leukocyte count >10 × 10⁶	73
Focal cerebral dysfunction	50	Protein >0.5 g/L	90
Evidence of increased intracranial pressure	43	Opening pressure >200 mm H_2O	53
Brain stem or cranial nerve disease	40		
Seizures	25		
Spinal cord disease	23		
Fever and sweats	20		
Anorexia and weight loss	20		

Figure 5-85. Clinical and laboratory findings of granulomatous angiitis of the nervous system (GANS). GANS is a rare, granulomatous, necrotizing arteritis of unknown cause. It is characterized by predominant or exclusive involvement of the central nervous system (CNS). Headache is found in 68% of patients. Global dysfunction of the CNS secondary to small vessel involvement, such as confusion, psychiatric disorder, memory disturbance, and lethargy is common. Occasionally, large vessel involvement may cause ischemic stroke and focal deficit [166]. The erythrocyte sedimentation rate is usually normal or minimally elevated. Spinal fluid is almost always abnormal, and the most consistent abnormality is the elevated protein. Some patients have a moderate lymphocytic pleocytosis. Cranial angiogram is abnormal in 70% to 90% of cases; therefore, a normal angiogram does not exclude the diagnosis [167]. Angiographic findings include arterial narrowing and dilation, occlusion, aneurysm formation, and alteration of circulation time in the affected vascular distribution [167,168]. (*Adapted from* Vollmer and colleagues [166].)

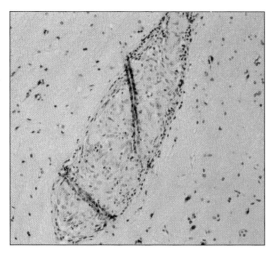

Figure 5-86. Brain biopsy specimen obtained from cerebral cortex showing an inflammatory process in the vascular wall with extensive granulomatous reaction from a patient with granulomatous angiitis. The cellular infiltrations are mainly composed of lymphocytes, plasma cells, and granuloma with multinucleated giant cells. A brain leptomeningeal biopsy is suggested in all cases when the diagnosis of granulomatous angiitis is suspected. In most cases, the duration of illness to death is less than 6 months. There is no standard treatment for this disease. Remission has been reported in a patient who was treated with a combination of prednisolone and cyclophosphamide. (*From* the case record of Massachusetts General Hospital [169]; with permission. Copyright © 1989 Massachusetts Medical Society. All rights reserved.)

Complications of Cocaine Use

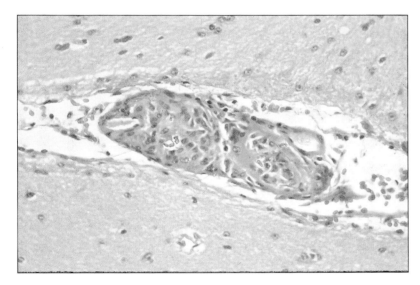

Figure 5-87. Histologic slide of a brain specimen showing vasculitis with foreign body giant cell reaction in a patient who had stroke secondary to intravenous cocaine use. Cocaine is a highly addictive drug that can cause a variety of neurovascular complications, including subarachnoid hemorrhage, intracerebral hemorrhage, cerebral infarction, seizures, and cerebral vasculitis. These complications are sometimes fatal and can occur at first use. Ischemic cerebrovascular complications are found in about half the patients with complications. The infarcts are usually located in the subcortical area in the middle cerebral artery territory. The mechanism of cocaine-induced ischemia is still poorly understood, but vasculitis, vasospasm, and effect of the drug on the hemostatic system have been proposed. Some reports found that hemorrhage is more common than infarction. It can occur within seconds or up to 12 hours after cocaine use. It may or may not be associated with underlying vascular malformations. In patients with subarachnoid hemorrhage, associated berry aneurysms and arteriovenous malformations are the common findings on angiogram. The intracranial hemorrhages in these patients are thought to be secondary to transient elevation of blood pressure due to cocaine [170,171]. (*Courtesy of* Jean Paul G. Vonsattel, MD, C.S. Kubik Laboratory for Neuropathology, Massachusetts General Hospital.)

Dissection of the Cervicocerebral Arteries

Carotid Dissection

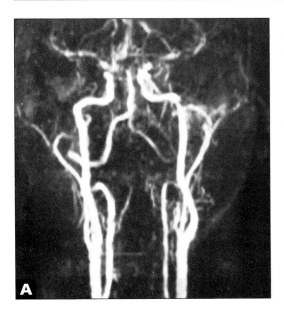

Figure 5-88. Carotid dissection. A 54-year-old man presented with headache described as a sharp band from the forehead to the right ear and involving the right side of the neck. Twelve hours after the onset of headache, he noticed that his voice became hoarse. When he licked ice cream, he found it to be bitter. He also reported pulsatile tinnitus, which started 2 weeks before the headache. On examination, a right-sided Horner's syndrome was noted. Loss of taste sensation on the anterior part of the tongue was also demonstrated. The remainder of the examination was normal. No evidence of a cerebral infarct was seen on the magnetic resonance image performed on the day of admission. **A,** Cerebral angiography showing narrowing of right internal carotid artery from its origin at the bifurcation of the common carotid artery to the base of the skull.

(*Continued on next page*)

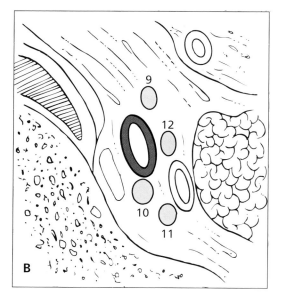

Figure 5-88. (*Continued*) **B**, Drawing of an anatomic section through the neck at the level of the first cervical vertebral body demonstrating the close relation between the internal carotid artery cranial nerves 9, 10, 11, and 12 [172]. Although cranial nerve manifestation is rare, involvement of cranial nerves 3, 5, 6, 7, 9, 10, 11, and 12 has been reported [173]. The abnormal taste sensation (dysgeusia) found in this patient is believed to be secondary to a compression of the chorda tympani nerve or a disturbance of the glossopharyngeal nerve as it passes forward in the neck. Hemilingual paralysis and atrophy are thought to be caused by compression of the hypoglossal nerve immediately below its exit through the anterior condylar canal. Involvement of the sixth cranial nerve suggests an extension of the dissection into the intracavernous portion of the internal carotid artery.

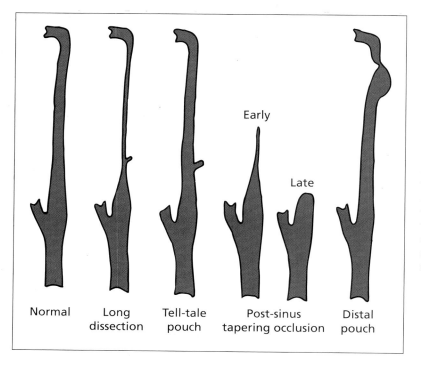

Figure 5-89. Angiographic features of the internal carotid artery (ICA) dissection as reported by Fisher [174]. These are features other than the most common findings at angiography, which is a narrowing of the ICA in the neck and then widening of the distal ICA, usually referable to the area between C1 and the skull base. The most distinctive angiographic finding in carotid dissection is the string sign, a long, irregular filling defect that develops when blood in the vessel wall compresses the lumen. It is usually noted no more than 2 to 3 cm above the common carotid bifurcation and extends upward to the distal part of the extracranial ICA. In most cases, the dissection begins at or above the base of the skull and extends downward. Less commonly, it extends upward through the petrous canal. In an acutely occluded artery, the lumen may become tapered as the dissection extends upward. Another pathognomonic feature is the double-barrel lumen with mural flap, which is found in only 4% of cases. Occasionally, dissection of the artery can cause a pseudoaneurysm, an outpouching due to thinning of the vascular wall. Pseudoaneurysms are usually found in the cervical portion of the artery between C1 and the base of the skull. In many cases, the dissection resolves spontaneously, and full restoration of the lumen can be demonstrated on follow-up angiogram [175,176].

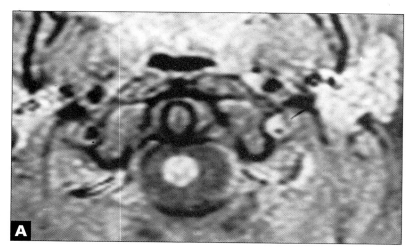
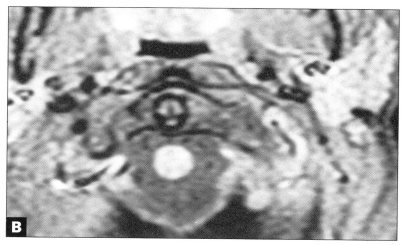

Figure 5-90. Standard spin echo magnetic resonance images showing a perivascular hematoma as a crescent-shaped hyperintense signal around the vessel, with a narrowed vessel lumen (**A, B**). Magnetic resonance imaging is becoming the most reliable modality for identifying carotid artery dissection. Magnetic resonance angiography (MRA) of the neck may be the only definitive diagnostic test in cases in which the dissection is in the subadventitial space instead of the subintimal space and does not alter the lumen diameter. Horizontal MRA sections in the horizontal dimension are often helpful when a long segment of the internal carotid artery is visible, but the high signal of subacute clot in its wall may simulate flow in the reconstructed images [177,178].

Vertebral Dissection

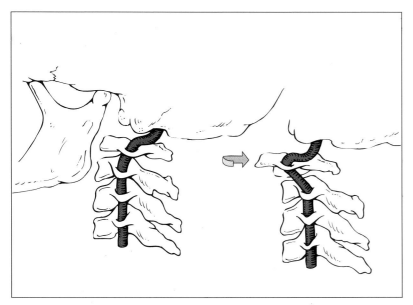

Figure 5-91. Vertebral artery dissections are increasingly recognized as a cause of ischemic stroke and less commonly as a cause of subarachnoid hemorrhage. Dissection of the cervical vertebral artery usually occurs spontaneously or is associated with sudden mechanical injury of the artery from rotational forces [173,178–182]. Most cases have been associated with chiropractic or other neck manipulation, minor falls, automobile accidents, sudden head turning, or extensive coughing [182]. Spontaneous dissections associated with cystic medial degeneration, arteritis, fibromuscular dysplasia, Marfan syndrome, and migraine have been reported [182]. Symptoms are usually characterized by the sudden onset of severe pain localized to the craniocervical region. The onset of ischemic symptoms may begin hours to weeks after the pain. The most common ischemic presentation is a partial or complete lateral medullary syndrome [183]. Isolated intracranial dissections arising in the vertebral artery between the posterior internal carotid artery and the basilar artery more frequently present with subarachnoid hemorrhage, but this is uncommon. The most common sight of origin of vertebral dissection is at C1 and C2. The vertebral artery is most mobile and thus most susceptible to mechanical injury at the C1 and C2 level as it leaves the transverse foramen and abruptly turns to enter the intracranial cavity [184]. Dissections at this site are more common in women, whereas intracranial dissections are more common in men. Either can occur throughout life from the first through the eighth decades.

Clinical Differences Between Intracranial and Extracranial Dissections

	Intracranial dissection	Extracranial dissection
Clinical presentation	Subarachnoid hemorrhage in more than half of cases; ischemic infarction in remainder	Ischemic infarction
Gender	More common in men	More common in women (2.5 times)
Pathology	Subadventitial or transmural dissection	Subintimal dissection

Figure 5-92. Clinical, gender, and pathologic differences between intracranial and extracranial vertebral artery dissections.

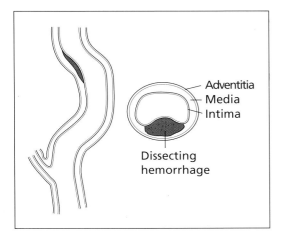

Adventitia
Media
Intima

Dissecting hemorrhage

Figure 5-93. Cross-section and longitudinal section of a vessel showing different types of vertebral dissections [179,181,182,185]. Generally, vertebral artery dissections occur between the internal elastic lamina and the media. The hematoma may occlude the lumen, giving rise to a lateral medullary infarction. In rare instances, the plane of dissection lies within the media or between the media and adventitia, and subarachnoid hemorrhage often develops. Small gap defects of the internal elastic lamina have been reported. It is clear from their histologic appearance that gaps have been present long before the episode of dissection, probably since birth. Intimal tears are of importance in spontaneous dissection.

Algorithm for Therapy of Acute Vertebral Dissection

Extracranial	Intracranial
Presents with ischemic symptoms or neck pain	Presents with SAH or infarction in the lateral medulla (distal vertebral artery dissection)
Diagnosis with MRA or conventional angiography	Diagnosis with MRA or conventional angiography
Heparin followed by warfarin for 3–6 months until the residual lumen stabilizes, improves, or occludes	Consider anticoagulation if ischemic symptoms occur; surgical or interventional neuroradiologic actions are considered, supportive treatment
Follow-up MRA at 3–6 months; if normal, discontinue therapy; if the lumen remains irregular, treat with antiplatelet therapy	

Figure 5-94. Algorithm for the therapy of acute vertebral dissection. MRA—magnetic resonance angiogram; SAH—subarachnoid hemorrhage.

Hematologic Causes of Ischemic Cerebrovascular Disease

Coagulation Defects

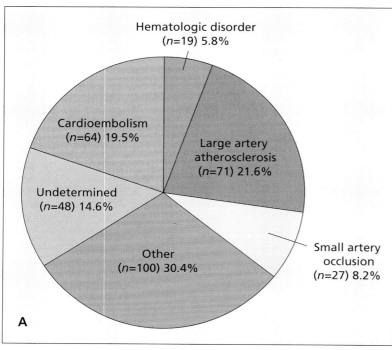

B. Hematologic and Coagulation Defects Associated With Stroke

Factor deficiencies
  Protein S
  Protein C
  Antithrombin III
  Heparin Cofactor II
Elevation in Factor VIII
Erythrocyte disorders
  Polycythemia vera
  Sickle cell anemia
  Thalassemia
  Paroxysmal nocturnal hemoglobinuria
  Tissue plasminogen activator deficiency
Platelet disorders
  Essential thrombocytosis
  Polycythemia vera
  Thrombotic thrombocytopenic purpura
Dysfibrogenemias
Fibrinolytic disorders
  Plasminogen deficiency
Antiphospholipid antibodies
Homocystinuria
Trousseau's syndrome

Figure 5-95. Hypercoagulable conditions. **A,** Hypercoagulable conditions are an important cause of ischemic stroke, particularly in the young. Strokes due to hematologic causes account for about 6% of strokes in young adults [186]. **B,** Hypercoagulable disorders should be suspected in any stroke patient who lacks conventional vascular risk factors, has a family history of thrombotic disorders, or has a past history of recurrent thrombotic episodes. Hypercoagulable states may account for a significant portion of the 10% to 25% of strokes of unknown cause in patients of all ages. Protein C is a vitamin K–dependent protein that is activated when thrombin binds to thrombomodulin, inactivating Factors Va and VIIIa. In patients with thromboembolic disease, the prevalence of protein C deficiency is 2% to 5%. Heterozygotes have about 50% normal protein C. Patients may present with amaurosis fugax, transient ischemic attacks, venous infarcts, or arterial infarcts. There are both dominant and recessive patterns of inheritance. The severity of thrombotic disease appears to depend on other factors, such as Factor V–Leiden mutation [187,188]. Deficiencies may be due to quantitative or qualitative defects. Patients with protein C deficiency have higher levels of activation of the homeostatic system as measured by the F_{1+2} level, which is a byproduct of thrombin generation [189]. Warfarin has been shown to reduce F_{1+2} levels in protein C–deficient patients. Normal physiology of fibrin formation and degradation. Patients with abnormal fibrinogen often are predisposed to hemorrhage; however, dysfibrogenemias have caused production of fibrin resistant to fibrinolysis, resulting in recurrent thromboembolic events. (Panel A *adapted from* Adams and colleagues [186].)

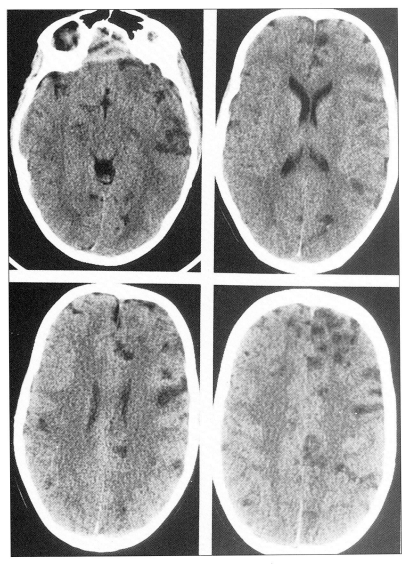

Figure 5-96. Noncontrast computed tomography scans of the brain of a 9-year-old girl with protein C deficiency who presented with multiple ischemic infarcts and seizures. Infants born with homozygous protein C deficiency present with purpura fulminans and do not survive the neonatal period.

Possible Implications of Abnormal Coagulation Tests

Result	Implications
Prolonged PT	Decreased Factor VII (uncommon)
	Warfarin therapy
Prolonged PTT	Bleeding
	Decreased Factor VIII
	Decreased Factor IX
	Decreased Factor XI
	Heparin therapy
	No bleeding
	Antiphospholipid antibody
	(for example, lupus anticoagulant)
	Decreased Factor XII
	Heparin therapy
Prolonged PT and PTT	Decreased Factor X
	Decreased Factor V
	Decreased prothrombin
	Decreased fibrinogen
	Vitamin K deficiency
	Warfarin therapy (higher doses)
	Disseminated intravascular coagulation
	Liver disease
	Thrombolytic agents (higher doses)

Figure 5-97. Possible implications of abnormal coagulation studies. Although heparin cofactor II deficiency and plasminogen deficiency have not been linked to cerebrovascular events, they have been shown to be causes of systemic thromboembolic events and may be considered in patients suspected of being hypercoagulable.

Elevated serum Factor VIII levels have been associated with venous thromboembolism, but there has also been a report of bilateral middle cerebral artery thrombosis attributed to elevated plasma Factor VIII [190]. PT—prothrombin time; PTT—partial thromboplastin time. (*Adapted from* Brott and colleague [191].)

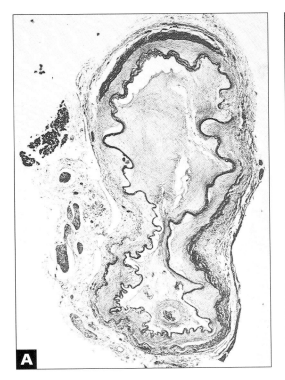

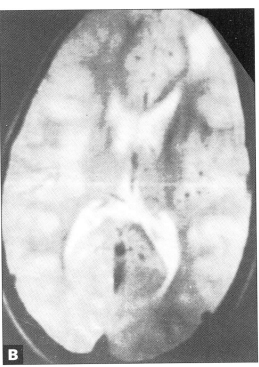

Figure 5-98. Sickle cell anemia. **A**, Microscopic specimen of a patient with sickle cell disease. **B**, Magnetic resonance image showing watershed infarcts. Sickle cell disease causes hemoglobin S to become more aggregable. Hypoxic states cause red blood cell deformation and increased aggregation. Patients with sickle cell disease have increased serum viscosity. Cerebral infarcts may be venous or arterial. Arterial infarcts are often in watershed zones, but may also involve small perforating arteries [192,193]. Acute therapy should be directed at reducing hypoxia and acidosis with hydration and oxygenation. Exchange transfusion may help by reducing the quantity of hemoglobin S and can significantly reduce the risk of recurrent stroke. (*From* Rothman and colleagues [193]; with permission.)

Antiphospholipid Antibody

Laboratory Evaluation and Clinical Features of Antiphospholipid Antibody

Laboratory diagnosis
  Prolonged phospholipid-dependent coagulation screening test
  Failure to correct with mixing studies
  Demonstration of phospholipid specificity
Laboratory studies
  Prothrombin time
  Activated partial thromboplastin time (aPTT)
  Tissue thromboplastin inhibition
  Platelet neutralization procedure
  Dilute antiphospholipid aPTT
  Kaolin clotting
  Russell's viper venom time
  Dilute Russell's viper venom time
  Anticardiolipin enzyme-linked immunosorbent assay
Clinical features
  Arterial thrombosis
    Cerebral, ocular, peripheral, myocardial, dermal, pulmonary, mesenteric

Venous thrombosis
  Deep vein, hepatic, retinal, cerebral, adrenal
Miscarriages
Livedo reticularis
Pulmonary hypertension
Cardiac lesions
  Verrucous endocarditis, myxomatous mitral valve
    degeneration, intracardiac thrombi
Chorea
Laboratory abnormalities
  Prolonged aPTT
  False-positive Veneral Disease Research Laboratory
  Thrombocytopenia
  Hemolytic anemia
  Positive antinuclear antibodies
  Reduced C4
  Increased complement fragment SC5b-9

Figure 5-99. Laboratory evaluation and clinical features of antiphospholipid antibody. Antiphospholipid antibodies are found in about 2% to 5% of healthy young people. The prevalence of antiphospholipid antibodies increases with age. About 40% of patients with systemic lupus erythematosus have antiphospholipid antibody. The presence of antiphospholipid antibody conveys a stroke risk 10 times that seen in patients without the antibody. Although the antibody is nonspecific and may be due to a coexisting illness or medication, patients with acquired antibodies do not manifest the antiphospholipid syndrome. Cerebral infarcts are more often due to arterial occlusion than venous thrombosis. Middle cerebral artery branch occlusions are most common, although small vessel infarcts occur as well.

Homocystinuria is a disorder of amino acid metabolism that may be due to one of three enzyme disorders: vitamin B_6, folate, or vitamin B_{12} deficiency.

Elevated homocysteine levels may also be secondary to renal insufficiency, acute lymphoblastic leukemia, psoriasis, or medications (eg, methotrexate, anticonvulsant drugs, colestipol, niacin, nitrous oxide, and vitamin B_6 antagonists). Patients who are homozygotes for the disorder have a marfanoid body type, ectopic lentis, and mental retardation. One third also have thromboembolic events—usually venous, but arterial thromboses have been reported as well. The diagnosis can be made by cyanide–nitroprusside reaction in the urine or prenatally by measuring cystathionine synthetase activity in cultured amniotic fluid cells. The proposed mechanism of infarction may be related to abnormal collagen cross-links causing abnormalities in vessel walls and increased platelet adhesion. Activated protein C resistance is considered the most common cause of familial thrombosis and is usually due to a missense mutation altering the cleavage site. (*Adapted from* Levine and colleague [194].)

Laboratory Tests for Trousseau's Syndrome

Test	Diagnosis
Complete blood count	Thrombocytosis
	Polycythemia vera
Prothrombin time	Factor VII deficiency
	Dysfibrogenemia or afibrogenemia
Activated thromboplastin time	Dysfibrogenemia or afibrogenemia
	Antiphospholipid syndrome
Hemoglobin electrophoresis	Sickle cell anemia
Functional factor assays	Protein C deficiency
	Protein S deficiency
	Antithrombin III deficiency
	Activated protein C resistance
Factor levels	Factor V deficiency, Factor VII deficiency
Fibrinogen level	Fibrinogen deficiency
Plasminogen level	Plasminogen deficiency
Fibroblast cystathione–β synthetase	Homocystinuria
Vitamin B_{12} and folate	Acquired homocystinuria
Lupus anticoagulant	Antiphospholipid antibody syndrome
Anticardiolipin antibody	Antiphospholipid antibody syndrome

Figure 5-100. Laboratory tests for Trousseau's syndrome (malignancy-associated hypercoagulable states). These are the recommended tests for evaluating cancer patients for a hypercoagulable state. About 7% of patients with a malignancy have an ischemic stroke during their illness [195]. The most common causes are nonbacterial thrombotic endocarditis, disseminated intravascular coagulation, and septic emboli. Atherosclerotic disease may also be a cause of stroke, particularly in older patients [196]. These patients have a low rate of recurrent stroke. The prognosis is poor, with death resulting from the underlying malignancy. The studies to date have not fully assessed the stroke mechanism responsible for the infarction.

Patients with malignant tumors may have any one of a number of hematologic abnormalities. Elevated fibrin degradation products and prolonged partial thromboplastin time were the most common abnormalities in one series [197], consistent with a chronic state of low-grade disseminated intravascular coagulation. The tumors most commonly associated with thromboembolic events are lung, pancreas, stomach, and colon [198]. Although cancer patients who have thromboembolic events are often resistant to heparin (fibrinopeptide A values remain high), fibrinopeptide A levels decrease on warfarin therapy in 67% of patients [198].

Experimental Hematologic Studies

Experimental Clotting Studies

Fibrinopeptide A

F_{1+2}

Factor V–Leiden

Activation of the hemostatic system

Familial thrombophilia

Figure 5-101. Experimental clotting studies. Although these tests are now used for research purposes, they may be part of the routine evaluation of patients with stroke in the future. Fibrinopeptide A is a byproduct of the conversion of fibrinogen to fibrin. The preceding step, the cleavage of prothrombin to thrombin, liberates the F_{1+2} fragment. Elevations in F_{1+2} values thus represent increased activity of the hemostatic system by either the intrinsic or extrinsic pathway. Factor V–Leiden is a genetic mutation that results in a substitution in the amino acids at the cleavage site for Factor V, causing activated protein C resistance. Although both homozygotes and heterozygotes are at increased risk for thromboembolic events, heterozygotes may develop symptoms only if there is a superimposed condition such as another factor deficiency of an acquired hypercoagulable state [199].

Acute Stroke Evaluation and Management

Goals of Evaluation and Management of Acute Stroke

Minimize the extent of brain injury

Prevent and treat the medical complications that frequently occur in patients with impaired motor, sensory, or cognitive function

Prevent secondary stroke

Maximize functional outcome

Figure 5-102. Goals of evaluation and management of acute stroke. Stroke affects approximately 500,000 Americans per year and is a major cause of prolonged, often permanent disability. The current standard of care will change drastically in the next decade as emerging therapies are shown to improve stroke outcome. The goals that guide acute stroke care will not change, but more powerful tools will be available to achieve these goals.

Pathophysiology

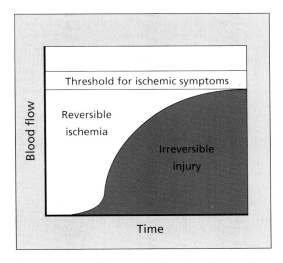

Figure 5-103. Degree and duration of ischemia. Returning blood flow, or thrombolysis, is necessary to salvage ischemic tissue. If the ischemia is severe and its duration prolonged, however, then reperfu-

sion likely brings with it the potential for intracerebral hemorrhage. Infarction is considered to occur due to the combined effects of the degree and duration of ischemia. The duration can be estimated from the onset of symptoms. Clinical signs of brain ischemia occur almost immediately when tissue perfusion drops below a certain level, which varies among brain regions. In some patients, the degree of ischemia sufficient to disturb brain function and cause the neurologic symptom or sign may not be sufficient to cause infarction unless sustained for hours. In others, the ischemia is so profound that brain injury occurs within a few minutes. Most patients have a gradient to their ischemic insult with severely impaired blood flow in the core and less severe reduction in the surrounding penumbra. The primary effort in modern acute stroke management is to salvage the penumbra from the processes that are triggered by ischemia and that eventuate in tissue infarction.

Most of the energy supply in brain tissue is used to maintain neuronal ionic gradients. In ischemia, adenosine triphosphate (ATP) is no longer available to maintain these gradients; there is widespread loss of membrane potential, opening of voltage activated channels, marked influx of water and ions into neurons, and dramatic elevation of intracellular calcium. Increased calcium causes widespread release of neurotransmitters, including the major excitatory transmitter, glutamate. Calcium flowing through voltage-gated and glutamate receptor–linked ion channels activates a myriad of potentially damaging intracellular processes. Mitochondria attempt to sequester calcium but can be damaged in these extreme conditions. Oxygen delivered to damaged mitochondria results in destructive free radical production. Various gene programs are activated after an ischemic insult; some are protective, others result in programmed cell death. Each of these potentially injurious processes are targets for neuroprotective drugs in clinical or preclinical investigations. The figure demonstrates the general targets of neuroprotective therapies currently undergoing clinical trial (Fig. 5-114).

Imaging Acute Stroke

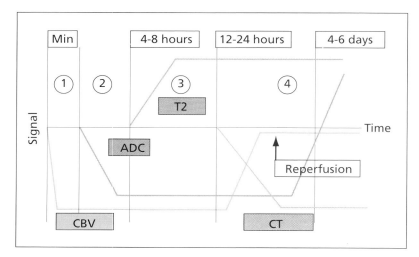

Figure 5-104. Staging acute stroke patients with magnetic resonance imaging (MRI). In addition to new therapies, exciting new methods are being developed to detect and follow ischemic brain injury. Their use will revolutionize care of the acute stroke patient. Standard imaging techniques are unable to detect ischemic tissue consistently in the first 6 to 12 hours of stroke. Most neuroprotective strategies require that treatment begin before 6 hours. Advanced diffusion or perfusion MRI is much more sensitive to ischemic injury in the first hours of stroke. Perfusion imaging detects brain regions that are less accessible to a bolus injection of intravenous contrast than normally perfused brain tissue. Diffusion imaging detects ischemic brain regions with lowered diffusibility of water. Water moves intracellularly when adenosine triphosphate (ATP) levels fall and ion gradients deteriorate. Intracellular water is ordered in a colloid matrix and is less diffusible. In addition, movement of water inside cells is dependent in large part on ATP. For these reasons, the apparent diffusion coefficient becomes less when ATP levels fall in ischemic brain. Diffusion imaging detects this change as increased signal intensity within minutes in animal models of stroke. Increased total water is detected as increased T2 signal. Computed tomography (CT) scan is less sensitive but also detects increased total water in stroke after a number of hours. The radiologic signature can be used to stage the progression of ischemic injury. Because the pathologic stage of the injury, and not time from onset of deficit, influences the potential for a positive response to therapy, we expect that magnetic resonance staging will determine future treatment decisions. ADC—apparent diffusion coefficients; CBV—cerebral blood volume.

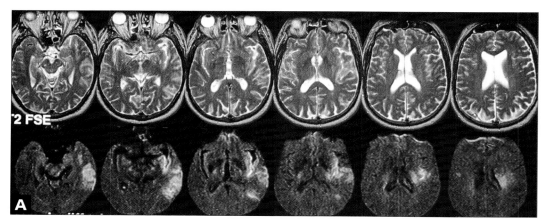

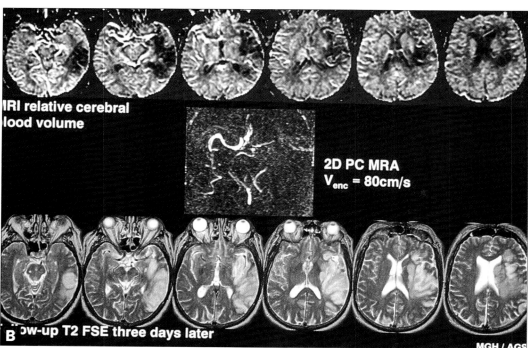

Figure 5-105. T2-weighted images in a patient taken 7 hours after onset of a left hemisphere ischemic deficit showing a hazy abnormality in the perisylvian and temporal cortex. **A,** Diffusion-weighted image (DWI) shows the lesion more clearly as it contains signal due to low water diffusibility as well as T2. **B,** Perfusion imaging shows a wider region of ischemia. Signs of ischemic injury enlarged into the entire ischemic zone in this patient. In many cases studied within hours of onset, the initial DWI abnormality is seen to enlarge over time (24 to 48 hours). In our experience, the patient's initial DWI lesion defines the minimal expected stroke size. The initial perfusion abnormality is generally larger than the final size of the stroke and generates the upper bounds of tissue damage. These techniques may be able to define a core (DWI abnormality) and penumbra (abnormal perfusion with normal diffusion) in the emergency ward, and therapies can be tested for their ability to preserve the penumbral region. Animal studies suggest that timely and effective neuroprotective therapy can even salvage tissue with abnormal DWI. Current efforts are devoted to testing thrombolytic and neuroprotective agents for their ability to minimize the growth of the DWI abnormality into the region with abnormal perfusion.

Evaluation and Management of Acute Stroke

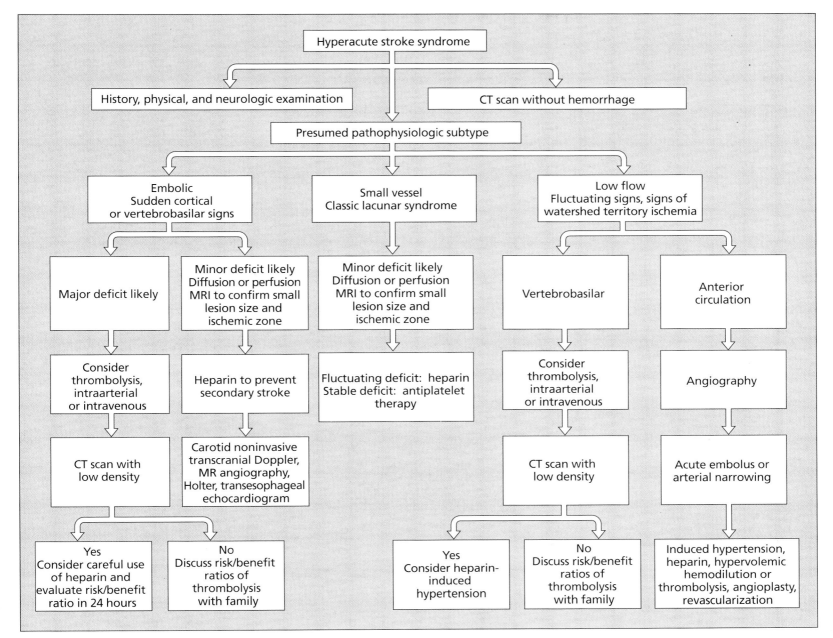

Figure 5-106. Hyperacute stroke syndrome. Classification of the patho-physiologic stroke type is important in determining which therapy is appropriate in a given patient. For patients presenting for emergency evaluation within hours of onset of ischemic symptoms with hyperacute stroke, our practice is governed by the simplified decision tree seen here. The overriding concern in this algorithm is the risk-to-benefit ratio of acute thrombolysis. This is motivated by animal studies showing decreased stroke size with timely reperfusion, better than expected outcome in patients with severe vertebrobasilar occlusive disease after intraarterial thrombolysis [200] and the National Institute of Neurological Disorders and Stroke intravenous reteplase tissue plasminogen activator (rt-PA) study results [201] on intra-arterial thrombolysis (Fig. 5-111). An attempt is made to discuss both the potential for improved outcome and the risk of fatal intracerebral hemorrhage in counseling the patient and family before deciding on thrombolysis. CT—computed tomography; MRI—magnetic resonance imaging.

Treatments and Complications in Acute Stroke

Treatments to consider	Complications to avoid
Respiratory support: Aspiration, partial airway obstruction, and hypoventilation lead to hypoxia that can increase the extent of brain injury. In addition to clearing airway, artificial ventilation should be considered if necessary. $Paco_2$ should be kept in physiologic limits.	Hypercapnia: Increases tissue acidosis and intracranial pressure ($Paco_2$ >30 mm Hg). Hypocapnia: Cerebral blood flow falls by 50% at $Paco_2$ levels below 20 mm Hg.
Control of blood pressure: Regional blood flow becomes dependent on perfusion pressure with loss of autoregulation in cerebral ischemia. Some patients have ischemic symptoms that worsen when systemic blood pressure falls below a specific level. Pressors, hypervolemic hemodilution, and hyperosmolar therapy (triple H therapy) are used in similar situations in patients with vasospasm after subarachnoid hemorrhage.	Hypotension: Blood pressure is generally elevated above the patient's baseline. This elevation may improve collateral flow to ischemic brain regions. Ischemic symptoms frequently worsen if blood pressure is lowered iatrogenically. Hypertension: Blood pressure above 220/130 mm Hg may be harmful to the vital organs and may be complicated with hypertensive encephalopathy. According to our experience, mean arterial pressure of about 150 to 160 mm Hg should be treated cautiously without causing more than 15 mm Hg decrease.
Correction of blood glucose: Blood glucose may increase due to acute stress response, especially in patients with impaired glucose tolerance. Ischemic damage is exacerbated by hyperglycemia. Administration of hypoosmolar glucose solutions should be avoided unless hypoglycemia is suspected.	Hyperglycemia: Blood glucose levels greater than 250 to 300 are associated with worse outcome in stroke. Hypoglycemia: Energy failure may be exacerbated by blood glucose levels falling below normal.
Mild hypothermia: The cerebral metabolic rate is proportional to body temperature. Lowering brain temperature by 2° to 3°C consistently decreases ischemic damage in animal stroke models, and hypothermia is successfully used to prevent infarction during surgical procedures requiring global or regional brain ischemia. Acetaminophen to treat fever and cooling blankets can affect normothermia or slight hypothermia without severe discomfort.	Fever: Elevated brain temperature is clearly associated with worsened ischemic brain injury in animal stroke models and exacerbates edema by increasing blood–brain barrier permeability.
Mannitol: Ischemic brain edema peaks 2 to 4 days after stroke and rarely is a clinical problem in the hyperacute phase. Progressive decline in consciousness associated with mass effect on computed tomography should trigger concern for fatal swelling. Raising serum osmolality with intermittent mannitol boluses can lead to clinical improvement. There is risk of relapse when discontinued. Mannitol improves cerebral blood flow by reducing viscosity.	Hyponatremia: Low serum osmolarity may exacerbate ischemic brain edema. Restricting free water while maintaining normal volume status is important. Cardiac and renal failure: Causes further decrease in cerebral blood flow.
Hyperventilation: Respiratory alkalosis can quickly and effectively reduce intracranial pressure.	
Decompressive surgery: Hemicraniectomy can be life-saving in patients with large cerebral infarctions. Ischemic cerebellar swelling can cause obstructive hydrocephalus requiring ventricular drainage, or brain stem compression requiring cerebellar decompression.	
Endarterectomy: The safety and efficacy of emergent carotid endarterectomy in acute stroke is controversial. It should be considered in patients with carotid stenosis and recurrent symptomatic ischemia.	
Hypervolemia or hemodilution: In patients with polycythemia and stroke, reducing hematocrit below 46% improves cerebral blood flow and blood viscosity [202]. Clinical benefit in stroke due to other conditions has not been established. Viscosity improves with lowering hematocrit, but values below 30% may impair tissue oxygenation.	Hypovolemia: Dehydration worsens cerebral perfusion and exacerbates clotting.
Heparin and low molecular weight heparins: Use in acute stroke is controversial. There is some evidence that it can decrease the risk of early recurrent embolism, especially in craniocervical arterial dissection, and that it can stop deterioration in progressive stroke, especially in cases of threatening vertebrobasilar occlusion.	Parenchymal hematoma: Anticoagulation and thrombolysis each can increase the risk of clinically significant hemorrhagic transformation and hematoma formation. Clear correlation has been shown with extension of brain infarction, advanced age, hypertension, and preexisting coagulopathy.
Intraarterial or intravenous thrombolysis	

Figure 5-107. Treatments to consider and complications to avoid in acute stroke.

Treatment

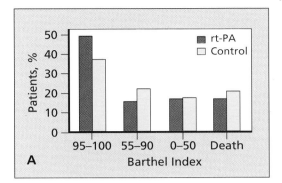 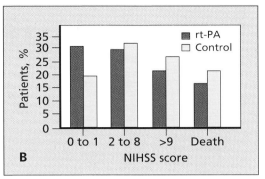

Figure 5-108. National Institute of Neurological Disorders and Stroke (NINDS) trial of reteplase tissue plasminogen activator (rt-PA). **A, B,** The NINDS trial of rt-PA, a fibrinolytic agent, is the first study to show positive effect on outcome as measured by functional outcome (Barthel Index) with hyperacute treatment of the stroke patient. A controlled trial from Hong Kong has also shown benefit on outcome after treatment with

low molecular weight heparin in the days after stroke [203]. Patients in the NINDS trial were selected according to strict criteria and managed according to protocol (Fig. 5-109). Emphasis was directed at very early treatment; all patients were treated within 3 hours, and half were treated within 90 minutes of stroke onset. NIHSS—National Institutes of Health Stroke Service.

NINDS rt-PA Protocol

Eligibility	Treatment
Less than 85 years old	rt-PA initiated within 3 hours
Acute stroke syndrome but not with rapidly improving deficit	Sites were obliged to treat half the patients within 90 minutes of stroke onset
No hemorrhage on computed tomography scan	
No seizure	Monitor blood pressure and neurologic examination q 15 minutes for 2 hours, then q 30 minutes for 6 hours, then q hour for 1 day
No history of stroke, trauma, or surgery within 3 months	
Systolic blood pressure (SBP) <180 mm Hg	Blood pressure controlled with intravenous labetolol or, if DBP >140 mm Hg, with intravenous nitroprusside
Diastolic blood pressure (DBP) <120 mm Hg	
Not on warfarin or heparin	BP goals SBP <180 mm Hg and DBP <120 mm Hg
	In case of hemorrhage, treat with cryoprecipitate and platelets
	No heparin or aspirin for 24 hours

Figure 5-109. National Institute of Neurological Disorders and Stroke (NINDS) reteplase tissue plasminogen activator (rt-PA) protocol. Eleven previous trials of other fibrinolytic agents reported negative results owing to the increased incidence of fatal hemorrhage in the treated group. Combined analysis of these results revealed a significant excess in death in the treated group, 23% versus 19% in the control subjects. There was a 10% reduction in combined death or dependency at follow-up evaluation in the treated

group. The European Cooperative Acute Stroke Study (ECASS) [204] of rt-PA also reported negative results owing to increased incidence of hemorrhage in the treated group. In the ECASS, however, there was evidence that the risk of hemorrhage occurred primarily in treated patients enrolled despite early signs of stroke on computed tomography. Excluding those with early signs of stroke on computed tomography, there was an outcome benefit in the targeted treatment group.

Comparison of NINDS and ECASS rt-PA Studies

	ECASS	NINDS
rt-PA dose	1.1 mg/kg, 100 mg maximum	0.9 mg/kg, 90 mg maximum
Time window	6 h	3 h
Median time to treat	4.4 h	1.5 h
Mortality in control group	16%	22%
Mortality in treated group	23%	17%
Hemorrhage in control group	7%	3.5%
Hemorrhage in treated group	20%	11%

Figure 5-110. Comparison of the National Institute of Neurological Disorders and Stroke (NINDS) and European Cooperative Acute Stroke Study (ECASS) reteplase tissue plasminogen activator (rt-PA). Unlike the other trials, the NINDS trial was designed to enroll the hyperacute stroke patient. The median time between onset of symptoms and treatment was only 90 minutes. An analysis of published results indicates that very early intravenous thrombolytic therapy can improve the chance of a good functional outcome in stroke patients. However, the benefit comes at the expense of an increased incidence of symptomatic brain hemorrhage. The risk of hemorrhage into the ischemic region increases as ischemic brain tissue progresses toward infarction. Intracerebral hemorrhage complicates thrombolytic therapy even in the treatment of patients with myocardial infarction. Further data are needed to determine in which patient group the risk-to-benefit ratio favors treatment. Currently we reserve thrombolysis for patients in whom the natural history of the stroke suggests that there is high likelihood that death or severe permanent disability will ensue if the ischemic injury is not reversed. The latter remains controversial because patients with small vessel strokes also benefited from rt-PA in the NINDS trial.

Comparison of Intraarterial and Intravenous Thrombolysis

	Intraarterial rt-PA or urokinase	Intravenous rt-PA
Recanalization rate		
Internal carotid artery	Low	8% [206]
M_1 segment	80% to 90% [205]	24% [206]
M_2, M_3 segments	80% to 90%	38% [206]
Basilar	80% to 90% [201]	—
Time to initiate treatment	Delayed until angiography performed, 1–2 h Recanalization occurs soon after treatment	Immediately after decision to treat; recanalization may be delayed
Probability of treating patient without stroke	Negligible—treat only if occlusion found at angiography	Considerable—hysteria, migraine, postictal state, transient ischemic attacks, overdose
Probability of treating patient with small stroke	Low—treat only major arterial occlusion seen on angiogram	Considerable, but evidence suggests it improves outcome; still questionable whether improvement is balanced by risk of hemorrhage in single penetrator stroke
Probability of failed treatment attempt	Considerable if unable to cannulate the intracranial clot because of proximal stenosis or occlusion	Negligible
Incidence of hemorrhage	18% to 25%	11% (NINDS) to 20% (ECASS); higher in patients >75 years old and NIHSS >20
Improved outcome	Suggested by data in patients with vertebrobasilar occlusion not known for anterior circulation	Yes, following NINDS criteria and procedures
Access of thrombolytic drug to clot	Good to excellent	Potentially poor
Systemic dose of thrombolytic drug	Low to moderate	Higher

Figure 5-111. Comparison of intraarterial and intravenous thrombolysis. Intraarterial thrombolysis has certain advantages and disadvantages compared with intravenous reteplase tissue plasminogen activator (rt-PA). With intraarterial thrombolysis, angiography is used to locate the clot, and thrombolytic drugs are injected through microcatheters placed distal to, within and in front of the clot. This has not yet been tested conclusively in a controlled trial. ECASS—European Cooperative Acute Stroke Study; NIHSS—National Institutes of Health Stroke Service; NINDS—National Institute of Neurological Disorders and Stroke.

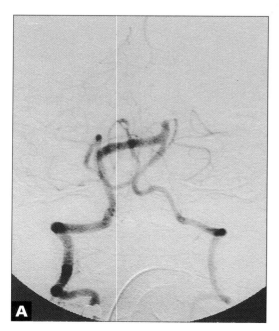 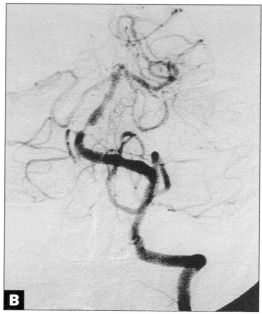

Figure 5-112. Intraarterial thrombolysis in a patient who presented after 6 hours of fluctuating brain stem signs. Before treatment, the patient had become stuporous and decerebrate bilaterally. **A,** Pretreatment angiogram shows mid-basilar occlusion. **B,** Posttreatment angiogram shows recanalization of the basilar artery with a mid-basilar stenosis. Hours after the procedure, the patient had a normal neurologic examination. He left the hospital healthy, with no stroke seen on follow-up magnetic resonance imaging. The case attests to the almost miraculous sudden improvements seen in cases of successful thrombolysis.

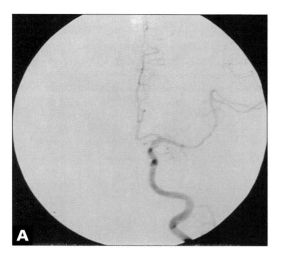
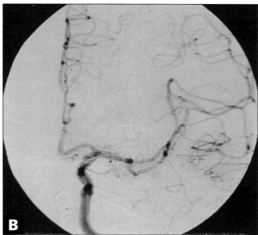

Figure 5-113. A patient whose superior division of the middle cerebral artery was recanalized 6 hours after onset of sudden hemispheric stroke. **A**, Pretreatment angiogram shows absent filling of vessels supplying the frontal and anterior temporal lobes. **B**, Posttreatment angiogram shows recanalization of these vessels. No clinical change in condition was seen, and follow-up computed tomography showed hemorrhage into the stroke. The case illustrates the increased risk of hemorrhage into stroke after thrombolysis.

Clinical Trials of New Drugs for the Treatment of Acute Stroke

Drug	Action
Fiblast	Basic fibroblast growth factor
Aptiganel hydrochloride	NMDA receptor ion-channel blocker
Selfotel (Ciba-Geigy Corp., Summit, NJ)	NMDA receptor antagonist
CV 150-526A	NMDA receptor glycine site blocker
YM90K	AMPA receptor antagonist
Tirilazad (Upjohn Co., Kalamazoo, MI)	Fe^{3+}-generated free radical scavenger
Pergorgotein	Polyethylene glycol superoxide dismutase
Enlimomab (Boehringer Ingelheim, Ridgefield, CT)	Granulocyte adhesion blocker
Lubeluzole	Na^+-channel blocker
Riluzole	Na^+-channel blocker
Phosphenytoin	Na^+-channel blocker
SNX111	N type Ca^+-channel blocker
Nimodipine	L type Ca^+-channel blocker
Citicoline	Phospholipid precursor
Clomethiazole	Potentiates GABA
Prourokinase	Fibrinolytic (intraarterial)
Ancrod	Defibrinogenation (intravenous)
Nadroparin	Low molecular weight heparin
Org 10172	Heparinoid

Figure 5-114. Partial list of new drugs in clinical trials for the treatment of acute stroke. Neuroprotective therapies slow and limit ischemic tissue injury in animal stroke models. Others decrease stroke size because they limit "reperfusion injury." Some important general themes cross multiple stroke types: 1) blood flow—is there ongoing ischemia? 2) minimal ischemic stage—are there brain regions that are ischemic but salvageable by a neurointervention? 3) maximal ischemic stage—are there regions that have progressed toward infarction and are not salvageable by current therapies? New therapies, developed in animal stroke models, target specific biologic processes activated in ischemic brain. Their effective application will be enhanced by information about the extent, location, and pathophysiologic stage of the ischemic brain injury. The incorporation of advanced neuroimaging technology into the emergency evaluation of the stroke patient will improve the therapeutic decision process. AMPA—α-amino-3-hydroxy-5-methyl-4 isoxazole-proprionic acid; GABA—γ-aminobutyric acid; NMDA—*N*-methyl-D-aspartate.

Stroke Recovery

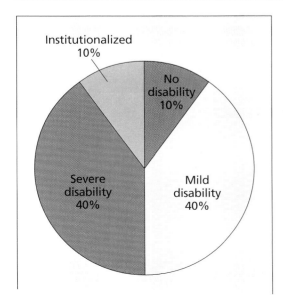

Figure 5-115. Range of disability after stroke. About 400,000 patients survive stroke each year, surviving an average of 7 years. The range of recovery for these patients is broad. Stallones and colleagues [202] concluded that as many patients were institutionalized after stroke (10%) as were free of disability (10%). Most stroke patients were left with mild (40%) or severe (40%) disability. As a rule, however, the more severe the deficit at onset, the more substantial is the residual neurologic dysfunction. This relation holds for dysfunction as measured both in neurologic and in functional terms. (*Adapted from* Stallones and colleagues [206].)

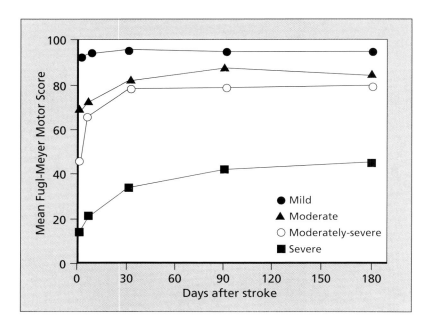

Figure 5-116. Rates of recovery after stroke. A number of different processes contribute to improvement of neurologic function, from resolution of edema and the ischemic cascade to reorganization of the function of surviving neurons. As a result, different patterns of recovery are apparent. Age, brain atrophy, size of lesion, severity of deficit, depression, specific cognitive deficits, and other variables have been found to influence the outcome after stroke [207]. In a study measuring motor recovery in upper and lower extremities after stroke, Duncan and colleagues [208] found that more severe motor deficit at onset predicted more severe deficit 6 months later, as measured by a standard scale (Fugl-Meyer) of motor recovery. Patients experienced the most recovery within the first 30 days after strokes of all levels of severity. Recovery continued for 90 days among patients with moderate and most severe strokes. (*Adapted from* Duncan and colleagues [208].)

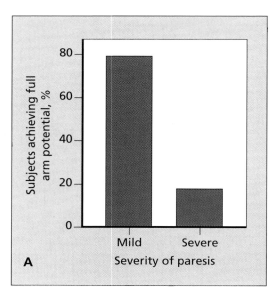

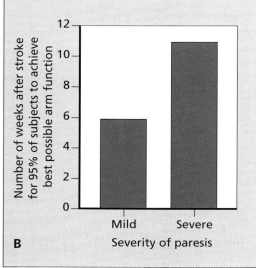

Figure 5-117. Functional versus neurologic assessment of recovery from stroke. Neurologic assessments measure objective parameters such as strength and tone, whereas functional assessments measure performance of certain tasks such as those pertinent to activities of daily living. In addition to neurologic gains, functional gains reflect expanded use of intact limbs, development of strategies, and more. Use of functional outcomes as measures of poststroke recovery confirms the same trends described in Figure 5-116. Nakayama and colleagues [209] used a subsection of the Barthel Index, a functional measure, to make serial assessments of the upper extremity during recovery from stroke. Initial poststroke arm paresis was classified into mild and severe categories using a neurologic measure, the Scandinavian Stroke Scale. Those patients with milder arm paresis on admission were more likely to achieve full arm function (**A**) and to do so earlier (**B**). (*Adapted from* Nakayama and colleagues [209].)

Stages of Motor Function Restoration After Hemiplegia

Loss of voluntary movement, with a decrease in tone and deep tendon reflexes

Hyperactivity of deep tendon reflexes

Increase in tone

First willed movements, usually proximal muscles preceding distal

Willed flexion movements achieved only as part of a flexion synergy

Extensor synergy apparent

Increase in power, accompanied by decrease in tone

Movement of a single digit possible

Complete recovery of willed effort with retained hyperactive deep tendon reflexes

Figure 5-118. The stages of motor function recovery after hemiplegia. Despite varying outcomes among patients, there is a commonality to the pattern of recovery. In a seminal study, Twitchell [210] described the general course of events in humans during recovery from hemiplegic stroke. Although there was a wide variation in the outcome of the 25 patients studied, recovery in each was found to follow the same general pattern of stages until a plateau was reached or full recovery attained. These stages are summarized in the figure. Twitchell emphasized that stages developed gradually with a great deal of overlap.

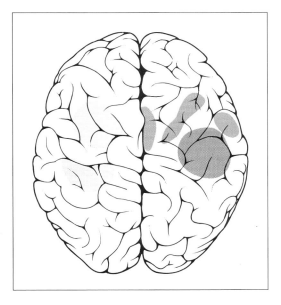

Figure 5-119. Mechanisms of recovery after stroke. Studies in animals and humans have suggested possible mechanisms by which recovery may take place in the brain. Evidence supports three principal contributing processes, which may occur in combination. They are reorganization of the map of the body within the cortex neighboring a lesion, referred to as *plasticity* (*red*); recruitment of secondary motor areas in the hemisphere ipsilateral to a lesion (*green*); and activation of homologous regions of the unaffected hemisphere (*yellow*). The area shaded gray represents a nonfunctional region of brain damaged by ischemia to the cortex or its underlying efferents.

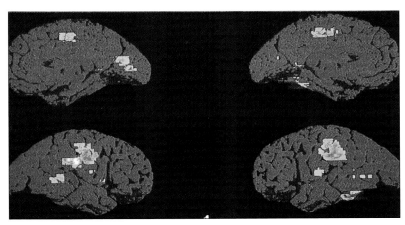

Figure 5-120. Positron-emission tomography (PET) studies of the post-stroke recovered state. Studies using PET have confirmed the activity of several mechanisms in patients who have recovered from stroke. Weiller and colleagues [211] measured regional cerebral blood flow (CBF) in patients who recovered from a single, small, deep stroke. A regional increase in CBF reflects enhanced neural activity in a given brain area. Using PET to measure regional CBF during movement of the recovered hand, the brain areas of each patient were identified that exhibited an increase in blood flow significantly greater than that seen in control subjects. Although the pattern of functional reorganization varied among individual patients, all patients showed significantly more activation of bilateral brain structures than did control subjects. The pattern of these activations largely corresponded to the processes described in Figure 5-119.

The PET scan from patient 1 from this study is shown here. There are four views of the brain: right medial view (*top left*), left medial view (*top right*), right lateral view (*bottom left*), and left lateral view (*bottom right*). The recovered hand was on the right. The highlighted pixels represent significantly activated pixels; the scale is arbitrary and thresholded to the level of statistical significance. All of the brain recovery mechanisms listed in Figure 5-119 were in evidence. Areas activated with movement of the recovered hand in this patient include the face area of the sensorimotor cortex in the infarcted hemisphere, consistent with cortical map reorganization. The contribution to recovery of the undamaged hemisphere was highlighted by significant activation in the primary sensorimotor and premotor cortices. The supplementary motor area, here projected onto the medial surface of the brain, is activated. This is consistent with the role of secondary motor areas in achieving restitution of function. (*From* Weiller and colleagues [211]; with permission.)

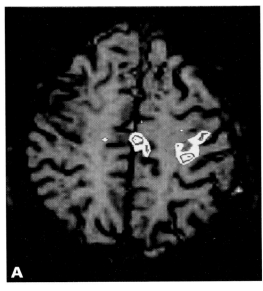 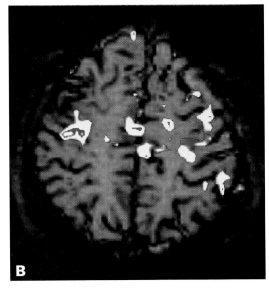

Figure 5-121. Functional magnetic resonance imaging (MRI) studies of the poststroke recovered state. A 66-year-old right-handed woman sustained a cortical infarct in the right frontotemporal cortex, resulting in moderate left hemiplegia, with minimal movement of the left hand. By 15 months poststroke, full motor function had returned to the hand. A functional MRI scan was performed with the patient opening and closing one fist at 1 Hz. Voxels of brain ($3 \times 3 \times 7$ mm) significantly activated at *P* less than 10^{-6}, shown in yellow after smoothing, have been superimposed onto T1-weighted axial brain images taken in the same plane as the functional scan. Activated voxels represent an increase in cerebral blood flow coincident with performance of the task. **A,** Opening and closing of the right (unaffected) hand is associated with activation in the left (contralateral) precentral gyrus and supplementary motor areas. **B,** Opening and closing of the left (recovered) hand is associated with activation in the contralateral (right) precentral gyrus and supplementary motor area as well as in the left (ipsilateral) postcentral gyrus, precentral gyrus, and premotor area. Images such as these provide further evidence for a contribution of bilateral hemispheres to recovery. Functional MRI is a technique that relies on cerebral vasoreactivity to depict neuronal activation; its ability to depict changes in cerebral function after a cerebrovascular accident is under investigation. The potential value of this modality to the understanding of stroke recovery is great. As knowledge is gained about the cellular and molecular mechanisms of poststroke recovery processes, defining the time course of these processes with serial functional images in individual patients will be key to effective therapeutic intervention.

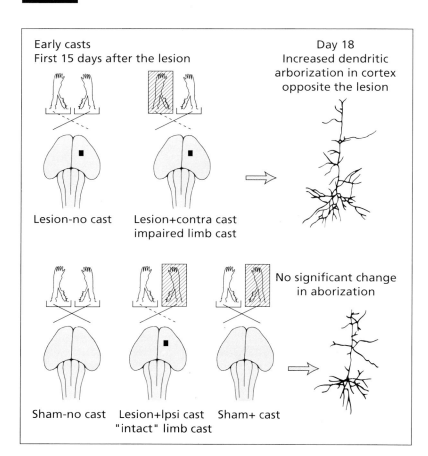

Early casts
First 15 days after the lesion

Lesion-no cast

Lesion+contra cast
impaired limb cast

Day 18
Increased dendritic
arborization in cortex
opposite the lesion

Sham-no cast

Lesion+Ipsi cast
"intact" limb cast

Sham+ cast

No significant change
in aborization

Figure 5-122. Cellular correlates of recovery. A further understanding of stroke recovery is achieved by reviewing cellular and molecular studies related to the restorative brain mechanisms demonstrated by functional neuroimaging. Jones and Schallert [212] studied dendritic arborization patterns in the undamaged hemisphere 18 days after producing lesions in the sensorimotor cortices of rats. Unilateral lesions resulted in an increase in the number of basilar dendritic branches of layer V pyramidal neurons in the undamaged hemisphere. Importantly, immobilization of the intact limb resulted in a significant reduction in dendritic branching, an effect not seen with immobilization of the paretic limb (*ie*, the limb contralateral to the damaged hemisphere). Furthermore, restricting the use of the intact limb also caused a mild but generalized decrement in bilateral performance on tests of sensorimotor function. Such a difference in sensorimotor function was not found, however, in animals with a restriction placed on the use of the paretic limb. Studies such as this one are important in defining the cellular correlates and molecular targets of stroke recovery interventions. (*Adapted from* Jones and colleague [212].)

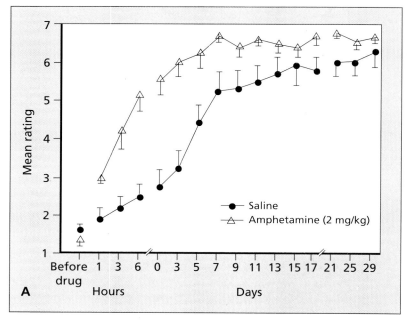

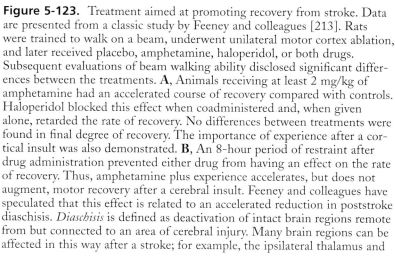

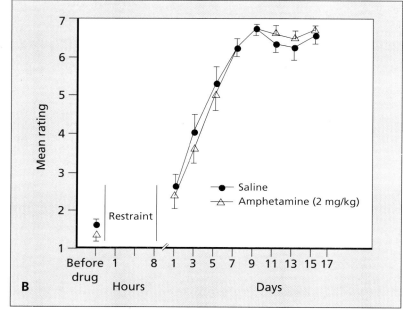

Figure 5-123. Treatment aimed at promoting recovery from stroke. Data are presented from a classic study by Feeney and colleagues [213]. Rats were trained to walk on a beam, underwent unilateral motor cortex ablation, and later received placebo, amphetamine, haloperidol, or both drugs. Subsequent evaluations of beam walking ability disclosed significant differences between the treatments. **A**, Animals receiving at least 2 mg/kg of amphetamine had an accelerated course of recovery compared with controls. Haloperidol blocked this effect when coadministered and, when given alone, retarded the rate of recovery. No differences between treatments were found in final degree of recovery. The importance of experience after a cortical insult was also demonstrated. **B**, An 8-hour period of restraint after drug administration prevented either drug from having an effect on the rate of recovery. Thus, amphetamine plus experience accelerates, but does not augment, motor recovery after a cerebral insult. Feeney and colleagues have speculated that this effect is related to an accelerated reduction in poststroke diaschisis. *Diaschisis* is defined as deactivation of intact brain regions remote from but connected to an area of cerebral injury. Many brain regions can be affected in this way after a stroke; for example, the ipsilateral thalamus and

contralateral cerebellum may show a decrease in regional blood flow after an infarct in the cerebral cortex. Whether resolution of diaschisis is a contributor to, or merely a reflection of, stroke recovery remains unclear.

Similar results have been obtained in several species, including humans. Goldstein [214] identified a significant impairment in upper extremity motor function 7 to 84 days after stroke among patients receiving drugs deemed detrimental to motor recovery, such as haloperidol, benzodiazepines, and α_2-receptor agonists. In a study of eight patients recovering from stroke, Crisostomo and colleagues [215] demonstrated a significant improvement in motor function in patients examined 1 day after amphetamine administration plus physical therapy, as compared with those receiving placebo plus physical therapy; a larger study has confirmed these findings [216]. These studies emphasize the susceptibility of the recovery process to pharmacologic and environmental influences.

The goal of current studies is to identify a treatment capable of augmenting the final degree of recovery. Several other strategies are under active investigation to enhance recovery from stroke, including neurotrophic growth factors and neural transplantation. (*Adapted from* Feeney and colleagues [213].)

Hypertensive Intracerebral Hemorrhage

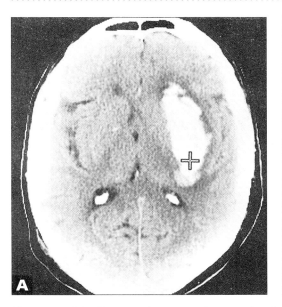
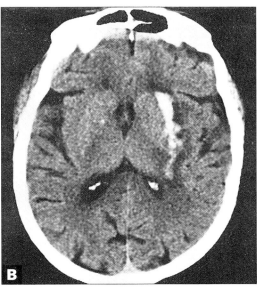

Figure 5-124. Computed tomography scan showing a large left putamen hemorrhage (**A**) in a 68-year-old woman who collapsed at the dinner table, becoming aphasic and hemiplegic on the right side. She had a history of hypertension. She was taken emergently to the operating room, where a stereotactic aspiration of the hematoma was performed. The postoperative CT scan (**B**) is shown. At the time of discharge, the patient was able to ambulate and had only moderate residual expressive aphasia. In this case, the patient was seen in the emergency room within 1 hour of her ictus and was

taken for emergent clot removal within 2 hours. Whether this contributed to her ultimate improvement and outcome has yet to be determined. Putamen hemorrhage is characterized by progressive onset in almost two thirds of patients. Small hemorrhages cause moderate contralateral motor and sensory deficits. Moderate-sized hemorrhages can present with flaccid hemiplegia, hemisensory deficit, conjugate eye deviation toward the side of the lesion, and aphasia if the dominant hemisphere is involved. Large hemorrhages produce almost immediated coma [217].

Hypertensive cerebrovascular disease accounts for 70% to 90% of cases of spontaneous intracerebral hemorrhage [218]. The most common sources of hemorrhage are small penetrating arteries (less than 300 μm), including the thalamoperforating and lenticulostriate arteries and paramedian branches of the basilar artery [219]. There appears to be hypertension-induced degeneration of the media of the arterial wall, resulting in progressive development of microaneurysms [219]. This pathoanatomic factor accounts for the characteristic locations of hypertensive hemorrhages: basal ganglia (35% to 45%), subcortical white matter (25%), thalamus (20%), cerebellum (15%), and pons (5%) [220,221].

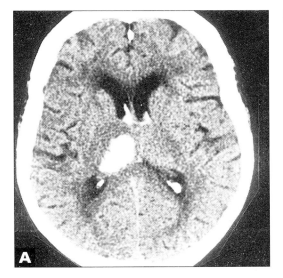
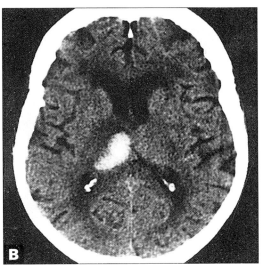

Figure 5-125. Thalamic hemorrhage.
A, Computed tomography scan showing a right thalamic hemorrhage from a 68-year-old woman with a history of hypertension who collapsed at home. During subsequent weeks, she remained drowsy, following only simple commands. **B**, Follow-up computed tomography scan demonstrating mild resolution of the hematoma with clearing of the intraventricular hemorrhage. Thalamic hemorrhages produce hemiplegia and hemisensory deficit. Visual field deficits, aphasia (dominant hemisphere), and contralateral neglect (nondominant hemisphere) may also be seen. Because of their near-midline location and extension into the subthalamus and brain stem, thalamic hemorrhages are more likely to lead to ocular palsies and alterations of consciousness. The classic presentation of obtundation associated with downward and inward deviation of the contralateral eye is well known.

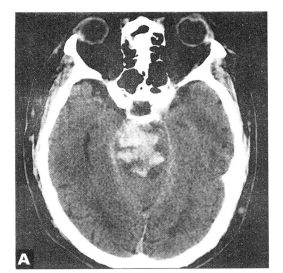
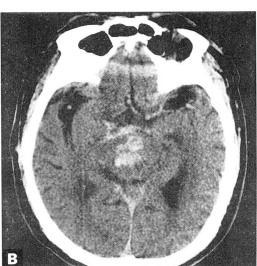

Figure 5-126. Emergent head computed tomography scans (**A, B**) showing a large pontine hemorrhage in a 67-year-old hypertensive man who collapsed at home and became completely unresponsive. On initial neurologic evaluation, he had no brain stem reflexes. Comfort measures were offered and the patient expired the following day. Pontine hemorrhages are the most devastating of all brain hemorrhages. Even small hemorrhages lead to coma, small but reactive pupils, lateral gaze paresis, cranial nerve abnormalities, and quadraparesis [222].

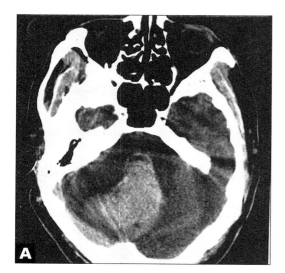 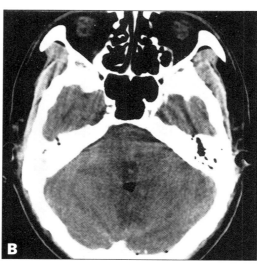

Figure 5-127. Cerebellar hemorrhage. A patient developed sudden onset of nausea, vomiting, and difficulty walking. Within 20 minutes, she became unresponsive. On examination, she was comatose with severely impaired brain stem reflexes and bilateral up-turning toes. **A**, Emergent computed tomography (CT) scans showed a large cerebellar hematoma. Despite her poor neurologic condition, the patient was taken to the operating room for clot evacuation. **B**, Postoperative CT scans. The patient had a good neurologic outcome. At discharge, she was awake and alert, with some dysarthria. Despite severe bilateral dysmetria, she was able to sit unattended. Cerebellar hematoma can be a surgical emergency. If decompressed rapidly, it can be associated with a favorable outcome. Characteristically, cerebellar hemorrhage presents with a sudden onset of nausea, vomiting, and an inability to walk [223]. It is therefore imperative to test gait in patients with vomiting and dizziness. As the hemorrhage enlarges, a conjugate gaze palsy develops. Dysarthria and mild ipsilateral facial weakness may be present. When these signs of brain stem dysfunction occur, mentation is found to be altered. Although this alteration may be subtle initially, it can progress rapidly to frank coma, pinpoint pupils, and decerebration.

Cerebral Amyloid Angiopathy

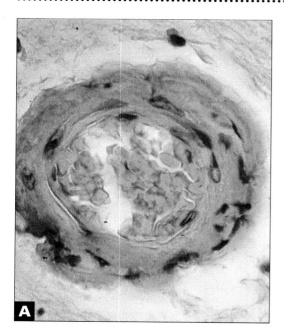 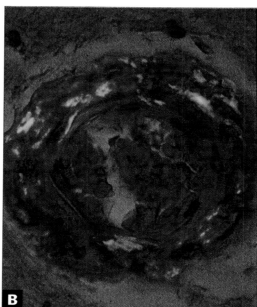

Figure 5-128. Cerebral amyloid angiopathy (CAA) in a cortical vessel stained with Congo red (**A**). The term *amyloid* refers to protein deposits that, because of their physical structure, possess specific staining properties, such as the green birefringence to polarized light (**B**). Amyloid in this vessel has largely replaced the media layer, resulting in thickening of the vessel wall. Vascular amyloid in CAA is almost entirely restricted to the cortex, largely sparing the penetrating vessels of the white and deep gray matter. CAA is an important cause of spontaneous intracerebral hemorrhage in the elderly [224,225]. The presence of at least some cerebrovascular amyloid in the elderly is common, occurring in 20% or more of patients older than 70 years [224]. In most of these patients, the amyloid deposits have no evident effect on the patency of the vessel or integrity of the vessel wall. In a subset of patients, however, CAA initiates a cascade of steps that includes death of vascular smooth muscle cells (perhaps due to direct toxic properties of β-amyloid [226]), cracking and necrosis of cerebral vessel walls [227–229], and ultimately intracerebral hemorrhage. (*Courtesy of* Jean Paul Vonsattel, MD, C.S. Kubik Laboratory for Neuropathology, Massachusetts General Hospital, Boston, MA.)

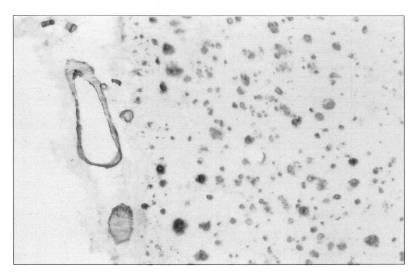

Figure 5-129. Immunostain with a monoclonal antibody to the β-amyloid peptide shows the close relation between the material in the vessel wall in cerebral amyloid angiopathy (CAA) and in the senile plaques that characterize Alzheimer's disease. CAA generally occurs in the absence of systemic amyloidosis but often in conjunction with the other major amyloidosis of the brain, Alzheimer's disease. The β-amyloid peptide comprising the deposits in these two disorders is a 39- to 43-amino acid fragment of the β-amyloid precursor protein (β-APP), a 695- to 770-amino acid glycoprotein expressed throughout the body. Cerebrovascular amyloid has been reported to contain both the 39- to 40-amino acid form of β-amyloid and the longer 42- to 43-amino acid form [230,231], which may have specific pathogenic properties [232]. Despite the close molecular relation and significant overlap between CAA and Alzheimer's disease, it is worth considering them as separate diseases with distinct pathologies, genetics (Fig. 5-136), and clinical presentations. (*Courtesy of* Jean Paul Vonsattel, MD, C.S. Kubik Laboratory for Neuropathology, Massachusetts General Hospital, Boston, MA.)

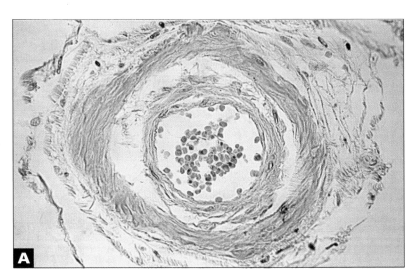

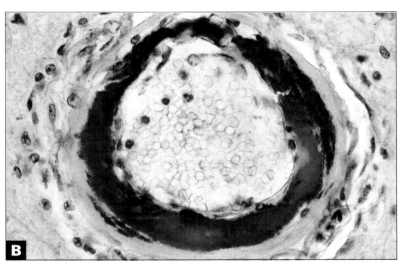

Figure 5-130. Cerebral amyloid angiopathy (CAA)-related vasculopathic changes. Several pathologic changes in the amyloid-laden vessels identify those cases of CAA that are sufficiently severe to raise the risk of hemorrhage [227–229]. These vasculopathic changes include cracking of the vessel wall, producing a vessel-within-vessel appearance (**A**) and fibrinoid necrosis of the vessel wall, demonstrated by staining with phosphotungstic acid hematoxylin (**B**). The presence of severe CAA (defined by vessel wall fragmentation and at least one paravascular focus of blood leakage) and fibrinoid necrosis is significantly more common in patients with CAA-related intracerebral hemorrhage than in those with CAA and no hemorrhage [231]. Still unknown are the factors that determine which patients with CAA will develop the vasculopathic changes leading to hemorrhage. (*Courtesy of* Jean Paul Vonsattel, MD, C.S. Kubik Laboratory for Neuropathology, Massachusetts General Hospital, Boston, MA.)

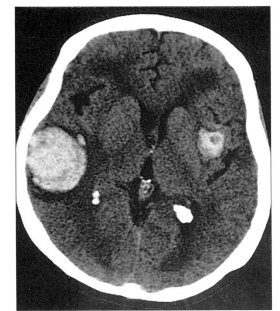

Figure 5-131. Unenhanced computed tomography image from a 69-year-old woman who presented with hemorrhages in the right parietotemporal and left temporal lobes. Pathologic examination of cortical tissue obtained from evacuation of the right-sided hematoma demonstrated cerebral amyloid angiopathy (CAA). The hemorrhages in this patient illustrate the characteristic lobar location and multifocality of CAA-related hemorrhage.

Although concerns have been raised about the risk of surgical trauma provoking further hemorrhage from the amyloid-laden vasculature, surgical experience with CAA has generally been good [233–235]. Surgical indications for CAA-related hemorrhage (*eg*, acute neurologic deterioration of an otherwise stable patient) are thus similar to those for other types of hemorrhage. Examination of vessels in the wall of the hematoma or within the hematoma itself can provide important diagnostic information in support of CAA [236].

This patient was taking warfarin at the time of her hemorrhages. CAA appears to be an important contributor to warfarin-related intracerebral hemorrhages, particularly those in lobar brain regions [237]. Other than avoiding anticoagulation, however, there are no known treatments for preventing hemorrhage due to CAA.

Boston Criteria for Diagnosis of CAA-Related Intracerebral Hemorrhage

Definite CAA

Full postmortem examination demonstrating:
 Lobar, cortical, or corticosubcortical hemorrhage
 Severe CAA with vasculopathy [228]
 Absence of other diagnostic lesion

Probable CAA with supporting pathology

Clinical data and pathologic tissue (evacuated
 hematoma or cortical biopsy) demonstrating:
 Lobar, cortical, or corticosubcortical hemorrhage
 Some degree of CAA in specimen
 Absence of other diagnostic lesion

Probable CAA

Clinical data and magnetic resonance imaging (MRI) or computed tomography (CT) demonstrating:
 Multiple hemorrhages restricted to lobar, cortical, or corticosubcortical
 regions (cerebellar hemorrhage allowed)
 Age ≥55 years
 Absence of other causes of hemorrhage*

Possible CAA

Clinical data and MRI or CT demonstrating:
 Single lobar, cortical, or corticosubcortical hemorrhage
 Age ≥55 years
 Absence of other cause of hemorrhage*

For the purposes of these criteria, other causes of intracerebral hemorrhage include the following: excessive warfarin (International Normalized Ratio (INR) above 3.0); antecedent head trauma or ischemic stroke; central nervous system tumor, vascular malformation, or vasculitis; and blood dyscrasia or coagulopathy. INRs above 3.0 or other nonspecific laboratory abnormalities permitted for diagnosis of possible CAA.

Figure 5-132. Boston criteria for diagnosis of cerebral amyloid angiopathy (CAA)-related intracerebral hemorrhage. Cerebral amyloid angiopathy-related hemorrhage has historically been a diagnosis reached only after pathologic examination of tissue. The criteria presented here were developed by the Boston Cerebral Amyloid Angiopathy Research Group (Steven M. Greenberg, MD, PhD, Daniel S. Kanter, MD, Carlos S. Kase, MD, Michael S. Pessin, MD) to formalize the clinical and pathologic diagnosis of CAA. By these criteria, diag-nosis of definite CAA-related hemorrhage requires full postmortem examination, while the diagnoses of probable and possible CAA-related hemorrhage can be applied to patients for whom only clinical and radiographic data are available. The clinical criteria are based on the predilection of CAA-related hemorrhage for the cortical or corticosubcortical (lobar) regions and its tendency to occur at multiple foci. In a series of 13 patients with hemorrhage clinically diagnosed with probable CAA, all 13 demonstrated CAA pathologically [238].

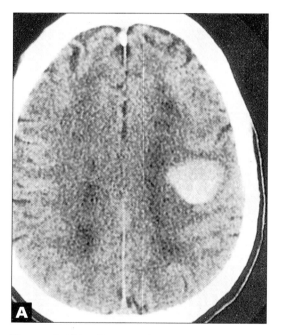 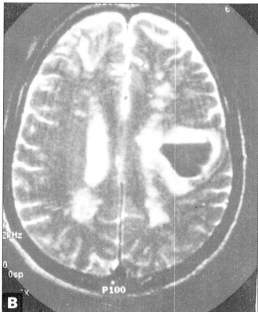 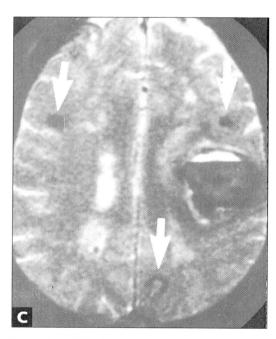

Figure 5-133. Computed tomography (CT) scan (**A**), T2-weighted magnetic resonance image (MRI) (**B**), and gradient-echo MRI (**C**) from a 69-year-old man who presented with left frontal lobar hemorrhage. The gradient-echo MRI demonstrates, in addition to the large lobar hemorrhage, multiple small corticosubcortical hemorrhages (*arrows*) not detected by the other techniques. In a prospective study, gradient-echo MRI detected accompanying small hemorrhages in 12 of 15 elderly patients presenting with lobar hemorrhage, compared with 3 of 15 detected by CT and 5 of 15 by T2-weighted MRI [239]. No similar lesions were seen on gradient-echo studies in 10 elderly control patients.

CAA can cause small, clinically silent hemorrhages in addition to large lobar hemorrhages. These small hemorrhages can often be detected by the sensitive technique of gradient-echo MRI. Gradient-echo MRI enhances the signal dropout produced by foci of chronic hemorrhage, increasing the sensitivity of detection. Applied to patients presenting with large lobar hemorrhage, this technique frequently identifies accompanying petechial hemorrhages scattered in the lobar regions [239], thereby aiding in the clinical diagnosis of CAA.

The technique of gradient-echo MRI is designed to enhance the magnetic susceptibility and resultant signal dropout produced by chronic blood products. It requires neither additional hardware nor software relative to conventional fast spin-echo MRI and can thus serve as a useful tool in the diagnostic evaluation of cerebral hemorrhage.

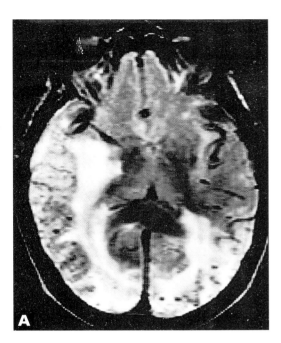 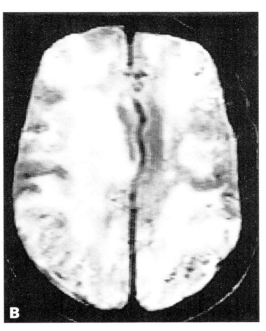

Figure 5-134. T2-weighted magnetic resonance images (MRI) from a 75-year-old man with dramatic deterioration in global cognition over several days (**A, B**). The study demonstrates diffuse, confluent hyperintensity in the white matter with mass effect and right-to-left midline shift. There are also multiple small corticosubcortical foci of hypointensity consistent with hemorrhage. Pathologic examination revealed severe cerebral amyloid angiopathy (CAA) with patchy loss of myelin and axons in the white matter and multiple small cortical hemorrhages of various ages. The pathologic changes in the white matter in cases such as this resemble those seen in Binswanger's disease [240], and may represent white matter ischemia due to diffuse CAA-related narrowing of penetrating cortical vessels. CAA has been implicated in several neurologic syndromes other than lobar hemorrhage, including a syndrome of transient spreading neurologic symptoms [241].

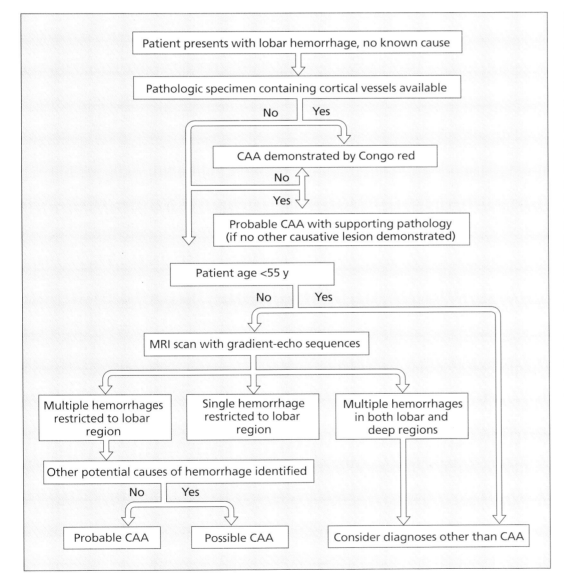

Figure 5-135. Algorithm for evaluation of lobar hemorrhage. An approach to the diagnostic evaluation of lobar hemorrhage is outlined based on the criteria presented in Figure 5-132. In the absence of pathologic data, the evaluation is predicated on the age of the patient, the distribution of hemorrhages seen radiographically, and the presence or absence of other potential causes of hemorrhage (Fig. 5-132). The categories of probable cerebral amyloid angiopathy (CAA) with supporting pathology, probable CAA, possible CAA, and consideration of other diagnoses are designed to reflect the relative likelihood of CAA as the cause of hemorrhage, but should be considered tentative diagnoses in the absence of postmortem pathologic data. A large number of other processes can cause lobar hemorrhage, including trauma, lobar extension of hypertensive hemorrhage, vascular malformation, hemorrhagic tumor, hemorrhagic transformation of ischemic stroke, vasculitis, sympathomimetic agents, rupture of mycotic or sacular aneurysm, and coagulopathy.

Risk factors for CAA include advanced age and the presence of Alzheimer's disease but apparently not hypertension [224,225]. The gene for apolipoprotein E (apoE), identified as an important determinant of a patient's risk for Alzheimer's disease, appears to exert an independent effect on the risk for CAA. Evidence from pathologic and clinical series of patients suggests that both the ϵ2 and ϵ4 alleles of apoE are risk factors for the presence and earlier onset of CAA-related hemorrhage [242–245]. Despite this relationship, the presence of the ϵ2 and ϵ4 alleles is neither necessary nor sufficient for CAA-related hemorrhage. Determination of apoE genotype is therefore not recommended as part of the clinical evaluation for CAA. MRI—magnetic resonance imaging.

Genetic Causes of CAA With Hemorrhage

Gene	Amino acid change	Clinical phenotype
β-Amyloid precursor protein	693 Glu changes to Gln	CAA with hemorrhage (HCHWA-D)
	692 Ala changes to Gly	CAA with hemorrhage *or* AD
	694 Asp changes to Asn	CAA with dementia
Cystatin C	68 Glu changes to Leu	CAA with hemorrhage (HCHWA-I)

Figure 5-136. Genetic causes of hereditary cerebral hemorrhage with amyloidosis (HCHWA). Four genetic causes have been identified for CAA with hemorrhage. Three are mutations within the β-amyloid peptide segment of the β-amyloid precursor protein, one associated primarily with CAA

(referred to as the Dutch type, or HCHWA-D) [246,247], and two affecting adjacent amino acid residues that can cause CAA as well as pathologic changes characteristic of Alzheimer's disease [248,249]. The other genetic mutation affects cystatin C, an inhibitor of enzymatic proteases normally present in cerebrospinal fluid. This mutation (referred to as the Icelandic type, or HCHWA-I) [250,251] causes hemorrhage as early as the second or third decade of life. Each of the described mutations is associated with a familial, autosomal dominant syndrome of early-onset cerebral hemorrhage. Most patients with nonfamilial CAA-related hemorrhage appear not to carry any of these mutations [252,256]. Ala—alamine; Asn—asparagine; Asp—asparaginase; Gln—glutamine; Glu—glutamic acid; Gly—glycine; Leu—leucine.

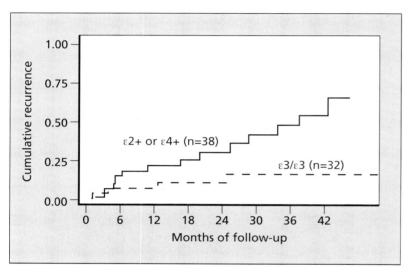

Figure 5-137. Association of apolipoprotein E (apoE) genotype with risk of recurrent lobar hemorrhage. ApoE is a normal constituent of plasma and cerebrospinal fluid lipoprotein. The gene coding for apoE has three major alleles: apoE ε2, apoE ε3, and apoE ε4; ε3 is the most common. Among 70 consecutive patients age 55 years or older who survived an initial lobar hemorrhage, those who carried the apoE ε2 or ε4 alleles were at significantly increased risk for recurrent hemorrhage [257]. Using the Kaplan-Meier estimates of rate of hemorrhage occurrence, two-year cumulative recurrence was 28% among patients with ε2 or ε4 compared with 10% for patients with the common apoE ε3/ε3 genotype. The risk ratio associated with these alleles was 3.8 (95% CI, 1.2–11.6). Another risk factor for recurrence in this cohort was a history of hemorrhagic stroke before entry into the study, with an associated two-year recurrence rate of 61% and risk ratio of 6.4 (95% CI, 2.2–18.5). Age, sex, and history of hypertension did not appear to affect risk of hemorrhage recurrence.

Subarachnoid Hemorrhage

Hunt and Hess Grading System

Grade 0 Unruptured
Grade 1 Asymptomatic or minimal headache, nuchal rigidity
Grade 2 Moderate to severe headache, nuchal rigidity, no
        neurologic deficit other than cranial nerve palsy
Grade 3 Drowsiness, mild neurologic deficit
Grade 4 Stupor, moderate to severe hemiparesis, possible
        early decerebrate rigidity, vegetative disturbances
Grade 5 Deep coma, decerebrate rigidity, moribund appearance

Figure 5-138. Hunt and Hess grading system for subarachnoid hemorrhage. The grading system according to Hunt and Hess [257] is widely used to standardize the clinical classification based on the initial neurologic examination. The initial clinical grade is strongly related to the severity of the hemorrhage and to the acute and long-term prognosis.

Subarachnoid hemorrhage (SAH) has several causes. Rupture of saccular aneurysms of the basal vessels of the brain is the cause of about 80% of cases of SAH [258]. Other causes include arteriovenous malformations and other vascular malformations, central nervous system infections, head trauma, brain tumors, and diverse blood disorders. About 28,000 cases of aneurysmal SAH are encountered annually in the United States, making this a significant public health problem [259]. As many as 12% of patients die from the initial injury [260], and up to one quarter die within 3 months after hemorrhage [259]. Aneurysmal obliteration is the initial crucial goal in the management of SAH. Although initial experience with early surgery produced discouraging results, more recent experience has demonstrated an advantage to early operation [261]. Microsurgery has become the main technique for treatment of intracranial aneurysms, but endovascular treatment with detachable coil therapy may offer an effective alternative to surgery. Neurologic complications of SAH are frequent, can be devastating, and must be prevented and treated aggressively. These include diffuse ischemic injury, rehemorrhage, cerebrovascular vasospasm, hydrocephalus, and seizures.

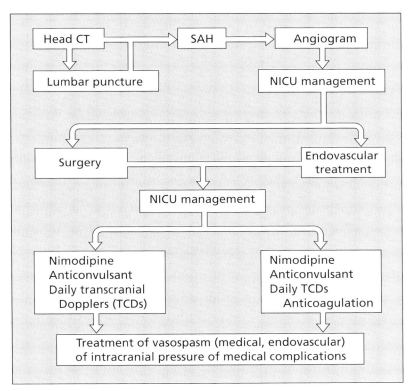

Figure 5-139. Algorithm for management of patients in good clinical condition after subarachnoid hemorrhage (SAH) (Hunt and Hess grades 1 and 2). A head computed tomography (CT) scan is obtained that confirms the presence of subarachnoid blood. If the head CT scan does not show subarachnoid blood and the patient has symptoms consistent with SAH (*ie*, intense headache, nausea, vomiting, and photophobia), a lumbar puncture is performed to confirm the diagnosis. Once the diagnosis is confirmed a four-vessel angiogram is obtained. The angiogram delineates the anatomy of the lesion, diagnoses the presence of multiple aneurysms (seen in up to 20% of patients), and helps to plan for subsequent therapy. Once the angiogram is performed, the patient is observed in the neurology and neurosurgery intensive care unit (NICU) with invasive central monitoring. After multidisciplinary discussion, the lesion is obliterated using surgical or endovascular techniques. The patient is monitored in the NICU for the development of vasospasm, hydrocephalus, or any of the other multiple medical complications associated with SAH. Early surgery in good grade aneurysm patients (Hunt and Hess grades 1 to 3) is a generally accepted treatment with a satisfying outcome in most patients. The results of large series of good grade aneurysm patients lie in the 70% to 90% good neurologic recovery range, with a mortality rate of 1.7% to 8% [262].

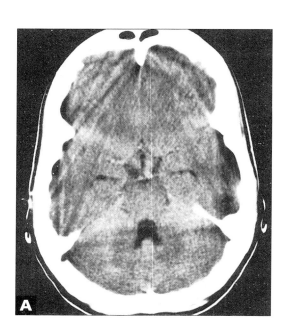
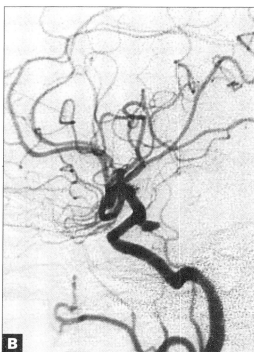
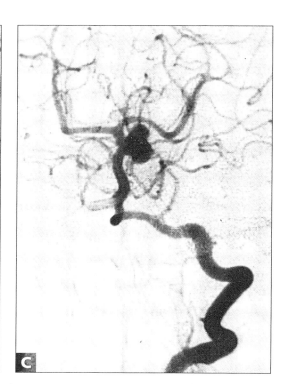

Figure 5-140. Good grade aneurysm. **A,** Computed tomography scan showing a small amount of subarachnoid hemorrhage from a patient who presented with intense headache, nausea, and vomiting (Hunt and Hess grade 2). **B, C,** Angiograms showed two separate intracranial aneurysms.

A lesion was present on the posterior communicating artery (*B*), and a second lesion was seen on the right superior cerebellar artery (SCA) (*C*). The lesions were obliterated during surgery.

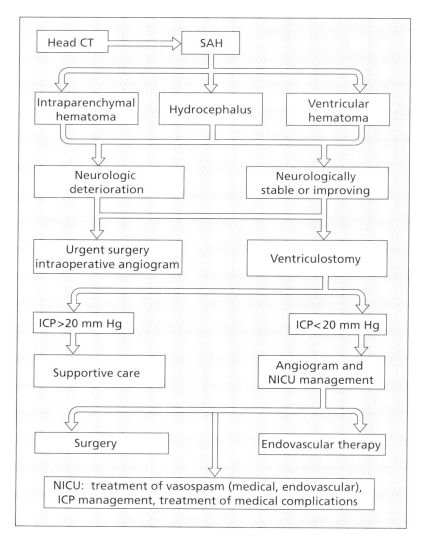

Figure 5-141. Management algorithm for patients presenting with clinical Hunt and Hess grade 3 subarachnoid hemorrhage (SAH). A head computed tomography (CT) scan is obtained to confirm the diagnosis of SAH. If the patient is stable neurologically, a four-vessel angiogram is performed and, as with good grade patients, the lesion is rapidly treated using surgical or endovascular techniques to prevent subsequent rehemorrhage. If neurologic deterioration due to the presence of an intraparenchymal hematoma occurs, urgent surgery is considered with an intraoperative angiogram or CT angiogram. If the initial head CT scan shows hydrocephalus or an intraventricular hematoma, or if neurologic deterioration is due to the development of hydrocephalus, a ventriculostomy is rapidly placed to monitor intracranial pressure. If neurologic improvement follows the placement of a ventriculostomy, or if the intracranial pressure is controlled to less than 20 mm Hg, the patient is treated according to standard procedures. If the intracranial pressure is uncontrollable (greater than 20 mm Hg), then supportive care only is offered. Once the aneurysm is obliterated, the patient is followed closely in the neurology and neurosurgery intensive care unit (NICU) with serial clinical examination and daily transcranial Dopplers to detect development of vasospasm. ICP—intracranial pressure.

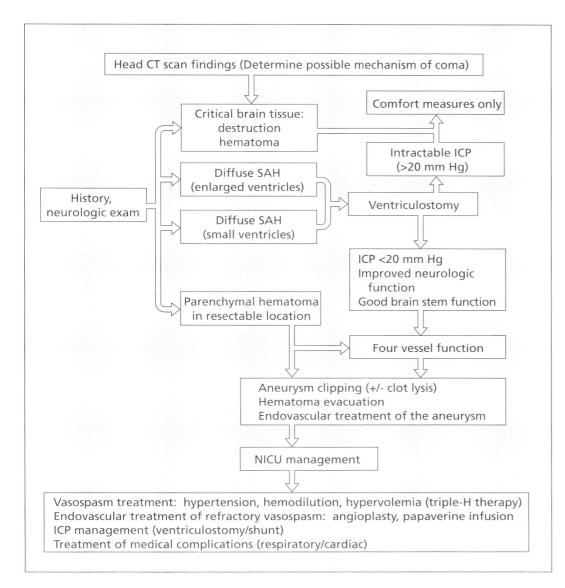

Figure 5-142. Management of poor grade patients (Hunt and Hess grade 4 and 5) with subarachnoid hemorrhage (SAH). After review of the patient's clinical condition, a computed tomography scan is obtained, and some attempt is made to define the overall mechanism of induced poor clinical grade. All patients, except those who show radiographic evidence of significant brain destruction or destruction of critical areas such as the thalamus or the brain stem, have a ventriculostomy placed to measure the intracranial pressure (ICP). Patients with significant tissue destruction are treated with comfort measures only. If after placement of the ventriculostomy, the ICP can be controlled below 20 mm Hg, or if the patient's condition is stable or improves, angiographic diagnosis is the next step. The aneurysm is then treated with surgery or an endovascular procedure. If the patient's poor clinical condition is the result of a surgically resectable intraparenchymal hemorrhage, we generally proceed with surgery without further delay. After surgery, the patient is managed in the neurology and neurosurgery intensive care unit (NICU). Continuous monitoring for the possible development of medical complications is performed. Daily transcranial Doppler measurements and clinical observations are used to detect the development of vasospasm. Traditionally, the outlook for patients presenting with SAH in Hunt and Hess grade 4 or 5 has been dismal. More recently, a few groups have reported a good outcome in 40% to 50% of selected patients who presented in poor clinical grade [263] and who were treated with early surgery or endovascular techniques. Our experience in treating patients in poor grade is similar to that reported by other groups. Based on our and other experience, it appears that there is a population of patients who initially present in poor neurologic condition but who have the potential to make a meaningful recovery.

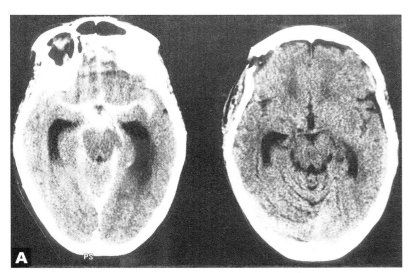 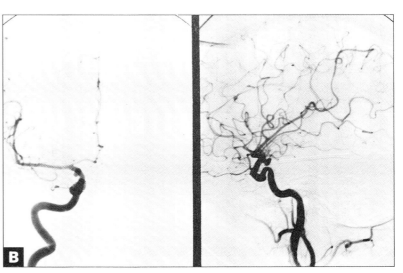

Figure 5-143. Poor grade aneurysm (Hunt and Hess grade 4). **A,** Computed tomography (CT) scans of a patient who presented with Hunt and Hess grade 4 subarachnoid hemorrhage (SAH). The initial CT scan (*left*) shows a dense SAH. Tissue plasminogen activator was used after clipping of the aneurysm, and a follow-up CT scan (*right*) shows complete resolution of the blood within 3 days of surgery. **B,** Anteroposterior (*left*) and lateral (*right*) angiograms of the right internal carotid artery demonstrating the posterior communicating artery that caused the SAH. The patient was a 55-year-old woman who was initially comatose. Within 3 weeks, she was able to respond appropriately to questions and over 6 months made an excellent recovery, returning to a normal life-style.

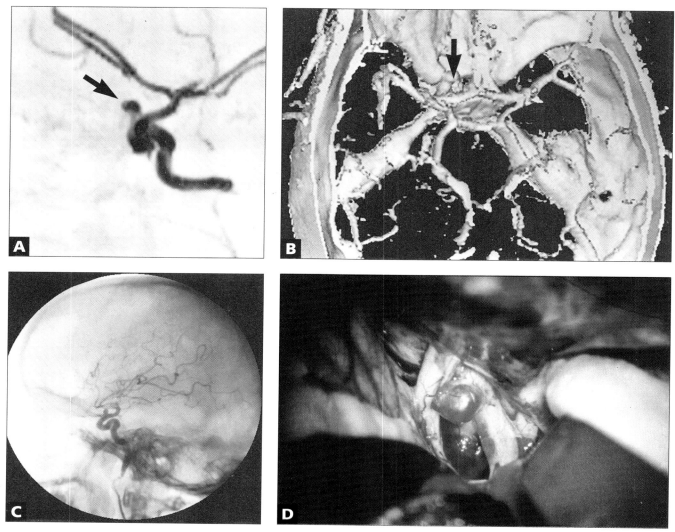

Figure 5-144. Unruptured aneurysm. With improved neuroradiologic diagnostic techniques (*eg,* magnetic resonance angiogram, computed tomography [CT] angiogram) unruptured aneurysms are discovered more frequently. Autopsy series have reported that about 5% of patients have intracranial aneurysms. The annual risk of unruptured aneurysm is about 1% to 2% [264]. The decision about whether to treat an unruptured aneurysm depends on the patient's age, the size of the lesion, and other concurrent medical conditions. Lesions larger than 1 cm are at a fairly significant risk of hemorrhage [265], especially in patients who are younger than 50 years old. Of patients who present with subarachnoid hemorrhage (SAH), 70% have an aneurysm less than 1 cm in size, with an average size of 5 to 7 mm. This discrepancy remains unresolved. In the young patients with lesions 8 to 10 mm in diameter, such as in the 22-year-old woman shown here, we favor aneurysmal obliteration.

A, Magnetic resonance angiogram of the circle of Willis in a 22-year-old woman who presented with left eye pain. An aneurysm can be seen in the paraclinoid region of the left side (*arrow*). **B,** CT angiogram confirms the location of the lesion and demonstrates the relation of the aneurysm to the skull base and anterior clinoid process (*arrow*). **C,** Lateral angiogram of the left internal carotid artery demonstrates the aneurysm in association with the ophthalmic artery. **D,** The aneurysm was exposed surgically and can be seen pressing against the optic nerve. The aneurysm was obliterated with aneurysm clips. The patient made an excellent recovery and was discharged 3 days after surgery.

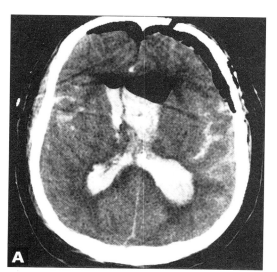

Figure 5-145. Acute hydrocephalus. Acute hydrocephalus is a known complication of subarachnoid hemorrhage (SAH). Dramatic improvement of consciousness has been observed after immediate drainage of cerebrospinal fluid (CSF) [266]. Commonly, acute hydrocephalus may develop as a result of dense blood in the basal cisterns, or it may be due to direct intraventricular hemorrhage with interference of CSF pathways at the foramen of Monro or at the level of the fourth ventricle, with obstruction of the foramina of Luschka and Magendie. The incidence of acute hydrocephalus after SAH has been reported to be from 12% to 63% [267]. It may present as the relatively abrupt onset of lethargy, stupor, or coma. Urgent placement of unilateral or bilateral ventriculostomy can be beneficial in reversing the process and rapidly improving the neurologic condition of the patient.

This 72-year-old man suffered an aneurysmal subarachnoid and intraventricular hemorrhage from a left posterior communicating artery aneurysm. Surgery was performed to clip the aneurysm, and tissue plasminogen activator was instilled in the subarachnoid space. Although the subarachnoid blood partially resolved, a computed tomography scan performed 2 days after surgery (**A**) demonstrated dense intraventricular hematoma.

(*Continued on next page*)

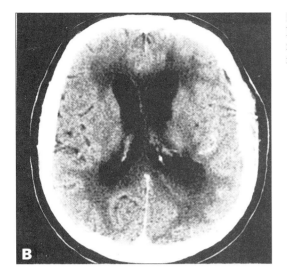

Figure 5-145. (*Continued*) With ventricular drainage, the hematoma resolved (**B**), yet the patient had persistent hydrocephalus, as can be seen with transependymal flow of CSF in the paraventricular region. A ventriculoperitoneal shunt was placed, and the patient had good improvement in neurologic function and associated decreased ventricular size.

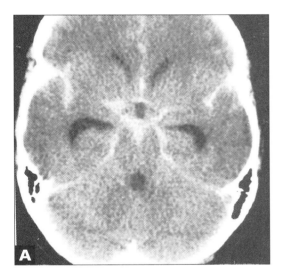

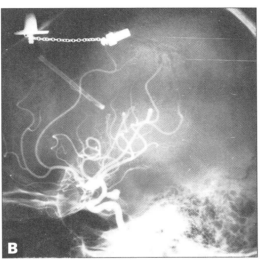

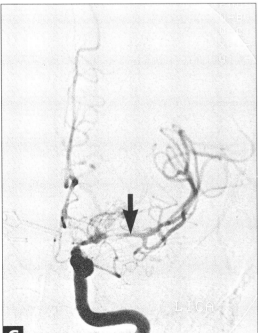

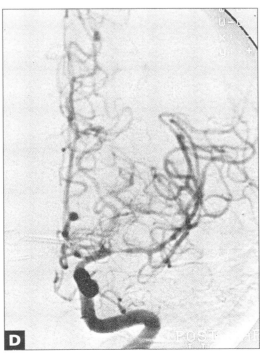

Figure 5-146. Vasospasm. A 25-year-old woman presented with dense subarachnoid hemorrhage (SAH) in clinical grade 1. **A**, Computed tomography scan showing a significant amount of SAH, which is known to correlate with an increased risk of developing vasospasm [268]. **B**, A four-vessel angiogram demonstrated a right posterior communicating artery aneurysm. **C**, The patient underwent successful surgery, but 3 days after the operation developed right hemiparesis and was found to have significant narrowing of the left internal carotid artery consistent with cerebral vasospasm (*arrow*). **D**, A supraselective angiogram was performed, and papaverine was infused intraarterially, which relaxed the intracranial portion of the internal carotid artery. The patient had immediate neurologic improvement with resolution of the right-sided weakness. She required subsequent papaverine treatments and had an excellent neurologic recovery. Papaverine is a potent vasodilator, and intraarterial high-dose infusion of papaverine dilates areas of severe vasospasm [269]. Its effects depend on adequate dose and adequate delivery to a vasospastic vessel. The vasodilatory effects of papaverine are transient [270], and often multiple serial treatments are required.

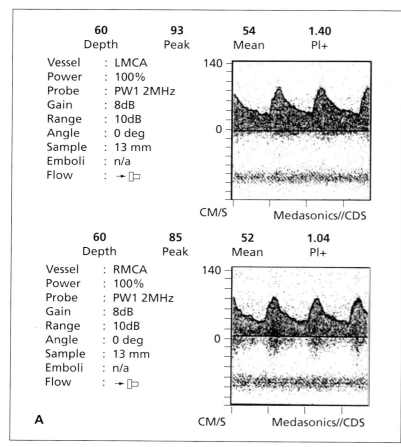

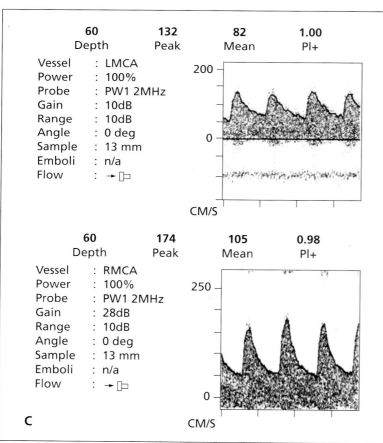

A

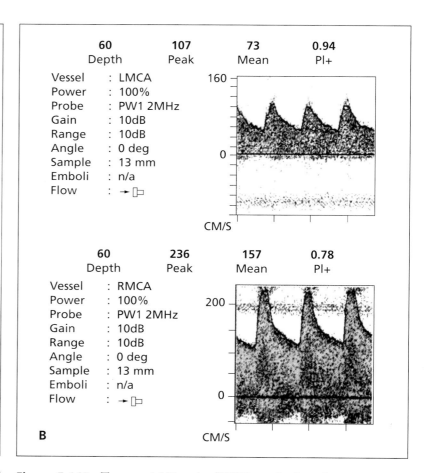

B

Figure 5-147. Transcranial Doppler (TCD) monitoring of vasospasm. The Doppler probe must be tuned to the appropriate depth for the vessel in question. **A,** TCD recordings from a patient 4 days after subarachnoid hemorrhage (SAH) with normal velocities in the left middle cerebral artery (LMCA) and right middle cerebral arteries (RMCAs). **B,** The patient developed vasospasm and by day 8 had significant elevation of TCD velocities in the right MCA. **C,** At day 15, the velocities in the right MCA improved and were almost back to baseline. TCD technique can detect changes in blood flow velocity in the proximal segments of the internal carotid artery, MCA, anterior cerebral artery, and vertebral and basilar arteries that presumably are caused by vessel lumina restricted by vasospasm. TCD is an effective screening tool for detection of vasospasm [271]. It can detect changes in flow velocities that precede the appearance of neurologic signs by 24 to 48 hours so that therapies can be started before ischemia begins. PI+—pulsatile index; PW—power.

Medical Treatment of Vasospasm

Hypervolemia
  Central venous pressure elevated
  Colloid used to expand central volume
  Selective use of pulmonary artery catheter to monitor
    cardiac function and help management
Hemodilution
  Hematocrit kept at 30% to 32% to reduce viscosity while
    maintaining oxygen-carrying capacity
Hypertension
  Pressors used alone or in combination to induce hypertension

Figure 5-148. Medical treatment of vasospasm. About 20% to 30% of patients with recent subarachnoid hemorrhage (SAH) develop clinical features of symptomatic vasospasm [272]. The clinical course is variable and usually peaks at 7 to 10 days [273]. Symptoms gradually evolve, with waxing and

waning of neurologic deficits, including new headache, seizures, or decreased alertness. Focal neurologic signs depend on the affected vessel. Several measures can help to prevent ischemic complications of vasospasm. The classic strategy, which is the standard at most medical centers, involves prophylactic management with nimodipine and maintenance of normovolemia, augmented by aggressive hypervolemic hemodilution and systemic arterial hypertension only when patients develop the clinical signs of ischemic neurologic deficit. Clinical experience with this strategy indicates that symptomatic vasospasm can be treated effectively in many cases but that neurologic improvement fails in as many as 25% to 40% of patients [274]. Because the development of vasospasm is strongly associated with thick collections of blood in the subarachnoid space, evacuation of blood may lessen the likelihood of severe vasospasm. Intracisternal administration of thrombolytic drugs at the time of clipping of the aneurysm improves the removal of subarachnoid clot. Clinical trials with tissue plasminogen activator have shown that vasospasm can be prevented in some patients [275]. Blood deposited after SAH degrades with the conversion of oxyhemoglobin to methemoglobin, releasing an activated form of oxygen that catalyzes free radical reactions, including lipid peroxide formation. Limiting the effects of lipid peroxidation may lessen the effects of cerebral ischemia. Preliminary clinical studies report a lessening of clinical ischemia and lower mortality rates with the use of tirilazad mesylate, a 21-aminosteroid that has been shown to inhibit lipid peroxidation.

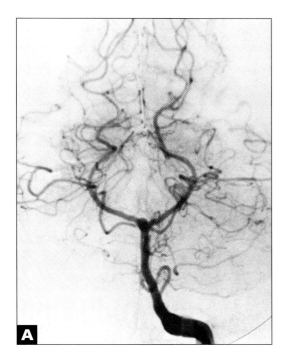
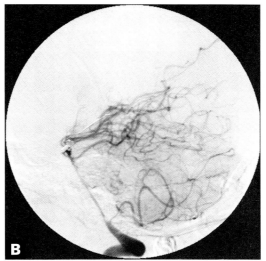
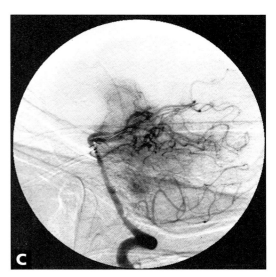

Figure 5-149. Angioplasty of the basilar artery. A 56-year-old woman presented with a dense subarachnoid hemorrhage (SAH) around the basal cisterns. Angiography demonstrated a small basilar tip aneurysm (**A**). Four days after surgery,

the patient became obtunded and transcranial Doppler suggested severe vasospasm of the basilar artery, which was confirmed by angiography (**B**). The patient was treated with intraarterial papaverine and balloon angioplasty of the basilar artery. An angiogram shows the improvement of the caliber of the basilar artery after treatment (**C**). The patient was awake after the treatment and able to follow commands. She gradually improved neurologically and eventually had an excellent recovery. The risks of angioplasty include vessel rupture and thrombosis. Several small studies have reported marked clinical improvement of ischemic deficits as well as angiographic resolution of vasospasm in patients refractory to standard medical therapy with angioplasty treatment [276]. Balloon angioplasty can dilate proximal segments of vessels but is not well suited for dilation of the distal vasculature. This therapy should be reserved for patients who have not responded to other interventions.

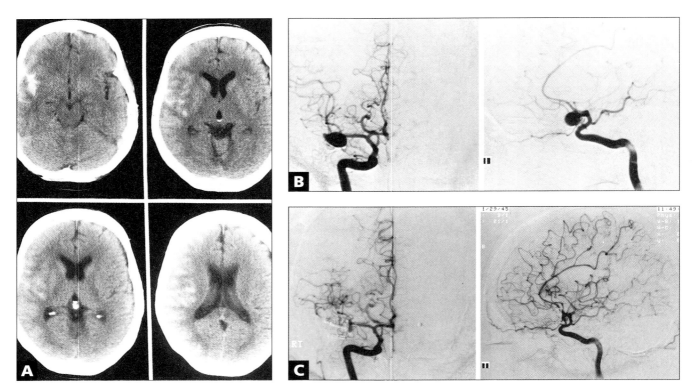

Figure 5-150. Anterior circulation aneurysm. **A,** Computed tomography scans of a 48-year-old woman who presented with Hunt and Hess grade 3 subarachnoid hemorrhage (SAH). Dense subarachnoid blood can be seen in the right sylvian fissure. **B,** Anteroposterior (*left*) and lateral cerebral (*right*) angiograms show a large right middle cerebral artery (MCA) bifurcation aneurysm. **C,** Anteroposterior (*left*) and lateral (*right*) postoperative angiograms demonstrate complete obliteration of the aneurysm with nor-mal filling of the MCA branches. After an extended stay in the neurology and neurosurgery intensive care unit, the patient had an excellent recovery. About 85% of these aneurysms occur in the anterior circulation [277]. The most common sites of ruptured aneurysms are the internal carotid artery, including the posterior communicating artery junction (41%), the anterior communicating artery (34%), and the MCA (20%).

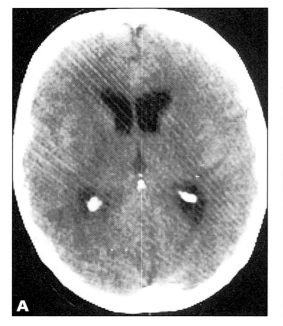

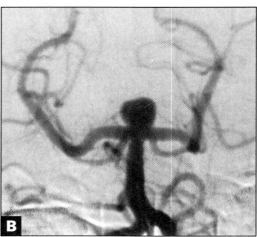

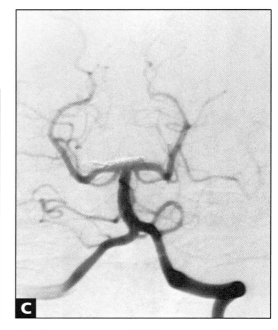

Figure 5-151. Posterior circulation aneurysm. Four percent of aneurysms are seen in the posterior circulation at the level of the vertebral or basilar artery. **A,** Computed tomography scan of a patient who presented with Hunt and Hess grade 3 subarachnoid hemorrhage (SAH). **B,** Vertebral artery angiogra-phy demonstrating a 1.1-cm basilar tip aneurysm. **C,** The patient underwent a right frontotemporal craniotomy for microsurgical clip obliteration of the lesion, with excellent angiographic result. The patient was treated for vasospasm and had an excellent recovery, returning to a normal life-style.

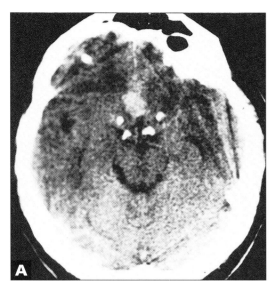
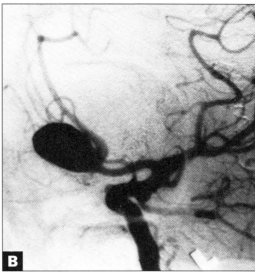
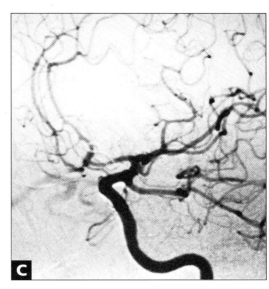

Figure 5-152. Giant aneurysm. **A,** Computed tomography scan showing a large interhemispheric hyperdensity consistent with an aneurysm in a patient with subarachnoid hemorrhage (SAH). **B,** Angiogram showing a giant aneurysm at the level of the anterior communicating artery. **C,** Angiograms showing the postoperative result with preservation of normal patent vasculature and complete obliteration of the aneurysm using a fenestrated clip. The term *giant aneurysm* is used for lesions exceeding 25 mm in greatest diameter [278]. Lesions of this size account for about 5% of all intracranial aneurysms. Patients usually present with SAH or with signs and symptoms of mass lesions. Embolic transient ischemic attacks and stroke have also been reported because these aneurysms contain extensive intramural thrombus. The management of such lesions pose special problems. The neck may be wide and incorporate the origins of adjacent vessels, or the calcification of the neck from partial thrombosis of the aneurysm may make the clipping extremely hazardous.

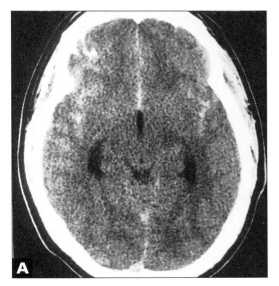
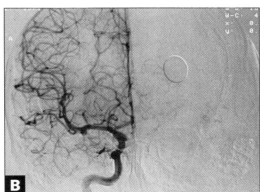
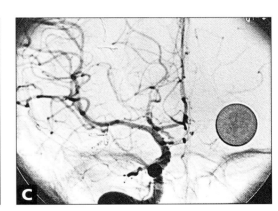
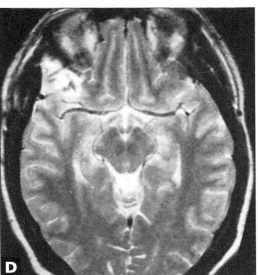

Figure 5-153. Presumed infectious aneurysm. A 22-year-old man with a history of intravenous drug use was admitted with severe headache and fever. **A,** Computed tomography scan showed diffuse subarachnoid hemorrhage (SAH) and a possible lesion in the right frontal lobe. **B,** Angiography confirmed the presence of a fusiform aneurysm of a frontal branch of the right middle cerebral artery. Surgery was performed to trap the lesion with small aneurysm clips, and **C,** the postoperative angiogram confirmed complete resection of the aneurysm. The patient made an excellent recovery after surgery and a prolonged course of antibiotics. **D,** The follow-up magnetic resonance image shows the area of abnormality. Mycotic aneurysms are usually fusiform and located on small distal vascular branches, whereas saccular aneurysms tend to be found primarily on the large vessels at the base of the brain. They constitute about 5% of cerebral aneurysms and occur primarily as a complication of subacute bacterial endocarditis (SBE). About 4% of patients with SBE present with mycotic aneurysms. Angiographic evaluation is recommended for patients with SBE and symptoms suggestive of cerebral embolic events [279]. Patients who harbor an unruptured bacterial aneurysm should be treated with high doses of the appropriate antibiotic, and the aneurysm should be followed with repeat angiography. If the aneurysm thromboses or disappears, no further treatment is necessary. If the aneurysm enlarges or remains unchanged, it should be treated surgically.

Vascular Malformations

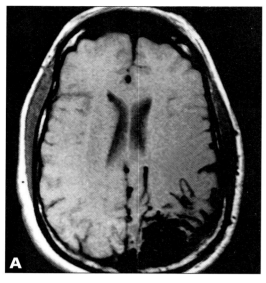

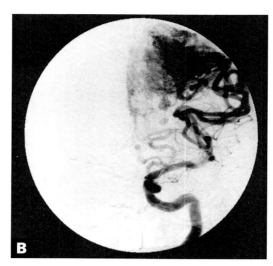

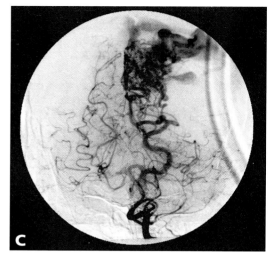

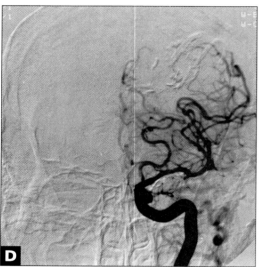

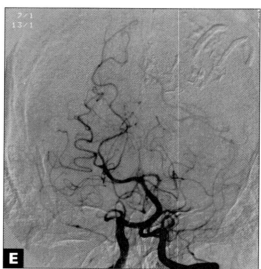

or deep. **C**, Vertebral angiogram showing a large left posterior cerebral artery feeding supply to the AVM. After preoperative partial transarterial embolization, it was possible to resect the lesion in its entirety. The patient had no neurologic deficit. **D**, Carotid angiogram showing complete resection of the AVM with no residual arterial-to-venous shunting. **E**, Anteroposterior vertebral arteriograms showing complete resection of the lesion. AVM can present with hemorrhage, seizure, or progressive neurologic deficit. The lesions typically present in patients between 20 and 50 years old. When deciding whether to treat an AVM, the risks of treatment have to be carefully weighed against the natural history of the disease. AVMs have the potential for hemorrhage at a rate of about 4% per year [280]. Other risk factors can modify the actual hemorrhage rate, however, including intranidal aneurysms, deep venous drainage, paraventricular location, and single draining vein. AVM accounts for 6% to 13% of spontaneous intracerebral hematomas [281]. They are congenital abnormalities that develop between the 4th and 8th weeks of embryonic life [282]. AVMs are located predominantly in the cerebral hemispheres (70% to 93%) and most commonly involve branches of the middle cerebral artery.

Figure 5-154. Hemispheric arteriovenous malformation. A 44-year-old man had a seizure and was found to have a large left occipitoparietal arteriovenous malformation (AVM). **A**, T1-weighted magnetic resonance image shows the typical flow voids associated with AVMs. The flow voids are low density on the T1-weighted images. The lesion can be seen extending about 4 cm into the parietal cortex. **B**, Carotid anteroposterior arteriogram showing large middle cerebral artery feeding vessels to this AVM. The lesion was drained by the superior sagittal sinus. The risk with resection of AVMs is known to be associated with the size of the lesion, the eloquence of involved brain tissue, and whether the venous drainage is superficial

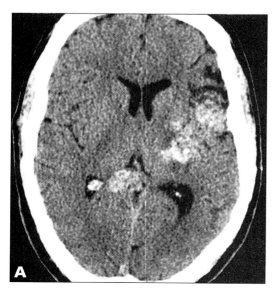

Figure 5-155. Cavernous malformations. Cavernous malformations are blood vessel malformations of the central nervous system that can occur anywhere in the cerebrum, brain stem, or spinal cord. The lesions consist of thin-walled channeled vessels that have no muscular layer and that can hypertrophy with time. With the advent of magnetic resonance imaging (MRI), diagnosis of angiographically occult lesions has led to a clearer understanding of the natural history of the disease [283,284]. These lesions most commonly present with headache, seizures, or focal neurologic deficit [283,284]. Although MRI usually shows evidence of occult bleeding, overt hemorrhage is infrequent. The actual incidence of cavernous malformation hemorrhage is not known. Several series in the literature have documented hemorrhage rates from 7.5% to 20% per year. Once the lesion hemorrhages, the potential for future hemorrhage appears to be greater. The estimated risk of clinically significant hemorrhage is 0.25% to 0.7% per person-year of exposure [283,284].

    A, Unenhanced computed tomography (CT) scan of a patient who had a significant parietal hemorrhage at the age of 1 year. By the age of 19 years, when this CT scan was obtained, he had had several more hemorrhages, rendering his contralateral arm plegic. The patient also began to have as many as eight simple partial seizures a day. Surgery is indicated in such lesions for seizure control and prevention of future bleeding. This patient had multiple lesions, as can be seen on the CT scan, with a right lesion posterior to the pulvinar on the right side.

(Continued on next page)

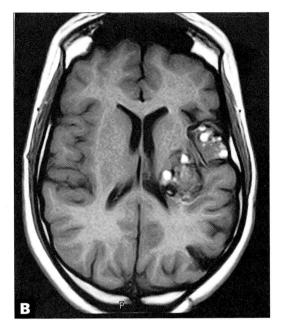 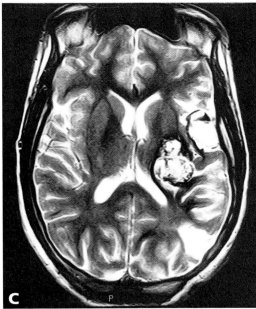 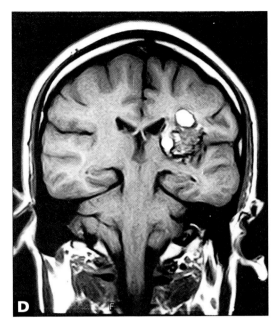

Figure 5-155. (*Continued*) **B,** The T1-weighted and **C,** T2-weighted axial MRI scans show two cavernous malformations in close association. These lesions at times can be resected from seemingly critical areas without incurring neurologic deficit. These lesions had hemorrhaged on multiple occasions, and therefore it seemed appropriate to proceed with surgical resection. **D,** Coronal T1-weighted MRI showing the typical appearance of cavernous malformation. The lesions are heterogeneous in appearance, with areas of acute and subacute hemorrhage. This lesion can be seen at the base of the sylvian fissure.

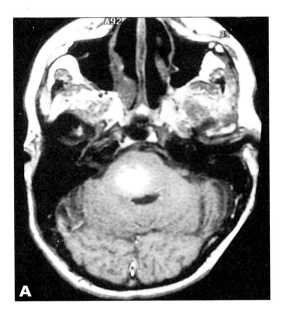 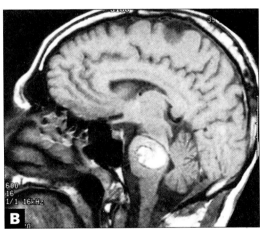 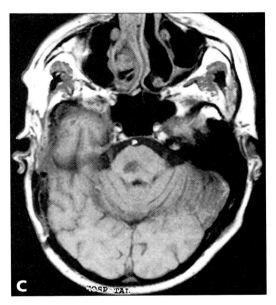

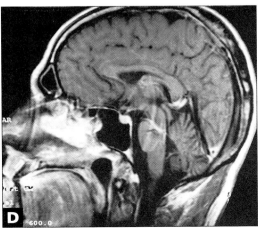

Figure 5-156. Brain stem cavernous malformation. A 32-year-old man presented after two episodes of unsteadiness of gait. **A, B,** Magnetic resonance images (MRIs) showing a large hematoma mixed with cavernous malformation of the brain stem and associated venous anomaly. Surgery was decided on, and the patient had an excellent recovery. **C, D,** Postoperative MRIs.

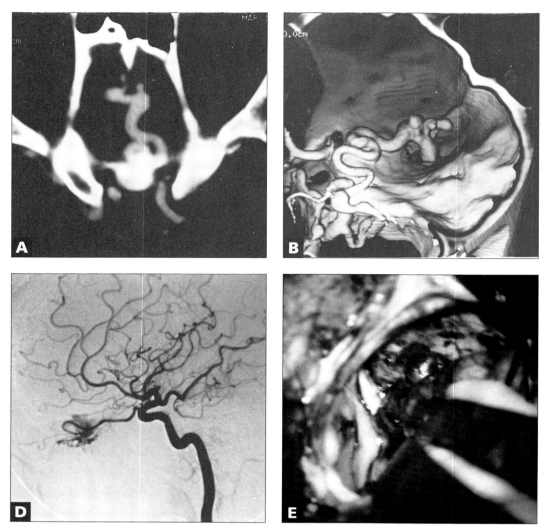
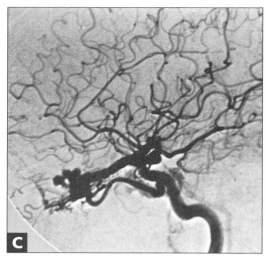

B, three-dimensional reconstruction that shows the draining vein from this ethmoidal plate dural AVM. **C**, Cerebral angiogram showing branches of the ophthalmic artery and ethmoidal artery, which feed the dural AVM. The large draining vein can be seen posteriorly. **D**, Injection of the right carotid artery that also has arterial feeders to the dura. **E**, During surgery, the large draining vein can be seen emanating from the dural base and projecting superiorly. We recommend surgical or endovascular treatment of these lesions because of the high morbidity rates associated with hemorrhage. These hemorrhages are thought to be due to the venous ectasias and aneurysms, which are prone to hemorrhage. Endovascular treatment usually involves a transarterial approach to inject glue or coils into the arterial input. Otherwise, a transvenous approach can be taken and the veins obliterated, thereby completely halting inflow and obliterating the AVM. These lesions can also cause progressive neurologic deficit owing to venous hypertension.

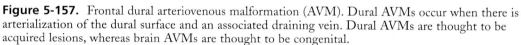

Figure 5-157. Frontal dural arteriovenous malformation (AVM). Dural AVMs occur when there is arterialization of the dural surface and an associated draining vein. Dural AVMs are thought to be acquired lesions, whereas brain AVMs are thought to be congenital.
   A, Computed tomography angiogram with contrast from a 22-year-old woman who was found to have a vascular abnormality, showing the lesion in association with the cribriform plate, and

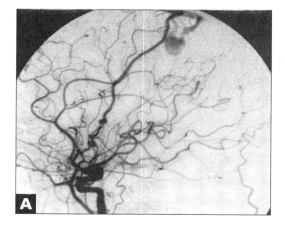
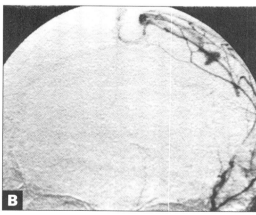
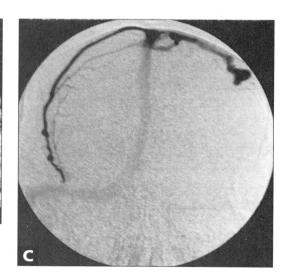

Figure 5-158. Convexity dural arteriovenous malformation. A 63-year-old woman presented with headache, and a magnetic resonance imaging study showed a flow void in the left cerebral hemisphere. **A**, Follow-up angiography shows a dural AVM with a large draining varix into the superior sagittal sinus and venous aneurysm. **B**, Left external carotid angiogram shows the fistula present on the lateral edge of the sagittal sinus. **C**, Selective injection of the left middle meningeal artery with filling to the arteriovenous shunt present on the left side of the superior sagittal sinus.

(Continued on next page)

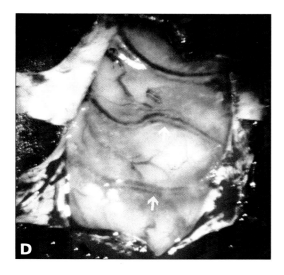
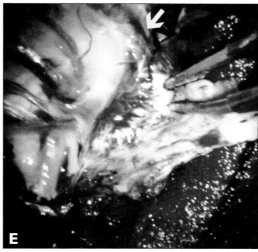

Figure 5-158. (*Continued*) **D,** Intraoperative view. There are two large arterialized veins that drain the arteriovenous fistula at the dural sinus (*arrows*) edge adjacent to the superior sagittal sinus. **E,** By elevating the dura further, it is possible to see the tiny vessels entering the dural abnormality and draining into the draining veins (*arrow*).

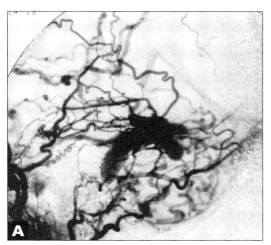
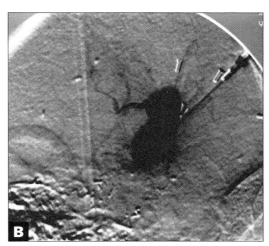

Figure 5-159. Transverse sinus dural arteriovenous malformation (AVM). A 55-year-old woman presented with progressive memory problems and ataxia. **A,** External carotid artery (ECA) angiogram shows an isolated segment of the transverse sigmoid sinus on the left side. There is venous hypertension in the transverse sinus and retrograde flow with hypertension into the parietal cortex as well as the cerebellum. **B,** Lateral angiogram shows the same approach with direct puncture of the lesion and injection of glue. **C,** Angiogram performed 1 year later with continued dural AVM of the transverse sigmoid sinus. This segment of sinus is isolated and therefore does not connect with the normal venous system. The lesion was exposed surgically, and a catheter was inserted. A number of coils were inserted through the catheter to obliterate the transverse sigmoid sinus. **D,** The lesion was obliterated in its entirety, as can be seen by the common carotid injection. The arrow shows the coils in the sinus.

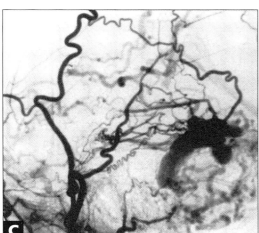
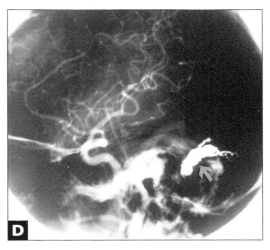

References

1. Kistler JP: Cerebrovascular Disease. In *Atherosclerosis and Coronary Artery Disease.* Edited by Fuster V, Ross R, Topol EJ. Philadelphia: Lippincott-Raven; 1996:463–474.

2. Kistler JP, Ropper AH, Martin JB: Cerebrovascular Diseases. In *Harrison's Principles of Internal Medicine,* edn 13. Edited by Isselbacher KJ, Braunwald E, Wilson JD, *et al.* New York: McGraw-Hill; 1994:2233–2256.

3. Sacco RL, Ellenberg JH, Mohr JP, *et al.*: Infarcts of undetermined cause: The NINCDS stroke data bank. *Ann Neurol* 1989, 25:382–390.

4. Fisher CM, Gore I, Okabe M, *et al.*: Atherosclerosis of the carotid and vertebral arteries: Extracranial and intracranial. *J Neuropathol Exp Neurol* 1965, 24:455–476.

5. Adams RD, Sidman RL: Cerebrovascular Diseases. In *Introduction to Neuropathology.* New York: McGraw-Hill; 1968:197.

6. Kistler JP, Buonanno FS, Gress DR: Carotid endarterectomy—specific therapy based on pathophysiology. *N Engl J Med* 1991; 325:505–507.

7. Kistler JP, Furie KL: Carotid endarterectomy revisited. *N Engl J Med* 2000, 342:1743–1745.

8. Wechsler LR, Kistler JP, Davis KR, *et al.*: The prognosis of carotid siphon stenosis. *Stroke* 1986, 17:714–718.

9. Caplan LR, Babikian C, Helgason C, *et al.*: Occlusive disease of the middle cerebral artery. *Neurology* 1985, 35:975–982.

10. Fisher CM, Karnes WE, Kubik CS: Lateral medullary infarction: the pattern of vascular occlusion. *Neuropathol Exp Neurol* 1961, 20:323–379.

11. Kubik CS, Adams RD: Occlusion of the basilar artery: a clinical and pathological study. *Brain* 1946, 69:73–121.

12. Watanabe T, Sato K, Yoshimoto T: Basilar artery occlusion caused by thrombosis of atherosclerotic fusiform aneurysm of the basilar artery. *Stroke* 1994, 25(5):1068–1070.

13. Levine RL, Turski PA, Grist TM: Basilar artery dolichoectasia: review of the literature and six patients studied with magnetic resonance angiography. *J Neuroimaging* 1995, 5(3):164–170.

14. Besson G, Bogousslavsky J, Moulin T, *et al.*: Vertebrobasilar infarcts in patients with dolichoectatic basilar artery. *Acta Neurol Scand* 1995, 91(1):37–42.

15. Kistler JP, Ojemann RG, Crowell RM: Atherothrombotic Disease of the Carotid Circulation: Pathophysiology, Evaluation and Management. In *Surgical Management of Neurovascular Disease*, edn 3. Edited by Ojemann RG, Ogilvy CS, Crowell RM, *et al.* Baltimore: Williams & Wilkins; 1995:3–24.

16. Suwanwela N, Can U, Furie K, *et al.*: Carotid Doppler ultrasound criteria for internal carotid artery stenosis based on residual lumen diameter calculated from en block carotid endarterectomy specimens. *Stroke* 1996, 27:1965–1969.

17. Can U, Furie KL, Suwanwela N, *et al.*: Transcranial Doppler ultrasound criteria for hemodynamically significant carotid artery stenosis based on residual lumen diameter calculated from en bloc endarterectomy specimens. *Stroke* (in press).

18. Furie KL, Suwanwela N, Can U, *et al.*: Magnetic resonance angiography criteria for predicting hemodynamically significant carotid artery stenosis. Work in progress.

19. Couderc R, Mahieux F, Bailleul S, *et al.*: Prevalence of apolipoprotein E phenotypes in ischemic cerebrovascular disease: a case-control study. *Stroke* 1993, 24:661–664.

20. North American Symptomatic Carotid Endarterectomy Trial Collaborators. Beneficial effect of carotid endarterectomy in symptomatic patients with high-grade carotid stenosis. *N Engl J Med* 1991, 325:445–453.

21. Barnett HJ, Taylor DW, Eliasziw M, *et al.*: Benefit of carotid endarterectomy in patients with symptomatic moderate or severe stenosis. *N Engl J Med* 1998, 339:1415–1425.

22. European Carotid Surgery Trialists' Collaborative Group. MRC European Carotid Surgery Trial: Interim results for symptomatic patients with severe (70-99%) or with mild (0-29%) carotid stenosis. *Lancet* 1991, 337:1235–1243.

23. Mayberg MR, Wilson SE, Yatsu F, *et al.*: Carotid endarterectomy and prevention of cerebral ischemia in symptomatic carotid stenosis. *JAMA* 1991, 266:3289–3294.

24. Kistler JP, Buonanno FS, Gress DR: Carotid endarterectomy: specific therapy based on pathophysiology. *N Engl J Med* 1991, 325:505–507.

25. Hobson RW II, Weiss DG, Fields WS, *et al.*: Efficacy of carotid endarterectomy for asymptomatic carotid stenosis. *N Engl J Med* 1993, 328:221–227.

26. Executive Committee for the Asymptomatic Carotid Atherosclerosis Study. Endarterectomy for symptomatic carotid stenosis. *JAMA* 1995, 273:1421–1428.

27. Eagle KA, Coley CM, Newell JB, *et al.*: Combining clinical and thallium data optimizes preoperative assessment of cardiac risk before major vascular surgery. *Ann Intern Med* 1989, 110:859–866.

28. Beebe HG, Archie JP, Baker WH, *et al.*: Concern about safety of carotid angioplasty. *Stroke* 1996, 27:197–198.

29. The Warfarin-Aspirin Recurrent Stroke Study (WARSS), The Antiphospholipid Antibodies and Stroke Study (APASS), The Patent Foramen Ovale in Cryptogenic Stroke Study (PICSS), The Hemostatic System Activation Study (HAS), The Genes in Stroke Study (GENESIS): The feasibility of a collaborative double-blind study using an anticoagulant. *Cerebrovasc Dis* 1997, 7:100–112.

30. The EC/IC Bypass Study Group. Failure of extracranial-intracranial arterial bypass to reduce the risk of ischemic stroke: results of an international randomized trial. *N Engl J Med* 1985, 313:1191–1200.

31. Mohr JP, Kase CS, Wolf PA: Lacunes in the NINCDS pilot stroke data bank [Abstract]. *Ann Neurol* 1982, 12:84.

32. Fisher CM: Lacunar stroke and infarcts: a review. *Neurology* 1982, 32:871–876.

33. Fisher CM: Capsular infarcts; the underlying vascular lesion. *Arch Neurol* 1979, 36:65–73.

34. Mohr JP: Lacunes. *Stroke* 1982, 13:3–11.

35. Fisher CM: Lacunar infarcts: a review. *Cerebrovasc Dis* 1991, 1:311–320.

36. Fisher CM: The arterial lesions underlying lacunes. *Acta Neuropathol* 1969, 12:1–15.

37. Fisher CM, Caplan LR: Basilar artery branch occlusion: a cause of pontine infarction. *Neurology* 1971, 21:900–903.

38. Pullicino PM: Pathogenesis of Lacunar Infarcts and Small Deep Infarcts. In *Advances in Neurology*. Edited by Pullicino PM, Caplan LR, Hommel M. New York: Raven Press; 1991:125–139.

39. Fisher CM: Thalamic pure sensory stroke: a pathological study. *Neurology* 1978, 28:1141–1144.

40. Fisher CM, Caplan LR: Basilar artery branch occlusion: a cause of pontine infarction. *Neurology* 1971, 21:900–905.

41. Fisher CM: Bilateral occlusion of basilar artery branches. *J Neurol Neurosurg Psychiatry* 1977, 40:1182–1189.

42. Fisher CM: Pure sensory stroke involving face, arm, and leg. *Neurology* 1965, 15:76–80.

43. Fisher CM: Pure sensory stroke and allied conditions. *Stroke* 1982, 13:434–447.

44. Orgogozo JM, Bogousslavsky J: Lacunar Syndromes. In *Handbook of Clinical Neurology*. Edited by Toole JF. New York: Elsevier Science Publishers; 1989:235–269.

45. Besson G, Hommel M: Lacunar Syndrome. In *Advances in Neurology*. vol 62. Cerebral Small Artery Disease. Edited by Pullicino PM, Caplan LR, Hommel M. New York: Raven Press; 1993:141–159.

46. Ropper AH, Fisher CM, Kleinman GM: Pyramidal infarction in the medulla: a cause of pure motor hemiplegia sparing face. *Neurology* 1979, 29:91–95.

47. Fisher CM, Cole M: Homolateral ataxia with crural paresis: a vascular syndrome. *J Neurol Neurosurg Psychiatry* 1965, 28:48–55.

48. Fisher CM: A lacunar syndrome: the dysarthria-clumsy hand syndrome. *Neurology* 1967, 17:614–617.

49. Fisher CM: Ataxic hemiparesis: a pathologic study. *Arch Neurol* 1978, 35:126–128.

50. Mohr JP, Kase CS, Meckler RJ, *et al.*: Sensorimotor stroke due to thalamocapsular ischemia. *Arch Neurol* 1977, 34:739–741.

51. Marie P: Des foyers lacunaire de desintegration et de differents aytres etats cavitaires du cerveau. *Rev Med* 1901, 21:281.

52. Mori E., Yoneda Y: Early Spontaneous Recanalization of Thromboembolic Stroke. In *Thrombolytic Therapy in Acute Ischemic Stroke*, vol 2. Edited by del Zoppo GJ, Mori E, Hacke. Berlin: Springer-Verlag, 1993:129–137.

53. Bladin PF: A radiologic and pathologic study of embolism of the internal carotid-middle cerebral arterial axis. *Radiology* 1964, 82:615–625.

54. Irino T, Yaneda M, Takaku M: Angiographic manifestations in postrecanalized cerebral infarction. *Neurology* 1977, 27:471–475.

55. Kistler JP, Ropper AH, Martin JB: Cerebrovascular Diseases. In *Harrison's Principles of Internal Medicine*, edn 13. Edited by Isselbacher KJ, Martin JB, Braunwald E, *et al.*: New York: McGraw-Hill; 1994:2233–2256.

56. Kistler JP, Ropper AH, Heros RC: Therapy of ischemic cerebral vascular disease due to atherothrombosis. *N Engl J Med* 1984, 311:27–34, 100–105.

57. Sacco RL, Ellenberg JH, Mohr JP, *et al.*: Infarcts of undetermined cause: the NINCDS Stroke Data Bank. *Ann Neurol* 1989, 25:382–390.

58. Melo TP, Bogousslavsky J, Van Melle G, *et al.*: Pure motor stroke: a reappraisal. *Neurology* 1992, 42:789–798.

59. Adams RD, Victor M: Cerebrovascular Diseases. In *Principles of Neurology*. Edited by Adams RD, Victor M. New York: McGraw-Hill; 1993:669–748.

60. Helgason CM: Anterior Choroidal Artery. In *Stroke Syndromes*. Edited by Bogousslavsky J, Caplan L. New York: Cambridge University Press; 1995:270–275.

61. Mohr JP, Steinke W, Timsit SG, *et al.*: The anterior choroidal artery does not supply the corona radiata and the lateral ventricular wall. *Stroke* 1991, 22:1502–1507.

62. Mohr JP, Gautier JC, Pessin MS: Internal Carotid Artery Disease. In *Stroke: Pathophysiology, Diagnosis and Management*, edn 2. Edited by Barnett HJM, Bennett MS, Mohr JP, *et al.*: New York: Churchill Livingstone; 1992:285–335.

63. Kistler JP: Cerebral embolism. *Compr Ther* 1996, 22(8):515–530.

64. Orsinelli DA, Pearson AC: Detection of prosthetic valve strands by transesophageal echocardiography: clinical significance in patients with suspected cardiac source of embolism. *J Am Coll Cardiol* 1995, 26:1713–1718.

65. Hacke W: Thrombolysis: Stroke Subtypes and Embolus Type. In *Thrombolytic Therapy in Acute Ischemic Stroke II*. Edited by del Zoppo GJ, Mori E, Hacke W. Berlin: Springer-Verlag; 1993:153–159.

66. Barnett HJM, Jones MW, Boughner DR, *et al.*: Cerebral ischemic events associated with prolapsing mitral valve. *Arch Neurol* 1976, 33:777–782.

67. Gilon D, Buonanno FS, Kistler JP, *et al.*: Mitral valve prolapse: Is it associated with acute ischemic neurologic events? *Circulation* 1995, 92(suppl I):1–284.

68. Marks AR, Choong CY, Chir MB, *et al.*: Identification of high-risk and low-risk subgroups of patients with mitral valve prolapse. *N Engl J Med* 1989, 320:1031–1036.

69. Nishimura RA, McGoon MD, Shu C, *et al.*: Echocardiographically documented mitral valve prolapse: long-term follow-up of 237 patients. *N Engl J Med* 1985, 313:1305–1309.

70. Finkelhor RS, Lamont WE, Ramanavarapu SK, *et al.*: Spontaneous echocardiographic contrast in the thoracic aorta: factors associated with its occurrence and its association with embolic events. *Am Heart J* 1995, 130:1254–1258.

71. Mikell FL, Asinger RW, Elsperger KJ, *et al.*: Regional stasis of blood in the dysfunctional left ventricle: echocardiographic detection and differentiation from early thrombus. *Circulation* 1982, 66:755–763.

72. Mahony C, Spain C, Spain M, *et al.*: Spontaneous contrast and intravascular platelet aggregation. *J Ultrasound Med* 1994, 13:443–450.

73. Chimowitz MI, DeGeorgia MA, Poole M, *et al.*: Left atrial spontaneous echo contrast is highly associated with previous stroke in patients with atrial fibrillation or mitral stenosis. *Stroke* 1993, 24:1015–1019.

74. Mounier-Vehier F, Leys D, Rondepierre PH, *et al.*: Silent infarcts in patients with ischemic stroke are related to age and size of the left atrium. *Stroke* 1993, 24:1347–1351.

75. Jones HR Jr, Caplan LR, Come PC, *et al.*: Cerebral emboli of paradoxical origin. *Ann Neurol* 1983, 13:314–319.

76. Lechat PH, Mas JL, Lascault G, *et al.*: Prevalence of patent foramen ovale in patients with stroke. *N Engl J Med* 1988, 318:1148–1152.

77. DiTullio MR, Sacco RL, Venketasubramanian N, *et al.*: Comparison of diagnostic techniques for the detection of a patent foramen ovale in stroke patients. *Stroke* 1993, 24:1020–1024.

78. Homma S, DiTullio MR, Sacco RL, *et al.*: Characteristics of patent foramen ovale associated with cryptogenic stroke: a biplane transesophageal echocardiographic study. *Stroke* 1994, 25:582–586.

79. DiTullio MR, Sacco RL, Gopal A, *et al.*: Patent foramen ovale as a risk factor for cryptogenic stroke. *Ann Intern Med* 1992, 117:461–465.

80. Hanna JP, Sun JP, Furlan AJ, *et al.*: Patent foramen ovale and brain infarct: echocardiographic predictors, recurrence and prevention. *Stroke* 1994, 25:782–786.

81. Cabanes L, Mas JL, Cohen A, *et al.*: Atrial septal aneurysm and patent foramen ovale as risk factors for cryptogenic stroke in patients less than 55 years of age: a study using transesophageal echocardiography. *Stroke* 1993, 24:1865–1873.

82. Kistler JP, Furie KL: Patent foramen ovale diameter and embolic stroke: a part of the puzzle? *Am J Med* 2000, 109:506–507.

83. Ranoux D, Cohen A, Cabanes L, *et al.*: Patent foramen ovale: is stroke due to paradoxical embolism? *Stroke* 1993, 24:31–34.

84. Bridges ND, Hellenbrand W, Latson L, *et al.*: Transcatheter closure of patent foramen ovale after presumed paradoxical embolism. *Circulation* 1992, 86:1902–1908.

85. Rome JJ, Keane JF, Perry SB, *et al.*: Double-umbrella closure of atrial defects: initial clinical applications. *Circulation* 1990, 82:751–758.

86. Falk RH: A plea for a clinical trial of anticoagulation in dilated cardiomyopathy. *Am J Cardiol* 1990, 65:914–915.

87. Fuster V, Gersh BJ, Giuliani ER, *et al.*: The natural history of idiopathic dilated cardiomyopathy. *Am J Cardiol* 1981, 47:525–530.

88. Roberts WC, Siegel RJ, McManus BM: Idiopathic dilated cardiomyopathy: analysis of 152 necropsy patients. *Am J Cardiol* 1987, 60:1340–1355.

89. Cheng JWM, Spinler SA: Should all patients with dilated cardiomyopathy receive chronic anticoagulation? *Ann Pharmacother* 1994, 28:604–609.

90. Laupacis A, Albers G, Dunn M, *et al.*: Antithrombotic therapy in atrial fibrillation. *Chest* 1992, 102(suppl 4):S426–S433.

91. Lopez JA, Ross RS, Fishbein MC, *et al.*: Nonbacterial thrombotic endocarditis: a review. *Am Heart J* 1987, 113:773–784.

92. Biller J, Challa VR, Toole JF, *et al.*: Nonbacterial thrombotic endocarditis a neurologic perspective of clinicopathologic correlations of 99 patients. *Arch Neurol* 1982, 39:95–98.

93. Kooiker JC, MacLean JM, Sumi SM: Cerebral embolism, marantic endocarditis, and cancer. *Arch Neurol* 1976, 33:260–264.

94. Lehto VP, Stenman S, Somer T: Immunohistochemical studies on valvular vegetations in nonbacterial thrombotic endocarditis (NBTE). *Acta Pathol Microbiol Immunol Scand (A)* 1982, 90:207–211.

95. Meltzer RS, Visser CA, Fuster V: Intracardiac thrombi and systemic embolization. *Ann Intern Med* 1986, 104:689–698.

96. Chesebro JL, Fuster V: Antithrombotic therapy for acute myocardial infarction: mechanisms and prevention of deep venous, left ventricular, and coronary artery thromboembolism. *Circulation* 1986, 74(suppl III):1–10.

97. Halperin JL, Fuster V: Left ventricular thrombus and stroke after myocardial infarction: toward prevention or perplexity? *J Am Coll Cardiol* 1989, 14:912–914.

98. Smith P, Arnesen H, Holme I: The effect of warfarin on mortality and reinfarction after myocardial infarction. *N Engl J Med* 1990, 323:147–152.

99. Kupper AJF, Verheugt FWA, Peels CH, *et al.*: Left ventricular thrombus incidence and behavior studied by serial two-dimensional echocardiography in acute anterior myocardial infarction: left ventricular wall motion, systemic embolism and oral anticoagulation. *J Am Coll Cardiol* 1989, 13:1514–1520.

100. Tramarin R, Pozzoli M, Febo O, *et al.*: Two-dimensional echocardiographic assessment of anticoagulant therapy in left ventricular thrombosis early after acute myocardial infarction. *Eur Heart J* 1986, 7:482–492.

101. Cregler LL: Antithrombotic therapy in left ventricular thrombosis and systemic embolism. *Am Heart J* 1992, 123:1110–1114.

102. Hess DC, D'Cruz IA, Adams RJ, *et al.*: Coronary Artery Disease, Myocardial Infarction, and Brain Embolism. In *Neurologic Clinics: Neurocardiology*, vol 11. Edited by Brillman J. Philadelphia: WB Saunders; 1993:399–417.

103. Case Records of the Massachussetts General Hospital weekly clinico-pathological exercises. Case 451970. *N Engl J Med* 1970, 283:982–990.

104. Fourth ACCP Consensus Conference on Antithrombotic Therapy. Edited by Dalen JE, Hirsh J. *Chest* 1995, 108(suppl 4):225S–522S.

105. Szekely P: Systemic embolism and anticoagulant prophylaxis in rheumatic heart disease. *Br Med J* 1964, 1:1209–1212.

106. Becker RC, Ansell J: Antithrombotic therapy: an abbreviated reference for clinicians. *Arch Intern Med* 1995, 155:149–161.

107. Wolf PA, Abbott RD, Kannel WB: Atrial fibrillation: a major contributor to stroke in the elderly. The Framingham study. *Arch Intern Med* 1987, 147:1561–1564.

108. Wolf PA, Abbott RD, Kannel WB: Atrial fibrillation as an independent risk factor for stroke: the Framingham study. *Stroke* 1991, 22:983–988.

109. Petersen P, Godtfredsen J, Boysen G, *et al.*: Placebo-controlled, randomized trial of warfarin and aspirin for prevention of thromboembolic complications in chronic atrial fibrillation: the Copenhagen AFASAK study. *Lancet* 1989, 1:175–179.

110. Stroke Prevention in Atrial Fibrillation Investigators: stroke prevention in atrial fibrillation study: final results. *Circulation* 1991, 89:527–539.

111. Boston Area Anticoagulation Trial for Atrial Fibrillation Investigators: The effect of low dose warfarin on the risk of stroke in patients with nonrheumatic atrial fibrillation. *N Engl J Med* 1990, 323:1505–1511.

112. CAFA Study Investigators: Canadian atrial fibrillation (CAFA) study. *J Am Coll Cardiol* 1991, 18:349–355.

113. Ezekowitz MD, Bridgers SL, James KE, *et al.*: Warfarin in the prevention of stroke associated with nonrheumatic atrial fibrillation. *N Engl J Med* 1992, 327:1406–1412.

114. Laupacis A, Boysen G, Connolly S, *et al.*: Atrial fibrillation: risk factors for embolization and efficacy of anti-thrombotic therapy. *Arch Intern Med* 1994, 154:1449–1457.

115. Turpie AGG, Gunstensen J, Hirsh J, *et al.*: Randomized comparison of two intensities of oral anticoagulant therapy after tissue heart valve replacement. *Lancet* 1988, 1:1242–1245.

116. Fourth ACCP Consensus Conference on Antithrombotic Therapy. Edited by Dalen JE, Hirsh J. *Chest* 1995, 108(suppl 4):225S–522S.

117. Becker RC, Ansell J: Antithrombotic therapy: an abbreviated reference for clinicians. *Arch Intern Med* 1995, 155:149–161.

118. Kistler JP, Singer DA, Millenson MM, *et al.*, for the BAATAF investigators: Effect of low intensity warfarin anticoagulation on level of activity of the hemostatic system in patients with atrial fibrillation. *Stroke* 1993, 24:1360–1365.

119. Rosenberg RD, Aird WC: Vascular-bed–specific hemostasis and hypercoagulable states. *N Engl J Med* 1999, 340:1555–1564.

120. Kistler JP, Bauer KA: The Level of Activity of the Hemostatic System, the Rate of Embolic Stroke, and Age: Is There a Correlation? In *Cerebrovascular Diseases*. Edited by Moskowitz MA, Caplan LR. Boston: Butterworth-Heinemann; 1995:437–442.

121. Pruitt AA, Rubin RH, Karchmer AW, *et al.*: Neurologic complications of bacterial endocarditis. *Medicine* (Baltimore) 1978, 57:329–343.

122. Salgado AV, Furlan AJ, Keys TF, *et al.*: Neurologic complications of endocarditis: a 12-year experience. *Neurology* 1989, 39:173–178.

123. Francioli P: Central Nervous System Complications of Infective Endocarditis. In *Infections of the Central Nervous System*. Edited by Scheld WM, Whitley RJ, Durack DJ. New York: Raven Press; 1991:515–559.

124. Roeltgen DP, Syna DR: Neurologic Complications of Cardiac Tumors. In *Handbook of Clinical Neurology*, vol 19. Edited by Goetz CG, Tanner CM, Aminoff MJ. Amsterdam: Elsevier Science Publishers; 1993:93–109.

125. Peters MN, Hall RJ, Cooley DA, *et al.*: The clinical syndrome of atrial myxoma. *JAMA* 1974, 230:695–700.

126. Wold LE, Lie JT: Atrial myxomas: a clinicopathological profile. *Am J Pathol* 1980, 101:219–240.

127. Thompson J, Kapoor W, Wechsler LR: Multiple strokes due to atrial myxoma with a negative echocardiogram. *Stroke* 1988, 19:1570–1571.

128. Knepper LE, Biller J, Adams HP Jr, Bruno A: Neurologic manifestations of atrial myxoma: a 12 year experience and review. *Stroke* 1988, 19:1435–1440.

129. Reynen K: Cardiac myxomas. *N Engl J Med* 1995, 333:1610–1617.

130. Amarenco P, Cohen A, Baudrimont M, *et al.*: Transesophageal echocardiographic detection of aortic arch disease in patients with cerebral infarction. *Stroke* 1992, 23:1005–1009.

131. Amarenco P, Duyckaerts C, Tzourio C, *et al.*: The prevalence of ulcerated plaques in the aortic arch in patients with stroke. *N Engl J Med* 1992, 326:221–225.

132. Amarenco P, Cohen A, Tzourio C, *et al.*: Atherosclerotic disease of the aortic arch and the risk of ischemic stroke. *N Engl J Med* 1994, 331:1474–1479.

133. Khatibzadeh M, Mitusch R, Stierle U, *et al.*: Aortic atherosclerotic plaques as a source of systemic embolism. *J Am Coll Cardiol* 1996, 27:664–669.

134. Kistler JP: The risk of embolic stroke another piece of the puzzle. *N Engl J Med* 1994, 331:1517–1519.

135. French Study of Aortic Plaques in Stroke Group: Atherosclerotic disease of the aortic arch as a risk factor for recurrent ischemic stroke. *N Engl J Med* 1996, 334:1216–1221.

136. Moore PM, Cupps TR: Neurological complications of vasculitis. *Ann Neurol* 1983, 14:155–167.

137. Fauci AS, Haynes BF, Katz P: The spectrum of vasculitis. *Ann Intern Med* 1978, 89:660–676.

138. Kurent JE, Moore PM: Vasculitis of the Nervous System. In *Systemic Vasculitis, the Biological Basis*. Edited by LeRoy EC. New York: Marcel Dekker; 1992:451–482.

139. Biller J, Sparks LH: Diagnosis and Management of Cerebral Vasculitis. In *Handbook of Cerebrovascular Diseases*. Edited by Adams HP. New York: Marcel Dekker; 1993:549–568.

140. Giang D: Central nervous system vasculitis secondary to infections, toxins, and neoplasms. *Semin Neurol* 1994, 14:313–319.

141. Suwanwela C, Suwanwela N, Charuchinda S, *et al.*: Intracranial mycotic aneurysm of extravascular origin. *J Neurosurg* 1972, 36:552–559.

142. Reshef E, Greenberg SE, Jancovic J: Herpes zoster ophthalmicus followed by contralateral hemiparesis: report of two cases and review of literature. *J Neurol Neurosurg Psychiatry* 1985, 48:122–127.

143. Brown MM, Swash M: Polyarteritis Nodosa and Other Systemic Vasculitides. In *Handbook of Clinical Neurology*, vol 11, no. 5. Edited by Toole JF. Amsterdam: Elsevier Science Publishers; 1989:353–367.

144. Kissel JT: Neurologic manifestations of vasculitis. *Neurol Clin* 1989, 7:655–673.

145. Ferris EJ, Levine HL: Cerebral arteritis. *Radiology* 1972, 109:327–341.

146. Moore PM, Calabrese LH: Neurologic manifestations of systemic vasculitides. *Semin Neurol* 1994, 14:300–306.

147. Jennette JC, Falk RJ, Milling DM: Pathogenesis of vasculitis. *Semin Neurol* 1994, 14:291–299.

148. Tunkel AR, Scheld WM: Bacterial meningitis: Pathogenic and Pathophysiologic Mechanisms. In *Infections of the Central Nervous System*. Edited by Lambert HP. Philadelphia: BC Decker; 1991:1–15.

149. Igarashi M, Gilmartin RC, Gerald B, *et al.*: Cerebral arteritis and bacterial meningitis. *Arch Neurol* 1984, 41:531–535.

150. Simon RP: Neurosyphilis. *Arch Neurol* 1985, 42:606–613.

151. Case record of Massachusetts General Hospital. *N Engl J Med* 1991, 325:414–422.

152. Teoh R, Humphries M: *Tuberculous Meningitis*. In *Infections of the Central Nervous System*. Edited by Lambert HP. Philadelphia: BC Decker; 1991:189–206.

153. Hsieh E, Chia L, Shen W: Location of cerebral infarctions in tuberculous meningitis. *Neuroradiology* 1992, 34:197–199.

154. Saravia-Gomez J: Aspergillosis of the Central Nervous System. In *Handbook of Clinical Neurology*. Part III. Infection of the Nervous System. Edited by Vinken PJ, Bruyn GW. Amsterdam: North-Holland; 1978:531–539.

155. Walsh TJ, Hier DB, Caplan LR: Aspergillosis of the central nervous system: clinicopathological analysis of 17 patients. *Ann Neurol* 1985, 18:574–582.

156. Cook GC: Protozoan and Helminthic Infections. In *Infections of the Central Nervous System*. Edited by Kass EH, Weller TH, Wolff SM, *et al.* Philadelphia: BC Decker; 1991:264–282.

157. Del Brutto OH, Sotelo J: Neurocysticercosis: an update. *Rev Infectious Dis* 1988, 10:1075–1087.

158. Suwanwela N, Piyachon C: Takayasu arteritis in Thailand: clinical and imaging features. *Int J Cardiol* (in press).

159. Matsubara O, Yoshimura N, Tamura A, *et al.*: Heart Vessels 1992, 7(suppl):18–25.

160. Caselli RHJ, Hunder GG, Whisnant JP: Neurologic disease in biopsy-proven giant cell arteritis. *Neurology* 1988, 38:352–359.

161. Hunder GG, Lie JT, Goronzy JJ, *et al.*: Pathogenesis of giant cell arteritis. *Arthritis Rheum* 1993, 36:757–761.

162. Turnbull J: Temporal arteritis and polymyalgia rheumatica: nosographic and nosologic considerations. *Neurology* 1996, 46:901–906.

163. Kansa T, Corbett JJ, Savino P, *et al.*: Giant cell arteritis with normal sedimentation rate. *Arch Neurol* 1977, 34:624–625.

164. Procter CD, Hollier LH, Trosclair CM: Temporal arteritis, clinical implications for the vascular surgeon. *J Cardiovasc Surg* 1992, 33:599–603.

165. Case record of Massachusetts General Hospital. *N Engl J Med* 1986, 315:631–639.

166. Vollmer TL, Guanaccia J, Harrington W, *et al.*: Idiopathic granulomatous angiitis of the central nervous system: diagnostic challenges. *Arch Neurol* 1993, 50:925–930.

167. Alhalabi M, Moore PM: Serial angiography in isolated angiitis of the central nervous system. *Neurology* 1994, 44:1221–1226.

168. Hurst RW, Grossman RI: Neuroradiology of central nervous system vasculitis. *Semin Neurol* 1994, 14:320–340.

169. Case record of Massachusetts General Hospital. *N Engl J Med* 1989, 320:514–524.

170. Brown E, Prager J, Lee H, *et al.*: CNS complications of cocaine abuse: prevalence, pathophysiology and neuroradiology. *AJR* 1992, 159:137–147.

171. Daras M, Tuchman AJ, Koppel BS, *et al.*: Neurovascular complications of cocaine. *Acta Neurol Scand* 1994, 90:124–129.

172. Sturzenegger M, Huber P: Cranial nerve palsies in spontaneous carotid artery dissection. *J Neurol Neurosurg Psychiatry* 1993, 56(11):1191–1199.

173. Mas J-L, Henin D, Bousser MG, *et al.*: Dissecting aneurysm of the vertebral artery and cervical manipulation: a case report with autopsy. *Neurology* 1989, 39:512–515.

174. Fisher CM: The headache and pain of spontaneous carotid dissection. *Headache* 1982, 22(2):60–65.

175. Selky AK, Pascuzzi R: Reader's paratrigeminal syndrome due to spontaneous dissection of the cervical and petrous internal carotid artery. *Headache* 1995, 35(7):423–424.

176. Mokri B, Sundt TM, Houser OW, *et al.*: Spontaneous dissection of the cervical internal carotid artery. *Ann Neurol* 1986, 19:126–138.

177. Sturzenegger M, Mattle HP, Rivoir A, *et al.*: Ultrasound findings in carotid artery dissection: analysis of 43 patients. *Neurology* 1995, 45(4):691–698.

178. Nguyen Bui L, Brant-Zawadzki M, Verghese P, *et al.*: Magnetic resonance angiography of cervicocranial dissection. *Stroke* 1993, 24(10):126–131.

179. Frisoni GB, Anzola GP: Vertebrobasilar ischemia after neck motion. *Stroke* 1991, 22:1452–1460.

180. Frumkin LR, Baloh RW: Wallenberg's syndrome following neck manipulation. *Neurology* 1990, 40:1990:611–615.

181. Sherman DG, Hart RG, Easton JD: Abrupt change in head position and cerebral infarction. *Stroke* 1981, 12:2–6.

182. Saver JL, Easton JD, Hart RG: Dissections and Trauma of Cervicocerebral Arteries. In *Stroke: Pathophysiology, Diagnosis and Management*, edn 2. Edited by Barnett HJM, Bennett MS, Mohr JP, *et al*. New York: Churchill Livingstone; 1992:671–688.

183. Caplan LR, Baquis GD, Pessin MS, *et al.*: Dissection of the intracranial vertebral artery. *Neurology* 1988, 38:868–877.

184. Barnett HJM: Progress towards stroke prevention. Robert Wartenberg Lecture. *Neurology* 1980, 30:1212–1225.

185. Hinse P, Thie A, Lachenmayer L: Dissection of the extracranial vertebral artery: Report of four cases and review of the literature. *J Neurol Neurosurg Psychiatry* 1991, 54:863–869.

186. Adams HP, Kappelle LJ, Biller J, *et al.*: Ischemic stroke in young adults. *Arch Neurol* 1995, 52:491–495.

187. Bovill EG, Bauer KA, Dickerman JD, *et al.*: The clinical spectrum of heterozygous protein C deficiency in a large New England kindred. *Blood* 1989, 73:712–717.

188. Miletich J, Sherman L, Broze G: Absence of thrombosis in patients with heterozygous protein C deficiency. *N Engl J Med* 1987, 317:991–996.

189. Bauer KA, Broekmans AW, Bertina RM, *et al.*: Hemostatic enzyme generation in the blood of patients with hereditary protein C deficiency. *Blood* 1988, 71:1418–1426.

190. Kosik KS, Furie B: Thrombotic stroke associated with elevated plasma factor VIII. *Ann Neurol* 1980, 8:435–437.

191. Brott T, Stump D: Overview of hemostasis and thrombosis. *Semin Neurol* 1991, 11:305–313.

192. Pavlakis SG, Bello J, Prohovnik I, et al.: Brain infarction in sickle cell anemia: magnetic resonance imaging correlates. *Ann Neurol* 1988, 23:125–130.

193. Rothman SM, Fulling KH, Nelson JS: Sickle cell anemia and central nervous system infarction: a neuropathological study. *Ann Neurol* 1986, 20:684–690.

194. Levine SR, Brey RL: Antiphospholipid antibodies and ischemic cerebrovascular disease. *Semin Neurol* 1991, 11:329–338.

195. Graus F, Rogers LR, Posner JB: Cerebrovascular complications in patients with cancer. *Medicine* 1985, 64:16–35.

196. Chaturvedi S, Ansell J, Recht L: Should cerebral ischemic events in cancer patients be considered a manifestation of hypercoagulability? *Stroke* 1994, 25:1215–1218.

197. Sun NC, McAfee WM, Hum GJ, *et al.*: Hemostatic abnormalities in malignancy: a prospective study of one hundred eight patients. *Am J Clin Pathol* 1979, 71:10–16.

198. Rickles FR, Edwards RL: Activation of blood coagulation in patients with cancer. Fibrinopeptide A generation and tumor growth. *Cancer* 1983, 51:301–307.

199. Mandel H, Brenner B, Berant M, *et al.*: Coexistence of hereditary homocystinuria and factor V Leiden: effect on thrombosis. *N Engl J Med* 1996, 334:763–768.

200. Hacke W, Zeumer H, Ferbert A, *et al.*: Intra-arterial thrombolytic therapy improves outcome in patients with acute vertebrobasilar occlusive disease. *Stroke* 1988, 19:1216–1222.

201. National Institute of Neurological Disorders and Stroke rt-PA Stroke Study Group: Tissue plasminogen activator for acute ischemic stroke. *N Engl J Med* 1995, 333:1581–1587.

202. Thomas DJ, du Boulay GH, Marshall J, *et al.*: Effect of haematocrit on cerebral blood flow in men. *Lancet* 1977, 2:941–943.

203. Kay R, Wong KS, Yu YL, *et al.*: Low molecular weight heparin for the treatment of acute ischemic stroke. *N Engl J Med* 1995, 333:1588–1593.

204. European Cooperative Acute Stroke Study: Intravenous thrombolysis with recombinant tissue plasminogen activator for acute hemispheric stroke. *JAMA* 1995, 274:1017–1025.

205. del Zoppo GJ, Poeck K, Pessin MS, *et al.*: Recombinant tissue plasminogen activator in acute thrombotic and embolic stroke. *Ann Neurol* 1992, 32:78–86.

206. Stallones RA, Dyken ML, Fang HCH, *et al.*: Epidemiology for stroke facilities planning. *Stroke* 1972, 3:360–371.

207. Jeffery DR, Good DC: Rehabilitation of the stroke patient. *Curr Opin Neurol* 1995, 8:62–68.

208. Duncan PW, Goldstein LB, Matchar D, *et al.*: Measurement of motor recovery after stroke. *Stroke* 1992, 23:1084–1089.

209. Nakayama H, Jørgensen HS, Raaschou HO, *et al.*: Recovery of upper extremity function in stroke patients: the Copenhagen stroke study. *Arch Phys Med Rehabil* 1994, 75:394–398.

210. Twitchell TE: Restoration of motor function following hemiplegia in man. *Brain* 1951, 74:443–480.

211. Weiller C, Ramsay SC, Wise RJS, *et al.*: Individual patterns of functional reorganization in the human cerebral cortex after capsular infarction. *Ann Neurol* 1993, 33:181–189.

212. Jones TA, Schallert T: Use-dependent growth of pyramidal neurons after neocortical damage. *J Neurosci* 1994, 14:2140–2152.

213. Feeney DM, Gonzalez A, Law WA: Amphetamine, haloperidol, and experience interact to affect rate of recovery after motor cortex injury. *Science* 1982, 217:855–857.

214. Goldstein LB: Common drugs may influence motor recovery after stroke: The Sygen In Acute Stroke Study Investigators. *Neurology* 1995, 45:865–871.

215. Crisostomo EA, Duncan PW, Propst M, *et al.*: Evidence that amphetamine with physical therapy promotes recovery of motor function in stroke patients. *Ann Neurol* 1988, 23:94–97.

216. Walker-Batson D, Smith P, Curtis S, *et al.*: Amphetamine paired with physical therapy accelerates motor recovery after stroke. *Stroke* 1995, 26:2254–2259.

217. Ojeman R, Mohr J: Hypertensive brain hemorrhage. *Clin Neurosurg* 1975, 23:220.

218. Mohr J, Caplan L, Melski J, *et al.*: The Harvard Cooperative Stroke Registry: a prospective registry. *Neurology* 1978, 28:754–762.

219. Fisher C: Pathological observations in hypertensive cerebral hemorrhage. *J Neuropathol Exp Neurol* 1971, 30:536–550.

220. Freytag E: Fatal hypertensive intracerebral hematomas: a survey of the pathological anatomy in 393 cases. *J Neurol Neurosurg Psychiatry* 1968, 31:616–620.

221. Ojeman R, Mohr J: Hypertensive brain hemorrhage. *Clin Neurosurg* 1975, 23:220–244.

222. Ojeman R, Heros R: Spontaneous brain hemorrhage. *Stroke* 1983, 14:468–475.

223. Fisher C, Picard E, Polak A, *et al.*: Acute hypertensive cerebellar hemorrhage: diagnosis and surgical treatment. *J Nerv Ment Dis* 1965, 140:38–45.

224. Kase CS: Cerebral Amyloid Angiopathy. In *Intracerebral Hemorrhage*. Edited by Kase CS, Caplan LR. Boston: Butterworth-Heinemann; 1994:179–200.

225. Vinters HV: Cerebral amyloid angiopathy: a critical review. *Stroke* 1987, 18:311–324.

226. Yankner BA, Dawes LR, Fisher S, *et al.*: Neurotoxicity of a fragment of the amyloid precursor associated with Alzheimer's disease. *Science* 1989, 245:417–420.

227. Mandybur TI: Cerebral amyloid angiopathy: the vascular pathology and complications. *J Neuropathol Exp Neurol* 1986, 45:79–90.

228. Vonsattel JP, Myers RH, Hedley-Whyte ET, *et al.*: Cerebral amyloid angiopathy without and with cerebral hemorrhages: a comparative histological study. *Ann Neurol* 1991, 30:637–649.

229. Maeda A, Yamada M, Itoh Y, *et al.*: Computer-assisted three-dimensional image analysis of cerebral amyloid angiopathy. *Stroke* 1993, 24:1857–1864.

230. Roher AE, Lowenson JD, Clarke S, *et al.*: β-Amyloid-(1-42) is a major component of cerebrovascular amyloid deposits: implications for the pathology of Alzheimer disease. *Proc Natl Acad Sci USA* 1993, 90:10836–10840.

231. Gravina SA, Ho LB, Eckman CB, *et al.*: Amyloid β protein (a-β) in Alzheimer's disease brain: biochemical and immunocytochemical analysis with antibodies specific for forms ending at a-β-40 or a-β-42(43). *J Biol Chem* 1995, 270:7013–7016.

232. Suzuki N, Cheung TT, Cai XD, *et al.*: An increased percentage of long amyloid β protein secreted by familial amyloid β protein precursor (β APP717) mutants. *Science* 1994, 264:1336–1340.

233. Greene GM, Godersky JC, Biller J, *et al.*: Surgical experience with cerebral amyloid angiopathy. *Stroke* 1990, 21:1545–1549.

234. Matkovic Z, Davis S, Gonzales M, *et al.*: Surgical risk of hemorrhage in cerebral amyloid angiopathy. *Stroke* 1991, 22:456–461.

235. Izumihara A, Ishihara T, Iwamoto N, Ito H: Postoperative outcome of 37 patients with lobar intracerebral hemorrhage related to cerebral amyloid angiopathy. *Stroke* 1999, 30:29–33.

236. Greenberg SM, Vonsattel JP: Diagnosis of cerebral amyloid angiopathy. Sensitivity and specificity of cortical biopsy. *Stroke* 1997, 28:1418–1422.

237. Rosand J, Hylek EM, O'Donnell HC, Greenberg SM: Warfarin-associated hemorrhage and cerebral amyloid angiopathy. A genetic and pathological study. *Neurology* 2000, 55:947–955.

238. Knudsen KA, Rosand J, Karluk D, Greenberg SM: Clinical diagnosis of cerebral amyloid angiopathy. Validation of the Boston criteria [abstract]. *Neurology* 2000, 54:A467.

239. Greenberg SM, Finklestein SP, Schaefer PW: Petechial hemorrhages accompanying lobar hemorrhages: Detection by gradient-echo MRI. *Neurology* 1996, 46:1751–1754.

240. Caplan LR: Binswanger's disease—revisited. *Neurology* 1995, 45:626–633.

241. Greenberg SM, Vonsattel JP, Stakes JW, *et al.*: The clinical spectrum of cerebral amyloid angiopathy: Presentations without lobar hemorrhage. *Neurology* 1993, 43:2073–2079.

242. Greenberg SM, Rebeck GW, Vonsattel JPV, *et al.*: Apolipoprotein E e4 and cerebral hemorrhage associated with amyloid angiopathy. *Ann Neurol* 1995, 38:254–259.

243. Premkumar DR, Cohen DL, Hedera P, *et al.*: Apolipoprotein E-ε4 alleles in cerebral amyloid angiopathy and cerebrovascular pathology associated with Alzheimer's disease. *Am J Pathol* 1996, 148:2083–2095.

244. Nicoll JA, Burnett C, Love S, *et al.*: High frequency of apolipoprotein E ε2 allele in hemorrhage due to cerebral amyloid angiopathy. *Ann Neurol* 1997, 41:716–721.

245. Greenberg SM, Vonsattel JP, Segal AZ, *et al.*: Association of apolipoprotein E ε2 and vasculopathy in cerebral amyloid angiopathy. *Neurology* 1998, 50:961–965.

246. Levy E, Carman MD, Fernandez Madrid IJ, *et al.*: Mutation of the Alzheimer's disease amyloid gene in hereditary cerebral hemorrhage, Dutch type. *Science* 1990, 248:1124–1126.

247. Van Broeckhoven C, Haan J, Bakker E, *et al.*: Amyloid β protein precursor gene and hereditary cerebral hemorrhage with amyloidosis (Dutch). *Science* 1990, 248:1120–1122.

248. Hendriks L, van Duijn CM, Cras P, *et al.*: Presenile dementia and cerebral haemorrhage linked to a mutation at codon 692 of the β-amyloid precursor protein gene. *Nat Genet* 1992, 1:218–221.

249. Cho HS, Grabowski TJ, Rebeck GW, Greenberg SM: APP mutation at a novel site. The Iowa Mutation (D694N) associated with cognitive decline and severe cerebral amyloid angiopathy. *Soc Neurosci Abs* 2000, in press.

250. Palsdottir A, Abrahamson M, Thorsteinsson L, *et al.*: Mutation in cystatin C gene causes hereditary brain hemorrhage. *Lancet* 1988, 2:603–604.

251. Levy E, Lobez-Otin C, Ghiso J, *et al.*: Stroke in Icelandic patients with hereditary amyloid angiopathy is related to a mutation in the cystatin C gene, an inhibitor of cysteine proteases. *J Exp Med* 1989, 169:1771–1778.

252. Graffagnino C, Herbstreith MH, Roses AD, Alberts MJ: A molecular genetic study of intracerebral hemorrhage. *Arch Neurol* 1994, 51:981–984.

253. Anders KH, Wang ZZ, Kornfeld M, *et al.*: Giant cell arteritis in association with cerebral amyloid angiopathy: immunohistochemical and molecular studies. *Hum Pathol* 1997, 28:1237–1246.

254. Itoh Y, Yamada M: Cerebral amyloid angiopathy in the elderly: the clinicopathological features, pathogenesis, and risk factors. *J Med Dent Sci* 1997, 44:11–19.

255. Nagai A, Kobayashi S, Shimode K, *et al.*: No mutations in cystatin C gene in cerebral amyloid angiopathy with cystatin C deposition. *Mol Chem Neuropathol* 1998, 33:63–78.

256. McCarron MO, Nicoll JA, Stewart J, *et al.*: Absence of cystatin C mutation in sporadic cerebral amyloid angiopathy-related hemorrhage. *Neurology* 2000, 54:242–244.

257. O'Donnell HC, Rosand J, Knudsen KA, *et al.*: Apolipoprotein E genotype and the risk of recurrent lobar intracerebral hemorrhage. *N Engl J Med* 2000, 342:240–245.

258. Hunt W, Hess R: Surgical risk as related to time of intervention in the repair of intracranial aneurysms. *J Neurosurg* 1968, 28:14–20.

259. Wirth F: Surgical Treatment of Incidental Intracranial Aneurysms. In *Clinical Neurosurgery*. Edited by Wirth F. Baltimore: Williams & Wilkins; 1985.

260. Garaway W, Whinant J, Drury I: The continuing decline in the incidence of stroke. *Mayo Clin Proc* 1983, 58:520–523.

261. Weir B: Intracranial Aneurysms and Subarachnoid Hemorrhage. In *Neurosurgery*. Edited by Wilkins RH, Rengachray SS. New York: McGraw-Hill; 1985:1308–1329.

262. Haley E, Kassell N, Torner J, *et al.*: Early versus delayed surgery for ruptured aneurysm [Abstract]. *Stroke* 1992, 23:30.

263. Adams HJ, Kassel N, Torner J, *et al.*: Early management of aneurysmal subarachnoid hemorrhage: a report from the Cooperative Aneurysm Study. *J Neurosurg* 1981, 54:141–145.

264. Bailes J, Spetzler R, Hadley M, *et al.*: Management morbidity and mortality of poor grade aneurysm patients. *J Neurosurg* 1990, 72:559–566.

265. Jane J, Kassell N, Torner J, *et al.*: The natural history of aneurysms and arteriovenous malformations. *J Neurosurg* 1985, 62:321–323.

266. Dell S: A symptomatic cerebral aneurysm: assessment of its risk of rupture. *Neurosurgery* 1982, 10:162–166.

267. Black P: Hydrocephalus and vasospasm after subarachnoid hemorrhage from ruptured intracranial aneurysm. *Neurosurgery* 1986, 18:12–16.

268. Kusske J, Turner P, Ojemann G: Ventriculostomy for the treatment of acute hydrocephalus following subarachnoid hemorrhage. *J Neurosurg* 1973, 38:591–595.

269. Fisher C, Kistler J, Davis J: Relation of cerebral vasospasm to subarachnoid hemorrhage visualized by computerized tomographic scanning. *Neurosurgery* 1980, 6:1–9.

270. Kaku Y, Yonekawa Y, Tsukabara T, *et al.*: Supraselective intraarterial infusion of papaverine for the treatment of cerebral vasospasm after subarachnoid hemorrhage. *J Neurosurg* 1992, 77:847–848.

271. Marks M, Steinberg G, Lane B: Intraarterial papaverine for the treatment of vasospasm. *Am J Neuroradiol* 1993, 14:822–826.

272. Newell D, Winn H: Transcranial Doppler in cerebral vasospasm. *Neurosurg Clin North Am* 1990, 1:319–328.

273. Sundt T, Whisnant J: Subarachnoid hemorrhage from intracranial aneurysms. *N Engl J Med* 1978, 299:116–122.

274. Fisher C, Roberson G, Ojeman R: Cerebral vasospasm with ruptured saccular aneurysm: the clinical manifestations. *Neurosurgery* 1977, 1:245–248.

275. Awad I, Carter L, Spetzler R, *et al.*: Clinical vasospasm after subarachnoid hemorrhage: response to hypervolemic hemodilution and arterial hypertension. *Stroke* 1987, 18:365–372.

276. Findlay J, Kassell N, Weir B, *et al.*: A randomized trial of intraoperative, intracisternal tissue plasminogen activator for the prevention of vasospasm. *Neurosurgery* 1995, 37:168–178.

277. Newell D, Eskridge J, Mayberg M, *et al.*: Angioplasty for treatment of symptomatic vasospasm. *J Neurosurg* 1989, 71:654–660.

278. Weir B: *Epidemiology*. In *Aneurysms Affecting the Nervous System*. Baltimore: Williams & Wilkins, 1987:19–53.

279. Morley T, Barr H: Giant intracranial aneurysms: diagnosis, course and management. *Clin Neurosurg* 1969, 16:73–94.

280. Zabramski J, Spetzler R: Management of Mycotic Aneurysms. In *Stroke*. Edited by Barnett H, Mohr J, Stein B, *et al.* New York: Churchill Livingstone; 1992:1065–1066.

281. Ondra S, Troupp H, George E, *et al.*: The natural history of symptomatic arteriovenous malformations. *J Neurosurg* 1990, 73:387–391.

282. Tsementzis S: Surgical management of intracerebral hematomas. *Neurosurgery* 1985, 16:562–572.

283. McCormick WF: The pathology of vascular ("arteriovenous") malformations. *J Neurosurg* 1966, 24:807–816.

284. Curling OJ, Kelly DJ, Elster A, *et al.*: An analysis of the natural history of the cavernous angioma. *Neurosurgery* 1991, 75:702.

285. Robinson J, Award I, Little J: Natural history of cavernous angioma. *J Neurosurg* 1991, 75:709–714.

6

Dementias

Thomas J. Grabowski, Jr • Antonio R. Damasio

APPROXIMATELY 2 million people in the United States suffer from severe dementia, and an additional 5 million have mild to moderate dementia. As life expectancy and the proportion of older individuals in the population continue to increase, dementia will become an ever more significant health problem, one that is compounded by its effects on the families of affected individuals. If the course of dementia is not modified by treatment, the number of individuals who will be affected by degenerative dementia in the coming decades will increase dramatically [1,2].

The term *dementia* indicates a progressive cognitive deterioration with memory impairment as a salient feature. This definition of the term, based mainly on the natural history of Alzheimer's disease, is incorporated in standard diagnostic criteria, such as those found in the Diagnostic and Statistical Manual of Mental Disorders (DSM-IV) [3] or the International Classification of Diseases (ICD-10) [4]. From the clinical point of view, however, it is useful to define dementia in broader terms to encompass any acquired and persistent impairment of intellectual faculties that occurs in an alert individual and affects several cognitive domains, which is sufficiently severe to impair social or occupational competence. Although most cases of dementia result from degenerative brain processes, this definition makes no reference to pathologic correlates and, indeed, leaves open the possibility that dementia can occur without recognized structural alterations in the brain (such as the pseudodementia of depression); nor does this definition specify there be progression or prominent memory impairment. Dementia may be a relatively static condition, as occurs after cumulative large vessel cerebral infarcts or head injury. In some cases, as in Pick's disease or unusual variants of Alzheimer's disease, memory disturbance may not be prominent or may appear later in the course of the illness. The term dementia does not apply to isolated impairments of memory, language, visuospatial abilities, or higher visual processes (best denoted by the terms *amnesia*, *aphasia*, *visual agnosia*, and so forth), or to the fluctuating encephalopathy known as the "confusional state" or delirium, in which impaired attention and level of consciousness are the critical defects. Such fluctuating conditions are usually caused by a metabolic disturbance. Dementia should be distinguished from developmental encephalopathies, which do not permit a fully developed level of intellectual function, and from benign age-associated cognitive change, which does not impair social or occupational competence.

Although the differential diagnosis of dementia includes many conditions, the contemporary clinical approach is straightforward. Most dementias, especially the degenerative dementias, are neither reversible nor treatable, given our current knowledge. The clinician who encounters such a patient, therefore, concentrates first on determining the presence of potentially treatable causes of dementia. Dementia secondary to medical diseases, the adverse effects of medication, depression, or certain space-occupying brain lesions is often treatable with a high degree of efficacy. Alzheimer's disease, which causes most cases of dementia, has a fairly characteristic presentation, and a relatively small number of diseases account for most of the remaining cases.

The classification of dementia into one of several clinical categories facilitates recognition of cases requiring further evaluation or referral to a specialist. Another priority in dementia management is the recognition and treatment of psychiatric symptoms, which are not only common but often the immediate reason for institutionalization of patients with dementia.

Evaluation of Dementia

ICD-10 Criteria for the Diagnosis of Dementia

Impairment of short- and long-term memory (more accurately, of anterograde memory)

At least one of the following:

Impairment of abstract thinking

Impaired judgment

Other disturbances of higher cortical function

Personality change

Memory impairment and intellectual impairment causing significant social and occupational impairment

Absence of occurrence exclusively during the course of delirium

Either of the following:

Evidence of an organic factor causing this impaired memory and intellect

Impaired memory and intellect that cannot be accounted for by any nonorganic mental disorder

Figure 6-1. International Classification of Diseases (ICD-10) criteria for the diagnosis of dementia [4].

Clinical Dementia Rating (CDR) Scale

	Healthy (CDR 0)	Questionable dementia (CDR 0.5)	Mild dementia (CDR 1)	Moderate dementia (CDR 2)	Severe dementia (CDR 3)
Memory	No memory loss or slight irregular forgetfulness	Mild, consistent, "benign" forgetfulness; partial recall of events	Moderate memory loss, especially for recent events; loss interferes with daily activities	Severe memory loss; only highly learned material retained; new material rapidly lost	Severe memory loss; only fragments remain
Orientation	Fully oriented		Oriented for place and person at examination; may have geographic disorientation; some difficulty with time relationships	Usually disoriented in time, often to place	Orientation to person only
Judgment/problem solving	Solves everyday problems well; judgment consistent with past performance	Doubtful impairment in similarities, differences, solving problems	Moderate difficulty in handling complex problems; social judgment usually maintained	Severely impaired in handling problems, similarities, differences; social judgment usually impaired	Unable to make judgments, solve problems
Community affairs	Independent function at usual level in business, financial, and social affairs	Doubtful or mild impairment if any	Unable to function independently at these activities; may still appear normal to casual inspection	No pretense of independent function outside home	
Home/hobbies	Well maintained	Well maintained or only slightly impaired	Mild but definite impairment of function; more difficult chores and complicated hobbies abandoned	Only simple chores preserved; very restricted interests, poorly sustained	No significant function outside of own room
Personal care	Fully capable of self care		Needs occasional prompting	Requires assistance in dressing, hygiene, keeping of personal effects	Often incontinent; requires much help with personal care

Score as 0.5, 1, 2, 3 only if impairment is due to cognitive loss.

Figure 6-2. Grading the severity of dementia. The presence and severity of dementia are assessed in terms of functional and neuropsychologic consequences. The label *dementia* is not applied without evidence of a decline in competence in daily living. The Washington University Clinical Dementia Rating Scale (CDR) assesses performance in the areas of memory, orientation, judgment, community affairs, home and hobbies, and personal care, using a five-point scale [5]. Functional impairment short of mild dementia is designated CDR 0.5, "questionable dementia," which is indeterminate with respect to the presence of degenerative disease. (*Adapted from* Hughes and colleagues [5].)

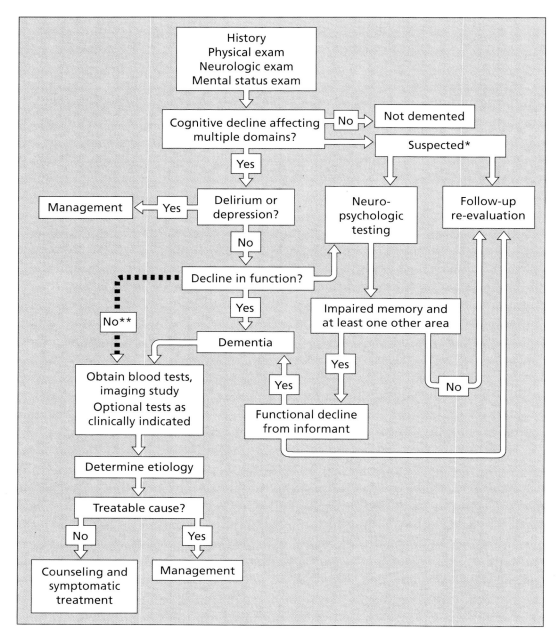

Figure 6-3. The clinical evaluation of dementia. The American Academy of Neurology has suggested this algorithm for the clinical evaluation and diagnosis of dementia [6,7]. Note that despite the absence of detection of abnormalities with office mental status testing (*eg*, Folstein Mini-Mental Status Examimation) [8,9], dementia may be suspected (*) on the basis of the history or a threat to employment. In these cases, neuropsychologic evaluation is especially helpful. Note also that some neurologists do not recommend neuropsychologic testing in patients without functional decline (**). (*Adapted from* Corey-Bloom and colleagues [6].

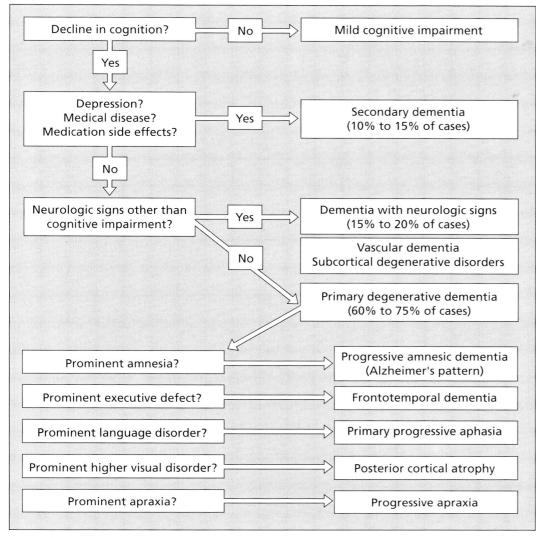

tia plus"), and primary degenerative dementia. Patients who complain of memory decline but have normal neuropsychologic test results may have mild cognitive impairment [10] (MCI) (Fig. 6-5). The clinician may reassure these patients that dementia has not been detected. However, because some patients prove to have incipient dementia, follow-up evaluation for a year or more is advised. Cases of secondary dementia are frequently "treatable" (Figs. 6-8–6-10). Cases of primary degenerative dementia are characterized by a prominent impairment in cognitive function in the *absence* of defects in primary sensory and motor function [11]. Aside from mental status, the neurologic examination is normal. This is the most common category of dementia, and usually is the result of degenerative disease. The diagnosis in progressive amnesic dementia is usually Alzheimer's disease (AD), and this profile is sometimes referred to as dementia of the Alzheimer type. These patients can often be managed exclusively by the primary caregiver, although as specific therapies become available, the involvement of a specialist may be useful. Syndromes of primary degenerative dementia, which depart from the usual Alzheimer's pattern, are distinctly unusual. These syndromes may have a different natural history than AD, raise special clinical issues, and are best handled with the assistance of a specialist. The presence of noncognitive neurologic signs in patients with dementia often indicates the presence of significant subcortical structural pathology or involvement of parts of the cortex that are usually spared in primary degenerative dementia. Often, a "subcortical" pattern of dementia is present (Fig. 6-5) [12,13]. Such cases of dementia with neurologic signs call for comprehensive neurologic evaluation and generally require the assistance of a specialist.

Figure 6-4. Clinical classification of dementia. A useful clinical classification of dementia distinguishes mild cognitive impairment, secondary dementia, dementia with neurologic signs (or "dementia plus"),

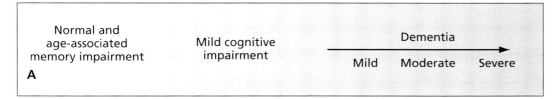

Figure 6-5. Cognitive changes associated with aging. **A,** The clinical assessment of cognitive function involves classification of patients' states along a continuum from a state reflecting common effects of aging through mild cognitive impairment (MCI) to dementia. Patients do not necessarily progress from one stage to the next. MCI is defined as cognitive impairment of insufficient degree to interfere with daily functioning. It bears a close but not one-to-one relationship with clinical dementia rating (CDR) 0.5, "questionable dementia" [5].

(*Continued on next page*)

B. Cognitive Neurologic Changes in Aging

Function	Finding	Clinical significance
Speed of mental processing	Slows with age for perception, reaction time, and choice reaction time	Pervasive effects on cognitive function
Attention	Sustained attention preserved into eighth decade; selective attention preserved into ninth decade	Marked decline in ability to sustain attention should be recognized as evidence of disease
Visuospatial functions	Decline in perceptual and constructional abilities	Evident on testing but not typically functionally significant
Memory	Immediate and long-term memory begins to decline as early as the sixth decade	Deficits not functionally significant in the absence of frank dementia
Language	Syntax and word usage are preserved, while naming and verbal fluency begin to decline in eighth decade	Language problems beyond mild naming difficulty should be recognized as evidence of disease

Figure 6-5. (*Continued*) **B,** Both CDR 0.5 and MCI should be distinguished from "age-associated memory impairment" [14,15] and the older term "benign senescent forgetfulness." The latter terms designate nonprogressive and non-impairing conditions that reflect universal effects of aging, including mild changes in the efficiency of memory encoding (but not retrieval) and of word retrieval (but not syntax or comprehension of speech), and diminished speed of mental processing [16]. Standardized neuropsychological assessment is the most reliable way to make these distinctions, and also provides the necessary baseline for measuring the progression of cognitive impairment. There is evidence that the pathologic changes of Alzheimer's disease (AD) occur years before patients become symptomatic; therefore, some patients with MCI have early AD. Neither MCI nor CDR 0.5 is synonymous with incipient AD, because not all patients with MCI have progressive impairment and not all progressive syndromes are caused by AD. Some patients with MCI have treatable conditions like depression; other patients have normal age-associated cognitive changes. Prospective studies have estimated the proportion of patients with CDR 0.5 or MCI who progress to overt dementia/probable AD at 20% to 75% over several years [10]. Risk factors for progression include parkinsonism [17,18], possession of an apolipoprotein €4 allele [19], the presence of some functional impairment [20], the presence of mesial temporal lobe atrophy as measured with magnetic resonance imaging [21,22], and performance on certain neuropsychologic tests [20,23,24]. However, no test is available to predict those who will progress to dementia; follow-up after 9 to 12 months is advisable, including standardized neuropsychologic assessment. MCI is currently a matter of intense research interest, as are treatment approaches that may slow the course of AD in its early stages. (Panel B *adapted from* Kaye and colleagues [16].)

Relative Frequency of Causes of Dementia

Disease	Frequency (%)	
Alzheimer's	63	
Pure		40
+VaD		12
+Lewy		10
+IPD		1
VaD (pure)	10	
DLB (pure)	5	
FTLA	10	
DLDH		7
Pick's		2
CBD		1
IPD	2	
Reversible	5	
Others	5	
NPH		1
CJD		1
Hippocampal sclerosis		1
Remainder		2

Figure 6-6. Relative frequency of causes of dementia. Hospital-based studies and autopsy series indicate the approximate incidences shown. The relative frequencies of the leading causes of dementia are unclear because some conditions have only been recognized recently or have had diagnostic criteria redefined, and some of the disease processes can be superimposed [25,26]. The most prevalent cause of dementia by far is Alzheimer's disease (AD), which accounts for at least half of all cases. The vascular dementias (VaDs) account collectively for 10% to 20% of cases, and constitute the second most common cause. Dementia complicating idiopathic Parkinson's disease (IPD) and dementia with cortical Lewy bodies (DLB) [27] constitute the other important cluster of "dementia plus." The substantial proportion of patients who present with both vascular disease *and* AD or combined DLB and AD pose diagnostic challenges to the clinician. The cluster of conditions causing frontotemporal lobar atrophy (FTLA), sometimes termed "Pick complex" [28], is the other leading form of degenerative dementia. Cases of AD outnumber FTLAs by a ratio of approximately 5 to 1, and FTLA is frequently misdiagnosed by inexperienced clinicians. Dementia secondary to medical or psychiatric illness, despite its clinical importance, is apparently less common [29], although hospital-based studies may underestimate its incidence. All other causes of dementia, most of them degenerative, are quite uncommon. Among these, hydrocephalic dementia and spongiform encephalopathy have distinctive presentations. CBD—corticobasal degeneration; CJD—Creutzfeld-Jakob disease; DLDH—dementia lacking distinctive histopathology; NPH—normal pressure hydrocephalus.

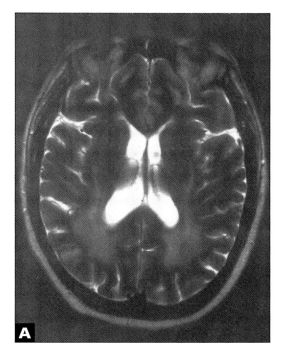 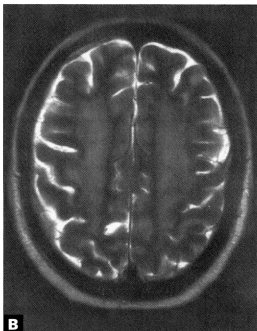

Figure 6-7. Subcortical dementia. **A, B,** T2-weighted magnetic resonance imaging scan of a 49-year-old man who developed a diffuse leukoencephalopathy after treatment of non-Hodgkin's lymphoma with chemotherapy and bone marrow transplantation. He had cognitive impairment conforming to a subcortical profile. **C,** The major features distinguishing cortical and subcortical patterns of dementia are summarized. Subcortical dementia is characterized by a slowing of cognition, poor problem solving, poor memory, apathy, and depression [12,13]. The amnesia is characterized primarily by defective *retrieval* of material, distinguishing it from the anterograde learning deficit so characteristic of Alzheimer's disease and other cortical dementias. Although acquisition of new material may be slowed because of a defective learning strategy, these patients benefit more from retrieval cues and manifest better recognition of learned material than patients with cortical dementia. Similarly, the executive and emotional dysfunction that characterizes subcortical dementia is distinguishable from the executive dysfunction that accompanies damage to the frontal lobes, because such features as personality change, lost insight, socially inappropriate behavior, and perseveration are not prominent. Agnosia, apraxia, and aphasia are not prominent features of subcortical dementia. **D,** The major causes of subcortical dementia are listed.

C. Subcortical Patterns of Dementia

	Cortical dementia	Subcortical dementia
Memory	Anterograde amnesia, agnosia	Poor retrieval, preserved recognition
Executive function	Poor insight, judgment, abstraction	Poor problem solving, slowed thought
Affect	Disinhibited	Apathy, depression
Visuospatial	Poor visuoconstruction	Normal
Language	Aphasia, anomia	Normal
Motor system	Apraxia	Extrapyramidal signs, gait disturbance

D. Major Causes of Subcortical Dementia

Diseases of subcortical gray matter	Diseases of white matter
Parkinson's disease	Small vessel vascular disease
Huntington's disease	Multiple sclerosis
Progressive supranuclear palsy	Head injury
Small vessel vascular disease	Human immunodeficiency virus encephalopathy
Wilson's disease	Hydrocephalus
	Binswanger's encephalopathy

Secondary Causes of Dementia

Medication encephalopathy
Pseudodementia of depression
Normal pressure hydrocephalus
Hypothyroidism
Hypovitaminosis B$_{12}$
Other metabolic disorders
Resectable intracranial tumors
Subdural hematomas
Chronic meningitis

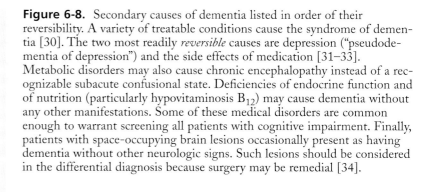

Figure 6-8. Secondary causes of dementia listed in order of their reversibility. A variety of treatable conditions cause the syndrome of dementia [30]. The two most readily *reversible* causes are depression ("pseudodementia of depression") and the side effects of medication [31–33]. Metabolic disorders may also cause chronic encephalopathy instead of a recognizable subacute confusional state. Deficiencies of endocrine function and of nutrition (particularly hypovitaminosis B$_{12}$) may cause dementia without any other manifestations. Some of these medical disorders are common enough to warrant screening all patients with cognitive impairment. Finally, patients with space-occupying brain lesions occasionally present as having dementia without other neurologic signs. Such lesions should be considered in the differential diagnosis because surgery may be remedial [34].

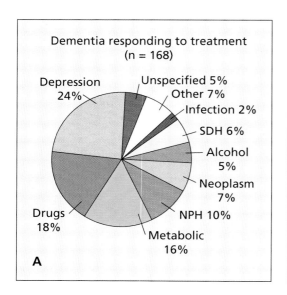

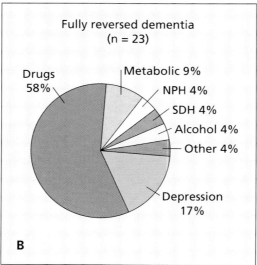

Figure 6-9. Reversibility of secondary dementia. Although about 10% to 20% of cases of dementia are associated with medically- or surgically-treatable conditions, only 10% of these cases (*ie*, about 1% overall) will actually be reversed with specific treatment [35]. More often, the treatable condition is only one component of the dementia, superimposed on another condition, usually Alzheimer's disease. **A**, In a meta-analysis of studies of 1551 cases of dementia, Weytingh and colleagues reported that 15% of all cases were potentially reversible and 11% had at least partial response to treatment [29]. **B**, Dementia was fully reversed in 1.5% of cases. Depression, medication encephalopathy, and metabolic disorders dominated the reversible cases. Full responders outnumber partial responders among cases of medication encephalopathy. NPH—normal pressure hydrocephalus; SDH—subdural hematoma.

Medications Causing Encephalopathy

Cholinergic antagonists
Sedative-hypnotics (benzodiazepines, barbiturates)
Narcotics
Histamine$_2$ antagonists
Digoxin
Dopaminergic antagonists (neuroleptics)

Figure 6-10. Medications causing encephalopathy. Medication encephalopathy is frequently underappreciated as a cause of, or contributor to, dementia in elderly patients [36–38]. Among medications that have this unintended effect, perhaps the most likely to be overlooked are cholinergic antagonists. Medications with recognized and unrecognized anticholinergic properties are commonplace, and patients may take more than one such agent concurrently. In addition, some anticholinergic agents are readily available to patients over-the-counter as antispasmodics, sedatives, and motion sickness preparations. These agents can have catastrophic effects in patients with dementia, probably because of the central cholinergic deficiency that has been documented in Alzheimer's disease, Parkinson's disease, and dementia with Lewy bodies [39].

Ancillary Studies to Evaluate Dementia

All patients
  General medical evaluation
  CBC, general metabolic screen, CXR, UA, ECG, TSH, vitamin B$_{12}$
  Brain imaging (CT or MRI)
  Neuropsychologic testing (repeated 9–12 months later)
Selected patients
  EEG (periodic complexes, asymmetric slowing, metabolic encephalopathy)
  CSF evaluation (inflammatory processes)
  Syphilis serology
  Functional imaging (SPECT, PET)
  Fibrinogen, plasma viscosity (vascular dementia)
  Drug levels, heavy metal screening, HIV serologic screen, ceruloplasmin levels, other tests as needed
  Muscle, nerve biopsy (mitochondrial encephalopathy, leukodystrophy)
  Brain and leptomeningeal biopsy (cerebral vasculitis)
  Ophthalmic examination (Kayser-Fleischer rings, pigmentary changes)

Figure 6-11. Useful ancillary studies in the standard evaluation of dementia. In the standard laboratory evaluation for dementia, the primary goals are the detection of secondary dementia and the detection of cerebrovascular disease [7]. (See Figs. 6-9–6-12 for elaboration.) Evidence of abnormalities in other systems, departures from the common demographic profile (*eg*, dementia in a young patient), rapid worsening of dementia, or a family history of a similar disorder should trigger more extensive evaluation. CBC—complete blood count; CSF—cerebrospinal fluid; CT—computed tomography; CXR—chest roentgenogram; ECG—electrocardiogram; EEG—electroencephalogram; MRI—magnetic resonance imaging; PET—positron emission tomography; SPECT—single photon emission computed tomography; TSH—thyroid-stimulating hormone; UA—urinalysis.

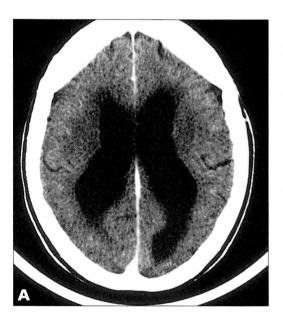

A

Figure 6-12. A, Cranial computed tomography (CT) scan of a patient with dementia and normal pressure hydrocephalus (NPH). Neuroimaging is used in the evaluation of dementia to detect space-occupying abnormalities, such as hydrocephalus, subdural hematomas, or tumors; to provide evidence of cerebrovascular disease; and to detect disproportionate regional atrophy. In this case, the ventricles are enlarged out of proportion to the cerebral sulci, indicating the possibility that the ventricles are under tension and impinging on the adjacent white matter. The low X-ray absorption in the white matter represents reversible transependymal edema. After shunting, this patient's urinary incontinence and cognition improved markedly, and ventricular size was reduced.

"Normal pressure hydrocephalus," a condition first described by Adams and colleagues and Fisher [40,41], is characterized by the symptom triad of dementia, usually conforming to a "subcortical" profile; urinary incontinence; and gait disturbance, characterized by short steps and a "magnetic" quality. The gait disturbance is the most specific feature of the triad, and the one whose change best predicts a favorable response to a shunting procedure. Because ventriculoperitoneal shunts are risky procedures in the elderly, owing to complicating subdural hemorrhage, additional evidence for NPH is usually sought; such evidence usually comes from a therapeutic lumbar puncture (resulting in gait improvement) or overnight monitoring of intracranial pressure [42,43]. Although the cerebrospinal fluid pressure is usually normal at the time of lumbar puncture, transitory pressure elevations do occur in NPH.

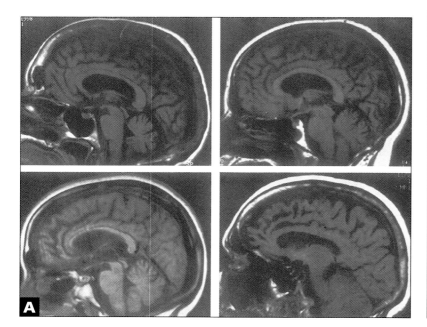

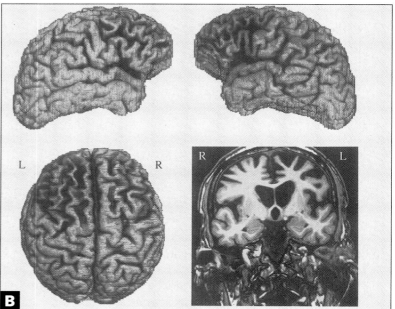

Figure 6-13. Disproportionate regional atrophy on structural brain images. The cerebral cortex does not atrophy homogeneously in degenerative conditions; the pattern varies across conditions and even among cases of the same degenerative condition. For example, the two leading causes of primary degenerative dementia, frontotemporal lobar degeneration and Alzheimer's disease (AD), have differing patterns of atrophy. **A**, Parasagittal T1-weighted magnetic resonance imaging (MRI) scans of patients with AD (*upper tier*) and frontotemporal dementia (*lower tier*). Note the relative widening of posterior sulci, especially the parieto-occipital and posterior cingulate sulci in AD and the relative widening of anterior sulci and thinning of the rostrum of the corpus callosum in frontotemporal dementia. **B**, Asymmetric cerebral cortical atrophy in a patient with frontotemporal dementia, displayed in 2D and 3D T1-weighted MRI scans. The atrophy is more pronounced in the left hemisphere. Right–left asymmetry is very common in the frontotemporal lobar atrophies. Note that the atrophy is predominant in association regions, with relative sparing of the primary sensorimotor cortex.

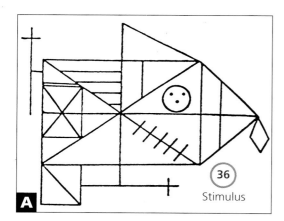

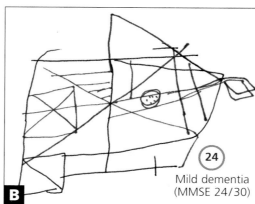

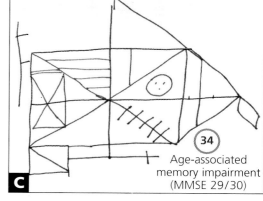

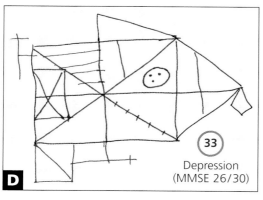

Figure 6-14. Neuropsychologic testing in the evaluation of dementia. Standardized neuropsychologic assessment [44] is a valuable adjunct in the evaluation of virtually all cases of dementia. The purposes of neuropsychologic testing are to distinguish mild dementia from age-associated memory impairment; to detect focal neuropsychologic manifestations; to distinguish organic dementia from depression; to characterize cognitive capacity comprehensively and in detail; to make appropriate recommendations regarding competence for such activities as financial responsibility and the operation of vehicles and machinery; and to provide longitudinal assessment, including assessments of the rate of decline and the efficacy of medical interventions. Visually mediated performances, such as copying complex figures or the immediate reproduction of recently viewed geometric figures, are useful in discriminating between depression or age-associated memory impairment, on the one hand, and dementia on the other. Displayed here are reproductions of the Rey-Osterrieth complex figure (**A**), as copied while in view by three patients with complaints of memory difficulty: one with mild dementia (**B**), one with age-associated memory impairment (AAMI) (**C**), and one with depression (**D**). Patients with AAMI give normal performances on all tests. Although verbally mediated performances do not discriminate well between patients with depression and patients with dementia, visually mediated abilities are usually well preserved in patients with depression ("pseudodementia") [45]. The circled numbers represent each patient's score out of a possible score of 36. MMSE—Folstein Mini Mental Status Examination. (*Courtesy of* the Benton Laboratory of Neuropsychology, Department of Neurology, The University of Iowa.)

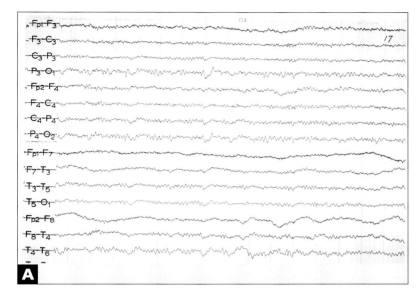

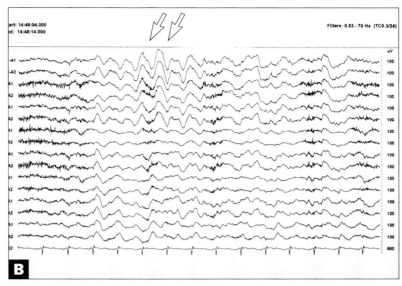

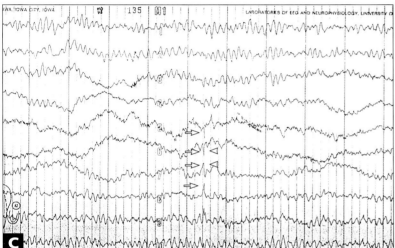

Figure 6-15. Electroencephalography in the evaluation of dementia. **A,** In early Alzheimer's disease (AD), the electroencephalogram (EEG) is either normal or shows irregular theta slowing in the temporal regions. In more advanced AD, pronounced slowing may occur but does not correlate consistently with the degree of dementia. Because these findings are nonspecific, EEG has a limited role in the evaluation of most cases of dementia. EEG, however, can be quite helpful in cases of recent onset or subacute cognitive impairment, and in cases in which symptoms are reported to fluctuate with time [46]. **B,** EEG of a 61-year-old woman with a history of imbalance and memory impairment for several months. The EEG shows delta waves, a degree of slowing out of proportion to the degree of cognitive impairment. This pattern strongly suggests a metabolic cause for the dementia. (Conversely, a normal EEG in the presence of severe dementia strongly suggests degenerative rather than metabolic disease). The EEG also gives the clue to the cause in this case: some of the slow waves have a distinct *triphasic* contour (*arrows*), a pattern seen in hepatic encephalopathy. The serum ammonia was 138 ng/dL. The final diagnosis was hepatic encephalopathy caused by cryptogenic cirrhosis. **C,** EEG of an 80-year-old man with fluctuating cognitive impairment. Although serial neuropsychologic testing documented *stable* cognitive deficits, he experienced periods, particularly at night, during which he was unable to recognize his immediate family, including his wife. The initial EEGs were normal, but this EEG, taken immediately after an episode, discloses epileptiform activity. Note the spike wave (*arrows*) with a phase reversal (*arrowheads*) indicating an origin in the right anterior temporal region. After administration of carbamazepine, such episodes became infrequent and his mental state improved. (Panel A, *courtesy of* Thoru Yamada, MD, Department of Neurology, The University of Iowa; Panel B, *courtesy of* the Laboratory of Human Neuroanatomy and Neuroimaging, Department of Neurology, The University of Iowa.)

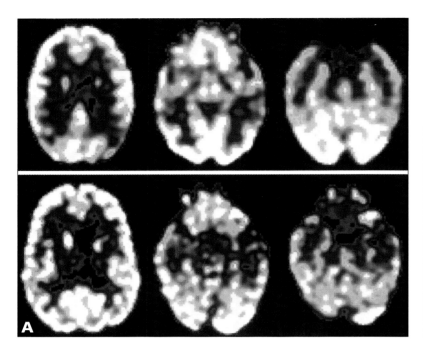

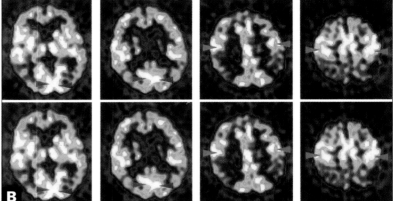

Figure 6-16. Functional imaging in the evaluation of dementia. Functional imaging creates images of the brain's physiologic state on the basis of the distribution of radiopharmaceutical agents. In degenerative dementia, images of glucose metabolism (positron-emission computed tomography [PET]) or cerebral blood flow (single photon emission computed tomography [SPECT]) frequently demonstrate regionalized metabolic defects. Currently, functional imaging is most helpful in evaluating cases of atypical primary dementia not dominated by amnesia; the pattern of regional hypometabolism may or may not depart from the classic Alzheimer's pattern [47]. **A,** [18]F fluorodeoxyglucose (FDG) PET images of the brain of two patients with dementia featuring conspicuous aphasia. In both cases, low metabolism is seen in multifocal locations. *Upper tier,* The patient has reductions in parietal and posterior temporal cortex, more pronounced on the left side of the brain. This pattern of reductions strongly suggests Alzheimer's disease (AD) [48,49]. *Lower tier,* The patient has anterior and polar temporal reductions, more pronounced on the left side of the brain, a pattern suggestive of frontotemporal lobar degeneration presenting with progressive aphasia. **B,** *Upper tier,* [18]F FDG PET images of the brain of a third patient with aphasic dementia also showing multifocal reduction of tracer uptake. Note the low metabolism in left primary visual cortex and left sensorimotor cortex (*arrows*). Reductions in these areas are not characteristic of either AD or frontotemporal lobar degenerations, in which reductions occur mainly in association cortex. This patient proved to have Creutzfeld-Jakob disease. *Lower tier,* [18]F FDG PET images from a patient with a typical case of moderately advanced AD.

Alzheimer's Disease

Important Milestones in the Understanding of Alzheimer's Disease

1907 Alzheimer describes neurofibrillary tangles and senile neuritic plaques in a patient, aged 51

1910 Kraepelin applies the eponym "Alzheimer's disease" (AD)

1962 Corsellis recognizes the identity of "Alzheimer's disease" in the presenium and "senile dementia"

1963 Kidd describes the ultrastructure of neurofibrillary tangles with electron microscopy

1976 Davies and Maloney report selective loss of central cholinergic neurons in AD

1983 Coyle, Price, and DeLong propose that AD is a disorder of cortical cholinergic innervation

1984 Research criteria for clinical diagnosis established

1984 Hyman, van Hoesen, and Damasio propose a disconnection hypothesis of amnesia in AD

1985 National Institute of Aging (Khachaturian) criteria for the pathologic diagnosis of AD

1991 Report of amyloid precursor gene mutation causing AD

1993 Strittmater, Roses, and colleagues describe the association of apolipoprotein E4 with late onset familial AD

1995 Presenilin 1 and presenilin 2 genes are identified

First cholinomimetic agent approved for treatment of AD

Development of transgenic mouse model of AD

1999 Report of reduced amyloid burden in transgenic mouse with Aβ immunization
Identification of β-secretase

Figure 6-17. Timeline of important milestones in the understanding of Alzheimer's disease [50–52]. Alzheimer's disease (AD) is a prevalent degenerative encephalopathy with distinctive histopathology that usually presents clinically as progressive amnesic dementia. The neuropathologic hallmarks of AD are intraneuronal neurofibrillary tangles and extraneuronal deposition of amyloid material, which accumulates focally in the form of neuritic or senile plaques. These signature lesions have a predilection for certain regions of the cerebral cortex and, within given regions, for certain layers. Although these lesions may occasionally be found in other disorders, in AD they occur in large quantity and with a characteristic topography that permits an unambiguous pathologic diagnosis [53,54].

NINCDS-ADRDA Criteria for Diagnosis of Alzheimer's Disease

Features supporting probable diagnosis of Alzheimer's disease

Dementia established by clinical examination and standardized brief mental status examination and confirmed by neuropsychologic tests

Deficits in two or more areas of cognition

Progressive worsening of memory and other cognitive function

No disturbance of consciousness

Onset between 40 and 90 years

Absence of other systemic or neurologic disorders sufficient to account for the progressive cognitive defects

Features supporting diagnosis of Alzheimer's disease

Progressive deterioration of specific cognitive functions such as language (aphasia), motor skills (apraxia), and perception (agnosia)

Impaired activities of daily living and altered patterns of behavior

Family history of a similar disorder, especially if confirmed neuropathologically

Normal lumbar puncture

Normal pattern or nonspecific changes in electroencephalogram

Evidence of cerebral atrophy on computed tomography, with progression on serial observation

Features against diagnosis of Alzheimer's disease

Sudden onset

Focal neurologic findings such as hemiparesis, sensory loss, visual field deficits, and incoordination early in the course of the illness

Seizures or gait disturbance at the onset or very early in the course of the illness

Figure 6-18. National Institute of Neurological and Communicative Disorders and Stroke—Alzheimer's Disease and Related Disorders Association (NINCDS-ADRDA) criteria for the clinical research and diagnosis of Alzheimer's disease, which were proposed in 1984 [55]. In contrast to the distinctive histopathologic features of AD, there are no pathognomonic clinical features, nor are there yet laboratory tests specific for AD. Nevertheless, these accepted clinical research criteria for the diagnosis of AD are highly accurate (approaching 90%).

Alzheimer's disease gradually progresses over 7 to 10 years. There are no remissions, although the rate of decline may vary. Most patients present with insidious anterograde memory impairment, which may be moderately severe before it is recognized. Other cognitive impairments ensue, especially agnosia and disorders of executive function. A striking clinical feature in many cases is the patient's lack of appreciation (insight) into the nature and severity of cognitive problems. Another striking clinical feature is the sparing of motor function and of primary touch, hearing, and sight.

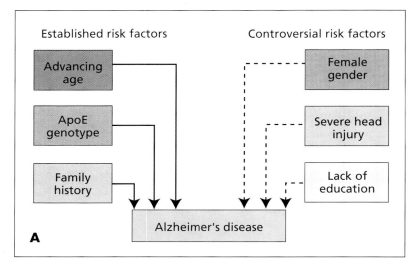

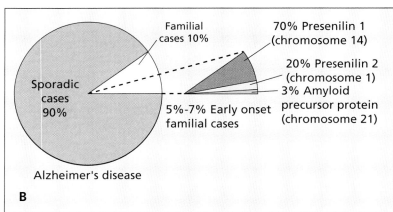

Figure 6-19. Risk factors for Alzheimer's disease (AD). **A,** Among the established risk factors [56] for the development of AD, the most important is advancing age. The prevalence approximately doubles in each subsequent 5-year increment, reaching about 10% by age 85 [57]. On the basis of the limited data available, it appears that the incidence tends to level off after age 85. Following age, the most important risk factors are genetic. Up to 10% of AD cases are transmitted genetically in an autosomal dominant manner. About 30% of persons with AD have an affected first-degree relative. In the EURODEM case control study, patients with a first-degree relative with AD had a relative risk (RR) of 3.5 for developing AD [58]. This risk was highest when the relative had the onset of dementia before

age 70. The presence of two first-degree relatives imparted an RR of 7.5. **B,** Three genes accounting for much of familial onset AD have now been identified. A defect in the amyloid precursor protein gene on chromosome 21 was the first to be delineated, accounting for a small proportion (3%) of cases [59]. Most recently discovered were the presenilin genes, which appear to encode proteins that participate in intracellular protein transport. Defects in presenilin 1 may account for almost half of all cases of autosomal dominant AD [60,61]. Weaker and controversial risk factors for the development of AD include past head injury, female gender, and limited degree of education [62]. Estrogen replacement may be a protective factor in postmenopausal women [63].

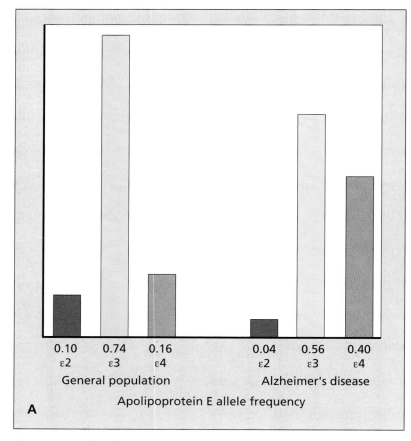

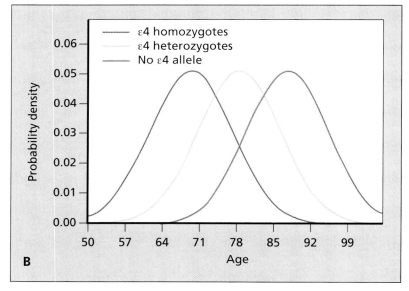

Figure 6-20. Apolipoprotein E and Alzheimer's disease (AD). **A,** In addition to the gene mutations displayed in Figure 6-19, which invariably lead to the clinical manifestation of AD, the genotype for

apolipoprotein E, specifically the dose of the ε4 allele, confers susceptibility to AD, tending to shift onset to an earlier age. Thus, patients with sporadic and familial late-onset AD have an excess of the ε4 allele [64–66]. The gene dose of the ε4 allele confers susceptibility to AD, tending to shift onset to an earlier age in susceptible patients. **B,** Three probability distributions of age of onset of AD for ε4 homozygotes, ε4 heterozygotes, and those without an ε4 allele [67]. However, individuals carrying an ε4 allele do not necessarily develop dementia, which indicates that apolipoprotein genotyping has a limited value in diagnosis and prognosis [68,69]. Current experimental evidence suggests that apoE (and especially apoε4) has a chaperone function and promotes aggregation of Aβ [70]. The ε4 allele is also present in excess in patients with other dementing illnesses [71]. (Panel B *adapted from* Breitner [67].)

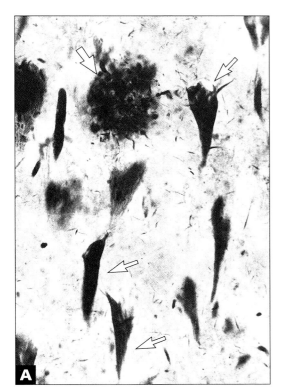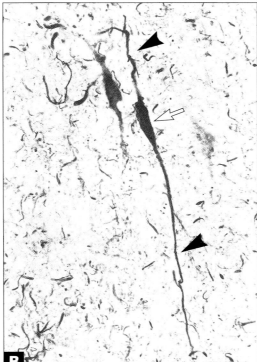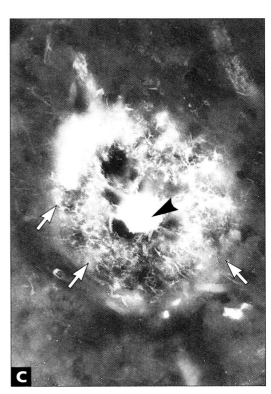

Figure 6-21. Pathologic hallmarks of Alzheimer's disease (AD). The principal lesions associated with AD are neurofibrillary tangles (NFTs) and senile or neuritic plaques (SPs). **A**, Neurofibrillary tangles (*thin arrows*, silver stain) are insoluble intracellular structures composed of the microtubule-associated protein tau, in the form of paired 10-nm helical filaments with a characteristic periodicity. **B**, In addition to NFTs, neuropil threads also appear frequently in the distal processes of tangle-bearing neurons (*arrowheads*). **C**, The dystrophic neurites that surround senile plaques are also tau-positive. SPs (Panel *A, wide arrows*; Panel *C*, thioflavin-S stain), in fully developed form, are characterized by a focal deposit of amyloid material, surrounded by dystrophic neurites (Panel *C, thin arrows*), reactive astrocytes,

and microglia. The core of the plaque (Panel *C, wide arrow*) is composed of the β-amyloid protein, a hydrophobic fragment of a transmembrane glycoprotein (amyloid precursor protein). Other substances found in SPs include apolipoprotein E, lipoprotein receptor-related protein, and cytokines. Although important advances have been made, the pathogenesis of AD remains a mystery. In particular, the relationship between neurofibrillary pathology and amyloid deposition, and the relationship between these observable structural alterations and the clinical symptomatology, remain unexplained. (*Courtesy of* Gary Van Hoesen, PhD, Department of Anatomy, The University of Iowa.)

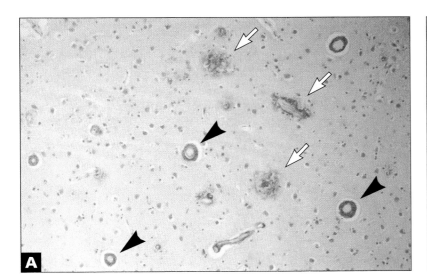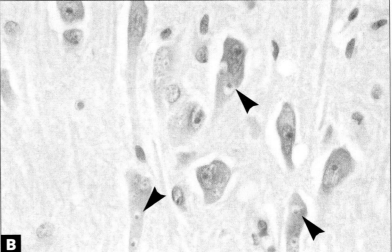

Figure 6-22. Histopathologic features of Alzheimer's disease (AD). **A**, In addition to its presence in plaques in the neuropil (*arrows*), β-amyloid is also found in leptomeningeal and cortical arterioles (β-amyloid stain) in about 85% of cases of AD [72] (*arrowheads*). The role of amyloid angiopathy in the dementia of AD is incompletely understood. Occasionally, amyloid angiopathy causes severe

leukoencephalopathy (Fig. 6-40). **B**, Other important histopathologic features of AD include granulovacuolar degeneration in hippocampal pyramidal cells (hematoxylin and eosin stain) (*arrowheads*) and changes in white matter, which remain incompletely characterized. (*Courtesy of* Lee Reed, MD, Department of Pathology, The University of Iowa.)

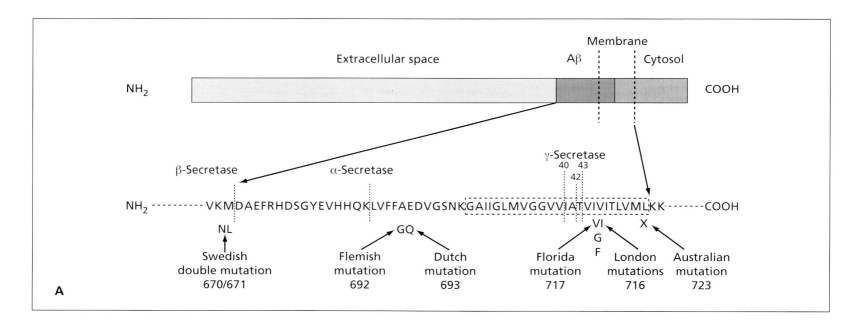

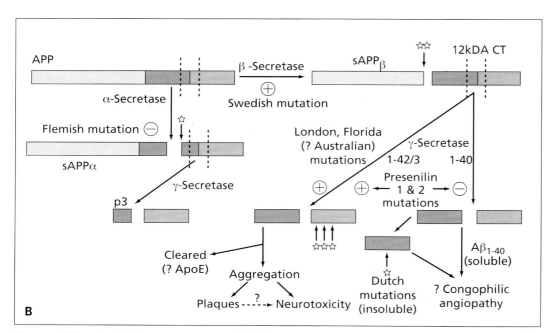

Figure 6-23. Amyloid precursor protein (APP) processing. **A,** APP is processed in neurons by three proteases, known as *secretases* [73]. Cleavage by α-secretase produces sAPPα, a peptide whose normal function remains obscure, while precluding production of the amyloidogenic peptide Aβ42. Mutations of the APP gene near the α-secretase cleavage site (Flemish and Dutch mutations) have been associated with hereditary cerebral amyloid angiopathy. In normal cells, not all APP is cleaved at the alpha site; action of β-secretase and γ-secretase produces Aβ40 and/or Aβ42. **B,** Mutations near the β (Swedish mutation) or γ (London, Florida, and Australian mutations) cleavage sites are associated with familial Alzheimer's disease (AD), presumably because of altered APP proteolysis. Aβ42 is relatively insoluble and becomes the major component of senile plaques, primarily as diffuse plaques. Aβ40 is incorporated in mature plaques and is the chief form of Aβ in amyloid-laden vessel walls [74].

The relationship between neurofibrillary and amyloid pathology in AD has not yet been fully explained. The specificity of plaques for AD, the alterations in amyloid metabolism that arise from mutations of the APP and presenilin genes, and data from the transgenic mouse model have focused attention on amyloid deposition as the inciting event [75], while neurofibrillary tangles (NFTs) mark dysfunctional neural systems that correlate with cognitive manifestations of the disease.

(Continued on next page)

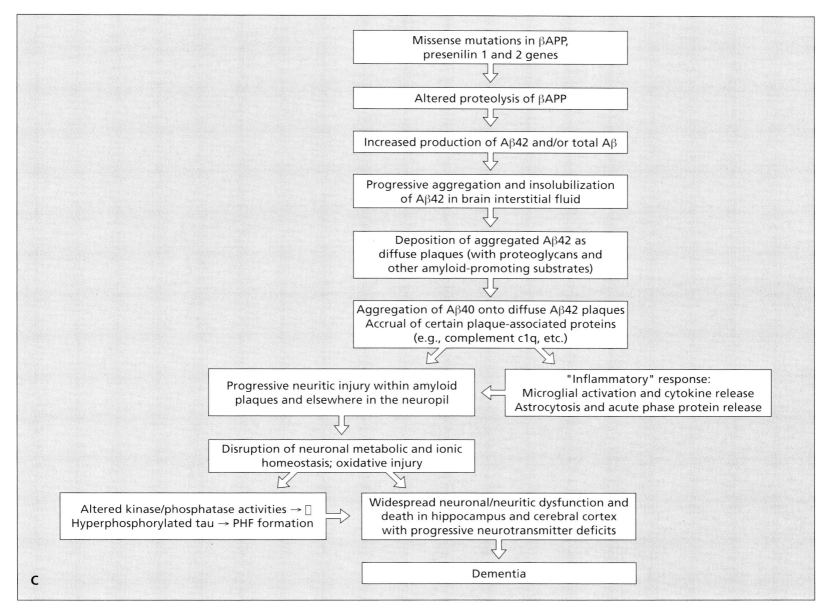

Figure 6-23. *(Continued)* **C,** The amyloid cascade hypothesis of Alzheimer pathogenesis suggests that altered amyloidogenesis leads to neurotoxicity, characterized by astrogliosis, activation of microglia, and the appearance of dystrophic neurites. A cascade of events follows that culminates in hyperphosphorylation of tau, NFT formation, and, ultimately, neural degeneration. (Panels A and B *adapted from* Storey and colleague [73]; Panel C *adapted from* Selkoe [75].)

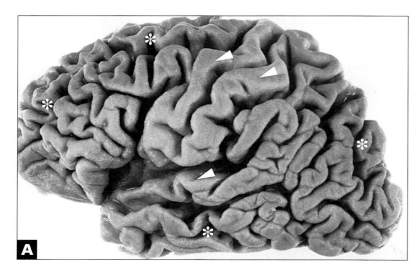

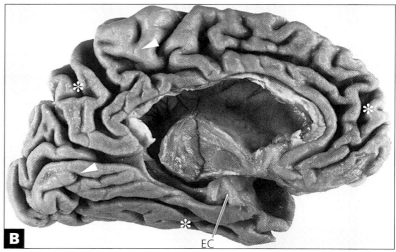

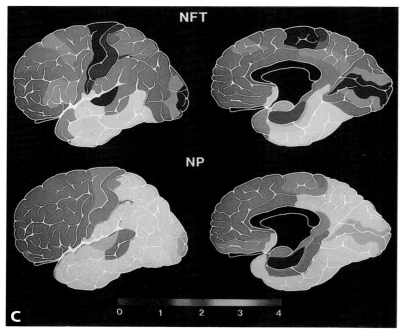

Figure 6-24. Gross pathologic specimen of a brain with Alzheimer's disease (AD). The meninges have been stripped from the lateral (**A**) and the mesial (**B**) surfaces of the cerebrum to reveal more clearly the pattern of atrophy in AD. Although all lobes are affected, the degree of atrophy is not homogeneous. The entorhinal cortex (EC), overlying the uncus, has a granular appearance, reflecting the devastation of the cellular islands in layer II. The frontal, parietal, and inferotemporal association cortices are highly atrophic (*asterisks*). In contrast, the primary sensorimotor areas (calcarine region, Heschl's gyri, precentral and postcentral gyri, and paracentral lobule (*arrowheads*) are relatively spared. Note the consistency between the gross pattern of atrophy and the topographic distribution of neurofibrillary tangles (NFTs). NFTs occur in highly characteristic locations, specifically in the limbic and association regions. **C**, Arnold and colleagues [76] surveyed the distribution of NFTs (*top*) finding the greatest numbers in the limbic periallocortex and allocortex. Tangles become progressively less numerous in the nonlimbic periallocortex, the nonprimary association cortex, and the primary association cortex. Neuritic plaques (NPs), on the other hand, have a somewhat different distribution (*bottom*) than NFTs. For example, they are relatively uncommon in the limbic periallocortex and the allocortex and they tend to be distributed more evenly throughout the cortex than are tangles. Most investigators have reported that NPs have less specific regional and laminar distributions. (Panels A and B *courtesy of* Gary Van Hoesen, PhD, Department of Anatomy, The University of Iowa; Panel C *from* Arnold and colleagues [76]; with permission.)

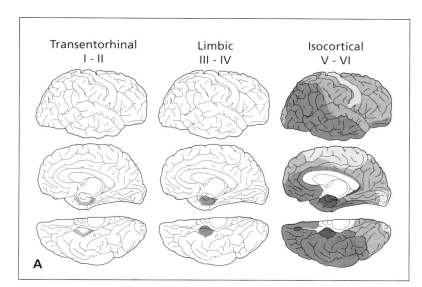

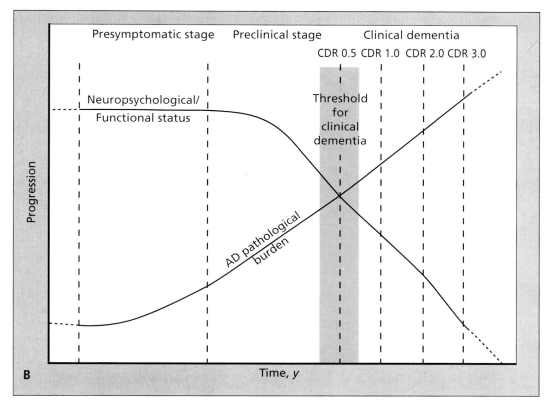

Figure 6-25. Pathologic staging of Alzheimer's disease (AD). **A,** The Braak staging system reflects the temporal order of involvement of different brain regions in AD [77]. Stages I and II (transentorhinal stages) are associated with neurofibrillary tangles (NFTs) limited to perirhinal cortex (Brodman area 35). Stages III and IV (limbic stages) are characterized by increasingly numerous NFTs in the hippocampal formation and other limbic structures. Stages V and VI (isocortical stages) are associated with tangles in neocortical regions, beginning in the inferior temporal lobe. The earliest stage of neurofibrillary pathology that has been correlated with dementia is late limbic/early isocortical pathology [78,79]. Braak stages I and II are presymptomatic and may last for years [77]. **B,** This time line for the progression of AD suggests that patients can display mild cognitive impairment years before the development of dementia [24,80]. There is a period when Alzheimer pathology accumulates, without apparent symptoms, followed by a preclinical stage during which there may be subtle alteration in cognition, progressing to mild cognitive impairment, and later to dementia [80]. Establishing the existence and duration of the presymptomatic and preclinical stages are crucial elements in formulating an approach to the prevention of AD. (Panel A *adapted from* Braak and colleague [77]; Panel B *adapted from* Daffner and colleague [80].)

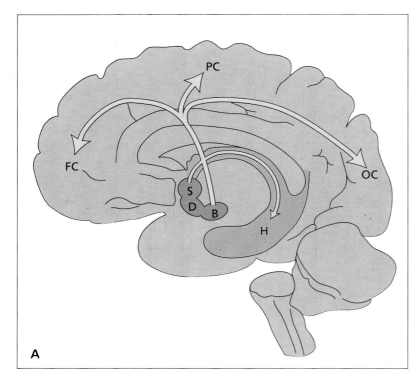

A

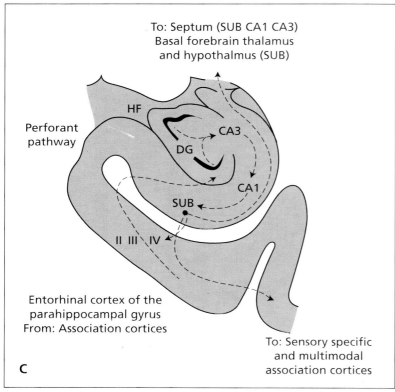

To: Septum (SUB CA1 CA3)
Basal forebrain thalamus
and hypothalmus (SUB)

HF

Perforant
pathway

CA3

DG

CA1

SUB

II III IV

Entorhinal cortex of the
parahippocampal gyrus
From: Association cortices

To: Sensory specific
and multimodal
association cortices

C

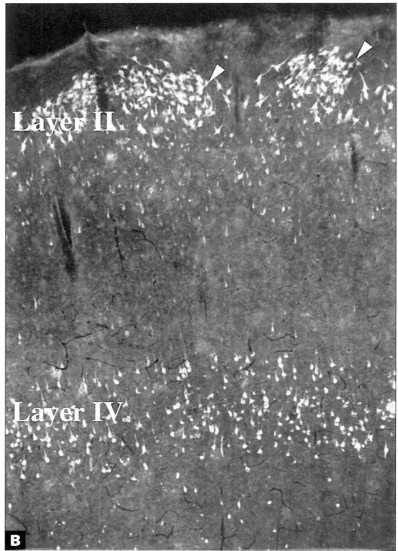

Layer II

Layer IV

B

nuclei in the basal forebrain that diffusely innervate the cortex and are thought to play an important role in attentional processes. The cholinergic hypothesis, however, overlooks the neural degeneration that occurs in other systems. Perhaps not surprisingly, replacement pharmacotherapy based on this paradigm has been only modestly successful [84,85]. More recent work on cholinergic systems in AD has emphasized an intriguing regional variation in the degree of cholinergic deficiency and the covariance of cholinergic deficiency and quantity of neurofibrillary tangles [86].

B, The second theory, cortical disconnection, was advanced by Hyman, Van Hoesen, and Damasio in 1984 [87]. The disconnection theory correlates the salient anterograde amnesia in AD with the early appearance of neurofibrillary tangles in layers II and IV of entorhinal cortex (EC).

C, The EC, which sits at the apex of the convergence of neural projections from all posterior cortices, is the only cortical portal into the hippocampus. Cells in layers II and III of EC (Panel *B, arrowheads*) give rise to the perforant pathway, the only cortical afferent pathway, and cells in layer IV receive the output of the hippocampal formation. Thus, the hippocampus, which is essential for the encoding of new declarative knowledge, may be functionally isolated by the neurofibrillary pathology in AD. B—basal nucleus of Meynert; CA—cornu ammonis; D—diagonal band of Broca; DG—dentate gyrus; FC—frontal cortex; H—hippocampus; HF—hippocampal formation; OC—occipital cortex; PC—parietal cortex; S—septal nuclei; SUB—subiculum. (Panel A *adapted from* Coyle and colleagues [83]; Panel B *courtesy of* Gary Van Hoesen, PhD, Department of Anatomy, The University of Iowa; Panel C *adapted from* Hyman and colleagues [78].)

Figure 6-26. Two theories of anterograde amnesia in Alzheimer's disease (AD). The first theory to explain memory impairment in AD was the *cholinergic hypothesis*, advanced in 1976 by Davies and Maloney and subsequently elaborated by other investigators [81–83]. Evidence showed early vulnerability of the nucleus basalis, which is the source of cortical afferent cholinergic projections. Cholinergic markers are deficient in brains afflicted with AD, and neurites surrounding senile plaques are cholinesterase-positive. Moreover, cholinergic blockade causes anterograde memory impairment in young normal human subjects. **A,** The cholinergic hypothesis postulates that amnesia in AD is caused by cholinergic deafferentation of the cortex owing to degeneration in the nucleus basalis and other cholinergic

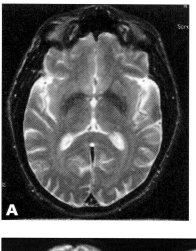
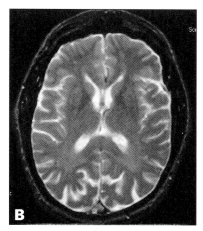
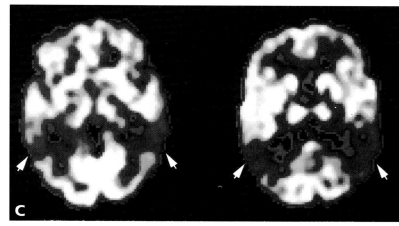

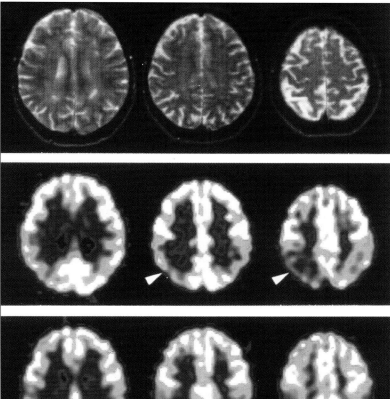

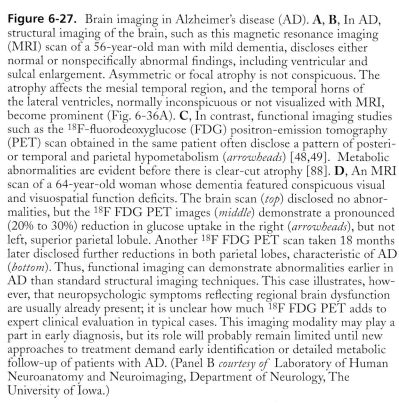

Figure 6-27. Brain imaging in Alzheimer's disease (AD). **A, B,** In AD, structural imaging of the brain, such as this magnetic resonance imaging (MRI) scan of a 56-year-old man with mild dementia, discloses either normal or nonspecifically abnormal findings, including ventricular and sulcal enlargement. Asymmetric or focal atrophy is not conspicuous. The atrophy affects the mesial temporal region, and the temporal horns of the lateral ventricles, normally inconspicuous or not visualized with MRI, become prominent (Fig. 6-36A). **C,** In contrast, functional imaging studies such as the ^{18}F-fluorodeoxyglucose (FDG) positron-emission tomography (PET) scan obtained in the same patient often disclose a pattern of posterior temporal and parietal hypometabolism (*arrowheads*) [48,49]. Metabolic abnormalities are evident before there is clear-cut atrophy [88]. **D,** An MRI scan of a 64-year-old woman whose dementia featured conspicuous visual and visuospatial function deficits. The brain scan (*top*) disclosed no abnormalities, but the ^{18}F FDG PET images (*middle*) demonstrate a pronounced (20% to 30%) reduction in glucose uptake in the right (*arrowheads*), but not left, superior parietal lobule. Another ^{18}F FDG PET scan taken 18 months later disclosed further reductions in both parietal lobes, characteristic of AD (*bottom*). Thus, functional imaging can demonstrate abnormalities earlier in AD than standard structural imaging techniques. This case illustrates, however, that neuropsychologic symptoms reflecting regional brain dysfunction are usually already present; it is unclear how much ^{18}F FDG PET adds to expert clinical evaluation in typical cases. This imaging modality may play a part in early diagnosis, but its role will probably remain limited until new approaches to treatment demand early identification or detailed metabolic follow-up of patients with AD. (Panel B *courtesy of* Laboratory of Human Neuroanatomy and Neuroimaging, Department of Neurology, The University of Iowa.)

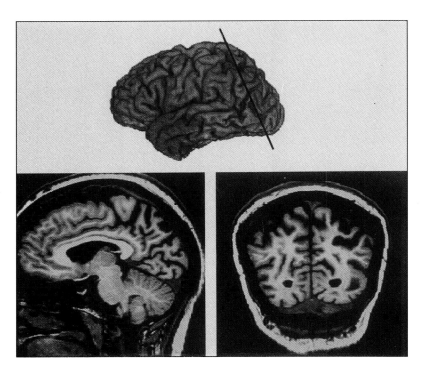

Figure 6-28. Posterior cortical atrophy. A small proportion of cases of dementia present with a salient defect of higher vision featuring visual disorientation, resembling the Balint syndrome [89,90]. These patients usually present to a neurologist after unproductive standard ophthalmic assessment. This figure shows a three-dimensional magnetic resonance image reconstruction and selected coronal sections of the brain of a patient with posterior cortical atrophy. Note the prominent widening of the parietal and lateral occipital sulci. The syndrome of posterior cortical atrophy usually turns out to be caused by Alzheimer's disease (AD), although cases of progressive subcortical gliosis and Creutzfeldt-Jakob disease have also been reported [91]. In contrast to classic AD, abundant neurofibrillary tangles are found in early visual association areas and even in primary visual cortex, with smaller numbers in the classic limbic areas. Although impairments of memory and executive function are also present, these may be relatively mild at the time of diagnosis, and the disease may pursue a relatively protracted course before severe dementia develops.

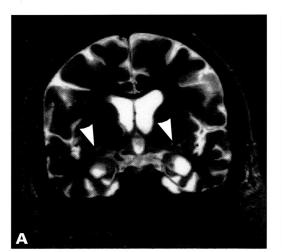
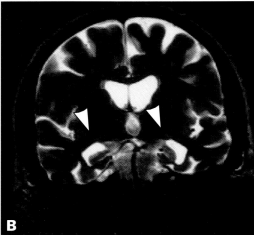
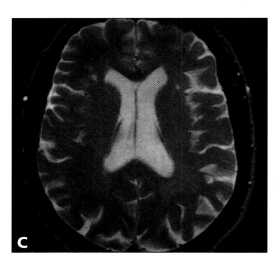

Figure 6-29. Accuracy of diagnosis of Alzheimer's disease (AD) at autopsy. Several large series indicate that autopsy confirms most (85% to 90%) of the cases of probable AD, according to National Institute of Neurological Disorders and Stroke (NINDS) criteria [92–95]. Among the unconfirmed cases, the most frequent misdiagnoses are idiopathic Parkinson's disease (about 30%); hippocampal sclerosis (15%) [96,97]; frontal lobe dementia (15%); and dementia with Lewy bodies (5%). About 10% of these cases have *no* recognized pathology. **A–C,** A magnetic resonance scan of a 60-year-old woman who presented with circumscribed anterograde memory impairment is shown here. Note the pronounced, disproportionate mesial temporal atrophy, implied by the dilation of the temporal horns of the lateral ventricles (*arrowheads*). The patient subsequently developed other cognitive impairments and more widespread atrophy and was given a diagnosis of probable AD, but neurofibrillary tangles and senile plaques were not found at autopsy. Instead, focal neuronal loss and gliosis were found in the hippocampal formation and the amygdala bilaterally, histopathologic features which are not distinctive.

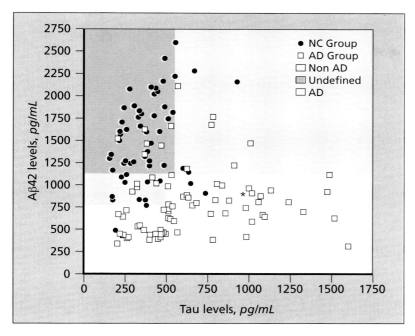

Figure 6-30. Biomarkers of Alzheimer's disease (AD). The existence of a presymptomatic phase for AD has focused attention on early diagnosis and a search for biomarkers. The ideal biomarker should detect a fundamental feature of neuropathology of AD, have sensitivity and specificity in excess of 80%, and be noninvasive, simple, and reliable [98]. Candidate biomarkers include cerebrospinal fluid (CSF) tau, Aβ42, presenilin 1, and neuronal thread protein [99,100]. A study of two CSF biomarkers illustrates the promise and uncertainties of currently available tests [99]. The study tested 216 subjects: 82 patients with probable AD, 74 patients with clinically-diagnosed non-AD degenerative conditions, and 60 normal control patients. CSF levels of Aβ42 were lower in patients with AD than in the control group, and CSF tau levels were higher. Aβ42 levels at or below 1125 pg/mL and tau levels at or above 558 pg/mL identified patients with AD with greater than 85% specificity; Aβ42 levels at or above 1125 pg/mL and tau levels at or below 558 pg/mL identified normal controls with greater than 85% specificity. The remaining patients and controls could not be classified. Of 24 very mild cases of AD (Folstein Mini-Mental State Examination score at or above 24), 15 were classified as AD by CSF markers and 3 were classified as non-AD; the remaining patients were classified as indeterminate. Although these results are encouraging, specificity was reduced when the non-AD degenerative conditions were included. Of these 74 patients, 26 were classified as having AD; these patients had cognitive impairment and an apolipoprotein ε4 frequency comparable to the AD group. Some of these patients may therefore actually have AD or a combination of AD and another degenerative condition. Assessment of the utility of these tests awaits autopsy follow-up. (*Adapted from* Galasko and colleagues [99].)

Vascular Dementias

NINDS-AIREN Criteria for the Diagnosis of Vascular Dementia

Probable vascular dementia

Dementia

Cerebrovascular disease (CVD): neurologic signs and evidence of relevant CVD by imaging

A relationship between dementia and cerebrovascular disease

Onset of dementia within 3 months of a recognized stroke

Abrupt onset or fluctuating, stepwise progression of dementia

Features supporting a diagnosis of vascular dementia

Early gait disturbance

Unsteadiness or frequent, unprovoked falls

Early urinary incontinence or other urinary symptoms

Pseudobulbar palsy

Subcortical encephalopathy: personality change, abulia, depression, pseudobulbar affect

Features against a diagnosis of vascular dementia

Early/prominent amnesia, aphasia, apraxia, or agnosia without focal imaging correlates

Absence of focal signs

Absence of cerebrovascular lesions on computed tomography or magnetic resonance imaging

Definite vascular dementia

Presence of clinical criteria for probable vascular dementia

Histopathologic evidence of cerebrovascular disease from biopsy or autopsy

Absence of neurofibrillary tangles and neuritic plaques exceeding those expected for age

Absence of other clinical or pathologic disorder capable of producing dementia

Figure 6-31. National Institute of Neurological Disorders and Stroke—Association Internationale pour la Recherche et l'Enseignement en Neurosciences (NINDS-AIREN) criteria for the diagnosis of vascular dementia (VaD). The contemporary view is that vascular conditions are the second leading cause of dementia [101]. The classic concept of VaD as a diffuse, continuous, chronic process has given way to the modern concept of a quantal and episodic process related to the accumulation of infarcts, which impact cognition because of their location as well as their volume [102–104]. The problem is still imprecisely understood, as exemplified by the lack of consensus on standard diagnostic criteria [101,105–107]. Indeed the term "vascular dementia" has been criticized on the one hand as too broad, because sundry mechanisms of disease are included, and on the other hand as too narrow, because cognitive impairment short of dementia is excluded.

Several sets of diagnostic criteria for VaD have been proposed. These criteria improve on the Hachinski score (Fig. 6-32) mainly because of the availability of neuroimaging techniques. In a series of 27 patients diagnosed with VaD by the Erkinjuntti criteria, 85% of cases were confirmed at autopsy [108,109]. Though similar, these various sets of criteria are not equivalent to one another [107]. Recognizing the valuable role that the widely accepted National Institute of Neurologic and Communicative Disorders and Stroke (NINCDS) criteria for the diagnosis of AD have played in facilitating research into that entity, a joint task force of NINDS and AIREN published research criteria for the diagnosis of VaD in 1993 [101]. Note that the criteria call for evidence of cerebrovascular disease by both imaging and neurologic signs; neuroimaging studies alone are not sufficient. These criteria have yet to be evaluated thoroughly. Although studies must be interpreted cautiously because of the lack of standard criteria, one study found that patients hospitalized for a first ischemic stroke have a ninefold relative risk of developing dementia in the subsequent year 8.4 cases/100 per year, with the relative risk falling to twofold thereafter [110–111]. The relative risk increases steeply with the age of the patient. The prevalence of dementia 3 months after a first stroke is 15% to 30%. One third of these patients were diagnosed with pre-existing AD, one third was diagnosed with dementia owing to cumulative strokes, and one third was diagnosed with dementia caused by a large or strategically located infarct. The establishment of standard criteria for diagnosis will no doubt permit and encourage many more such studies in this important area. Criteria such as these will also facilitate systematic work on the treatment of VaD. As yet, no convincing studies have demonstrated successful modification of the natural history of VaD by any treatment, once cerebral vasculitis and cerebral vascular malformations are excluded.

The Hachinski Ischemic Score

Abrupt onset	2
Stepwise deterioration	1
Fluctuating course	2
Nocturnal confusion	1
Preservation of personality	1
Depression	1
Somatic complaints	1
Emotional incontinence	1
History/presence of hypertension	1
History of strokes	2
Evidence of atherosclerosis	1
Focal neurologic symptoms	2
Focal neurologic signs	2

Figure 6-32. Hachinski Ischemic Score. The Hachinski Ischemic Score is a clinical system aimed at distinguishing between vascular dementia (VaD) and Alzheimer's disease (AD) and other degenerative dementias [112,113]. VaD is recognized clinically by a stroke-like course of illness and the presence of atherosclerotic vascular disease, hypertension, and signs of focal brain damage. The most useful signs are those indicating asymmetric dysfunction in primary motor and sensory regions, regions that are commonly affected by infarcts but not by AD and most other degenerative dementias. Before the advent of computer-assisted tomography, these clinical criteria were formalized in the Hachinski Ischemic Score. On this scale, a score of more than 7 points suggests a diagnosis of VaD; less than 4, AD. Several studies have investigated the efficacy of this score in diagnosis [114,115]. Sensitivity and specificity are estimated at 70% to 80%. The ischemic score does not help to distinguish cases of VaD from cases with combined vascular and degenerative disorders. When neuroimaging is included in the evaluation of dementia, sensitivity improves, but the detection of cases of combined VaD and AD remains challenging. Such cases of "mixed dementia" are approximately as common as pure VaD.

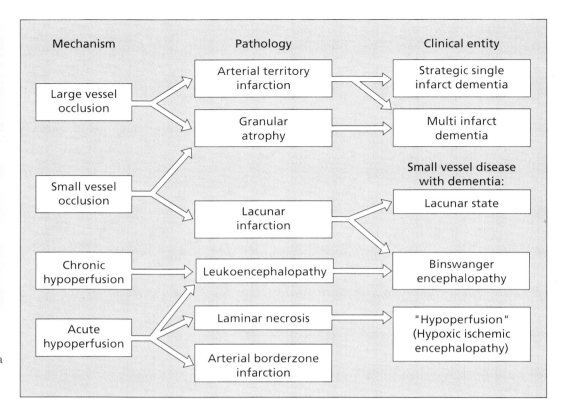

Figure 6-33. Subtypes of ischemic vascular dementia (VaD). The National Institute of Neurological Disorders and Stroke—Association Internationale pour la Recherche et l'Enseignement en Neurosciences (NINDS-AIREN) workshop recognized four subtypes of ischemic VaD as well as hemorrhagic dementia [101]. The relationships between the ischemic subtypes, the underlying mechanisms of injury, and their histopathologic correlates are illustrated.

Although one or a few strategic infarcts may cause dementia, VaD commonly results from an accumulation of infarcts. These infarcts may affect the territories of large cerebral vessels, a condition referred to as "multi-infarct dementia." Large vessel thromboembolism, however, may not be the dominant mechanism of VaD. A more common scenario is cumulative infarction of the territories of small penetrating arterioles. Such small vessel infarcts tend to complicate poorly controlled hypertension and diabetes. A less frequent presentation of VaD is Binswanger's encephalopathy, which is associated with diffuse leukoencephalopathy and ventriculomegaly and is thought to occur by an ischemic mechanism. Other cerebrovascular mechanisms leading to dementia are hypoxic-ischemic encephalopathy and cerebral hemorrhage.

The natural history of VaD is difficult to summarize, because the precise mechanisms of infarction and the topographic pattern of infarct accumulation vary among cases. The rate of progression is often uneven, punctuated by datable events, rebounds, and fluctuations [116]. The overall course in many cases, however, may be more rapid than that of AD. Ischemic VaD may have predominantly "subcortical" features: impaired executive function, impaired speed of thought, depression, and apathy. Spotty or mild impairment of classic "cortical" faculties, such as language, praxis, and visuospatial function, is the rule. Gait impairment and urinary incontinence are common.

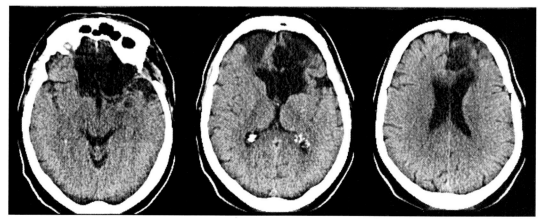

Figure 6-34. Computed tomography (CT) scans of a 47-year-old man with a history of "strategic infarct" dementia. Single-stroke vascular dementia may result from strategically placed infarcts in the dominant posterior cerebral artery territory, bilateral or dominant anterior cerebral artery territory, bilateral or dominant thalamus, or basal forebrain. This patient sustained a subarachnoid hemorrhage caused by the rupture of an anterior communicating artery aneurysm. Delayed ischemic damage ensued in the territories of the anterior cerebral arteries. One year after the event, the patient had marked defects in memory and executive control, including poor behavioral organization, initiation, altered social behavior, and impaired insight. He improved slowly but incompletely; 6 years after the event, impairments of verbal memory and verbal associative fluency persisted, but other cognitive abilities were normal. (*Courtesy of* Laboratory of Human Neuroanatomy and Neuroimaging, Department of Neurology, The University of Iowa.)

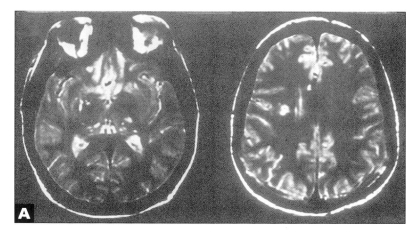

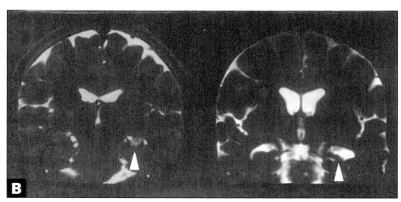

Figure 6-35. Dementia caused by small-vessel cerebrovascular disease. **A,** Magnetic resonance images of a 39-year-old man with type I diabetes mellitus who was admitted with complaints of subjective weakness of the left limbs and problems with gait and memory. Several small infarcts are present in the right corona radiata, the left hippocampal formation, and, most notably, in the territories supplied by penetrating arterioles: thalamus, basal ganglia, and basis pontis. Severe dementia was present, with maximal deficits in verbal memory, attention, and expressive language. Marked slowing of speech and thought were evident. Right limb ataxia and left extensor plantar response were also present. Carotid duplex ultrasonography and echocardiography were unremarkable. **B,** Two years later, his neuropsychologic profile was stable. Note the interim atrophy of the left hippocampal formation (*arrowheads*). Such accumulation of infarcts in the territories of small cerebral vessels is probably the most common mechanism of vascular dementia.

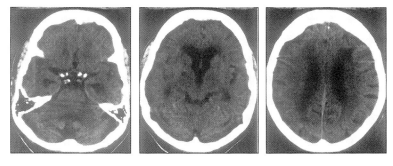

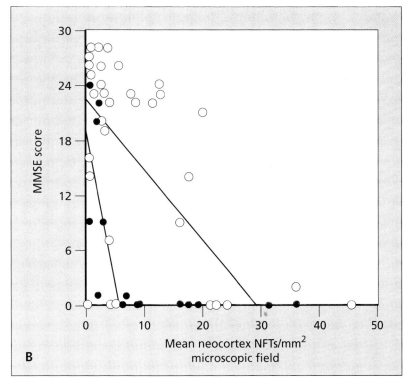

Figure 6-36. Mixed Alzheimer's disease (AD) and vascular dementia (VaD). **A,** Noncontrast computed tomography (CT) scans of an 84-year-old woman with progressive amnesic dementia who met the National Institute of Neurological Disorders and Stroke—Alzheimer's Disease and Related Disability Association (NINDS-ADRDA) criteria for probable AD. The CT scans disclosed low periventricular absorption and a few focal deep gray matter lacunar infarcts, indicating the presence of significant small vessel cerebrovascular disease, and severe mesial temporal atrophy consistent with AD. Mixed pathology is common in dementia, with mixed Alzheimer and small vessel VaD constituting one of the most important overlaps. The presence of infarcts appears to increase the severity of the associated cognitive impairment [117,118]. **B,** Data expressing the relationship between the number of neurofibrillary tangles (NFTs) in the neocortex and the Folstein Mini-Mental State Examination (MMSE) score for patients with deep lacunar infarcts (closed circles, thick regression line) and for patients without such infarcts (open circles, thin regression line). All patients met the neuropathologic criteria for AD. Note that the presence of a small vessel infarcts was associated with markedly lower MMSE scores, for any degree of neurofibrillary pathology. (Panel B *adapted from* Snowdon and colleagues [117].)

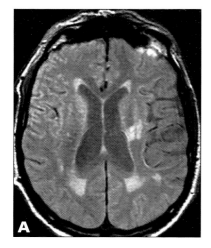 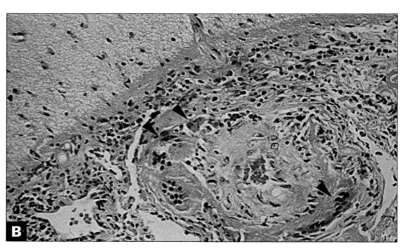 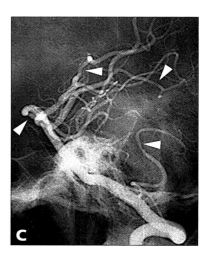

Figure 6-37. Dementia caused by cerebral vasculitis. **A**, Cranial computed tomography scan of a patient with granulomatous angiitis of the central nervous system [119], who presented with subacute dementia. The cerebral arteriogram was normal. **B**, However, brain and lepto-meningeal biopsy specimens confirmed the presence of a mononuclear infiltrate in the cortical and meningeal vessels, with multinucleated giant cells (*arrowheads*), prominent eosinophilia, and obliteration of small vascular lumina. **C**, Cerebral angiogram in a similar case displays diagnostic multi-segmental narrowing of branches of the posterior cerebral arteries (*arrowheads*). Primary angiitis of the central nervous system is uncommon, but it frequently enters the differential diagnosis of subacute dementia because it is amenable to treatment [119]. (Panel B *courtesy of* Lee Reed, MD, Department of Pathology, The University of Iowa.)

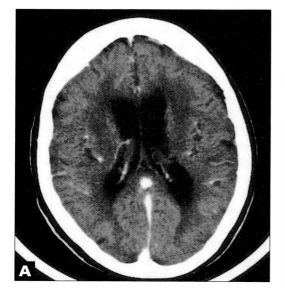 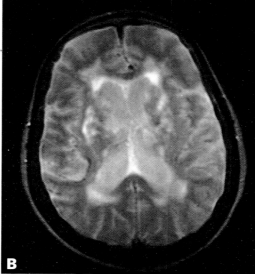 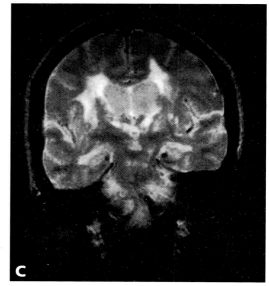

Figure 6-38. Binswanger's encephalopathy. Computed tomography scan (**A**) and cranial magnetic resonance scans (**B, C**) of a 61-year-old woman with suspected Binswanger's encephalopathy, who presented with hypertension, gait deterioration of frontal type, pseudobulbar palsy, pseudobulbar affect, and urinary incontinence. Note ventricular enlargement, periventricular low X-ray absorption, patchy but generally symmetric involvement of white matter, and numerous lacunar infarcts. Binswanger's encephalopathy [120,121] is associated with progressive leukoencephalopathy caused by patchy, multifocal demyelination and infarction in the cerebral white matter, especially in periarteriolar zones. The lateral ventricles are always enlarged and the small penetrating arteries are always abnormal, with thickened walls, fibrous intimal proliferation, adventitial fibrosis, and splitting of the internal elastic membrane. In some cases, the vessels reveal prominent amyloid deposits (congophilic amyloid angiopathy). Although ischemia has been proposed as an explanation of leukoencephalopathy, the precise mechanism by which this occurs remains elusive. The main clinical features are hypertension, "subcortical" dementia, frontal gait disturbance, pseudobulbar signs, and urinary incontinence—a constellation reminiscent of normal pressure hydrocephalus, which often enters the differential diagnosis.

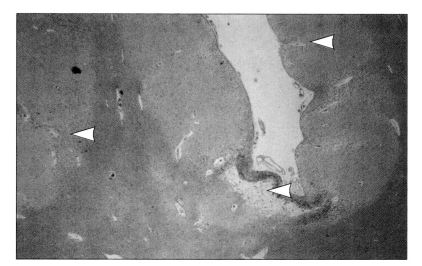

Figure 6-39. Granular cortical atrophy. Granular cortical atrophy is an unusual pattern of multiple foci of infarction (*arrowheads*) located entirely in the cerebral cortex, thought to be associated with occlusion or embolization of small leptomeningeal vessels. Multifocal small infarcts affect the cortex and spare the underlying white matter (trichrome stain). (*Courtesy of* Lee Reed, MD, Department of Pathology, The University of Iowa.)

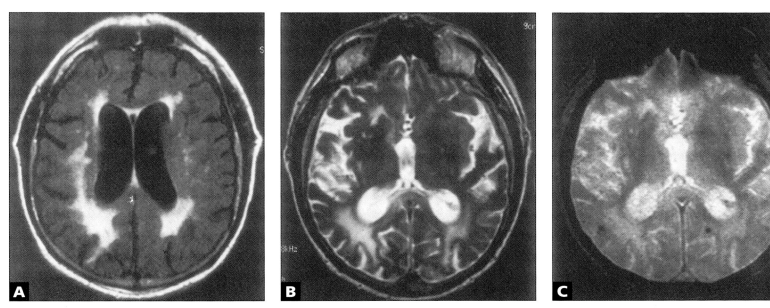

Figure 6-40. Cerebral amyloid angiopathy (CAA). CAA is present in about 85% of patients with Alzheimer disease, and is of severe degree in about 25% [72]. Conversely, most cases of CAA also have parenchymal amyloid deposition and other pathology typical of Alzheimer's disease. In CAA, Aβ is deposited in the walls of cortical and meningeal vessels, disrupting the normal architecture of the vessels. Amyloid-laden vessels are prone to rupture, causing cerebral lobar hemorrhage. Small, covert petechial cortical hemorrhages occur more often. Amyloid angiopathy is also associated with cortical microinfarcts (Fig. 6-39) and diffuse leukoencephalopathy, presumably related to chronic white matter ischemia [123]. **A, B,** Fluid-attenuated inversion recovery (FLAIR) and T2-weighted images may display small vessel territory signal change or diffuse leukoencephalopathy. **C,** The presence of small foci of signal dropout on T2* (gradient echo)-weighted images (*arrowheads*), caused by residual hemosiderin from previous cortical petechial hemorrhage, is more useful in diagnosing CAA [122].

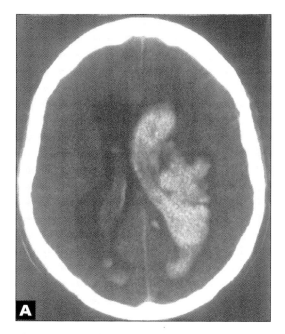 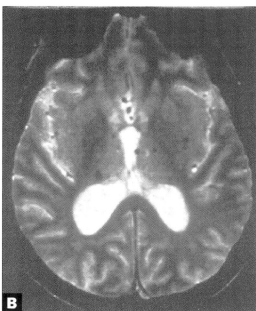 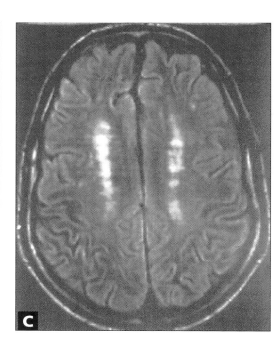

Figure 6-41. Typical neuroimaging findings in cerebral autosomal dominant arteriopathy with subcortical infarcts and leukoencephalopathy (CADASIL). **A,** Proton density-weighted magnetic resonance image showing deep white matter ischemic change. **B,** Gradient echo T2*-weighted image showing punctate signal dropout caused by prior deep hemorrhages. **C,** Cranial computed tomography scan showing multifocal subcortical hemorrhage. This condition is a non-amyloid, non-atherosclerotic microangiopathy that occurs as an autosomal dominant condition, due to a mutation of the Notch 3 gene. The mean age of onset is about 45, though many patients have prodromal migrainous episodes before then. Subcortical transient ischemic attacks and strokes occur; gait disturbance, urinary incontinence, and pseudobulbar palsy are common. About 30% of patients exhibit dementia. A systemic disease, CADASIL can be diagnosed by skin biopsy, although genetic testing is more straightforward [124,125].

Degenerative Dementias of Non-Alzheimer's Type

Principal Causes of Non-Alzheimer's Degenerative Dementia

Frontotemporal lobar degeneration
 Pick's disease
 Corticobasal degeneration
 Dementia lacking distinctive histopathologic features
 Frontotemporal dementia with parkinsonism linked to
   chromosome 17
Degenerative conditions with parkinsonism
 Dementia with Lewy bodies
 Idiopathic Parkinson's disease
 Progressive supranuclear palsy
 Corticobasal degeneration
Spongiform encephalopathies
 Creutzfeldt-Jakob disease

Figure 6-42. Principal classes of non-Alzheimer's degenerative dementia. A significant number of cases of degenerative dementia are atypical by virtue of the unusual profile of cognitive impairment, the presence of motor signs, or the rapid rate of decline. Many such cases, along with 10% to 15% of typical cases (those that meet National Institute of Neurological and Communicative Disorders and Stroke—Alzheimer's Disease and Related Disorders Association [NINCDS-ADRDA] criteria for probable Alzheimer's disease) are associated with non-Alzheimer's histopathologic features. Diagnostically, such cases are challenging, and surprises at autopsy are not infrequent.

Frontotemporal Dementia

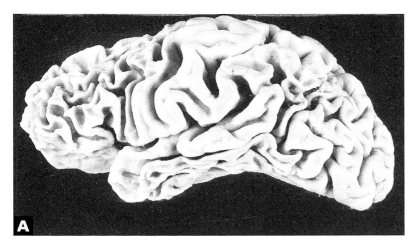

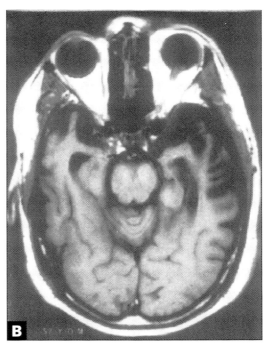

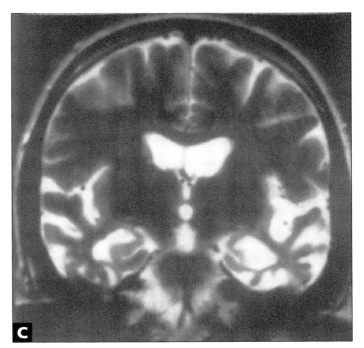

Figure 6-43. Gross pathologic specimen and magnetic resonance imaging (MRI) scans of the brain in frontotemporal lobar degeneration. **A,** In frontotemporal lobar degeneration, cerebral atrophy is more striking than that seen in Alzheimer's disease (AD) (compare to Fig. 6-24A). A pattern of *lobar atrophy* involving both cortex and subjacent white matter involves the frontal and anterior temporal lobes. Note the "knife-edge" gyri (ulegyria) in these regions and the abrupt transition between mildly and severely involved sectors (*eg,* between the anterior and posterior segments of the superior temporal gyrus). These findings differ from those in AD, and since they may also be apparent on MRI, they are useful in differential diagnosis. Degenerative diseases of the nervous system usually display an early predilection for certain neural structures, and most dementias also have a focus of maximal neuropsychologic impairment in their early stages. In early AD, for example, anterograde amnesia is the leading impairment; other forms of cognitive deterioration follow, reflecting the involvement of many sectors of the brain. In cases of frontotemporal lobar degeneration, impairments of executive function are quite prominent (frontotemporal dementia). The process begins in the frontal lobes, asymmetrically, and then progresses to the opposite side and the temporal regions (Fig. 6-13B). **B, C,** Frontotemporal lobar degeneration may also begin in the temporal region, again often asymmetrically. If the disease affects the dominant temporal lobe first, the presentation is one of progressive aphasia without dementia (or with late dementia). Other atypical profiles of dementia include progressive visuospatial impairment (Fig. 6-28) and progressive apraxia (Fig. 6-50). The clinical manifestations of lobar atrophy are determined by the brain regions affected. The "anterior" syndromes (*ie,* those involving the frontal and temporal lobes: frontotemporal dementia, progressive aphasia) usually have histopathologic findings compatible with Pick's disease, ballooned neurons without Pick bodies, or nonspecific changes such as superficial spongiosis and cortical gliosis. Only rarely are these presentations due to AD, and almost never to a secondary medical cause. By contrast, the posterior cortical atrophy syndrome is usually a variant presentation of AD (see Fig. 6-28) [89,90]. Progressive apraxia with extrapyramidal signs is usually caused by corticobasal degeneration. (*Courtesy of* Gary Van Hoesen, PhD, Department of Anatomy, The University of Iowa.)

Clinical Criteria for Frontotemporal Dementia

Core diagnostic features

Insidious and slowly progressive behavior disorder
  Early loss of personal and social awareness
  Disinhibition, impulsivity, utilization behavior, hyperorality
  Mental rigidity and inflexibility
  Stereotyped and perseverative behavior
  Distractibility, motor impersistence
Affective symptoms
  Depression, anxiety, excessive sentimentality, hypochondriasis,
    bizarre somatic preoccupation, emotional unconcern,
    inertia, aspontaneity
Speech disorder
  Progressive reduction in speech; late mutism
  Stereotypy, echolalia and perserveration
Preserved spatial orientation and praxis

Physical signs
  Early primitive reflexes
  Early incontinence
  Late akinesia, rigidity, tremor
  Low and labile blood pressure
Investigations
  Normal electroencephalogram
  Brain imaging: predominant frontal and/or anterior
    temporal abnormality
  Neuropsychology: profound defect on tests of executive
    function

Features supporting diagnosis of frontotemporal dementia

Onset before age 65
Family history of similar disorder in a first-degree relative
Signs of motor neuron disease

Features against diagnosis of frontotemporal dementia

Abrupt onset, ictal events
Head trauma related to onset
Early severe amnesia, spatial disorientation, or apraxia
Myoclonus, cerebellar ataxia, choreoathetosis
Early, severe, pathologic electroencephalogram

Figure 6-44. Clinical manifestations of frontotemporal dementia. **A,** Summary of the consensus clinical criteria for the diagnosis of frontotemporal dementia published by the Lund and Manchester centers [126,127]. Frontotemporal dementia is the syndrome of primary degenerative dementia with an early and prominent disorder of executive function and social behavior. Patients with pathologic diagnoses of Pick's disease, frontal lobe degen- eration [128], and motor neuron disease [129] may present with this syndrome. In the Manchester series of 150 patients, the usual age at onset was 45 to 60 years; no difference in incidence occurred between men and women. The median duration of illness was 8 years. About 40% of the patients had a first-degree relative with dementia, mostly in dominant kindreds [130].

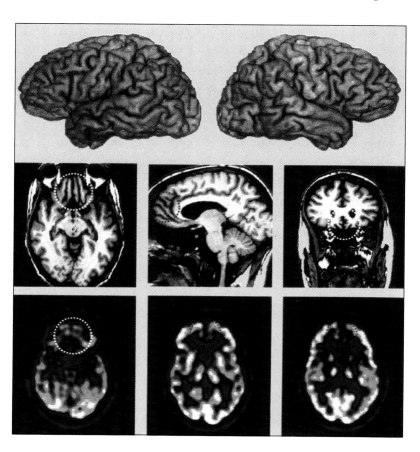

Figure 6-45. Early frontotemporal dementia. T1-weighted magnetic resonance imaging and ^{18}F fluorodeoxyglucose positron-emission tomography (FDG PET) scans of a 52-year-old man with a two-year history of decline in social competence, progressive apathy, and poor insight. His Mini-Mental State Examination score was 29. Atrophy is more or less limited to the orbitofrontal (*yellow circles*) and medial prefrontal regions (*green circles*). Patients with frontotemporal dementia at such an early stage, when personality change, declining interpersonal skills, or affective disturbances dominate, are frequently not recognized to have a neurological condition.

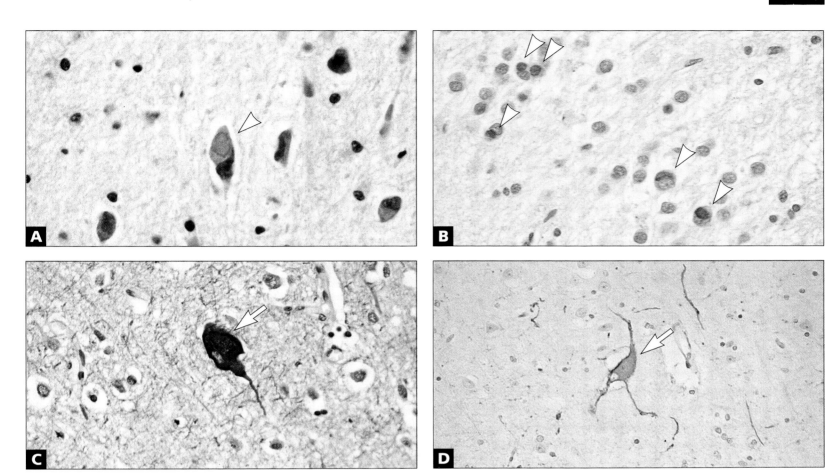

Figure 6-46. Histopathologic specimens of Pick's disease [131]. The pathognomonic inclusions known as Pick bodies (*arrowheads*) occur in neurons of the cerebral cortex, concentrating in cortical layer II (**A,** hematoxylin and eosin stain) and in the dentate gyrus of the hippocampus (**B,** tau-2 stain, counterstained with Nissl). They are argyrophilic cytoplasmic inclusions composed of straight filaments. Pale, ballooned neurons (*arrows*), sometimes called "Pick cells" (**C,** stained with SMI-31 monoclonal antibody and **D,** stained with crystallin) are also seen, typically in the frontal lobes. Note the eccentric nuclei and the large size of these neurons relative to their neighbors.

Intense reactive astrocytosis is found in both the cortex and the white matter.

Not all cases of dementia with prominent defects in executive function share all these histopathologic features, and no criteria are universally accepted for the diagnosis. Some authors reserve the diagnosis "Pick's disease" for those cases in which all of the classic features including Pick bodies, are found. In this conservative scheme, as few as 10% of patients presenting with the syndrome of frontotemporal dementia would be classified as having Pick's disease. (*Courtesy of* Lee Reed, MD, Department of Pathology, The University of Iowa.)

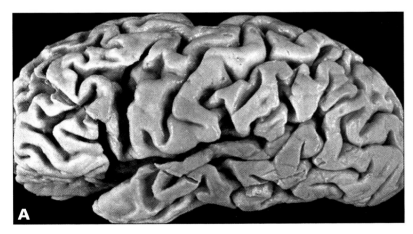
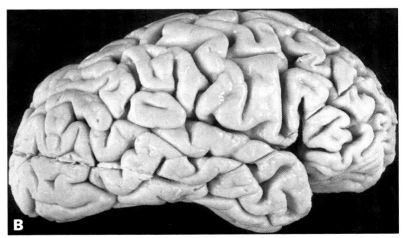

Figure 6-47. Progressive nonfluent aphasia (PNFA). Pathologic specimens of the left (**A**) and right (**B**) hemispheres of the brain of a patient with progressive nonfluent aphasia. Note the asymmetric temporal and perisylvian atrophy, affecting mainly the left hemisphere. In the initial report of Pick's disease in 1892, Arnold Pick concluded that "a more or less circumscribed type of aphasia could result from a single circumscribed atrophic process." Contemporary interest in this phenomenon began in 1982, with Mesulam's report of six cases of slowly progressive language disorder with preserved intellect, visually-mediated abilities, and insight [132]. Although dementia

with disproportionate aphasia occurs fairly frequently, PNFA is rare. The Manchester group estimates the relative frequencies of progressive aphasia and dementia of Alzheimer's type at a ratio of 1 to 40 (versus a ratio of 1 to 5 for frontotemporal dementia and dementia of Alzheimer's type) [133]. The early disturbance is often characterized by anomia, word-finding difficulties in running speech, dysfluency, and frustration [134]. As the disease progresses, apraxia is common, and depression is likely. Other cognitive deficits eventually emerge, but perhaps not always.

(Continued on next page)

C. Criteria for Progressive Nonfluent Aphasia

Core features
    Insidious onset, gradual progression
    Nonfluent spontaneous speech with agrammatism
    Phonemic paraphasia, or anomia
 Supportive features
  Speech and language
    Stuttering or oral apraxia
    Impaired recognition
    Alexia, agraphia
    Early preservation of word meaning
    Late mutism
  Behavior
    Early preservation of social skills
    Later behavioral changes similar to FTD
  Physical signs
    Late contralateral primitive reflexes, akinesia, rigidity
      and tremor
  Investigations
    Neuropsychology: nonfluent aphasia in the absence of
      severe amnesia, or perceptuospatial disorder
    EEG: normal or minor asymmetric slowing
    Imaging: asymmetric abnormality of dominant hemi-
      sphere

Figure 6-47. *(Continued)* **C**, Criteria for the diagnosis of progressive nonfluent aphasia [127]. (Panels A and B *courtesy of* Gary Van Hoesen, PhD, Department of Anatomy, the University of Iowa.)

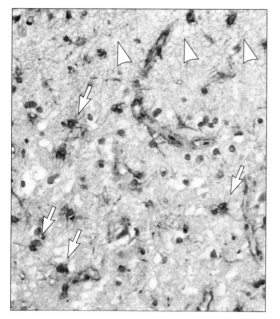

Figure 6-48. Dementia lacking distinctive histopathology (DLDH). Histopathologic section (glial fibrillary acid protein [GFAP] stain) of the frontal lobe cortex of a patient with progressive nonfluent aphasia. The only salient microscopic changes are spongiosis in the superficial layers (*arrowheads*), abundant reactive astrocytes (*arrows*), and neuronal loss. These findings are all nonspecific [135]. Several variants of DLDH have been described: a cortical type (the most important variant, corresponding to Brun's frontal lobe degeneration [128]; a thalamostriate type; a motor neuronopathy type; and a leukogliotic type, also known as progressive subcortical gliosis. Some cases of DLDH are familial, but their genetic basis remains obscure. The pathologic picture sometimes varies among members of the same family. Diverse genetic and pathophysiologic mechanisms will likely be found responsible for DLDH [136–138]. (*Courtesy of* Lee Reed, MD, Department of Pathology, The University of Iowa.)

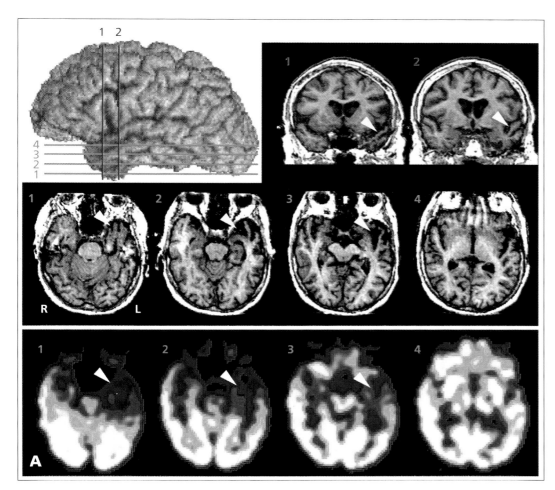

Figure 6-49. Primary progressive aphasia and semantic dementia. **A**, Magnetic resonance images (*top tiers*) and coregistered ^{18}F-fluorodeoxyglucose positron-emission tomograms (*bottom tier*) of the brain of a 73-year-old woman with progressive anomic aphasia and visual agnosia. Note the circumscribed atrophy of the left temporal and perisylvian areas (*arrowheads*) and the accompanying hypometabolism in these regions. The bilateral posterior temporoparietal metabolic deficits characteristic of Alzheimer's disease are absent. This less common variant of progressive aphasia, *semantic dementia*, is described in Panel B [139,140].

In most cases, the pathologic findings are those of Pick's disease (Fig. 6-46), Pick-spectrum pathology lacking Pick bodies, or nonspecific histopathologic findings characterized by neuronal loss, cortical gliosis, and spongiform change in the superficial cortical layers. (Panel A *courtesy of* Laboratory of Human Neuroanatomy and Neuroimaging, Department of Neurology, The University of Iowa.)

B. Core Features of Semantic Dementia

Insidious onset, gradual progression
Language disorder characterized by
  Progressive fluent empty spontaneous speech
  Loss of word meaning, manifest by impaired naming and comprehension
  Semantic paraphasias
      and/or
Perceptual disorder, characterized by
  Prosopagnosia *and/or*
  Associative agnosia
Preserved perceptual matching and drawing reproduction
Preserved single word repetition
Preserved ability to read aloud and write to dictation orthographically regular words
Supportive features
  Speech and language
    Press of speech
    Idiosyncratic word usage
    Absence of phonemic paraphasias
    Surface dyslexia and dysgraphia
    Preserved calculation
  Behavior
    Loss of sympathy and empathy
    Narrowed preoccupations
    Stinginess
  Physical signs
    Absent or late primitive reflexes
    Akinesia, rigidity, tremor
  Investigations
    Neuropsychology: profound semantic loss, preserve phonology and syntax, elementary perceptual processing, spatial skills, and memory
    EEG: normal
    Imaging: predominant anterior temporal abnormality

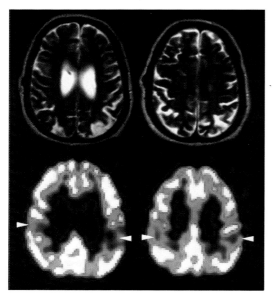

Figure 6-50. Progressive apraxia. Progressive apraxia is a primary dementia with prominent and progressive apraxia, which is associated with circumscribed atrophy of the parietal lobes. As is the case with primary progressive aphasia, progressive apraxia can remain a relatively focal syndrome for several years before other cognitive deficits become severe. In the magnetic resonance imaging (*top tier*) and positron-emission tomography (*bottom tier*) scans of the brain of a patient with progressive apraxia, note the asymmetric widening of parietal sulci, worse on the left side of the brain. In progressive apraxia, unlike standard Alzheimer's disease, the atrophy and reductions also prominently involve the postcentral gyrus, accounting for the cortical sensory loss that frequently accompanies these cases. Progressive apraxia without extrapyramidal signs, which is rare, has been associated with both Alzheimer's and Pick's diseases. It may be accompanied by some degree of progressive aphasia. More often, progressive apraxia occurs as a cardinal feature of corticobasal degeneration (CBD), together with asymmetric parkinsonism (poorly responsive to levodopa), action myoclonus, alien limb phenomena, and cortical sensory loss [141–143]. (*Courtesy of* Laboratory of Human Neuroanatomy and Neuroimaging, Department of Neurology, The University of Iowa.)

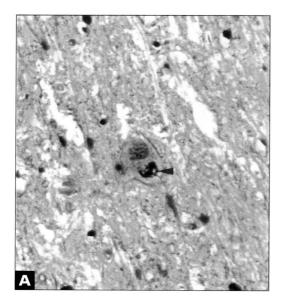

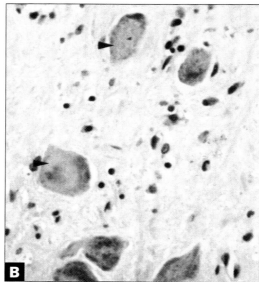

Figure 6-51. Tauopathies. **A**, Globose neurofibrillary tangle (NFT) (*arrowhead*) in a neuron in the globus pallidus of a patient with progressive supranuclear palsy (Bielschowsky stain). **B**, Corticobasal body in the substantia nigra of a patient with corticobasal degeneration (hematoxylin and eosin stain). Both these inclusion bodies are composed of microtubule-associated protein tau, as are Pick bodies and NFTs of Alzheimer's disease (AD). The central role of tau in many forms of neurodegeneration became clear with the discovery of dominant kindreds with point mutations in the tau gene who presented with frontotemporal dementia with parkinsonism linked to chromosome 17 (FTDP-17) [144,145]. Symptoms of FTDP-17 are varying degrees of parkinsonism, executive dysfunction, and subcortical dementia, together with tau deposition in neural tissue.

(*Continued on next page*)

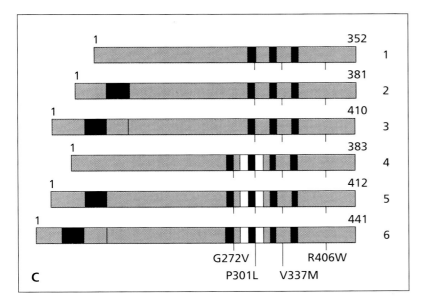

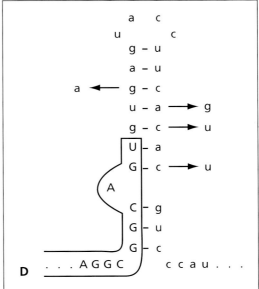

Figure 6-51. *(Continued)* **C,** The tau transcript is differentially spliced into six tau isoforms. The resulting peptides have 3 or 4 microtubule binding domains depending on whether exon 10 is spliced in or out. **D,** In most cases of FTDP-17, mutations in the stem-loop structure flanking exon 10 prevent the production of 4-repeat isoforms and alter the normal stoichiometry of 3- to 4-repeat tau. Tau deposits in FTDP-17 and Pick bodies are composed of 3-repeat tau; corticobasal bodies and globose tangles are composed of 4-repeat tau. NFTs in AD are composed of both 3- and 4-

repeat tau. Many genetic and environmental factors can lead to a final common pathway of tau-based neurodegeneration, involving hyperphosphorylation of tau, disruption of microtubule function, and, ultimately, neuronal dysfunction. The topographic distribution of these effects and the clinical phenotype appear to be influenced heavily by the particular tau mutation, normal polymorphism of tau, stoichiometry of tau isoforms, and other factors [146–148]. (Panel C *adapted from* Spillanti and colleague [146].)

Dementia with Lewy Bodies

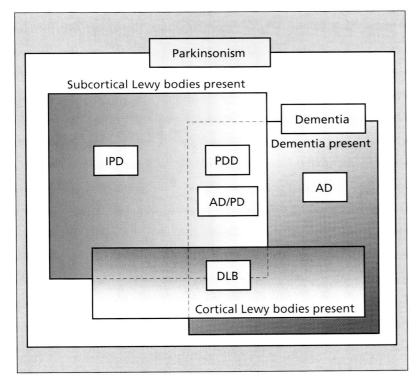

Figure 6-52. Dementia with parkinsonism. An important class of non-Alzheimer's degenerative dementias is that in which subcortical nuclei are affected and extrapyramidal motor signs are a prominent feature. The most common such disorders are idiopathic Parkinson's disease (IPD) [149–151], dementia with Lewy bodies (DLB) [27], progressive supranuclear palsy (PSP) [148], and corticobasal degeneration (CBD) [141,142]. In some cases (*eg*, IPD, PSP), the pathologic changes are mostly subcortical and the dementia has the *subcortical* pattern, characterized by slowing of thought, reduction in drive, apathy, and personality change, but not prominent amnesia, aphasia, agnosia, or apraxia [12] (Fig. 6-7). In other cases (*eg*, DLB, CBD), the cortex is involved and amnesia and apraxia are prominent.

Most cases of dementia with parkinsonism are due to IPD, Alzheimer's disease (AD), DLB, or a combination of these. This figure diagrams the relationships between these entities.

Of patients with IPD, 20% to 40% have dementia. Most cases of dementia associated with IPD are probably due to IPD itself, rather than to superimposed Alzheimer's pathology or cortical Lewy bodies. The profile is subcortical, and distinguishable in some degree from the Alzheimer's pattern.

DLB is characterized by the presence of Lewy bodies in cortical neurons. In addition, it is usually associated with subcortical Lewy bodies and some degree of parkinsonism that is generally responsive to levodopa. Cortical Lewy bodies can occur concurrently with neurofibrillary tangles (NFTs) and senile plaques (SPs), which may or may not be present in sufficient quantity to allow a pathologic diagnosis of AD. The overlap of pathologic features of cortical Lewy body disease with AD has led to a confusing set of terms, including senile dementia of Lewy body type (SDLT), in which cortical Lewy bodies coexist with SPs and NFTs but are not numerous enough to make a concurrent diagnosis of AD and the Lewy body variant of AD (LBV), in which pathologic criteria for AD are fulfilled. The currently preferred term is *dementia with Lewy bodies* (DLB), but concurrent AD is common.

Many (30% to 50%) AD patients have mild extrapyramidal signs. The presence of mild extrapyramidal signs in patients with dementia presages a more severe course, possibly because it indicates superimposed Alzheimer and Lewy body pathology. It also predicts the development of dementia in patients with subclinical cognitive impairment. These patients tend to be more sensitive to the side effects of neuroleptics and anticholinergic agents. Psychiatric symptoms, including depression, are also much more common in these patients, further exacerbating the disability. At autopsy 20% to 25% are found to have subcortical pathology characteristic of IPD. Approximately 20% of AD cases have coincident cortical Lewy bodies. Clearly, AD and DLB are frequently superimposed. But some cases of dementia of Alzheimer type and parkinsonism lack cortical or subcortical Lewy bodies [152]. In these cases, AD itself is held to be responsible for the extrapyramidal signs [153]. PDD—Parkinson's disease dementia. (*Courtesy of* Laboratory of Human Neuroanatomy and Neuroimaging, Department of Neurology, The University of Iowa.)

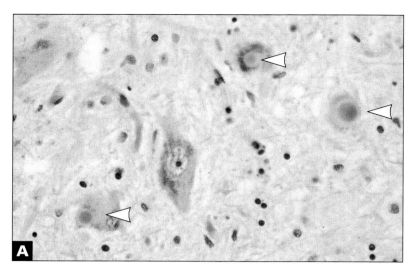

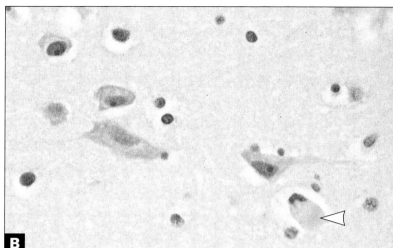

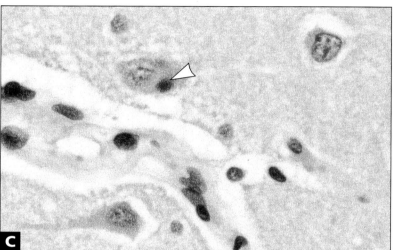

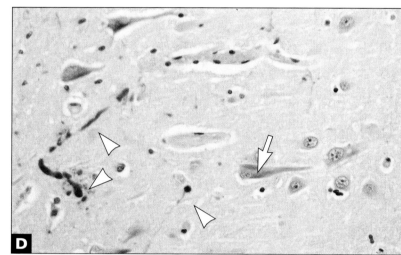

Figure 6-53. Histopathologic changes in dementia with Lewy bodies (DLB). When they occur in cortical neurons, the eosinophilic cytoplasmic inclusions called Lewy bodies are much less conspicuous than those occurring in classic subcortical locations. **A,** Midbrain section (hematoxylin and eosin stain) from a patient with DLB, showing three classic Lewy bodies (*arrowheads*). **B,** In contrast, cortical Lewy bodies (*arrowhead*) may not be detected with standard stains because they lack the pale halo and are sparsely distributed. They are detectable after immunostaining with antibodies to ubiquitin. **C,** Ubiquitin-stained cortical Lewy body (*arrowhead*) in the same patient. Cortical Lewy bodies occur most frequently in the anterior cingulate gyrus, anterior frontal, anterior temporal, and insular cortices [27]. Another characteristic pathologic feature of DLB is the presence of dystrophic neurites in sectors CA2 and CA3 of the hippocampus. **D,** CA2 and CA3 hippocampal region in the same patient (ubiquitin stain). Note the extracellular ubiquitinated dystrophic neurites (*arrowheads*) and the coincidental neurofibrillary tangle (*arrow*) [154–156]. (*Courtesy of* Lee Reed, MD, Department of Pathology, The University of Iowa.)

Criteria for Dementia with Lewy Bodies (DLB)

Dementia *and*
Probable DLB: two of three cardinal features (Possible DLB: one of three)
  Fluctuating sensorium/cognition
  Parkinsonism
  Visual hallucinations
Supporting features
  Repeated falls
  Syncope
  Transient LOC
  Neuroleptic sensitivity
  Systematized delusions
  Hallucinations in other modalities
Other reported associations
  REM sleep behavior disorder
  Depression
  Slow EEG

Figure 6-54. Consensus criteria for dementia with Lewy bodies (DLB). The formal criteria for DLB presented here incorporated retrospective analysis of case records. These criteria have good specificity (90%) but limited sensitivity (50% to 75%). However, sensitivity is better in prospective than in retrospective ones; the primary difficulty in retrospective analysis is in defining and quantifying fluctuation. DLB is commonly misdiagnosed as vascular dementia [157–164].

Spongiform Encephalopathies

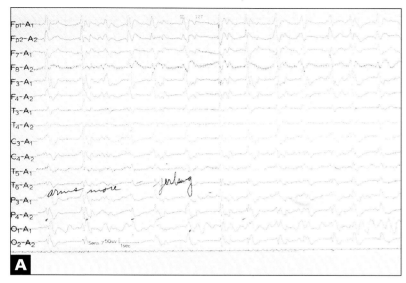

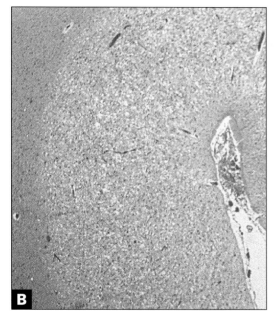

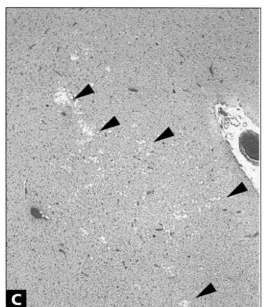

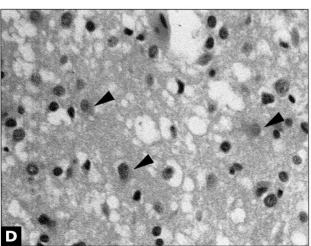

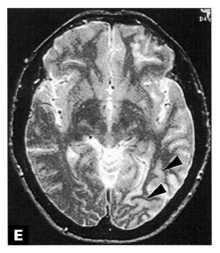

Figure 6-55. Subacute spongiform encephalopathy. Another important class of non-Alzheimer degenerative dementias is the spongiform encephalopathies, which are characterized by the rapidity of their clinical course and the presence of myoclonus [165]. They include Creutzfeldt-Jakob disease (CJD), Gerstmann-Sträussler-Scheinker disease (GSS), fatal familial insomnia, and kuru [153]. The most important clinical example is CJD, which occurs sporadically worldwide. Spongiform encephalopathies, also known as prion diseases, are distinctive among degenerative diseases because they are transmissible in experimental settings, though transmission is *not* involved in most clinical cases. Transmission apparently occurs by a unique mechanism that does not involve nucleic acids, hence the term *prion*, which stands for *p*roteinaceous *i*nfectious u*n*it. Even more remarkably, the prion protein is a normal component of the mammalian nervous system; thus, the disease can also be transmitted genetically, as it is in GSS.

Creuzfeldt-Jakob disease (CJD) is a rapidly progressive dementia, with a mean duration of about 6 months until death. Most cases of CJD are sporadic, with an annual incidence of about $1/10^6$ per year, although the disease has been unintentionally communicated to others by means of corneal transplants, dural grafts, and pituitary extracts. The recent appearance of new variant CJD in the United Kingdom has also raised the possibility of oral transmission (Fig. 6-59). Insidious in onset, CJD evolves rapidly to a characteristic stage in which myoclonic jerks and a prominent startle response are present. **A,** Highly characteristic periodic sharp waves are seen on the electroencephalogram (EEG), and are so specific that a brain biopsy is not needed [166,167]. When EEG findings are inconclusive, cerebrospinal fluid assay for the 14-3-3 antigen has excellent predictive value [168]. At autopsy, spongiform changes affect the full thickness of the cerebral cortex. **B, C,** Hematoxylin and eosin sections of the calcarine and perirhinal cortex, respectively, in a patient with CJD, who presented with complex visual impairment (a presentation known as the Heidenhain variant). Note that the spongiform change is present in all cortical layers and is patchy, with devastation of the calcarine region but only mild involvement of the perirhinal cortex (*arrowheads, C*). **D,** Reactive astrocytosis is present (*arrowheads*), but there is little sign of inflammation. Because of the absence of inflammation, cerebrospinal fluid examination can be helpful in distinguishing CJD from rapidly evolving inflammatory encephalopathies such as granulomatous angiitis, limbic encephalitis, and basal meningitides. **E,** Note that heavily involved cortical regions can be visualized as regions of hyperintense T2-weighted signal with magnetic resonance imaging (MRI) (*arrowheads*); however, MRI scans usually show no abnormalities. (Panel A *courtesy of* Thoru Yamada, MD, Department of Neurology, The University of Iowa; Panels B–D *courtesy of* Lee Reed, MD, Department of Pathology, The University of Iowa.)

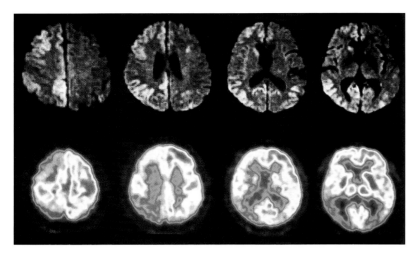

Figure 6-56. Neuroimaging in Creutzfeldt-Jakob disease (CJD). Diffusion-weighted magnetic resonance imaging (MRI) (*top tier*) and fluorodeoxyglucose positron-emission tomography (bottom tier) of a patient with CJD. Conventional MRI scans often show no clear-cut abnormalities in CJD; in such cases functional imaging will usually demonstrate widespread and multifocal metabolic reductions (Fig. 6-16B). It has been demonstrated that diffusion-weighted MRI locates abnormalities concordant with the results of functional imaging [169]. (From Na and colleagues [169].)

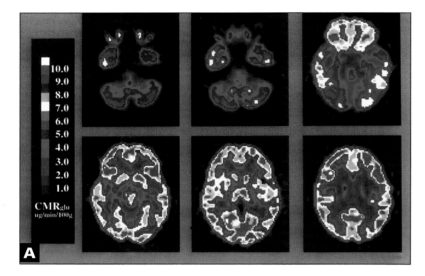

Figure 6-57. Genetic effects on prion diseases. **A**, ^{18}F fluorodeoxyglucose positron-emission tomography scan of a 40-year-old woman who is a member of a kindred with Gerstmann-Sträussler-Scheinker (GSS) disease. The patient presented with progressive ataxia and oscillopsia. There is a striking decrease in cerebellar glucose uptake. Owing to a mutation in the prion protein (PrP) gene, GSS is autosomal dominant, presents as progressive ataxia and dysarthria, and runs a 4- to 10-year course. Cognitive impairment is a relatively late feature. A striking feature of the neuropathology of GSS is prominent cerebellar (PrP) plaques. Approximately 10% of cases of Creutzfeld-Jakob disease (CJD) are also autosomal dominant [170].

(Continued on next page)

B. Molecular and Phenotypic Features of Sporadic Creutzfeld-Jakob Disease (sCJD) Variants

sCJD variant	Previous classification	% of cases	Duration (mo)	Clinical features	Neuropathologic features
MM1 or MV1	Myoclonic, Heidenhain variants	70	3.9	Rapidly progressive dementia, early and prominent myoclonus, typical EEG; visual impairment or unilateral signs at onset in 40% of cases	Classic CJD distribution of pathology; often prominent involvement of occipital cortex; synaptic type PrP staining; in addition, one-third of cases shows confluent vacuoles and perivacuolar PrP staining
VV2	Ataxic variant	16	6.5	Ataxia at onset, late dementia, no typical EEG in most cases	Prominent involvement of subcortical, including brain stem nuclei; in neocortex, spongiosis is often limited to deep layers; PrP staining shows plaque-like focal deposits as well as prominent perineuronal staining
MV2	Kuru-plaques variant	9	17.1	Ataxia in addition to progressive dementia, no typical EEG, long duration (>2 y) in some cases	Similar to VV2 but with amyloid-kuru plaques in the cerebellum, and more consistent plaque-like focal PrP deposits
MM2-thalamic	Thalamic variant	2	15.6	Insomnia and psychomotor hyperactivity in most cases, in addition to ataxia and cognitive impairment, no typical EEG	Prominent atrophy of the thalamus and inferior olive (no spongiosis) with little pathology in other areas; spongiosis may be absent or focal, and PrP^{Sc} is detected in lower amount than in other variants
MM2-cortical	Not established	2	15.7	Progressive dementia, no typical EEG	Large confluent vacuoles with perivacuolar PrP staining in all cortical layers; cerebellum is relatively spared
VV1	Not established	1	15.3	Progressive dementia, no typical EEG	Severe pathology in the cerebral cortex and striatum with sparing of brain stem nuclei and cerebellum; no large confluent vacuoles; very faint synaptic PrP staining

Figure 6-57. *(Continued)* **B,** Although no disease-causing mutations at codon 129 in the PrP gene have been reported, a polymorphism at this codon significantly affects the clinical manifestation of prion diseases. Either methionine (M) or valine (V) is encoded at this location, with a ratio of 0.625 to 0.375 in the normal population. Patients with CJD who are homozygous for methionine (MM) at 129 develop the classic myoclonic or Heidenhain variants, manifest periodic sharp waves on electroencephalogram (EEG), have a disease course lasting 3 to 6 months, and are reliably diagnosed with cerebrospinal fluid (CSF) 14-3-3 antigen assay. Cases with genotype Val-Met or Val-Val tend to an ataxic presentation, a longer course, and are less reliably detected with EEG or 14-3-3 antigen CSF assay. Interestingly, the 129 polymorphism also determines whether a specific PrP mutation (D178N) causes familial CJD (129 Val) or fatal familial insomnia (129 Met) [171]. PrP^{Sc}—protease-resistant PrP. (Panel B *adapted from* Parchi and colleagues (171).)

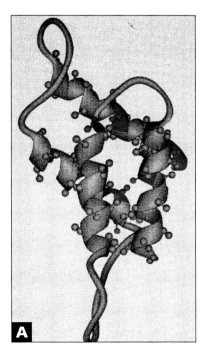

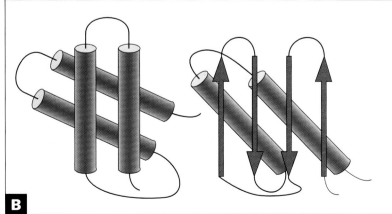

B

A

Figure 6-58. Current model of pathogenesis of spongiform encephalopathies. The common factor in all spongiform encephalopathies, including Creutzfeldt-Jakob disease (CJD), fatal familial insomnia, and Gerstmann-Sträussler-Scheinker disease, is a defect in the human prion protein (PrP), a molecule shown in the ribbon model (**A**). The PrP in sporadic cases of CJD differs from that in nondiseased individuals only in *conformation*; in disease it assumes an insoluble form. All mutations that cause or confer risk for prion diseases (red sites on the ribbon model) give rise to protein sequences that promote folding of the PrP into a β-pleated sheet conformation (**B**) (*arrows* in the hypothetical conformation on the *right*) rather than α helices (*cylinders* in the normal conformation on the *left*). Current thinking is that once transmitted or arising spontaneously, the malignant conformation of molecules can induce molecules in the native conformation to convert to the malignant form. The mechanism that triggers the cascade, however, has not been elucidated [170,172]. (Panel A *from* Prusiner [165]; with permission.)

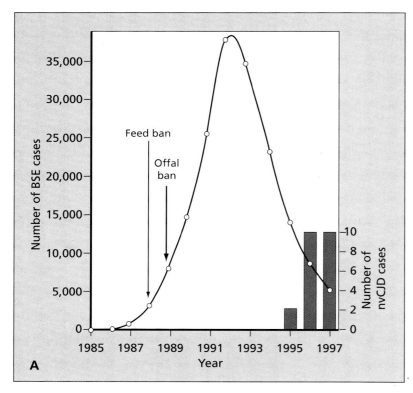

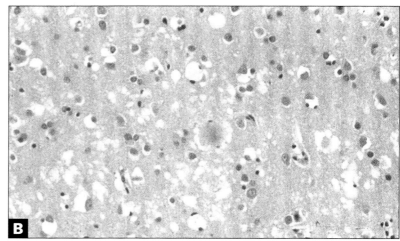

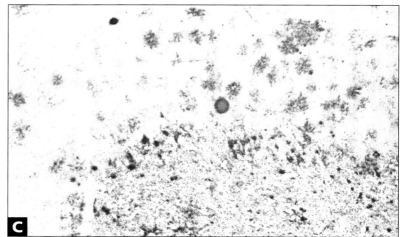

Figure 6-59. New variant Creutzfeld-Jakob disease (nvCJD). In 1996 a new form of prion disease was identified among 17 patients by a British Creutzfeld-Jakob disease (CJD) surveillance unit established to monitor the population for signs that an epidemic of prion disease in cattle, bovine spongiform encephalopathy (BSE), might lead to human prion disease. **A,** Incidence of BSE and nvCJD in the United Kingdom from 1985 to 1997. The BSE epidemic, which began in 1986, was attributed to feed contaminated with prions from scrapie-affected sheep or BSE-affected cattle. It peaked in 1992 after the use of these products in cattle feed was banned. A ban on use of cattle offal in human food products was imposed in 1989. The median age of the patients reported in 1996 was 29, and their clinical presentation featured ataxia, sensory loss, and an absence of periodic sharp waves on electroencephalogram. At autopsy, these patients were all Met-Met homozygous at codon 129, and had no prion protein (PrP) mutations. **B, C,** The pathology was striking for extensive PrP plaques, surrounded by intense spongiform degeneration. nvCJD is thought to be caused by oral transmission of prions from BSE-infected cattle. It is too soon to know whether these cases represent the start of a human epidemic [173,174].

Limbic Encephalitis

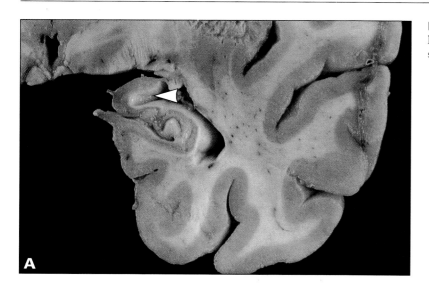

Figure 6-60. Limbic encephalitis. **A,** Gross pathologic specimen of the left mesial temporal region in a patient with limbic encephalitis. Note the sclerotic, granular appearance of the hippocampal formation (*arrowhead*).

(Continued on next page)

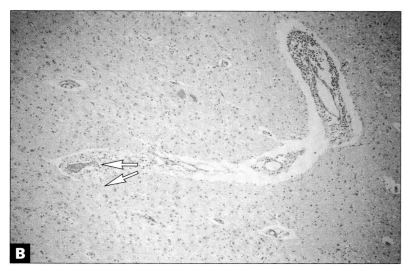

Figure 6-60. *(Continued)* **B,** Microscopic features (hematoxylin and eosin stain), in this case, include the characteristic perivenular lymphocytic infiltrates, neuronal loss, and reactive astrocytosis (*arrows*). Paraneoplastic limbic encephalitis is a rare remote effect of systemic tumors, especially small cell carcinoma of the lung. The patient usually presents with a subacute, severe, and relentless dementia, beginning with amnesia or behavioral disturbance. The disorder has a striking predilection for limbic cortices, especially those in the mesial temporal area. Limbic encephalitis may occur as the only remote effect or else as part of a complex of sensory neuronopathy and encephalomyelitis. In the latter case, antibodies to the antigen Hu are usually present in blood and cerebrospinal fluid, which may otherwise be normal or else show an inflammatory profile. Antibodies to Hu are not reliably present in cases of isolated limbic encephalitis [175]. The primary tumor may be miniscule or even undetectable at the onset of the neurologic disorder. (*Courtesy of* Cheryl Ann Palmer, MD, Department of Neuropathology, University of Alabama, Birmingham.)

References

1. Schoenberg BS: Epidemiology of Alzheimer's disease and other dementing illnesses. *J Chronic Dis* 1986, 39:1095–1104.

2. Hagnell O, Ojesjo L, Rorsman B: Incidence of dementia in the Lundby study. *Neuroepidemiology* 1992, 11:61–66.

3. *Diagnostic and Statistical Manual of Mental Disorders: DSM-IV.* Washington, DC: American Psychiatric Association; 1994.

4. *The ICD-10 Classification of Mental and Behavioural Disorders: Clinical Descriptions and Diagnostic Guidelines.* Geneva: World Health Organization; 1992.

5. Hughes CP, Berg L, Danziger WL, *et al.*: A new clinical scale for the staging of dementia. *Brit J Psychiatry* 1982, 140:566–572.

6. Corey-Bloom J, Thal LJ, Galasko D, *et al.*: Diagnosis and evaluation of dementia. *Neurology* 1995, 45:211–218.

7. Practice parameter for diagnosis and evaluation of dementia (summary statement): report of the Quality Standards Subcommittee of the American Academy of Neurology. *Neurology* 1994, 44:2203–2206.

8. Tombaugh TN, McIntyre NJ: The mini-mental state examination: a comprehensive review. *JAGS* 1992, 40:922–935.

9. Folstein MF, Folstein SE, McHugh PR: "Mini-mental state." A practical method for grading the cognitive state of patients for the clinician. *J Psychiatr Res* 1975, 12:189–198.

10. Petersen RC, Smith GE, Waring SC, *et al.*: Mild cognitive impairment: clinical characterization and outcome. *Arch Neurol* 1999, 56:303–308.

11. Marsden CD: Assessment of dementia. In *Handbook of Clinical Neurology* vol 46. Edited by Frederiks JAM. Amsterdam: Elsevier Science Publishers; 1985:221–231.

12. Albert ML, Feldman RG, Willis AL: The 'subcortical dementia' of progressive supranuclear palsy. *J Neurol Neurosurg Psych* 1974, 37:121–130.

13. Cummings JL, Benson DF: Subcortical dementia. *Arch Neurol* 1984, 41:874–879.

14. Larrabee GJ, McEntee WJ: Age-associated memory impairment: sorting out the controversies. *Neurology* 1995, 45:611–614.

15. Koivisto K, Reinikainen KJ, Hanninen MA, *et al.*: Prevalence of age-associated memory impairment in a randomly selected population from eastern Finland. *Neurology* 1995, 45:741–747.

16. Kaye J, Quinn J: Clinical changes associated with normal aging. In *Neurodegenerative Dementias*. Edited by Clark CM, Trojanowski JQ. New York: McGraw-Hill; 2000.

17. Richards M, Stern Y, Mayeux R: Subtle extrapyramidal signs can predict the development of dementia in elderly individuals. *Neurology* 1993, 43:2184–2188.

18. Chui HC, Lyness SA, Sobel E, Schneider LS: Extrapyramidal signs and psychiatric symptoms predict faster cognitive decline in Alzheimer's disease. *Arch Neurol* 1994, 51:676–681.

19. Petersen RC, Smith GE, Ivnik RJ, *et al.*: Apolipoprotein E status as a predictor of the development of Alzheimer's disease in memory-impaired individuals. *JAMA* 1995, 273:1274–1278.

20. Daly E, Zaitchik D, Copeland M, *et al.*: Predicting conversion to Alzheimer disease using standardized clinical information. *Arch Neurol* 2000, 57:675–680.

21. Jack CR Jr, Petersen RC, Xu YC, *et al.*: Medial temporal atrophy on MRI in normal aging and very mild Alzheimer's disease. *Neurology* 1997, 49(3):786–794.

22. Killiany RJ, Gomez-Isla T, Moss M, *et al.*: Use of structural magnetic resonance imaging to predict who will get Alzheimer's disease. *Ann Neurol* 2000, 47:430–439.

23. Albert MS: Cognitive and neurobiologic markers of early Alzheimer disease. *Proc Natl Acad Sci U S A* 1996, 93:13547–13551.

24. Fox NC, Warrington EK, Seiffer AL, *et al.*: Presymptomatic cognitive deficits in individuals at risk of familial Alzheimer's disease. A longitudinal prospective study. *Brain* 1998, 121:1631–1639.

25. van Duijn CM: Epidemiology of the dementias: recent developments and new approaches. *J Neurol Neurosurg Psych* 1996, 60:478–488.

26. Brayne C, Gill C, Huppert FA, *et al.*: Incidence of clinically diagnosed subtypes of dementia in an elderly population. *Br J Psychiatr* 1995, 167:255–262.

27. Perry E, McKeith I, Perry R, eds.: *Dementia with Lewy Bodies: Clinical, Pathologic, and Treatment Issues.* Cambridge: Cambridge University Press; 1996.

28. Kertesz A, Munoz D: Pick's disease, frontotemporal dementia, and Pick complex: emerging concepts. *Arch Neurol* 1998, 55(3):302–304.

29. Weytingh MD, Bossuyt PMM, van Crevel H: Reversible dementia: more than 10% or less than 1%? A quantitative review. *J Neurol* 1995, 242:446–471.

30. Mahler ME, Cummings JL, Benson DF: Treatable dementias. *West J Med* 1987, 146:705–712.

31. Caine ED: Pseudodementia: current concepts and future directions. *Arch Gen Psychiatry* 1981, 38:1359–1364.

32. Nussbaum PD: Pseudodementia: a slow death. *Neuropsychol Rev* 1994; 4(2):71–90.

33. Abramowicz M: Drugs that cause psychiatric symptoms. *Medical Letter* 1993, 30:65–70.

34. Alexander EM, Wagner EH, Buchner DM, *et al.*: Do surgical brain lesions present as isolated dementia? A population-based study. *J Am Geriatr Soc* 1995, 43:138–143.

35. Clarfield AM: The reversible dementias: do they reverse? *Ann Intern Med* 1988, 109:476–486.

36. Sunderland T, Tariot PN, Cohen RM, *et al.*: Anticholinergic sensitivity in patients with dementia of the Alzheimer type and age-matched controls. *Arch Gen Psychiatry* 1987, 44:418–426.

37. Blazer DG, Federspiel CF, Ray WA, Schaffner W: The risk of anticholinergic toxicity in the elderly: a study of prescribing practices in two populations. *J Gerontology* 1983, 38:31–35.

38. Cantu TG, Korek JS: Central nervous system reactions to histamine-2 receptor blockers. *Ann Intern Med* 1991, 114:1027–1034.

39. Tiraboschi P, Hansen LA, Alford M, *et al.*: Cholinergic dysfunction in diseases with Lewy bodies. *Neurology* 2000, 54:407–411.

40. Adams RD, Fisher CM, Hakim S, *et al.*: Symptomatic occult hydrocephalus with "normal" cerebrospinal-fluid pressure. *N Engl J Med* 1965, 273:117–126.

41. Fisher CM: Hydrocephalus as a cause of disturbances of gait in the elderly. *Neurology* 1982, 32:1358–1363.

42. Wikkelso C, Andersson H, Blomstrand C, *et al.*: Normal pressure hydrocephalus: predictive value of the cerebrospinal fluid tap-test. *Acta Neurol Scand* 1986, 73:566–573.

43. Graff-Radford NR, Godersky JC, Jones MP: Variables predicting surgical outcome in symptomatic hydrocephalus in the elderly. *Neurology* 1989, 39:1601–1604.

44. Benton AL: Neuropsychological assessment. *Annu Rev Psychol* 1994, 45:1–23.

45. Jones RD, Tranel D, Benton A, Paulsen J: Differentiating dementia from "pseudodementia" early in the clinical course: utility of neuropsychological tests. *Neuropsychology* 1992, 6:13–21.

46. Harner RN: EEG evaluation of the patient with dementia. In *Psychiatric Aspects of Neurologic Disease.* Edited by Benson DF, Blumer D. New York: Grune & Stratton; 1975:63–82.

47. Caselli RJ, Jack CR, Petersen RC, *et al.*: Asymmetric cortical degenerative syndromes: clinical and radiologic correlations. *Neurology* 1992, 42:1462–1468.

48. Duara R, Grady C, Haxby J, *et al.*: Positron emission tomography in Alzheimer's disease. *Neurology* 1986, 36:879–887.

49. Powers WJ, Perlmutter JS, Videen TO, *et al.*: Blinded clinical evaluation of positron emission tomography for diagnosis of probable Alzheimer's disease. *Neurology* 1992, 42:765–770.

50. Alzheimer A: On a peculiar disease of the cerebral cortex. *Allgemeine Zeitschrift* 1907, 64:146–148.

51. Khachaturian ZS: Diagnosis of Alzheimer's disease. *Arch Neurol* 1985, 42:1097–1105.

52. Consensus recommendations for the postmortem diagnosis of Alzheimer's disease. The National Institute on Aging, and Reagan Institute Working Group on Diagnostic Criteria for the Neuropathological Assessment of Alzheimer's disease. *Neurobiol Aging* 1997, 18:S1–S2.

53. Mirra SS, Heyman A, McKeel D, *et al.*: The consortium to establish a registry for Alzheimer's disease (CERAD). Part II. Standardization of the neuropathologic assessment of Alzheimer's disease. *Neurology* 1991, 41:479–486.

54. Gearing M, Mirra SS, Hedreen JC, *et al.*: The consortium to establish a registry for Alzheimer's disease (CERAD). Part X. Neuropathology confirmation of the clinical diagnosis of Alzheimer's disease. *Neurology* 1995, 45:461–466.

55. McKhann G, Drachman D, Folstein M, *et al.*: Clinical diagnosis of Alzheimer's disease: report of the NINCDS-ADRDA Work Group under the auspices of Department of Health and Human Services Task Force on Alzheimer's Disease. *Neurology* 1984, 34:939–944.

56. Katzman R, Kawas C: The epidemiology of dementia and Alzheimer disease. In *Alzheimer Disease.* Edited by Terry RD, Katzman R, Bick KL. New York: Raven Press; 1994:105–122.

57. Jorm AF, Korten E, Henderson AS: The prevalence of dementia: a quantitative integration of the literature. *Acta Psychiatr Scand* 1987, 76:465–479.

58. van Duijn CM, Stijnen T, Hofman A: Risk factors for Alzheimer's disease: overview of the EURODEM collaborative re-analysis of case-control studies. *Int J Epidemiol* 1991, 20:S4–S12.

59. Goate A, Chartier-Harlin MC, Mullan M, *et al.*: Segregation of a missense mutation in the amyloid precursor protein gene with familial Alzheimer's disease. *Nature* 1991, 349:704–706.

60. Levy-Lahad E, Wasco W, Poorkaj P, *et al.*: Candidate gene for the chromosome 1 familial Alzheimer's disease locus. *Science* 1995, 269:(5226)973–977.

61. Alzheimer's Disease Collaborative Group: The structure of the presenilin 1 (S182) gene and identification of six novel mutations in early onset AD families. *Nat Genet* 1995, 11:(2)219–222.

62. Cummings JL, Vinters HV, Cole GM, Khachaturian ZS: Alzheimer's disease: etiologies, pathophysiology, cognitive reserve, and treatment opportunities. *Neurology* 1998, 51(1 Suppl 1):S2–17.

63. Tang M-X, Jacobs D, Stern Y, *et al.*: Effect of estrogen during menopause on risk and age at onset of Alzheimer's disease. *Lancet* 1996, 348:429–432.

64. Strittmatter WJ, Roses AD: Apolipoprotein E and Alzheimer disease. *Proc Natl Acad Sci U S A* 1995, 92:4725–4727.

65. Myers RH, Schaefer EJ, Wilson PWF, *et al.*: Apolipoprotein E4 association with dementia in a population-based study: The Framingham Study. *Neurology* 1996, 46:673–677.

66. Welsh-Bohmer KA, Gearing M, Saunders AM, *et al.*: Apolipoprotein E genotypes in a neuropathological series from the consortium to establish a registry for Alzheimer's disease. *Ann Neurol* 1997, 42:319–325.

67. Breitner JCS: The end of Alzheimer's disease? *Int J Geriatr Psychiatry* 1999, 14:577–586.

68. Hyman BT, Gomez-Isla T, Briggs M, *et al.*: Apolipoprotein E and cognitive change in an elderly populations. *Ann Neurology* 1996, 40:55–66.

69. Mayeux R, Saunders AM, Shea S, *et al.*: Utility of the apolipoprotein E genotype in the diagnosis of Alzheimer's disease. *N Engl J Med* 1998, 338:506–511.

70. Strittmatter WJ, Saunders AM, Schmechel D, *et al.*: Apolipoprotein E: high-avidity binding to beta-amyloid and increased frequency of type 4 allele in late-onset familial Alzheimer disease. *Proc Natl Acad Sci U S A* 1993, 90:1977–1981.

71. Pickering-Brown SM, Mann DMA, Bourke JP, *et al.*: Apolipoprotein E4 and Alzheimer's disease pathology in Lewy body disease and in other beta-amyloid-forming diseases. *Lancet* 1994, 343:1155.

72. Ellis RJ, Olichney JM, Thal LJ, *et al.*: Cerebral amyloid angiopathy in the brains of patients with Alzheimer's disease: the CERAD experience, part XV. *Neurology* 1996, 46:1592–1596.

73. Storey E, Cappai R: The amyloid precursor protein of Alzheimer's disease and the Aβ peptide. *Neuropathol Appl Neurobiol* 1999, 25:81–97.

74. Selkoe DJ: Alzheimer's disease: a central role for amyloid. *J Neuropathol Exp Neurol* 1994, 53:438–447.

75. Selkoe DJ: The pathophysiology of Alzheimer's disease. In *Early Diagnosis of Alzheimer's Disease.* Edited by Scinto LFM, Daffner KR. Totowa, NJ: Humana Press; 2000:83–104

76. Arnold SE, Hyman BT, Flory J, *et al.*: The topographical and neuroanatomical distribution of neurofibrillary tangles and neuritic plaques in the cerebral cortex of patients with Alzheimer's disease. *Cereb Cortex* 1991, 1:103–116.

77. Braak H, Braak E: Neuropathological staging of Alzheimer-related changes. *Acta Neuropathologica* 1991, 82:239–259.

78. Hyman BT, Arriagada PV, McKee AC, *et al.*: The earliest symptoms of Alzheimer disease: anatomic correlates. *Soc Neurosci Abstr* 1991, 15:352.

79. Hof PR, Bierer LM, Perl DP, *et al.*: Evidence for early vulnerability of the medial and inferior aspects of the temporal lobe in an 82-year-old patient with preclinical signs of dementia. *Arch Neurol* 1992, 49:946–953.

80. Scinto LFM, Daffner KR: *Early Diagnosis of Alzheimer's Disease.* Totowa, NJ: Humana Press; 2000.

81. Davies P, Maloney AJF: Selective loss of central cholinergic neurons in Alzheimer's disease. *Lancet* 1976, 1403.

82. Bartus RT, Dean RLI, Beer B, Lippa AS: The cholinergic hypothesis of geriatric memory dysfunction. *Science* 1982; 217:408–414.

83. Coyle JT, Price DL, DeLong MR: Alzheimer's disease: a disorder of cortical cholinergic innervation. *Science* 1983, 219:1184–1190.

84. Knapp MJ, Knopman DS, Solomon PR, *et al.*: A 30-week randomized controlled trial of high-dose tacrine in patients with Alzheimer's disease. *JAMA* 1994, 271:985–991.

85. Mayeux R, Sano M: Treatment of Alzheimer's disease. *N Engl J Med* 1999, 341:1670–1679.

86. Geula C, Mesulam MM: Systematic regional variations in the loss of cortical cholinergic fibers in Alzheimer's disease. *Cerebral Cortex* 1996, 6:165–177.

87. Hyman BT, Van Hoesen G, Damasio AR, Barnes CL: Alzheimer's disease: cell-specific pathology isolates the hippocampal formation. *Science* 1984, 225:1168–1170.

88. Reiman EM, Caselli RJ, Yun LS, *et al.*: Preclinical evidence of Alzheimer's disease in persons homozygous for the (epsilon) 4 allele for apolipoprotein E. *N Engl J Med* 1996, 334:752–758.

89. Hof PR, Bouras C, Constantinidis J, Morrison JH: Selective disconnection of specific visual association pathways in cases of Alzheimer's disease presenting with Balint's syndrome. *J Neuropathol Exp Neurol* 1990, 40:168–184.

90. Levine DN, Lee JM, Fisher CM: The visual variant of Alzheimer's disease. *Neurology* 1993, 43:305–313.

91. Victoroff J, Webster R, Benson F, *et al.*: Posterior cortical atrophy. Neuropathologic correlations. *Arch Neurol* 1994, 51:269–274.

92. Joaquim CL, Morris JH, Selkoe DJ: Clinically diagnosed Alzheimer's disease: autopsy results in 150 cases. *Ann Neurol* 1988, 24:50–56.

93. Wade JPH, Mirsen TR, Hachinski VC, *et al.*: The clinical diagnosis of Alzheimer's disease. *Arch Neurol* 1987, 44:24–29.

94. Molsa PK, Paljarvi L, Rinne JO, *et al.*: Validity of clinical diagnosis in dementia: a prospective clinicopathological study. *J Neurol Neurosurg Psychiatr* 1985, 48:1085–1090.

95. Klatka LA, Schiffer RB, Powers JM, Kazee AM: Incorrect diagnosis of Alzheimer's disease: a clinicopathologic study. *Arch Neurol* 1996, 53:35–42.

96. Dickson DW, Davies P, Bevona C, *et al.*: Hippocampal sclerosis: a common pathological feature of dementia in very old (over 80 years of age) humans. *Acta Neuropathol* 1994, 88:212–221.

97. Ala TA, Beh GO, Frey II WH: Pure hippocampal sclerosis. *Neurology* 2000, 54:843–848.

98. Consensus report of the Working Group on: "Molecular and Biochemical Markers of Alzheimer's Disease". The Ronald and Nancy Reagan Research Institute of the Alzheimer's Association and the National Institute on Aging Working Group. *Neurobiol Aging* 1998, 19:109–116.

99. Galasko D, Clark C, Chang L, *et al.*: Assessment of CSF levels of tau protein in mildly demented patients with Alzheimer's disease. *Neurology* 1997, 48:632–635.

100. Kahle PJ, Jakowec M, Teipel SJ, *et al.*: Combined assessment of tau and neuronal thread protein in Alzheimer's disease CSF. *Neurology* 2000, 54:1498–1504.

101. Roman GC, Tatemichi TK, Erkinjuntti T, et al: Vascular dementia: diagnostic criteria for research studies. Report of the NINDS-AIREN International Workshop. *Neurology* 1993, 43:250–260.

102. Tatemichi TK: How acute brain failure becomes chronic: a view of the mechanisms of dementia related to stroke. *Neurology* 1990, 40:1652–1659.

103. Tatemichi TK, Desmond DW, Paik M, *et al.*: Clinical determinants of dementia related to stroke. *Ann Neurol* 1993, 33:568–575.

104. Erkinjuntti T, Hachinski VC: Rethinking vascular dementia. *Cerebrovasc Dis* 1993, 3:3–23.

105. Chui HC, Victoroff JI, Margolin D, *et al.*: Criteria for the diagnosis of ischemic vascular dementia proposed by the state of California Alzheimer's disease diagnostic and treatment centers. *Neurology* 1992, 42:473–480.

106. Rockwood K, Parhad I, Hachinski V, *et al.*: Diagnosis of vascular dementia: consortium of Canadian Centres for clinical cognitive research consensus statement. *Can J Neurol Sci* 1994, 21:358–364.

107. Verhey FRJ, Lodder J, Rozendaal N, Jolles J: Comparison of seven sets of criteria used for the diagnosis of vascular dementia. *Neuroepidemiology* 1996, 15:166–172.

108. Erkinjuntti T, Haltia M, Palo J, *et al.*: Accuracy of the clinical diagnosis of vascular dementia: a prospective clinical and post-mortem neuropathological study. *J Neurol Neurosurg Psychiatr* 1988, 51:1037–1044.

109. Gold G, Giannakopoulos P, Montes-Paixao C, *et al.*: Sensitivity and specificity of newly proposed clinical criteria for possible vascular dementia. *Neurology* 1997, 49:690–694.

110. Tatemichi TK, Desmond DW, Mayeux R, *et al.*: Dementia after stroke: baseline frequency, risks, and clinical features in a hospitalized cohort. *Neurology* 1992, 42:1185–1193.

111. Hebert R, Brayne C: Epidemiology of vascular dementia. *Neuroepidemiology* 1995, 14:240–257.

112. Hachinski V, Lassen NA, Marshall J: Multi-infarct dementia: a cause of mental deterioration in the elderly. *Lancet* 1974, 1:207–210.

113. Hachinski VC, et al: Cerebral blood flow in dementia. *Arch Neurol* 1975, 32:632–637.

114. Rosen WG, Terry RD, Fuld PA, et al.: Pathological verification of ischemic score in differentiation of dementias. *Ann Neurol* 1980, 7:486–488.

115. Fischer P, Jellinger K, Gatterbi G, Danielczyk W: Prospective neuropathological validation of Hachinski's ischaemic score in dementias. *J Neurol Neurosurg Psychiatr* 1991, 54:580–583.

116. Hershey LA, Modic MT, Jaffe DF, Greenough PG: Natural history of the vascular dementias: a prospective study of seven cases. *Can J Neurol Sci* 1986, 13:559–565.

117. Snowdon DA, Greiner LH, Mortimer JA, *et al.*: Brain infarction and the clinical expression of Alzheimer disease. The Nun study. *JAMA* 1997, 277:813–817.

118. Esiri MM, Nagy Z, Smith MZ, *et al.*: Cerebrovascular disease and threshold for dementia in the early stages of Alzheimer's disease. *Lancet* 1999, 354:919–920.

119. Lie JT: Primary (granulomatous) angiitis of the central nervous system: a clinicopathologic analysis of 15 new cases and a review of the literature. *Hum Pathol* 1992, 23:164–171.

120. Caplan LR: Binswanger's disease–revisited. *Neurology* 1995, 45:626–633.

121. Fisher CM: Binswanger's encephalopathy: a review. *J Neurol* 1989, 236:65–79.

122. Greenberg SM, Finklestein SP, Schaefer PW: Petechial hemorrhages accompanying lobar hemorrhage: detection by gradient-echo MRI. *Neurology* 1996, 46:1751–1754.

123. Greenberg SM, Vonsattel JPG, Stakes JW, *et al.*: The clinical spectrum of cerebral amyloid angiopathy: presentations without lobar hemorrhage. *Neurology* 1993, 43:2073–2079.

124. Hutchinson, M, O'Riordan J, Javed M, *et al.*: Familial hemiplegic migraine and autosomal dominant arteriopathy with leukoencephalopathy (CADASIL). *Ann Neurol* 1995, 38:817–824.

125. Dichgans M, Mayer M, Uttner I, *et al.*: The phenotypic spectrum of CADASIL: clinical findings in 102 cases. *Ann Neurol* 1998, 44:731–739.

126. The Lund and Manchester Groups: Clinical and neuropathological criteria for frontotemporal dementia. *J Neuro Neurosurg Psychiatry* 1994, 57:416–418.

127. Neary D, Snowden JS, Gustafson L, *et al.*: Frontotemporal lobar degeneration: a consensus on clinical diagnostic criteria. *Neurology* 1998, 51:1546–1554.

128. Brun A: Frontal lobe degeneration of non-Alzheimer type. I. Neuropathology. *Arch Gerontol Geriatr* 1987, 6:193–208.

129. Neary D, Snowden JS, Mann DMA, *et al.*: Frontal lobe dementia and motor neuron disease. *J Neurol Neurosurg Psychiatry* 1990, 53:23–32.

130. Chow TW, Miller BL, Hayashi VN, Geschwind DH: Inheritance of frontotemporal dementia. *Arch Neurol* 1999, 56(7):817–822.

131. Tissot R, Constantinidis J, Richard J: Pick's Disease. In *Handbook of Clinical Neurology* vol 46. Edited by Frederiks JAM. Amsterdam: Elsevier Science Publishers; 1985:233–246.

132. Mesulam MM: Slowly progressive aphasia without generalized dementia. *Ann Neurol* 1982, 11:592–598.

133. Snowden JS, Neary D, Mann DMA: Fronto-Temporal Lobar Degeneration: Fronto-Temporal Dementia, Progressive Aphasia, Semantic Dementia. New York: Churchill Livingstone; 1996.

134. Kertesz A, Hudson L, Mackenzie IRA, Munoz DG: The pathology and nosology of primary progressive aphasia. *Neurology* 1994, 44:2065–2072.

135. Turner RS, Kenyon LC, Trojanowski JQ, *et al.*: Clinical, neuroimaging, and pathologic features of progressive nonfluent aphasia. *Ann Neurol* 1996, 39:166–173.

136. Knopman DS, Mastri AR, Frey II WH, *et al.*: Dementia lacking distinctive histologic features: a common non-Alzheimer degenerative dementia. *Neurology* 1990, 40:251–256.

137. Knopman DS: Overview of dementia lacking distinctive histology: pathological designation of a progressive dementia. *Dementia* 1993, 4:132–136.

138. Giannakopoulos P, Hof PR, Bouras C: Dementia lacking distinctive histopathology: clinicopathological evaluation of 32 cases. *Acta Neuropathol* 1995, 89:346–355.

139. Graff-Radford NR, Damasio AR, Hyman BT, *et al.*: Progressive aphasia in a patient with Pick's disease: a neuropsychological, radiologic, and anatomic study. *Neurology* 1990, 40:620–626.

140. Hodges JR, Patterson K, Oxbury S, Funnell E: Semantic dementia. Progressive fluent aphasia with temporal lobe atrophy. *Brain* 1992, 115:1783–1806.

141. Gibb WRG, Luthert PJ, Marsden CD: Corticobasal degeneration. *Brain* 1989, 112:1171–1192.

142. Boeve BF, Maraganore DM, Parisi JE, *et al.*: Pathologic heterogeneity in clinically diagnosed corticobasal degeneration. *Neurology* 1999, 53:795–800.

143. Grimes DA, Lang AE, Bergeron CB: Dementia as the most common presentation of cortical-basal ganglionic degeneration. *Neurology* 1999, 53:1969–1974.

144. Foster NL, Wilhelmsen K, Sima AAF, *et al.*: Frontotemporal dementia and Parkinsonism linked to chromosome 17: a consensus conference. *Ann Neurol* 1997, 41:706–715.

145. Spillantini, MG, Bird TD, Ghetti B: Frontotemporal dementia and parkinsonism linked to chromosome 17: a new group of tauopathies. *Brain Pathology* 1998, 8:387–402.

146. Spillantini MG, Goedert M: Tau protein pathology in neurodegenerative diseases. *Trends Neurosci* 1998, 21:428–433.

147. Bennet P, Bonifati V, Bonuccelli U, *et al.*: Direct genetic evidence for involvement of tau in progressive supranuclear palsy. European Study Group on Atypical Parkinsonism Consortium. *Neurology* 1998, 51:982–985.

148. Gearing M, Olson DA, Watts RL, Mirra SS: Progressive supranuclear palsy: neuropathologic and clinical heterogeneity. *Neurology* 1994, 44:1015–1024.

149. de Vos RA, Jansen EN, Stam FC, Swaab DF: 'Lewy body disease': clinicopathological correlations in 18 consecutive cases of Parkinson's disease with and without dementia. *Clin Neurol Neurosurg* 1995, 97:13–22.

150. Hughes AJ, Daniel SE, Blankson S, Lees AJ: A clinicopathologic study of 100 cases of Parkinson's disease. *Arch Neurol* 1993, 50:140–148.

151. Hughes AJ, Daniel SE, Kilford L, Lees AJ: Accuracy of clinical diagnosis of idiopathic Parkinson's disease: a clinico-pathological study of 100 cases. *J Neurol Neurosurg Psychiatry* 1992, 55:181–184.

152. Hulette C, Mirra S, Wilkinson W, *et al.*: The Consortium to Establish a Registry for Alzheimer's Disease (CERAD). Part IX. A prospective cliniconeuropathologic study of Parkinson's features in Alzheimer's disease. *Neurology* 1996, 45:1991–1995.

153. Ditter SM, Mirra SS: Neuropathologic and clinical features of Parkinson's disease in Alzheimer's disease patients. *Neurology* 1987, 37:754–760.

154. Dickson DW, Ruan D, Crystal H, *et al.*: Hippocampal degeneration differentiates diffuse Lewy body disease (DLBD) from Alzheimer's disease: light and electron microscopic immunocytochemistry of CA2-3 neurites specific to DLBD. *Neurology* 1991, 41:1402–1409.

155. Kim H, Gearing M, Mirra SS: Ubiquitin-positive CA2/3 neurites in hippocampus coexist with cortical Lewy bodies. *Neurology* 1995, 45:1768–1770.

156. Lippa CF, Johnson R, Smith TW: The medial temporal lobe in dementia with Lewy bodies: a comparative study with Alzheimer's disease. *Ann Neurol* 1998, 43:102–106.

157. McKeith IG, Fairbairn AF, Bothwell RA, *et al.*: An evaluation of the predictive validity and inter-rater reliability of clinical diagnostic criteria for senile dementia of Lewy body type. *Neurology* 1994, 44:872–877.

158. McKeith IG, Ballard CG, Perry RH, *et al.*: Prospective validation of consensus criteria for the diagnosis of dementia with Lewy bodies. *Neurology* 2000, 54:1050–1058.

159. Verghese J, Crystal HA, Dickson DW, Lipton RB: Validity of clinical criteria for the diagnosis of dementia with Lewy bodies. *Neurology* 1999, 53:1974–1982.

160. McKeith IG, Perry EK, Perry RH: Report of the second dementia with Lewy body international workshop. *Neurology* 1999, 53:902–905.

161. Boeve BF, Silber MH, Ferman TJ, *et al.*: REM sleep behavior disorder and degenerative dementia: an association likely reflecting Lewy body disease. *Neurology* 1998, 51:363–370.

162. McKeith I, Fairbairn A, Perry R, *et al.*: Neuroleptic sensitivity in patients with senile dementia of Lewy body type. *BMJ* 1992, 305:673–678.

163. Ballard C, Grace J, McKeith I, Holmes C: Neuroleptic sensitivity in dementia with Lewy bodies and Alzheimer's disease. *Lancet* 1998, 351:1032–1033.

164. Walker MP, Ayre GA, Cummings JL, *et al.*: Quantifying fluctuation in dementia with Lewy bodies, Alzheimer's disease, and vascular dementia. *Neurology* 2000, 54:1616–1624.

165. Prusiner SB: The prion diseases. *Sci Am* 1995, 272:48–57.

166. Bortone E, Bettoni L, Giorgi C, *et al.*: Reliability of EEG in the diagnosis of Creutzfeldt-Jakob disease. *Electroencephalogr Clin Neurophysiol* 1994, 90:323–330.

167. Steinhoff BJ, Racker S, Herrendorf G, *et al.*: Accuracy and reliability of periodic sharp wave complexes in Creutzfeldt-Jakob disease. *Arch Neurol* 1996, 53:162–166.

168. Zerr I, Bodemer M, Gefeller O, *et al.*: Detection of 14-3-3 protein in the cerebrospinal fluid supports the diagnosis of Creutzfeldt-Jakob disease. *Ann Neurol* 1998, 43:32–40.

169. Na DL, Suh CK, Choi SH, *et al.*: Diffusion-weighted magnetic resonance imaging in probable Creutzfeldt-Jakob disease: a clinical-anatomic correlation. *Arch Neurol* 1999, 56(8):951–957.

170. DeArmond SJ, Prusiner SB: Etiology and pathogenesis of prion diseases. *Am J Pathol* 1995, 146:785–811.

171. Parchi P, Giese A, Capellari S, *et al.*: Classification of sporadic Creutzfeldt-Jakob disease based on molecular and phenotypic analysis of 300 subjects. *Ann Neurol* 1999, 46:224–233.

172. Mestel R: Putting prions to the test. *Science* 1996, 273:184–189.

173. Will RG, Ironside JW, Zeidlee M, *et al.*: A new variant of Creutzfeldt-Jakob disease in the UK. *Lancet* 1996, 347:921–925.

174. Johnson RT, Gibbs CJ: Creutzfeldt-Jakob disease and related transmissible spongiform encephalopathies. *N Engl J Med* 1998, 339:1994–2004.

175. Gultekin SH, Rosenfeld MR, Voltz R, *et al.*: Paraneoplastic limbic encephalitis: neurological symptoms, immunological findings and tumour association in 50 patients. *Brain* 2000, 123:1481–1494.

7

Behavioral Neurology

Daniel Tranel • Thomas J. Grabowski, Jr
Hanna Damasio

BEHAVIORAL neurology encompasses a variety of diseases and disorders of higher brain functions, related to focal cortical and subcortical brain disease. "Higher" here refers to the fact that the domain of behavioral neurology covers the most complex and advanced aspects of human cognition and behavior, including functions such as memory, language, problem-solving, complex perception, social behavior, planning and decision-making, and personality. In general, behavioral neurology is concerned with disorders of these functions that occur as a consequence of acquired brain disease in adults who previously were normal. Hence, developmental conditions, psychiatric diseases, and disorders attributable to progressive dementia conditions (see Chapter 6) are not included here.

There is considerable overlap, conceptually and practically, between the fields of behavioral neurology, neuropsychiatry, and neuropsychology. In fact, most of the disorders described in this chapter are properly known as neuropsychologic disorders, while some could be referred to as neuropsychiatric disorders. Behavioral neurology, though, remains a useful term, because it conveys accurately the notion that the approach to the patient is from the perspective of neurology, and the diagnosis and management of the patient are couched in the tradition and technology of medicine. However, accurate diagnosis and optimal management of many of the conditions covered in this chapter require the combined expertise of behavioral neurology and neuropsychology, and the neurologist should not hesitate to consult a neuropsychologist when confronted with patients with conditions such as those described here. In particular, with regard to the *measurement* of higher-order cognition and behavior, the neuropsychologist has access to a rich armamentarium of well-standardized tests that allow precise quantification of complex functions such as memory and language. Availing oneself of such measurement will help avoid pitfalls in diagnosis that occur when seemingly reasonable but overly observer-dependent "clinical intuition" is applied.

The neuropsychological disorders covered in this chapter are most frequently caused by one of the following conditions: cerebrovascular disease; traumatic brain injury; cerebral tumors; and viral infections of the central nervous system, especially herpes simplex encephalitis. These processes and conditions affect selectively different brain areas and occur preferentially in particular age groups. This means that not all conditions have the same potential to produce the same types of disorders. For example, most disorders of language are caused by stroke, due to the fact that stroke is the primary cause of dysfunction in the perisylvian territory of the left hemisphere. The result is that most patients with aphasia are middle-aged or elderly. By contrast, acquired disorders of personality, which are associated with dysfunction of the ventromedial prefrontal region, are much more common in patients with traumatic brain injury and in patients who have undergone surgical treatment of brain tumors in this region; most of the victims are relatively young. Memory dysfunction is a hallmark feature of viral brain infections, especially herpes simplex encephalitis.

Some of the conditions described in this chapter are relatively uncommon. For example, a practitioner may rarely encounter a clear-cut case of prosopagnosia, auditory agnosia, or Balint's syndrome. However, a working understanding of such conditions is essential to the practice of neurology, because many of these conditions do occur with some regularity, particularly in patients with focal cortical and subcortical lesions. Also, in many neuropsychologic conditions there is ample opportunity for the patient to be misdiagnosed as having psychiatric disease, given the unusual, and even bizarre, nature of presenting signs and symptoms. A psychiatric approach to these patients is rarely helpful in the long run, and may be quite counterproductive. Thus, it is imperative that the neurologist have a sufficient base of knowledge to reach an accurate and timely diagnosis.

As a final introductory comment, it should be noted that scientific study of many of the conditions described below has yielded numerous pathbreaking discoveries regarding the neural basis of complex human behavior. Behavioral neurology and neuropsychology have a long tradition of furnishing revealing cases in which it has been possible to establish new insights into the neural underpinnings of higher-order functions such as language, memory, and decision-making. Even with the recent advent of functional neuroimaging techniques, such as positron emission tomography and functional magnetic resonance imaging, which can be applied to normal individuals, the tenets of behavioral neurology continue to guide the empirical thrust of cognitive neuroscience, and the scientific value of cases in the domain of behavioral neurology should not be underestimated.

Agnosia

Principal Agnosic Conditions

Modality or capacity	Subtypes	Neuroanatomical correlates
Vision	Visual object agnosia	Bilateral occipitotemporal, right or left occipitotemporal
	Associative prosopagnosia	Bilateral occipitotemporal
	Apperceptive prosopagnosia	Right occipitotemporal and occipitoparietal; bilateral "early" visual association cortices
Audition	Auditory agnosia	Bilateral posterosuperior temporal
	Environmental sound agnosia	Bilateral posterosuperior temporal
	Amusia	Right posterior temporal, inferior parietal
Somatosensory perception	Tactile object agnosia (complete)	Right and left parietal operculum; posterior insula
	Tactile object agnosia (nonmanipulable stimuli)	Right superior mesial parietal
Perception of disease	Anosognosia	Right inferior parietal; bilateral ventromedial prefrontal

Figure 7-1. Principal agnosic conditions. The term *agnosia* signifies lack of knowledge, and denotes an impairment of recognition. In the traditional literature, two types of agnosia were described [1]. One, termed *associative* agnosia, referred to a failure of recognition that results from defective activation of information pertinent to a given stimulus. The other, termed *apperceptive* agnosia, referred to a disturbance of the integration of otherwise normally perceived components of a stimulus. The term agnosia should not be used for conditions in which perceptual problems are so severe as to preclude the patient's apprehension of meaningful information. In patients with associative agnosia, perception is largely intact, and the recognition defect is strictly or primarily a disorder of memory. In patients with apperceptive variety, the problem can be traced, at least in part, to faulty perception, usually in reference to higher-order aspects of perception. It should be understood, though, that the core feature in designating a condition as agnosia is that there is a recognition impairment that cannot be attributed simply or entirely to faulty perception. Thus, the following operational definitions can be used [2,3]. Associative agnosia is a modality-specific impairment of the ability to recognize previously known stimuli (or new stimuli for which learning would normally have occurred) that occurs in the absence of disturbances of perception, intellect, or language and is the result of acquired cerebral damage. The designation apperceptive agnosia applies when the patient meets the above definition in all respects except that *perception is altered*. The terms associative and apperceptive

agnosia remain useful, even if the two conditions overlap to some extent. Most patients with recognition impairments can be classified as having primarily a disturbance of memory (associative agnosia) or primarily a disturbance of perception (apperceptive agnosia). Such classification has important implications for patient management (*eg*, what rehabilitation should be applied), and it also maps onto different sites of neural dysfunction.

The term agnosia should be restricted to situations in which recognition impairments are confined to one sensory modality, for example, vision, audition, or touch. When recognition defects extend across two or more modalities, the appropriate designation is *amnesia*. Also, the term agnosia should be reserved for conditions that develop suddenly, after the onset of acquired cerebral dysfunction. In principle, agnosia can occur in any sensory modality, relative to any type of entity or event. In practice, however, some types of agnosia occur much more frequently. *Visual agnosia*, especially agnosia for faces (*prosopagnosia*), is the most commonly encountered recognition disturbance. The condition of *auditory agnosia*, which includes subtypes of *environmental sound agnosia* and *amusia*, is rarer, followed by the even less frequent *tactile agnosia*. One relatively frequent condition that conforms to the designation of agnosia is *anosognosia*, which is a disturbance in the recognition of illness. Some agnosic patients preserve recognition at a nonconscious level. For example, patients can produce discriminatory autonomic responses, such as a skin conductance response, to familiar stimuli, even though they cannot recognize those stimuli at a conscious level.

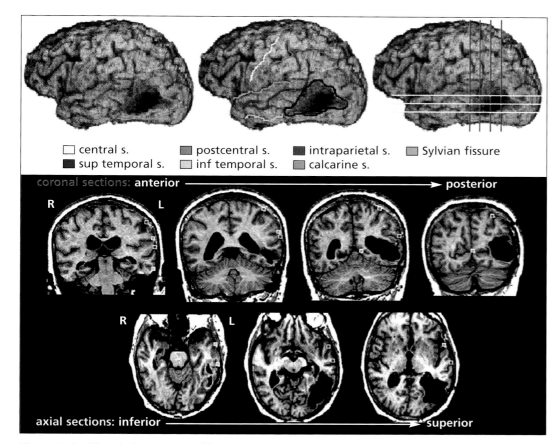

central s. **postcentral s.** **intraparietal s.** **Sylvian fissure**
sup temporal s. **inf temporal s.** **calcarine s.**

coronal sections: **anterior** ⟶ **posterior**

R   L

R   L

axial sections: **inferior** ⟶ **superior**

Figure 7-2. Visual object agnosia. Three-dimensional brain reconstruction of a patient with visual object agnosia.* Magnetic resonance imaging (MRI) data from a subject with a left occipitotemporal lesion and visual object agnosia. The MRI data are reconstructed in three dimensions in the pictures in the top row. The first image in the top row shows the left lateral view of a three-dimensional reconstruction of contiguous coronal MRIs, after digital deletion of extracerebral structures, using Brainvox (a three-dimensional visualization and analysis system developed in the Human Neuroanatomy and Neuroimaging Laboratory at The University of Iowa) [4,5]. The surface extent of the lesion in the region of the left occipitotemporal junction is apparent. In the middle image, major cerebral sulci have been marked with traces that are color-coded, according to the key provided. The right image in the top row shows the orientations of the four coronal (red) and three axial (yellow) cuts depicted in the bottom two thirds of the figure, corresponding to the images in the middle and lower rows, respectively. (Coronal sections are displayed in anterior to posterior order, left to right. Axial [transverse] sections are displayed in inferior to superior order, left to right.) The colored traces of the sulci have been transferred (automatically) to coronal and axial sections (*middle* and *lower rows*). These images make the extent and location of the lesion apparent. In this case, the lesion extends from the cortical surface to the ventricular surface, beginning at the midportion of the middle and inferior temporal gyri, and continuing to the lateral occipital region, sparing the calcarine cortex, the superior temporal gyrus, and the parietal lobe. The full extent of the lesion was traced on the two-dimensional slices and then projected to the surface. The surface projection of the lesion is outlined with a black trace in the middle image of the upper row, to give some idea of its subcortical extent.

Visual object agnosia is a disorder of recognition confined to the visual realm, in which a patient cannot arrive at the meaning of some or all categories of previously known nonverbal visual stimuli, despite normal or near-normal visual perception and intact alertness, attention, intelligence, and language. Most patients also have an impairment in learning new visual stimuli. The condition is associated with bilateral or unilateral right or left occipitotemporal lesions. The profile of this patient with a left-sided lesion includes impaired recognition of tools and utensils and normal recognition of animals. (*Courtesy of* Laboratory of Human Neuroanatomy and Neuroimaging, Department of Neurology, The University of Iowa.)

*The display conventions used in this figure apply throughout the chapter.

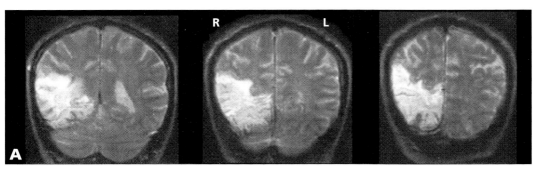

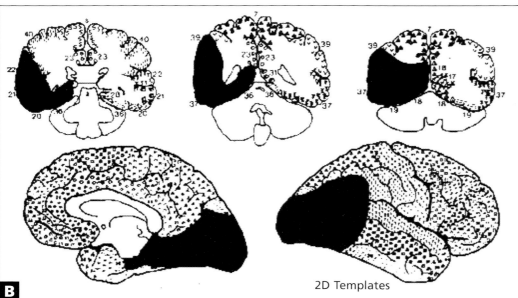

2D Templates

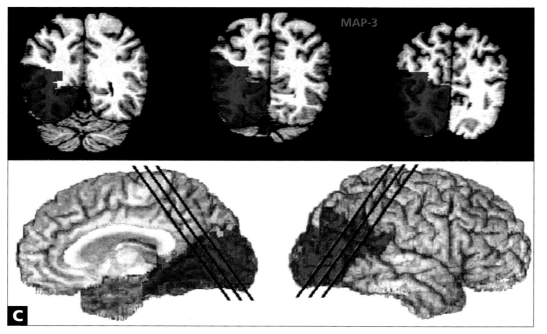

MAP-3

Figure 7-3. Visual object agnosia. Two methods to interpret lesions when three-dimensional imaging data are not available are shown here. **A**, Three coronal magnetic resonance image (MRI) sections of a patient with a right occipitotemporal lesion and visual object agnosia. **B**, These data have been mapped onto a set of standard coronal brain templates (*top row*) and the mesial and lateral views of the right hemisphere (*bottom row*) of a standard brain. These templates and surface views were derived from sliced postmortem specimens. In this method, the best fitting template set is identified, and the contour of the lesion is transferred with respect to a Cartesian coordinate system and any identifiable anatomic landmarks. **C**, A more recent and flexible approach is shown (*two rows*), in which the lesion has been transferred to a three-dimensional MR reconsruction of a standard normal brain, a process known as MAP-3 [5]. The standard three-dimensional brain is sliced to match the slices in the available two-dimensional images, improving the fit of template to target (compare coronal images in *A*, *B*, and *C*). The contour of the lesion is then transferred, as in the two-dimensional template system described previously. Once transferred, the lesion and standard brain can be rendered in three dimensions. In the MAP-3 technique, the lesion is depicted in red. (The display conventions used in this figure apply throughout this chapter.) These images make it possible to appreciate the extent and location of this lesion, which involves virtually all of the right occipital cortex and the posterior parts of the right occipitotemporal and parahippocampal gyri.

Visual object agnosia rarely affects all types of visual stimuli with equal magnitude [6–10]. In this patient with a right-sided occipitotemporal lesion, the profile of visual recognition impairment includes a major defect in recognizing entities from categories of living things, especially animals, but normal recognition of entities from categories of artifactual things (*eg*, tools and utensils). The varied patterns of visual object agnosia reflect the fact that different types of stimuli are mapped by different neural systems [11]. (*Courtesy of* Laboratory of Human Neuroanatomy and Neuroimaging, Department of Neurology, The University of Iowa.)

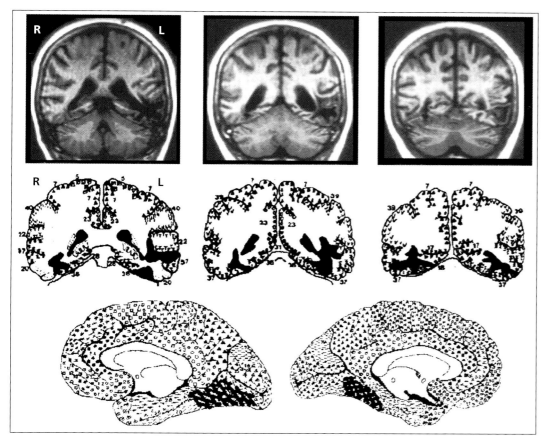

Figure 7-4. Associative prosopagnosia. T1-weighted magnetic resonance image (MRI) (*top row*) of a 67-year-old right-handed woman, showing bilateral occipitotemporal lesions caused by cerebral infarcts. The lesions are mapped onto standard brain templates in the middle and bottom rows. The patient developed associative prosopagnosia. Most cases of prosopagnosia are due to cerebral infarcts caused by occlusion in posterior cerebral artery branches, and this patient is an example of such pathophysiology. Head injury and cerebral tumors, especially gliomas originating in one occipital lobe and traversing into the opposite hemisphere, can also produce prosopagnosia.

Associative prosopagnosia, which is an inability to recognize familiar faces, is the most frequent and well established of the visual agnosias [12]. Associative prosopagnosia is caused by bilateral damage in inferior occipital and temporal visual association cortices, that is, the inferior component of areas 18 and 19 and the adjacent portion of area 37.

As is typical of prosopagnosia, the face recognition defect in this patient covered both the retrograde and anterograde compartments. The patient could no longer recognize the faces of previously

known people and was unable to learn new faces. The patient was unable to recognize the faces of family members, close friends, and even herself. On seeing those faces, the patient failed to experience any sense of familiarity and had no inkling that those faces were known to her. She could not conjure up any pertinent information that would trigger recognition. In associative prosopagnosia, the recognition impairment is relatively pure in the sense that it is confined to the visual modality and occurs in the setting of normal or near-normal visual perception. This patient performed normally on standard neuropsychologic tests of visuoperceptual discrimination and visuospatial judgment. Recognition by other modalities was unaffected. Thus, upon hearing the voices of people whose faces were unrecognized, the patient instantly recognized the identities of those people. Even within the visual modality, the defect was highly circumscribed. For instance, the patient had no problem recognizing people on the basis of a distinctive feature (*eg*, hairstyle, gait, or posture).

Prosopagnosia must be distinguished from disorders of *naming*. It is *not* an inability to name faces of people who are otherwise recognized as familiar. There are numerous examples of face naming failure from both brain-injured populations and from the realm of normal everyday experience, but in such instances, the unnamed face is invariably detected as familiar, and the precise identity of the possessor of the face is usually apprehended accurately. Conversely, patients with recognition defects may not have naming defects. In fact, the patient shown here remained capable of naming a wide range of familiar people, provided the naming did not depend on visual input—for example, she answered correctly questions such as "Which former President has Alzheimer's disease?" (*Courtesy of* Laboratory of Human Neuroanatomy and Neuroimaging, Department of Neurology, The University of Iowa.)

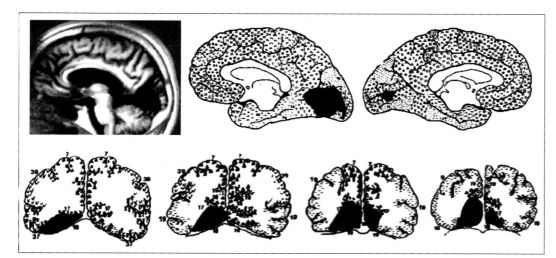

Figure 7-5. Apperceptive prosopagnosia. Depiction of brain lesions in a 28-year-old right-handed man who suffered a severe closed head injury with resultant damage to the mesial ventral occipital region bilaterally. A T1-weighted magnetic resonance imaging (MRI) scan is shown in the upper left corner. The other top row pictures show the lesions plotted on mid-sagittal standard brain templates; the bottom row

shows the lesions plotted on coronal templates. The patient had apperceptive prosopagnosia, which denotes face agnosia in the setting of visuoperceptual disturbance. The patient had defects in visual perception, demonstrable on neuropsychologic testing, which compromised abilities such as matching of unfamiliar faces, judgment of line orientations, and mental manipulation of pictures and picture fragments. The apperceptive face agnosia in this patient is associated with damage in mesial aspects of the ventral occipital cortices. Another cause is damage to the right visual association cortices within the occipitotemporal and occipitoparietal regions. The damage generally involves both the inferior and superior components of posterior visual association cortices (areas 18 and 19), mesially and laterally, for severe and lasting face agnosia to develop. In most cases, parts of areas 39 and 37 on the right are also damaged. (*Courtesy of* Laboratory of Human Neuroanatomy and Neuroimaging, Department of Neurology, The University of Iowa.)

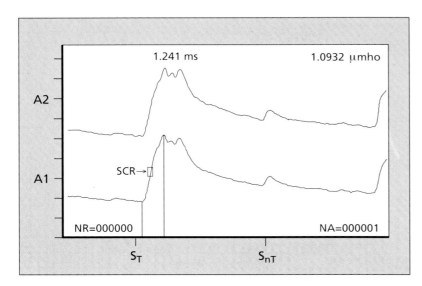

Figure 7-6. Nonconscious discrimination of familiar faces. Skin conductance polygraph recording for the right hand (*top trace, A2*) and left hand (*bottom trace, A1*) of a prosopagnosic patient. The patient is passively viewing slides of familiar (S_T) and unfamiliar (S_{nT}) faces. Note that the patient generated a large-amplitude skin conductance response (SCR) to the familiar face (the SCR amplitude is circumscribed by the *black vertical bars* on the A1 trace) but only a small response to the unfamiliar face. This outcome indicates clearly that the patient can discriminate familiar faces on the basis of an autonomic index, even though the patient is completely unable to provide any overt indication of familiar face recognition. Many prosopagnosic patients show this accurate *covert* or *nonconscious* discrimination of familiar faces, despite their complete inability to recognize those faces at an *overt* level [13,14]. Preserved covert face discrimination has been demonstrated in other experimental paradigms, such as reaction time tasks and forced-choice procedures. In the electrodermal paradigm, covert face discrimination has been demonstrated for faces from the anterograde compartment, suggesting that the brain can continue to learn new visual information even without conscious influence [15]. (*Courtesy of* the Psychophysiology Laboratory, Division of Behavioral Neurology and Cognitive Neuroscience, Department of Neurology, The University of Iowa.)

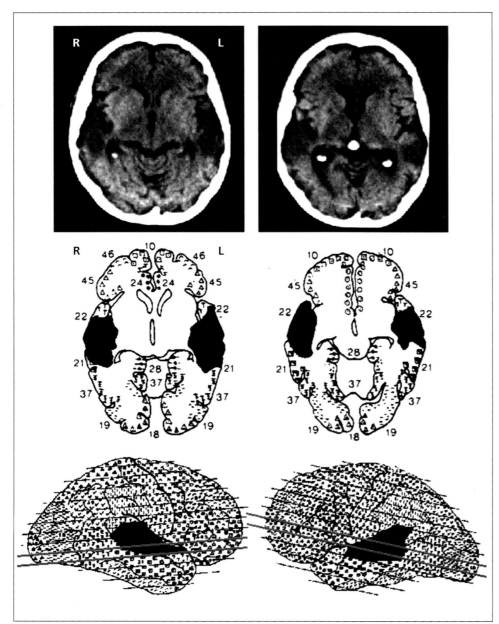

Figure 7-7. Auditory agnosia. A 37-year-old right-handed woman had bilateral lesions in the posterior portion of the superior temporal gyrus, which produced the condition of auditory agnosia. The top row shows two transverse computed tomographic cuts, and the lesions are indicated by hypointense signal. The lesions are plotted on standard brain templates in the middle and bottom rows.

Auditory agnosia is a disorder of recognition confined to the auditory realm, in which a patient cannot arrive at the meaning of some or all categories of previously known auditory stimuli, despite normal or near-normal auditory acuity and intact alertness, attention, and intelligence. Strictly speaking, the term should be reserved for an inability to recognize nonverbal sounds, such as environmental sounds, melodies, and timbres, and the term *aphasia* should apply to the verbal component of auditory agnosia. In fact, some degree of aphasia (related to the left temporal lobe lesion) is virtually always present. This patient had a fluent aphasia, but language capacities through the visual modality were preserved, and she remained capable of reading and writing. The defining characteristic of auditory agnosia is a defect in the recognition of common environmental sounds. The patient could not determine the meaning of sounds such as knocking on the door, a telephone ringing, a baby crying, or a bird chirping. The defect is modality specific, and the patient had normal recognition of entities presented visually, even though the sounds of those stimuli were unrecognized.

The auditory agnosia started acutely. The patient suddenly became almost entirely deaf. The patient also became speechless, failing to realize, owing to the sudden loss of auditory feedback, that she could speak. By writing, the patient complained of near-complete loss of hearing. The appropriate label at this point is *cortical deafness*. This improved rapidly and within a few weeks, the patient could hear sounds, and audiometry became normal. At this juncture, when the audiometric pattern normalized and the patient continued to report an inability to recognize sounds, the diagnosis of auditory agnosia was applied. In the acute phase, it is common for auditory agnosic patients to manifest severe behavioral disturbances, including anxiety, agitation, and even disorderly behavior. These behavioral features are attributable to the sudden and seemingly inexplicable deprivation of auditory feedback. It is important at this time to understand the reasons for the patient's behavior and to provide continual reassurance and support. These behaviors may prompt a psychiatric evaluation, but a psychiatric approach to the condition usually proves frustrating for both the patient and the examiner.

This presentation is strongly associated with bilateral lesions in the posterior one third of the superior temporal gyrus, as exemplified by this patient. The damage involves auditory association cortices (posterior area 22), while sparing to some extent the primary auditory cortices (areas 41 and 42). Invariably, such lesions are caused by stroke. We have often observed a staged presentation of this condition, whereby the patient suffers a unilateral lesion that may fail to produce noticeable, permanent defects, and then sustains a second lesion in the other hemisphere. The combined lesions produce the full-blown unfolding of cortical deafness evolving into auditory agnosia. Unilateral lesions in either the left or right auditory cortex rarely produce auditory agnosia or environmental sound agnosia. (*Courtesy of* Laboratory of Human Neuroanatomy and Neuroimaging, Department of Neurology, The University of Iowa.)

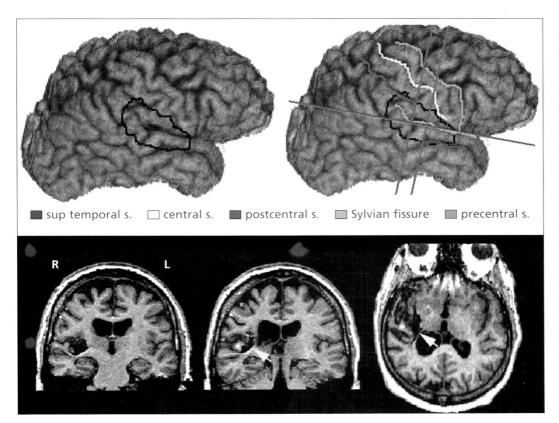

sup temporal s. ☐ central s. ■ postcentral s. ☐ Sylvian fissure ■ precentral s.

Figure 7-8. Auditory amusia. Auditory amusia, in which a patient loses the ability to recognize the unique timbres of singing voices, as well as the identities of familiar melodies, is a rare condition that can occur with or without other components of auditory agnosia. The condition is difficult to evaluate in patients who lack a musical education or regular musical activities. In the few cases that have been reported, the evidence suggests that the condition is caused by a right inferior parietal or posterior temporal lesion that disconnects right auditory association cortices from other important parts of the auditory processing system, including portions of the temporal and parietal lobes on the right, and homologous areas on the left. Interestingly, this patient with auditory amusia showed covert discrimination of familiar singing voices, demonstrated by large-amplitude skin conductance responses to familiar voices in a manner analogous to the covert recognition of familiar faces in prosopagnosic patients described in Figure 7-6 [13]. The lesion in this case (*yellow arrows*) is subcortical, its surface projection outlined with the black trace. It involves the insular cortex and white matter of the superior temporal lobe, undercutting the primary auditory cortex in Heschl's gyrus (*asterisk*). (*Courtesy of* Laboratory of Human Neuroanatomy and Neuroimaging, Department of Neurology, The University of Iowa.)

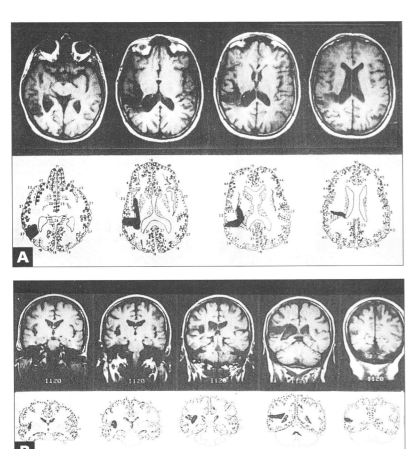

Figure 7-9. Tactile agnosia. T1-weighted transverse magnetic resonance images (MRIs) (**A**) and coronal MRIs (**B**) and accompanying templates from a patient with tactile agnosia. Lesions in somatosensory-related cortices can produce *tactile agnosia*, an impairment of recognition of entities presented in the somatosensory (tactile) channel, not attributable to defective perception, nor to alterations of intellect, language, or attention. There is a fundamental difference between tactile agnosia and visual agnosia, owing to different task demands; many visual stimuli, including things such as unique faces and landmarks, require recognition at the most specific level, *ie*, a precise identification of the individual stimulus. In the tactile modality, few items are learned at the most specific, unique level, and for most things it is sufficient to recognize the item at the basic object level (*eg*, a stapler as a "stapler" [as opposed to *my* stapler]; a screwdriver as a "screwdriver" [as opposed to *my* screwdriver]). Hence, tactile agnosia is more or less tantamount to the notion of tactile object agnosia, referring to defective recognition of objects such as tools, musical instruments, fruits, and animals. The defect is restricted to the tactile modality, and patients can easily recognize these stimuli when they are presented visually. The condition has been associated with damage to temporoparietal cortices, especially in and near the region of the inferior parietal operculum and posterior insula, possibly including the second somatosensory cortex, in either hemisphere [16]. A restricted form of tactile object agnosia, in which the patient could not recognize nonmanipulable entities (*ie*, stimuli that are learned and operated exclusively through the visual modality, such as large animals, buildings, vehicles) but was capable of recognizing manipulable entities (*eg*, tools, utensils), has been described in connection with a mesial superior parietal lesion in the right hemisphere [17]. The most frequent neuropathologic factor is cerebral infarction, followed by a few cases attributable to tumor, head injury, or herpes simplex encephalitis. (*From* Caselli [16]; with permission.)

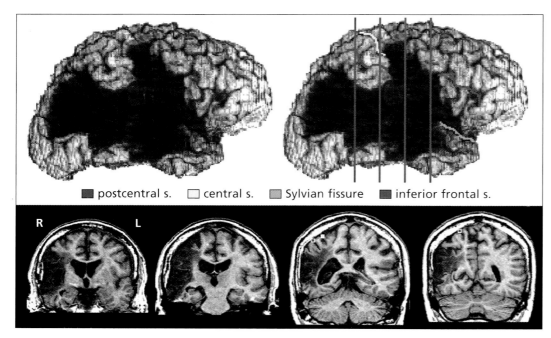

■ postcentral s.   □ central s.   ▨ Sylvian fissure   ■ inferior frontal s.

Figure 7-10. Anosognosia. A lesion in the right hemisphere involving a significant portion of the inferior parietal lobule (areas 39 and 40), shown in lateral three-dimensional brain reconstructions (*top*) and in coronal T1-weighted magnetic resonance imaging (MRI) cuts (*bottom*) in a patient with anosognosia. The patient, a 34-year-old right-handed woman, sustained an infarct in the territory of the right middle cerebral artery and developed severe anosognosia in connection with this lesion.

Anosognosia denotes a condition in which patients lose the ability to recognize disease states in themselves; the term was first applied to a patient who denied a left hemiplegia [18]. The condition is in essence a disturbance of recognition, and in that sense, it conforms to the designation of agnosia. In the most extreme and paradigmatic examples, patients fail to recognize major disabilities such as a complete hemiplegia or hemianesthesia; marked pain may be ignored; and the gravity of heart disease or cancer may go unacknowledged. Anosognosia also occurs in relation to cognitive and behavioral deficits. Patients give little indication of understanding that their cognition and behavior are compromised and fail to appreciate the ramifications of their disabilities. The term anosognosia can be applied

whenever there is a significant discrepancy between the patient's report of his or her disabilities and the objective evidence regarding the patient's level of functioning.

Anosognosia is strongly associated with damage to the right somatosensory cortices in the parietal and insular regions, as exemplified by this patient. The condition is rarely observed in connection with left-hemisphere damage. This reflects the fact that the right hemisphere has a relative specialization for the processing of somatic information, in keeping with its relative specialization in emotional and affective processing. Typical neuropsychologic correlates include defects in spatial abilities (visuoperceptual and visuoconstructional skills) and left-sided neglect, that is, an impairment in attention to and acknowledgment of stimuli presented to the left hemispace. The ventromedial prefrontal region, including the orbital and lower mesial frontal cortices, is another frequent neural correlate of anosognosia [19]. Damage to this area is commonly produced by head injury, rupture of anterior cerebral or anterior communicating artery aneurysms, or tumors. Patients manifest severe anosognosia for acquired defects in social conduct and decision making. For example, they are unaware that their poor decisions have produced a trail of personal catastrophes in terms of interpersonal relationships, social rank, and occupational endeavors. Patients evidence little insight into the relationship between their own behavior and the responses of those around them [20] (Figs. 7-33 to 7-37.) (*Courtesy of* Laboratory of Human Neuroanatomy and Neuroimaging, Department of Neurology, The University of Iowa.)

Disorders of Visual Perception

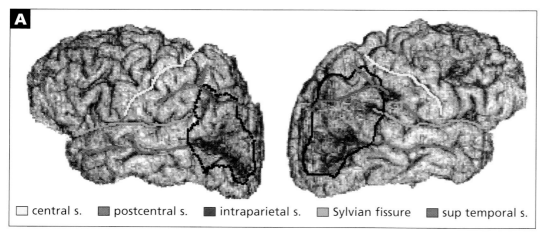

□ central s.   ■ postcentral s.   ■ intraparietal s.   ▨ Sylvian fissure   ■ sup temporal s.

Figure 7-11. Balint's syndrome. **A,** Three-dimensional magnetic resonance imaging (MRI) reconstruction of the left and right hemispheres of a 74-year-old right-handed man who sustained bilateral infarcts in the superior occipital region. **B,** Coronal T1-weighted MR images of the patient. The lesions involve the association cortices of areas 18 and 19 and encroach into the adjacent parietal areas 39 and 7. The patient developed Balint's syndrome in connection with these lesions, which were caused by borderzone infarcts, a common cause of this lesion pattern.

When situated in the primary visual cortex of area 17 or its connections, lesions to the dorsal sector of the occipital region lead to a loss of form vision (*ie*, blindness) in the inferior visual field contralateral to

the lesion. When the lesions spare the primary visual cortex and involve the association cortices of areas 18 and 19, the condition known as *Balint's syndrome* develops. The dorsal visual system is sometimes referred to as the *where* system, owing to its specialization for locating of objects in space and aspects of motion processing [21].

Balint's syndrome is based on the presence of three components: visual disorientation (also known as simultanagnosia); ocular apraxia (also known as psychic gaze paralysis); and optic ataxia. The key constituent in the syndrome is visual disorientation, and there is considerable variability in the emphasis placed on the other components [22,23].

Visual disorientation (simultanagnosia) can be conceptualized as an inability to attend to more than a limited sector of the visual field at any given moment. Patients report that they can see clearly in only a small part of the field, the rest being out of focus and "foggy." The sector of clear vision is unstable and may shift without warning in any direction, so that patients experience a literal jumping about of their visual perception.

(*Continued on next page*)

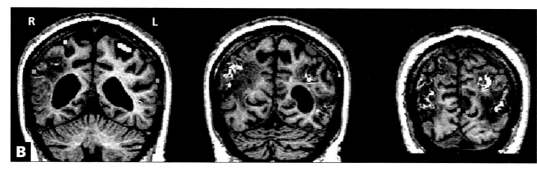

Figure 7-11. (*Continued*) Patients are incapable of constructing a spatially coherent visual field, and they cannot follow trajectories of stimuli or place stimuli in their proper locations in space. Perception of motion is often impaired, so that patients fail to notice objects that have moved in their visual field or the meaning of movements they have otherwise perceived correctly [24]. Patients may fail to recognize a familiar gait or stride or to understand pantomime [12]. Patients with visual disorientation can perceive color and shape normally if the objects are appreciated within a clear sector of the visual field [23,28].

Ocular apraxia (psychic gaze paralysis) is a deficit of visual scanning. It consists of an inability to direct one's gaze voluntarily toward a stimulus located in peripheral vision to bring it into central vision. Thus, patients fail to direct saccades toward stimuli that have appeared in the panorama of their visual fields, or they produce saccades that are inaccurate and miss the target. Ocular apraxia is not necessary for the development of visual disorientation, but it always occurs with either visual disorientation or optic ataxia. The neural substrates for the processing of actions and motions are only recently beginning to be understood [25–27].

Optic ataxia is a disturbance of visually guided reaching behavior. Patients are not able to point accurately at a target, under visual guidance. They cannot point precisely to the examiner's fingertip or to items such as a cup or coin. Pointing to targets on one's own body can be accomplished on the basis of somatosensory information and thus does not pose a problem. Also, these patients have no difficulty pointing to sound sources [29]. Optic ataxia can occur in isolation, particularly when lesions are at the border of the occipital and parietal regions, or in the parietal region exclusively.

Balint's syndrome is generally associated with bilateral occipitoparietal lesions, although a unilateral lesion, especially on the right, can also produce the syndrome. When lesions are confined to the superior occipital cortices without extension into the parietal region, visual disorientation is likely to occur without associated ocular apraxia or optic ataxia. The defects in motion perception that are frequent in patients with Balint's syndrome are probably related to damage in the lower parietal or lateral occipital region [30]. Many patients with Balint's syndrome have an impairment of stereopsis, that is, the process of depth perception from visual information dependent on binocular visual interaction, although complete astereopsis is seen only in the setting of bilateral lesions [28,31]. (*Courtesy of* Laboratory of Human Neuroanatomy and Neuroimaging, Department of Neurology, The University of Iowa.)

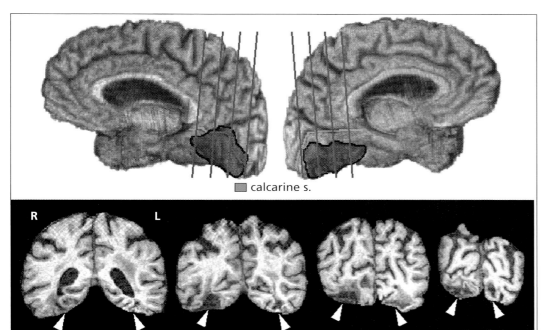

calcarine s.

Figure 7-12. Acquired achromatopsia. Mesial views of a three-dimensional magnetic resonance imaging (MRI) reconstruction of a 67-year-old right-handed woman who sustained bilateral infarcts in the infracalcarine visual association cortices (*top*). Coronal sections (*bottom*) have been digitally edited to remove extracerebral structures, and the lesions are marked (*arrowheads*). The patient had bilateral superior quadrantanopia. In the lower fields, form vision was normal, but she was unable to see color, that is, she had achromatopsia. The lesions were caused by two separate infarcts, which occurred several months apart. A staged stroke presentation is common in patients who sustain bilateral lesions of this type. The patient had prosopagnosia as well, and this is a common correlate of achromatopsia (Fig. 7-4).

Acquired (central) achromatopsia is a disorder of color perception with preservation of form vision, caused by damage to the inferior visual association cortex or its subjacent white matter [32,33]. Patients lose color vision in a quadrant, a hemifield, or the entire visual field. The loss may be partial, with patients complaining that colors appear washed out or dirty, or entire, with patients seeing all forms in shades of black and white. Perception of form is unaltered, and depth and motion perception are also normal. This disorder is *acquired*. It is not a hereditary (retinal) disorder of color vision, such as the red-green color blindness that is common in males; thus the designation *central* achromatopsia. Also, the inability to *name* colors is not part of the disorder but rather is associated with *color anomia*. Patients with color anomia can pass basic color perception tests such as the Ishihara Color Plate Test and the Farnsworth-Munsell 100-Hue Test. Nor is achromatopsia a disturbance of color association (a disorder known as *color agnosia*); achromatopsic patients can answer prompts, such as "the color of grass is _____ [green]," or "the color of blood is _____ [red]."

The most precise anatomic studies based on the lesion method have indicated that the middle third of the lingual gyrus is the most common site of damage in patients with central achromatopsia, followed by the white matter immediately behind the posterior tip of the lateral ventricle [34]. Studies using functional neuroimaging techniques have corroborated the lesion-based work. When subjects are given tasks requiring inspection or searching for colored stimuli, there are areas of activation in the region of the lingual and fusiform gyri, or putative human area V4, essentially the same area implicated by lesion work [35–37]. The functional imaging and lesion studies are also consistent with neurophysiology work in animals [38,39] and with event-related potential (ERP) studies [40]. The work in nonhuman primates has indicated that separate cellular channels within area 17 are differently dedicated to the processing of color, form, and motion [38,39], and that some visual association cortices have an important specialization for color processing.

A disorder closely related to achromatopsia involves defective color imagery, that is, the inability to imagine objects in color. Functional imaging studies have shown that imagining and naming the colors associated with various entities activate a region in the fusiform gyrus, bilaterally, but more strongly on the left [41]. (*Courtesy of* Laboratory of Human Neuroanatomy and Neuroimaging, Department of Neurology, The University of Iowa.)

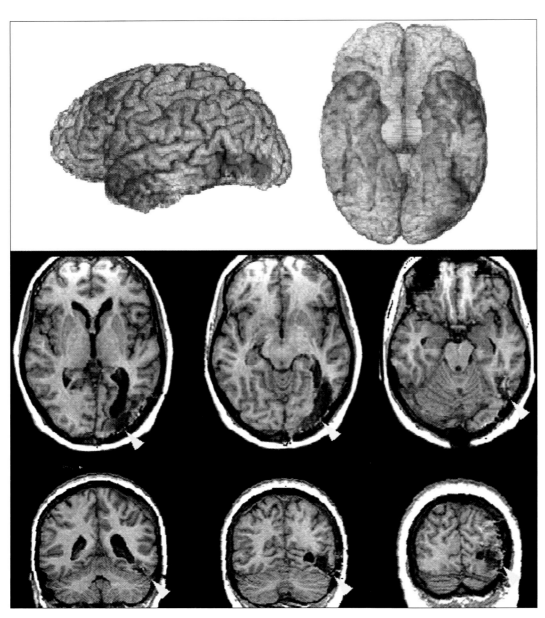

Lesions such as the one exemplified here disconnect both visual association cortices from the dominant, language-related temporoparietal cortices, and produce an impairment in reading known as *acquired*, or pure, *alexia*. Pure alexia can be caused by a single lesion strategically placed in the region behind, beneath, and under the occipital horn of the left lateral ventricle, damaging pathways from the callosum and from the left visual association cortex; such is the case here. Another setting is the combination of a lesion in the corpus callosum, which disconnects right to left visual information transfer, and a lesion in the left occipital lobe, which disconnects left visual association cortex from left language cortex. Such lesions are likely to produce a right hemianopia, and this sign is a frequent, although not invariable, accompaniment of pure alexia. A common neuropsychologic correlate of pure alexia is color anomia.

The "purity" of the condition stems from the fact that some patients with this type of lesion do not develop disturbances in writing or in other aspects of speech and linguistic functioning, separating this type of alexia from the types of reading defects that are common in aphasic patients. (Alexia occurs commonly in the setting of aphasia, often with a coexistent disturbance of writing. This pattern is common with lesions in traditional language regions of the left hemisphere, especially in the territory around the sylvian fissure.) In this sense, pure alexia can be construed as a disturbance of visual pattern recognition. Pure alexia is also known as *alexia without agraphia* or *pure word blindness*.

Patients with pure alexia are unable to read most words and sentences, and in severe cases, even reading of single letters is impaired. The problem is not one of visual acuity; the fact that patients can *see* the sentences, words, and letters they cannot read can be readily demonstrated by having patients copy those stimuli, a task that is executed normally. Most patients with pure alexia have normal visual acuity, although a quadrantanopia or hemianopia may be present. (*Courtesy of* Laboratory of Human Neuroanatomy and Neuroimaging, Department of Neurology, The University of Iowa.)

Figure 7-13. Acquired ("pure") alexia. Three-dimensional magnetic resonance imaging (MRI) reconstruction (*top*) of a standard brain (left lateral and ventral views), onto which has been plotted (in red, using MAP-3 [Fig. 7-2]) the left occipitotemporal infarct sustained by a 43-year-old right-handed woman. T1-weighted MRI scans of the patient's brain in transverse (*middle*) and coronal (*bottom*) sections, on which the lesion is designated by the yellow arrows, are also shown. The patient developed alexia after this lesion. Acutely, she also had transcortical sensory aphasia, but this resolved (Fig. 7-20).

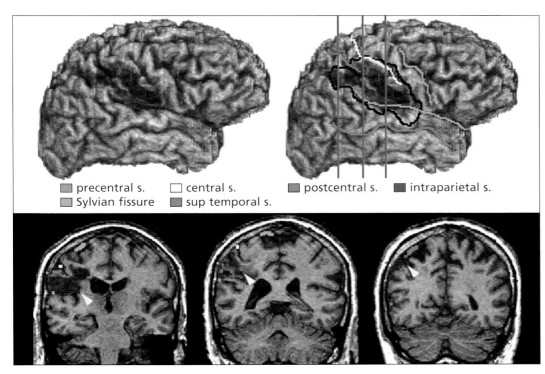

□ precentral s.   □ central s.   ■ postcentral s.   ■ intraparietal s.
□ Sylvian fissure   ■ sup temporal s.

Figure 7-14. Visual neglect. Three-dimensional magnetic resonance imaging (MRI) reconstruction of a 44-year-old right-handed man who sustained a right parietal infarct. Lateral hemispheric (*top*) and coronal (*bottom*) orientations are depicted. The lesion (*arrows*) resulted from a middle cerebral artery infarct and includes portions of the postcentral gyrus and the inferior parietal lobule (Brodmann's areas 39 and 40). The patient had severe left-sided visual neglect.

The patient was unable to shift his attention to the left half of extrapersonal and intrapersonal space. When asked to draw a picture of a clock, the patient produced a drawing that had all the numbers on the right side of the clock face. The patient also neglected the left side of his own body, failing to acknowledge limbs on that side, to shave the left side of his face, and to dress the left side. Practical remedies can be helpful in managing these patients; for example, making sure to interact with the patient from the patient's right side, and situating the patient's bed so that visitors will approach from the patient's right.

Several features of left hemispace neglect warrant emphasis. The condition is strongly associated with right posterior lesions. It is highly uncommon to observe the development of right-sided neglect in connection with a left hemisphere lesion (about as uncommon as the development of aphasia in connection with a right hemisphere lesion). Also, the phenomenon is often fairly short-lived; in many cases, it manifests immediately after the onset of brain damage and resolves quickly and completely. Finally, neglect is strongly associated with disturbances of spatial processing, including visuoperceptual and visuoconstructional defects, defects in visuospatial memory, and impairments in nonverbal intellectual abilities [42]. (*Courtesy of* Laboratory of Human Neuroanatomy and Neuroimaging, Department of Neurology, The University of Iowa.)

Aphasia

Disorders of Language

Disorder	Examples of neural correlates
Aphasia	
Broca's	Left frontal operculum (Broca's area)
Wernicke's	Left posterosuperior temporal gyrus (Wernicke's area)
Global	Entire perisylvian region on left, including frontal operculum, parietal operculum, and posterior temporal region
Conduction	Parietal operculum, supramarginal gyrus, and insula
Transcortical	Left prefrontal (motor version); left posterior temporal, inferior to Wernicke's area (sensory version)
Subcortical	Left basal ganglia; thalamus
Anomic	Left inferotemporal; temporal pole
Crossed	Right perisylvian (frontal, parietal, temporal)
Aprosody	Right perisylvian region, including posterosuperior temporal, inferior parietal, frontal operculum

Figure 7-15. Disorders of language. The study of language impairments associated with focal brain damage is one of the most extensively developed areas of research in neuropsychology, and much has been learned about the neural systems related to functions such as comprehension, speech production, lexical retrieval, and reading and writing [43]. Our understanding of brain–language relations has been facilitated by multidisciplinary approaches to language disorders, and scientists from fields such as cognitive psychology and linguistics, together with neuropsychologists and neurologists, have made important contributions to the investigation of speech and language [44–46].

Aphasia is an acquired disturbance of the comprehension and formulation of verbal messages caused by dysfunction in a set of language-related cortical and subcortical structures in the left hemisphere. Aphasia can be further specified as a defect in the two-way translation mechanism between thought processes and language, that is, between the nonverbal mental representations whose organized manipulation constitutes thought, and the verbal symbols and grammatical rules whose organized processing constitutes sentences. Aphasia can compromise either the *formulation* or *comprehension* of language, or both, and it can affect *syntax* (the grammatical structure of sentences), the *lexicon* (the dictionary of words that denote meanings), or *word morphology* (the combination of phonemes that results in word structure).

Deficits in various subcomponents of language occur with different severity and in different patterns, producing a number of distinctive syndromes of aphasia. Each syndrome has a fairly regular set of neuropsychologic manifestations and a typical site of neural dysfunction. Cerebrovascular disease is the most common cause. Head injury and tumors are other common causes, and aphasia may also occur in the setting of progressive degenerative diseases, particularly Pick's disease and sometimes Alzheimer's disease. Several of the classic subtypes of aphasia are reviewed in this chapter.

Of the aphasia syndromes most common in neurologic patients, the Broca, Wernicke, and global subtypes are most frequent. Focal damage to neural sectors in the territory of the left middle cerebral artery is relatively common, and these aphasia syndromes, all related to dysfunction of various sectors in the vicinity of the sylvian fissure, occur with regularity in neurologic patients with focal lesions.

Well-developed treatment programs can have a major beneficial effect on recovery from aphasia [47]. In general, patients whose aphasia is caused by head injury fare better than patients whose aphasia is due to vascular causes, and younger age and higher premorbid intelligence are also related to better recovery. Most studies have found that the more severe the initial aphasia, the poorer is the recovery, and patients with global aphasia typically show the least recovery [48,49].

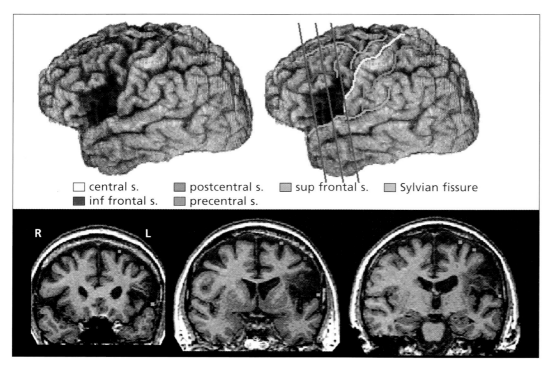

Figure 7-16. Broca's aphasia. Three-dimensional magnetic resonance imaging (MRI) reconstruction of a 76-year-old right-handed man who developed Broca's aphasia after a left frontal infarct. The lesion, shown in lateral (*top*) and coronal (*bottom*) images, includes the precentral gyrus and Broca's

area (pars opercularis and triangularis of the inferior frontal gyrus), formed by Brodmann's areas 44 and 45. In addition to aphasia, the patient had a right hemiparesis, with the face and arm affected most severely, a sign that is typical of Broca's aphasia. No visual field impairment was present. Patients with Broca's aphasia are *nonfluent*, and their speech production is effortful, sparse, and agrammatic. Paraphasias (word substitutions) are common, usually involving omission of phonemes or substitution of incorrect phonemes (*eg*, "hostapil" for "hospital"). Verbatim repetition is defective, and naming and writing are also impaired. However, patients with Broca's aphasia have relatively normal comprehension of language, in both its aural and written forms. Also, even a severely nonfluent patient may be able to *sing*, because the production of singing is mediated by brain regions other than Broca's area (probably homologous right hemisphere structures). As exemplified here, the syndrome of Broca's aphasia is related to damage in the frontal operculum. When the lesion extends into subcortical structures and the anterior insula, the aphasia is more severe and resolves less. It is not uncommon for global aphasia (Fig. 7-18) to resolve into Broca's aphasia. (*Courtesy of* Laboratory of Human Neuroanatomy and Neuroimaging, Department of Neurology, The University of Iowa.)

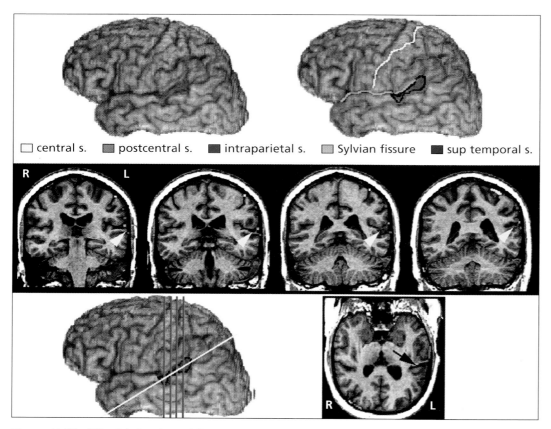

Figure 7-17. Wernicke's aphasia. Three-dimensional magnetic resonance imaging (MRI) reconstruction of a 56-year-old right-handed man who developed Wernicke's aphasia after a small left posterior temporal infarct. The lesion, shown in lateral (*top; bottom left*), coronal (*middle*), and transverse (*bottom right*) images, involves the posterior third of the superior temporal gyrus, in the heart of what is known as *Wernicke's area*. The lesion shown here is quite circumscribed; commonly, lesions producing Wernicke's aphasia will also involve nearby structures in the inferior parietal lobule (supramarginal gyrus) and temporal lobe (angular gyrus).

Wernicke's aphasia can be considered a counterpart to Broca's aphasia. Affected patients, in contrast to patients with Broca's aphasia, produce fluent, well-articulated speech. Effort is normal; in fact, the patient may be hyperfluent, producing copious responses to simple questions. Phrase length,

most aspects of grammatical structure, and articulation and prosody are normal. However, the speech is dominated by paraphasic errors, both *semantic* (*eg*, "bacon" for "pig") and *phonemic* (*eg*, "peepas" for "people"). Or the speech may be virtually devoid of nouns, and composed of pronouns, prepositions, and other nonspecific words. A distinctive feature of Wernicke's aphasia is a severe impairment of comprehension for both aural and written forms of language. Verbatim repetition and naming are also defective. Wernicke's aphasia is related to damage in the left posterosuperior temporal gyrus (Wernicke's area) and nearby regions in the temporal and lower parietal cortices.

The development of Wernicke's aphasia may be accompanied by a right-sided visual field defect (homonymous hemianopia) due to interruption of the optic radiations, but other neurologic manifestations, such as motor or sensory changes, are often absent. In fact, there may be no other neurologic signs besides the aphasia. Thus, a patient may present with an isolated and rather striking disturbance of speech, which can easily lead to misdiagnosis, particularly as psychiatric disease. Consideration of the age and history of the patient can help steer the diagnosis in the correct direction, and neuroimaging (MRI or computed tomography) confirms the neurologic basis for the presentation. Patients with Wernicke's aphasia tend to recover considerably, especially with speech therapy. Lesion size is a factor, and smaller lesions can be expected to result in better recovery. Two years after lesion onset, this patient had only a mild word-finding defect and a mild impairment in confrontation naming. (*Courtesy of* Laboratory of Human Neuroanatomy and Neuroimaging, Department of Neurology, The University of Iowa.)

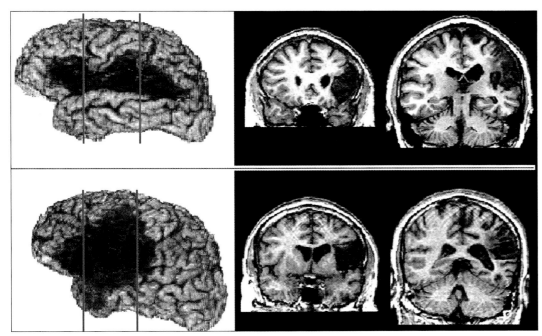

coronal (*right*) orientations. As is typical of global aphasia, these patients had right hemiplegia affecting face, arm, and leg, right hemisensory impairment, and right homonymous hemianopia.

As the term implies, global aphasia involves virtually complete dilapidation of speech and linguistic capacities. The patient is rendered incapable of both comprehending and producing verbal messages. Verbatim repetition, naming, reading, and writing are all severely impaired. The patient may, however, retain the capacity for singing, and it is worth testing for this, because the production of fluent singing can be highly encouraging in a patient who is otherwise virtually mute. As exemplified in both these patients, the syndrome is related to extensive destruction of the perisylvian region, including Broca's area, the inferior parietal cortices, Wernicke's area, and underlying white matter and subcortical structures. Rarely, global aphasia may result from two noncontiguous lesions, one involving Broca's area and the other involving Wernicke's area. In this presentation, the patient does *not* have a right hemiparesis, owing to the sparing of motor cortex between the two lesions, and the prognosis for recovery of some linguistic abilities is considerably better [50]. Otherwise, global aphasia has a worse prognosis for recovery than any of the other aphasia syndromes. (*Courtesy of* Laboratory of Human Neuroanatomy and Neuroimaging, The University of Iowa).

Figure 7-18. Global aphasia. Three-dimensional magnetic resonance imaging (MRI) reconstructions of two patients with global aphasia. The top row depicts a 74-year-old right-handed man who suffered a large infarct in the territory of the left middle cerebral artery, which damaged all language-related regions in the perisylvian sector, including Broca's area, Wernicke's area, and the parietal opercular region. The other patient, a 68-year-old right-handed man, is shown in the bottom row. The patient had a similar presentation; virtually all of the regions in the immediate vicinity of the sylvian fissure are damaged, although there is some sparing of the more posterior aspects of the region. Both lesions are shown in lateral (*left*) and

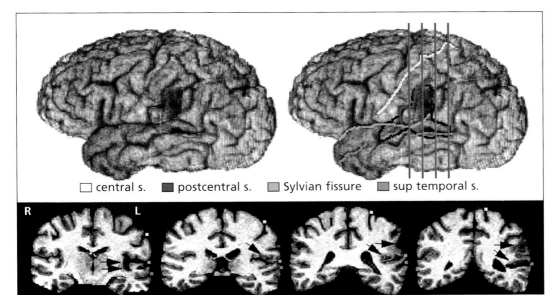

Figure 7-19. Conduction aphasia. Three-dimensional magnetic resonance imaging (MRI) reconstruction of a 35-year-old right-handed woman who developed conduction aphasia after a left middle cerebral artery territory infarct. The lesion, shown in lateral (*top*) and coronal (*bottom*) images, is in the left supramarginal gyrus (Brodmann's area 40), the parietal operculum, and the posterior insula (*arrows*). The lesion spares the primary auditory cortex and the main part of Wernicke's area (posterior Brodmann's area 22), and it also spares entirely the frontal operculum (Broca's area). The woman

had conduction aphasia, which is hallmarked by a severe defect in verbatim repetition. Other aspects of language, including fluency and comprehension, were relatively less affected. Phonemic paraphasic errors were common, and naming was impaired. The patient was unable to write to dictation (a defect parallel to the repetition impairment) but could write much better when copying another script or when producing spontaneous compositions. Conduction aphasia is related to damage either to the supramarginal gyrus (Brodmann's area 40) in the lower parietal region, or to the primary auditory cortices with extension into the insular cortex and underlying white matter. The primary auditory association cortices in posterior Brodmann's area 22 are spared, allowing the preservation of comprehension. Neurologic signs vary considerably; many patients manifest some degree of motor or sensory impairment (including visual field defects) in the acute phase, but neurologic abnormalities may recover quickly and completely, leaving a relatively isolated disturbance of language. Conduction aphasia tends to respond well to speech therapy. (*Courtesy of* Laboratory of Human Neuroanatomy and Neuroimaging, Department of Neurology, The University of Iowa.)

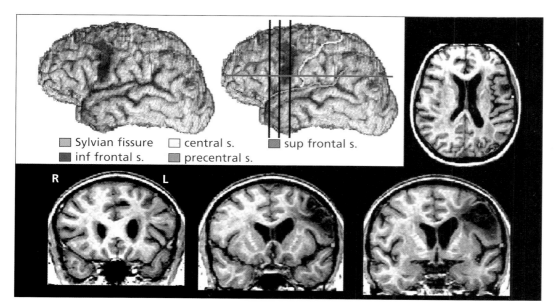

Figure 7-20. The transcortical aphasias. The four aphasia subtypes shown in Figure 7-16 through 7-19 share the feature that *verbatim repetition* is impaired, and all are associated with damage to some part of the perisylvian region on the left. In fact, impaired repetition is a reliable sign pointing to dysfunction in cortices in and around the sylvian fissure. When the lesion is situated either anterior (in front of or above Broca's area) or posterior (behind and below Wernicke's area) to the perisylvian region, the aphasias that develop, known as the *transcortical aphasias*, lack the feature of impaired repetition.

Three-dimensional magnetic resonance imaging (MRI) reconstruction in lateral (*top left* and *middle*), transverse (*top right*), and coronal (*bottom*) views from a 49-year-old right-handed man who sustained a lesion in the left premotor region. The damage is in the left frontal operculum just anterior to the precentral

sulcus, but most of Broca's area is spared. The man had transcortical motor aphasia. This is a Broca-like aphasia, except that the patient can repeat verbatim. Thus, the speech is nonfluent, effortful, and sparse; comprehension is relatively preserved; reading and writing are usually disturbed. Confrontation naming may be spared, especially for specific objects (noun retrieval), although it has been shown that naming of actions (verb retrieval) can be impaired [51]. Patients with this type of aphasia have a good prognosis if the lesion is fairly circumscribed, but when substantial white matter involvement is present (as is the case in the patient shown here), recovery is poorer.

A lesion in the left inferotemporal region, situated primarily in the angular gyrus, produces a Wernicke-like aphasia, except that verbatim repetition is spared (Fig. 7-13). This syndrome is known as *transcortical sensory aphasia*. This aphasia subtype is fairly uncommon, although a number of patients who present acutely with Wernicke's aphasia gradually evolve into a transcortical sensory profile. Speech is fluent, with normal grammar, articulation, and prosody; comprehension is at least somewhat impaired. There is some impairment of confrontation naming, although the defect may be much greater for certain categories of items (*eg*, tools and utensils) than for others (*eg*, animals) [52]. (*Courtesy of* Laboratory of Human Neuroanatomy and Neuroimaging, Department of Neurology, The University of Iowa.)

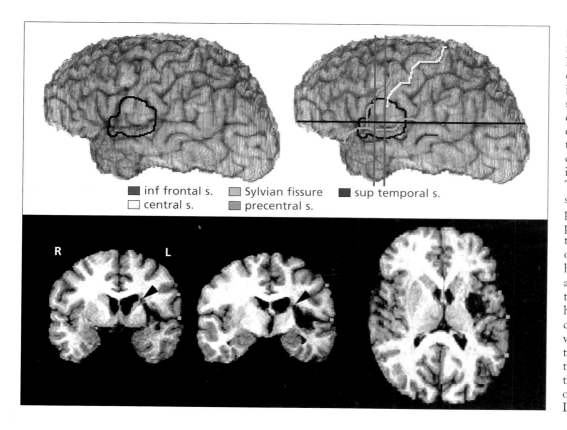

Figure 7-21. Subcortical aphasia. Three-dimensional magnetic resonance imaging (MRI) reconstruction in lateral (*top*) and coronal (*bottom*) depictions of a 35-year-old right-handed woman who sustained a subcortical intracerebral hemorrhage. The lesion involves the left striatum, including part of the head of the caudate nucleus (*arrowhead*) and part of the putamen. On the lateral views, there is no evidence of the lesion, and all of the perisylvian cortices are intact. The patient had a characteristic *basal ganglia* or *subcortical*, aphasia, which is marked in particular by severe dysarthria [53,54]. There are mixed linguistic impairments. Patients with subcortical aphasia usually have variably fluent, paraphasic, and highly dysarthric speech accompanied by poor auditory comprehension and, in some cases, repetition impairment. This profile does not conform to any of the typical cortical-related aphasia subtypes. Right hemiparesis or hemisensory impairment is a frequent accompanying neurologic sign. Subcortical aphasia tends to have good recovery, especially when caused by hemorrhagic lesions. Disorders of speech and language can also follow lesions to the left thalamus, especially when damage involves the ventrolateral and anteroventral nuclei. The aphasia associated with left anterior thalamic lesions shares several of the characteristics of the transcortical aphasias [55]. (*Courtesy of* Laboratory of Human Neuroanatomy and Neuroimaging, Department of Neurology, The University of Iowa.)

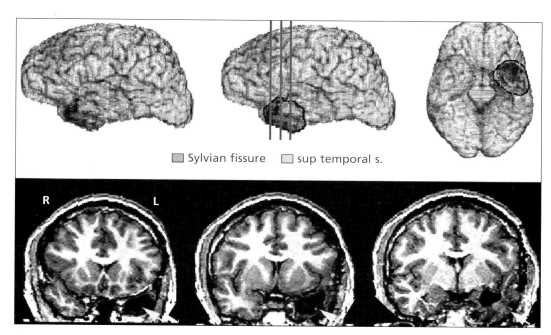

Sylvian fissure   sup temporal s.

Figure 7-22. Anomic aphasia. Three-dimensional magnetic resonance imaging (MRI) reconstruction of a 25-year-old right-handed man who suffered a hemorrhage and surgical intervention in the region of the left anteroinferior temporal lobe. The lesion, shown in lateral (*top left* and *middle*), ventral (*top right*), and coronal (*bottom*) views, involves the temporal lobe at the pole (*arrows*), with extension posteriorly and ventrally into the anterior part of the inferotemporal region. The patient had a severe impairment of confrontation naming (anomia), but no other speech or language impairment. This profile conforms to the designation of *anomic aphasia*. Naming defects are common in all of the classic aphasia subtypes [56–58]. Anomia can occur in isolation, however, as demonstrated here. In this presentation, a left inferotemporal or polar temporal lesion, outside the classic language regions, is the typical neural correlate.

Different profiles of naming impairment have been associated with different patterns of brain damage. Damage to the inferotemporal region, particularly in Brodmann's areas 20 and 21 and the anterior part of Brodmann's area 37, produces defects in the retrieval of common nouns; for example, the patient cannot name entities such as various animals, fruits, and vegetables, and tools and utensils [52,58]. A further distinction is possible, whereby naming of animals is more affected by anterior inferotemporal damage, and naming of tools and utensils is more affected by posterior inferotemporal damage. In contrast, damage to the temporal polar region (Brodmann's area 38) produces an impairment of proper naming, that is, naming of unique entities such as famous people and well-known landmarks. In the case shown here, the naming impairment affected the categories of people and animals, but naming of tools and utensils was normal. Evidence suggests that patients with anomia caused by damage to the inferotemporal region do *not* have impaired naming of actions; that is, retrieval of verbs is normal. If damage is in the left premotor or prefrontal region, however, patients may have naming defects for actions, but not for concrete entities [51,59]. (*Courtesy of* Laboratory of Human Neuroanatomy and Neuroimaging, Department of Neurology, The University of Iowa.)

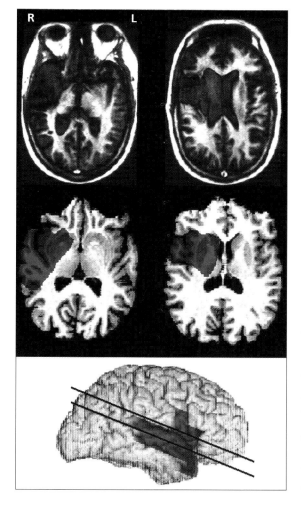

Figure 7-23. Crossed aphasia. Aphasia is associated almost exclusively with lesions in the left hemisphere, in keeping with the fact that nearly all right-handed people (about 98%) have left hemisphere dominance for speech, and even most left-handed people (about 70%) also have left hemisphere dominance for speech. Rare exceptions occur, however, and one of these is illustrated in this figure. The patient is a 73-year-old *right-handed* man who developed severe aphasia after this infarct in the *right* perisylvian region. The lesion is shown in red on a lateral MAP-3 reconstruction (*bottom*) and on axial T1-weighted magnetic resonance imaging (MRI) cuts of this reconstruction (*middle*). The area of abnormal signal on the MRI cuts is shown in the T2-weighted axial MRI cuts (*top*). This presentation—aphasia in a right-handed person after a right hemisphere lesion—has been termed *crossed aphasia* [60]. The disorder is rare, and subtypes have not been specified in detail. This patient had nonfluent, effortful speech; impaired naming, reading, and writing, and a mild comprehension defect. As is typical with crossed aphasia, the patient had significant defects in a number of spatial, nonverbal capacities, including visuoperceptual discrimination, visuoconstruction, and nonverbal memory. This profile suggests that the neural organization in the patient did not involve a mere reversal of hemispheric dominance, but rather the addition of language mediation to right hemisphere structures that were also subserving many spatial functions. (*Courtesy of* Laboratory of Human Neuroanatomy and Neuroimaging, Department of Neurology, The University of Iowa.)

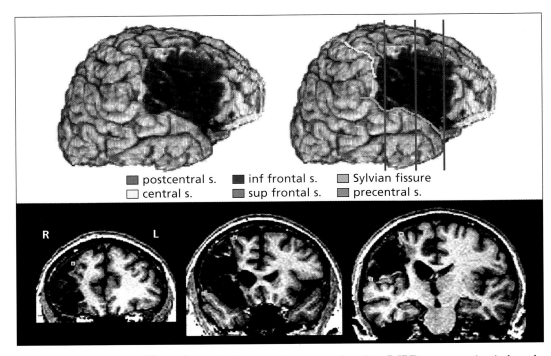

Figure 7-24. Aprosodia. Three-dimensional magnetic resonance imaging (MRI) reconstruction in lateral (*top*) and coronal (*bottom*) views of the right hemisphere. The patient is a 49-year-old right-handed man who suffered this lesion as the result of an infarct in the territory of the right middle cerebral artery. Damage to frontal and parietal structures occurred, including the right frontal operculum, that is, the right-hemisphere homologue of Broca's area. This patient had normal speech and language, with a prominent exception: he had a severe defect in *prosody*, that is, the melody, stress, and intonation applied to spoken language that help communicate attitudes and emotions. Prosody comprises a vital part of speech production, allowing the differentiation of statements, questions, and exclamations, and the emotional coloring of speech. Aprosodia, which can occur in the absence of defects in other aspects of speech and language, as exemplified by the patient shown here, involves a flat, amelodic speech production that resembles a monotone, devoid of emotional overtones [61]. Aprosodia is common with right frontoparietal lesions of the type shown here. It is frequently accompanied by spatial cognitive impairments and defects in affective behavior (*eg*, disturbed emotion, impaired social conduct, anosognosia), but *not* by defects in propositional speech, as are characteristic of left hemisphere aphasias. (*Courtesy of* Laboratory of Human Neuroanatomy and Neuroimaging, Department of Neurology, The University of Iowa.)

Amnesia

Disorders of Memory

Type of memory disorder	Examples of neural correlates
Anterograde (declarative)	
Verbal	Left mesial temporal region
	Left thalamus
	Basal forebrain
Nonverbal	Right mesial temporal region
	Right thalamus
	Basal forebrain
Retrograde	
Verbal	Left nonmesial anterotemporal
Nonverbal	Right nonmesial anterotemporal
Working memory	Dorsolateral prefrontal
Nondeclarative	Basal ganglia
	Cerebellum

Figure 7-25. Disorders of memory. The term *amnesia* refers to conditions in which patients lose, partially or completely, the ability to learn new information or to retrieve previously acquired knowledge. Amnesia is one of the most common types of cognitive impairment suffered by brain-injured patients [62,63]. In patients with degenerative disease (*eg*, Alzheimer's disease) or head injury, which constitute two of the most frequent causes of brain damage, memory defects are virtually ubiquitous. Other common causes include seizure disorder, particularly when this condition is treated surgically with temporal lobectomy, and herpes simplex encephalitis. Cerebral anoxia, produced frequently by conditions such as cardiopulmonary arrest, carbon monoxide poisoning, and near-drowning, is also a common cause of amnesia [64].

Several fundamental distinctions can be made among different types of memory and among the different neural systems related to these types of memory.

Anterograde and retrograde memory. Anterograde memory refers to the capacity to learn new information, that is, to acquire new facts, skills, and other types of knowledge. Anterograde memory for declarative knowledge is dependent on mesial temporal lobe structures, including the hippocampus and interconnected structures, such as the entorhinal and perirhinal cortices, amygdala, and other parts of the parahippocampal gyrus. Retrograde memory refers to the retrieval of information that was acquired previously, that is, retrieval of facts, skills, and other knowledge learned in the recent or remote past. Retrograde memory for declarative knowledge is related to nonmesial sectors of the temporal lobe, including the polar and inferotemporal regions [65]. Some evidence indicates that aspects of retrograde memory are related to dorsolateral sectors of the frontal lobes [66]. *Verbal and nonverbal memory.* Knowledge can be divided into that which exists in verbal form, such as words (written or spoken) and names, and that which exists in nonverbal form, such as faces, geographic routes, and complex musical patterns. Memory systems in the two hemispheres of the brain are specialized differently for verbal and nonverbal material. Systems in the left hemisphere are dedicated primarily to verbal material, and systems in the right hemisphere are dedicated primarily to nonverbal material [67,68]. *Declarative and nondeclarative memory.* Declarative, or explicit, memory refers to knowledge that can be declared and brought to mind for conscious inspection. For example, facts, words, names, and faces can be retrieved from memory, placed in the "mind's eye," and reported. Declarative memory is linked to the functioning of the hippocampus and related mesial temporal lobe structures. Nondeclarative, or implicit, memory refers to forms of memory that cannot be declared or brought into the mind's eye, such as sensorimotor skills, autonomic conditioning, and habits. Skating and skiing are examples of motor skills that constitute forms of nondeclarative memory. Nondeclarative memory depends on the neostriatum, cerebellum, and sensorimotor cortices. In many conditions of amnesia (*eg*, those caused by Alzheimer's disease, temporal lobectomy, or herpes simplex encephalitis), declarative memory is impaired and nondeclarative memory is normal [69,70]. *Short-term and long-term memory.* Short-term, or primary, memory designates a time-span of memory that covers from about 0 to 45 seconds, a brief period during which a limited amount of information (7 ± 2 "chunks") can be held without rehearsal. Short-term memory is linked to neural systems related to attention and concentration and does not depend on the hippocampal system. Note that *short-term* does not mean *anterograde*, although anterograde memory (learning) does depend on intact short-term memory. Long-term, or secondary,

(*Continued on next page*)

Figure 7-25. (*Continued*) memory refers to a time expanse that covers everything beyond short-term memory; knowledge that is held for days, years, and even decades, in more or less permanent form. The capacity of long-term memory is enormous. The acquisition of knowledge into long-term memory is dependent on the hippocampal system; retrieval of knowledge from long-term memory depends on memory systems in other parts of the temporal lobe and elsewhere. *Unique and nonunique memory.* Unique knowledge refers to material that constitutes a class of one, such as a particular person (*eg*, "Bill Clinton"), a particular place (*eg*, "Devil's Tower"), or a particular animal (*eg*, my daughter's horse "Rowdy"). Nonunique knowledge refers to material that belongs to a class of more than one, such as "politicians," "landmarks," or "horses." The terms *unique* and *nonunique* roughly correspond, respectively, with the older terms *episodic* and *semantic*, original-

ly suggested by Tulving [71]. A detailed explication of these concepts has been provided [11,72]. *Working memory.* This refers to a short time period during which the brain can hold several pieces of information in an active register and perform operations on them. Working memory is akin to short-term memory, but implies a somewhat longer time frame (several minutes) and more emphasis on the operational features of the mental process rather than merely the acquisition of information. Working memory is an "on-line" processing of and operating of knowledge that is being held in activated form. Working memory has been linked to the dorsolateral prefrontal lobes, with material-specific hemispheric specialization: the left dorsolateral prefrontal lobe is linked to verbal material, and the right dorsolateral prefrontal lobe is linked to nonverbal material [73].

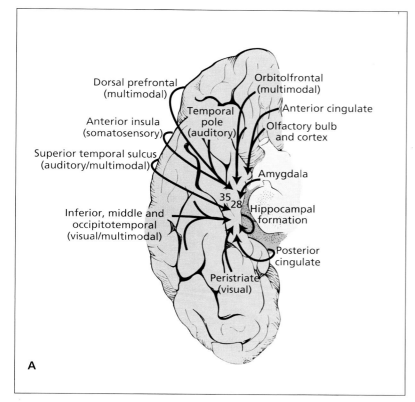

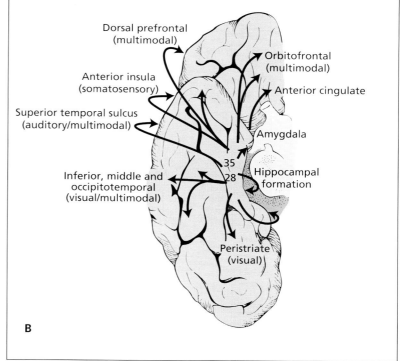

Figure 7-26. Neuroanatomic connectivity between the hippocampal complex and various parts of the cerebral cortices. The hippocampal system has extensive bidirectional connections with unimodal and polymodal association cortices throughout the brain. Ventral views of the human brain depict likely input (**A**) and output (**B**) relations of the entorhinal (area 28) and perirhinal (area 35) cortices as gleaned from nonhuman primate neuroanatomic research [74]. These areas probably receive extensive direct or indirect sensory-specific (unimodal) association input (visual, auditory, somatosensory, and olfactory) as well as multimodal sensory input from the prefrontal, superotemporal, and occipitotemporal regions of the cortex. Limbic system input from the amygdala, hippocampal system, and temporal polar and cingulate areas is

also a probable neuroanatomic feature. In all instances, the input structures receive direct or indirect feedback from areas 28 and 35. The powerful interconnections between the entorhinal or perirhinal cortices and the hippocampal formation ensure widespread cortical and hippocampal interactions in a multitude of neural systems. This places the hippocampal system in a highly favorable position to send and receive signals from throughout the entire brain, an arrangement that provides the neural substrate needed for the acquisition of new information. (*Adapted from* Tranel and colleague [63]; and from original drawings of Gary Van Hoesen; *courtesy of* Neuroanatomy Laboratory, Department of Anatomy, University of Iowa.)

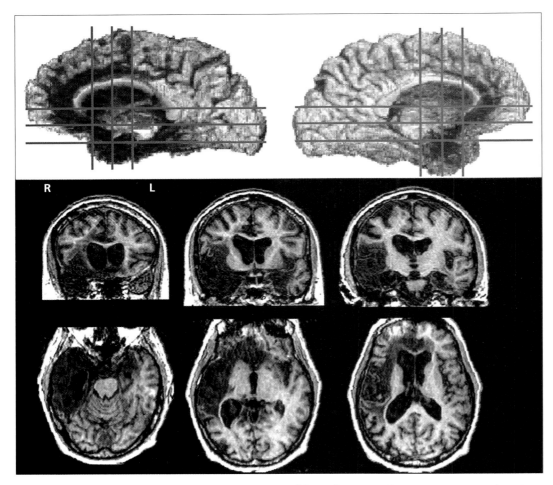

Figure 7-27. Amnesia following temporal lobe lesions. Three-dimensional magnetic resonance imaging (MRI) reconstruction in mid-sagittal views of the right (*upper left*) and left (*upper right*) hemispheres, and coronal (*middle*) and transverse (*bottom*) T1-weighted MRI cuts. The patient is a 48-year-old right-handed man who developed severe global amnesia after suffering these lesions, which were caused by herpes simplex encephalitis. The lesions include the anterotemporal regions (amygdala, hippocampus, parahippocampal gyrus, and temporal pole [Brodmann's area 38]) and the anterior portion of the inferior, middle, and superior temporal gyri (Brodmann's areas 20, 21, and anterior 22). Damage is more extensive in the right hemisphere.

The mesial temporal lobe, formed by the hippocampal system (amygdala, entorhinal cortex, and hippocampus proper) and adjoining parahippocampal gyrus, has been linked to memory function for several decades. Several relations have been firmly established. First, there is a consistent correspondence between the side of damage and the type of learning impairment. Left-sided lesions produce defects in the learning of verbal information (*eg*, words and written material), but learning of nonverbal information is spared; conversely, damage to the right hippocampus produces a defect in the learning of nonverbal material (*eg*, complex visual and auditory patterns), but verbal information is spared. A second consistent finding is that, although the hippocampus is critical for the acquisition of new information (anterograde memory), it is much less important for the retrieval of previously learned knowledge (retrograde memory). Even when there is extensive bilateral hippocampal damage, the ability to retrieve information that was acquired before

the onset of the lesion is largely spared. A third finding is that the hippocampus plays a role in the acquisition of *declarative* information; however, the hippocampus does *not* appear to be needed for the acquisition of *nondeclarative* information.

Damage confined to the mesial temporal lobes produces anterograde amnesia. If the damage extends into nonmesial structures in the anterior region, including various higher-order association cortices, the memory defect invades the *retrograde* compartment as well [75–78], as is the case here. The patient is not only incapable of learning new information but also is unable to retrieve information that was acquired before the onset of brain injury. More specific and unique levels of knowledge tend to be most affected, while nonunique types of information are less affected. For instance, the patient has difficulty retrieving detailed information about episodes such as the birth of children, weddings, and the purchase of a home, but remains capable of retrieving knowledge about the meanings of words, the locations of different countries, and the names of major cities in various states. The right nonmesial temporal region may have a more dominant role in retrograde memory than the left nonmesial temporal cortices.

One of the most common causes of damage to the hippocampal system is Alzheimer's disease, in which the first onset of pathology typically occurs in the entorhinal cortex and hippocampus (Fig. 6-27B). This fact accords well with the finding that anterograde memory impairment is the hallmark neuropsychologic feature of Alzheimer's disease. Another frequent cause of mesial temporal damage, illustrated in this case, is herpes simplex encephalitis, which produces various patterns of unilateral and bilateral damage, with or without extension into nonmesial temporal structures, and with a number of distinctive neuropsychologic profiles [64]. Head injury is another common cause of mesial temporal damage [79]. One other cause that should be mentioned is surgical resection of anterior and mesial temporal structures for control of intractable seizure disorders; such operations not infrequently extend into the entorhinal cortex and even the anterior hippocampus, and material-specific anterograde memory defects may ensue. (*Courtesy of* Laboratory of Human Neuroanatomy and Neuroimaging, Department of Neurology, The University of Iowa.)

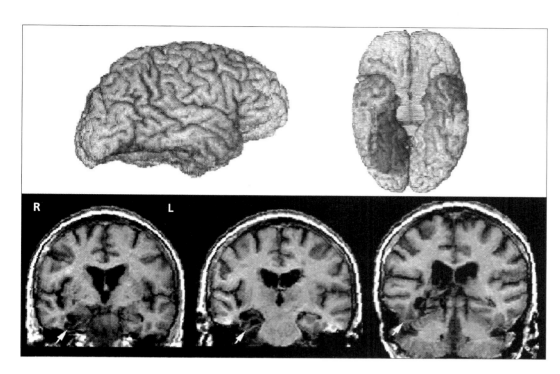

Figure 7-28. Amnesia for nonverbal material following a right temporal lobe lesion. Three-dimensional magnetic resonance imaging (MRI) reconstruction of a standard brain from lateral (*upper left*) and ventral (*upper right*) views, onto which has been transferred (using the MAP-3 technique; see Fig. 7-2) the lesion (*red*) of a patient who suffered a stroke in the right mesial temporal region. Coronal T1-weighted MRI cuts (*bottom*) also illustrate the lesion (*arrows*), especially the involvement of the hippocampus and parahippocampal gyrus. The patient, a 59-year-old right-handed woman, developed a severe impairment in anterograde memory for nonverbal material after this lesion. As noted in Figure 7-27, unilateral mesial temporal lesions produce material-specific learning impairments. The patient featured in Figure 7-27 had bilateral lesions; hence, learning was impaired for both verbal and nonverbal material. In this case, the lesion is unilateral and on the right; thus, the learning defect affects nonverbal material (faces, spatial patterns, and complex geographic routes) [80], but learning of verbal material is spared. Also, because the lesion has minimal extension into nonmesial temporal structures, retrieval of previously acquired knowledge (retrograde memory) is normal. The patient had normal learning of sensorimotor skills. (*Courtesy of* Laboratory of Human Neuroanatomy and Neuroimaging, Department of Neurology, The University of Iowa.)

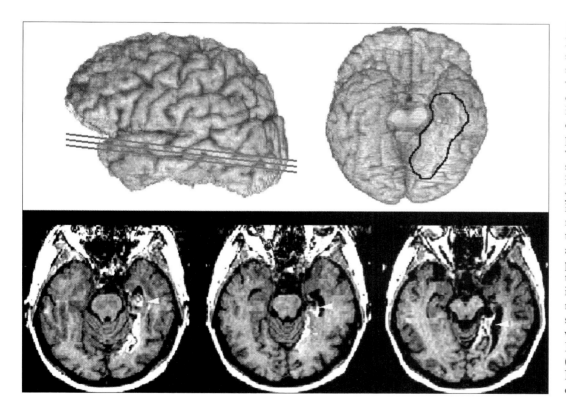

Figure 7-29. Amnesia for verbal material following a left temporal lobe lesion. Three-dimensional magnetic resonance imaging (MRI) reconstruction of a 66-year-old right-handed woman who suffered a posterior cerebral artery infarct, causing damage in the left mesial temporal region, including parts of the entorhinal cortex, hippocampus, and parahippocampal gyrus. The surface projection of the lesion is outlined on a ventral view of the brain (*top right*). On the left top are shown lines of cut for the three axial slices depicted in the bottom row, and the lesion is marked by yellow arrows. The patient developed a severe impairment in anterograde memory for verbal material after this lesion. She had normal short-term memory and normal working memory. After a brief delay of several minutes, however, the patient showed a complete loss of information, that is, a complete inability to transfer information into long-term memory. The impairment was most pronounced for words and sentences, and she had relatively better performances for nonverbal material such as geometric designs. Retrograde memory was relatively spared. (*Courtesy of* Laboratory of Human Neuroanatomy and Neuroimaging, Department of Neurology, The University of Iowa.)

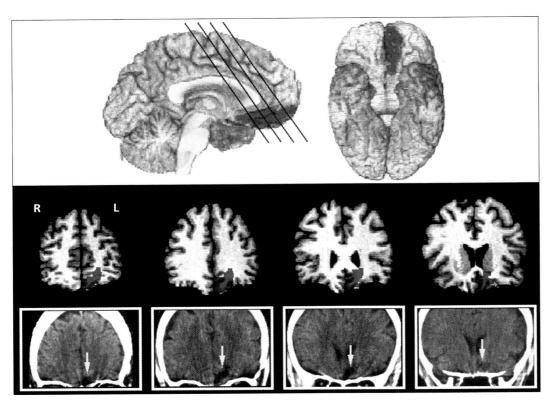

Figure 7-30. Amnesia following basal forebrain damage. A 32-year-old right-handed man suffered rupture of an anterior communicating artery aneurysm. The lesion is shown in red on a MAP-3 reconstruction displayed from mesial (*upper left*) and ventral (*upper right*) perspectives, and on oblique sections (*middle*) corresponding to the lines marked on the upper left view. The lower row shows the lesion in black on oblique computed tomographic sections, and it can be seen that the damage involves the left gyrus rectus and the left basal forebrain (*arrows*). The patient had a distinctive amnesic syndrome, with

anterograde and retrograde deficits and confabulation. The basal forebrain, situated immediately posterior to the orbital prefrontal cortices, comprises a set of bilateral paramidline gray nuclei, including the septal nuclei, the diagonal band of Broca, the nucleus accumbens, and the substantia innominata. Damage to this region is common in the setting of ruptured aneurysms of the anterior communicating artery or of the anterior cerebral artery. A characteristic amnesia develops in connection with basal forebrain lesions. Patients are able to acquire some new information, and they can remember most information from the past; however, they have difficulty associating specific subcomponents of memory episodes with one another. They may recall a particular family event, for example, but place the event entirely out of context with respect to other events that occurred in the same time period. This problem affects new learning as well—for example, the patient may learn new faces but associate these with incorrect names. A related phenomenon is what has been termed *source amnesia*. A patient may learn a particular fact or piece of information accurately but be unable to recall the circumstances under which the learning took place. The patient recalls the content, but not the source, of the learning experience. Basal forebrain amnesic patients also tend to produce wild confabulations, particularly in the acute phase, for example, making up stories about various bizarre adventures that have no basis in fact [64]. (*Courtesy of* Laboratory of Human Neuroanatomy and Neuroimaging, Department of Neurology, The University of Iowa.)

Figure 7-31. Amnesia following diencephalic lesions. Three-dimensional magnetic resonance imaging (MRI) reconstruction (*top*), with surface projection of a left thalamic lesion marked on the lateral left

hemisphere (*top right*). The lesion (*arrows*) is shown in the bottom row on T1-weighted MRI cuts (coronal, transverse, and sagittal, from *left* to *right*). The patient is a 68-year-old right-handed woman who suffered this thalamic lesion as the result of a lacunar infarct. The woman developed a severe memory impairment in connection with this lesion. The amnesia affected primarily verbal material, in keeping with standard left hemisphere dominance for verbal information. Diencephalic lesions generally produce a severe anterograde amnesia that resembles the amnesia associated with mesial temporal damage, specifically, a major defect in the acquisition of *declarative* knowledge, with sparing of learning of *nondeclarative* information. Usually, some impairment occurs in the retrograde compartment as well. The retrograde amnesia associated with diencephalic lesions tends to have a *temporal gradient*, which means that retrieval of recently acquired memories is more defective, while retrieval of remote memories is much better preserved. Severe alcoholism and stroke are two frequent causes of damage to portions of the diencephalon, especially the mammillary bodies and the dorsomedial nucleus of the thalamus [81]. (*Courtesy of* Laboratory of Human Neuroanatomy and Neuroimaging, Department of Neurology, The University of Iowa.)

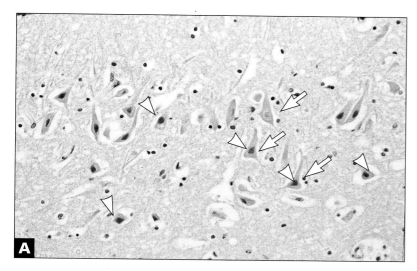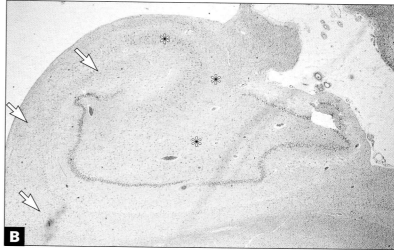

Figure 7-32. Amnesia following cerebral anoxia. **A,** Characteristic histologic features of recent anoxic injury to the pyramidal cells of the hippocampus. The characteristic features include eosinophilia, angulated borders (*arrows*), and pycnosis (small, compacted appearance; *arrowheads*) of the nuclei. **B,** Characteristic sclerotic appearance of the hippocampus in the chronic epoch after an anoxic or ischemic injury. Note that the well-defined pyramidal cell layer (*asterisks*) is absent in the vulnerable CA1 region (*arrows*). Cerebral anoxia is a relatively frequent condition, typically caused by cardiopulmonary arrest, carbon monoxide poisoning, or near drowning. The condition often leads to the selective destruction of cellular groups within the hippocampal formation, with the extent of damage linked to the number of minutes of anoxia or ischemia. Brief periods of anoxia or ischemia may cause minimal damage, but after several minutes, bilateral damage to the hippocampus is likely, and resultant memory impairment is probable. In fact, memory impairment is often the sole consequence of these conditions. The amnesia associated with cerebral anoxia is essentially an anterograde amnesia (learning defect) affecting both verbal and nonverbal material, although there may be some asymmetry whereby the verbal or nonverbal domain is relatively more involved. Retrograde defects are minimal or absent. Also, learning of nondeclarative material is spared. Histologic studies indicate that the critical site of damage is in the CA1 field of the hippocampus, as seen here [82,83]. (*Courtesy of* Laboratory of Human Neuroanatomy and Neuroimaging, Department of Neurology, The University of Iowa.)

Acquired Disorders of Social Conduct, Emotion, and Affect

Disorders of Social Conduct, Emotion, and Affect

Disorder	Examples of neural correlates
Acquired sociopathy	Ventromedial prefrontal
Akinetic mutism	Cingulate gyrus; supplemental motor area (mesial area 6)
Depression	Left prefrontal
Impaired emotional processing	Bilateral amygdala

Figure 7-33. Disorders of social conduct, emotion, and affect. Disturbances of social conduct, emotion, and affect are common in brain-injured patients. Many patients develop depression and related manifestations, such as anxiety and withdrawal. Often, these disturbances are a reaction on the part of the patient to the experience of having newly acquired and often debilitating defects in movement, sensation, and cognition. Other disorders of emotion and social conduct are linked directly to damage in particular neural regions. These disorders develop reliably in connection with damage to specific brain areas, and they are not directly attributable to factors such as psychological reaction to illness or the stress of coping with disability. Several kinds of disturbances of social conduct, emotion, and affect are associated with acquired brain damage. Akinetic mutism is a related condition. Many of these conditions, especially acquired disorders of social conduct, are frequently accompanied by a marked anosognosia (Fig. 7-10). Affected patients appear oblivious to the consequences of their behavior, and they may adamantly deny the existence of problems. This feature is a major consideration in rehabilitation and management because it can seriously encumber efforts to direct patients in a more constructive path.

Throughout the history of neuropsychology, investigators have called attention to the seemingly bizarre development of abnormal social behavior after brain injury, especially damage to the ventromedial prefrontal sector [84–86]. These patients have a number of features in common, including an inability to organize future activity and hold gainful employment, diminished capacity to respond to punishment, a tendency to present an unrealistically favorable view of themselves, stereotyped but correct manners, a tendency to display inappropriate emotional reactions, and normal intelligence [87,88]. The personality and behavioral profile develops *after* the onset of frontal lobe damage in patients with previously normal personalities and socialization. Other investigators have called attention to similar characteristics in patients with ventromedial prefrontal lobe damage. For example, Blumer and Benson [89] noted a personality type that characterized patients with orbital damage (which the authors termed *pseudo-psychopathic*). Salient features were puerility, a jocular attitude, sexually disinhibited humor, inappropriate and near-total self-indulgence, and complete lack of concern for others. Stuss and Benson [90] emphasized that such patients demonstrate a remarkable lack of empathy and general lack of concern about others. The patients tend to show callous unconcern, boastfulness, and unrestrained and tactless behavior. Other descriptors include impulsiveness, facetiousness, and diminished anxiety and concern about the future.

Damasio [91] articulated a theory of emotion and feeling, which can be used to account for the somewhat enigmatic neuropsychologic profiles of ventromedial damaged patients. The theory posits that patients with ventromedial damage have a defect in the activation of *somatic markers* that must accompany the internal and automatic processing of possible response options. The patients are deprived of a somatic marker that normally assists, both consciously and covertly, with response selection. This reduces their chances of responding in the most advantageous manner and increases their chances of generating responses that lead to negative consequences.

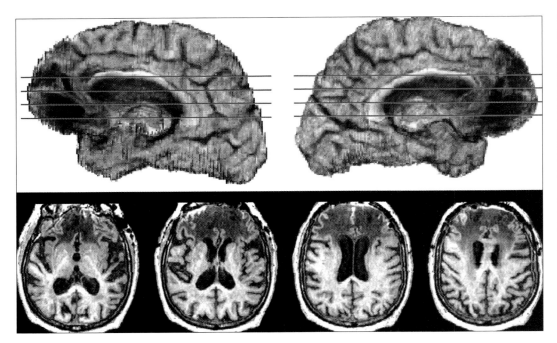

Figure 7-34. Disorders of social conduct (acquired sociopathy). Mesial hemisphere views (*top*) of the three-dimensional magnetic resonance imaging (MRI) reconstruction of a 74-year-old right-handed man who suffered a bilateral ventromedial prefrontal lesion caused by a stroke. The lesions are also shown on the transverse MRI scans (*bottom*), corresponding to the levels marked by the colored lines on the mesial hemispheres. The damage includes bilateral destruction of the orbital and lower mesial frontal cortices, or what is termed the *ventromedial prefrontal region*. The basal forebrain is spared. The patient developed severe changes in personality, but did not manifest defects in conventional neuropsychologic abilities.

The ventromedial prefrontal region plays a critical role in the domain of behaviors that can be grouped under the rubric of *social conduct*. Lesions in this region frequently lead to a severe disruption of social conduct; remarkably, the patients are free of impairments in most basic domains of cognition, such as intellectual capacity, memory, speech and language, perception, and attention. Affected patients have drastic changes in personality and show profound defects in planning, judgment, and decision making. These changes occur against the background of a normal premorbid personality and few if any defects in basic neuropsychologic function. This disorder has been termed *acquired sociopathy* [19,92]. The term captures well the proclivity of these patients to engage in decisions and behaviors that have repeated negative consequences for their well-being. The patients are usually not destructive and harmful to others in society (a feature that distinguishes the *acquired* form of the disorder from the standard *developmental* form); however, they repeatedly select courses of action that are not in their best interest in the long run. They make poor decisions about interpersonal relationships, occupational endeavors, and finances. Recently, it has been shown that ventromedial prefrontal lesions acquired early in life produce a similar profile of defective social conduct, perhaps even more severe than that evidenced by patients with adult-onset lesions; the early-onset patients also manifest defects in moral reasoning [93].

Misdiagnosis of these patients is not uncommon—they may be labeled as psychopaths, or even malingerers, and it is often hard to convince caretakers and family members that the patient's behavior is the result of a brain injury. The fact that there are no neurologic defects (outside of anosmia, which is typical) and few obvious neuropsychologic impairments makes it difficult to establish that the patients will not be able to hold gainful employment in conventional settings; this is further exacerbated by the patient's own lack of acknowledgment of limitations (anosognosia). In short, these patients can present very challenging management issues. Clarifying the organic basis for the behavior and the fact that the behavior has a neurobiological explanation is important. (*Courtesy of* Laboratory of Human Neuroanatomy and Neuroimaging, Department of Neurology, The University of Iowa.)

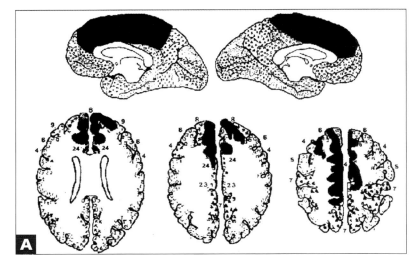

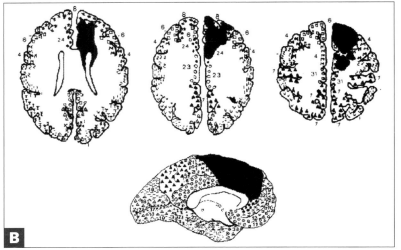

Figure 7-35. Akinetic mutism. Bilateral mesial frontal lesions in a 43-year-old right-handed woman (**A**). The patient developed akinetic mutism, which was severe and persistent. The lesions, plotted on standard brain templates in mesial hemispheric views (*top section of A*) and axial sections (*bottom part of A*), involve the anterior cingulate (area 24) and supplementary motor area (area 6), bilaterally. An infarct of the anterior cerebral artery was the cause. Lesions in the cingulate gyrus or the supplementary motor area often cause a combination of *akinesia* and *mutism*. The patient produces no speech, even when spoken to, and makes few facial expressions. Movements are also lacking, except for a few automatic types of behaviors, such as adjusting the bedcovers. Unlike patients with aphasia, who invariably struggle to produce language even when they are having severe difficulty, patients with akinetic mutism make no attempt to communicate. They act, in short, as though they have lost the will to interact verbally and kinetically with their environments. In this sense, akinetic mutism can be conceptualized as a disorder of motivation.

Akinetic mutism tends to be more severe and long-lasting when there is bilateral damage to the anterior cingulate or supplementary motor region.

Unilateral lesions produce a more transient condition (**B**). The side of damage does not appear to be critical because the same syndrome develops in relation to lesions on either the right or left side. This is consistent with the notion that the cingulate and supplementary motor area structures are dedicated primarily to motivation and affective control and not to language processes. The condition is most pronounced in the acute phase, immediately after the onset of brain injury, and most patients demonstrate good recovery, especially if the lesion is unilateral.

Depiction of the lesion in a 40-year-old right-handed man, marked in black on axial templates (*top section of B*) and on the mesial left hemisphere (*bottom section of B*). The lesion involves the mesial aspect of the left supplementary motor area (area 6) and part of the left anterior cingulate gyrus (area 24). Initially, the patient had severe akinetic mutism, but 3 months after onset, he demonstrated excellent recovery. (*Courtesy of* Laboratory of Human Neuroanatomy and Neuroimaging, Department of Neurology, The University of Iowa.)

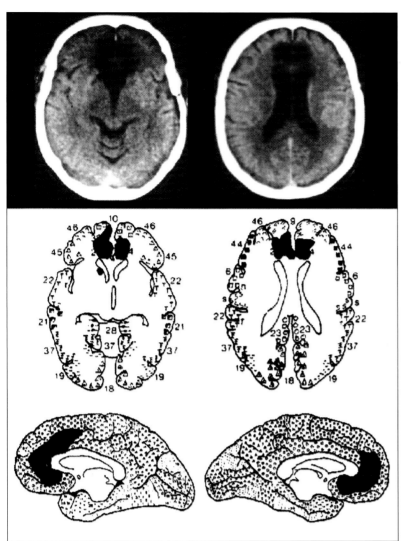

Figure 7-36. Acquired personality disorder and amnesia. Two axial computed tomography scans (*top*) and the template plotting (*middle* and *bottom*) of bilateral mesial lesions caused by rupture of an anterior communicating artery aneurysm. The patient is a 58-year-old right-handed woman who demonstrated a significant change in personality, impaired decision-making, and amnesia. The lesion involves the anterior cingulate below and in front of the rostrum of the corpus callosum and some mesial frontal structures; the basal forebrain also is likely damaged. The patient had flat (blunted) affect and impaired emotional expression, giving the appearance of depression (see [94] for a PET study relevant to these observations); however, she also evidenced considerable lack of concern for her condition and anosognosia. She reported that she had memory "problems," but at the same time, she expressed virtually no affect congruent with this complaint—she did not appear distressed or concerned. Her memory defect was marked by a prominent impairment in placing memories correctly in *time*. The patient could remember many personal and public events and could recall correctly the *content* of these memories; however, she could not order events correctly in the context of her autobiography. For example, she could recall many details regarding a factory job that she had held for many years, but she was unable to remember that several major life events had occurred after she retired from this job, including a move, the death of her parents, and the births of several grandchildren. The same type of defect was evident in the anterograde compartment. This profile of memory impairment has been linked to basal forebrain damage. (*Courtesy of* Laboratory of Human Neuroanatomy and Neuroimaging, Department of Neurology, The University of Iowa.)

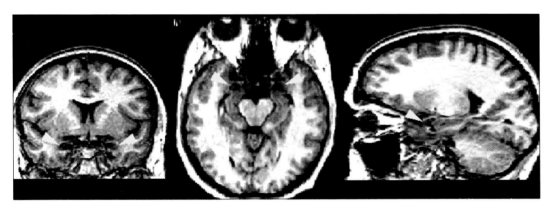

Figure 7-37. Impaired emotional processing. Coronal (*left*), axial (*middle*), and sagittal (*right*) cuts from a T1-weighted magnetic resonance imaging (MRI) scan in a patient with a rare selective, bilateral damage to the amygdala. The patient is a 28-year-old right-handed woman who has a number of impairments in emotional processing related to the bilateral amygdala damage. The patient had Urbach-Wiethe disease, one characteristic of which is bilateral calcification of the amygdala. The arrowheads mark the location of mineralization of the amygdala on both sides. A positron emission tomographic study confirmed that these regions were severely hypometabolic [95].

She is impaired in recognizing certain emotional facial expressions, particularly *fear* [96]. She cannot perceive multiple emotions in a single facial expression, and she has difficulty detecting similarities and differences among facial expressions. The patient cannot acquire conditioned autonomic responses to neutral stimuli that are paired with an aversive event [97]. The patient has no impairment in recognition of identity from faces, and she can learn new faces normally. Also, most of her defects in emotional processing are related to stimuli that have negative affective valence (*eg*, fear, anger, disgust), and she performs much better with positive stimuli (*eg*, happiness). The presentation of this patient is consistent with the idea that the amygdala is specialized for the processing of stimuli with emotional significance, especially negatively valenced stimuli that are related directly to basic survival mechanisms ("flight-or-fight" responses). Impairments of the type described here have been noted in other patients with bilateral amygdala damage, including patients with bilateral amygdalectomy or bilateral damage from herpes simplex encephalitis [98]. (*Courtesy of* Laboratory of Human Neuroanatomy and Neuroimaging, Department of Neurology, The University of Iowa.)

References

1. Lissauer H: Ein fall von Seelenblindheit nebst einem Beitrag zur theorie der-selben. *Arch Psychiatr Nervenkr* 1890, 21:22–70.

2. Bauer RM: Agnosia. In *Clinical Neuropsychology*, edn 3. Edited by Heilman KM, Valenstein E. New York: Oxford University Press; 1993:215–278.

3. Tranel D, Damasio AR: The Agnosias and Apraxias. In *Neurology in Clinical Practice*, edn 2. Edited by Bradley WG, Daroff RB, Fenichel GM, *et al.* Stoneham, MA: Butterworth, 1996:119–129.

4. Damasio H, Frank RJ: Three-dimensional in vivo mapping of brain lesions in humans. *Arch Neurol* 1992, 49:137–143.

5. Frank RJ, Damasio H, Grabowski TJ: Brainvox: an interactive, multimodal visualization and analysis system for neuroanatomical imaging. *Neuroimage* 1997, 5:13–30.

6. Damasio AR, Damasio H, Tranel D, *et al.*: Neural regionalization of knowl-edge access: preliminary evidence. *Symp Quant Bio* 1990, 55:1039–1047.

7. Caramazza A, Shelton JR: Domain-specific knowledge systems in the brain: The animate-inanimate distinction. *J Cog Neurosci* 1998, 10:1–34.

8. Humphreys GW, Forde EME: Hierarchies, similarity and interactivity in object recognition: On the multiplicity of "category-specific" deficits in neu-ropsychological populations. *Behav Brain Sci* 2001, in press.

9. Warrington EK, McCarthy RA: Multiple meaning systems in the brain: a case for visual semantics. *Neuropsychologia* 1994, 32:1465–1473.

10. Tranel D, Damasio H, Damasio AR: A neural basis for the retrieval of con-ceptual knowledge. *Neuropsychologia* 1997, 35:1319–1327.

11. Damasio AR: Time-locked multiregional retroactivation: a systems-level pro-posal for the neural substrates of recall and recognition. *Cognition* 1989, 33:25–62.

12. Damasio AR, Tranel D, Damasio H: Face agnosia and the neural substrates of memory. *Annu Rev Neurosci* 1990, 13:89–109.

13. Tranel D, Damasio AR: Knowledge without awareness: an autonomic index of facial recognition by prosopagnosics. *Science* 1985, 228:1453–1454.

14. Tranel D, Damasio AR: Nonconscious face recognition in patients with face agnosia. *Behav Brain Res* 1988, 30:235–249.

15. Tranel D: Electrodermal activity in cognitive neuroscience: Neuroanatomical and neuropsychological correlates. In *Cognitive Neuroscience of Emotion*. Edited by Lane RD, Nadel L. New York: Oxford University Press; 2000:192–224.

16. Caselli RJ: Ventrolateral and dorsomedial somatosensory association cortex damage produces distinct somesthetic syndromes in humans. *Neurology* 1993, 43:762–771.

17. Damasio H, Tranel D, Bellugi U, *et al.*: Selective impairment of concept retrieval through a tactile channel. *Soc Neurosci* 1992, 18:1207.

18. Babinski J: Contribution a l'etude des troubles mentaux dans l'hemiplegie organique cerebrale (agnosognosie). *Rev Neurol* 1914, 27:845–847.

19. Damasio AR, Tranel D, Damasio H: Individuals with sociopathic behavior caused by frontal damage fail to respond autonomically to social stimuli. *Behav Brain Res* 1990, 41:81–94.

20. Barrash J, Tranel D, Anderson SW: Acquired sociopathy: A syndrome of per-sonality changes associated with damage to the ventromedial frontal lobes. *Dev Neuropsych* 2001, in press.

21. Ungerleider LG, Mishkin M: Two cortical visual systems. In *Analysis of Visual Behavior*. Edited by Ingle DJ, Goodale MA, Mansfield RJW. Cambridge, MA: MIT Press; 1982:549–586.

22. Rizzo M: "Balint's syndrome" and associated visuospatial disorders. In *Bailliere's International Practice and Research*. Edited by London KC. Philadelphia: WB Saunders; 1993:415–437.

23. Damasio AR, Tranel D, Rizzo M: Disorders of complex visual processing. In *Principles of Behavioral and Cognitive Neurology*, edn 2. Edited by Mesulam MM. New York: Oxford University Press; 2000:332–372.

24. Zihl J, Von Cramon Z, Mai N: Selective disturbances of movement vision after bilateral brain damage. *Brain* 1983, 106:313–340.

25. Decety J, Grezes J, Costes N, *et al.*: Brain activity during observation of actions: influence of action content and subject's strategy. *Brain* 1997, 120:1763–1777.

26. Fadiga L, Fogassi L, Gallese V, Rizzolatti G: Visuomotor neurons: ambiguity of the discharge or "motor" perception? *Int J Psychophysiol* 2000, 35:165–177.

27. Kourtzi Z, Kanwisher N: Activation in human MT/MST by static images with implied motion. *J Cogn Neurosci* 2000, 12:48–55.

28. Rizzo M, Hurtig R: Looking but not seeing: attention, perception, and eye movements in simultanagnosia. *Neurology* 1987, 37:1642–1648.

29. Damasio AR, Benton AL: Impairment of hand movements under visual guid-ance. *Neurology* 1979, 29:170–174.

30. Tranel D, Adolphs R, Damasio H, Damasio AR: A neural basis for the retrieval of words for actions. *Cogn Neuropsych*. [Submitted for publication.]

31. Rizzo M: Astereopsis. In *Handbook of Neuropsychology*, vol 2. Edited by Boller F, Grafman J. Amsterdam: Elsevier; 1989:415–427.

32. Damasio AR, Yamada T, Damasio H, *et al.*: Central achromatopsia: behav-ioral, anatomical and physiologic aspects. *Neurology* 1980, 30:1064–1071.

33. Meadows JC: Disturbed perception of colors associated with localized cerebral lesions. *Brain* 1974, 97:615–632.

34. Rizzo M, Nawrot M: Human visual cortex and its disorders. *Curr Opin Ophthalmol* 1993, 4:38–47.

35. Corbetta M, Miezin FM, Dobmeyer S, *et al.*: Attentional modulation of neur-al processing of shape, color, and velocity in humans. *Science* 1990, 248:1556–1559.

36. Lueck CJ, Zeki S, Friston KJ, *et al.*: The color centre in the cerebral cortex of man. *Nature* 1989, 340:386–389.

37. Zeki SM, Watson JDG, Lueck CJ, *et al.*: A direct demonstration of functional specialization in human visual cortex. *J Neurosci* 1991, 11:641–649.

38. Hubel DH, Livingstone MS: Segregation of form, color, and stereopsis in pri-mate area 18. *J Neurosci* 1987, 7:3378–3415.

39. Livingstone MS, Hubel DH: Segregation of form, color, movement, and depth: anatomy, physiology, and perception. *Science* 1988, 240:740–749.

40. Rosler F, Heil M, Henninghausen E: Distinct cortical activation patterns dur-ing long-term memory retrieval of verbal, spatial, and color information. *J Cogn Neurosci* 1995, 7:51–65.

41. Martin A, Haxby JV, Lalonde FM, *et al.*: Discrete cortical regions associated with knowledge of color and knowledge of action. *Science* 1995, 270:102–105.

42. Benton AL, Tranel D: Visuoperceptual, visuospatial, and visuoconstructive dis-orders. In *Clinical Neuropsychology*, edn 3. Edited by Heilman KM, Valenstein E. New York: Oxford University Press; 1993:165–213.

43. Damasio AR, Damasio H: Brain and language. *Sci Am* 1992, 267:88–95.

44. Goodglass H: *Understanding Aphasia*. New York: Academic Press; 1993.

45. Brown CM, Hagoort P: *The Neurocognition of Language*. New York: Oxford University Press; 1999.

46. Levelt WJ, Roelofs A, Meyer AS: A theory of lexical access in speech produc-tion. *Behav Brain Sci* 1999, 22:1–75.

47. Sarno MT: Recovery and Rehabilitation in Aphasia. In *Acquired Aphasia*, edn 3. Edited by Sarno MT. New York: Academic Press; 1998:595–631.

48. Basso, A: Therapy of Aphasia. In *Handbook of Neuropsychology*, vol 2. Edited by Boller F, Grafman J. Amsterdam: Elsevier; 1989:67–82.

49. Holland AL: Recovery in aphasia. In *Handbook of Neuropsychology*, vol 2. Edited by Boller F, Grafman J. Amsterdam: Elsevier; 1989:83–90.

50. Tranel D, Biller J, Damasio H, *et al.*: Global aphasia without hemiparesis. *Arch Neurol* 1987, 44:304–308.

51. Damasio AR, Tranel D: Nouns and verbs are retrieved with differently distrib-uted neural systems. *Proc Nat Acad Sci* 1993, 90:4957–4960.

52. Damasio H, Grabowski TJ, Tranel D, *et al.*: A neural basis for lexical retrieval. *Nature* 1996, 380:499–505.

53. Naeser MA, Alexander MP, Helm-Estabrooks N, *et al.*: Aphasia with pre-dominantly subcortical lesion sites. *Arch Neurol* 1982, 39:2–14.

54. Damasio H, Eslinger P, Adams HP: Aphasia following basal ganglia lesions: new evidence. *Semin Neurol* 1984, 4:151–161.

55. Alexander MP: Clinical-Anatomical Correlations of Aphasia Following Predominantly Subcortical Lesions. In *Handbook of Neuropsychology*, vol 2. Edited by Boller F, Grafman J. Amsterdam: Elsevier; 1989:47–66.

56. Goodglass H, Wingfield A: Word-finding deficits in aphasia: brain-behavior relations and clinical symptomatology. In *Anomia: Neuroanatomical and Cognitive Correlates*. Edited by Goodglass H, Wingfield A. New York: Academic Press; 1997:3–27.

57. Zingeser LB, Berndt RS: Retrieval of nouns and verbs in agrammatism and anomia. *Brain Lang* 1990, 39:14–32.

58. Tranel D, Damasio H, Damasio AR: On the Neurology of Naming. In *Anomia*: Neuroanatomical and cognitive correlates. Edited by Goodglass H, Wingfield A. New York: Academic Press; 1997:67–92.

59. Daniele A, Giustolisi L, Silveri MC, *et al.*: Evidence for a possible neuroanatomical basis for lexical processing of nouns and verbs. *Neuropsychologia* 1994, 32:1325–1341.

60. Joanette Y: Aphasia in Left-Handers and Crossed Aphasia. In *Handbook of Neuropsychology*, vol 2. Edited by Boller F, Grafman J. Amsterdam: Elsevier; 1989:173–183.

61. Ross ED: The aprosodias: functional-anatomic organization of the affective components of language in the right hemisphere. *Arch Neurol* 1981, 38:561–569.

62. Baddeley AD: The Psychology of Memory. In *Handbook of Memory Disorders*. Edited by Baddeley AD, Wilson BA, Watts FN. New York: John Wiley & Sons; 1995:3–25.

63. Tranel D, Damasio AR: Neurobiological foundations of human memory. In *Handbook of Memory Disorders*. Edited by Baddeley AD, Wilson BA, Watts FN. Chichester, England: John Wiley & Sons; 1995:27–50.

64. Tranel D, Damasio AR, Damasio H: Amnesia caused by herpes simplex encephalitis, infarctions in basal forebrain, and anoxia/ischemia. In *Handbook of Neuropsychology*, edn 2, vol 1. Edited by Boller F, Graman J. Amsterdam: Elsevier Science; 2000:37–62.

65. Kopelman MD: The Neuropsychology of Remote Memory. In *Handbook of Neuropsychology*, vol 8. Edited by Boller F, Grafman J. Amsterdam: Elsevier; 1993:215–238.

66. Schacter DL, Tulving E: What Are the Memory Systems of 1994? In *Memory Systems 1994*. Edited by Schacter DL, Tulving E. Cambridge, MA: MIT Press; 1994:1–38.

67. Milner B: Disorders of learning and memory after temporal lobe lesions in man. *Clin Neurosurg* 1972, 19:421–446.

68. Tranel D: Dissociated verbal and nonverbal retrieval and learning following left anterior temporal damage. *Brain and Cognition* 1991, 15:187–200.

69. Tranel D, Damasio AR, Damasio H, *et al.*: Sensorimotor skill learning in amnesia: additional evidence for the neural basis of nondeclarative memory. *Learning and Memory* 1994, 1:165–179.

70. Gabrieli JDE, Corkin S, Mickel SF, *et al.*: Intact acquisition and long-term retention of mirror-tracing skill in Alzheimer's disease and in global amnesia. *Behav Neurosci* 1993, 107:899–910.

71. Tulving E: Episodic and Semantic Memory. In *Organization of Memory*. Edited by Tulving E, Donaldson W. New York: Academic Press; 1972.

72. Damasio AR: The brain binds entities and events by multiregional activation from convergence zones. *Neural Computation* 1989, 1:123–132.

73. Smith EE, Jonides J, Koeppe RA, *et al.*: Spatial versus object working memory: PET investigations. *J Cognitive Neurosci* 1995, 7:337–356.

74. van Hoesen GW: The parahippocampal gyrus: new observations regarding its cortical connections in the monkey. *Trends Neurosci* 1982, 5:345–350.

75. Cohen NJ, Squire LR: Retrograde amnesia and remote memory impairment. *Neuropsychologia* 1981, 19:337–356.

76. De Renzi E, Lucchelli F: Dense retrograde amnesia, intact learning capability and abnormal forgetting rate: a consolidation deficit? *Cortex* 1993, 29:449–466.

77. Kapur N: Focal retrograde amnesia in neurological disease: a critical review. *Cortex* 1993, 29:217–234.

78. Markowitsch HJ, Calabrese P, Haupts M, *et al.*: Searching for the anatomical basis of retrograde amnesia. *J Clin Exp Neuropsychol* 1993, 15:947–967.

79. Rizzo M, Tranel D: *Head Injury and Postconcussive Syndrome*. New York: Churchill Livingstone; 1995.

80. Barrash J, Damasio H, Adolphs R, Tranel D: The neuroanatomical correlates of route learning impairment. *Neuropsychologia* 2000, 38:820–836.

81. Graff-Radford NR, Tranel D, van Hoesen GW, *et al.*: Diencephalic amnesia. *Brain* 1990, 113:1–25.

82. Zola-Morgan S, Squire LR, Amaral DG: Human amnesia and the medial temporal region: enduring memory impairment following a bilateral lesions limited to field CA1 of the hippocampus. *J Neurosci* 1986, 6:2950–2967.

83. Rempel-Clower NL, Zola SM, Squire LR, Amaral DG: Three cases of enduring memory impairment after bilateral damage limited to the hippocampal formation. *J Neurosci* 1996, 16:5233–5255.

84. Ackerly SS, Benton AL: Report of a case of bilateral frontal lobe defect. Research Publication of the Association for Research in Nervous and Mental Disease. 1948, 27:479–504.

85. Harlow JM: Recovery from the passage of an iron bar through the head. *Publications of the Massachusetts Medical Society* 1868, 2:327–347.

86. Hebb DO, Penfield W: Human behavior after extensive bilateral removals from the frontal lobes. *Arch Neurol Psychiatry* 1940, 44:421–438.

87. Damasio AR, Anderson SW: The frontal lobes. In *Clinical Neuropsychology*, edn 4. Edited by Heilman KM, Valenstein E. New York: Oxford University Press; 2001, in press.

88. Barrash J, Tranel D, Anderson SW: Acquired sociopathy: A syndrome of personality changes associated with damage to the ventromedial frontal lobes. *Dev Neuropsychol* 2001, in press.

89. Blumer D, Benson DF: Personality Changes with Frontal and Temporal Lobe Lesions. In *Psychiatric Aspects of Neurologic Disease*. Edited by Benson DF, Blumer D. New York: Grune & Stratton; 1975:151–169.

90. Stuss DT, Benson DF: *The Frontal Lobes*. New York: Raven Press; 1986.

91. Damasio AR: *Descartes' Error: Emotion, Reason, and the Human Brain*. New York: Grossett/Putnam; 1994.

92. Tranel D: "Acquired Sociopathy": The Development of Sociopathic Behavior Following Focal Brain Damage. In *Progress in Experimental Personality and Psychopathology Research*, vol 17. Edited by Fowles DC, Sutker P, Goodman SH. New York: Springer; 1986:285–311.

93. Anderson SW, Bechara A, Damasio H, *et al.*: Impairment of social and moral behavior related to early damage in the human prefrontal cortex. *Nat Neurosci* 1999, 2:1032–1037.

94. Drevets WC, Price JL, Simpson JR, *et al.*: Subgenual prefrontal cortex abnormalities in mood disorders. *Nature* 1997, 386:824–827.

95. Adolphs R, Tranel D, Damasio H, *et al.*: Fear and the human amygdala. *J Neurosci* 1995, 15:5879–5891.

96. Adolphs R, Tranel D, Damasio H, *et al.*: Impaired recognition of emotion in facial expressions following bilateral damage to the human amygdala. *Nature*, 1994, 372:669–672.

97. Bechara A, Tranel D, Damasio H, *et al.*: Double dissociation of conditioning and declarative knowledge relative to the amygdala and hippocampus in humans. *Science*, 1995, 269:1115–1118.

98. Adolphs R, Tranel D, Hamann S, *et al.*: Recognition of facial emotion in nine individuals with bilateral amygdala damage. *Neuropsychologia* 1999, 37:1111–1117.

8

Neuro-oncology

Karen L. Fink • Elisabeth J. Rushing
S. Clifford Schold, Jr

THE field of neuro-oncology is a relatively young one. Most of the advances in neurologic diagnosis and therapy relevant to neuro-oncology have occurred within the last 85 years. Before the development of theories of neurologic localization, the presence of a brain tumor could be suspected, but treatment was impossible. Once preoperative localization using clinical examination techniques was possible, surgery for diagnosis and treatment of brain tumors was an option, but successful brain tumor surgery required the development of aseptic surgical techniques, anesthetics, antibiotics, and corticosteroids. Nonsurgical treatments for brain tumors were also developed in the twentieth century, including radiotherapy and chemotherapy. Refinements of these treatments are still being developed, and include γ-knife radiosurgery, radiosensitizers, localized chemotherapy using polymer wafers, gene therapy, and multiagent chemotherapy regimens for specific brain tumors.

Imaging of central nervous system (CNS) tumors in living patients became possible early in the twentieth century with the introduction of skull radiographs, angiography, myelography, and pneumoencephalography. These techniques have been replaced by computed tomography (CT) and magnetic resonance imaging (MRI) over the last two decades. These newer, noninvasive imaging techniques allow accurate anatomic localization of CNS tumors and are used to plan surgery and to follow response to treatment. Other CNS imaging methods include functional MRI, MR spectroscopy, and positron-emission tomography (PET). These techniques provide functional images of cerebral blood flow or metabolism, rather than anatomic information. PET or MR spectroscopy scans may be used to resolve diagnostic dilemmas in patients with brain tumors. For instance, PET may help differentiate recurrent tumor from radionecrosis.

Tumors involving the CNS are an important cause of morbidity and mortality throughout the world. They account for 2% of solid tumors in adults and for 15% of solid tumors in children. Although primary CNS malignancies account for only 2% of all cases of cancer, they account for 7% of years of life lost due to cancer before age 70 [1]. Each year in the United States, 60,000 to 80,000 metastatic intracranial tumors and 10,000 to 20,000 primary brain tumors are diagnosed. There are 30,000 to 40,000 deaths from brain tumors in the United States each year.

Advances in histopathologic classification of brain tumors began in the early nineteenth century and continue today. The presence of necrosis in glioblastomas was identified as a grave prognostic feature early in the 1900s, and correlations between histopathologic features of brain tumors and patient outcomes continue to be identified. Classification of brain tumors by histologic criteria allows predictions regarding prognosis to be made, and it identifies patients who require additional treatment following total or subtotal resection of a CNS tumor. Recently, immunohistochemical stains and electron microscopy have clarified the lineage of some neoplastic cells, allowing the identification of some previously obscure tumors.

Studying the epidemiology of brain tumors is difficult. Many CNS tumors are not confirmed histologically, and many series collect epidemiologic information on brain tumor patients without regard to histology. Thus, population studies may combine malignant gliomas with usually benign meningiomas, giving a skewed idea of survival rates in patients with brain tumors. Hospital series suffer from referral bias, and population studies often do not provide adequate histologic data. Attempts to define causative factors for brain tumors suffer from inadequate case control and the low incidence of these tumors. Despite these problems, increasingly accurate figures regarding brain tumor incidence and mortality are becoming available worldwide. From these data it is clear that the incidence of brain tumors increases with age, rising to 10 to 35 cases per 100,000 population in the eighth decade of life. In addition, the incidence of brain tumors is rising with time in the United States. This increase does not appear to be entirely the result of improvements in imaging technology or access to medical care. As the US "baby-boomers" age, physicians will see more patients with metastatic and primary brain tumors.

Epidemiology of Brain Tumors

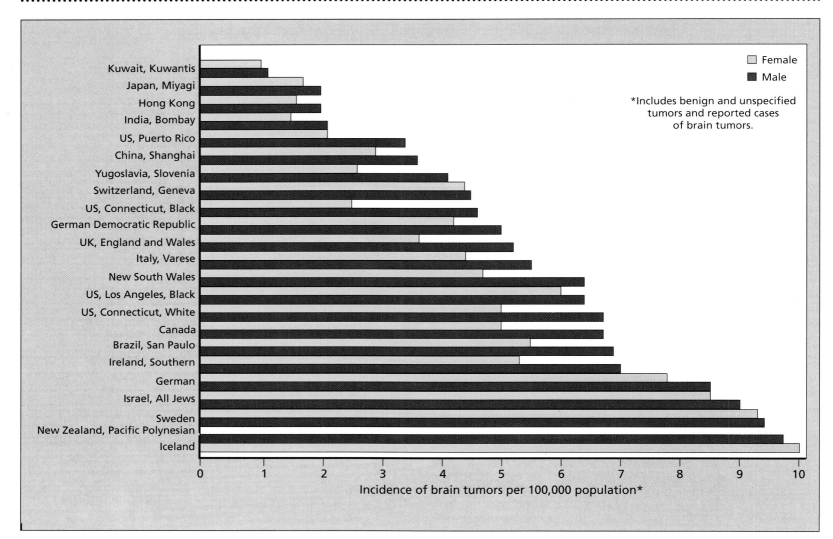

Figure 8-1. Incidence of brain tumors per 100,000 population, age-standardized to the world population, in selected countries worldwide. The data are compiled from tumor registries and population studies and reported in *Patterns of Cancer in Five Continents* [2]. The worldwide annual incidence of brain tumors ranges from a low of 1 per 100,000 population in Kuwait to a high of 10 per 100,000 women in Iceland.

The incidence of brain tumors tends to be lowest in Asian populations, and highest in white populations. Genetic and environmental differences undoubtedly contribute to this variance. The availability of computed tomography and magnetic resonance imaging in industrialized nations may explain some of the apparent difference in incidence of brain tumors, but interestingly, in Japan and in the United States, two countries with high levels of medical technology, the incidence of brain tumors is different.

The incidence of brain tumors in men is usually slightly higher than in women within a population. The average male to female ratio is 1.4 to 1 when all histologic types are considered together. When race is considered within a population, white people have the highest rate of brain tumors, and black and Asian people have lower rates [3,4].

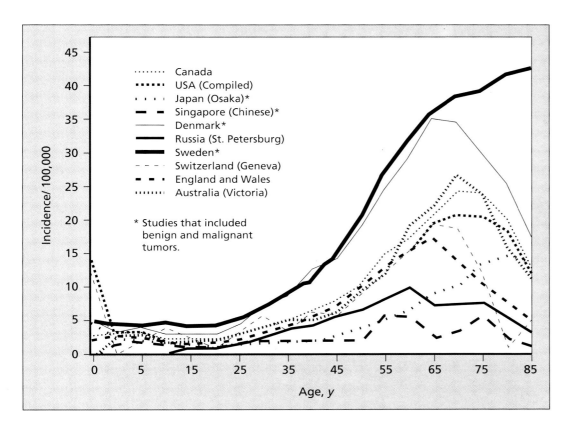

Figure 8-2. Incidence of primary brain tumors related to age. The incidence of primary brain tumors increases in older adults. Population studies in widely separated areas of the world have shown similar increases in brain tumor incidence with age, although there is some variation among ethnic and geographic groups [4]. Some studies show a peak of brain tumor incidence in early childhood, which decreases to low levels in late childhood and adolescence. The frequency of brain tumors then increases up to at least age 75. A decrease in brain tumor incidence after age 75 is seen in many studies, but may represent incomplete ascertainment of cases in extreme old age [5]. In populations with a high autopsy rate and almost complete case ascertainment, the decline in brain tumor incidence in extreme old age does not occur. This pattern can be seen in the line representing brain tumor incidence in Sweden. Population studies from Rochester, Minnesota have shown a similar continuous increase in incidence of brain tumors with age [5–7]. Both of these population studies included benign tumors such as meningiomas in their incidence figures, which may also change the shape of the incidence versus age curve.

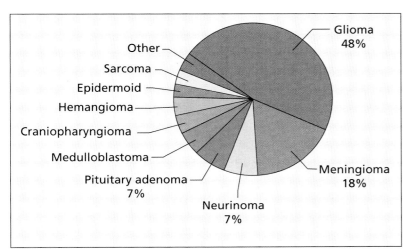

Figure 8-3. Relative frequency of primary intracranial tumors and gliomas. Gliomas are the most common primary intracranial neoplasm, comprising 48% of all primary intracranial tumors when all age groups are considered. Meningiomas are the second most common primary intracranial tumor. Medulloblastomas are the most common nongliomatous intracranial tumor in children, and thus account for a significant proportion of intracranial tumors when all ages are considered. Other types of intracranial tumors occur less frequently. When gliomas are considered alone, tumors derived from astrocytes are most common. Astrocytic tumors, which include astrocytomas and glioblastomas, account for 71% of all gliomas. Oligodendroglial and ependymal tumors are less common.

This chart includes only primary brain tumors, not intracranial metastases. In some series, intracranial metastases are the most frequent intracranial tumor, and can account for 50% of all intracranial tumors [8]. In autopsied patients with cancer, 20% to 40% have intracranial metastases [9,10]. (*Adapted from* Evans [11].)

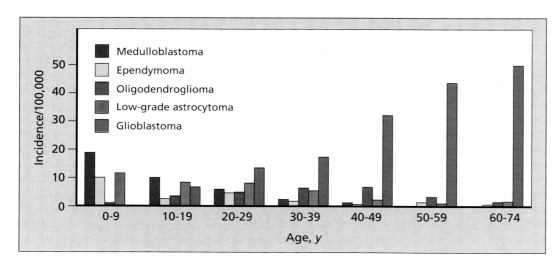

Figure 8-4. Incidence of several types of primary brain tumors in different age groups. Although the overall incidence of brain tumors increases with age, different histologic types have different age distributions. Medulloblastomas are most common in early childhood, and are rare in adulthood. Ependymomas are also more common in childhood. Oligodendrogliomas are most frequently diagnosed in young adults. Low grade astrocytomas are common in young adults, but become less frequent with age, when glioblastoma multiforme becomes the most common astrocytic tumor. The high incidence of glioblastomas in older adults accounts for the overall increase in brain tumors with age seen in Figure 8-2. (*Adapted from* Evans [11]; DeVita and colleagues [12].)

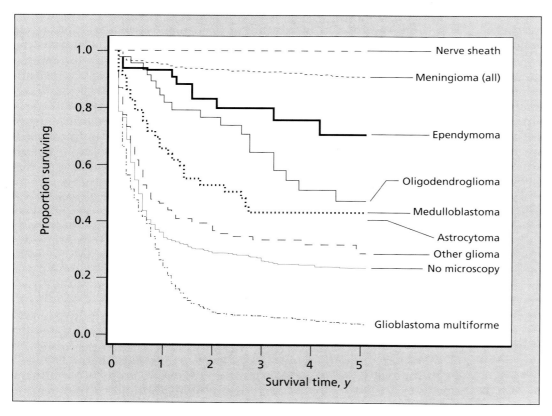

Figure 8-5. Kaplan-Meier survival curves for patients with various types of central nervous system tumors. The data are from the Victorian Cancer Registry in Victoria, Australia, from 1982 to 1991 [1]. As the survival curves show, glioblastoma multiforme is almost invariably lethal, and survival time is short, with less than 5% of patients surviving 5 years. Meningioma, on the other hand, has little effect on the survival of the patient. (This curve includes both benign and malignant meningiomas.) Patients with ependymoma, low-grade astrocytoma, or oligodendroglioma have intermediate survival curves and can live for years after their initial diagnosis. The astrocytoma curve includes anaplastic and well-differentiated tumors. The curve indicating "no microscopy" refers to tumors that were identified on clinical and radiologic study only.

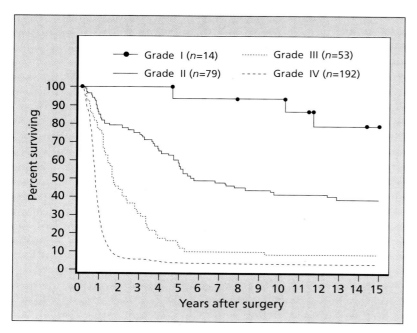

Figure 8-6. Survival curves for patients with astrocytoma grades I to IV. The histology of astrocytomas can vary from mildly atypical cells infiltrating normal brain parenchyma to highly cellular tumors with many mitoses, pleomorphism, and necrosis. There is some disagreement regarding which histologic criteria are most appropriate for grading astrocytomas (Fig. 8-33), but within each grading system, patients with higher grade tumors have shorter survival [13]. Patients with low grade astrocytomas have fairly long survival, with up to 68% surviving 5 years [14,15]. Patients with higher grade astrocytomas do not do as well. The 2-year survival for grade III astrocytoma ranges from 38% to 50%, while for grade IV astrocytoma patients, the 2-year survival is only 8% to 12%. Most of the patients with grade III or IV astrocytomas were treated with surgery and radiation. (*Adapted from* Daumas-Duport and colleagues [13].)

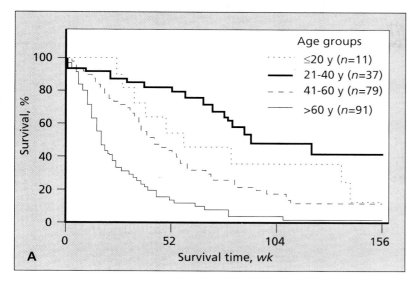

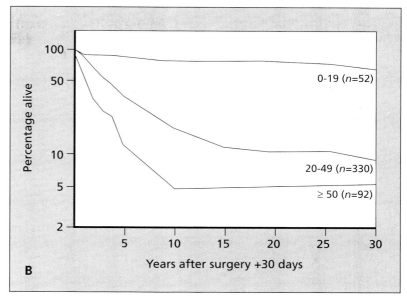

Figure 8-7. Age as an important prognostic factor in patients with both high- and low-grade gliomas. Even when patients have the same grade of glioma, younger patients survive longer [14,16–21]. **A,** The Kaplan-Meier survival curves of patients in different age groups from a retrospective study of malignant gliomas conducted by Devaux, O'Fallon, and Kelly [16]. Patients in the older age groups do not survive as long as younger patients (*P* is less than 0.0001). Even when grade III and grade IV gliomas were plotted separately, younger patients survived significantly longer than older patients (*P* is 0.005 or less).

B, Survival data in patients with low-grade supratentorial gliomas treated from 1915 to 1975 at the Mayo Clinic, Rochester, Minnesota [17]. These gliomas were grades 1 and 2, using the Kernohan grading system (Fig. 8-33). Again, younger patients survived longer. The number of patients in each group is included in parentheses. (Panel A *adapted from* Devaux and colleagues [16]; Panel B *adapted from* Laws and colleagues [17].)

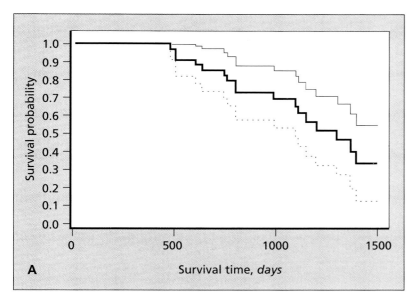

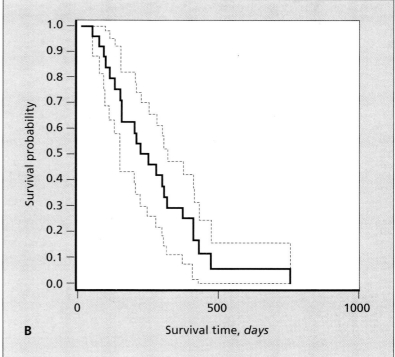

Figure 8-8. Wide variability in survival in patients with brain tumors. The prognosis of a patient with a brain tumor depends on the histology of the tumor, the patient's age, and his or her functional status [18–21]. **A,** Survival curve for a cohort of brain tumor patients who were younger than age 40, had a Karnofsky performance status (KPS) of greater than 70, and had a favorable histologic diagnosis. **B,** Dramatically different survival curve for patients who were older than age 40, with a KPS of less than 70, and a more malignant histology. The patients with all three favorable prognostic factors survived much longer [22]. Other factors such as extent of tumor resection may also affect prognosis, but are more difficult to demonstrate.

Diagnosis of Brain Tumors

Symptoms of Brain Tumors

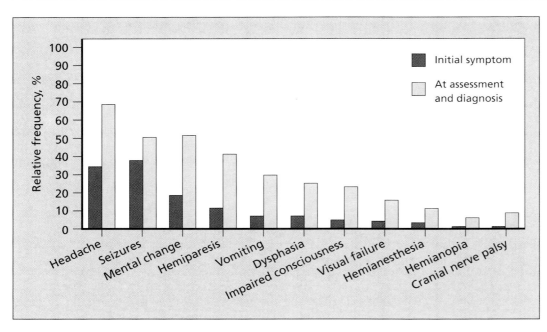

Figure 8-9. Initial symptoms and symptoms at diagnosis in patients with brain tumors. The most common initial symptoms in patients with primary malignant gliomas are headaches (35%) and

seizures (38%). Patients with brain tumors usually develop additional symptoms before definitive diagnosis. Many patients have noticeable mental status changes (52%) or hemiparesis (43%) by the time a diagnosis is made [23,24].

Brain tumor patients who present with seizures may have a better prognosis than those who present with other signs and symptoms. Tumors that cause seizures tend to be located peripherally and supratentorially, and are thus more surgically accessible. In addition, seizures occur more often in patients with low-grade gliomas than in patients with high-grade tumors [25]. The onset of seizures after 25 years of age should be investigated with magnetic resonance imaging (MRI). Up to 60% of patients presenting with new seizures after age 25 will have an abnormality detected on MRI, and 13% to 18% of these patients will have a brain tumor [26].

This information was collected from a series of 653 patients with cerebral gliomas seen at the National Hospital in London, from 1955 to 1975 [23,24]. Therefore most of these patients received their diagnosis before computed tomography or MRI became available.

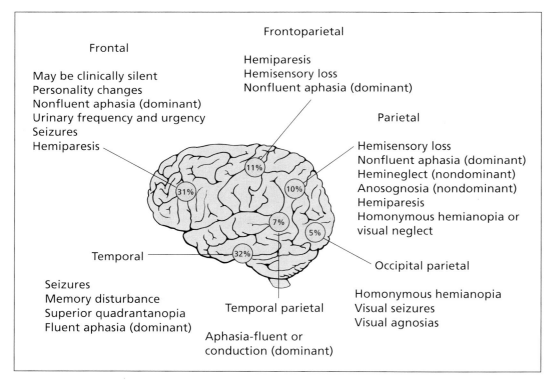

Figure 8-10. Distribution of malignant gliomas in adults and clinical symptoms associated with specific locations. Gliomas can occur anywhere within the brain, but some sites are more frequently involved than others [27]. Most supratentorial tumors occur in the frontal or frontoparietal area (42%), which comprise a larger volume of brain tissue than most of the other lobes. These frontal

lobe tumors can be clinically silent, especially if they occur in the nondominant hemisphere, or they may produce personality changes, seizures, incontinence, or nonfluent (Broca's) aphasia [28].

Gliomas also commonly involve the temporal lobe (32%). These tumors may present with simple or complex partial seizures that may include olfactory or gustatory hallucinations or déjà vu. A superior quadrantanopia may occur, and memory difficulties are often encountered. Fluent aphasia (Wernicke's) also occurs in patients with gliomas in the dominant temporal lobe [28].

Parietal lobe gliomas produce hemisensory loss, especially impairment of joint position sense and two-point discrimination, graphesthesia, and stereognosis. Gliomas in the dominant parietal lobe cause aphasia, while lesions in the nondominant parietal lobe can lead to contralateral neglect, various agnosias and apraxias, including anosognosia, or the inability to acknowledge a deficit. Homonymous hemianopia, or contralateral visual field neglect may also occur. Occipital gliomas are infrequent, probably related to the small size of the occipital lobe. These gliomas usually cause homonymous hemianopia, and may cause visual seizures [28]. Tumors arising in the posterior fossa produce neurologic syndromes that are too detailed to present here. (*Adapted from* Salcman and colleague [27]; Kraemer and colleague [29].)

Neurologic Examination

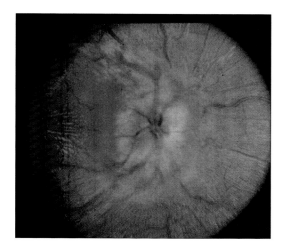

Figure 8-11. Funduscopic photo showing a patient's well-developed papilledema. The funduscopic examination is important in any patient with headache, and can be an important indicator of the presence of a brain tumor. This patient presented at age 11 with retro-orbital headaches, nausea, and vomiting. Her general examination and neurologic examination were normal except for papilledema and enlargement of her blind spot. The optic disc seen here is blurred and elevated. Exudates are present in the retina, and the nerve fiber layer is visible in the right eye, as yellow streaks directed from the optic disc toward the macula.

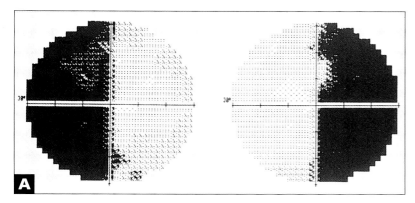

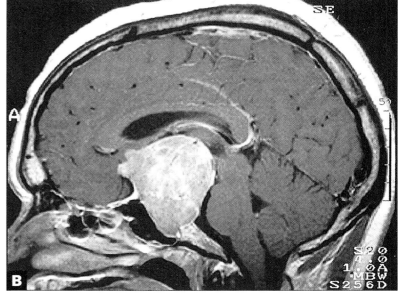

Figure 8-12. Humphrey visual field results showing bitemporal hemianopia due to a pituitary adenoma. Examination of the visual fields is an often omitted portion of the physical and neurologic examination, but is an inexpensive and noninvasive way to detect a brain tumor. This 33-year-old man presented with progressive visual loss over 1 year. Bitemporal visual field deficits were found on clinical examination. **A**, Patient's Humphrey visual field results are shown. **B**, Sagittal, T1-weighted postcontrast magnetic resonance image showing a large enhancing mass arising in the pituitary fossa, with suprasellar extension. Transphenoidal resection revealed a pituitary adenoma.

Bitemporal visual field loss is a helpful localizing sign, because it indicates dysfunction of the optic chiasm. The optic chiasm is very small, and the most common tumors that present in this region are pituitary adenomas with suprasellar extension, optic chiasm gliomas, and craniopharyngiomas.

Formal visual field testing may uncover subtle visual deficits in a patient with a tumor that threatens the optic nerves, chiasm, or tracts, and provides a tool for followup of these patients. (*Courtesy of* C. S. Zimmerman, MD, Department of Ophthalmology, University of Texas Southwestern Medical Center, Dallas, TX.)

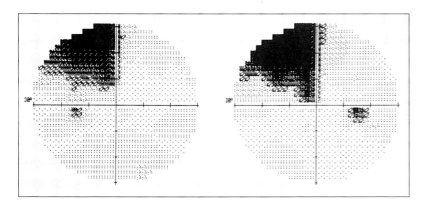

Figure 8-13. Superior quadrantanopia secondary to glioma in the right temporal lobe. More subtle visual field defects can also occur in patients with brain tumors. This patient had the "pie in the sky" visual field cut—a superior quadrantanopia. The nerve fibers that serve the inferior retina (superior visual field) divide from those that serve the superior retina, and course through the temporal lobe. A lesion involving the optic radiations in the temporal lobe produces a superior quadrantanopia, while a lesion involving the optic radiations in the parietal lobe produces an inferior quadrantanopia. (*Courtesy of* C. S. Zimmerman, MD, Department of Ophthalmology, University of Texas Southwestern Medical Center, Dallas, TX.)

Cerebrospinal Fluid Evaluation

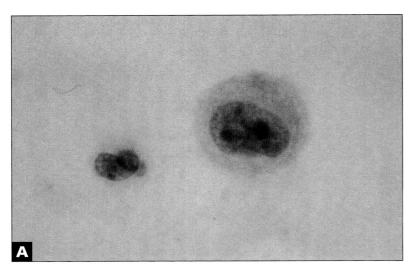

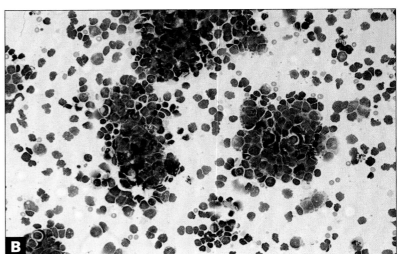

Figure 8-14. Malignant cells in cerebrospinal fluid (CSF). Occasionally, gliomas or metastatic tumors can be detected by studying CSF. **A,** CSF sample obtained from a patient with a history of breast carcinoma who presented with new headaches but had a negative head computed tomography scan. A Papanicolaou stain performed on the cellular pellet of centrifuged spinal fluid shows malignant cells. The malignant cell has a high nuclear to cytoplasm ratio, and large nucleoli.

Medulloblastoma is one intracranial tumor that frequently seeds the leptomeninges, and is often disseminated in the CSF at diagnosis. **B,** CSF sample showing clumps of small cells with some nuclear molding. The clumps of cells on cytologic examination are characteristic of solid tumors rather than leukemic infiltrates. Medulloblastomas are classically composed of "small blue cells," and thus this cytologic picture is characteristic.

Malignant cells in the CSF occur most often in patients with systemic cancer, but may also be found in patients with gliomas. The CSF cytologic specimen may contain malignant cells in as many as 15% to 40% of patients with gliomas [30,31], but these cells rarely form clinically significant leptomeningeal metastases. A recent study found spinal metastases in 0.14% of brain tumor patients undergoing treatment [32]. Today, with the high sensitivity of magnetic resonance imaging (MRI) scans, leptomeningeal disease can be detected with contrast MRI scans, and fewer spinal taps are done specifically to detect central nervous system malignancies or CSF spread.

Electroencephalographic Findings

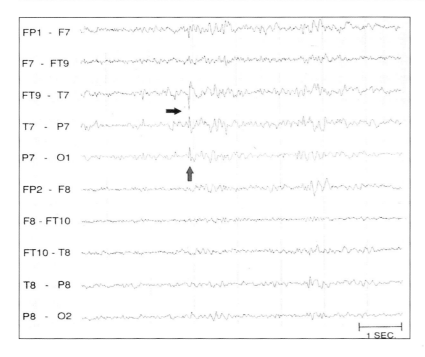

Figure 8-15. Focal spikes on an electroencephalogram (EEG) secondary to a left temporal lobe ganglioglioma. This patient presented with seizures that began with difficulty understanding speech and progressed to complex partial seizures. EEG tracing shows a focal spike, with a phase reversal near the T7 electrode (*red* and *blue arrows*), indicating a seizure focus in the left temporal area. A subtotal resection revealed a ganglioglioma. The patient's seizure control improved following resection.

Angiographic Studies

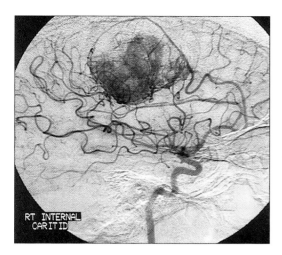

Figure 8-16. Arterial phase angiogram with a tumor blush following injection of the right internal carotid artery. Before the availability of computed tomography and magnetic resonance scanning, angiography was the only way to directly visualize intracranial tumors. The most helpful findings on angiography are abnormal vessels feeding a tumor, or a "tumor blush" of contrast indicating a hypervascular tumor. This patient had a very vascular tumor, a hemangiopericytoma. The tumor was fed by both internal carotid arteries, by the posterior circulation, and by the left external carotid artery. In some patients, the arterial phase of the angiogram is normal, but a tumor blush appears during the venous phase.

Imaging Studies

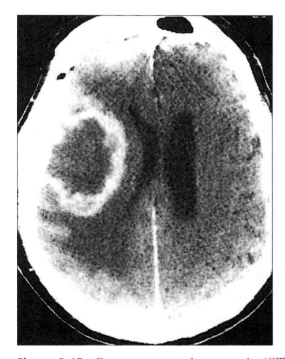

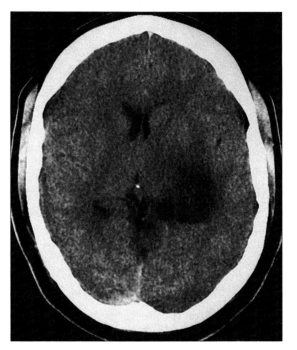

Figure 8-17. Contrast computed tomography (CT) scan with right posterior frontal glioblastoma multiforme in a 56-year-old man with a 2-month history of left-sided clumsiness and headache. There is a large ring-enhancing lesion high in the right frontal lobe and mass effect, with deformation of the right lateral ventricle and effacement of cerebral sulci on the right. Edema surrounding the tumor has decreased attenuation and involves the entire right hemisphere at this level. Subtotal resection revealed glioblastoma multiforme. Despite steroids and radiation therapy, the patient survived only 7 months.

Brain tumors are probably diagnosed earlier in their course since the advent of CT and magnetic resonance imaging (MRI). Before the development of these imaging techniques, brain tumors were recognized based on history, clinical examination, skull films, angiography, radionuclide scanning, and pneumoencephalography. CT and MRI have virtually replaced these modalities except for the history and clinical examination. Occasionally angiography is performed in patients with known or suspected tumors, for preoperative planning.

Figure 8-18. Contrasted computed tomography scan showing a low-density area deep in the left temporoparietal area in a patient with a low-grade glioma. There is mass effect on the frontal horn of the left lateral ventricle, but no appreciable midline shift, and no contrast enhancement. This 39-year-old man presented with seizures and headaches, but had no other neurologic impairment. Biopsy showed oligodendroglioma without anaplastic features.

In general, tumors that do not enhance are less likely to be anaplastic or clinically aggressive. These low-grade gliomas are more likely to occur in young adults rather than older adults, and often present with seizures.

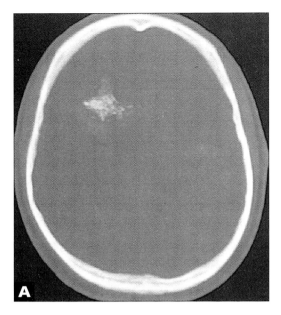

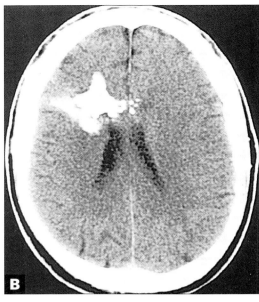

C. Frequency of Calcification Within Different Types of Tumors

Type of tumor	Percent that calcify
Astrocytomas	20
Oligodendrogliomas	50–60
Craniopharyngiomas	70–80
Ependymomas	50
Gangliogliomas	35
Meningiomas	10

Figure 8-19. Calcium within a brain tumor on computed tomography (CT) scan. CT scan is particularly useful for detecting calcification within brain tumors. Calcium can be difficult to distinguish from blood products or flow voids on magnetic resonance imaging, but is obvious as increased attenuation on CT scans. **A,** "Bone window" CT scan of a patient with a right posterior frontal tumor. Speckles of increased attenuation in an infiltrating pattern are present in the right cerebral hemisphere. Their visibility on bone window settings, and their distribution, suggest calcification within a brain tumor.

B, Standard CT soft tissue windows in the same patient following contrast administration. Without the bone windows, and without an unenhanced CT scan, the bright lesion in the right hemisphere might be considered enhancement rather than calcification.

The presence of calcification within a brain tumor can suggest its histologic subtype. **C,** Frequency of calcification within different types of tumors. Craniopharyngiomas and oligodendrogliomas are the primary brain tumors that are most likely to contain calcium. Nevertheless, since astrocytomas outnumber other primary brain tumors by a large margin, most tumors containing calcium are astrocytic [33].

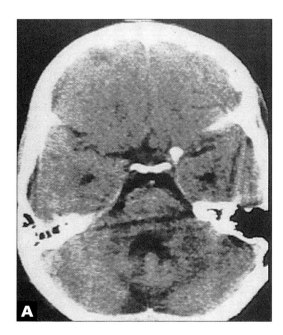

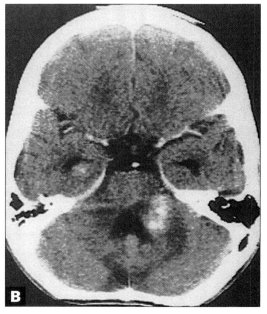

Figure 8-20. Contrast-enhanced computed tomography (CT) scans. Occasionally, brain tumors are isodense with brain on CT scans. If there is no mass effect distorting local structures, these tumors may be difficult to detect on an unenhanced CT scan. **A,** An 8-year-old boy had a CT scan done to investigate progressive ataxia when he presented in 1983. The initial noncontrast scan was essentially normal, although the fourth ventricle was not exactly symmetric. **B,** Two days later, a contrast-enhanced CT scan was performed, and clearly showed an enhancing mass in the right cerebellar peduncle. The contrast also revealed a second enhancing lesion adjacent to the temporal horn of the left lateral ventricle (not shown). The tumor was a medulloblastoma, and the presence of two distinct lesions indicated that it had disseminated via the cerebrospinal fluid.

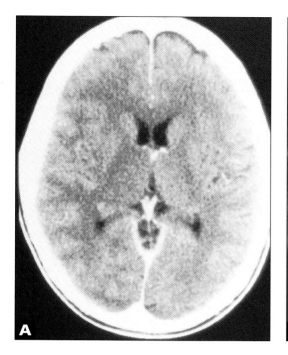

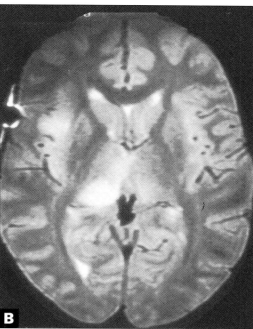

Figure 8-21. Magnetic resonance imaging (MRI) compared with computed tomography (CT). A 47-year-old woman presented with a left hemisensory deficit at a time when CT scan was the primary diagnostic technique used to visualize intracranial pathology. MRI scans were then prohibitively expensive. **A,** The contrast-enhanced CT scan failed to show any intracranial lesions. **B,** Because of the high index of suspicion, an MRI was done. The T2-weighted MRI scan clearly shows increased signal within the right thalamus. The lesion was nonenhancing (scans not shown). Stereotactic biopsy revealed anaplastic astrocytoma.

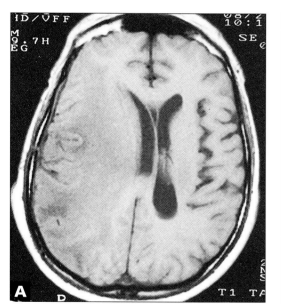

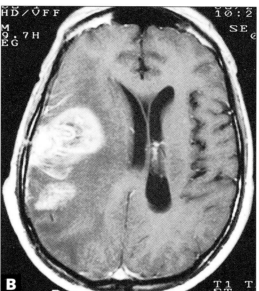

Figure 8-22. High-grade glioma on magnetic resonance imaging (MRI) with and without contrast, showing cystic areas and an infiltrating border. **A,** Precontrast T1-weighted axial MRI in a patient with headaches, personality change, and seizures. There is decreased T1 signal throughout the right hemisphere and mass effect on the right lateral ventricle. **B,** The administration of gadolinium contrast produces dramatic enhancement of the mass that is obviously infiltrating. The tumor is a glioblastoma multiforme (see Fig. 8-36 for gross and histologic correlation).

Glioblastomas are heterogeneous both microscopically and grossly. These scans demonstrate the infiltrating nature of these high-grade astrocytic neoplasms. Malignant cells can be found beyond the area of enhancement on MRI. The area of decreased T1 signal surrounding the enhancing lesion represents both edema and infiltrating nonenhancing tumor [34]. It is difficult to surgically remove all of the malignant cells in an infiltrating glioma, even when the area of contrast enhancement can be completely resected. This explains the tendency of these tumors to recur near the borders of a surgical resection.

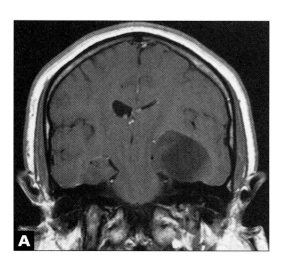

Figure 8-23. Magnetic resonance imaging (MRI) findings in low grade gliomas. Low-grade tumors often do not appear as aggressive as glioblastomas on MRI scans. They may appear circumscribed, usually have less mass effect, and may not enhance. This 38-year-old man presented with a seizure. **A,** Coronal T1-weighted, gadolinium-enhanced MRI scan shows a mass in the left temporal lobe that has low signal on T1-weighted images, and no enhancement with gadolinium. Left anterior temporal lobectomy revealed a low grade mixed oligoastrocytoma.

(*Continued on next page*)

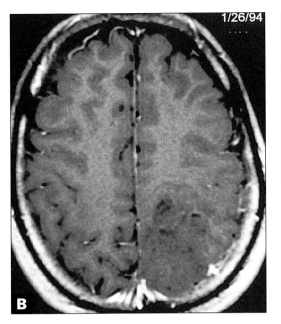
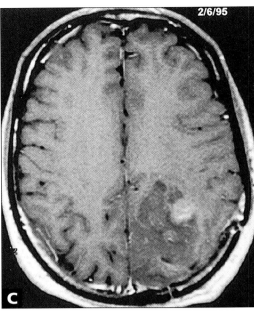

Figure 8-23. (*Continued*) Sometimes a change in the MRI characteristics of a glioma heralds a change in its biologic behavior as seen in these serial MRI scans from a patient whose low-grade oligodendroglioma progressed to anaplastic oligodendroglioma. **B,** The T1-weighted gadolinum-enhanced MRI shows a low signal area in the left occipital lobe that does not enhance. The histology was an oligodendroglioma without anaplastic features. **C,** One year later, the MRI scan shows a small area of enhancement within the tumor. The volume of the tumor is essentially unchanged, but stereotactic biopsy of the enhancing lesion revealed anaplastic oligodendroglioma.

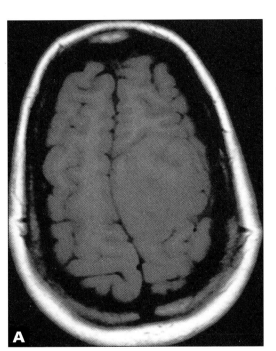
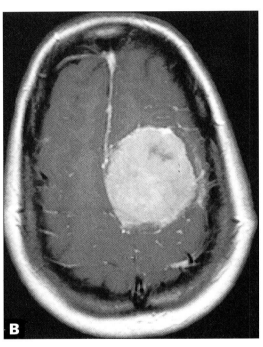
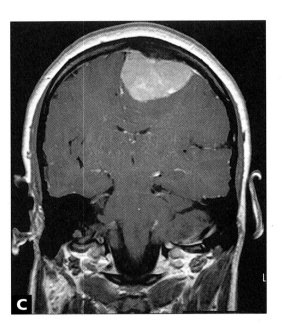

Figure 8-24. Characteristics of meningiomas on magnetic resonance imaging (MRI). Meningiomas often have a characteristic MRI appearance. They are usually isointense to slightly hypointense compared to the cortex on T1-weighted MRI scans. Nearly all meningiomas enhance intensely with gadolinium [35]. There may be a cerebrospinal fluid cleft visible around a meningioma, separating it from brain parenchyma, and confirming the extra-axial location. An extension of contrast enhancement along the dura at the margins of the tumor ("dural tail") may be present in 60% of meningiomas [36]. This finding suggests meningioma, but is not entirely specific [37]. Peritumoral edema may be present in two thirds of meningiomas, but does not correlate with tumor size or histologic subtype [38,39].

A young woman presented after a single focal onset seizure, and an MRI scan revealed a large densely enhancing tumor high in the parietal lobe. **A,** The tumor distorts the normal cerebral sulci on the T1-weighted MRI. **B,** Gadolinium administration produces bright, nearly uniform enhancement of the tumor. **C,** Coronal MRI with gadolinium shows the intimate association of the tumor with the overlying dura. Meningioma was suspected, and was confirmed on craniotomy. A complete resection was achieved. The patient is tumor-free and her MRI with contrast is normal 1 year following resection.

When meningiomas can be completely resected, long-term survival is the rule. A recent study reported overall survival rates of 83% at 5 years, 77% at 10 years, and 69% at 15 years. The recurrence-free survival is affected by the extent of resection and by the presence of atypical histologic features. The recurrence rate of benign meningiomas following complete resection was 19% in a population study in Finland [40]. The same author showed that atypical meningiomas carried a higher risk of recurrence (38% at 5 years) [41].

Meningiomas can occur anywhere meningothelial cells are found. **D,** Distribution of anatomic locations of meningiomas. (Panel C *from* DeMonte and colleague [42]; with permission.)

D. Distribution of Anatomic Locations of Meningiomas

Site	Relative incidences, %
Parasagittal/falcine	25
Convexity	19
Sphenoid ridge	17
Suprasellar (tuberculum)	9
Posterior fossa	8
Olfactory groove	8
Middle fossa/Meckel's cave	4
Tentorial	3
Peritorcular	3
Lateral ventricle	1–2
Foramen magnum	1–2
Orbit/optic nerve sheath	1–2

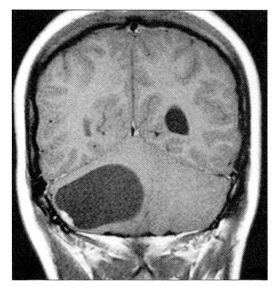

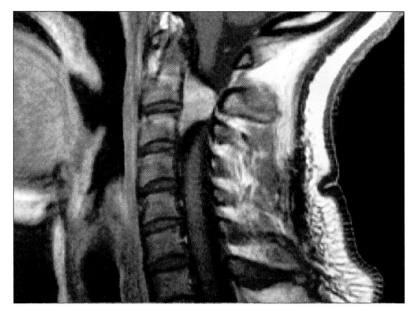

Figure 8-25. Contrast-enhanced coronal T1-weighted magnetic resonance imaging (MRI) scan showing a hemangioblastoma of the right cerebellar hemisphere. As discussed earlier, meningiomas have many features that help identify their benign nature based on MRI scans (Fig. 8-24). Hemangioblastoma is another tumor that has a characteristic MRI appearance. This tumor usually occurs in the posterior fossa within a cerebellar hemisphere (80% to 85%) [43]. In 60% of cases, there is a small mural nodule that enhances, surrounded by a variably sized cyst [43]. Pilocytic astrocytomas may also have this appearance [44].

Hemangioblastomas usually occur in young adults, and most occur sporadically, but some hemangioblastomas are associated with a genetic condition known as von Hippel-Lindau syndrome (VHL). Some VHL patients (42%) have multiple hemangioblastomas or retinal hemangioblastomas (60%) [45].

Figure 8-26. Sagittal T1-weighted magnetic resonance imaging (MRI) scan with gadolinium showing brightly enhancing, apparently dural-based tumor that severely narrows the cervical spinal canal. The patient was a 36-year-old black female who presented with a month-long history of gait instability and new bladder incontinence. Examination revealed left upper extremity weakness with deltoid muscle atrophy and lower extremity spasticity. MRI provides a noninvasive method to evaluate the spinal cord. The neurologic examination remains important in these patients, because localization to a spinal cord level allows a more focused, less time-consuming MRI examination. The tumor was resected, and proved to be a schwannoma.

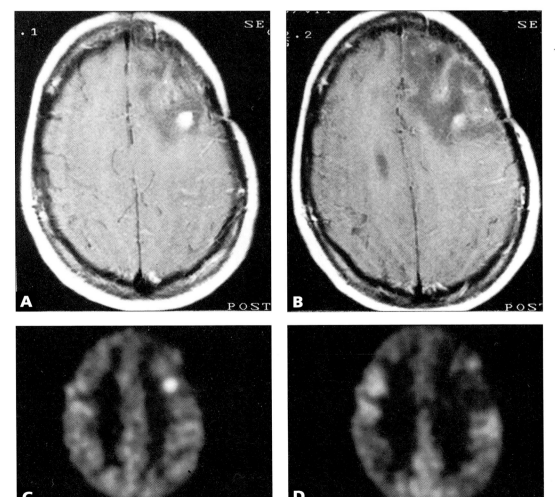

Figure 8-27. The use of positron-emission tomography (PET) to differentiate radionecrosis and tumor recurrence. **A, B,** Axial T1-weighted gadolinium-enhanced magnetic resonance imaging (MRI) scans in a patient who had an anaplastic astrocytoma removed from his left frontal lobe 9 months before this scan. He received postoperative radiation therapy to 5900 cGy. The MRIs show a low density area within the left frontal lobe with a small focus of enhancement. Radionecrosis and tumor recurrence were both diagnostic possibilities. Radionecrosis can look exactly like tumor recurrence on MRI scans, with enhancement, mass effect, and progression on serial scans. Radiation necrosis usually occurs 6 to 24 months following radiation therapy [46]. **C, D,** PET scans showing an area of increased metabolic activity in the same region as the area of contrast enhancement on MRI, making a diagnosis of tumor recurrence more likely than radionecrosis. An area of enhancement that does not have increased metabolic activity on a PET scan is more likely to represent radiation necrosis [47–50]. Often, however, the PET scan is inconclusive. When reoperation is performed for presumed radiation necrosis after I^{125} interstitial implants, 66% of patients have a mixture of radiation necrosis and recurrent tumor. Only 5% have radiation necrosis alone, and only 29% have tumor alone [51].

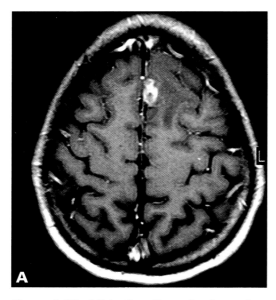 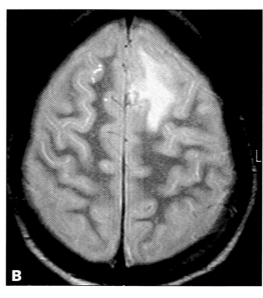

Figure 8-28. Misleading diagnosis of central nervous system tumor using imaging studies. Despite the exquisite anatomic detail provided by magnetic resonance imaging (MRI) scans, they are not entirely specific. Cerebral abscesses, severe acute demyelination, progressive multifocal leukoencephalopathy, toxoplasmosis, and occasionally cerebral infarctions with mass effect can resemble brain tumors on computed tomography or MRI. The clinical course and other associated findings can narrow the differential diagnosis, but a biopsy is sometimes required to differentiate these conditions. **A,** Axial contrast-enhanced MRI scan of a 32-year-old man who presented with a subacute history of headache, nausea, and vomiting. The MRI scan shows a small nodule of enhancement. **B,** Axial proton-density scan highlighting the abnormal white matter surrounding the enhancing lesion. The patient underwent a stereotactic biopsy, which recovered only inflammatory infiltrates, consistent with a cerebral abscess. Bacterial and fungal stains and cultures were negative, and an echocardiogram was also normal. Abscesses can closely mimic tumors on modern imaging, but the clinical history of acute to subacute onset of symptoms, or the presence of systemic signs and symptoms (*eg,* fever) suggests the correct diagnosis. The patient's MRI scan was normal 2 weeks following treatment with antibiotics.

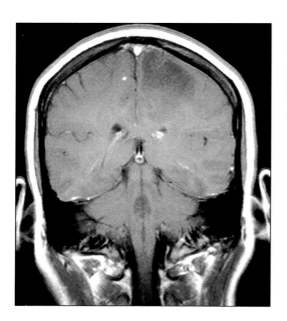

Figure 8-29. Coronal T1-weighted magnetic resonance imaging (MRI) scan showing a low-signal area with mass effect in the white matter of the left hemisphere in a young patient who presented with chronic headache and right-sided clumsiness of approximately 1 week's duration. An examination revealed a mild right hemiparesis. On admission, this MRI scan was performed, and the patient received steroids for a presumptive diagnosis of intracranial tumor. The following week, the patient's hemiparesis improved. She later experienced an episode of optic neuritis, making the correct diagnosis of multiple sclerosis more obvious.

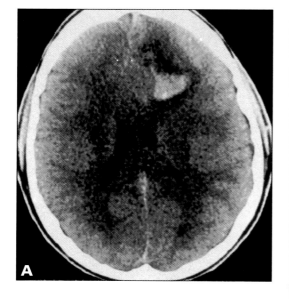

B. Frequency of Bleeding as a Complication of Primary Intracranial Tumors

Tumor	Bleeding, %
Glioblastoma	6.3
Astrocytoma	2.5
Oligodendroglioma	8.3
Ependymoma	6.6
Meningioma	1.3
Schwannoma	0.0
Medulloblastoma	1.4
Hemangioblastoma	0.0
Craniopharyngioma	3.3
Pituitary adenoma	15.8
Choroid plexus papilloma	16.7

Figure 8-30. Glioma presenting with intracranial hemorrhage. Although the clinical history is very helpful in making a diagnosis of intracranial tumor, sometimes it provides a red herring. This child presented with sudden onset of headache and vomiting followed by somnolence. **A,** Computed tomography scan shows a large frontal lobe hemorrhage. There is a low-density area adjacent to the bright hemorrhage. A follow-up magnetic resonance imaging scan showed persistent mass effect after the hemorrhage resolved, and biopsy showed anaplastic astrocytoma.

Acute symptoms suggest a diagnosis of cerebrovascular ischemia or hemorrhage rather than brain tumor. Nevertheless, tumor is present in 4.6% of intracranial hemorrhages [52]. Metastatic tumors are more likely to bleed than primary brain tumors, but hemorrhage has been reported in nearly every histologic type of primary brain tumor as well. **B,** The frequency of bleeding as a complication of primary intracranial tumors. (Panel A, *courtesy of* S. Roach, MD, Department of Pediatric Neurology, University of Texas Southwestern, Dallas, TX; Panel B *adapted from* Salcman [52].)

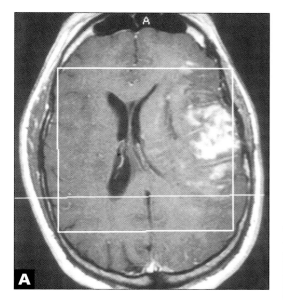

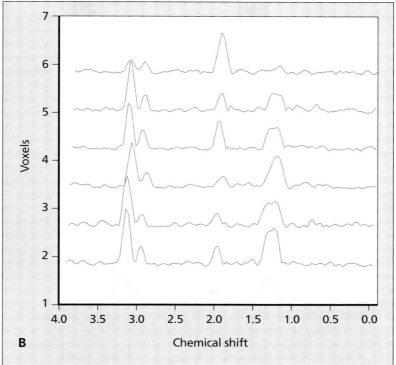

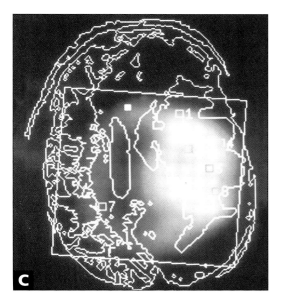

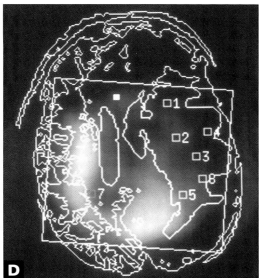

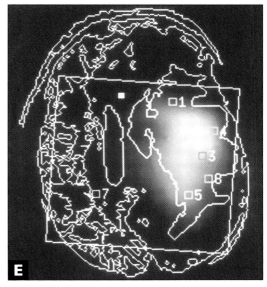

Figure 8-31. A, An axial T1-weighted, contrast-enhanced magnetic resonance imaging (MRI) scan in a patient with recurrent hemiparesis 22 months after radiation therapy for an anaplastic mixed glioma. Magnetic resonance (MR) spectroscopy was performed to help differentiate radiation necrosis from recurrent tumor. MR spectroscopy is a new tool that can detect several molecular species within a given area of the brain on an MRI scan. It can be helpful in differentiating radiation necrosis from recurrent tumor, although studies regarding the specificity and sensitivity of MR spectroscopy for this purpose are ongoing. Sampling error is a major problem with single voxel MR spectroscopy, but multiple voxel images are now available, and are being used clinically. **B,** Line spectra at various voxels throughout the brain. The lines show the four characteristic peaks seen on brain MR spectroscopy. The first peak, at chemical shift 3.1, represents choline. As a major component of cell membranes, choline is increased in areas of high cellularity, and is usually larger than the second peak in higher grade brain tumors. The second peak is due to creatinine, which does not usually change intensity in tumors. The third peak on most MR spectra is due to N-acetyl aspartate (NAA), a component of neurons. This peak is highest in areas of normal brain. The fourth and broader peak around chemical shift 1.1 is due to lactate, and can be increased in radiation necrosis or high grade tumor. The most normal spectrum in this patient is seen in the top line. The choline and creatinine peaks are about equal in height, and there is a large NAA peak. This spectra is obtained from voxel 7, which is located in the hemisphere opposite the patient's tumor. The spectra obtained from all of the other voxels (1 through 6) show an elevated choline peak compared to creatinine, and reduced NAA (neurons). The excess of choline is better demonstrated in the multiple voxel image (**C**). The bright signal within the line diagram of the brain shows where choline is elevated. The area of choline elevation indicates probable high-grade tumor, and involves an even larger area than the enhancing area on the MRI scan. **D,** Decreased DNA within the same area. **E,** Smaller zone of increased lactate in the middle of the tumor, consistent with high grade tumor, confirming the clinical suspicion that the enhancement represents recurrent tumor. Radiation necrosis usually does not have an elevated choline peak, although elevated lactate can be seen.

Histologic Classification of Primary Central Nervous System Tumors

WHO Histologic Typing of CNS Tumors

1	Tumors of Neuroepithelial Tissue
1.1	*Astrocytic tumors*
1.1.1	Astrocytoma
1.1.1.1	Variants: Fibrillary
1.1.1.2	Protoplasmic
1.1.1.3	Gemistocytic
1.1.2	Anaplastic (malignant) astrocytoma
1.1.3	Glioblastoma
1.1.3.1	Variants: Giant cell glioblastoma
1.1.3.2	Gliosarcoma
1.1.4	Pilocytic astrocytoma
1.1.5	Pleomorphic xanthoastrocytoma
1.1.6	Subependymal giant cell astrocytoma (tuberous sclerosis)
1.2	*Oligodendroglial tumors*
1.2.1	Oligodendroglioma
1.2.2	Anaplastic (malignant) oligodendroglioma
1.3	*Ependymal tumors*
1.3.1	Ependymoma
1.3.1.1	Variants: Cellular
1.3.1.2	Papillary
1.3.1.3	Clear cell
1.3.2	Anaplastic (malignant) ependymoma
1.3.3	Myxopapillary ependymoma
1.3.4	Subependymoma
1.4	*Mixed gliomas*
1.4.1	Oligo-astrocytoma
1.4.2	Anaplastic (malignant) oligo-astrocytoma
1.4.3	Others
1.5	*Choroid plexus tumors*
1.5.1	Choroid plexus papilloma
1.5.2	Choroid plexus carcinoma
1.6	*Neuroepithelial tumors of uncertain origin*
1.6.1	Astroblastoma
1.6.2	Polar spongioblastoma
1.6.3	Gliomatosis cerebri

1.7	*Neuronal and mixed neuronal-glial tumors*
1.7.1	Gangliocytoma
1.7.2	Dysplastic gangliocytoma of cerebellum (Lhermitte-Duclos)
1.7.3	Desmoplastic infantile ganglioglioma
1.7.4	Dysembryoplastic neuroepithelial tumor
1.7.5	Ganglioglioma
1.7.6	Anaplastic (malignant) ganglioglioma
1.7.7	Central neurocytoma
1.7.8	Paraganglioma of the filum terminale
1.7.9	Olfactory neuroblastoma (Aesthesioneuroblastoma)
1.7.9.1	Variant: Olfactory neuro-epithelioma
1.8	*Pineal parenchymal tumors*
1.8.1	Pineocytoma
1.8.2	Pineoblastoma
1.8.3	Mixed / transitional pineal tumors
1.9	*Embryonal tumors*
1.9.1	Medulloepithelioma
1.9.2	Neuroblastoma
1.9.2.1	Variant: Ganglioneuroblastoma
1.9.3	Ependymoblastoma
1.9.4	Primitive neuroectodermal tumors (PNETs)
1.9.4.1	Medulloblastoma
1.9.4.1.1	Variants: Desmoplastic medulloblastoma
1.9.4.1.2	Medullomyoblastoma
1.9.4.1.3	Melanotic medulloblastoma
2	Tumors of cranial and spinal nerves
2.1	*Schwannoma (neurilemmoma, neurinoma)*
2.1.1	Variants: Cellular
2.1.2	Plexiform
2.1.3	Melanotic
2.2	*Neurofibroma*
2.2.1	Circumscribed (solitary)
2.2.2	Plexiform

(Table continued on next page)

Figure 8-32. Histologic classification of central nervous system (CNS) tumors from the World Health Organization (WHO) Histologic Typing of Tumors of the Central Nervous System [53,54]. The CNS and related structures are affected by a variety of primary and metastatic neoplasms. Glial neoplasms, which are derived from cells of neuroectodermal origin, are the most common primary tumors in the CNS. Glial cells include astrocytes, oligodendrocytes, ependymal cells, and choroid plexus cells. Recent advances in therapies for specific tumor types, such as effective chemotherapy for anaplastic oligodendroglioma, underscore the importance of recognizing prognostically significant pathologic phenotypes of glial tumors. Other less common intrinsic CNS tumors, including neuronal, embryonal, and lymphoid neoplasms, are also named according to their presumed cell of origin.

(Continued on next page)

WHO Histologic Typing of CNS Tumors (*continued*)

2.3	*Malignant peripheral nerve sheath tumor (MPNST) (neurogenic sarcoma, anaplastic neurofibroma, "malignant schwannoma")*
2.3.1	Variants: Epithelioid
2.3.2	MPNST with divergent mesenchymal and/or epithelial differentiation
2.3.3	Melanotic

3   Tumors of the meninges

3.1   *Tumors of meningothelial cells*
3.1.1   Meningioma
3.1.1.1   Variants: Meningothelial
3.1.1.2   Fibrous (fibroblastic)
3.1.1.3   Transitional (mixed)
3.1.1.4   Psammomatous
3.1.1.5   Angiomatous
3.1.1.6   Microcystic
3.1.1.7   Secretory
3.1.1.8   Clear cell
3.1.1.9   Chordoid
3.1.1.10   Lymphoplasmacyte-rich
3.1.1.11   Metaplastic
3.1.2   Atypical meningioma
3.1.3   Papillary meningioma
3.1.4   Anaplastic (malignant) meningioma

3.2   *Mesenchymal, non-meningothelial tumors*

Benign neoplasms
3.2.1   Osteocartilaginous tumors
3.2.2   Lipoma
3.2.3   Fibrous histiocytoma
3.2.4   Others

Malignant neoplasms
3.2.5   Hemangiopericytoma
3.2.6   Chondrosarcoma
3.2.6.1   Variant: Mesenchymal chondrosarcoma
3.2.7   Malignant fibrous histiocytoma
3.2.8   Rhabdomyosarcoma
3.2.9   Meningeal sarcomatosis
3.2.10   Others

3.3   *Primary melanocytic lesions*
3.3.1   Diffuse melanosis
3.3.2   Melanocytoma
3.3.3   Malignant melanoma
3.3.3.1   Variant: Meningeal melanomatosis

3.4   *Tumors of uncertain histogenesis*
3.4.1   Haemangioblastoma (Capillary haemangioblastoma)

4   Lymphomas and haemopoietic neoplasms

4.1   Malignant lymphomas
4.2   Plasmacytoma
4.3   Granulocytic sarcoma
4.4   Others

5   Germ cell tumors

5.1   Germinoma
5.2   Embryonal carcinoma
5.3   Yolk sac tumor (endodermal sinus tumor)
5.4   Choriocarcinoma
5.5   Teratoma
5.5.1   Immature
5.5.2   Mature
5.5.3   Teratoma with malignant transformation
5.6   Mixed germ cell tumors

6   Cysts and tumor-like lesions

6.1   Rathke cleft cyst
6.2   Epidermoid cyst
6.3   Dermoid cyst
6.4   Colloid cyst of the third ventricle
6.5   Enterogenous cyst
6.6   Neuroglial cyst
6.7   Granular cell tumor (choristoma, pituicytoma)
6.8   Hypothalamic neuronal hamartoma
6.9   Nasal glial heterotopia
6.10   Plasma cell granuloma

7   Tumors of the sellar region

7.1   Pituitary adenoma
7.2   Pituitary carcinoma
7.3   Craniopharyngioma
7.3.1   Variants: Adamantinomatous
7.3.2   Papillary

8   Local extensions from regional tumors

8.1   Paraganglioma (chemodectoma)
8.2   Chordoma
8.3   Chondroma
       Chondrosarcoma
8.4   Carcinoma

9   Metastatic tumors

10   Unclassified tumors

Figure 8-32. (*Continued*)

Kernohan	Ringertz/Burger	WHO	Daumas-Duport-Scheithauer
			Histologic features: pleomorphism, mitoses, vascular proliferation, necrosis
1 Normal-appearing astrocytes without anaplasia	**Astrocytoma** Mild pleomorphism and hypercellularity; mitoses and vascular proliferation rare	**I** Pilocytic astrocytoma	**1** No features present (negligibly rare)
2 Most cells show mild anaplasia with no mitosis		**II** Diffuse growth of well-differentiated astrocytes	**2** One feature present (pleomorphism)
3 Moderate anaplasia of 50% of cells; mitoses present; vascular proliferation and necrosis may be seen; foci of hypercellularity	**Anaplastic astrocytoma** Moderate pleomorphism and hypercellularity; increased mitoses, vascular proliferation common	**III** Anaplastic features present: pleomorphism, increased mitoses, vascular proliferation	**3** Two features present (usually pleomorphism and mitoses)
4 Most cells show marked anaplasia; numerous mitoses; vascular proliferation and necrosis may be prominent	**Glioblastoma multiforme** Features of anaplastic astrocytoma plus zones of necrosis	**IV** Undifferentiated or primitive-appearing cells predominate	**4** Three or four features present (pleomorphism, mitoses, and vascular proliferation and/or necrosis)

Figure 8-33. Comparison of histologic grading systems for astrocytomas. Astrocytic tumors are the most common glial neoplasms. Several classification systems for primary infiltrating central nervous system (CNS) astrocytic tumors have been proposed, each of which has advantages and limitations [55]. The grading systems compared are the Kernohan, Ringertz-Burger [55–57], World Health Organization (WHO) [53,54], and Daumas-Duport-Scheithauer [58] grading systems. Histologic features of anaplasia that form the basis of current classification systems include degree of cellularity, mitoses, nuclear pleomorphism, endothelial proliferation, and necrosis. The Kernohan [56] and Daumas-Duport [58] histologic classification system for astrocytic tumors are both four-grade systems. The other commonly used classification systems [55,57,59], and the WHO Histologic Typing of Tumors of the Central Nervous System, whose classification scheme is used in this chapter [53,54], differ in the relative significance they assign to each histologic feature, and attempt to divide infiltrating astrocytomas into three categories. The overlap of Kernohan grade 2 and 3 astrocytomas with tumors that would be graded as 1 to 4 in other systems is illustrated with arrows. (*Adapted from* Coons and colleague [60].)

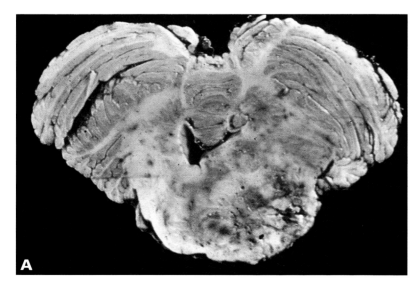

Figure 8-34. Brain stem glioma. A 7-year-old boy presented with a 5-month history of slurred speech, gait abnormalities, visual problems, and attention deficit. Magnetic resonance imaging (MRI) scan showed diffuse enlargement of the pons, hypointense on T1 images and hyperintense on T2 images and proton density images (Fig. 8-87). Chemotherapy and radiation therapy were initiated without a biopsy for the presumed diagnosis of brain stem glioma. After an initial positive response to therapy, the patient deteriorated, and died 12 months after initial diagnosis. **A,** Autopsy revealed symmetric nodular enlargement of the pons and medulla with extension into the midbrain and cerebellar white matter.

(*Continued on next page*)

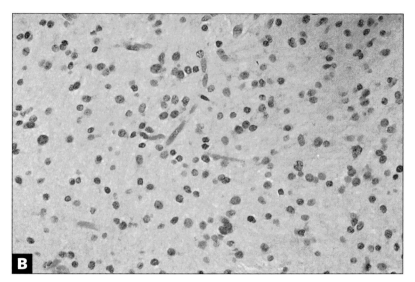

Figure 8-34. (*Continued*) **B**, Histologic examination disclosed a diffuse pontine fibrillary astrocytoma composed of widely dispersed small astrocytic cells.

Brain stem gliomas most commonly occur in males, with a 2.5 to 1 ratio of boys to girls, in the first decade of life (75%), and represent 10% to 15% of infratentorial central nervous system (CNS) neoplasms in the pediatric population. Brain stem gliomas are usually diffusely infiltrative and involve the pons, medulla, and less frequently, the midbrain. They can demonstrate exophytic growth into the cerebellopontine angle, cisterna magna, and perimesencephalic structures. These tumors are typically low grade, but may span the spectrum of histologic grades [61,62].

The differential diagnosis of brain stem glioma includes non-neoplastic processes such as encephalitis, tuberculoma, multiple sclerosis, vascular malformation, and hemorrhage [61]. According to a recent collaborative study by the Children's Cancer Group, diagnosis of brain stem gliomas by MRI scans is highly specific, and a characteristic MRI scan eliminates the need for biopsy before therapy is initiated. Histopathologic confirmation is recommended in the presence of a focal, enhancing, peripontine mass that is in the midbrain, medulla, or peduncle, or if there is a dorsally exophytic tumor protruding into the fourth ventricle [63,64].

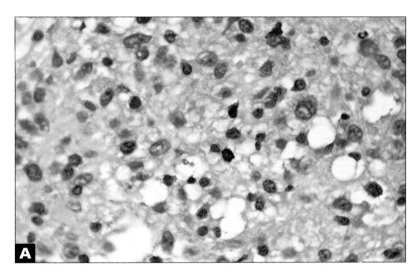

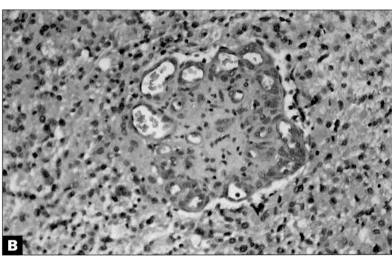

Figure 8-35. Photomicrographs showing the typical morphologic features of an anaplastic astrocytoma [54,55,61]. This neoplasm was removed from the frontal lobe of a 54-year-old man who presented with new focal motor seizures. The tumor is moderately cellular, with nuclear atypia, increased mitotic activity (**A**), and florid microvascular proliferation (**B**).

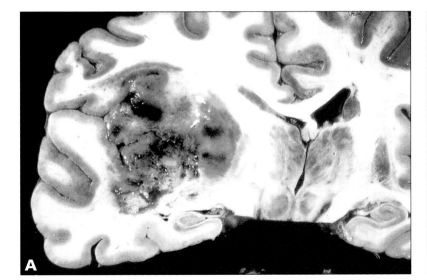

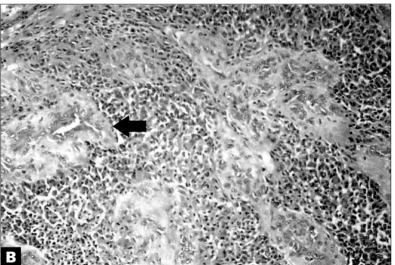

Figure 8-36. Glioblastoma multiforme. **A**, Coronal section from the brain of a 68-year-old man who was admitted for the evaluation of a change in personality noted by his family. He died several months later and an autopsy was performed. Grossly, the soft mass merges imperceptibly into surrounding brain parenchyma and appears hemorrhagic and necrotic. **B**, Microscopically, the tumor is characterized by a densely cellular infiltrating glial proliferation with astrocytic differentiation, moderate nuclear pleomorphism, microvascular hyperplasia (*arrow*), and **C**, widespread "pseudopalisading necrosis" (*arrows*). The features are consistent with a grade IV astrocytoma (World Health Organization classification) or glioblastoma multiforme.

(*Continued on next page*)

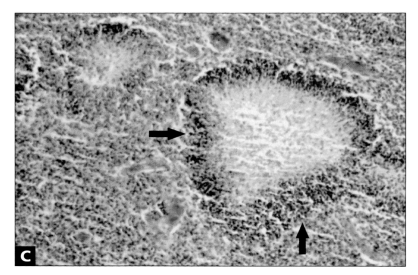

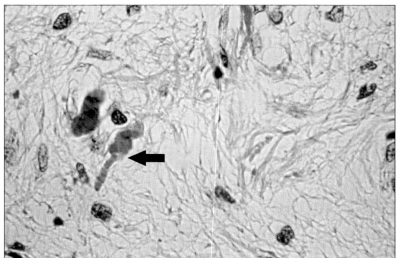

Figure 8-36. (*Continued*) Glioblastoma multiforme is an anaplastic astrocytic neoplasm in which microvascular proliferation and necrosis are requisite histologic features for diagnosis. Significant cellular pleomorphism, multinucleated giant cells, and enhanced mitotic activity often complete the histopathologic picture [54,55,61]. These highly aggressive tumors have a peak incidence between 45 and 60 years of age and are typically located in the cerebral hemispheres [61].

Figure 8-37. Photomicrograph from a contrast-enhancing hypothalamic mass in a 4-year-old boy. The histopathologic features consist of a loosely textured neoplasm containing Rosenthal fibers (*arrow*) and stellate astrocytes. Typically, the loosely textured spongy tissue alternates with more compact areas, resulting in a biphasic architecture.

Pilocytic astrocytomas are circumscribed and often cystic astrocytomas that are common in children and young adults. Although they can occur anywhere along the neuraxis, including the cerebral hemispheres and spinal cord, the cerebellum, optic nerve, and hypothalamus are favored. Pilocytic astrocytomas may contain microvascular proliferation, nuclear atypia, and an occasional mitotic figure. Despite the fact that these morphologic features are ominous findings in "diffuse" astrocytomas, they do not appear to affect prognosis adversely in pilocytic astrocytomas. Malignant degeneration has been reported, but it is rare [61,65,66].

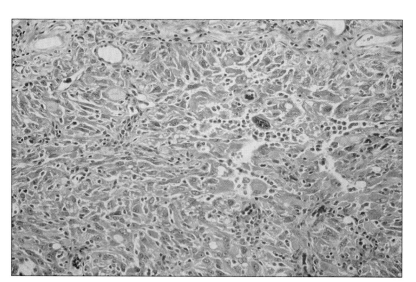

Figure 8-38. Microscopic features of a pleomorphic xanthoastrocytoma. A superficial, cystic temporal lobe neoplasm was excised from a 14-year-old girl with a long-standing history of seizures. The neoplasm consists of sheets of large, pleomorphic cells with abundant pink cytoplasm and focal perivascular collections of lymphocytes. Cytoplasmic vacuolization due to the presence of lipid accumulation is often present in the bizarre cells, although it is not a prominent feature of this case. Rosenthal fibers and eosinophilic granular bodies are sometimes found. Mitotic activity, microvascular proliferation, and necrosis are usually absent.

Pleomorphic xanthoastrocytomas (PXA) are uncommon but important astrocytic neoplasms to recognize because of the potential confusion with high-grade glioma. The absence of necrosis, significant mitotic activity, and microvascular proliferation in the setting of a highly pleomorphic neoplasm with perivascular inflammation, and cytoplasmic vacuolization suggest the diagnosis of PXA. Most cases occur in patients under 30 years of age, with a history of seizures. Superficial temporal or parietal lobes are the most frequent sites [63,67,68]. The prognosis of patients with PXA is much better than that for patients with high-grade glioma, especially if complete resection is achieved. Survival rates of 10 to 20 years are common [69].

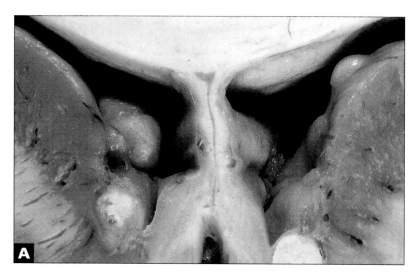

Figure 8-39. Subependymal giant cell astrocytoma associated with tuberous sclerosis. **A,** Coronal section of brain that shows a mass overlying the head of the caudate associated with an enlarged lateral ventricle and multiple smaller nodules from a 14-year-old girl with a 2-year history of headaches. She had poorly controlled seizures for 5 years prior to admission, and a malar rash on examination (adenoma sebaceum).

(*Continued on next page*)

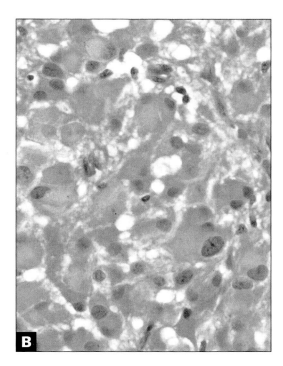

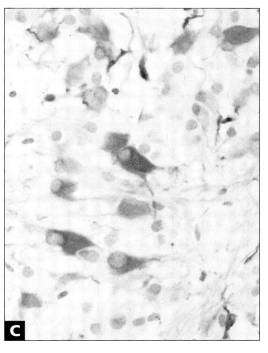

Figure 8-39. (*Continued*) **B,** Histologic study reveals large cells with eccentric round to oval nuclei, prominent nucleoli, and abundant glassy, eosinophilic cytoplasm extending into a few coarse processes. Individual tumor cells often show a perivascular orientation. **C,** Immuno-histochemical staining for glial fibrillary acidic protein (GFAP) highlights the large astrocytic cells and their processes. These features are consistent with a subependymal giant cell astrocytoma.

Tuberous sclerosis is an autosomal dominant disease characterized by Vogt's triad of seizures (90%), adenoma sebaceum (60% to 90%), and mental retardation (40% to 60%). Approximately 50% to 80% of cases are sporadic and *formes frustes* are common. The major central nervous system (CNS) mass lesions associated with tuberous sclerosis are cortical tubers, subependymal nodules, and subependymal giant cell astrocytoma [61,70,71].

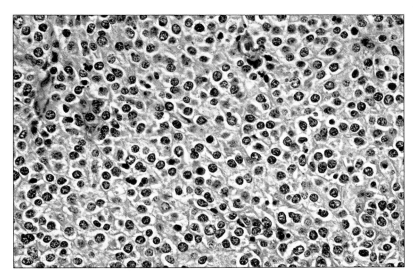

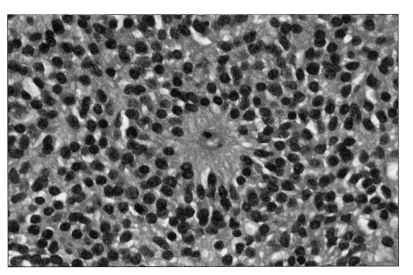

Figure 8-40. Classic histologic features of oligodendrogliomas. This soft, hemorrhagic tumor was excised from the temporal lobe of a 41-year-old man who presented with a 3-month history of olfactory hallucinations. The neoplasm is composed of sheets of uniform cells with round nuclei surrounded by clear cytoplasm or perinuclear halos imparting a "fried egg" appearance. Arborizing capillaries compartmentalize the neoplasm, corresponding to the "chicken-wire" background. Small foci of calcification are present.

Oligodendrogliomas account for approximately 4% to 7% of intracranial gliomas. Seizures and headaches are the most common presenting symptoms. Spontaneous hemorrhage is an uncommon, but important clinical manifestation. The frontal and temporal lobes are the most frequent sites. Microscopic calcification and microcyst formation are frequent histologic features. When glial neoplasms, in particular oligodendrogliomas, infiltrate the cerebral cortex, neoplastic cells aggregate around neurons, a phenomenon referred to as perineuronal satellitosis, and show a tendency to cuff blood vessels and collect under the pia [61,65].

Although grading schemes have been applied to oligodendrogliomas, the correlation between histologic features of anaplasia and biologic behavior is not as close as with infiltrating astrocytomas. Reports of effective therapeutic regimens for anaplastic oligodendroglioma have increased the importance of recognizing this entity as separate from other high-grade gliomas [65,72]. Identification of a specific immunohistochemical marker for neoplasms of oligodendroglial lineage would facilitate this categorization.

Figure 8-41. Low-power photomicrograph of a fourth ventricle ependymoma removed from a 23-year-old woman who complained of increasing headaches and clumsiness. The moderately cellular neoplasm is composed of generally uniform, round to oval cells that alternate with acellular, fibrillar zones around blood vessels. These characteristic "perivascular pseudorosettes" are a diagnostically helpful feature. True ependymal rosettes are much less common and consist of columnar epithelium surrounding a distinct membrane-lined lumen.

Histologic grading of ependymomas is problematic because specific morphologic features that reliably correlate with prognosis have not been identified [61]. For example, necrosis is a common finding in ependymomas, but does not indicate an ominous prognosis.

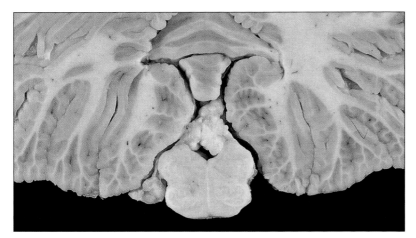

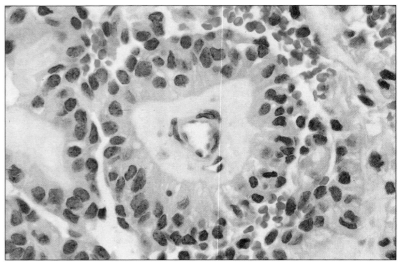

Figure 8-42. Subependymoma from the brain of a 28-year-old man who presented with a 1-year history of gait ataxia and persistent occipital headaches. Examination of cranial nerves revealed decreased elevation of the palate and left deviation of the uvula. Magnetic resonance imaging disclosed a lobulated mass located in the fourth ventricle and extending through the foramen of Lushka. A suboccipital craniectomy exposed a circumscribed, multilobulated mass arising from the floor of the fourth ventricle. The patient died 1 week later of unrelated causes, and an autopsy was performed. The gross specimen was soft, cystic, and contained focal calcifications. Microscopically, the neoplasm was hypocellular and consisted of clusters of oval cells with finely dispersed nuclear chromatin arranged in a fibrillary matrix.

Subependymomas are slow-growing, noninvasive tumors located most commonly in the ventricular system, followed by the septum pellucidum, cerebral aqueduct, or proximal spinal cord. Autopsy series estimate the incidence of these tumors to be 0.4%, whereas in surgical series, subependymomas account for 0.2% to 0.7% of all intracranial tumors. They may become symptomatic, most frequently in the fourth decade. Headache, gait ataxia, visual disturbances, memory deficits, and cranial nerve paresis are the most common symptoms. Hydrocephalus is present in 88% of symptomatic cases [61,62,73].

Figure 8-43. Microscopic examination of a myxopapillary ependymoma in a 30-year-old man who had a 2-year history of low back pain. One month before admission, he developed bilateral leg pain that progressed to paraparesis. An intramedullary spinal cord mass was detected on magnetic resonance imaging.

The microscopic examination showed a moderately cellular neoplasm composed of fibrillated cells with small, oval nuclei and mucin accumulation between islands of tumor cells and separating blood vessels from surrounding tumor cells, forming "myxopapillary rosettes." Grossly, the lesion was firm, lobulated, and appeared to be encapsulated.

Myxopapillary ependymoma is a distinct subtype of ependymoma that is usually restricted to the filum terminale or cauda equina (95%). The peak prevalence of these tumors is in the third and fourth decades. There is a male predominance. The 5-year survival rate is 85% to 100%, although recurrence has been reported with subtotal resection [61,62].

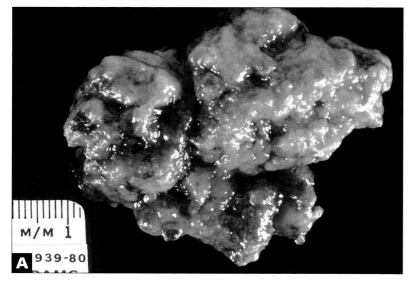

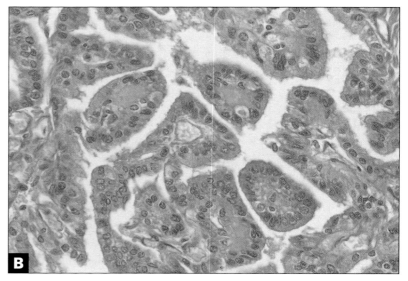

Figure 8-44. Choroid plexus papilloma. **A,** Papillary tumor removed from the fourth ventricle of a 5-year-old boy who developed severe ataxia and had bilateral papilledema on examination. **B,** The papillary fronds with vascular connective tissue cores are covered by a single layer of cuboidal epithelium resting on a basement membrane that is focally pseudostratified. Nuclear atypia is minimal and mitotic figures are absent.

This papillary neuroepithelial tumor represents a choroid plexus papilloma, a benign neoplasm that causes symptoms by obstructing cerebrospinal fluid pathways. They occur most frequently in the left lateral ventricle in children, while the fourth ventricle is the favored site in adults. Malignant transformation is infrequent, typically occurring in children under 10 years of age, and is manifest by histologic features of anaplasia and brain invasion. Because of the greater possibility of a metastatic papillary neoplasm, choroid plexus carcinoma is a diagnosis of exclusion in adults [61,62,74].

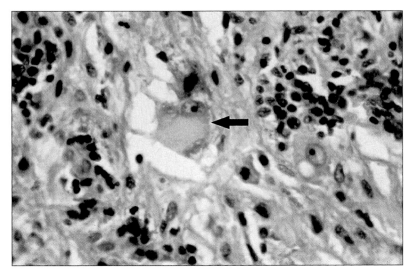

Figure 8-45. Microscopic findings in a ganglioglioma, a cystic cerebellar tumor that was completely excised from a 26-year-old man who presented with headaches. Grossly, the tumor was a circumscribed, cystic mass with a mural nodule. Microscopically, the neoplasm consists of a proliferation of large cells with prominent nucleoli with gangliocytic morphology within the cerebellum. Many of the ganglion cells are binucleate (*arrow*), which is consistent with a ganglion cell neoplasm. Interspersed among the clusters of ganglionic elements are abundant mildly atypical astrocytes, many of which have a bipolar or "piloid" morphology. There are also numerous Rosenthal fibers and prominent perivascular aggregates of small lymphocytes.

Gangliogliomas are generally indolent tumors composed of neoplastic neuronal and glial cells that represent less than 1% of all primary central nervous system (CNS) tumors, but account for 4.0% to 4.5% of pediatric CNS tumors. The majority of cases (60% to 80%) become symptomatic before the age of 30, not uncommonly manifesting as new-onset seizures [61,62,67]. Rarely, these neoplasms undergo anaplastic transformation of the glial component.

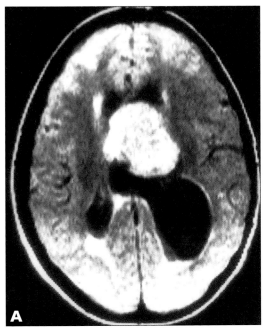

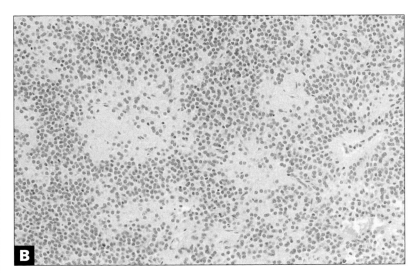

Figure 8-46. Central neurocytoma. A 25-year-old man presented with a 3-month history of headaches and diplopia. He had bilateral papilledema on neurologic examination. **A,** T1-weighted magnetic resonance imaging scan with contrast shows an irregular enhancing mass near the foramen of Monro. The mass is attached to the septum pellucidum, and has internal foci of low signal corresponding to calcification.

B, Microscopic examination of the mass revealed sheets of monotonous small cells with uniform, round nuclei surrounded by perinuclear halos.

An arborizing network of capillaries separated the tumor into lobules. No anaplastic features were noted. Acellular fibrillary areas were randomly scattered throughout the neoplasm. The cells expressed synaptophysin, signifying neuronal differentiation. Electron microscopy confirmed neuronal differentiation by the identification of neurosecretory granules, parallel bundles of microtubules, and synaptic vesicles.

The diagnosis of central neurocytoma was confirmed. This entity is a recently described tumor of neuroepithelial origin, which can mimic oligodendroglioma or ependymoma. Although experience is limited, available data suggest that these tumors follow a benign course following surgical excision [54,61]. (Panel A *courtesy of* James Smirniotopoulos, MD, Uniformed Services University of the Health Sciences, Department of Radiology/Nuclear Medicine, Bethesda, MD.)

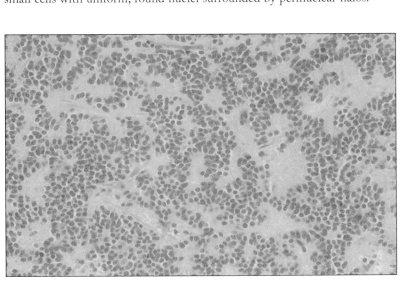

Figure 8-47. Microscopic appearance of a pineal gland tumor removed from a 42-year-old woman who complained of visual disturbances and headaches. Grossly, the neoplasm replaced the pineal gland and protruded into the third ventricle. Microscopically, the neoplasm is moderately cellular and compartmentalized by a delicate connective tissue stroma. The individual cells are small, relatively uniform, and contain coarsely clumped chromatin. In some areas, acellular "nuclear-free" zones representing pineocytomatous rosettes interrupt the cellular growth pattern. These morphologic features are consistent with a diagnosis of pineocytoma.

Pineal parenchymal tumors are uncommon modified neuronal tumors of the pineal gland that exhibit a range of differentiation from the poorly differentiated pineoblastoma to the well-differentiated pineocytoma. The intermediate grade is represented by the mixed pineoblastoma-pineocytoma. Pineoblastomas occur more frequently in children and pursue an aggressive course, whereas pineocytomas occur more frequently in adolescents and young adults [61,62,75].

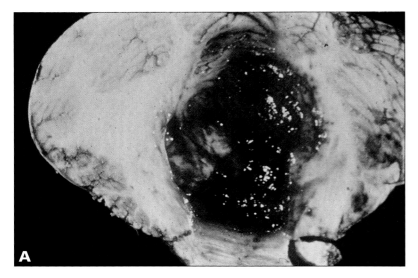

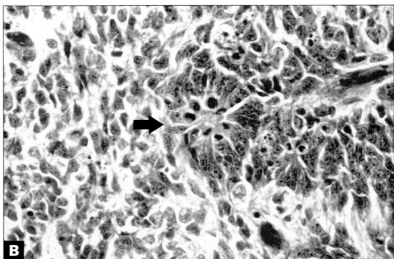

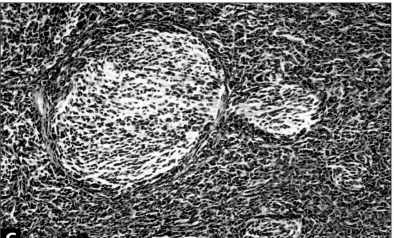

Figure 8-48. Medulloblastoma. **A,** A soft, hemorrhagic, necrotic mass in the expanded fourth ventricle of a 6-year-old boy who had a 6-month history of projectile vomiting and ataxia. The patient died the day of the craniotomy. There was extensive infiltration of the cerebellar meninges and multiple, gelatinous tumor nodules studded the surface of the spinal cord. **B,** Microscopic examination disclosed a highly cellular, necrotic tumor in the cerebellum composed of sheets of hyperchromatic, undifferentiated cells with scant cytoplasm and occasional neuroblastic Homer-Wright rosettes (*arrow*).

Medulloblastomas are malignant, embryonal tumors of childhood that occur in the cerebellum and are included under the rubric primitive neuroectodermal tumor (PNET) by some authors. Divergent differentiation, including neuronal, astrocytic, ependymal, and melanotic, has unresolved prognostic implications. These tumors are thought to arise from remnants of the external granular layer of the cerebellar vermis. **C,** The desmoplastic variant typically occurs in the cerebellar hemispheres in young adults and has a better prognosis [61,62,76]. Histologically, this variant is characterized by a dense, intercellular reticulin network that is punctuated by pale, reticulin-free islands.

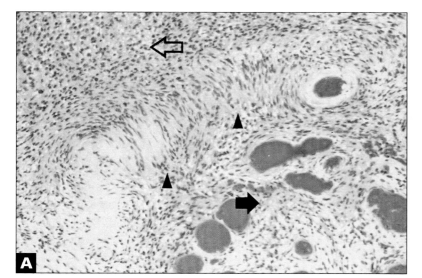

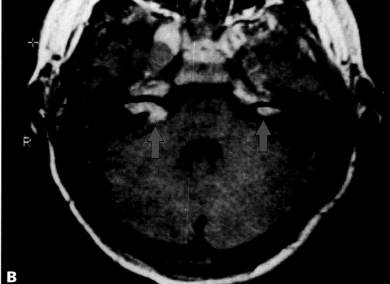

Figure 8-49. Schwannoma. A 39-year-old woman consulted her physician because of a 1-year history of progressive unilateral hearing loss and tinnitus. Neuroimaging studies showed a mass eroding the internal acoustic meatus. The tumor was completely excised and noted to be a tan-white, rubbery mass with a cystic cut surface. Microscopic examination confirmed the diagnosis of a schwannoma. **A,** Section showing a biphasic tumor composed of compact (Antoni A) (*open arrow*) and looser areas (Antoni B, *closed arrow*) in which the individual spindle-shaped cells are focally arranged in palisades (Verocay body, *arrowheads*).

Acoustic neuromas (also known as schwannoma or neurilemmoma) account for up to 10% of all intracranial neoplasms and up to 90% of all tumors of the cerebellopontine angle. Neurilemmomas are benign, slow-growing neoplasms that arise from Schwann cells immediately inside the

internal auditory canal. Although schwannomas may arise from any cranial nerve, they most frequently originate from the vestibular portion of the eighth cranial nerve, and less commonly from the fifth cranial nerve. Females are affected more often than males, usually in the fourth to seventh decades of life. Bilateral acoustic schwannomas are almost always associated with neurofibromatosis type 2 (NF2) (central), whereas over 95% of solitary vestibular and spinal schwannomas are sporadic [61,77–79]. **B,** Axial, contrast-enhanced magnetic resonance image (MRI) shows enhancing masses in both cerebellopontine angles (*blue arrows*) that are consistent with bilateral acoustic neuromas and a diagnosis of NF2.

(*Continued on next page*)

C. Comparison of Neurofibromatosis Type 1 and Neurofibromatosis Type 2

Neurofibromatosis Type 1	Neurofibromatosis Type 2
Peripheral	Central
Chromosome 17	Chromosome 22
Gliomas and meningiomas	Schwannomas
Cutaneous abnormalities	Minimal skin involvement
Skeletal abnormalities	No skeletal abnormalities

Figure 8-49. (*Continued*) **C**, Comparison of the salient features of neurofibromatosis type 1 and neurofibromatosis type 2. (Panel C *adapted from* Roach [80].)

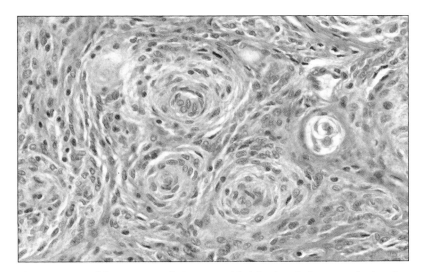

Figure 8-50. Meningioma. A 36-year-old right-handed woman had sudden onset of simple-partial seizures 6 weeks before admission. Computed tomography of the head revealed a hyperdense parasagittal mass that enhanced homogeneously with intravenous contrast dye. Magnetic resonance imaging (MRI) showed a mass, hypodense on both T1- and T2-weighted images that enhanced homogeneously with contrast. An MRI scan of a meningioma is shown in Figure 8-24.

The sharply demarcated dural-based mass was firm, lobular, tan-white, and gritty in consistency. Microscopically (seen here), the neoplasm displays lobular growth with tumor nests separated by a variable amount of fibrous tissue. Psammoma bodies and characteristic "whorls" composed of round to oval nuclei with pale-staining cytoplasm and indistinct cell borders are seen. Nuclei often have a punched-out or empty appearance from intranuclear cytoplasmic "pseudo-inclusions."

Meningiomas are typically slowly enlarging neoplasms that originate from cells of the arachnoid membrane (arachnoid cap cells). They constitute between 13% and 18% of all primary intracranial neoplasms and occur most commonly in women in the middle decades of life. The majority of meningiomas express hormone receptors, progesterone more often than estrogen. Fifty percent of intracranial meningiomas are parasagittal, others have orbital, intrapetrous, calvarial, and intraventricular (left more often than right) locations. Spinal meningiomas are much more common in women and occur most often at the thoracic level [54,61,81].

Although meningiomas tend not to infiltrate the brain, they can penetrate dura, surround soft tissue structures, or cause thickening of overlying bone (hyperostosis). All 11 World Health Organization (WHO) histologic subtypes of typical meningiomas show a similar biologic behavior corresponding to grade I. Atypical meningiomas have an increased incidence of recurrence, and exhibit hypercellularity, mitoses, necrosis, and "sheetlike" growth. Malignant (anaplastic) meningiomas generally manifest the same histologic features as atypical meningiomas, but often to a greater degree. Brain invasion alone is enough to classify a meningioma as atypical in the new WHO classification.

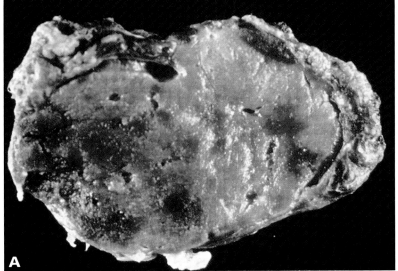

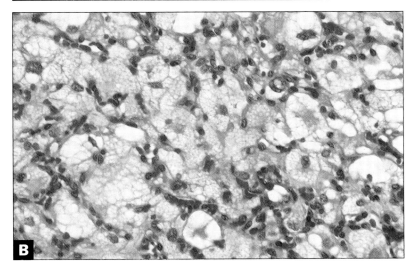

Figure 8-51. Capillary hemangioblastoma. **A**, Gross features of a sharply demarcated, mottled red-brown and yellow mass removed from the lateral wall of the fourth ventricle of a 38-year-old man who presented with progressive gait ataxia and memory impairment. **B**, Microscopic examination reveals a vascular neoplasm composed of delicate vascular channels arranged in lobules containing large, polygonal stromal cells with clear to foamy cytoplasm. The surrounding cyst wall is composed of compressed, gliotic brain parenchyma that can mimic an astrocytoma.

(*Continued on next page*)

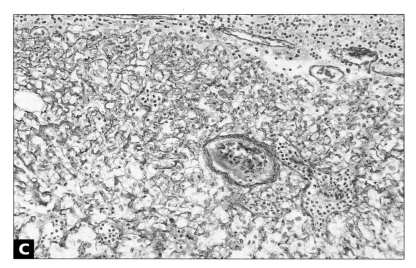

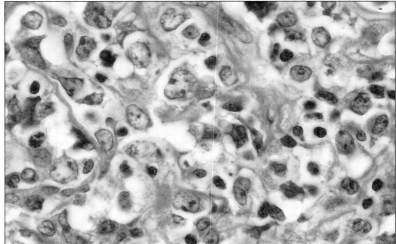

Figure 8-51. (*Continued*) **C,** A reticulin stain is useful in outlining the numerous thin-walled vascular channels in the tumor.

Capillary hemangioblastomas are benign, vascular, and usually cystic tumors of uncertain histogenesis that occur most frequently in the cerebellum of adults. A characteristic magnetic resonance image of a hemangioblastoma is shown in Figure 8-25. These tumors arise either in the setting of von Hippel-Lindau disease or, more often, as solitary sporadic lesions [61,62]. The differential diagnosis includes metastatic renal cell carcinoma, which may look similar histologically, but usually occurs in older patients. Patients with hemangioblastomas may have extramedullary hematopoiesis with associated polycythemia. The recurrence rate is approximately 25% [61,62]. Diagnosis at a younger age (less than 30), association with von Hippel-Landau syndrome, multicentricity, and lack of cyst formation are all adverse prognostic factors in patients with hemangioblastoma.

Figure 8-52. Photomicrograph from a 41-year-old HIV-positive man who presented with a personality change. Stereotactic biopsy of a frontal lobe lesion revealed an angiocentric and patchy infiltrative proliferation of atypical cells with vesicular nuclei and nucleolar prominence that showed immunoreactivity for B-cell lymphocytic markers.

Primary central nervous system (CNS) lymphoma frequently occurs in immunocompromised individuals, particularly in patients with acquired immunodeficiency syndrome (AIDS). Multifocal, deep parenchymal involvement is characteristic of AIDS, whereas single lesions occur more often in sporadic cases. Histologically, most cases of primary CNS lymphoma are high-grade B-cell lymphomas [61,82].

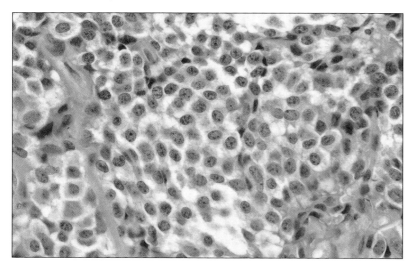

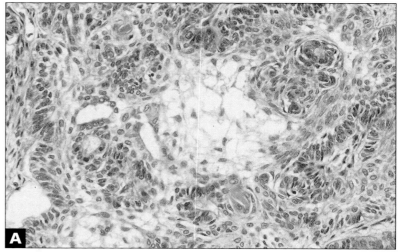

Figure 8-53. Microscopic features of a pituitary neoplasm removed by transsphenoidal resection from a 32-year-old woman who presented with amenorrhea. The neoplasm consists of a monomorphic proliferation of cells that show immunohistochemical staining for prolactin. The individual cells have an evenly dispersed or "salt and pepper" chromatin pattern characteristic of neuroendocrine tumors.

Pituitary adenomas represent 10% to 20% of intracranial neoplasms. Fifty percent to 80% are functional or symptomatic. Up to 3% are associated with multiple endocrine neoplasia syndromes. They most commonly present in women in the third to sixth decades, although they may occur at any age. Symptomatic adenomas less than 1 cm in diameter are referred to as "microadenomas," whereas tumors with diameters greater than 1 cm are known as "macroadenomas" [61,83].

Figure 8-54. Craniopharyngioma. **A,** Typical histologic features of a calcified, polycystic suprasellar neoplasm arising in a 10-year-old girl. This complex epithelioid neoplasm is composed of distinctive lobules of cuboidal to columnar epithelium blending into looser central zones containing stellate cells. Cystic spaces are lined by neoplastic cells arranged in palisaded profiles.

(*Continued on next page*)

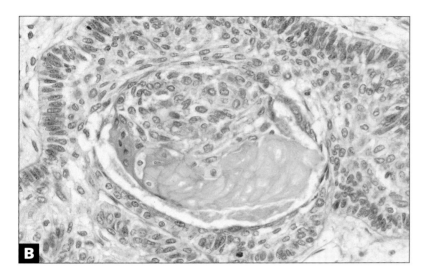

Figure 8-54. (*Continued*) **B**, Calcification and clumps of "wet keratin" consisting of ghosts of keratinized cells are a prominent feature of the classic or "adamantinomatous" variant of craniopharyngioma.

Craniopharyngiomas are the most common suprasellar neoplasms of childhood, but may occur at any age. Another less common variant, the papillary craniopharyngioma, occurs almost exclusively in adults, has a more solid growth pattern and usually lacks palisaded cells, keratin nodules, and calcification. Although craniopharyngiomas are histologically benign, they frequently invade local tissues and have high recurrence rates [61,84].

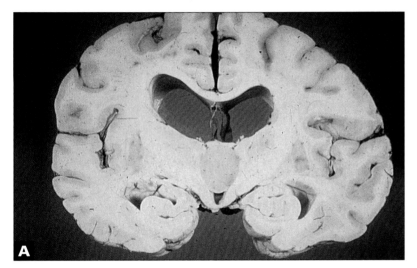

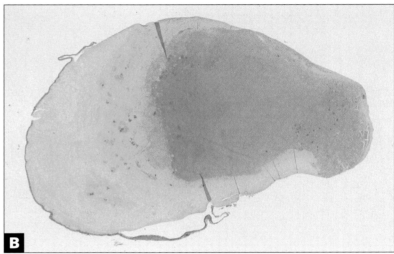

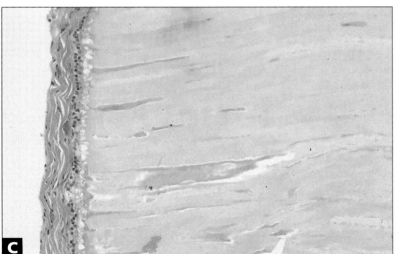

Figure 8-55. Colloid cyst. **A,** Cystic lesion in the third ventricle from a 30-year-old woman who presented with a 3-month history of bifrontal headaches and gait unsteadiness that were consistently precipitated by bending forward and were relieved by a change in posture. Neurologic examination was unremarkable; however, a magnetic resonance scan revealed a round mass, bright on T1-weighted images, in the anterior third ventricle, near the foramen of Monro. The patient refused hospital admission and was found dead at home a month after initial evaluation. **B,** Whole-mount histologic preparation of the mass showing a spherical mass filled with amorphous mucinous material characteristic of a colloid cyst. **C,** Higher power photomicrograph demonstrating the simple epithelial lining that may contain ciliated or goblet cells.

Colloid cysts are epithelial-lined cysts that produce symptoms by intermittent obstruction of cerebrospinal fluid flow. Although the histogenesis of these lesions is disputed, the most widely accepted evidence favors an endodermal origin. Surgical removal is curative, although sudden death has been reported secondary to acute hydrocephalus [61,62].

Treatment of Gliomas

Surgery

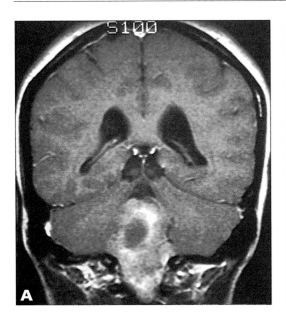

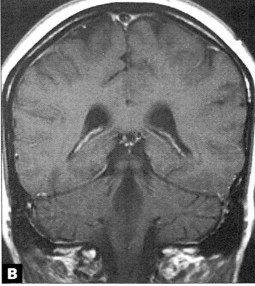

Figure 8-56. T1-weighted, coronal magnetic resonance imaging (MRI) scan showing an irregular, inhomogeneously enhancing mass filling the fourth ventricle (**A**) in a 34-year-old woman who presented with headaches and ataxia. A complete resection was accomplished at surgery, and the tumor was an ependymoma. A follow-up MRI scan done 2 years later shows no enhancing tumor (**B**).

Some brain tumors can be completely resected and not recur. Pilocytic astrocytomas in children and meningiomas in adults are good examples. Most gliomas, however, have an infiltrating border, and tumor cells are present beyond the enhancing tissue seen on imaging studies [34,85]. This makes them difficult to eradicate surgically. This patient had a good result with surgery for her ependymoma, but there is still a chance of recurrence, and serial scans will be needed for years.

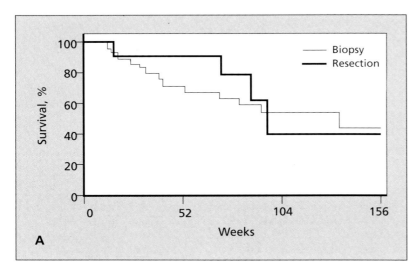

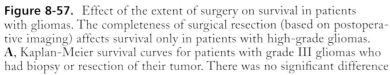

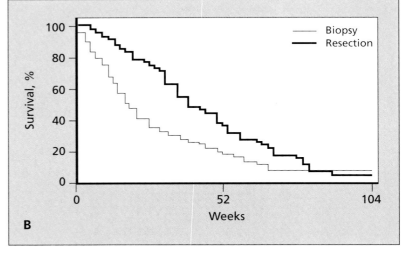

Figure 8-57. Effect of the extent of surgery on survival in patients with gliomas. The completeness of surgical resection (based on postoperative imaging) affects survival only in patients with high-grade gliomas. **A,** Kaplan-Meier survival curves for patients with grade III gliomas who had biopsy or resection of their tumor. There was no significant difference in survival between patients who had biopsy only compared with patients in whom all contrast-enhancing tumor was removed. **B,** In patients with grade IV gliomas there was a survival benefit for patients who had their tumors completely resected (*P* is 0.0016). (*Adapted from* Devaux and colleagues [86].)

Radiation Therapy

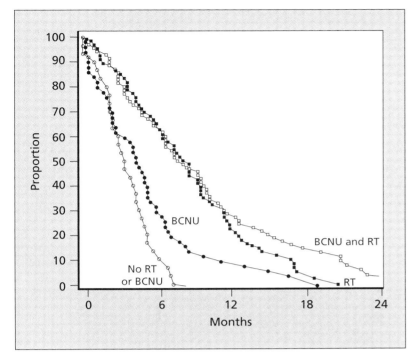

Figure 8-58. Effect of surgery, radiation, and carmustine chemotherapy on survival in patients with malignant glioma. One of the early studies, by Walker and colleagues [87], showed a beneficial effect of radiation therapy (RT) for patients with gliomas. Ninety percent of these patients had glioblastoma multiforme. The median survival of the group treated with supportive care was only 14 weeks, and it only increased to 18.5 weeks for patients treated with carmustine (a nitrosourea) without radiation. By contrast, patients with malignant gliomas who received radiation therapy (50 to 60 Gy) lived for 35 weeks. Chemotherapy with carmustine did not increase the median survival in patients who received radiation in this study. BCNU—bis-chlorethyl nitrosourea.

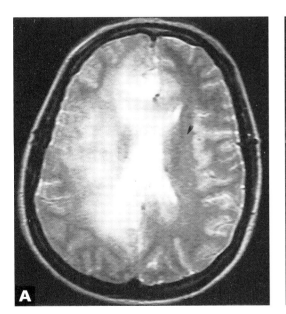
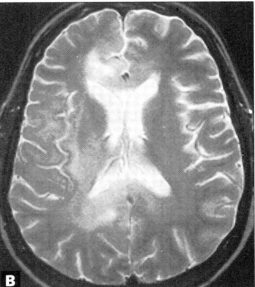

Figure 8-59. Response of gliomatosis cerebri to radiation therapy. A 30-year-old woman had chronic headaches and a minimal left hemiparesis. Her T1-weighted magnetic resonance imaging (MRI) scan was unremarkable (not shown) except for small ventricles and a "tight" appearance to the intracranial contents. **A,** T2-weighted MRI scan showing diffuse T2 signal changes throughout the right cerebral hemisphere, and within the left cerebral hemisphere as well. An open biopsy of the right frontal lobe revealed low-grade infiltrating cells that tended to cluster around neurons. The histologic picture was that of gliomatosis cerebri. The patient received radiation therapy and her headaches disappeared and her hemiparesis improved. **B,** MRI scan 6 months after radiation therapy showing a dramatic decrease in the T2 signal abnormalities.

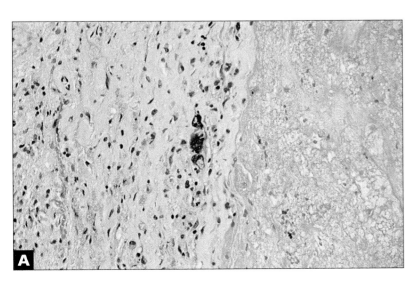

Figure 8-60. Histology of radiation change. Some complications of radiation therapy for gliomas are becoming more obvious as some patients experience prolonged survival. Radiation-induced brain necrosis or leukoencephalopathy may occur months to years after radiation therapy. Radiation is toxic to oligodendroglial cells, resulting in demyelination, and to vascular endothelium, resulting in hyaline necrosis of small blood vessels [80]. **A,** Bizzare nuclei that can be associated with radiation changes in the brain (centrally located). Necrosis is present throughout the right side of the specimen.

(*Continued on next page*)

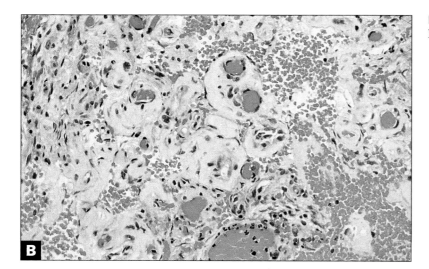

Figure 8-60. (*Continued*) **B,** Hyalinized vessels that occur in the brain following radiation.

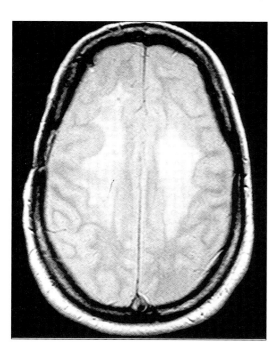

Figure 8-61. Radiation–induced leukoencephalopathy. Proton-density magnetic resonance imaging scan showing signal abnormalities throughout the white matter of both cerebral hemispheres in this patient who received whole-brain radiation therapy following subtotal resection of a right temporal anaplastic astrocytoma 7 years prior to this scan. The patient had mild cognitive deficits and hyperreflexia. Intellectual deficits have been identified in both children [89–91] and adults [92,93] following cranial irradiation. Endocrine disturbances are also common following prolonged survival after radiation therapy [94,95].

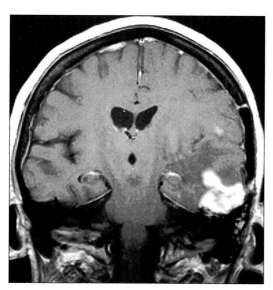

Figure 8-62. Magnetic resonance imaging (MRI) scan showing a mass lesion that represents radiation necrosis. Radiation necrosis usually occurs 8 to 20 months following radiation therapy, and can present exactly like a recurrent tumor, with focal neurologic findings, mass effect, and ring enhancement on MRI. In experienced hands, this complication occurs in less than 5% of patients treated for brain tumors. This patient had radiation therapy for a left temporal oligodendroglioma 5 years before this scan. A recurrence of her oligodendroglioma was treated with γ-knife radiosurgery. Twenty-seven months later, this ring-enhancing lesion with mass effect developed. Tumor recurrence was suspected, especially when a single photon emission computed tomography (SPECT) scan showed a "hot" area corresponding to the enhancing area on MRI. Biopsy showed only necrotic material and a few oligodendroglial cells that were not anaplastic. Thus the mass lesion was caused by radiation necrosis. A positron-emission tomography scan may help distinguish between radiation necrosis and recurrent tumor [96] but SPECT scans are less reliable. Patients with radiation necrosis may improve with steroids or with anticoagulation [97] but in severe cases they may require surgical decompression.

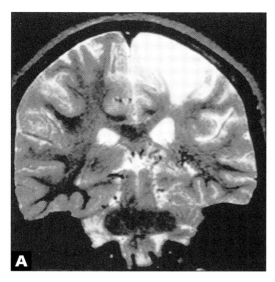
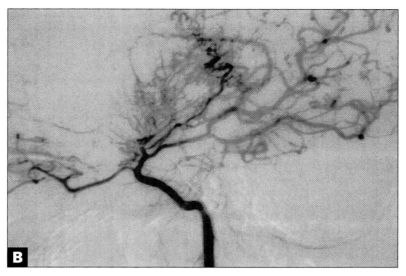

Figure 8-63. Radiation damage to larger intracranial vessels [98]. This patient received radiation therapy for a pituitary adenoma several years before this scan. When she suddenly developed right hemiparesis, a magnetic resonance imaging scan showed T2 signal changes in a wedge-shaped distribution consistent with a stroke (**A**). Angiography shows truncation of her intracranial vessels at the middle cerebral artery, with multiple smaller collateral vessels in a "puff of smoke" or "Moya-Moya" configuration (**B**). (*Courtesy of* S. Roach, MD, Department of Pediatric Neurology, University of Texas Southwestern, Dallas, TX.)

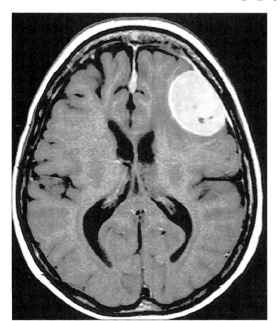

Figure 8-64. T1-weighted magnetic resonance imaging scan showing a typical homogeneously enhancing, dural-based meningioma in a patient who received radiation therapy for an intracranial ependymoma and developed focal-onset seizures 10 years later. Radiation therapy can induce secondary intracranial tumors. These secondary tumors include meningiomas [99] and sarcomas of the skull [100]. Most of the tumors ascribed to radiation therapy have occurred following low-dose cranial irradiation for tinea capitis, but they may also arise following high-dose radiation therapy, such as that performed for intracranial tumors [99].

Radiation-induced meningiomas usually occur 10 to 15 years following radiation therapy, and they arise in males and females equally, unlike spontaneous meningiomas, which occur more often in females.

Chemotherapy

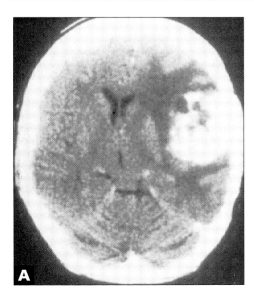
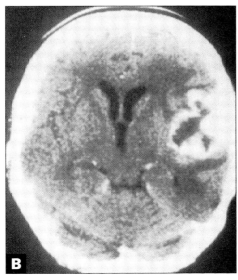

Figure 8-65. Computed tomography (CT) scan (**A**) showing a large ring-enhancing lesion consistent with a glioma in a patient who presented with increasing headache. He received steroids for two weeks, his headache resolved, and a follow-up CT scan (**B**) shows a decrease in the size of his enhancing lesion. Subsequent biopsy revealed glioblastoma multiforme. The administration of steroids can dramatically reduce edema and other neurologic signs and symptoms in patients with gliomas and have a direct cytotoxic effect on some tumor cells, but routine use of corticosteroids does not prolong survival [101].

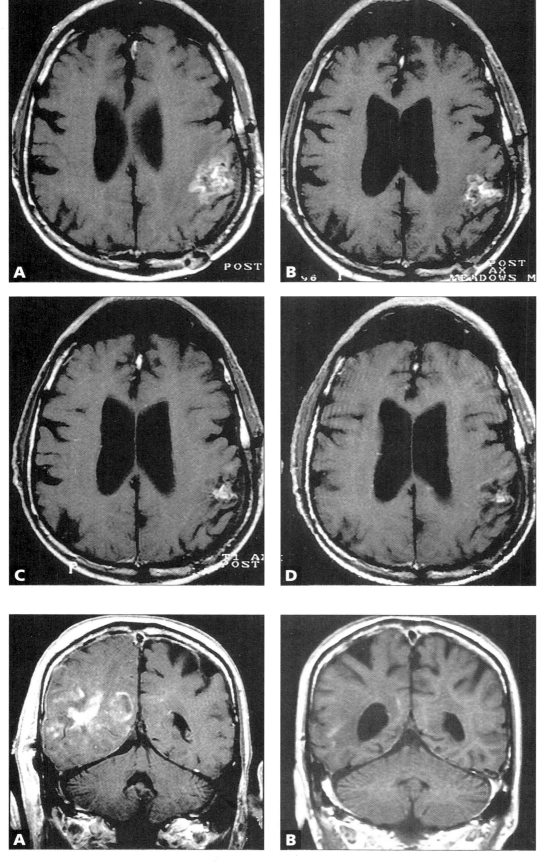

Figure 8-66. Response of glioblastoma multiforme to lomustine chemotherapy. This tumor was initially resected and treated with radiation therapy, but recurred. **A**, Magnetic resonance imaging (MRI) scan of contrast-enhancing lesion in the left parietal region. Biopsy confirmed recurrent glioblastoma multiforme. The patient received oral lomustine (150 mg/m^2) every 6 weeks for 1 year. **B**, **C**, During chemotherapy, there was a decrease in the size of the enhancing tumor. This response was sustained. **D**, MRI that was performed 14 months after the initial one.

Figure 8-67. Response of anaplastic oligodendroglioma to combination chemotherapy. Anaplastic oligodendrogliomas are particularly sensitive to chemotherapy. This patient had an anaplastic oligodendroglioma removed from his left hemisphere, and was subsequently treated with radiation therapy. His tumor recurred 1 year later. **A**, Magnetic resonance imaging (MRI) scan showing a large ring-enhancing lesion in his right hemisphere. **B**, He received combination chemotherapy with procarbazine, lomustine, and vincristine for 2 months, and his tumor practically disappeared.

Anaplastic oligodendrogliomas are increasingly recognized by pathologists. Many of these tumors were previously identified as glioblastomas because of the frequent presence of necrosis. The susceptibility of these tumors to chemotherapy makes their recognition important. Some patients achieve durable responses with relatively nontoxic chemotherapy. Currently a trial is underway to compare preradiation chemotherapy with radiation therapy alone in patients with anaplastic oligodendrogliomas.

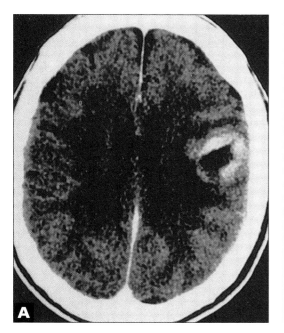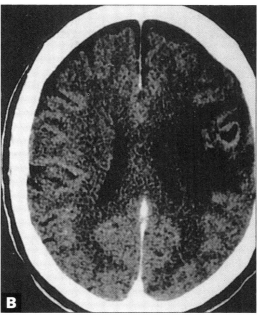

Figure 8-68. Intraarterial chemotherapy. **A**, Magnetic resonance imaging (MRI) scan of the brain of a patient who received intraarterial cisplatin for a malignant glioma. **B**, The tumor shrank significantly following one intraarterial treatment. Intraarterial treatment of gliomas must be performed by physicians who are experienced with angiography and intravascular therapy. Retinal toxicity can occur when chemotherapeutic agents are injected intraarterially, particularly if the injection is done below the origin of the ophthalmic artery. Auditory toxicity can also occur, and was seen in several patients during this study of intraarterial cisplatin [102].

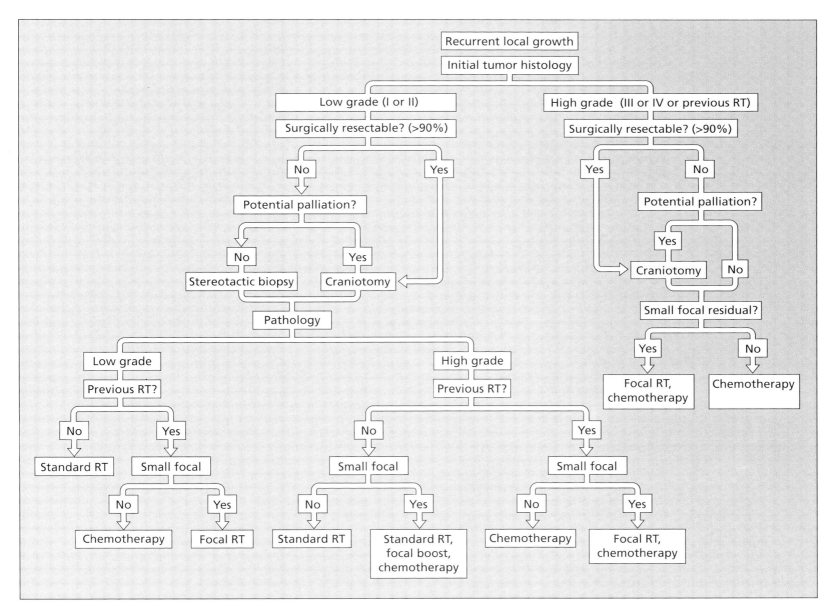

Figure 8-69. Management strategy for recurrent gliomas. Gliomas often recur or progress after surgical resection or radiation therapy (RT). Aggressive treatment of recurrent gliomas is warranted if the patient is in good medical and neurologic condition [103]. Most gliomas (80%) recur within 2 cm of the original margin of contrast-enhancing tumor [104].

The appropriate treatment is determined by the histologic grade of the tumor, its surgical resectability, and prior treatment the patient has received. In this paradigm, some patients undergo palliative surgery even when their tumor is not more than 90% resectable, usually relieve mass effect, and provide a smaller residual tumor that is more amenable to therapy.

Neurologic Complications of Systemic Cancer

Intracranial Metastases

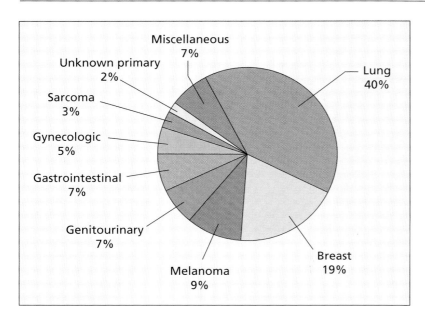

Figure 8-70. Sites of primary disease in patients with intracranial metastases. Lung cancer is the most common primary tumor in patients with intracranial metastases, and accounted for 40% of intracranial metastases seen at Memorial Sloan-Kettering Cancer Center (MSKCC) during 1994 (86% non–small cell, 14% small cell) [105]. Breast cancer is the second most common primary tumor in patients with intracranial metastases (19%). Melanoma represents only 1% of systemic cancers [106], yet accounted for nearly 10% of the intracranial metastases in this series. This suggests that melanoma may have a predilection for metastasizing to the brain. Less frequent systemic tumors producing intracranial metastases included genitourinary (7%—renal, testis, bladder, prostate), gastrointestinal (7%—colon, esophagus, gastric, pancreas), and gynecologic (5%—ovary, choriocarcinoma, cervix, endometrium).

In this series, 5% of the patients with histologically proved intracranial metastasis did not have an identifiable primary tumor. The percentage of patients with unknown primary tumors and intracranial metastases is lower in this series than it is in data generated from general hospitals, since MSKCC is a prominent cancer referral center. There are some cases in which a primary tumor is never discovered, although chest, abdominal, and pelvic computed tomography scans detect most systemic cancers producing intracranial metastases [105].

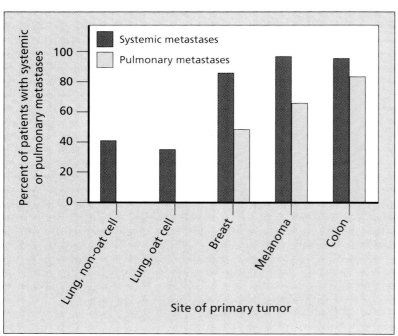

Figure 8-71. Extent of systemic disease in patients with intracranial metastases. Patients with intracranial metastases from nonlung primary tumors usually have systemic metastases when their intracranial metastases are discovered (80% to 98%). Pulmonary involvement is a very important risk factor in the development of intracranial metastases. Colon cancer almost never produces intracranial metastases without concomitant lung metastases, and most patients with intracranial metastases from breast cancer or melanoma also have pulmonary metastases when intracranial metastases are detected.

By contrast, patients with intracranial metastases from lung cancers do not necessarily have other systemic metastases. This illustrates the importance of tumor access to the pulmonary veins in patients with intracranial metastases. Tumor cells growing in the lungs can dislodge into the pulmonary veins, reach the systemic circulation via the heart, and enter the cerebral circulation to form cerebral metastases. This helps explain the high incidence of intracranial metastases in patients with lung cancer, and the high frequency of pulmonary metastases in patients with intracranial metastases arising from other tumors. More circuitous routes for metastatic cells must be postulated for intracranial metastases that occur without pulmonary involvement. (Data *from* J.B. Posner, MD, Memorial Sloan-Kettering Cancer Center, New York, NY.)

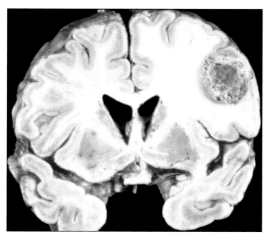

Figure 8-72. Gross pathology of a left hemisphere metastasis from a lung cancer. Intracranial metastases occur more often in the supratentorial compartment (85%) than infratentorially (15%). Infratentorial metastases seem to be more common in patients with gastrointestinal or pelvic primary tumors [107]. Supratentorial metastases lodge preferentially in the "watershed" zones of intracerebral vasculature, and typically form at the junction of the gray and white matter [107]. Intracerebral metastases are relatively well-demarcated from surrounding brain, but may produce a large area of adjacent cerebral edema. This metastasis from a primary lung cancer is located in the left hemisphere, and is surrounded by edematous white matter. (*Courtesy of* J.B. Posner, MD, Department of Neurology, Memorial Sloan-Kettering Cancer Center, New York, NY.)

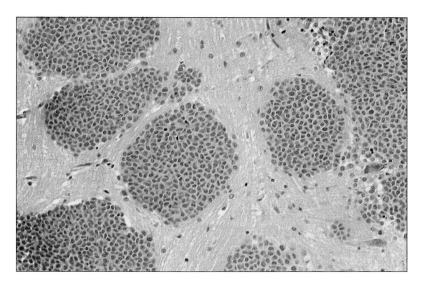

Figure 8-73. Tissue removed from a single supratentorial metastasis that occurred in a patient with a history of skin cancer. Intracranial metastases retain the histopathologic characteristics of the primary tumor. In some cases, biopsy material can indicate the source of the primary tumor. In this case, histology shows nests of tumor cells within brain parenchyma. The tumor cells stained with antibodies to HMB-45 (a melanoma marker), indicating that they arose from a melanoma.

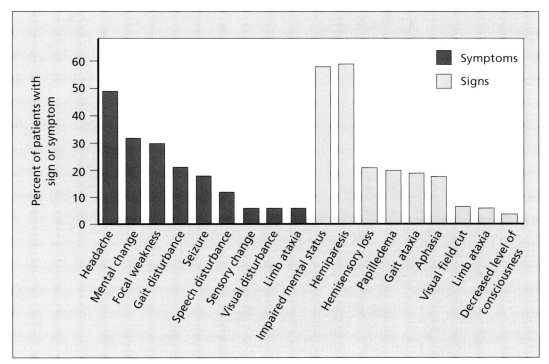

Figure 8-74. Initial signs and symptoms in patients with intracranial metastases. Headache is the most frequent complaint in patients with intracranial metastatic disease, and occurs in 49% of patients. When a focal headache is present, it has localizing value, but usually the headache is generalized. The classic "brain tumor headache," which is worst in the morning, is present in only a minority of cases. The most common presenting symptoms experienced by patients with intracranial metastases are

depicted in this bar graph, and include changes in mentation (32%), focal weakness (30%), gait ataxia (21%), and seizures (18%). Visual and sensory symptoms are unusual as a presenting complaint.

The most frequent signs on neurologic examination in patients with brain metastases are impaired mental status, which occurs in 58% of patients, and hemiparesis, which occurs in 59% of patients. Mental status changes in patients with brain metastases may be subtle, so the mental status examination is important in patients with a history of cancer who present with headache. Only 32% of patients with intracranial metastases complain of focal weakness, but 60% have hemiparesis on examination. Similarly, hemisensory loss can be demonstrated on examination in 21% of patients with brain metastases, yet only 6% of patients complain of sensory symptoms. Other neurologic signs such as papilledema (20%), gait ataxia (19%), aphasia (18%), visual field cuts (7%), and limb ataxia (6%) occur less frequently. When mental status changes, progressive headache, or focal neurologic signs are seen in a patient with a history of cancer, a contrast-enhanced computed tomography or magnetic resonance imaging scan of the head is indicated. (Data *from* Posner [105]; originally published in Cairncross and colleagues [108] and Young and colleagues [109].)

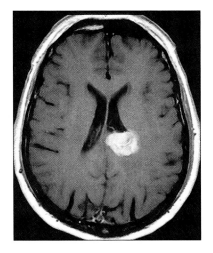

Figure 8-75. T1-weighted magnetic resonance imaging (MRI) scan with contrast showing a solitary enhancing lesion within the white matter just adjacent to the posterior horn of the lateral ventricle in a patient who presented with new, increasing headaches. MRI with contrast is the best currently available technique for demonstrating intracranial metastases. The administration of contrast is very important, since some metastases may appear to be solitary until contrast reveals other sites of involvement. This patient had no known systemic tumor, but abdominal computed tomography revealed a large mass arising from her left kidney that proved to be a renal cell carcinoma.

It is important to identify patients who have a solitary intracranial metastasis, because they may be candidates for surgery. Surgical removal of an accessible metastasis improves patients' quality of life and length of survival over conventional radiation therapy in patients with solitary intracranial metastases [110] (Fig. 8-77). Unfortunately, less than 50% of patients with intracranial metastases have a single lesion, and only about 50% of these patients are surgical candidates [110]. A recent study by Bindal [111] suggests that surgical removal of two or even three intracranial metastases can also improve survival.

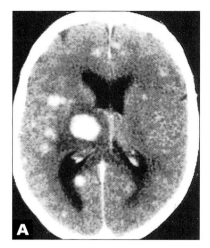 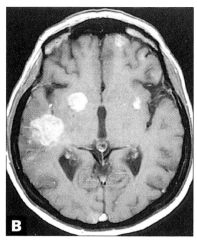 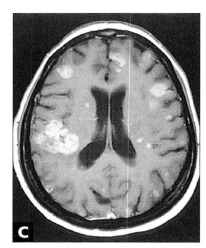

Figure 8-76. Computed tomography (CT) and magnetic resonance imaging (MRI) scans showing multiple intracranial metastases. An MRI scan with contrast is the diagnostic method of choice for demonstrating intracranial metastases. Patients may have normal CT scans, and have obvious metastatic disease when an MRI scan with gadolinium is performed [112–114]. When MRI scanning is not available, a CT scan with contrast can detect most symptomatic intracranial metastases. **A,** CT scan performed on a patient with lung cancer who developed headache and left-sided numbness. There is a large enhancing lesion in the right thalamus with surrounding edema. Other enhancing nodules are scattered through both hemispheres. Many of these nodules occur at the gray-white junction.

B, C, T1-weighted MRI scans with contrast enhancement from another patient with lung cancer. The patient had a chronic progressive headache, and had had a single seizure. The MRI scan reveals enhancing nodules in both cerebral hemispheres. In this case, the metastases are not associated with substantial mass effect. The ventricles remain nearly normal in shape and size. Again, many of the enhancing metastases are located at the junction between gray and white matter.

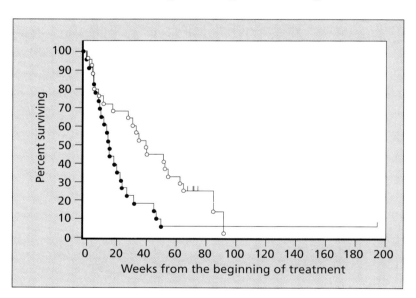

Figure 8-77. Data from a randomized trial of surgery for the treatment of single brain metastases. The top curve in this figure (*open circles*) represents the survival curve of patients treated with surgery followed by radiation. The bottom curve (*filled circles*) represents the survival curve of patients who received radiation therapy only. Patients who received surgery plus radiation for their single intracranial metastasis had a median survival of 40 weeks, while the patients treated with radiation alone had a median survival of only 15 weeks (P is less than 0.01) [110]. The patients in both treatment groups were well matched according to age, Karnofsky score, intracranial location of metastasis, and extent of systemic cancer. (*Adapted from* Patchel and colleagues [110].)

Intraspinal Metastases

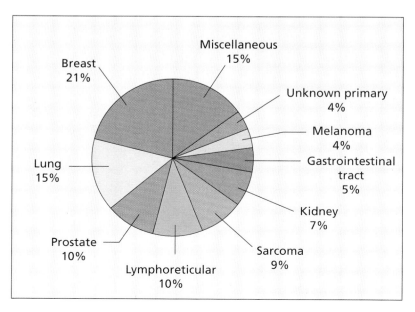

Figure 8-78. Distribution of primary tumors in patients with metastatic epidural spinal cord compression. In this series of 583 patients with metastatic spinal cord compression who were seen at the Memorial Sloan-Kettering Cancer Center (MSKCC), breast (21%) and lung cancer (15%) were the most frequent primary tumors. A wide variety of other primary tumors also produced metastatic spinal cord compression.

Metastatic spinal cord compression usually results from metastatic involvement of verterbral bones. The vertebral bones are particularly prone to the development of metastatic lesions, and are involved in 25% to 70% of patients with systemic cancer [115–117]. The thoracic vertebrae are the most frequently involved with metastatic disease [105]. Metastatic lesions to vertebral bones produce neurologic symptoms by expanding and compressing the spinal cord or nerve roots, or they may induce compression fractures that protrude anteriorly into the spinal canal.

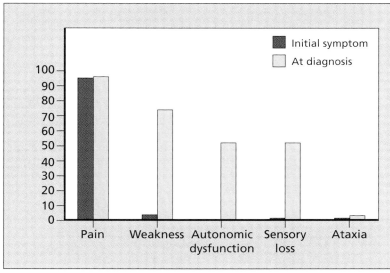

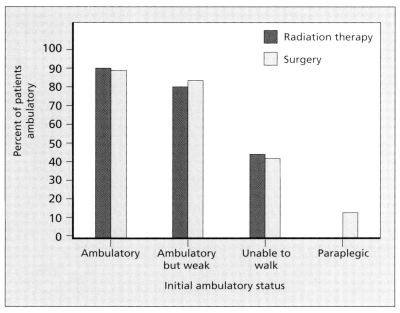

Figure 8-79. Signs and symptoms in patients with metastatic spinal cord compression. Pain is the most common initial symptom in patients with metastatic spinal cord compression. Over 90% of patients complain of pain, and the pain is usually localized to the site of the spinal metastasis. This pain may be worse in the recumbent position, unlike the pain from degenerative disc disease, which is usually exacerbated by standing up and by movement [105]. Most patients develop additional neurologic symptoms or signs by the time a diagnosis of spinal cord compression is made. Weakness is the most common neurologic sign, and occurs in 74% of patients. Well-localized back pain in patients with a history of systemic cancer should prompt evaluation. Plain films can detect metastatic vertebral lesions [118], but a magnetic resonance imaging scan with contrast provides valuable anatomic details, and is the procedure of choice for evaluating the spine for metastatic spinal cord compression [119–121].

It is very important to recognize the signs and symptoms of spinal cord compression. Treatment must be prompt to prevent neurologic deterioration. Diagnostic studies should be performed within 24 hours of presentation, and high-dose steroids should be given. The prognosis for ambulation depends on the patient's status prior to treatment (Fig. 8-80). These data are from a series of 211 patients with metastatic spinal cord compression seen at Memorial Sloan-Kettering Cancer Center [105].

Figure 8-80. Ambulation status after treatment in patients with intraspinal metastases by treatment modality and initial status. Patients who are ambulatory when their spinal metastasis is discovered are more likely to remain ambulatory regardless of whether radiation therapy (96%) or surgery (95%) is used as treatment. Ambulatory but weak patients retain ambulation 80% of the time with radiation therapy, and 84% of the time with surgery. Patients who are paraparetic and nonambulatory regain ambulation after treatment 47% of the time with radiation, and 45% of the time with surgery. Paraplegic patients rarely recover ambulation.

Patients who regain or retain ambulation survive longer than patients who do not [122]. This finding probably results from the more advanced stage of disease in patients who do not regain ambulation, and from complications of the paraplegic state. These data are derived from a series of 244 patients with intraspinal metastases who were treated at Memorial Sloan-Kettering Cancer Center [105].

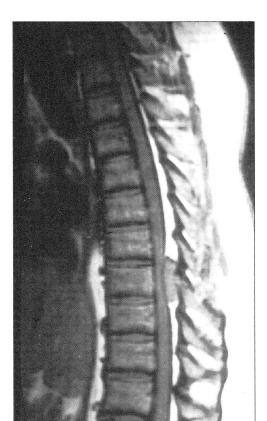

Figure 8-81. Sagittal T2-weighted magnetic resonance imaging scan showing a mass within the spinal canal that compresses the spinal cord. The patient presented with back pain, but had a normal neurologic examination. He had a history of prostate cancer. His back pain improved with radiation therapy. (*Courtesy of* Howard Morgan, MD, and Thomas Kopitnik, MD, Department of Neurosurgery, University of Texas Southwestern, Dallas, TX.)

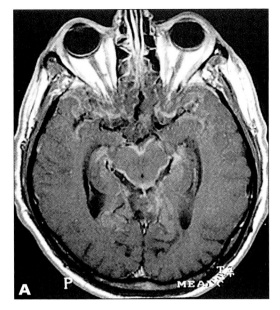
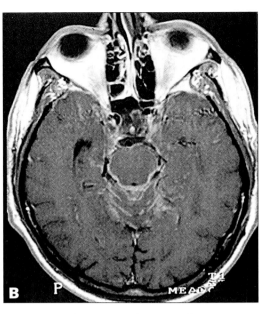

Figure 8-82. T1-weighted magnetic resonance imaging scans with contrast showing enhancement lining the perimesencephalic (**A**) and peripontine (**B**) cisterns, consistent with recurrent leptomeningeal carcinoma. This 56-year-old man developed lethargy and confusion over several weeks, and spinal fluid analysis revealed elevated protein, low glucose, and atypical cells on cytologic examination. Extensive investigations showed no infectious cause, and no systemic cancer, and a meningeal biopsy was obtained. Malignant cells containing melanin were seen in the meninges on histologic examination, but the precise primary carcinoma could not be determined. His leptomeningeal carcinoma was treated with intrathecal interleukin-2 (IL-2), as part of an experimental protocol. He survived for 2 years before the tumor recurred.

Only a small fraction of patients with systemic cancer develop symptomatic leptomeningeal carcinomatosis (0.8% to 8%) [105], but the frequency of this problem seems to be increasing [123]. Successful treatment of primary tumors may allow time for the development of leptomeningeal metastasis. Lung and breast cancer are the most common solid primary tumors in patients with leptomeningeal carcinomatosis. Lymphoma and leukemia can also seed the meninges. Findings on lumbar puncture may suggest the diagnosis of leptomeningeal carcinomatosis. Increased cells and protein concentration and decreased glucose concentration are usually present in the cerebrospinal fluid (CSF). Cytology may be initially negative in 50% of cases of leptomeningeal cancer [105], but when three or more large samples are collected (greater than 4 mL) and promptly processed, the sensitivity of CSF cytology is 91% [124].

Survival of patients with leptomeningeal carcinomatosis is currently dismal. Most patients die within 6 to 8 weeks from the initial diagnosis [125]. Current treatment for leptomeningeal carcinomatosis consists of radiation to symptomatic areas, and intrathecal methotrexate. Treatment can stabilize or improve neurologic symptoms in 75% of patients [105], but only minimally prolongs survival. The patient described here experienced a prolonged survival compared to most patients with leptomeningeal cancer.

Paraneoplastic Syndromes

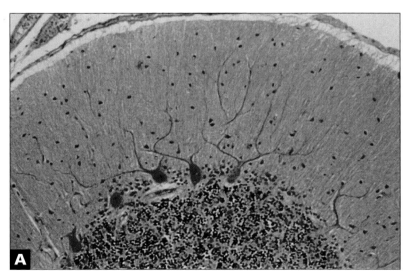
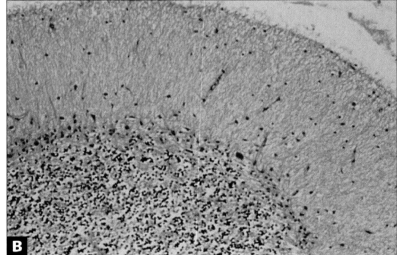

Figure 8-83. Paraneoplastic cerebellar degeneration (PCD). Systemic cancer can also cause neurologic symptoms without directly invading the nervous system, by inducing the production of antibodies directed against components of the nervous system, producing a paraneoplastic syndrome. **A,** Histologic features of normal cerebellar cortex. **B,** Clear loss of the large Purkinje cells compared with the normal cerebellar histology in panel *A*. Purkinje cells are preferentially destroyed in paraneoplastic cerebellar degeneration. Patients with PCD present with subacute pancerebellar dysfunction that becomes severe and disabling. PCD can occur with many types of cancer, but small cell lung cancer [126], ovarian or uterine cancer [127], and lymphomas (especially Hodgkin's disease) [128] are especially likely to cause the syndrome [105]. Several different antibodies have been associated with PCD. The antibody most closely associated with PCD is anti-Yo. This antibody occurs most frequently in patients with ovarian (46% of anti-Yo cases) or breast cancer (24%). Anti-Yo reacts with antigens on Purkinje cells and on the patient's primary tumor [129], and produces granular staining of neuronal cytoplasm. Female patients with subacute cerebellar degeneration without an obvious cause should be tested for anti-Yo antibodies, and if these are positive a thorough search for gynecologic or breast cancer should be made [130].

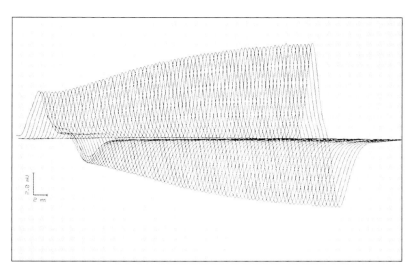

Figure 8-84. Electromyogram (EMG) in a patient with paraneoplastic Lambert-Eaton myasthenic syndrome (LEMS). This paraneoplastic syndrome produces progressive proximal weakness, and is most often associated with small cell lung cancer. The EMG is characteristic in patients with LEMS. At high frequencies of stimulation, the compound motor action potentials (CMAPs) become progressively larger with time, as seen in this patient with fatigability and a history of smoking. A computed tomography scan showed a nodule within the lung that was a small cell lung cancer on resection.

In most patients, LEMS is caused by an antibody directed toward presynaptic voltage-dependent calcium channels in the neuromuscular junction [131,132]. These antibodies prevent calcium from entering the nerve terminal when an action potential arrives, which leads to a decrease in the quantal release of acetylcholine into the neuromuscular junction. The CMAP increases at high rates of stimulation because eventually calcium builds up in the nerve terminal and allows greater release of acetylcholine. (*Courtesy of* T.H. Salmon, MD, Department of Neurology, University of Texas Southwestern Medical Center, Dallas, TX.)

Pediatric Central Nervous System Tumors

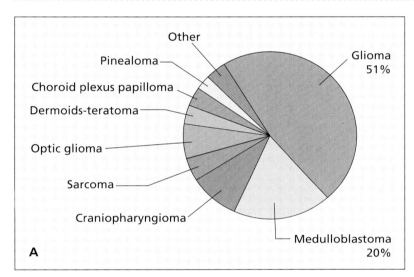

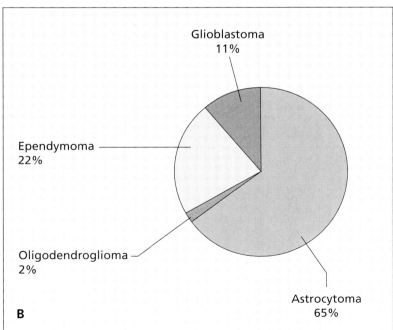

Figure 8-85. Distribution of primary intracranial tumors and gliomas in children less than 15 years old. **A,** As in adults, most intracranial tumors in children are gliomas (51%). The next most common intracranial tumor in children is the medulloblastoma, which seldom occurs in adults, but accounts for 20% of all intracranial tumors in children [133]. Craniopharyngiomas are also more common in children.

B, When medulloblastoma is excluded as of uncertain histogenetic origin, and only gliomas are considered, astrocytic tumors (astrocytomas and glioblastomas) are the most common histologic subtype in childhood brain tumors (65%). Glioblastomas are less frequent in children than they are in adults, accounting for only 11% of gliomas in children, compared with 35% of gliomas in adults. Ependymomas comprise a larger proportion of gliomas in childhood (22%) than they do in adults (10%). Oligodendrogliomas are also more common in adults (usually younger adults) (19%) than they are in children (2%). (Data *adapted from* Evans [134] and Thomas [135].)

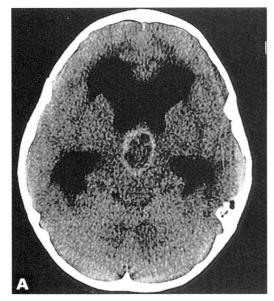
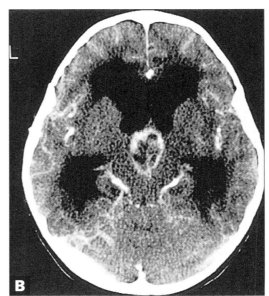
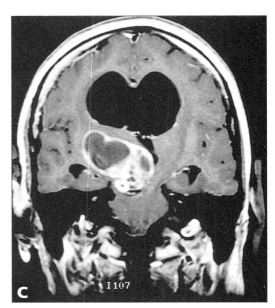

Figure 8-86. Hydrocephalus in children with brain tumors. Many childhood brain tumors present initially with hydrocephalus. Children with hydrocephalus may complain of headache, vomiting, and blurred or double vision. In younger children in whom the cranial sutures have not completely fused, head enlargement may occur. Papilledema is usually present on funduscopic examination (Fig. 8-11).

A, Computed tomography scan with and without contrast in a 4-year-old girl with headaches and papilledema. The noncontrast-enhanced scan shows a ring of calcium in the suprasellar region, and massive enlargement of the lateral ventricles. **B,** Enhancement is seen within the ring of calcium in the contrast-enhanced scan. A ventriculoperitoneal shunt was placed, and subtotal resection revealed a suprasellar germinoma. The patient responded well to radiation therapy.

C, Coronal T1-weighted, postgadolinium magnetic resonance imaging scan in a patient with chronic hydrocephalus secondary to a midline dermoid cyst, which was not completely resectable. The lesion has remained stable for almost 1 year, but the frontal horns of the lateral ventricles remain enlarged.

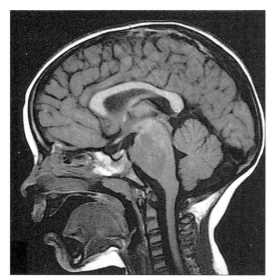

Figure 8-87. Sagittal T1-weighted magnetic resonance imaging (MRI) scan showing a hypointense mass lesion in the anterior pons in a 6-year-old boy who presented with diplopia. Biopsy revealed astrocytoma.

Brain stem gliomas are nearly as common as medulloblastomas in children [136]. Clinical features that predict a poor prognosis include short duration of symptoms (less than 6 months) and multiple brain stem signs. The computed tomography and MRI appearance of brain stem gliomas is characteristic, and has prognostic importance [137,138]. Exophytic lesions can sometimes be surgically removed [139]. Intrinsic lesions are much more difficult to resect safely, and stereotactic biopsy is usually employed. Biopsy provides useful prognostic information and occasionally identifies a non-neoplastic lesion [136,140,141]. See Figure 8-34 for histologic correlation.

Radiation therapy improves survival in patients with brain stem gliomas, but is rarely curative. There is a trend toward longer survival at higher doses of radiation [142]. Various chemotherapeutic agents and combinations have been employed, but the benefit has been small and short term [142].

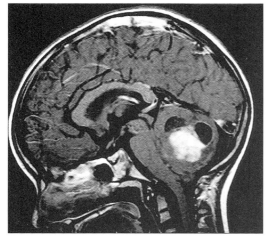

Figure 8-88. Sagittal T1-weighted magnetic resonance imaging scan with contrast from a patient who had chronic headaches and slowly progressive clumsiness (ataxia). There is a large multiloculated cystic mass in the cerebellum, with a brightly enhancing nodule anteriorly. Craniotomy revealed pilocytic astrocytoma.

Pilocytic astrocytomas occur most often in children, and can arise in the cerebellum, the hypothalamus, or the optic tracts (see Fig. 8-37 for histologic correlation). When a pilocytic astrocytoma occurs in the cerebellum, long survival is typical, particularly if complete resection can be achieved. Most of these tumors are cystic (80%), and they classically present as a cyst with a neoplastic mural nodule [143]. Young age at diagnosis and brain stem invasion predict a less favorable course [144,145]. The role of radiation therapy and chemotherapy for residual or recurrent pilocytic astrocytomas is under investigation [143].

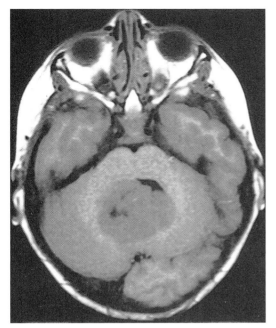

Figure 8-89. Axial T1-weighted, noncontrast magnetic resonance imaging scan from a 5-year-old boy with medulloblastoma. The tumor is in the midline of the cerebellum, and pushes the fourth ventricle forward and to the left. Medulloblastomas are the most common intracranial tumor in children. They arise most often in the midline of the cerebellum, and often spread via the cerebrospinal fluid (CSF) [146]. Medulloblastomas can even produce systemic metastases. Modern treatment with surgery, radiation therapy, and occasionally chemotherapy has resulted in improved survival of patients with medulloblastoma over the last several decades [133].

A complete surgical resection provides a better chance for long-term survival [147], but surgery alone provides poor disease control, with 12.5% 1-year and 4.2% 5-year survival rates [146]. Craniospinal irradiation improves survival in children with medulloblastoma to 65% at 5 years [148]. In children under 2 years old, chemotherapy has been used to postpone craniospinal radiation and decrease the risk of intellectual impairment [149]. Survival of patients with medulloblastoma has improved over the last two decades, and the addition of chemotherapy to standard craniospinal radiation therapy may have a lot to do with this improvement [150]. The most successful chemotherapy regimens for medulloblastoma include cisplatin [151,152]. (See Figure 8-48 for histologic correlation.)

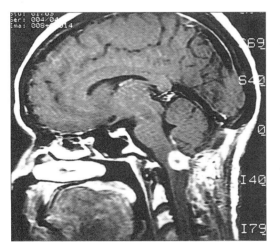

Figure 8-90. Sagittal T1-weighted magnetic resonance imaging (MRI) scan performed after contrast administration in a patient with a posterior fossa ependymoma. The contrast-enhancing mass just below the cerebellum was an ependymoma at surgical resection. Ependymomas comprise 8% to 10% of childhood brain tumors, with a mean age at diagnosis of 5 to 6 years [153]. They usually occur in relation to the ventricular system, but can occur anywhere within the brain. One third are supratentorial, and two thirds are infratentorial. Supratentorial ependymomas tend to have more anaplastic histology than ependymomas located in the posterior fossa [154]. Ependymomas are usually hyperintense to brain on computed tomography (CT) scans without contrast [155,156]. They do not have any distinctive signal intensity on MRI scans, but the anatomic details provided by MRI can sometimes suggest the diagnosis.

Ependymomas can spread via the cerebrospinal fluid (CSF), although the frequency of leptomeningeal seeding is uncertain. When myelography and CSF cytology are performed before treatment in patients with ependymomas, only 5% have evidence of CSF involvement [157]. Supratentorial ependymomas, and tumors with low-grade histology are unlikely to disseminate via the CSF. Posterior fossa ependymomas with malignant histology are especially likely to spread via the CSF, and craniospinal radiation is recommended for treatment. Supratentorial, low-grade ependymomas usually do not disseminate, so local radiation fields are used. The appropriate therapy for high-grade supratentorial ependymomas and for low-grade infratentorial ependymomas is more controversial [153]. At least 45 Gy is recommended for patients with ependymoma, since better survival has been obtained with higher doses [158]. Chemotherapy has been helpful in some cases. The most active reported chemotherapy regimens include platinum-based agents [159,160].

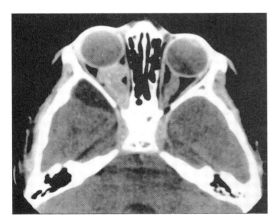

Figure 8-91. Computed tomography scan of the orbits showing thickened optic nerves, especially on the right, in a patient with neurofibromatosis type 1 (NF1) who had progressive visual loss. This appearance is characteristic for optic gliomas. These tumors occur more often in children with NF1. They usually have a pilocytic astrocytoma histology and an indolent course. Unilateral tumors may be removed surgically, but bilateral tumors, or tumors involving the optic chiasm or tracts are usually treated with radiation. (*Courtesy of* E.S. Roach, MD, Department of Pediatric Neurology, University of Texas Southwestern Medical Center, Dallas, TX; *from* Roach [161]; with permission.)

References

1. Giles GG, Gonzales MF: Epidemiology of Brain Tumors and Factors in Prognosis. In *Brain Tumors: An Encyclopedic Approach.* Edited by Kaye AH, Laws ER Jr. New York: Churchill Livingstone; 1994: 47–67.

2. Whelan SL, Parkin DM, Masuyer E: *Patterns of Cancer in Five Continents.* Edited by Whelan SL, Parkin DM, Masuyer E. Lyon: International Agency for Research on Cancer; 1990. [IARC Scientific Publications, vol 102.]

3. Bahemuka M: Worldwide incidence of primary nervous system neoplasms. Geographical, racial and sex differences, 1960–1977. *Brain* 1988, 111:737–755.

4. Velema JP, Walker AM: The age curve of nervous system tumor incidence in adults: common shape but changing levels by sex, race and geographical location. *Int J Epidemiol* 1987, 16:177–183.

5. Schoenberg BS, Christine BW, Whisnant JP: The resolution of discrepancies in the reported incidence of primary brain tumors. *Neurology* 1978, 28:817–823.

6. Annegers JF, Schoenberg BS, Okazaki H, *et al.*: Epidemiologic study of primary intracranial neoplasms. *Arch Neurol* 1981, 38:217–219.

7. Kurland LT, Schoenberg BS, Annegers JF, *et al.*: The incidence of primary intracranial neoplasms in Rochester, Minnesota, 1935–1977. *Ann N Y Acad Sci* 1982, 381:6–16.

8. Walker AE, Robins M, Weinfeld FD: Epidemiology of brain tumors: the national survey of intracranial neoplasms. *Neurology* 1985, 35:219–226.

9. Cairncross JG, Posner JB: The management of brain metastases. In *Oncology of the Nervous System.* Edited by Walker MD. Boston: Martinus Nijhoff; 1983:341–377.

10. Delattre JY, Krol G, Thaler HT, *et al.*: Distribution of brain metastases. *Arch Neurol* 1988, 45:741–744.

11. Evans RG: The role of radiation therapy in the treatment of brain tumors in children. In *Brain Tumors: A Comprehensive Text.* Edited by Morantz RA, Walsh JW. New York: Marcel Dekker; 1994: 659–677.

12. Levin VA, Sheline GE, Gutin PH: Neoplasms of the Central Nervous System. In *Cancer: Principles and Practice of Oncology*, vol 2. Edited by DeVita VT Jr, Hellman S, Rosenberg SA. Philadelphia: JB Lippincott; 1989:1557–1611.

13. Daumas-Duport C, Scheithauer BW, O'Fallon JR, *et al.*: Grading of astrocytomas: a simple and reproducible method. *Cancer* 1988, 62:2152–2165.

14. Shaw EG, Daumas-Duport C, Scheithauer BW, *et al.*: Radiation therapy in the treatment of low-grade supratentorial astrocytomas. *J Neurosurg* 1989, 70:853–861.

15. Guthrie BL, Laws ER Jr: Supratentorial low-grade gliomas. *Neurosurg Clin North Am* 1990, 1:37–48.

16. Devaux BC, O'Fallon JR, Kelly PJ: Resection, biopsy, and survival in malignant glial neoplasms. *J Neurosurg* 1993, 78:767–775.

17. Laws ER Jr, Taylor WF, Clifton MB, *et al.*: Neurosurgical management of low-grade astrocytoma of the cerebral hemisphere. *J Neurosurg* 1984, 61:665–673.

18. Burger PC, Vogel FS, Green SB, *et al.*: Glioblastoma multiforme and anaplastic astrocytoma: pathologic criteria and prognostic implications. *Cancer* 1985, 56:1106–1111.

19. Burger PG, Green SB: Patient age, histologic features, and length of survival in patients with glioblastoma multiforme. *Cancer* 1987, 59:1617–1625.

20. Salcman M: Malignant glioma management. *Neurosurg Clin North Am* 1990, 1:49–61.

21. Curran WJ Jr, Scott CB, Horton J, *et al.*: Recursive partitioning analysis of prognostic factors in three Radiation Therapy Oncology Group malignant glioma trials. *J Natl Cancer Inst* 1993, 85:704–710.

22. Schold SC Jr.: Unpublished data.

23. Pell MF, Thomas DGT: General Introduction to the Clinical Features of Malignant Brain Tumours. In *Malignant Brain Tumours.* Edited by Thomas DGT, Graham DI. London: Springer-Verlag; 1995:109–114.

24. McKeran RO, Thomas DGT: The clinical study of gliomas. In *Brain Tumours: Scientific Basis, Clinical Investigation and Current Therapy.* Edited by Thomas DGT, Graham DI. London: Butterworth; 1980:194–230.

25. Cascino GD: Epilepsy and brain tumours: implications for treatment. *Epilepsia* 1990, 31:537–544.

26. Henry C, Despland PA, Regli F: Initial epileptic crisis after the age of 60: aetiology, clinical aspect clind EEG. *Schweiz Med Wochenschr* 1990, 120:787–792.

27. Salcman M, Kaplan RS: Intracranial Tumors in Adults. In *Comprehensive Textbook of Oncology.* Edited by Moosa AR, Bobson MD, Schimpff SD. Baltimore: Williams & Wilkins; 1986: 617–629.

28. Black P, Wen PY: Clinical, Imaging and Laboratory Diagnosis of Brain Tumors. In *Brain Tumors: An Encyclopedic Approach.* Edited by Kaye AH, Laws ER Jr. Hong Kong: Churchill Livingstone; 1995:191–214.

29. Kraemer DL, Bullard DE: Clinical Presentation of the Brain Tumor Patient. In *Brain Tumors: A Comprehensive Text.* Edited by Morantz RA, Walsh JW. New York: Marcel Dekker; 1994:183–211.

30. Balhuizen JC, Bots GT, Schaberg A, *et al.*: The incidence of multifocal cerebral gliomas: a histologic study of large hemisphere sections. *Cancer* 1987, 60:1519–1531.

31. Bigner SH, Johnston WW: The diagnostic challenge of tumors manifested initially by the shedding of cells into cerebrospinal fluid. *Acta Cytol* 1984, 28:29–36.

32. Choucair AK, Leven VA, Gutin PH, *et al.*: Development of multiple lesions during radiation therapy and chemotherapy in patients with gliomas. *J Neurosurg* 1986, 65:654–658.

33. Segall HD, Destian S, Nelson Jr MD, *et al.*: CT and MR Imaging in Malignant Gliomas. In *Malignant Cerebral Glioma.* Edited by Apuzzo MLJ. Park Ridge, IL: American Association of Neurological Surgeons; 1991:63–78.

34. Kelly PJ, Daumas-Duport C, Kispert DB, *et al.*: Imaging-based stereotaxic serial biopsies in untreated intracranial glial neoplasms. *J Neurosurg* 1987, 66:865–874.

35. Fujii K, Fujita N, Hirabuki N, *et al.*: Neuromas and meningiomas: evaluation of early enhancement with dynamic MR imaging. *AJNR* 1992, 13:1215–1220.

36. Goldsher D, Litt AW, Pinto RS, *et al.*: Dural "tail" associated with meningiomas on Gd-DTPA–enhanced MR images: characteristics, differential diagnostic value, and possible implications of treatment. *Radiology* 1990, 176:447–450.

37. Tien RD, Yang PJ, Chu PK: "Dural tail sign": A specific MR sign for meningioma? *J Comput Assist Tomogr* 1991, 15:64–66.

38. Chen TC, Zee CS, Miller CA, *et al.*: Magnetic resonance imaging and pathological correlates of meningiomas. *Neurosurgery* 1992, 31:1015–1022.

39. Constantini S, Tamir J, Gomori MJ, *et al.*: Tumor prostaglandin levels correlate with edema around supratentorial meningiomas. *Neurosurgery* 1993, 33:204–211.

40. Jaaskelainen J: Seemingly complete removal of histologically benign intracranial meningioma: late recurrence rate and factors predicting recurrence in 657 patients. *Surg Neurol* 1986, 25:461–469.

41. Jaaskelainen J, Haltia M, Servo A: Atypical and anaplastic meningiomas: radiology, surgery, radiotherapy and outcome. *Surg Neurol* 1986, 25:233–242.

42. DeMonte F, Al-Mefty O: Meningiomas. In *Brain Tumors: An Encyclopedic Approach.* Edited by Kaye AH, Laws ER Jr. Hong Kong: Churchill Livingstone; 1995: 675–704.

43. Ho VB, Smirniotopoulos JG, Murphy FM, *et al.*: Radiologic-pathologic correlation: hemangioblastoma. *AJNR* 1992, 13:1343–1352.

44. Lee Y-Y, Van Tassel P, Bruner JM, *et al.*: Juvenile pilocytic astrocytomas: CT and MR characteristics. *AJNR* 1989, 10:363–370.

45. Neumann HPH, Eggert HR, Scheremet R, *et al.*: Central nervous system lesions in von Hippel-Lindau syndrome. *J Neurol Neurosurg Psychiatry* 1992, 55:898–901.

46. Leibel SA, Sheline GE: Radiation therapy for neoplasms of the brain. *J Neurosurg* 1987, 66:1–22.

47. DiChiro G, Hatazawa J, Katz DA, *et al.*: Diagnostic and Prognostic Value of Positron Emission Tomography Using [18F]-Fluorodeoxyglucose in Brain Tumors. In *Positron Emission Tomography.* Edited by Reivich M, Alavi A. New York: Alan R Liss; 1985:291–309.

48. Alavi JB, Alavi A, Chawluk J, *et al.*: Positron emission tomography in patients with gliomas. A predictor of prognosis. *Cancer* 1988, 62:1074–1078.

49. Valk PE, Budinger TF, Levin VA, *et al.*: PET of malignant cerebral tumors after interstitial brachytherapy. Demonstration of metabolic activity and correlation with clinical outcome. *J Neurosurg* 1988, 69:830–838.

50. Le Bihan D, Douek M, Argyropoulou M, *et al.*: Diffusion and perfusion magnetic resonance imaging in brain tumors. *Top Magnetic Resonance Imaging* 1993, 5:25–31.

51. Scharfen CO, Sneed PK, Wara WM, *et al.*: High activity iodine-125 interstitial implant for gliomas. *Int J Radiat Oncol Biol Phys* 1992, 24:583–591.

52. Salcman M: Intracranial hemorrhage caused by brain tumor. In *Intracerebral Hematomas.* Edited by Kaufman HH. New York: Raven Press; 1992:95–106.

53. Kleihues P, Burger PC, Scheithauer BW: The new WHO classification of brain tumors. *Brain Pathol* 1993, 3:255–268.

54. Kleihues P, Burger PC, Scheithauer BW: *Histological Typing of Tumours of the Central Nervous System*, edn 2. Berlin: Springer-Verlag; 1993.

55. Ringertz N: Grading of gliomas. *Acta Pathol Microbiol Scand* 1950, 27:51–64.

56. Svien HJ, Mabon RF, Kernohan JW, *et al.*: Astrocytomas. *Proc Staff Meet Mayo Clin* 1949, 24:54–63.

57. Burger PC, Vollmer RT: Histological factors of prognostic significance in glioblastoma multiforme. *Cancer* 1980, 46:1179–1186.

58. Daumas-Duport C, Scheithauer B, O'Fallon J, *et al.*: Grading of astrocytomas. A simple and reproducible method. *Cancer* 1988, 62:2152–2165.

59. Nelson JS, Tsukada Y, Schoenfeld D: Necrosis as a prognostic criterion in malignant, supratentorial astrocytic gliomas. *Cancer* 1983, 52:550–554.

60. Coons SW, Johnson P: Histopathology of astrocytomas: grading, patterns of spread and correlation with modern imaging modalities. *Semin Radiat Oncol* 1991, 1:2–9.

61. Berger PC, Scheithauer BW: *Atlas of Tumor Pathology: Tumors of the Central Nervous System*. Washington, DC: Armed Forces Institute of Pathology; 1994. [Third series; fascicle 10.]

62. Russell DS, Rubinstein LJ: *Pathology of Tumors of the Nervous System*, edn 5. Baltimore: Williams & Wilkins; 1989.

63. Albright AL, Packer RJ, Zimmerman R, *et al.*: Magnetic resonance scans should replace biopsies for the diagnosis of diffuse brain stem gliomas: a report from Children's Cancer Group. *Neurosurgery* 1993, 33:1026–1029.

64. Hoffman HJ, Soloniuk DS, Humphreys RP, *et al.*: Management and outcome of low-grade astrocytomas of the midline in children: a retrospective review. *Neurosurgery* 1993, 33:964–971.

65. Macdonald D: Low grade gliomas, mixed gliomas and oligodendrogliomas. *Semin Oncol* 1994, 21:236–248.

66. Sutton LN, Molloy PT, Sernyak H, *et al.*: Long-term outcome of hypothalamic/chiasmatic astrocytomas in children treated with conservative surgery. *J Neurosurg* 1995, 83:583–589.

67. Rushing EJ, Rorke LB, Sutton L: Problems in the nosology of desmoplastic tumors of childhood. *Pediatr Neurosurg* 1993, 19:57–62.

68. Vandenberg SR: Current diagnostic concepts of astrocytic tumors. *J Neuropathol Exp Neurol* 1992, 51:644–657.

69. Chen TC, Gonzalez-Gomez I, McComb JG: Uncommon Glial Tumors. In *Brain Tumors*. Edited by Kaye AH, Laws ER Jr. New York: Churchill Livingstone; 1995:525–557.

70. Hirose T, Scheithauer BW, Lopes MBS, *et al.*: Tuber and subependymal giant cell astrocytoma associated with tuberous sclerosis: an immunohistochemical, ultrastructural, and immunoelectron microscopic study. *Acta Neuropathol* 1995, 90:387–399.

71. Nixon JR, Miller GM, Okazaki H, *et al.*: Cerebral tuberous sclerosis: postmortem magnetic resonance imaging and pathologic anatomy. *Mayo Clin Proc* 1989, 64:305–311.

72. Cairncross G, Macdonald D, Ludwin S, *et al.*: Chemotherapy for anaplastic oligodendroglioma: National Cancer Institute of Canada Clinical Trials Group. *J Clin Oncol* 1994, 12:2013–2021.

73. Lombardi D, Scheithauer BW, Meyer FB, *et al.*: Symptomatic subependymoma: a clinicopathologic and flow cytometric study. *J Neurosurg* 1991, 75:583–588.

74. Ho DM, Wong TT, Liu HC: Choroid plexus tumors in childhood: histopathologic study and clinicopathological correlation. *Childs Nerv Sys* 1991, 7:437–441.

75. Mena H, Rushing EJ, Ribas JL, *et al.*: Tumors of pineal parenchymal cells: a correlation of histological features, including nucleolar organizer regions, with survival in 35 cases. *Hum Pathol* 1995, 26:20–30.

76. Sure U, Bertalanffy H, Isenmann St, *et al.*: Secondary manifestations of medulloblastoma: metastases and local recurrences in 66 patients. *Acta Neurochir* (*Wien*) 1995, 136:117–126.

77. National Institutes of Health Consensus Development Conference statement on acoustic neuroma. December 11-13, 1991. *Arch Neurol* 1994, 51:201–207.

78. Ng H, Lau K, Tse JYM, *et al.*: Combined molecular genetic studies of chromosome 22q and the neurofibromatosis type 2 gene in central nervous system tumors. *Neurosurgery* 1995, 37:764–773.

79. Sobel RA, Wang Y: Vestibular (acoustic) schwannomas: histologic features in neurofibromatosis 2 and unilateral cases. *J Neuropathol Exp Neurol* 1993, 52:106–113.

80. Roach, ES: Diagnosis and management of neurocutaneous syndromes. *Semin Neurol* 1988, 8:83–96.

81. Newman S: Meningiomas: a quest for the optimum therapy. *J Neurosurg* 1994, 80:191–194.

82. Sherman ME, Erozan YS, Mann RB, *et al.*: Stereotactic brain biopsy in the diagnosis of malignant lymphoma. *Am J Clin Pathol* 1991, 95:878–883.

83. Miller DC: Histopathologic Evaluation of Pituitary Tumors: Help for the Clinician. In: *Contemporary Diagnosis and Management of Pituitary Adenomas*. Edited by Cooper PR. Park Ridge, IL: American Association of Neurological Surgeons; 1991:37–45.

84. Brada M, Thomas DGT: Craniopharyngioma revisited. *Int J Radiat Oncol Biol Phys* 1993, 27:471–475.

85. Earnest F IV, Kelly PJ, Scheithauer BW, *et al.*: Cerebral astrocytomas: histopathologic correlation of MR and CT contrast enhancement with stereotactic biopsy. *Radiology* 1988, 166:823–827.

86. Devaux BC, O'Fallow JR, Kelly PJ: Resection, biopsy, and survival in malignant glial neoplasms. *J Neurosurg* 1993, 78:767–775.

87. Walker MD, Alexander E Jr, Hunt WE, *et al.*: Evaluation of BCNU and/or radiotherapy in the treatment of anaplastic gliomas—a cooperative clinical trial. *J Neurosurg* 1978, 49:333–343.

88. Schultheiss TE, Stephens LC, Jiang GL, *et al.*: Radiation myelopathy in primates treated with conventional fractionation. *Int J Radiat Oncol Biol Phys* 1990, 19:935–940.

89. Duffner PK, Cohen ME, Thomas PRM, *et al.*: The long-term effects of cranial irradiation on the central nervous system. *Cancer* 1985, 56:1841–1846.

90. Packer RJ, Sutton LN, Atkins TE, *et al.*: A prospective study of cognitive function in children receiving whole-brain radiotherapy and chemotherapy: 2-year results. *J Neurosurg* 1987, 70:707–713.

91. Cohen ME, Duffner PK: Long-term clinical effects. In *Brain Tumors in Children: Principles of Diagnosis and Treatment*. Edited by Cohen ME, Duffner PK. New York: Raven Press; 1994:455–481.

92. Twijnstra A, Boon PJ, Lormans ACM, *et al.*: Neurotoxicity of prophylactic cranial irradiation in patients with small cell carcinoma of the lung. *Eur J Cancer Clin Oncol* 1987, 23:983–986.

93. Hochberg FH, Slotnick B: Neuropsychologic impairment in astrocytoma survivors. *Neurology* 1980, 30:172–177.

94. Shalet SM: Irradiation induced growth failure. *Clin Endocrinol Metab* 1986, 15:591–606.

95. Constine LS, Woolf PD, Cann D, *et al.*: Hypothalamic-pituitary dysfunction after radiation for brain tumors. *N Engl J Med* 1993, 328:87–94.

96. Valk PE, Budinger TF, Levin VA, *et al.*: PET of malignant cerebral tumors after interstitial brachytherapy. Demonstration of metabolic activity and correlation with clinical outcome. *J Neurosurg* 1988, 69:830–838.

97. Glantz MJ, Burger PC, Friedman AH, *et al.*: Treatment of radiation-induced nervous system injury with heparin and warfarin. *Neurology* 1994, 44:2020–2027.

98. Valk PE, Dillon WP: Radiation injury of the brain. *AJNR* 1991, 12:45–62.

99. Soffer D, Gomori JM, Siegal T, *et al.*: Intracranial meningiomas after high-dose irradiation. *Cancer* 1989, 63:1514—1519.

100. Dodick DW, Mokri B, Shaw EG, *et al.*: Sarcomas of calvarial bones: rare remote effect of radiation therapy for brain tumors. *Neurology* 1994, 44:908–912.

101. Green SB, Byar DP, Walker MD, *et al.*: Comparisons of carmustine, procarbazine and high-dose methylprednisolone as additions to surgery and radiotherapy for the treatment of malignant glioma. *Cancer Treat Rep* 1983, 67:123–132.

102. Dropcho EJ, Rosenfeld SS, Morawetz RB, *et al.*: Pre-radiation intracarotid cisplatin treatment of newly diagnosed anaplastic gliomas. *J Clin Oncol* 1992, 10:452–458.

103. Salcman M, Kaplan RS, Samarns GM, *et al.*: Aggressive multimodality therapy based on a multicompartmental model of glioblastoma. *Surgery* 1982, 92:250–259.

104. Wallner KE, Galicich JH, Krol G, *et al.*: Patterns of failure following treatment for glioblastoma multiforme and anaplastic astrocytoma. *Int J Radiat Biol Oncol Phys* 1989, 16:1405–1409.

105. Posner JB: *Neurologic Complications of Cancer*. Philadelphia: FA Davis; 1995. Contemporary Neurology Series, vol 45.

106. DeVita VT Jr, Hellman S, Rosenberg SA: Edpidemiology of Cancer. In *Cancer Principles and Practice*. Edited by DeVita VT Jr, Hellman S, Rosenberg SA. Philadelphia: JB Lippincott; 1993:150–181.

107. Delattre JY, Krol G, Thaler HT, *et al.*: Distribution of brain metastases. *Arch Neurol* 1988, 45:741–744.

108. Cairncross JG, Kim J-H, Posner JB: Radiation therapy for brain metastases. *Ann Neurol* 1980, 7:529–541.

109. Young DF, Posner JB, Chu F, *et al.*: Rapid-course radiation therapy of cerebral metastases: results and complications. *Cancer* 1974, 4:1069–1076.

110. Patchel RA, Tibbs PA, Walsh JW, *et al.*: A randomized trial of surgery in the treatment of single metastases to the brain. *New Engl J Med* 1990, 322:494–500.

111. Bindal RK, Sawaya R, Leavens ME, *et al.*: Surgical treatment of multiple brain metastases. *J Neurosurg* 1993, 79:210–216.

112. Davis PC, Hudgins PA, Peterman SB, *et al.*: Diagnosis of cerebral metastases: double dose delayed CT vs contrast-enhanced MR imaging. *AJNR* 1991, 12:293–300.

113. Simpson RK Jr, Sirbasku DM, Baskin DS: Solitary brainstem metastasis: comparisons of x-ray computed tomography and magnetic resonance imaging to pathology. *J Neuro-oncol* 1987, 5:57–63.

114. Yuh WTC, Engelken JD, Muhonen MG, *et al.*: Experience with high-dose gadolinium MR imaging in the evaluation of brain metastases. *AJNR* 1992, 13:335–354.

115. Fornasier VL, Horne JG: Metastases to the vertebral column. *Cancer* 1975, 36:590–594.

116. Galasko CSB: The anatomy and pathways of skeletal metastases. In *Bone Metastasis.* Edited by Weiss L, Gilbert HA. Boston: GK Hall; 1981:49–63.

117. Wong DA, Fornasier VL, MacNab I: Spinal metastases: the obvious, the occult and the imposters. *Spine* 1990, 15:1–4.

118. Kamholtz R, Sze G: Current imaging in spinal metastatic disease. *Semin Oncol* 1991, 18:744–746.

119. Helweg-Larsen S, Wagner A, Kjaer L, *et al.*: Comparison of myelography combined with post-myelographic spinal CT and MRI in suspected metastatic disease of the spinal canal. *J Neuro-oncol* 1992, 13:231–237.

120. Li KC, Poon PY: Sensitivity and specificity of MRI in detecting malignant spinal cord compression and in distinguishing malignant from benign compression fractures of vertebrae. *Magn Reson Imaging* 1988, 6:547–556.

121. Smoker WR, Godersky JC, Knutzon RK, *et al.*: The role of MR imaging in evaluating metastatic spinal disease. *AJR* 1987, 149:1241–1248.

122. Greenberg HS, Kim J-H, Posner JB: Epidural spinal cord compression from metastatic tumor: results with a new treatment protocol. *Ann Neurol* 1980, 8:361–366.

123. Gasecki AP, Bashir RM, Foley J: Leptomeningeal carcinomatosis: a report of 3 cases and review of the literature. *Eur Neurol* 1992, 32:74–78.

124. Wasserstrom W, Glass JP, Posner JB: Diagnosis and treatment of leptomeningeal metastases from solid tumors: experience with 90 patients. *Cancer* 1982, 49:759–772.

125. Rosen ST, Aisner J, Makuch RW, *et al.*: Carcinomatous leptomeningitis in small cell lung cancer: a clinicopathologic review of the National Cancer Institute experience. *Medicine* 1982, 61:45–53.

126. Clouston PD, Saper CB, Arbizu T, *et al.*: Paraneoplastic cerebellar degeneration: III. Cerebellar degeneration, cancer and the Lambert-Eaton myasthenic syndrome. *Neurology* 1992, 42:1944–1950.

127. Peterson K, Rosenblum MK, Kotanides H, *et al.*: Paraneoplastic cerebellar degeneration: I. A clinical analysis of 55 anti-Yo antibody positive patients. *Neurology* 1992, 42:1931–1937.

128. Hammack J, Kotanides H, Rosenblum MK, *et al.*: Paraneoplastic cerebellar degeneration: II. Clinical and immunologic findings in 21 patients with Hodgkin's disease. *Neurology* 1992, 42:1938–1943.

129. Furneaux HM, Rosenblum MK, Dalmau J, *et al.*: Selective expression of Purkinje-cell antigens in tumor tissue from patients with paraneoplastic cerebellar degeneration. *N Engl J Med* 1990, 322:1844–1851.

130. Hetzel DJ, Stanhope CR, O'Neil BP, *et al.*: Gynecologic cancer in patients with subacute cerebellar degeneration predicted by anti-Purkinje cell antibodies and limited in metastatic volume. *Mayo Clin Proc* 1990, 65:1558–1563.

131. Hewett SJ, Atchison WD: Specificity of Lambert-Eaton myasthenic syndrome immunoglobulin for nerve terminal calcium channels. *Brain Res* 1992, 599:324–332.

132. Leys K, Lang B, Johnston I, *et al.*: Calcium channel autoantibodies in the Lambert-Eaton myasthenic syndrome. *Ann Neurol* 1991, 29:307–314.

133. Cohen ME, Duffner PK: Medulloblastomas. In *Brain Tumors in Children. Principles of Diagnosis and Treatment.* Edited by Cohen ME, Duffner PK. New York: Raven Press; 1995:177–201.

134. Evans RG: The role of radiation therapy in the treatment of brain tumors in children. In *Brain Tumors: A Comprehensive Text.* Edited by Morantz RA, Walsh JW. New York: Marcel Dekker; 1994:659–677.

135. Thomas DGT: *Neuro-oncology: Primary Malignant Brain Tumors.* Edited by Thomas DGT. Baltimore: Johns Hopkins University Press; 1990:165–167.

136. Punt J: Management of brain tumours in childhood. In *Malignant Brain Tumours.* Edited by Thomas DGT, Graham DI. London: Springer-Verlag; 1995:177–192.

137. Barkovich AJ, Krischer J, Kun L, *et al.*: Brain stem gliomas: a classification system based on magnetic resonance imaging. *Pediatr Neurosurg* 1991, 16:73–83.

138. Sanford RA, Freeman CR, Burger P, *et al.*: Prognostic criteria for experimental protocols in pediatric brain stem gliomas. *Surg Neurol* 1988, 30:276–280.

139. Hoffman HJ, Becker L, Craven MA: A clinically and pathologically distinct group of benign brain stem gliomas. *Neurosurgery* 1980, 7:243–248.

140. Frank F, Fabrizi AP, Frank-Ricci R, *et al.*: Stereotactic biopsy and treatment of brain stem lesions: combined study of 33 cases (Bologna-Marseille). *Acta Neurochir* 1988, 42:177–181.

141. Artigas J, Ferszt R, Brock M, *et al.*: The relevance of pathological diagnosis for therapy and outcome of brain stem gliomas. *Acta Neurochir* 1988, 42:166–169.

142. Cohen ME, Duffner PK: Brain stem tumors. In *Brain Tumors in Children. Principles of Diagnosis and Treatment.* Edited by Cohen ME, Duffner PK. New York: Raven Press; 1995:241–262.

143. Cohen ME, Duffner PK: Cerebellar Astrocytomas. In *Brain Tumors in Children. Principles of Diagnosis and Treatment.* Edited by Cohen ME, Duffner PK. New York: Raven Press; 1995:203–218.

144. Garcia DM, Latifi HR, Simpson JR, *et al.*: Astrocytomas of the cerebellum in children. *J Neurosurg* 1989, 71:661–664.

145. Undijian S, Marinov M, Georgiev K: Long-term follow-up after surgical treatment of cerebellar astrocytomas in 100 children. *Childs Nerv Syst* 1989, 5:99–101.

146. Farwell JR, Dohrmann GJ, Flannery JT: Medulloblastoma in childhood: an epidemiological study. *J Neurosurg* 1984, 61:593–664.

147. Tomita T, McClone DG: Medulloblastoma in childhood: results of radical resection and low-dose neuraxis radiation therapy. *J Neurosurg* 1986, 64:238–242.

148. Evans AE, Jenkin DT, Sposto R, *et al.*: The treatment of medulloblastoma. Results of prospective randomized trial of radiation therapy with and without CCNU, vincristine, and prednisone. *J Neurosurg* 1990, 72:572–582.

149. Duffner PK, Horowitz ME, Krischer JP, *et al.*: Postoperative chemotherapy and delayed radiation in children less than three years of age with malignant brain tumors. *N Engl J Med* 1993, 328:1725–1731.

150. Packer RJ, Sutton LN, Goldwein JW, *et al.*: Improved survival with the use of adjuvant chemotherapy in the treatment of medulloblastoma. *J Neurosurg* 1991, 74:433–440.

151. Packer RJ: Diagnosis, treatment, and outcome of primary central nervous system tumors of childhood. *Curr Opin Oncol* 1994, 6:240–246.

152. Kovnar EH, Kellie SJ, Horowitz ME, *et al.*: Preirradiation cisplatin and etoposide in the treatment of high-risk medulloblastomas and other malignant embryonal tumors of the central nervous system: A phase II study. *J Clin Oncol* 1990, 8:330–336.

153. Cohen ME, Duffner PK: Ependymomas. In *Brain Tumors in Children.* Edited by Cohen ME and Duffner PK. New York: Raven Press; 1995:219–239.

154. Dohrmann GJ, Farwell JR, Flannery JT: Ependymomas and ependymoblastomas in children. *J Neurosurg* 1976, 45:273–283.

155. Kingsley DPE, Kendall BE: The CT scanner in posterior fossa tumors of childhood. *Br J Radiol* 1979, 52:769–776.

156. Healey EA, Barnes PD, Kupsky WJ, *et al.*: The prognostic significance of postoperative residual tumor in ependymoma. *Neurosurg* 1991, 28:666–671.

157. Kovnar E, Kun L, Krischer J: Patterns of dissemination and recurrence in childhood ependymoma: preliminary results of Pediatric Oncology Group protocol #8532. *Ann Neurol* 1991, 30:457.

158. Goldwein JW, Leahy JM, Packer RJ, *et al.*: Intracranial ependymomas in children. *Int J Radiat Oncol Biol Phys* 1990, 19:1497–1502.

159. Bertolone SJ, Baum ES, Krivit W, *et al.*: A phase II study of cisplatin therapy in recurrent childhood brain tumors. *J Neuro-oncol* 1989, 7:5–11.

160. Gaynon PS, Ettinger LJ, Baum ES, *et al.*: Carboplatin in childhood brain tumors. *Cancer* 1990, 66:2465–2469.

161. Roach ES: Neurocutaneous syndromes. *Pediatr Clin North Amer* 1992, 39:591–619.

9

Movement Disorders

Stanley Fahn • Paul E. Greene
Blair Ford • Susan B. Bressman

MOVEMENT disorders can be defined as neurologic syndromes in which there is either an excess of movement (commonly referred to as *hyperkinesia, dyskinesia,* and *abnormal involuntary movement*), or a paucity of voluntary and automatic movements unrelated to weakness or spasticity. The latter group can be referred to as *hypokinesia* (decreased amplitude of movement), but *bradykinesia* (slowness of movement) and *akinesia* (loss of movement) are common alternatives. The parkinsonian syndromes are the most common cause of paucity of movement; other hypokinetic disorders represent only a small group of patients. Basically, movement disorders are conveniently divided into parkinsonism and all other types. Gait is affected by most types of movement disorders, including parkinsonism, dystonia, chorea, myoclonus, and cerebellar ataxia.

Most movement disorders are associated with pathologic alterations in the basal ganglia or their connections. The basal ganglia are a group of gray matter nuclei lying deep within the cerebral hemispheres (the caudate, putamen, and globus pallidus), the diencephalon (subthalamic nucleus), and the mesencephalon (substantia nigra). There are some exceptions to this general rule: Disorders of the cerebellum or its pathways typically result in impairment of coordination (asynergy, ataxia), misjudgment of distance (dysmetria), and intention tremor. Myoclonus and many forms of tremors do not appear to be related primarily to pathologic disorders of the basal ganglia, but often arise elsewhere in the central nervous system, including the cerebral cortex (cortical reflex myoclonus), the brain stem (reticular reflex myoclonus, hyperekplexia, and rhythmic brain-stem myoclonus such as palatal and ocular myoclonus), and the spinal cord (rhythmic segmental myoclonus and nonrhythmic propriospinal myoclonus). Moreover, many myoclonic disorders are associated with diseases that involve the cerebellum, such as those causing Ramsay Hunt syndrome. It is not known for certain which part of the brain is associated with tics, although the basal ganglia and the limbic structures have been implicated. Certain locales within the basal ganglia are classically associated with specific movement disorders: substantia nigra, with bradykinesia and rest tremor; subthalamic nucleus, with ballism; caudate nucleus, with chorea; and putamen, with dystonia. Some movement disorders derive from the peripheral nerves or their more proximal parts, the nerve roots, or motoneuron perikarya. Hemifacial spasms, myokymia, and the muscle spasms (stiff-muscles) of Isaacs syndrome are the most well recognized of such disorders. Others are the "jumpy stumps" seen in some amputees, and moving toes (fingers) and painful legs (arms) syndromes that occur as complications to injuries of peripheral nerves or roots.

Many movement disorders have a genetic cause, and some have now been mapped to specific regions of the genome or even localized to a specific gene. Neurogenetics is one of the fastest moving research areas in neurology.

Movement disorders are fairly common neurologic problems, but epidemiologic studies are lacking for many.

The first question to be answered when evaluating a patient for an abnormal movement disorder is whether or not an involuntary movement is actually present. One must decide if the suspected abnormal movements might be purposeful voluntary movements, such as exaggerated gestures, mannerisms, or compulsive movements, or if sustained contracted muscles might result from "involuntary" muscle tightness to reduce pain, as in guarding. As a general rule, abnormal involuntary movements are exaggerated with anxiety and diminished during sleep. They may or may not lessen with amobarbital administration or with hypnosis.

Having decided that abnormal involuntary movements are present and which body parts are involved, the next task is to determine the nature of the involuntary movements: chorea, dystonia, myoclonus, tics, and tremor. This requires the evaluation of such features as rhythmicity, speed, duration, pattern (*eg*, repetitive, flowing, continual, paroxysmal, diurnal), induction (*ie*, stimuli-induced, action-induced, exercise-induced), complexity of the movements (complex vs simple), suppressibility by volitional attention or sensory tricks, and whether the movements are accompanied by restlessness or the urge to release built-up tension.

Parkinsonism

Characteristics of Parkinsonism

| Major features | Variable features | | | |
	Motor	Autonomic	Cognitive	Other
Rest tremor	Freezing of gait	Urinary frequency	Slowness in thinking	Glabellar, palmomental, snout reflexes (frontal release signs)
Rigidity	Dystonia	Constipation	Dementia	
Bradykinesia	Muscle ache	Impotence in men	Depression	Limitation of upgaze
Loss of postural reflexes	Kyphosis			Interruption of smooth ocular pursuit
				Seborrhea

Figure 9-1. Characteristics of parkinsonism. The term *parkinsonism* is applied to neurologic syndromes in which patients exhibit some combination of rest tremor, rigidity, bradykinesia, and loss of postural reflexes. Patients with all these clinical features are likely to have a disturbance of the nigrostriatal dopamine system. In patients who lack one or two of these major features, the presence of dopaminergic dysfunction is less certain. Many patients with parkinsonism may also have other characteristic signs and symptoms. For example, in the "freezing" phenomenon, patients experience sudden transient inability to move one or both feet. This may happen on gait initiation, during turning, encountering boundaries (*eg*, curbs and doorways), upon reaching a destination, when startled, or under emotional pressure. Severe episodes of freezing can lead to frequent falls and are a major source of disability. Some patients who experience freezing in the lower extremities also have a similar phenomenon during speaking, or in the upper extremities while writing or performing other fine motor movements.

A. Classification of Parkinsonism

Idiopathic (Lewy body) parkinsonism

Parkinson's disease

Figure 9-2. Classification of parkinsonism (A–D). Parkinson's disease (PD) is the most common form of parkinsonism and occurs in about 200 of 100,000 people in the general population. A few patients with parkinsonism, however, have a disturbance in the nigrostriatal system from causes other than PD. Virtually every category of human disease can occasionally produce parkinsonism, including intoxication, tumors, infections, metabolic derangements, trauma, vascular disease, and degenerative diseases other than PD. Although many of these conditions produce signs and symptoms that do not occur in PD, up to 25% of patients with clinically diagnosed PD have been found to have another disease at autopsy [1]. PD-D-ALS—parkinsonian dementia–amyotrophic lateral sclerosis; PSP—progressive supranuclear palsy. (*Continued on next page*)

B. Classification of Parkinsonism

Parkinson-plus syndromes

Multiple System Atrophy syndromes (MSA)
  Striatonigral degeneration
  Shy-Drager syndrome
  Sporadic olivopontocerebellar atrophy
Steele-Richardson-Olszewski disease (SRO or PSP)
Cortical-basal ganglionic degeneration
Progressive pallidal atrophy
Lytico-Bodig (Guamanian PD-D-ALS)
Motor neuron disease-parkinsonism
Dementia syndromes
  Alzheimer's disease
  Cortical (diffuse) Lewy body disease
  Pick's disease

C. Classification of Parkinsonism

Heredodegenerative diseases

Hallervorden-Spatz disease
Huntington's disease
Lubag (Filipino X-linked dystonia-parkinson)
Machado-Joseph disease
Neuroacanthocytosis
Familial olivopontocerebellar atrophy
Frontotemporal dementia
Thalamic dementia syndrome
Mutant gene for α-synuclein on chromosome 4q21–q23
Mutant gene for parkin on chromosome 6q25–27

D. Classification of Parkinsonism

Secondary parkinsonism

Drug-induced
  Dopamine receptor blockers
    (neuroleptics, antiemetics)
  Dopamine depleters (reserpine,
    tetrabenazine)
  Lithium
  Flunarizine, cinnarizine, diltiazem
Hemiatrophy-hemiparkinsonism
Hydrocephalus
  Normal pressure hydrocephalus
  Noncommunicating hydrocephalus
Hypoxia

Infectious
  Fungal infection
  AIDS
  Subacute sclerosing panencephalitis
  Postencephalitic (encephalitis
    lethargica, other encephalitides)
  Creutzfeldt-Jakob disease
  Gerstmann-Straussler-Scheinker disease
Intranuclear hyaline inclusion disease
Metabolic
  Hypocalcemic parkinsonism
    (basal ganglia calcification)
  Chronic hepatocerebral degeneration
  Wilson's disease
  Ceroid lipofuscinosis
  GM_1 gangliosidosis
  Gaucher's disease
  Mitochondrial encephalomyopathies

Paraneoplastic parkinsonism
Psychogenic
Syringomesencephalia
Trauma (boxers' encephalopathy)
Toxin
  MPTP intoxication (1-methyl-4-phenyl-
    1,2,3,6-tetrahydropyridine)
  Carbon monoxide intoxication
  Manganese intoxication
  Cyanide
  Methanol
  Carbon disulfide intoxication
  Disulfiram
Tumor
Vascular
  Multi-infarct
  Binswanger's disease

Figure 9-2. (*Continued*) Classification of parkinsonism.

Clinical Manifestations of Parkinson's Disease

Unilateral onset (hemiparkinsonism)
Rest tremor
Absence of other neurologic signs, such as spasticity,
  Babinski signs, atypical speech disturbance
Absence of laboratory or radiologic abnormalities
Slow progression
Dramatic response to levodopa
Preservation of postural reflexes early in the illness

Figure 9-3. Clinical manifestations of Parkinson's disease. Usually, the diagnosis of Parkinson's disease (PD) is suggested by history, clinical examination, and the absence of incompatible clinical, laboratory, or radiologic abnormalities. However, no single feature absolutely guarantees or excludes the diagnosis of PD. Virtually all patients with PD respond dramatically to treatment with levodopa, but this response rarely occurs early in the course of other parkinsonism syndromes, such as olivopontocerebellar atrophy or progressive supranuclear palsy. Conversely, some patients with PD develop severe nausea, orthostatic hypotension, or psychosis while receiving moderate doses of levodopa, and are mistakenly diagnosed as having another parkinsonian syndrome on the basis of levodopa failure. At the onset of the disease, patients with PD usually have symptoms limited to one side of the body (hemi-PD), although symptoms eventually spread to both sides of the body. Occasionally PD begins with symmetric symptoms. In addition, mass lesions such as tumors may compress the substantia nigra or putamen and produce unilateral parkinsonism.

Motor Symptoms of Parkinson's Disease

Tremor
  "Inner motor"
  Rest tremor
  Rest tremor persisting
    with action
  Action tremor (in addition
    to rest tremor)
Rigidity
Akinesia/bradykinesia
  Decreased blink rate
  Facial masking
  Hypophonia
  Drooling
  Tachykinesia
  Terminal micrographia
  Festination

Loss of postural reflexes
Other motor features
  Dystonia
    Early morning dystonia,
      usually in the toes
    Hemidystonia
  Freezing
    Start hesitation
    Freezing of gait: during
      turning, at boundaries,
      at target, in mid-stride
    Freezing of other activities:
      speech (palilalia), writing

Figure 9-4. Motor symptoms of Parkinson's disease (PD). The broad categories of tremor, rigidity, and bradykinesia do not do justice to the complex motor difficulties of patients with PD. Tremor can affect most voluntary muscles, including those of the face, tongue, jaw, upper and lower extremities, and, less commonly, trunk and neck. The tremor is occasionally felt before it can be seen ("inner motor"), is present at rest, but may also be present with action. Tremors are sometimes so severe that they cause perspiration and weight loss. Rigidity contributes to slowness of movement, but patients with PD may be slow even when rigidity is minimal. Rigid muscles may be painful, and shoulder, calf, or thigh pain is sometimes the first symptom of PD.

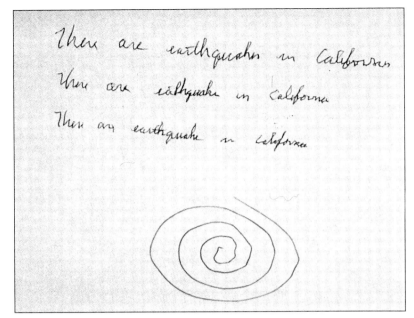

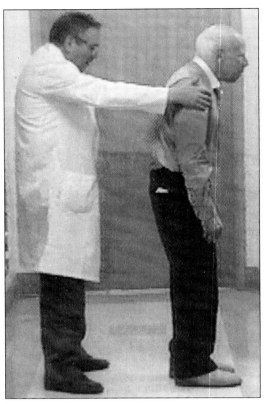

Figure 9-5. Handwriting sample of a patient with mild Parkinson's disease. The handwriting is slower and smaller, and the Archimedes spiral tends to be cramped and less open. Notice the progressive shortening of the length of the sentence as it is repeatedly written. If a tremor is present, it can usually be seen in the handwriting. Bradykinesia manifests in many other ways: decreased blinking and loss of facial expression (masked facies), decreased automatic swallowing leading to drooling, loss of arm swing while walking, and soft voice (hypophonia). During walking, some patients take faster and faster steps as the step size becomes smaller (festination).

Figure 9-6. Demonstration of the pull test. The examiner stands behind the patient and pulls the patient backwards. After explaining that the patient should take a step backwards to prevent falling, the examiner gives a quick pull on the shoulders and tests for retropulsion. On the first attempt, it is advisable to use only mild to moderate force when pulling. If the patient recovers well, then a stronger pull is used. The patient may require a practice with a mild pull to appreciate what is expected of him. The examiner needs to be prepared to catch the patient should he not recover his balance. If the patient is larger than the examiner, it is wise to have a wall behind the examiner to keep both the patient and examiner from falling.

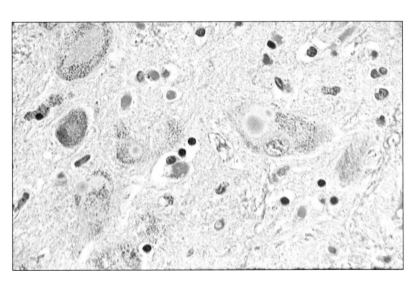

Figure 9-7. Lewy bodies in the substantia nigra (hematoxylin-eosin stain, magnification × 40). The major pathologic abnormalities in Parkinson's disease (PD) are neuronal cell loss, gliosis, and loss of pigment in the substantia nigra, especially in the ventrolateral portion projecting to the putamen, and the presence of abnormal intracytoplasmic neuronal inclusions called Lewy bodies. Lewy bodies consist of an amorphous central core with a halo of radially arranged neurofilaments measuring 10 to 20 nm in diameter. Lewy bodies stain with monoclonal antibodies to ubiquitin (a polypeptide associated with protein degradation) and to selected antigens from tubulin, paired helical filaments, and neurofibrillary tangle proteins. In many patients with PD, ubiquitin staining has revealed the presence of cortical intracytoplasmic inclusions that resemble Lewy bodies but have a homogeneous structure. Dopaminergic nuclei in the ventral tegmental area also show cell loss and Lewy body formation. Other neurotransmitter systems may undergo neuronal loss and Lewy body formation in PD, including noradrenergic neurons (in the locus ceruleus and the dorsal nucleus of the vagus), cholinergic neurons (in the nucleus basalis of Meynert and the Westphal-Edinger nucleus), and serotonergic neurons (in the dorsal raphe nucleus). Damage to these systems is usually less severe than that to the substantia nigra, and some symptoms of PD that respond poorly to dopamine replacement therapy may persist because of damage to non-dopaminergic systems.

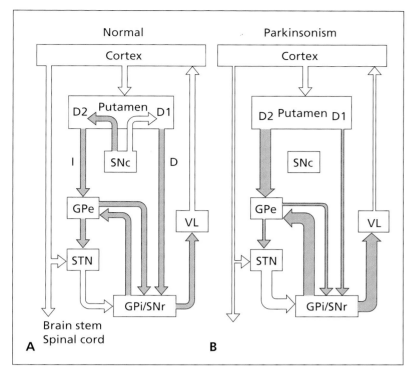

Figure 9-8. Pathophysiology of the basal ganglia in Parkinson's disease. **A,** Dopamine from the substantia nigra pars compacta innervates the neostriatum, with a mechanism affecting two distinct pathways, the "indirect" and the "direct" pathways. Dopamine inhibits the striatal neurons via D2 receptors belonging to the "indirect pathway." These striatal γ-aminobutyric acid (GABA) neurons send inhibitory output fibers to the globus pallidus externa (GPe); the GPe sends GABAergic inhibitory fibers to the subthalamic nucleus (STN); the STN sends glutamatergic excitatory fibers to the globus pallidus interna (GPi); the GPi sends GABAergic inhibitory fibers to the ventrolateral (VL) and ventral anterior nuclei of the thalamus. The net effect of dopamine via the "indirect" pathway is to inhibit the tonically active GPi. On the other hand, dopamine excites, via D1 receptors, the striatal neurons belonging to the "direct pathway." These striatal GABAergic neurons send inhibitory output fibers directly to the GPi. The net effect of dopamine via the "direct" pathway is to inhibit the tonically active GPi. Thus, by both the "indirect" and "direct" pathways, the GPi is inhibited by dopamine acting through the striatum. **B,** In Parkinson's disease, with loss of striatal dopamine due to degeneration of the substantia nigra pars compacta neurons, the net effect is to increase the activity of the GPi neurons by both the "indirect" and "direct" pathways. This has stimulated attempts to undo the effects of dopamine deficiency by surgical lesions in the STN and GPi. SNc—substantia nigra pars compacta; SNr—substantia nigra pars reticulata. (*Adapted from* Wichmann and colleague [2].)

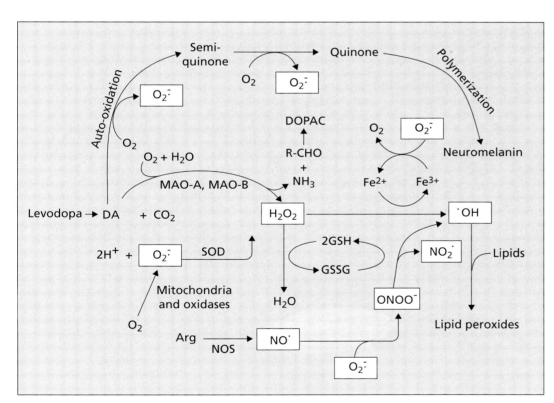

Figure 9-9. Dopamine metabolism pathways that can lead to the synthesis of hydrogen peroxide and the oxyradicals, superoxide and hydroxyl radical, and the possible contribution of nitric oxide in reacting with the superoxide radical to form other free radicals. The free radicals and H_2O_2 are highlighted within rectangles.

The cause of degeneration of the substantia nigra in Parkinson's disease (PD) remains unknown. Some explanations currently considered include intoxication by an endogenous or environmental toxicant, or a genetic predisposition. None of the current proposals explains all the features of PD as we know it, although each explains some aspects of the disease, and each hypothesis is actively being investigated by its proponents. The toxicant MPTP (1-methyl-4-phenyl-1,2,3,6-tetrahydropyridine)

produces a condition in people and animals that resembles PD both clinically and pathologically; no similar toxin in the environment has yet been identified. Oxidation of dopamine in the substantia nigra produces oxygen radicals that are toxic to cells. There is indirect evidence that patients with PD may not be able to detoxify these radicals adequately, and this might produce the ongoing neuronal damage that occurs in PD. Attempts to retard the progression of PD using antioxidants have not yet proven beneficial. A twin study in 1977 [3] indicated a low concordance of PD in monozygotic twins, which initially discouraged attempts to find a genetic basis for PD. Case-controlled studies, however, have shown that relatives of patients with PD have a higher risk of developing the disease than nonrelatives. Reanalysis of the original twin data, including abnormal positron emission tomography (PET) scans of apparently "asymptomatic" twins and subsequent development of PD in some originally asymptomatic twins, has renewed the search for a genetic component to PD. It has also been suggested that a combination of factors, such as an inherited predisposition to an environmental toxicant, may actually explain PD. Arg—arginine; CO_2—carbon dioxide; DA—dopamine; DOPAC—dihydroxyphenylacetic acid; Fe—iron; GSH—reduced glutathione; GSSG—oxidized glutathione; H_2O—water; H_2O_2—hydrogen peroxide; MAO—monoamine oxidase; NH_3—ammonia; NO·—nitric oxide radical; NO_2·—nitrogen dioxide radical; NOS—nitric oxide synthase; ·OH—hydroxyl radical; O_2—molecular oxygen; O_2·⁻—superoxide anion radical; ONOO⁻—peroxynitrite; R-CHO—aldehyde; SOD—superoxide dismutase.

Treatment of Motor Complications of Levodopa Therapy

Problems with response fluctuations	Possible solution
Wearing off	Controlled-release levodopa
	COMT inhibitors (entacapone, tolcapone)
	Dopamine agonist (bromocriptine, pergolide, pramipexole, ropinirole)
	Other long-acting agent (selegiline, amantadine, anticholinergic)
	More frequent doses, in smaller amounts to prevent dyskinesias
	Subthalamic nucleus stimulation
On/off	Treat as if wearing off, use liquid levodopa or apomorphine for rapid on
Yo-yo	Use dopamine agonist as main agent with tiny amounts of levodopa/carbidopa or even plain levodopa as "booster"
Dose failure	Crush levodopa/carbidopa and dissolve in large amount of liquid to promote transit through the stomach
Failure to respond after protein meal	Rearrange diet so that most protein is ingested at the end of the day—consult nutritionist to ensure balanced nutritional intake

Dyskinesias

Peak dose dyskinesias	Reduce the dose of carbidopa/levodopa and replace with other medications
Diphasic dyskinesias	Treat as for "yo-yo" above
Painful "off" dyskinesia/dystonia	Clozapine
	Amantadine
	Pallidotomy or pallidal stimulation

Figure 9-10. Treatment of motor complications of levodopa therapy. It has been suggested that levodopa itself promotes the development of complications of therapy. Although this has never been established, it seems prudent to use alternative medications when possible and minimize the dose of levodopa when it is needed. Patients with mild PD may not need any medications, although they may benefit from treatment of related conditions such as depression. In such patients, it would be ideal to prevent the progression of disease. The monoamine oxidase B (MAO-B) inhibitor selegiline was found to delay the need for levodopa in patients with mild PD, but this was probably due to its prolonged symptomatic effect rather than a true protective effect. For patients requiring symptomatic relief, but whose symptoms are still mild, a variety of other medications are available. Amantadine promotes release of dopamine from remaining nigral neurons, and provides relief of symptoms in about two-thirds of patients. Anticholinergic medications cause memory loss and confusion in older individuals but often reduce tremor when tolerated. Dopamine agonists provide modest but long-lasting symptomatic relief, especially when added to levodopa.

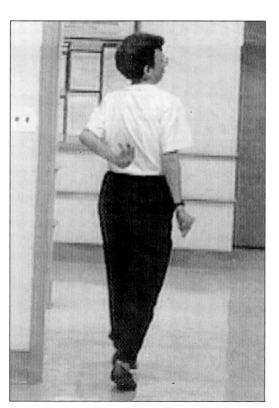

Figure 9-11. A patient with Parkinson's disease having peak levodopa dose choreic and dystonic movements. The left arm excessively swings and goes behind her back as the patient is walking. Dyskinesia is more pronounced on the side of the body that has more severe parkinsonism. Patients treated with levodopa initially generally experience long-lasting improvement in motor symptoms after each dose of levodopa. With time, many patients develop progressive reduction in the duration of benefit from each dose of medication ("wearing-off"). As wearing off develops, many also develop troublesome involuntary movements (dyskinesia or dystonia) in response to each dose of levodopa. These involuntary movements usually occur as the blood level of levodopa peaks ("peak dose" dyskinesia), or, less commonly, at the beginning and end of the dosing period (called DID for *Dyskinesia-Improvement-Dyskinesia*). As the dyskinesia or dystonia worsens, the threshold of appearance of levodopa-induced movements approaches the dose required to produce benefit, leaving an extremely narrow window between parkinsonian symptoms and excessive movement. In addition, some patients develop a variety of other fluctuations, including sudden loss of benefit ("on/off"), sudden change from severe dyskinesia to severe parkinsonian symptoms ("yo/yo"), loss of benefit after a protein meal, and failure of an occasional dose of levodopa to produce any benefit ("dose failure").

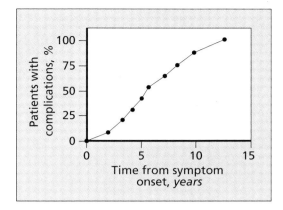

Figure 9-12. Time course for developing motor response complications in patients with Parkinson's disease (PD) treated with levodopa. In most patients with PD, symptoms of the disease respond well to levodopa, but the response becomes increasingly complex with time. Most commonly, the benefits of levodopa wear off—gradually or suddenly—a few hours after taking the medication. This can be circumvented by taking more frequent doses of levodopa. However, when dyskinesia becomes severe, the amount of levodopa taken at each dose must be decreased. To titrate the dose more accurately, levodopa can be given without carbidopa, or carbidopa/levodopa can be dissolved in water acidified with vitamin C. Sometimes, each dose of levodopa becomes so small that no benefit results. Some patients may do better using longer-acting agents, such as time-release carbidopa/levodopa or dopamine agonists. Patients with intolerable "off" periods may achieve a rapid response from the injectable medication apomorphine, or by crushing the pill and taking it with liquid to speed up entry into the small intestine. Since levodopa is not absorbed from the stomach, delay in gastric emptying may produce an apparent failure to respond to a dose of levodopa in a patient who otherwise does well, and this also may improve when the pill is dissolved in liquid. When patients do develop severe dyskinesias or dystonia, adding dopamine agonists and reducing the dose of levodopa often provide a smoother response and less severe involuntary movements than giving levodopa alone. When this fails, amantadine or the atypical neuroleptic clozapine sometimes reduces dyskinesia without worsening PD symptoms. Surgical pallidotomy or pallidal stimulation also may reduce levodopa-induced involuntary movements. The freezing phenomenon usually improves with increased medication, but occasionally it persists in someone who is otherwise adequately treated, and sometimes even worsens as medication is increased. Rarely, antiparkinsonian medications such as amantadine and levodopa may produce myoclonus severe enough to interfere with function. Patients with PD may have myoclonus even in the absence of medication, but these patients often have dementia as well, and the diagnosis of PD may be incorrect. (*Adapted from* Chase and colleagues [4].)

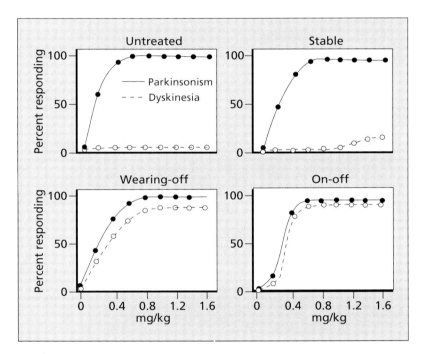

Figure 9-13. Levodopa dose-response curves in patients with Parkinson's disease who have never been treated, who have a stable response, who have "wearing-off," and who have "on-off." Curves with solid circles represent the parkinsonian motor responsiveness; curves with open circles represent the percentage of patients with dyskinesias. In patients without fluctuations, benefit appears before dyskinesias. Once patients develop wearing-off and on-off, most patients develop dyskinesias at the doses required to produce benefit. These patients have a narrow therapeutic window. (*Adapted from* Mouradian and colleagues [5].)

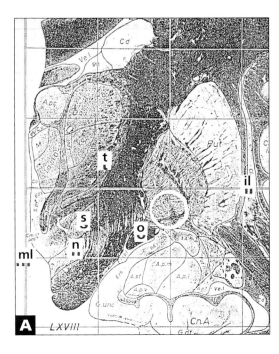

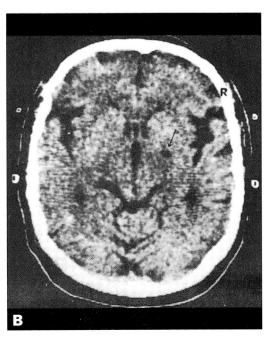

Figure 9-14. Pallidotomy in the posteroventral globus pallidus interna. **A,** Target for pallidotomy in the posteroventral globus pallidus interna. **B,** Computed tomography scan taken 6 months after pallidotomy showing the location of the lesion (*arrow*). Several neurosurgical procedures are used to treat Parkinson's disease (PD). Surgically created lesions in the output pathways from the basal ganglia have been used to treat PD since the 1950s. Stereotactically placed lesions in the ventrolateral thalamus (thalamotomy) may produce dramatic relief of tremor, but are less effective in reducing rigidity and bradykinesia. Bilateral thalamic lesions may produce speech and swallowing disturbances. Lesions made in the posteroventral globus pallidus (pallidotomy) dramatically reduce levodopa-induced dyskinesia, and may be more effective than thalamotomy in reducing bradykinesia. n—substantia nigra; o—optic tract; s—subthalamic nucleus; t—ventrolateral thalamus; ml—midplane of the third ventricle; il—intercommisural line. (*From* Laitinen and colleagues [6]; with permission.)

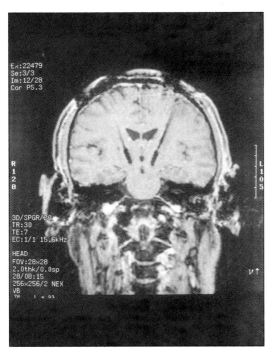

Figure 9-15. Magnetic resonance imaging scan showing bilateral subthalamic nucleus (STN) stimulator leads, with the tips of the leads in the subthalamic nucleus. Although lesioning procedures of the thalamus and pallidum can be effective for tremor and dyskinesias, they have significant risk, especially when bilateral procedures are performed. The group at Grenoble, France popularized high frequency stimulation of the brain as a safer alternative to lesioning. Deep brain stimulation is used in the thalamus for tremor and in the pallidum for levodopa-induced dyskinesias, but the most promising use is to interrupt the output of the STN [7], which is believed to normalize the "indirect pathway" of the basal ganglia. Stimulation of the STN reversibly inhibits STN neurons without destroying them. Patients with bilateral STN stimulation can reduce their intake of levodopa and at the same time have more sustained "on" periods with fewer dyskinesias. Although the initial reports have been promising, the effect of STN stimulation on cognition and such problems as gait, balance, speech, and freezing is still not clear.

Progressive Supranuclear Palsy

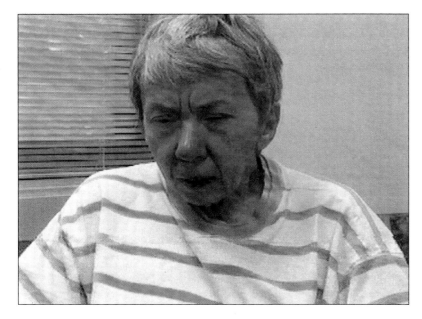

Figure 9-16. A patient with advanced progressive supranuclear palsy. In addition to not being able to voluntarily move her eyes, she has blepharospasm (eyelid closure), furrowed brow, deep nasolabial folds, and a flexed head.

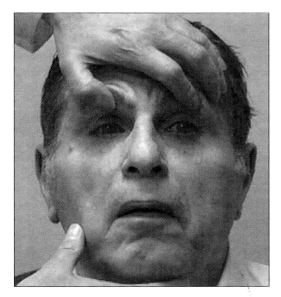

Figure 9-17. A patient with progressive supranuclear palsy (PSP) who is having his oculocephalic reflexes (doll's eyes) tested to determine whether the origin of the gaze palsy is supranuclear. The patient, who is unable to look down voluntarily, is asked to look straight ahead at an object while the examiner tilts the patient's head backwards and keeps the eyelids apart to look for downward movement of the eyes. If the eyes move downward, the origin of the gaze palsy is supranuclear.

The defining description of PSP appeared in 1964 in an article by Steele, Richardson, and Olszewski [8]. The prevalence of PSP has been estimated at 1.39 per 100,000. The mean age at onset is about 65 years, with a male preponderance in most series. Symptoms are steadily progressive, and death usually occurs 5 to 10 years after onset from aspiration or from the sequelae of multiple falls or bed sores. When supranuclear palsy (especially the loss of downgaze) appears early in the course of an akinetic-rigid syndrome, the diagnosis of PSP is likely.

PSP may be suspected in the absence of supranuclear palsy when other typical features are present. Frequent or continuous square wave jerks (small saccades alternately to the left and right in the horizontal plane) are often present. Patients with PSP lose postural reflexes early in the course of the disorder, and falling is an early feature. While walking, patients often assume a broad base, abduct the upper extremities at the shoulder and flex at the elbows, producing a characteristic gait that suggests PSP. Freezing (abrupt, transient interruption of motor activity) may be severe, and in some cases may be the major manifestation of PSP. Facial dystonia (deep nasolabial folds and furrowed brow) may create an angry or puzzled look when combined with a wide-eyed, unblinking stare. Axial rigidity is often more prominent than rigidity of the extremities, and in some cases, the limbs may have normal or reduced tone. Patients may be unable to open their lids even in the absence of orbicularis oculi spasms. This has been termed "apraxia of eyelid opening," but the phenomenon does not represent true apraxia; it might be the result of inappropriate inhibition of the levator palpebrae [9].

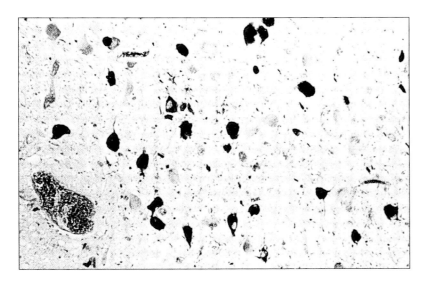

Figure 9-18. Neurofibrillary tangles in the locus ceruleus in a patient with progressive supranuclear palsy (PSP). This is a low power (magnification × 160) micrograph using a Gallyas (silver impregnation) technique. The pathology of PSP is characterized by cell loss and gliosis in the globus pallidus, the subthalamic nucleus, the red nucleus, the substantia nigra, the dentate nucleus, the periaqueductal gray matter, and the tectum of the brain stem. Neurofibrillary tangles consisting of 15-nm straight filaments—distinct from the tangles of Alzheimer's disease—are found in the same areas, but may also occur diffusely in the brain stem. Senile plaques are not found. Abnormal glia, with paired nuclei and fibrous inclusions, have been found in PSP but not in Parkinson's disease, striatonigral degeneration, or Alzheimer's disease. These inclusions, which stain with antibodies against the microtubule-associated protein tau, seem to differ from the glial inclusions described in multiple system atrophy. (*From* Lantos [10]; with permission.)

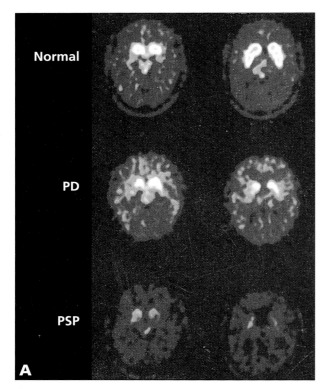

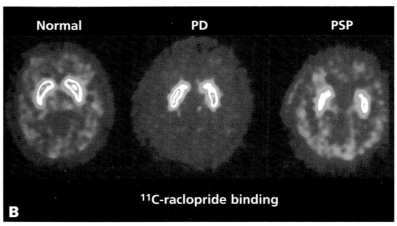

Figure 9-19. Positron emission tomographic (PET) scans comparing fluorodopa and raclopride uptake in a patient with progressive supranuclear palsy (PSP), a patient with Parkinson's disease (PD), and a normal control. **A,** Fluorodopa uptake is severely reduced in PSP, whereas some uptake occurs in the caudate nucleus in PD. **B,** Raclopride is a dopamine D2 receptor antagonist used to measure the number of available D2 receptors. PET scans show a loss of D2 receptors in the caudate nucleus and the putamen in the patient with PSP, but normal numbers of receptors in the patient with PD. Brain stem atrophy may be visualized on computed tomography (CT) or magnetic resonance imaging (MRI) of patients with PSP, but this finding is neither sensitive nor specific. A decreased signal in the putamen detected with high-field strength, T2-weighted MRI may distinguish PSP from normal scans, but is more characteristic of multiple system atrophy syndromes. PET scanning currently provides the most useful neuroimaging tool. Imaging of dopamine uptake with ^{18}F-fluorodopa reveals a decrease in fluorodopa uptake in both the anterior and the posterior putamen compared to uptake in PD, which is reduced in the posterior putamen but less so in the anterior putamen and the caudate nuclei. The overall severity of symptoms in PSP does not correlate with the reduction in fluorodopa uptake, highlighting the importance of pathologic changes outside the substantia nigra. PET scanning with ^{18}F-deoxyglucose reveals an anterior-to-posterior gradient, with the greatest hypometabolism occurring in the frontal cortex, and to a lesser degree in the striatum, thalamus, and cerebellum. Scanning with markers of dopamine D2 binding in the striatum, such as raclopride, demonstrates a moderate reduction in dopamine binding sites in PSP, but may be normal in some patients. (*From* Brooks [11]; with permission.)

Multiple System Atrophy

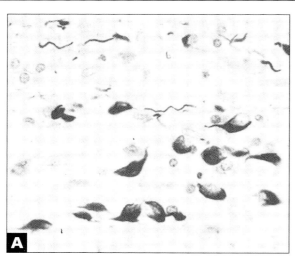

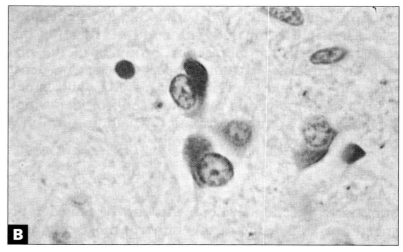

Figure 9-20. Multiple system atrophy (MSA). **A,** Low power, Gallyas silver-stained cytoplasmic inclusions and abnormal cell processes. **B,** High power, ubiquitin-stained inclusions in oligodendroglia in multiple system atrophy. The term *multiple system atrophy* was coined in 1969 by Graham and Oppenheimer in response to the observation that patients with a levodopa-unresponsive, akinetic-rigid syndrome plus cerebellar deficits or autonomic failure sometimes had widespread pathologic findings that could not be predicted on the basis of the clinical signs and symptoms [12]. These patients can be classified on clinical grounds as having Shy-Drager syndrome (SDS) if they have parkinsonism plus autonomic failure; olivopontocerebellar atrophy (OPCA) if they have parkinsonism plus cerebellar deficits; and striatonigral degeneration (SND) if they have levodopa-unresponsive parkinsonism without cerebellar signs, prominent autonomic dysfunction, or other abnormal neurologic findings. Although some patients classified as SDS, OPCA, or SND eventually develop signs associated with the other syndromes, these categories are still useful as clinical labels, and the terms persist in general clinical use.

The areas of pathologic involvement in MSA include Onuf's nucleus, pyramidal tracts, anterior horn cells, intermediolateral cell columns of the spinal cord, pontine nuclei, substantia nigra, locus ceruleus, inferior olives, dorsal motor nucleus of the vagus, vestibular nuclei, caudate, putamen, globus pallidus, and Purkinje cells. The involved areas show neuronal loss and gliosis, but neurofibrillary tangles and Lewy bodies are absent. Several reports have described cytoplasmic inclusions in glia and pontine neurons in the various MSA subtypes that may not occur in other degenerative diseases. (*From* Lantos and colleagues [13]; with permission.)

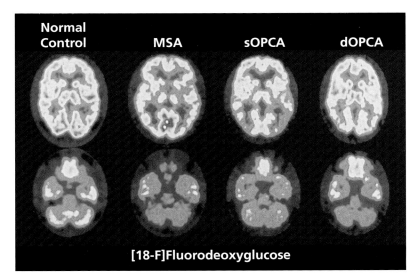

Figure 9-21. Positron-emission tomography (PET) scans using ^{18}F-fluorodeoxyglucose comparing a normal control; a patient with multiple system atrophy (MSA) who has parkinsonism, cerebellar, and autonomic dysfunction; a patient with sporadic olivopontocerebellar atrophy (sOPCA) who has parkinsonism and cerebellar dysfunction; and a patient with dominantly inherited OPCA (dOPCA) with cerebellar dysfunction. Metabolism in the cerebellum is decreased in the patients with MSA, sOPCA, and dOPCA. The cerebral cortex and basal ganglia have decreased glucose metabolism in MSA and sOPCA, but not in dOPCA.

Computed tomography (CT) scanning in MSA may reveal focal atrophy of the cerebellum and brachium pontis, and the pattern of atrophy may be useful in subdividing types of OPCA. In addition, magnetic resonance imaging (MRI) may detect demyelination of the transverse pontine fibers. One study reported decreased glucose metabolism of the brain stem and cerebellum on PET scanning. Striatonigral degeneration (SND) may be difficult to distinguish from Parkinson's disease (PD) early in the course, owing to the absence of marked cerebellar or autonomic deficits. Severe pathologic involvement of the putamen should be detectable in SND by neuroimaging techniques. Some reports have described decreased T2-weighted signals on MRI in the putamen, and decreased striatal glucose metabolism in patients with the SND variant of MSA. (*From* Gilman and colleagues [14]; with permission.)

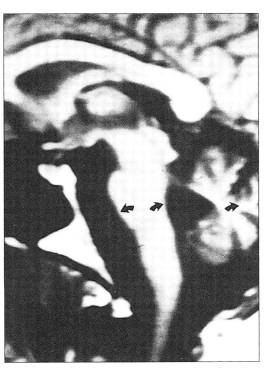

Figure 9-22. Magnetic resonance imaging (MRI) of a patient with olivopontocerebellar atrophy. The sagittal T1-weighted MRI demonstrates atrophy of the pons and cerebellum (*arrows*). (*From* Rutledge and colleagues [15]; with permission.)

Cortical-Basal Ganglionic Degeneration

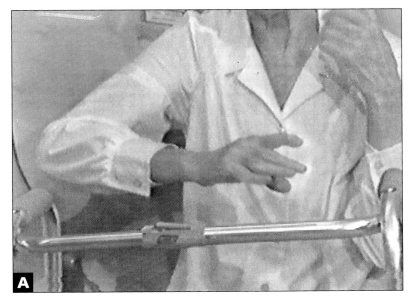

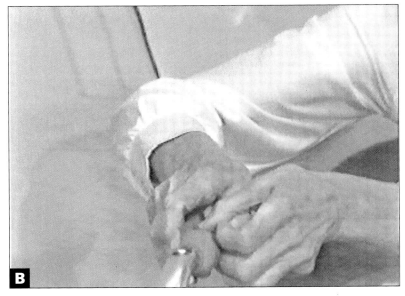

Figure 9-23. Unilateral dystonic and rigid right arm and hand in a patient with cortical-basal ganglionic degeneration. **A,** The patient has difficulty moving the right arm to the location she desires. **B,** To place or remove the apractic right hand onto or off of the handle of the walker, the patient must guide it with her left hand.

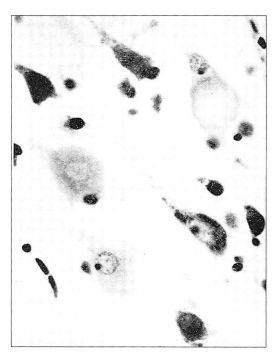

Figure 9-24. Achromatic, ballooned neurons with eccentric nuclei in cortical-basal ganglionic degeneration (CBGD) (cresyl violet stain, magnification × 650). CBGD was first described in 1968 by Rebeiz, Kolodny, and Richardson and was named "cortico-dentato-nigral degeneration with neuronal achromasia" after the characteristic pathologic finding. The disease was considered rare and not diagnosable during life until several unique features were recognized. To date, over 60 cases have been reported, most without pathologic verification, so that the full spectrum of the condition is not certain. Typical patients present with markedly asymmetric parkinsonism and cortical deficits. One limb, usually the upper but occasionally the lower, develops loss of dexterity, followed by athetotic posturing that progresses to dystonia, and then to a fixed posture that is sometimes painful. The cortical deficits include ideomotor apraxia, ideational apraxia, loss of graphesthesia or stereognosis, cortical focal myoclonus, and aphasia. The affected limb may have complex, unsuppressible movements, reminiscent of the "alien limb" phenomenon. Some patients have had prominent pseudobulbar palsy, with snout, palmomental, and grasp reflexes, and with emotional incontinence. In the characteristic speech disturbance, volume is preserved but speech becomes slurred and labored. Because of the speech and motor disturbances, communication becomes difficult. Although some patients have developed cognitive impairment, dementia has not been an early feature in most patients. Postural reflexes are lost early, resulting in falling. Supranuclear palsy may occur late in the course, and other disturbances of eye movement, characterized as apraxia, have been described. Rarely, apraxia of eyelid opening and lower motor neuron signs have been reported. CBGD progresses more rapidly than Parkinson's disease, with a mean survival time of about 4 to 7 years after onset of symptoms. (*From* Rebeiz and colleagues [16]; with permission.)

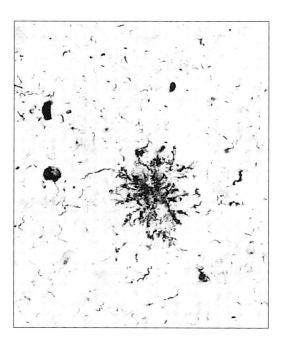

Figure 9-25. Cytoskeletal abnormalities in cortical-basal ganglionic degeneration (CBGD) (modified Gallyas stain, magnification × 300). Cytoplasm of the pyramidal neurons in the precentral cortex is densely stained. Star-like tufts and thread-like structures are visible. The pathologic findings of CBGD are characterized by cell loss, depigmentation, and gliosis in the substantia nigra with few, if any, Lewy bodies. Asymmetric cell loss and gliosis also occur in focal areas of the cerebral cortex. Involvement of other subcortical areas and the dentate nucleus is more variable. The putamen, globus pallidus, caudate, thalamus, dentate, and subthalamus may be involved. The characteristic histologic findings are ballooned, poorly staining (achromatic) neurons in any of the forementioned areas. These are similar, and may be identical, to abnormal cells found in Pick's disease, and a possible relationship between the two conditions has been suggested. New staining techniques have shown cytoskeletal abnormalities in cortical neurons of patients with CBGD that may be unique to this disease. (*From* Uchihara and colleagues [17]; with permission.)

Hemiparkinsonism-Hemiatrophy Syndrome

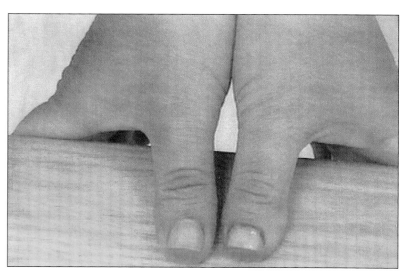

Figure 9-26. Patient with hemiparkinsonism-hemiatrophy syndrome, demonstrating the smaller-sized left thumb compared with the right thumb. In 1981, Klawans first identified patients with symptoms of Parkinson's disease (PD) limited to one side of the body and atrophy of the same side of the body (hemiparkinsonism-hemiatrophy syndrome or HP-HA) [18]. These patients were younger at onset of disease than most patients with PD; the course of PD tended to progress slowly, and symptoms remained limited to one side of the body. In subsequent reports, some patients with HP-HA have developed bilateral symptoms, but they often remain strikingly asymmetric. Many have had dystonia of the affected side prior to taking anti-parkinsonian therapy. The extent of atrophy varies: some patients have hemiatrophy of the face and upper and lower extremities, whereas others may have atrophy limited to one limb. Contralateral brain hemiatrophy may or may not accompany the body hemiatrophy. Some patients have a history of birth injury, suggesting possible asymmetric damage to the substantia nigra early in life. The response to levodopa in HP-HA has ranged from poor to excellent.

Parkinsonism-Dementia Syndromes

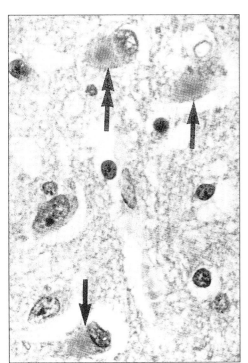

Figure 9-27. Cortical Lewy bodies (*arrows*) in specimen from a patient with diffuse Lewy body disease. Some patients with parkinsonism and dementia (or dementia alone) have diffuse Lewy body disease (DLBD) when examined pathologically, with Lewy bodies appearing in the neocortex and limbic regions in addition to the substantia nigra and other regions typical of Parkinson's disease (PD). These patients have a high prevalence of psychiatric symptoms (including agitation, hallucinations, and delusions), and tend to develop dementia before parkinsonism. The prevalence of DLBD is unknown.

The combination of parkinsonism and severe dementia is commonly encountered and presents a diagnostic challenge. Some dementia syndromes may include an akinetic-rigid state (eg, Creutzfeldt-Jakob disease, Pick's disease, Parkinson-dementia–amyotrophic lateral sclerosis complex of Guam), but account for only a small percentage of patients with parkinsonism and severe dementia. Concurrent Alzheimer's disease (AD) or a combination of AD with cortical Lewy bodies probably accounts for a larger percentage of patients in this category, as patients with PD are believed to have an increased risk for developing Alzheimer's disease. (*From Journal of the Neurological Sciences,* volume 95, Perry and colleagues, Senile dementia of lewy body type, pages 119 to 139, 1990, with permission from Elsevier Science.)

Normal Pressure Hydrocephalus

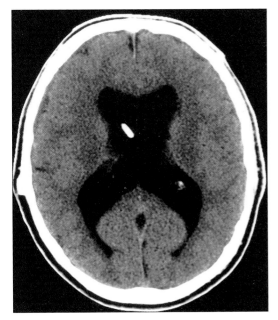

Figure 9-28. Computed tomography scan of a patient with normal-pressure hydrocephalus, which shows dilated ventricles. The patient had an excellent response to ventriculopleural shunting. In 1965, Hakim and Adams described patients with gait disturbance, dementia, and urinary incontinence caused by communicating hydrocephalus (large ventricles) with normal cerebrospinal fluid (CSF) pressure [20]. In some patients, trauma or subarachnoid-hemorrhage preceded the development of symptoms, but others had no apparent cause. Patients with this condition of normal pressure hydrocephalus (NPH) may improve temporarily after lumbar puncture and permanently after surgical diversion of CSF (eg, after ventriculoperitoneal shunting). Some patients with NPH seem to have their feet stuck to the ground, producing a "magnetic" gait, but other forms of gait disorder have also been observed. Patients with NPH may have facial masking, hypophonia, or other features of mild parkinsonism, so that NPH should be considered whenever gait disturbance is out of proportion to the other signs of parkinsonism. Enlarged ventricles and gait disorder, however, are not pathognomonic of NPH, and some patients with this combination do not improve after shunting. To identify patients who are candidates for surgical shunting, some clinicians have measured improvement after multiple daily lumbar punctures or several days of lumbar drainage. Attempts to establish other radiologic or laboratory criteria for identifying good candidates for shunting have not been successful.

Dystonia

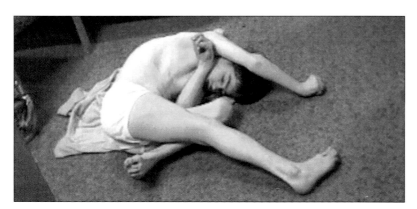

Figure 9-29. A patient with advanced childhood-onset generalized idiopathic torsion dystonia. This boy, who uses a wheelchair, is most comfortable lying on the floor in this position. The left hip, knee, elbow, and wrist are flexed; the right hip is flexed and the knee extended; the right arm is elevated with the elbow and wrist extended.

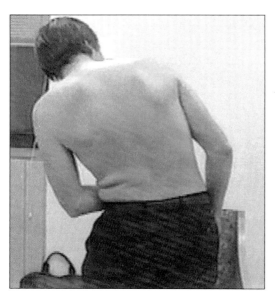

Figure 9-30. Scoliosis due to truncal dystonia. Dystonia is defined as a syndrome of sustained muscle contractions, frequently causing twisting and repetitive movements or abnormal postures. Dystonic movements vary, but certain features characterize dystonia and help distinguish it from other movement disorders: 1) the speed of contractions may be slow or rapid, but at the peak of movement, dystonia tends to be sustained; 2) whatever the speed, contractions almost always have a consistent directional or patterned character; and are predictably present in specific muscle groups; 3) dystonic contractions are usually aggravated during voluntary movement (action dystonia) and may only occur with specific actions such as writing.

The sustained, directional, patterned qualities of the movements distinguish dystonia from the simple shock-like contractions of myoclonus; the random, flowing, unsustained contractions characteristic of chorea; and the regular oscillations of tremor.

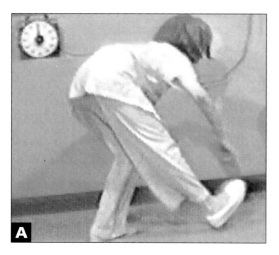

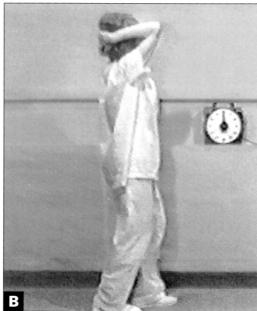

Figure 9-31. Patient with generalized dystonia (**A**) who has a lessening of the axial dystonia using a sensory trick (**B**). An almost unique characteristic of dystonia is the sensory trick, or *geste antagoniste*, performed by many patients. Sensory tricks consist of tactile or proprioceptive maneuvers by the patient to diminish dystonic movements. For example, patients with torticollis often place their hand on the chin, side of the face, or occiput to reduce nuchal contractions; patients with oromandibular dystonia may obtain relief by placing an object such as a toothpick in the mouth; and patients with writer's cramp often touch the affected hand with the other hand. The physiologic basis of sensory tricks is unknown.

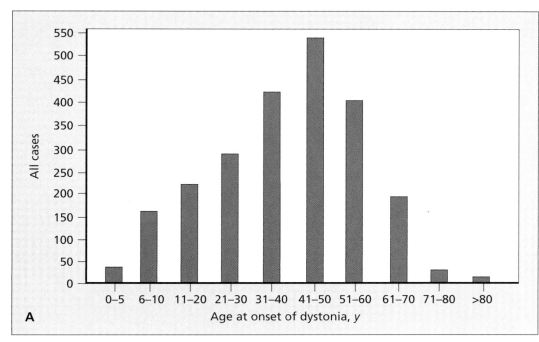

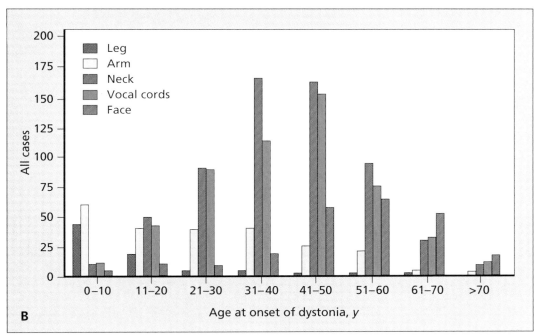

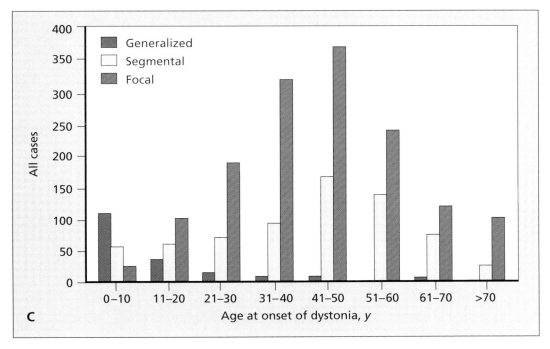

Figure 9-32. Age-of-onset distribution of primary dystonia. Age-at-onset distributions for (**A**) all cases, (**B**) for different sites at onset, and (**C**) for different distributions. The age-at-onset distributions of primary dystonia illustrates the different phenotypes observed in children and adults; the early-onset group consists primarily of limb-onset cases that frequently generalize; the late-onset group consists primarily of cervical and cranial-onset cases that remain localized as focal or segmental dystonia.

Classification of Dystonia

Age at onset	Distribution	Cause
Early-onset (<21 years) Usually starts in a leg or arm and frequently progresses to involve other limbs and the trunk Late-onset (>21 years) Usually starts in the neck, cranial muscles, or arm and tends to remain localized with restricted spread to adjacent muscles	Focal (eg, writer's cramp, blepharospasm, torticollis, spasmodic dysphonia) Segmental (contiguous body regions involved, eg, face and jaw, arm and neck, both arms) Multifocal (no contiguous body regions involved, eg, arm and leg, face and arm) Generalized (both legs or one leg and trunk and at least one other body region)	Primary (or idiopathic) dystonia is the only sign, and evaluation does not reveal an identifiable exogenous cause or other inherited or degenerative disease Secondary (or symptomatic)

Figure 9-33. Classification of dystonia. Dystonia is classified in three ways: age at onset, body regions affected, and cause. Clinical and genetic studies show that a strong relationship exists between the age at onset, which parts of the body are affected first, the progression or spread of dystonia to other body parts, and the cause (Fig. 9-41) [21]. Primary dystonia that begins in childhood and adolescence (early-onset) usually involves a leg or arm first, and then spreads to other limbs and the trunk within 5 years. A large proportion of childhood-onset dystonia is due to deletion of the trinucleotide GAG in the DYT1 gene, located on chromosome 9q34 [22]. Adult- or late-onset primary dystonia usually starts in the neck, cranial muscles (including the vocal cords), or arm; progression is limited and usually restricted to adjacent muscles. Leg involvement is rare in adult-onset primary dystonia, and this finding should raise the possibility that such dystonia occurs secondary to another disorder, such as early Parkinson's disease; similarly childhood-onset dystonia that begins in the cranial muscles is rare and again raises the issue that dystonia may be secondary or may represent another condition such as dystonic tics.

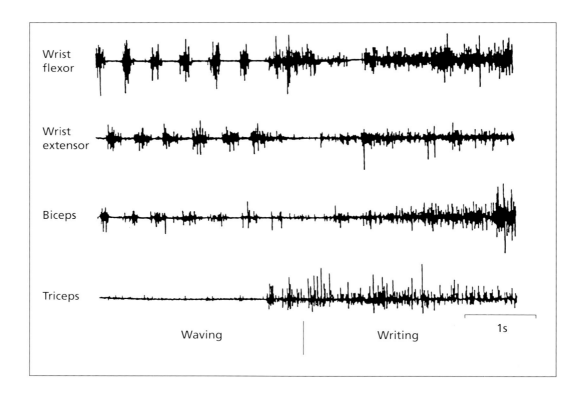

Figure 9-34. Normal reciprocal inhibition of wrist flexors and extensors during waving (*left*), and resumption of typical dystonic co-contraction when a patient with segmental dystonia of the arm stops to pick up a pen and write his name (*right*). This shows that the abnormal co-contraction may occur only with specific actions, such as brachial dystonia that is elicited with writing but not with activities such as waving.

Dystonic movements at rest and with activity are characterized by a pattern of co-contraction of agonist and antagonist muscles. Little or no activity may occur at rest or, in more severe cases, one or more of three types of electromyographic (EMG) patterns may appear: 1) long spasms that produce sustained postures; 2) repetitive, sometimes rhythmic, bursts of activity lasting 200 to 500 ms; 3) irregular brief jerks lasting less than 100 ms that resemble myoclonus. During voluntary movement, all three types of EMG activity may occur. Typically, patients have difficulty selectively activating the appropriate muscles and have co-contraction of antagonists; also contraction may spread to muscles not normally involved (overflow). Another abnormality detected in dystonia, related to the co-contraction just described, is a decrease in reciprocal inhibition. Normally antagonist muscles are actively inhibited during voluntary contraction of the agonist; this inhibition consists of an early phase, probably produced by spinal Ia inhibitory interneurons, and a later, longer-lasting phase produced by presynaptic inhibition of Ia afferent fibers. In dystonia, the degree of inhibition in the presynaptic (second) phase decreases. (*Adapted from* Rothwell and colleagues [23].)

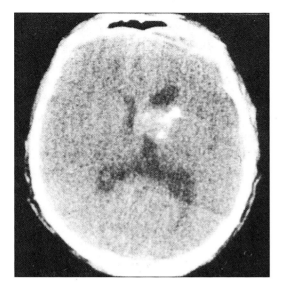

Figure 9-35. Computed tomography (CT) scan from a 38-year-old man with a 6-month history of left-turning torticollis. It shows a partially calcified enhancing lesion in the head of the right caudate nucleus that was identified as venous angioma during surgery. No pathologic disorder can be identified consistently in primary dystonia, but numerous anatomic studies implicate the basal ganglia (and rarely the brain stem) in secondary dystonia. Lesions have been found in the following: 1) striatum (both lentiform and caudate lesions, producing limb or neck dystonia); 2) cortex (producing dystonia of the limbs, torticollis, or cranial dystonia); 3) thalamus (producing limb dystonia, blepharospasm, or paroxysmal kinesigenic dystonia); 4) brain stem (producing blepharospasm); 5) cerebellum (producing torticollis); and 6) cervical cord (also producing torticollis). (*From* Marsden and colleagues [24]; with permission.)

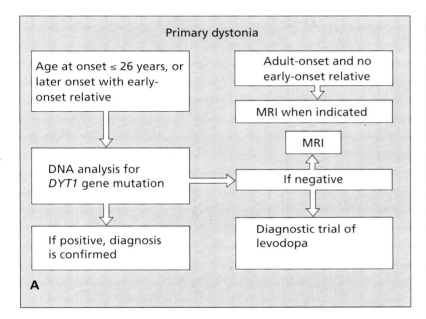

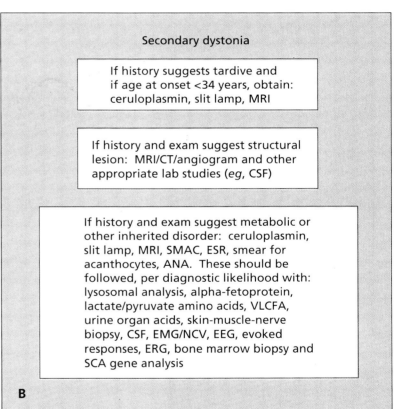

Figure 9-36. Diagnostic evaluation of dystonia. **A,** Primary dystonia. **B,** Secondary dystonia. ANA—antinuclear antibody; CSF—cerebrospinal fluid; CT—computed tomography; EEG—electroencephalogram; EMG—electromyogram; ERG—electroretinogram; ESR—erythrocyte sedimentation rate; MRI—magnetic resonance imaging; NCV—nerve conduction velocities; SMAC—serum chemistries including liver function tests; SCA—spinocerebellar atrophy; VLCFA—very long chain fatty acids.

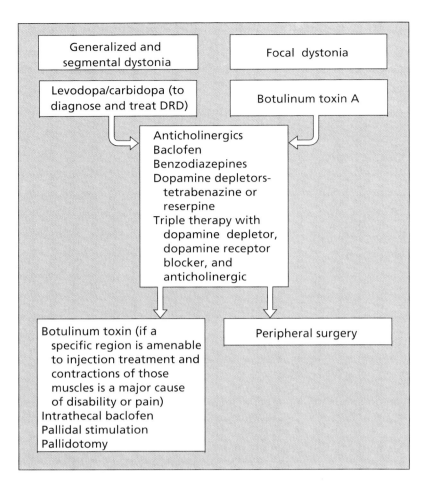

Generalized and segmental dystonia	Focal dystonia
Levodopa/carbidopa (to diagnose and treat DRD)	Botulinum toxin A

Anticholinergics
Baclofen
Benzodiazepines
Dopamine depletors-
    tetrabenazine or
    reserpine
Triple therapy with
    dopamine depletor,
    dopamine receptor
    blocker, and
    anticholinergic

Botulinum toxin (if a specific region is amenable to injection treatment and contractions of those muscles is a major cause of disability or pain)
Intrathecal baclofen
Pallidal stimulation
Pallidotomy

Peripheral surgery

Figure 9-37. Treatment of dystonia. Before initiating symptomatic treatment of dystonia, its etiology needs to be assessed for specific treatments. For example, Wilson's disease, acute drug-induced reactions, and tardive dystonia each call for a different treatment plan. Dopa-responsive dystonia (DRD) is diagnosed by the response to treatment. For most patients, including all those with primary dystonia and many with secondary forms of dystonia, symptomatic treatment can be ordered according to the distribution of muscle involvement.

Patients with early-onset generalized and segmental limb dystonia are treated first with levodopa; if no significant improvement occurs after slowly increasing the daily dose of 75 to 300 mg carbidopa/levodopa, the diagnosis of DRD is excluded and other medications are tried, beginning with anticholinergic agents. About 50% of all patients derive some benefit from current medical therapies, but few are totally relieved of their symptoms.

For most patients with focal dystonia, botulinum toxin injections can successfully ameliorate symptoms. About 90% of patients with blepharospasm and over 70% of patients with torticollis show moderate to marked improvement after botulinum toxin injections. Botulinum toxins are produced as fermentation products of the anaerobic bacterium *Clostridium botulinum*. Of the seven botulinum toxin (BTX) serotypes, BTX-A is the one used most widely in clinical practice. Injection of toxin into muscle causes temporary local muscle weakness by interfering with the release of acetylcholine from the presynaptic terminal at the neuromuscular junction.

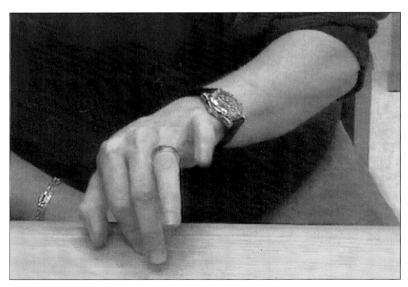

Figure 9-38. Musician's cramp, analogous to writer's cramp, is a focal dystonia of the arm induced with the action of playing a musical instrument. This patient has a pianist's cramp that is manifested when she attempts to perform piano-playing movements on top of the desk.

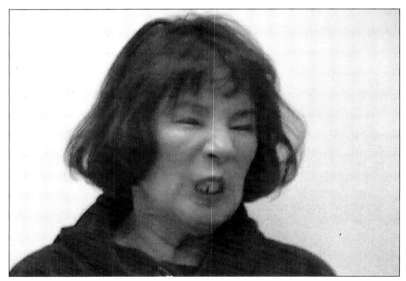

Figure 9-39. Cranial segmental dystonia, sometimes called Meige syndrome, with involvement of the facial and jaw muscles, which sometimes spreads to the neck muscles (cranial-cervical dystonia).

Primary Dystonia

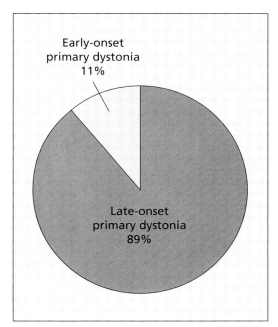

Figure 9-40. The causes of dystonia. Primary dystonias represent about 70% of patients, and secondary dystonias comprise only 30% of patients seen in movement disorder clinics. Early-onset dystonia (also known as dystonia musculorum deformans) represents about one ninth of the patients with primary dystonia. In the non-Jewish population, the prevalence of early-onset primary dystonia has been estimated at 1 to 4 per 100,000. It is about five times more common in persons of Eastern European Jewish ancestry [25]; a recent study suggests an even higher prevalence of 30 per 100,000 in this population [26]. The disorder is inherited in an autosomal dominant fashion, with reduced penetrance of 30% to 40% [27]. Because of the low penetrance, and because relatives may have mild signs never diagnosed as dystonia, patients are often the only one known to be affected in a family. Many cases of early-onset are caused by the *DYT1* gene, localized to chromosome 9q34 [22]. Direct testing for the DYT1 mutation is commercially available [28].

Late-onset dystonia represents the remainder of the patients with primary dystonia. The prevalence of late-onset primary dystonia is estimated to be 29.5 per 100,000. Family studies of patients with late-onset focal dystonias indicate that at least some cases are inherited in an autosomal dominant fashion with reduced penetrance [26]. Linkage studies in a few large non-Jewish families with late-onset of symptoms [29] or prominent cranial and cervical involvement [30] have excluded the *DYT1* gene. At least one gene locus on chromosome 18 has been identified to underlie torticollis [31]. (*Data from* the dystonia database on the Movement Disorder Group at Columbia Presbyterian Medical Center's Dystonia Clinical Research Center.)

Secondary Dystonia

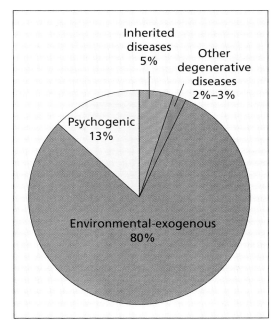

Figure 9-41. Causes of secondary dystonia. When evaluating patients for secondary dystonia, inherited diseases, degenerative disorders, environmental or exogenous factors, and psychogenic factors need to be considered. About 5% of cases of secondary dystonia are associated with inherited diseases, including dopa-responsive dystonia, myoclonic dystonia, ataxia telangiectasia, Wilson's disease, Huntington's disease, spinocerebellar ataxias, GM_1 and GM_2 gangliosidoses, metachromatic leukodystrophy, Lesch-Nyhan syndrome, homocystinuria, glutaric acidemia, methylmalonic aciduria, triosephosphate isomerase deficiency, mitochondrial cytopathies, dentatorubropallidoluysian atrophy, neuroacanthocytosis, Hallervorden-Spatz disease, dystonic lipidoses, X-linked Dystonia-Parkinsonism, intranuclear hyaline inclusion disease, juvenile ceroid-lipofuscinosis, Fahr's disease (calcification of the basal ganglia), rapid-onset dystonia-parkinsonism, Rett's syndrome, Pelizaeus-Merzbacher disease, and hereditary juvenile dystonia-parkinsonism.

Two percent to three percent of secondary dystonia cases are associated with degenerative disorders and disorders for which an inherited basis has not been established, such as Parkinson's disease, progressive supranuclear palsy (PSP), cortical-basal ganglia degeneration (CBGD), and multiple system atrophy (MSA).

Environmental or exogenous factors are associated with 80% of secondary dystonia cases. This is the largest group of secondary dystonia and includes tardive dystonia due to dopamine receptor blockers (40%), perinatal cerebral anoxia, signs of which may be delayed for years (15%), trauma (10%), stroke (cerebral infarction or hemorrhage) (5%), encephalitis (4%), tumor or vascular malformation (1%), and other conditions (5%). Psychogenic factors are associated with 13% of secondary dystonia cases.

A common cause of secondary dystonia, which is under-represented in tables of secondary causes of dystonia, is Parkinson's disease (PD) and other parkinsonism disorders (PSP, MSA, CBGD). Although "pure" dystonia as a presenting sign of PD is not common, dystonic posturing, such as action-induced foot flexion, is a frequent early complaint. Furthermore, trunk flexion and tilt that appear in the course of PD and dystonia occurring as a complication of levodopa therapy are common.

A. Clinical Signs Suggesting Secondary Dystonia

Parkinsonism	Neuropathy	Supranuclear oculomotor	Optic/Retinal	Ataxia
DRD	MLD	Dystonic-lipidoses	GM$_2$	Ataxia-telangiectasia
Wilson's	Neuroacanthocytosis	SCA1 and SCA3	HSD	Mitochondrial
Gangliosidosis	SCA1 and SCA3	Ataxia-telangiectasia	NCL	SCA1 and SCA3
HD	Mitochondrial	PSP	Mitochondrial	MLD
XPD		CBGD	LHON	Dystonic-lipidoses
RDP		HD	Homocystinuria	NCL
HSD		Pallidal degeneration		Hartnup's
SCA3/MJD				
Neuroacanthocytosis				
PD				
PSP				
CBGD				
Toxins: manganese, methanol, CS$_2$				
Anoxia				
Calcification of BG				
Hemiatrophy/hemiPD				

B. Clinical Clues That Dystonia Is Secondary

History of a possible etiologic factor
  Head trauma
  Peripheral trauma
  Encephalitis
  Drug exposure
  Toxin exposure
  Perinatal anoxia
Presence of neurologic abnormality other than dystonia
Presence of false weakness, false sensory findings, or inconsistent or incongruous movements to suggest a psychogenic basis
Onset at rest rather than with action
Site of onset does not fit usual pattern seen in primary dystonia, *eg*, cranial-onset in a child or leg-onset in an adult
Hemidystonia
Abnormal brain imaging
Abnormal laboratory work-up

Figure 9-42 Secondary dystonia. **A,** Clinical signs suggesting clinical dystonia. **B,** Clinical clues that dystonia is secondary. BG—basal ganglia; CBGD—cortical-basal ganglionic degeneration; CS$_2$—carbon disulfide; DRD—dopa-responsive dystonia; GM$_2$—gangliosidosis type 2; HD—Huntington's disease; HSD—Hallervorden-Spatz disease; LHON—Leber's hereditary optic atrophy; MJD—Machado-Joseph disease; MLD—metachromatic leukodystrophy; NCL—neuronal ceroid lipofuscinosis; PD—Parkinson's disease; PSP—progressive supranuclear palsy; RDP—Rapid-onset dystonia parkinsonism; SCA1—spinocerebellar ataxia type 1; SCA3—spinocerebellar ataxia type 3; XPD—X-linked parkinsonism dystonia.

Differential Features Among Juvenile Parkinsonism, Dopa-responsive Dystonia, and Childhood-onset Primary Dystonia

	Juvenile parkinsonism	Dopa-responsive dystonia	Primary dystonia
Age-onset, *y*	8–21	Average 6, infancy to 12, rarely to 16	>4 and <44, average 9
Gender	Male > female	Female > male	Male = female
Initial sign	Foot dystonia Parkinsonism	Leg dystonia Stiff-legged gait	Limb dystonia Rarely neck or voice dystonia
Diurnal	No	Often	Rare
Bradykinesia	Yes	Yes	No
Postural instability	Yes	Yes	No
Initial response to levodopa	Yes with moderate or high dose	Yes with very low dose (25/100 mg)	None or slight
Long-term levodopa response	Fluctuations with dyskinesias	Stable	Unknown
Fluorodopa PET	Decreased	Normal or slightly decreased	Normal
CSF HVA	Decreased	Decreased	Normal
CSF biopterin	Moderately decreased	Markedly decreased	Normal
Gene	*Parkin* mutations in most	GTP cyclohydrolase in many	*DYT1* gene in many
Genetic testing	Research only	Research only	Commercial testing
Prognosis	Progressive	Excellent with treatment	Usually progresses at first, then plateaus

Figure 9-43. Differential features among juvenile parkinsonism, dopa-responsive dystonia, and childhood-onset primary dystonia. About 5%–10% of patients with childhood-onset dystonia have dopa-responsive dystonia (DRD). This is an autosomal dominant condition with reduced penetrance that is influenced by gender (females are affected more commonly). Many cases appear to be caused by mutations in the gene for GTP cyclohydrolase 1; this is the first enzymatic step in the synthesis of tetrahydrobiopterin, a cofactor for tyrosine hydroxylase. Thus, partial deficiencies in this enzyme are thought to impair synthesis of dopamine [32].

DRD mimics early-onset primary dystonia, with leg involvement and an abnormal gait being the first and predominant features. Usually symptoms worsen as the day progresses and may improve after a nap. The gait is frequently stiff-legged and plantar flexion or eversion may occur. Dystonia may also involve the trunk and arms, and less commonly the neck. Signs of parkinsonism are usually present but may be subtle; these include postural instability, hypomimia, and bradykinesia. The patient may have hyperreflexia, particularly in the legs, and plantar extensor signs; because of the hyperreflexia and the stiff-legged gait, children with DRD are commonly misdiagnosed as having spastic diplegic cerebral palsy [33]. The diagnosis of DRD depends on both the examination findings and a dramatic response to low doses of levodopa. Treatment with as little as 50 to 200 mg of levodopa, together with a decarboxylase inhibitor, usually results in complete or nearly complete reversal of all signs and symptoms. Furthermore, patients do not develop fluctuations but maintain an excellent response to levodopa. In contrast, juvenile parkinsonism, which may begin with dystonia, requires higher doses of antiparkinson medication and typically is complicated by levodopa-related motor complications of dyskinesia and response fluctuations. CSF—cerebrospinal fluid; GTP—guanosine triphosphate; HVA—homovanillic acid; PET—positron-emission tomography.

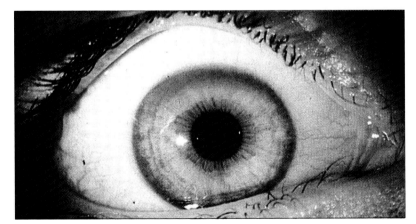

Figure 9-44. Early stage Kayser-Fleischer ring, located in the superior corneal pole only, in a patient with Wilson's disease. The rings consist of yellow-brown deposits of copper in Descemet's membrane in the cornea and may only be visible through a slit lamp. Usually they are most dense at the upper and lower poles of the corneal limbus. Because of the need for early recognition and treatment, Wilson's disease remains the most important diagnosis to consider when evaluating a patient with dystonia.

Neurologic signs of Wilson's disease usually manifest in the second or third decade, but may not become evident until the sixth decade. Dystonia, akinetic-rigid parkinsonism, and tremor with ataxia, titubation, and dysarthria are three common presenting syndromes. Drooling, "risus sardonicus" (a fixed grinning expression), clumsiness, and cognitive changes are usually present regardless of other signs. The responsible gene (a copper-transporting P-type ATPase) for this autosomal recessive condition has been cloned [34,35] and many different mutations in the gene have been identified [36]. Once a case is diagnosed, DNA analysis of linked markers can often be used to diagnose carrier status in a sibling, but direct DNA screening for mutations is not currently available. The diagnosis in a single patient, then, still rests upon finding a reduced serum ceruloplasmin level. About 5% of Wilson's patients have a normal ceruloplasmin level, and diagnosis then depends upon confirmatory evidence, including Kayser-Fleischer rings, typical computed tomographic and magnetic resonance imaging changes, low serum copper levels, increased urine copper levels, and, if necessary, liver biopsy for copper content. (*From* Wiebers and colleagues [37]; with permission.)

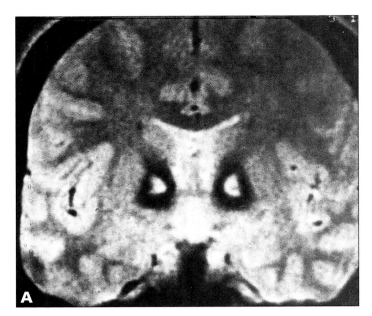
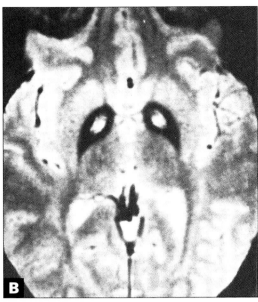

portion of patients. Onset usually occurs in childhood and adolescence, with progression to death by age 30; adult-onset and a more slowly progressive course, however, may occur. Pathologically, the basal ganglia degenerate, especially the zona reticulata of the substantia nigra and the internal segment of the globus pallidus. These areas contain pigment-bound iron and axonal spheroids. The diagnosis is supported by MRI. Early MRIs may show hyperintensity of the globus pallidus and substantia nigra on T2-weighted imaging; later in the course of disease, these lesions become target-like, with a central area of hyperintensity surrounded by a hypointense ring, as seen in this MRI scan. Another feature found in a subset of patients is the presence of acanthocytes on peripheral smear [38]. (*From* Sethi and colleagues [39]; with permission.)

Figure 9-45. T2-weighted magnetic resonance image (MRI) of Hallervorden-Spatz disease depicting the "eye of the tiger" sign, which shows a hyperintense signal (due to necrosis) surrounded by a hypointense signal (due to increased iron deposition) in the globus pallidus. **A,** Coronal view. **B,** Horizontal view.

Hallervorden-Spatz disease is a rare autosomal recessive disorder characterized by dystonia, dysarthria, pyramidal signs, parkinsonism, dementia, and psychiatric symptoms. Pigmentary retinopathy or optic atrophy is seen in a significant pro-

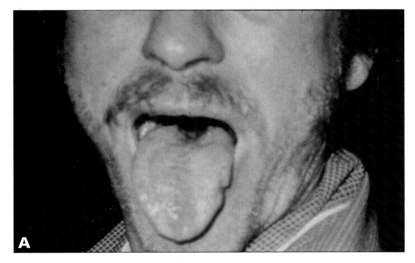

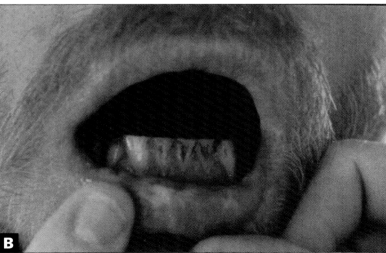

Figure 9-46. A 24-year-old man with neuroacanthocytosis and eating dystonia. He inflicted self-mutilations, which resulted in his biting off a piece of his tongue (**A**) and lip (**B**). A Wright-stained peripheral smear revealed acanthocytes (**C**), which are also depicted on scanning electron microscopy (**D**). The diagnosis of neuroacanthocytosis needs to be considered in patients with chorea, dystonia, tics, or parkinsonism. Symptoms usually begin in the third decade but age-at-onset ranges widely from 8 to 62 years. Typically, patients demonstrate lip and tongue biting (which may be mutilating), orolingual dystonia (with tongue protrusion) usually induced by eating, chorea, tics (including noisy smacking and hissing tics), parkinsonism, personality and cognitive changes, seizures, dysarthria, dysphagia, amyotrophy, and areflexia. Laboratory findings include elevated levels of creatine phosphokinase and caudate atrophy on imaging studies. The diagnosis is made by finding that more than 15% of red blood cells are acanthocytes. Various techniques have been recommended to detect acanthocytes, including diluting blood with normal saline, incubating a Wright-stained smear with EDTA, and using a scanning electron microscope [40]. (*Continued on next page*)

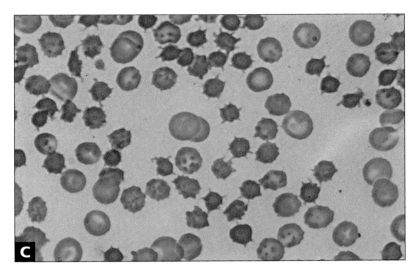

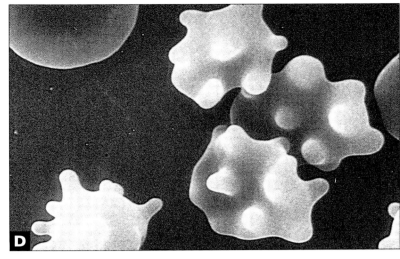

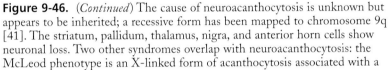

Figure 9-46. (*Continued*) The cause of neuroacanthocytosis is unknown but appears to be inherited; a recessive form has been mapped to chromosome 9q [41]. The striatum, pallidum, thalamus, nigra, and anterior horn cells show neuronal loss. Two other syndromes overlap with neuroacanthocytosis: the McLeod phenotype is an X-linked form of acanthocytosis associated with a particular erythrocyte Kell phenotype and clinical features of chorea, seizures, motor axonopathy, elevated creatine phosphokinase, hemolysis, and liver disease [42]; the other is a form of Hallervorden-Spatz syndrome, in which there appears hypo-prebetalipoproteinemia, acanthocytosis, retinitis pigmentosa, and pallidal degeneration (HARP syndrome) [43].

Huntington's Disease and Other Choreas

Causes of Chorea

Idiopathic
  Essential chorea
  Senile chorea
  Spontaneous oral dyskinesia
Hereditary
  Chorea is dominant feature
    Huntington's disease
    Hereditary nonprogressive chorea
    Neuroacanthocytosis
    Dentatorubropallidoluysian atrophy
  Chorea is not dominant feature
    Ataxia-telangiectasia
    Lesch-Nyhan syndrome
    Aminoacidurias, including glutaric
      acidemia, homocystinuria,
      phenylketonuria

Hereditary (*cont.*)
  Chorea is not dominant feature (*cont.*)
    Familial chorea and myoclonus
      epilepsy
    Wilson's disease
    Pyruvate decarboxylase deficiency
    Proprionic acidemia
    Cerebral lipidodoses, including GM$_1$
      and GM$_2$ gangliosidosis, ceroid lipo-
      fuscinosis and metachromatic
      leukodystrophy
    Spinocerebellar atrophies
    Mitochondrial cytopathies
Paroxysmal
  Paroxysmal kinesigenic choreoathetosis
  Paroxysmal nonkinesigenic (dystonic)
    choreoathetosis

(*Table continued on next page*)

Figure 9-47. Major causes of chorea. Chorea refers to an irregular, nonrhythmic, rapid, unsustained, involuntary movement that flows from one body part to another. Chorea is differentiated from other types of involuntary movements by its unpredictable quality. The timing, direction, and distribution of the movements are not patterned but random and changing. When infrequent, the brief, small-amplitude movements of chorea are difficult to distinguish from myoclonus. In Sydenham's and withdrawal emergent syndrome, the movements may be frequent and flowing, creating a picture of restlessness. Choreic movements can be suppressed partially, and patients often camouflage the movements by incorporating them into semipurposeful movements, known as parakinesias. Chorea is also distinguished by motor impersistence (or negative chorea). A common symptom of impersistence is dropping objects; on examination impersistence is elicited by asking the patient to sustain a contraction, such as protruding the tongue or gripping the examiner's hand (impersistence of gripping is known as a "milk maid" grip). (*Continued on next page*)

Causes of Chorea (*continued*)

Infectious
  Sydenham's chorea
  Encephalitides
    Epidemic, SSPE, arthropod-borne,
      syphilis, measles, varicella, pertussis,
      typhoid, mononucleosis, echovirus,
      AIDS, tuberculosis, Lyme disease
  Subacute bacterial endocarditis
  Creutzfeldt-Jakob disease
  Typhoid fever
Immunologic
  Systemic lupus erythematosus
  Primary antiphospholipid antibody
    syndrome
  Paraneoplastic
  Postvaccinal

Vascular
  Hemichorea/hemiballism secondary
    to stroke
  Polycythemia vera
  Henoch-Schönlein purpura
  Internal cerebral vein thrombosis
  Subdural hematoma
Chemicals/toxins
  Drugs
    Levodopa, neuroleptics, anticholiner-
      gics, antihistamines, oral contracep-
      tives, phenytoin, ethosuximide, carba-
      mazepine, valproate, imipramine,
      alpha methyldopa, methylphenidate,
      pemoline, methadone, cyprohepta-
      dine, cocaine
  Chemicals: CO, Hg, Li, azide
  Kernicterus

Metabolic and endocrine disorders
  Chorea gravidarum
  Birth control pills
  Idiopathic hypoparathyroidism
  Hypomagnesemia
  Addison's disease
  Hypernatremia
  Thyrotoxicosis
  Hypoglycemia
  Nonketotic hyperglycemia
  Chronic hepatocerebral degeneration
  Anoxic encephalopathy
Tumors, including metastases
Multiple sclerosis
Degeneration of centrum medianum
Postcardiac surgery

Figure 9-47. (*Continued*) Chorea has many causes, and the long list of inherited disorders and exogenous factors associated with chorea presents a daunting diagnostic challenge for the clinician. The lengthy list of causes is somewhat misleading, however; many are apparent on taking a history or produce other symptoms and signs that direct the order of a work-up. CO—carbon monoxide; Hg—mercury; Li—lithium; SSPE—subacute sclerosing panencephalitis.

Clinical Characteristics of Huntington's Disease

Age at onset
  Childhood–80s (peaks in 4th or
    5th decade)
Duration of illness
  15–20 years for adult onset
  10 years for juvenile onset
Chorea
  Upper and lower facial
  Limb and trunk
  Motor impersistence (negative chorea)
Other neurologic signs
  Abnormal saccades
  Clumsy fine motor movements
  Dancing or lurching gait
  Postural instability
  Dysarthria with abnormal rhythm and
    slurring
  Dysphagia
  Dystonia
  Tics (including noisy tics)
  Ataxia*
  Bradykinesia*
  Rigidity*
  Myoclonus*
  Seizures*

Psychiatric signs
  Apathy
  Social withdrawal
  Agitation
  Impulsiveness
  Hostility
  Depression
  Mania
  Paranoia
  Delusions
  Hallucinations
Cognitive decline
  Impaired attention
  Impaired recent memory
  Impaired judgment
  Impaired psychomotor and executive
    function (planning and initiation of
    activities and ability to switch from
    one plan to another)
  Apraxia
  Problems with verbal fluency

Figure 9-48. Clinical characteristics of Huntington's disease. The leading cause of adult-onset chorea is Huntington's disease. In children, infection and cardiac surgery are frequent causes. In all age groups, drug-induced chorea needs to be carefully investigated.

Especially likely to occur in those with juvenile onset before 20 years of age.

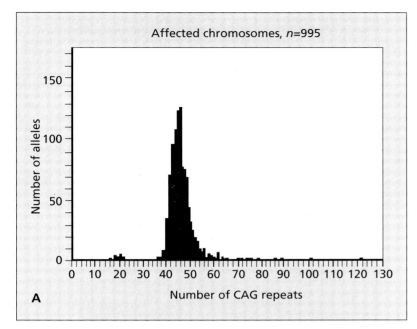

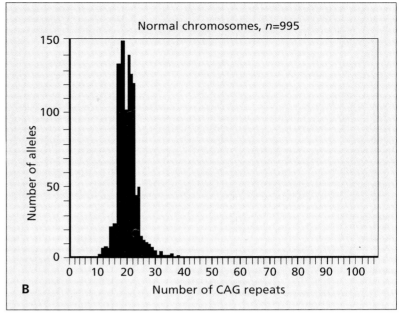

Figure 9-49. CAG triplet repeats. **A,** The number of CAG triplet repeats in chromosomes affected with Huntington's disease (HD) and **B,** 995 normal chromosomes. Huntington's disease is a true autosomal dominant condition, meaning that homozygotes and heterozygotes are clinically similar. The gene responsible for HD maps to chromosome 4p16.3 and codes a protein termed *huntingtin*. Huntingtin is found in neurons throughout the brain but its function is unknown. The gene mutation in HD consists of an unstable expansion of a CAG repeat within the coding region of the gene; this is translated into an expanded polyglutamine tract. The path-

ogenic mechanism of the enlarged polyglutamine stretch is not known, but may involve the accumulation of an associated protein. Normal individuals and people with other diseases have about 20 CAG repeats (varying from 6 to 39); HD patients have over 35 (with a range from 35 to 121), with most having more than 39 repeats. A few asymptomatic individuals have "intermediate" sized repeats of 30 to 39. The future development of HD in such patients and their risk for transmitting a further expansion still needs to be assessed [44,45]. (*Adapted from* Kremer and colleagues [46].)

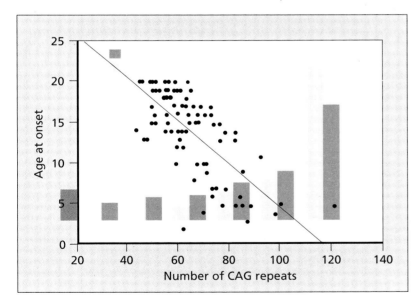

Figure 9-50. The negative correlation between CAG repeat size and age at onset of Huntington's disease (HD). There is a negative correlation between the CAG repeat size in HD and the age at onset of symptoms. The correlation is most dramatic in the range of larger repeats and much less so in the shorter range; individuals with the same number of repeats may vary widely in their ages at onset. Furthermore, the repeat size does not determine the type of symptoms at onset. Because there is significant variation in disease expression that cannot be explained by repeat size, caution needs to be exercised in the clinical interpretation of an expanded repeat other than predicting the eventual emergence of HD signs. The exception occurs in patients with very large repeats (greater than 80), in whom onset usually occurs in adolescence or childhood and the disorder is usually paternally inherited. (*Adapted from* Bressman and colleague [47].)

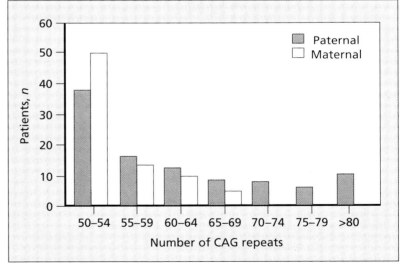

Figure 9-51. CAG repeat sizes of Huntington's disease gene on paternally inherited and maternally inherited chromosomes. Paternally inherited chromosomes have larger repeat sizes, particularly in the upper tail. CAG repeats enlarge from generation to generation, but are more unstable and more likely to undergo a large expansion during male meiosis. A corollary of this instability in male meiosis is that "sporadic cases" or new mutations arise from expansions of paternal repeats in the intermediate range [48]. (*Adapted from* Bressman and colleague [47].)

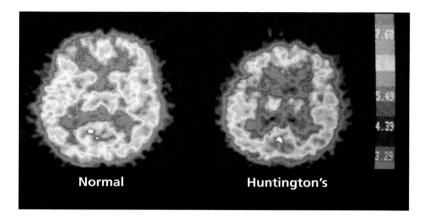

Figure 9-52. A normal fluorodeoxyglucose positron emission tomography (PET) scan (*left*) and one showing Huntington's disease (*right*). In the PET scan on the right striatal hypometabolism is seen. (*From* Martin and colleague [49]; with permission.)

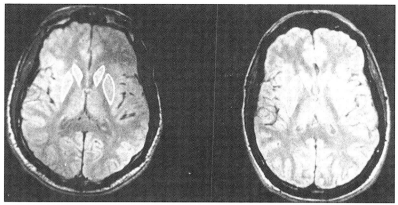

Figure 9-53. Magnetic resonance imaging (MRI) scan showing putaminal volume loss in a patient with early Huntington's disease (*left*) while the caudate appears normal when compared with the normal subject on the right. With disease progression caudate atrophy will be evident on computed tomography (CT) scan; detection of glucose hypometabolism on positron emission tomography (PET) may even precede that of caudate atrophy on CT. None of these imaging techniques, however, reliably detects asymptomatic gene carriers, which requires DNA testing. (*From* Harris and colleagues [50]; with permission.)

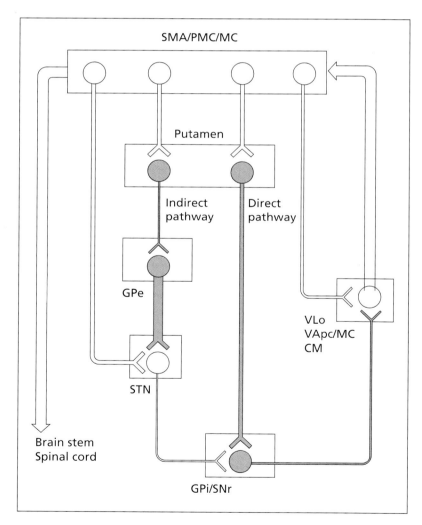

Figure 9-54. Pathophysiology of chorea. The selective loss of striatal γ-aminobutyric acid (GABA) neurons that project to the external segment of the pallidum results in decreased inhibition of pallidal inhibitory efferents to the subthalamic nucleus; the subthalamic nucleus is then over-inhibited, mimicking a subthalamic lesion. According to this model, the lack of subthalamic drive results in decreased output from the internal pallidum and thus less inhibition of the thalamus. The excessive thalamocortical drive to the premotor cortical regions results in chorea. Dopamine depletors and dopamine receptor blocking agents are the most effective drugs for suppressing choreic movements. CM—centromedian nucleus of thalamus; GPe—globus pallidus externa; GPi—globus pallidus interna; MC—motor cortex; PMC—premotor cortex; SMA—supplementary motor area; SNr—substantia nigra pars reticulata; STN—subthalamic nucleus; VAmc—nucleus ventralis anterior pars magnocellularis; VApc—nucleus ventralis anterior pars parvocellularis; VLo—nucleus ventralis lateralis pars oralis. (*Adapted from* DeLong [51].)

Tics

Classification of Tics

Primary tics
  Transient tic disorder (duration of
    tics <1 year)
  Chronic multiple motor or vocal tics
  Chronic single tic disorder
  Tourette syndrome
Secondary tics
  Infections
    Encephalitis
    Creutzfeldt-Jakob disease
    Syndenham's chorea
  Drugs
    Stimulants
      Methylphenidate
      Amphetamines
      Cocaine
    Levodopa
    Anticonvulsants
    Antipsychotics (tardive tics)
  Inherited disorders
    Huntington's disease
    Neuroacanthocytosis
  Toxins
    Carbon monoxide poisoning
  Perinatal injury
  Other causes
    Head injury
    Chromosomal abnormalities
    Autistic disorders
    Mental retardation
    Stroke
    Neurocutaneous syndromes

Figure 9-55. Classification of tics. Tics refer to spontaneous, purposeless, simple and complex movements or vocalizations that abruptly interrupt normal motor activity. The patient often experiences an associated sensation or urge to execute the tic and transient relief afterward. Tics are also temporarily suppressible.

Perhaps more than any other movement disorder, tics display the greatest range of phenomena and can resemble myoclonus, chorea, dystonia, or complex behaviors. A tic may consist of a fast (clonic), simple isolated jerk such as a blink, eye dart, or facial twitch; it may consist of a run of simple contractions such as repeated head nodding, shoulder shrugging, or blinking. Alternatively, the movement may be quite complex or sustained (*eg*, sustained eye deviation, jumping, copropraxia).

Most tics are primary and they are a common movement disorder; 5% to 24% of school-age children are estimated to have transient tics. The prevalence of Tourette syndrome (TS) is estimated to be 30 to 40 per 100,000. For the diagnosis of TS, both motor and vocal tics must be present for at least 1 year, and the age at onset must be less than 21 years (mean age at onset is 7 years and 96% of patients are affected by age 11). In TS tics generally wax and wane in severity, and one tic type is replaced by another; the tics usually begin in the face or neck (blinking and eye-rolling are common initial tics), but during the course of disease about half will involve the trunk or legs. Coprolalia, the most notorious sign in TS, is present in less than half of patients.

The etiologic (and specifically the genetic) relationship between TS, chronic tics, transient tics, and behavioral abnormalities such as obsessive-compulsive disorder (OCD), which occur with increased frequency in tic patients and their family members, is debated. Some family studies [52] suggest that TS, chronic motor tics, and obsessive-compulsive disorder are phenotypes of the same major gene, which is inherited in an autosomal dominant fashion with sex-influenced penetrance (it is higher in boys) and expression (girls are less likely to have TS and more likely to have OCD). Aside from OCD, other behavioral abnormalities associated with tics include attention deficit hyperactivity, depression, anxiety, and conduct disorders. Although most investigators believe that at least some OCD is genetically related to TS, the etiologic relationship of other behavioral disorders to tics is controversial. A gene for TS has not been localized; once it is, the phenotypic spectrum of TS can be studied more directly. The pathophysiology of TS is thought to involve a state of excess dopamine or hypersensitivity to dopamine. Dopamine receptors are not increased; however, dopamine hyperinnervation of the ventral striatum was suggested by one postmortem study [53].

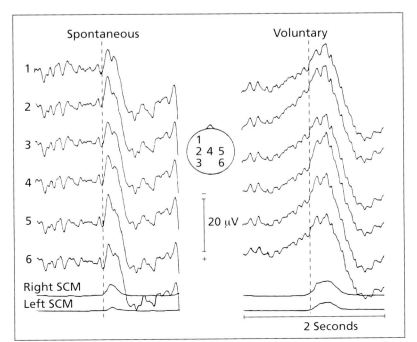

Figure 9-56. Recording of a Bereitschaftspotential showing averaged electroencephalographic (EEG) response time-locked to muscle jerks in the right sternocleidomastoid muscle of a patient with Tourette syndrome (TS). A characteristic feature of tics that helps distinguish them from most other movement disorders is an associated urge to execute the tic, or a localized preceding sensory experience (*eg*, burning in the eyes before blinking or rolling the eyes, shoulder aching before rotating the scapula, or muscle tension in the neck before nodding or jerking the head). Because of this associated sensory phenomena and the frequent relief of the sensation experienced with execution of the tic, and because tics can be transiently suppressed, patients often view their tics as intentional or semivoluntary. Electrophysiologic findings support the idea that tics are not normal voluntary actions; that is, normal planned voluntary movements are preceded on back-averaged EEG by a slow negative potential (the Bereitschaftspotential); these potentials are not observed before actual tics, but do occur when tics are voluntarily simulated. In this patient, the records on the left are from spontaneous tics and show that the Bereitschaftspotential is not present. The tracing on the right records the patient mimicking the tics. The vertical dotted line indicates the start of the muscle jerk. SCM—sternocleidomastoid muscle. (*Adapted from* Obeso and colleagues [54].)

Drugs Used to Treat Tic Disorders

Tics	Obsessive-compulsive disorder	Attention deficit disorder
Clonazepam	Imipramine	Clonidine
Clonidine	Fluoxetine	Imipramine
Baclofen	Sertraline	Desipramine
Tetrabenazine	Clomipramine	Selegiline
Risperidol	Clonazepam	Guanfacine
Fluphenazine	Carbamazepine	Methylphenydate
Pimozide		Pemoline
Haloperidol		
Trifluoperazine		
Thiothixene		
Botulinum toxin may be helpful for dystonic tics such as blinking/ blepharospasm and neck jerks		

Figure 9-57. Drugs used to treat tic disorders. The decision to treat tics is based on the degree to which the abnormal movements and sounds disrupt the patient's daily function. The benefits of tic suppression must be weighed against the risk of the medication's adverse effects. The magnitude of the tic's effect on the patient's school, work, and social life and whether the major problem is posed by the tics, attention deficit, or obsessions and compulsions must be considered.

If medication is prescribed, a drug that does not produce a tardive dyskinesia syndrome, although usually less effective, is appropriate. If this is not effective, a dopamine-receptor blocker may be necessary. All drugs should be started with a small dosage that is increased slowly, while monitoring for side effects. An adequate duration of drug trial on a sufficient dosage is necessary before deciding on efficacy—tics wax and wane and it is difficult to separate therapeutic effect from the natural history in a single patient. Changes should be made as a sequence of single steps and should always be tapered slowly. This is especially true for dopamine-receptor blockers—abrupt withdrawal can produce a withdrawal emergent syndrome.

Tremor

Types of Tremor, Etiology, Clinical, and Electrophysiologic Characteristics

Type of tremor	Etiology	Clinical and electrophysiologic characteristics
Rest	Parkinson's disease	3 to 6 Hz tremor occurring at rest, suppressed by posture-holding or action. Often most prominent during walking. The rest tremor of Parkinson's disease not infrequently returns with prolonged posture-holding, giving a "re-emergent rest tremor."
Action, posture-holding	Exaggerated physiologic tremor	8 to 12 Hz tremor occurring with action and posture-holding, often induced by specific stress, precipitant, or medication. Tremor frequency is reduced by inertial loading.
Posture-holding and action	Essential tremor	Symmetric postural and kinetic tremor of the arms, usually in the 4 to 10 Hz range, due to co-contracting antagonists. Essential tremor can be brought out by the tasks of the neurologic examination. It may interfere with activities of daily living, including handwriting.
Action, posture-holding, and sometimes at rest	Midbrain tremor	Classically described as an intention tremor, or sometimes ataxic tremor, midbrain tremor can manifest as a combination of rest, postural, and action tremors. The tremor frequency is usually between 2 to 5 Hz. The most common cause of this tremor is a focal lesion in the midbrain affecting cerebellothalamic and nigrostriatal pathways due to trauma, stroke, hemorrhage, and multiple sclerosis.
Kinetic and posture-holding	Dystonia	Irregular, asynchronous tremor, usually affecting arms or neck. Dystonic tremor has no specific electrophysiologic characteristics, but the dystonia manifests as co-contracting antagonists. Tremor may decrease with sensory trick or assumption of a "null point" posture. Includes primary writing tremor and task-specific tremor.

Figure 9-58. Types of tremor and their etiology and clinical and electrophysiological characteristics. A tremor describes the rhythmic oscillation of a body part produced by synchronous or alternating contractions of antagonist muscles. The clinical approach to tremor begins with an assessment of tremor characteristics. A *rest tremor* occurs when the limb is completely relaxed and supported. *Postural tremor* is present when the limb is maintaining a steady posture. *Kinetic tremors* occur during movement or tasks, such as water-pouring or handwriting. *Intention tremor* refers to a tremor that increases as the limb approaches the target on finger-to-nose testing. Intention tremor often implicates a lesion of the cerebellum or cerebellar outflow pathways. Postural and kinetic tremors are often considered together as *action tremors*.

Differential Diagnosis of Tremor

Tremors at rest		Action tremors
Parkinson's disease and other causes of parkinsonism	Postural tremors	Kinetic tremor
Heredodegenerative disorders	Physiologic tremors	Cerebellar disorders
Wilson's disease, neuroacanthocytosis, Hallervorden-Spatz disease, Gerstmann-Straussler-Scheinker disease, ceroid lipofuscinosis	Enhanced physiologic tremor	Multiple sclerosis, trauma, stroke, toxins, olivopontocerebellar atrophy (OPCA)
	Essential tremor	
	Postural tremor associated with Parkinson's disease, dystonia, myoclonus	Midbrain lesions
Severe essential tremor	Midbrain or rubral tremor	Task- or position-specific tremors
Midbrain or rubral tremor	Cerebellar tremor	Primary writing tremor
Myorhythmia	Neuropathy-associated tremor	Dystonic tremor
	Hereditary neuropathy, peripheral nerve injury, reflex sympathetic dystrophy, motor neuron disease	Orthostatic tremor
		Isometric tremor

Figure 9-59. Differential diagnosis of tremor. Tremor can be caused by a wide spectrum of neurologic and medical conditions. The differential diagnosis of tremor can be categorized into tremors at rest and action tremors.

Physiologic Tremor

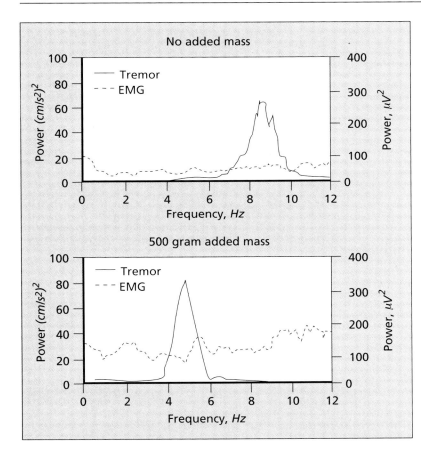

Figure 9-60. The frequency of physiologic tremor recorded at the wrist. Physiologic tremor is the oscillation of a body part resulting from the interaction of normal mechanical reflex mechanisms and a central oscillator. The usual frequency of physiologic tremor ranges between 8 to 12 Hz. The frequency of the mechanical component of the physiologic tremor is influenced by mechanical properties of the oscillating limb, including stiffness and inertia. Tremor amplitude is determined by synchronization of motor unit discharges, and is enhanced under certain conditions such as anxiety, stress, stimulants, fatigue, hypoglycemia, thyrotoxicosis, or pheochromocytoma. The frequency of physiologic tremor recorded at the wrist shown here decreases with mass loading, a mechanical phenomenon that does not typically occur with essential tremor or the tremor of Parkinson's disease. (*Adapted from* Elble [55].)

Factors That Enhance Physiologic Tremor

Psychological factors	Drugs (*cont.*)	Drugs (*cont.*)
Stress	Psychoactive drugs	Cardiac antiarrhythmic
Anxiety	Tricyclic antidepressants	agents
Excitement	Neuroleptics	Amiodarone
Fear	Lithium	Lidocaine
Metabolic factors	Dopamine agonists	Procainamide
Fatigue	Dopamine	Drug withdrawal
Fever	Amphetamine	Alcohol
Thyrotoxicosis	Anticonvulsants	Benzodiazepines
Hypoglycemia	Valproate	Opiates
Pheochromocytoma	Thyroxine	Toxins
Drugs	Nicotine	Bismuth
Beta-adrenergic agonists	Corticosteroids	Lead
Theophylline	Anticholinesterases	Arsenic
Metaproterenol	Calcium channel blockers	Methylbromide
Terbutaline	Nimodipine	Dietary factors
Epinephrine	Flunarizine	Caffeine
Pseudoephedrine		Monosodium glutamate

Figure 9-61. Factors that enhance physiologic tremor. Normal physiologic tremor may become prominent under certain circumstances ("exaggerated physiologic tremor"), including conditions known to enhance the activity of peripheral beta-adrenergic receptors, present in muscle fibers. Several drugs can induce or enhance tremor by direct peripheral receptor stimulation. Similarly, abrupt *withdrawal* of many drugs, including alcohol, beta-blockers, opioids, and nicotine, can cause tremor by increasing beta-adrenergic receptor activity. The mechanisms producing exaggerated physiologic tremor may enhance all types of pathologic tremor.

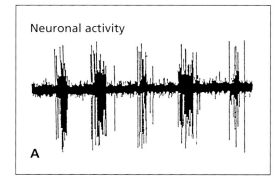

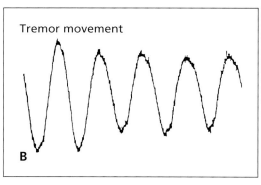

Figure 9-62. Parkinsonian tremor. Bursts of electrical spikes recorded in the subthalamic nucleus (**A**) of monkeys with parkinsonism who were treated with MPTP (1-methyl-4-phenyl-1,2,3,6-tetrahydropyridine) that are synchronous with tremor oscillations observed in the contralateral limb. **B,** The tremor of Parkinson's disease is predominantly a 3 to 6 Hz tremor of the limb at rest. Typically, the tremor reduces or disappears when the affected limb is engaged in an activity or posture-holding. The tremor appears to result from central oscillatory activity in parts of the basal ganglia. A parkinsonian tremor can be abolished by a contralateral lesion in the thalamic nucleus ventralis intermedius (Vim) or by electrical stimulation of the nucleus. (*Adapted from* Vitek and colleagues [56].)

Figure 9-63. Parkinson's disease versus essential tremor. One of the most frequent and important clinical problems in evaluating a patient with tremor is to decide whether it is due to Parkinson's disease or essential tremor.

Parkinson's Disease Versus Essential Tremor

	Parkinson's disease	Essential tremor
Tremor	Occurs at rest	Posture-holding and action
	Decreases with posture-holding or action	
	Increases with walking	
Distribution	Asymmetrical, sometimes unilateral	Symmetrical
Body part	Hands, legs	Hands, head, voice
Drawing a spiral	Micrographic	Tremulous
Age at onset	Middle age or elderly	All ages
Course	Progressive	Stable or slowly progressive
First-degree relatives	Usually unaffected	Often affected
Other neurologic signs	Bradykinesia, rigidity, postural instability	None
Tremor decreases with	Anticholinergics, levodopa	Alcohol, propranolol, primidone

Diagnostic Criteria for Essential Tremor

For *definite* essential tremor

- Patient exhibits a +2 postural tremor of at least one arm (head tremor may also be present but is not sufficient for diagnosis)
- Patient exhibits a +2 postural tremor during at least four tasks,* or a +2 kinetic tremor on one task and a +3 kinetic tremor on a second task
- If the tremor is present in the dominant hand, then it must interfere with at least one activity of daily living (eating, drinking, writing, or using the hands). If the tremor is not present in the dominant hand, then this criterion is irrelevant
- Medications, alcohol, parkinsonism, dystonia, other basal ganglionic disorders, and hyperthyroidism are not potential etiologic factors

All must be true

For *probable* essential tremor

- Patient exhibits a +2 postural tremor during at least four tasks, or a +2 kinetic tremor on one task and a +3 kinetic tremor on a second task; *or*
- Head tremor is present

Either must be true

- Medications, alcohol, parkinsonism, dystonia, other basal ganglionic disorders, and hyperthyroidism are not potential etiologic factors

Must be true

For *possible* essential tremor
A +2 kinetic tremor must be present on three tasks

Tremor ratings
0 = No visible tremor
+1 = Low amplitude, barely perceivable tremor, or intermittent tremor
+2 = Moderate amplitude (1–2 cm) tremor, usually present; clearly oscillatory
+3 = Large amplitude (> 2 cm), violent, jerky tremor that interferes with most activities

* Tasks include pouring water, drinking water from a glass or spoon, touching finger to nose, and drawing a spiral.

Figure 9-64. Diagnostic criteria for essential tremor. Essential tremor is the most common neurologic movement disorder, affecting more than 10 million people in the United States. (*Data from* Louis ED and colleagues [57].)

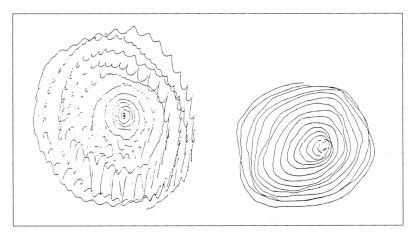

Figure 9-65. Spirals drawn by patients with essential tremor (*left*) and Parkinson's disease tremor (*right*). Essential tremor can interfere with drawing a smooth spiral, as seen in the left panel. The patient with Parkinson's disease typically has a tremor at rest that *decreases* upon action or writing; however, the spiral may be micrographic, as in the right panel. (*Courtesy of* Seth Pullman, MD, Columbia-Presbyterian Medical Center, New York, NY.)

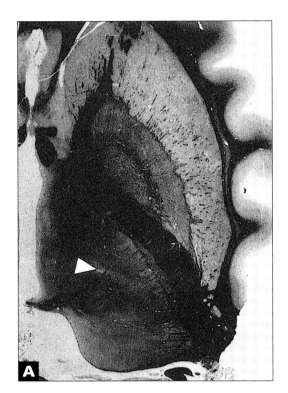

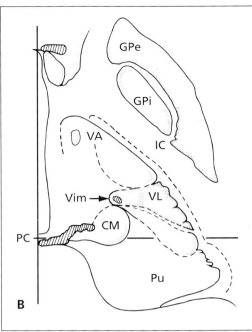

Figure 9-66. Thalamotomy for treatment of tremor in Parkinson's disease (PD) or essential tremor (ET). The tremor at rest in PD and the tremor of ET can be abolished by electrical stimulation or a lesion placed in the contralateral thalamic nucleus ventralis intermedius (Vim). **A,** Cross-section of the left thalamus in a patient with PD who had been treated with an implanted stimulator. The tip of the stimulator produced a 3.5 mm gliotic lesion within the Vim nucleus (*arrowhead*). **B,** Schematic representation of the cross-section shown in *A.* CM—centromedian nucleus; GPe—globus pallidus external segment; GPi—globus pallidus internal segment; IC—internal capsule; PC—posterior commisure; Pu—pulvinar; VA—ventral anterior nucleus; VL—ventral lateral nucleus. (*From* Caparros-Lefebvre and colleagues [58]; with permission.)

Midbrain Tremor

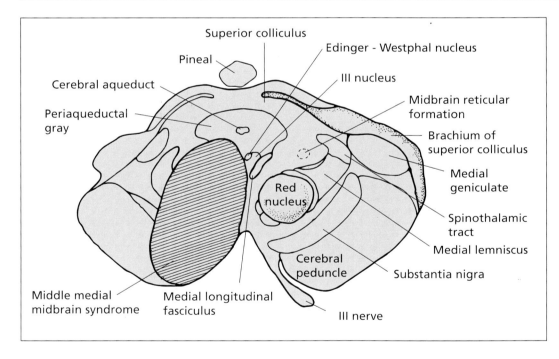

Figure 9-67. Paramedian infarction of the midbrain tegmentum produces a contralateral ataxia and intention tremor caused by damage in the red nucleus and brachium conjunctivum. *Claude syndrome* is a combination of midbrain tremor, ataxia, and ipsilateral third-nerve palsy; the additional presence of contralateral corticospinal tract signs is *Benedikt syndrome* [59]. (*Adapted from* Wall [60].)

Myoclonus

Etiologic Classification of Myoclonus

Physiologic myoclonus
 Sleep jerks (hypnic myoclonus)
 Hiccup (singultus)
 Benign infantile myoclonus
Essential myoclonus
 Unknown cause, no other neurologic abnormality
 Hereditary
 Sporadic
Epileptic myoclonus
 Clinical syndrome dominated by seizures
 Infantile myoclonus
 Lennox-Gastaut syndrome
 Myoclonic absences
 Epilepsia partialis continua
 Juvenile myoclonic epilepsy
Progressive myoclonic epilepsy
 Clinical syndrome dominated by progressive encephalopathy
 Mitochondrial encephalopathy—myoclonic epilepsy and
  ragged red fibers (MERRF)
 Ramsay Hunt syndrome
 Lafora body disease
 Sialidosis
 Neuronal ceroid lipofuscinosis
 Unverricht-Lundborg disease
Symptomatic causes of myoclonus
 Trauma
 Creutzfeldt-Jakob disease
 Viral encephalopathy—subacute sclerosis panencephalitis
  (SSPE)
 Degenerative disease—Alzheimer's
  disease, Parkinson's disease, atypical parkinsonism
 Metabolic encephalopathy—hepatic
  failure, renal failure
 Toxic encephalopathy—bismuth, heavy metals
 Post-hypoxic
 Brain tumor
 Stroke

Figure 9-68. Etiologic classification of myoclonus. Myoclonus is a brief, sudden, shock-like muscle jerk. It may have a physiologic or pathologic basis. Examples of physiologic myoclonus are sleep jerks ("hypnic jerk") and hiccoughs. It may be the primary symptom of a neurologic disease, or a minor symptom overshadowed by many others. Myoclonus is a feature of several epileptic syndromes, but can occur in many other conditions, including degenerative, toxic, metabolic, vascular, traumatic, and others. (*Adapted from* Weiner and colleague [61].)

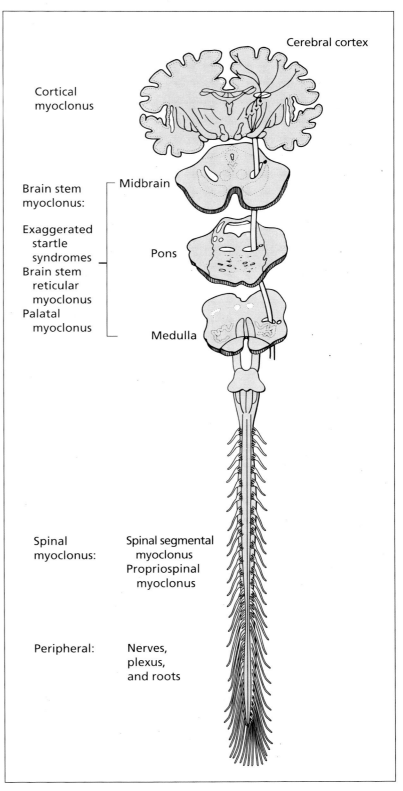

Figure 9-69. Localization of myoclonus. Myoclonus is a brief, sudden, shock-like muscle contraction. Electrophysiologically, a myoclonic jerk is due to a brief electromyographic (EMG) burst lasting 10 to 50 msec, rarely more than 100 msec. The diagnostic approach to myoclonus has a dual objective: identify the site of origin of myoclonus within the nervous system, and establish the cause. Myoclonus should be classified on the basis of its clinical characteristics (rest, action or reflex myoclonus); distribution (focal, segmental, multifocal, generalized); site of origin (cortical, brain stem, spinal cord, or peripheral nerve); and underlying cause. (*Adapted from* Carpenter [62].)

Localization, Electrophysiology, Clinical Manifestations, and Etiology of Myoclonus

Localization and type	Electrophysiology	Clinical manifestations	Etiology
Cortical myoclonus	Abnormal activity originates in the sensorimotor cortex and is transmitted to the spinal cord by the corticospinal tract; diagnostic features may include large amplitude SSEPs and a cortical focus identified by jerk-locked EMG to EEG back-averaging	Spontaneous muscle jerks, sometimes restricted to a body part, may have secondary generalization; jerks may be triggered by external stimuli (cortical reflex myoclonus) or may occur on movement (cortical action myoclonus)	*Focal myoclonus* may be due to a focal lesion in the cerebral cortex (tumor, trauma, vascular lesion), focal epilepsy, and epilepsia partialis continua *Multifocal or generalized myoclonus* may be due to primary generalized epilepsy, progressive myoclonic epilepsy, encephalitis, Creutzfeldt-Jakob disease, Alzheimer's disease, degenerative disease, hypoxia, toxic states, and various metabolic encephalopathies
Brain stem			
Exaggerated startle syndromes, or hyperekplexia	Diffuse brain stem abnormality	Generalized axial jerks and other motor responses triggered by unexpected external stimuli	Local brain stem pathology (anoxia, multiple sclerosis); hereditary hyperekplexia
Brain stem reticular myoclonus	Diffuse brain stem abnormality, utilizes pathways independent of startle reflex	Generalized axial muscle jerks, beginning in the muscles of the lower brain stem, and spreading both rostrally and caudally	Cerebral anoxia, uremia, and other toxic or metabolic states
Palatal myoclonus	Abnormal discharge due to brain stem disorder affecting dentato-olivary pathway in the central tegmental tract	Rhythmic palatal movements at 1.5 to 3 Hz, often accompanied by an audible click. Palatal myoclonus may persist during sleep	Focal brain stem lesion, usually due to stroke, multiple sclerosis, tumor, or trauma
Spinal cord			
Spinal segmental myoclonus	Abnormal discharge due to focal spinal cord lesion	Jerking of a body part, sometimes rhythmic, involving a few spinal segments	Focal lesion, such as trauma, tumor, multiple sclerosis, vascular lesion
Propriospinal myoclonus	Focal spinal cord generator, involves long propriospinal fibers distributed to axial musculature in an orderly sequence	Generalized axial jerks, usually beginning in abdominal muscles and spreading up and down the trunk	Focal lesion occasionally found
Peripheral nerve			
Focal myoclonus	Generator presumed to be a peripheral nerve or root	Focal myoclonic jerks restricted to a segment of the body, often a proximal limb, trunk musculature, or muscles innervated by the facial nerve (hemifacial spasm)	Focal neurovascular lesion, nerve compression, trauma, demyelination, radiation injury

Figure 9-70. Localization, electrophysiology, clinical manifestations, and etiology of myoclonus. EEG—electroencephalogram; EMG—electromyogram; SSEPs—somatosensory-evoked potentials.

Pharmacologic Treatment of Myoclonus

Medication	Dose range	Indication
ACTH	150 units/m²/d	Infantile spasms, opsoclonus
Clonazepam	0.5 to 20 mg/d	Most forms of myoclonus
5-Hydroxytryptophan	25 mg qid to 500 mg qid	Post-hypoxic myoclonus
Piracetam	400 mg tid to 16 g/d	Cortical myoclonus
Tetrabenazine	25 mg/d to 300 mg/d	Segmental myoclonus
Valproic acid	15 mg/kg/d to 2000 mg/d	Most forms of myoclonus
Gabapentin	100 mg tid to 600 mg tid	Most forms of myoclonus
Topiramate	200 mg bid	Most forms of myoclonus

Figure 9-71. Pharmacologic treatment of myoclonus. The pharmacologic treatment of myoclonus includes a variety of agents that are listed here with suggested dose ranges and indications. Doses are calculated for adults, except for adenocorticotropic hormone (ACTH).

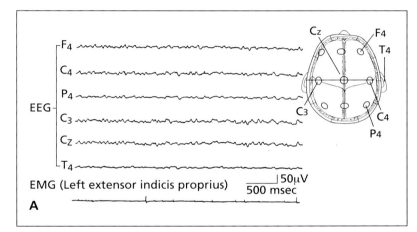

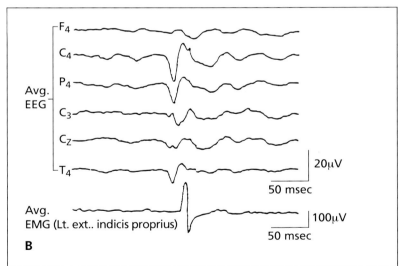

Figure 9-72. Cortical myoclonus. Jerk-locked electromyographic (EMG) to electroencephalographic (EEG) back-averaging is a helpful electrophysiologic technique in localizing myoclonus of cortical origin. Routine EEG recordings often do not reveal an abnormal cortical discharge in relation to a myoclonic jerk. **A,** EEG recording with simultaneous EMG activity from the left extensor indicis proprius (index finger muscle). No paroxysmal EEG activity is seen despite the frequent miniature myoclonic jerks recorded from the EMG. **B,** Averaged recording of 100 samples of EEG activity, each triggered by the electromyographic pulse of a single myoclonic jerk, and demonstrating an obvious biphasic spike over the right central hemisphere in close temporal relation to the EMG discharge. (*Adapted from* Shibasaki and colleague [63].)

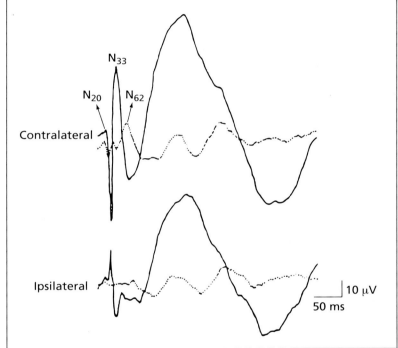

Figure 9-73. Giant somatosensory-evoked potentials (SSEPs) in progressive myoclonic epilepsy. SSEPs are useful in the study of myoclonus. The response consists of a characteristic waveform recorded from the cerebral cortex after an electrical stimulus is applied to a contralateral limb. In this diagram, the SSEP is recorded following an electrical stimulation of the median nerve just proximal to the wrist in a patient with progressive myoclonic epilepsy. The dotted tracing represents the normal response. The negative (upward) deflections are labeled N20, N33, and N62, corresponding to the time in milliseconds following the electrical stimulus. In the patient with myoclonus, the N33 peak has a mean amplitude of 41 μV, approximately 17 times larger than normal. The technique has consistently demonstrated giant SSEPs in patients with progressive myoclonic epilepsy, a syndrome that encompasses several rare disorders, including sialidosis, Lafora body disease, mitochondrial encephalomyopathy and ragged red fibers (MERRF), and neuronal ceroid lipofuscinosis (NCL). Most myoclonic disorders not in this disease category do not have giant SSEPs. (*Adapted from* Shibasaki and colleagues [64].)

Myoclonus in Creutzfeldt-Jakob Disease

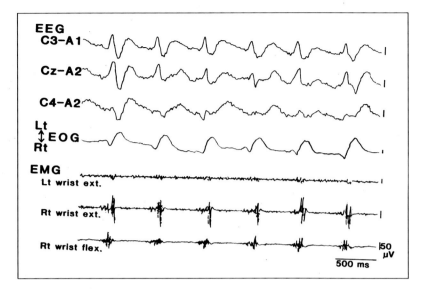

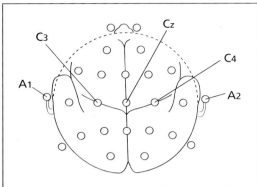

Figure 9-74. Electroencephalogram (EEG) and electrooculogram (EOG) in a patient with Creutzfeldt-Jakob disease. Creutzfeldt-Jakob disease (CJD) is a rare, fatal, transmissible encephalopathy characterized clinically by a rapidly progressive dementia and myoclonus. In this EEG recording, periodic sharp wave complexes predominate over the left hemisphere, corresponding to rhythmic myoclonic jerks of the right arm. The EOG records abrupt ocular deviations to the left, in synchrony with the periodic complexes and limb myoclonus. (*Adapted from* Shibasaki and colleagues [65].)

Asterixis

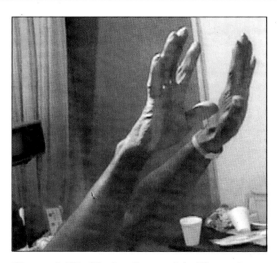

Figure 9-75. Testing for asterixis. The patient dorsiflexes the wrists to allow the hands to "flap" when the extensor muscles are suddenly inhibited. Asterixis is characterized by sudden brief lapses of posture. Asterixis can be demonstrated by having the patient extend the arms and dorsiflex the hands in a sustained posture.

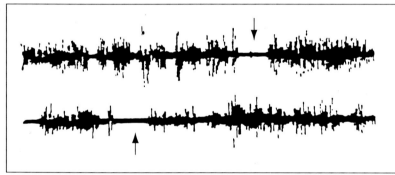

Figure 9-76. Electromyographic (EMG) tracing of forearm extensor activity using surface electrodes, with time calibrations of 250 ms, in a patient with asterixis. Electrophysiologically, asterixis consists of brief periods of EMG silence, usually lasting 50 to 200 ms, occurring against a background of tonic muscle contraction. On this tracing, periods of EMG silence are clearly seen at the arrows, corresponding to the sudden lapses in sustained hand posture.

Similarities between asterixis and myoclonus have led to the concept that asterixis is a form of negative myoclonus. The main clinical significance of asterixis is its frequent association with a toxic or metabolic encephalopathy. The typical clinical setting is uremia, hepatic encephalopathy, electrolyte imbalance, hypercarbia, anticonvulsant treatment, sedative use, or a similar condition. Associated features in a patient with asterixis generally include a depressed level of consciousness and slowing of the electroencephalogram. Posthypoxic myoclonus often includes negative myoclonus. (*Adapted from* Young and colleague [66].)

Drug-induced Movement Disorders

Movement Disorders Induced by Dopamine-Receptor Blocking Agents

Movement disorders	Time course	Description	Treatment
Acute dystonic reaction	Immediate, acute; usually within first days of treatment, sometimes following first dose	Abnormal sustained muscle contractions or postures, most often affecting eyes (oculogyric crisis), neck, face, or trunk	Administer parenteral anticholinergics or antihistamines; remove offending neuroleptic
Acute akathisia	Acute, immediate	Acute state of inner restlessness	Self-limited upon discontinuation of neuroleptics
Neuroleptic-induced parkinsonism	Subacute, insidious	Dose-related parkinsonism, with rigidity, bradykinesias, postural instability, and all other clinical features of idiopathic Parkinson's disease	Reduce or withdraw neuroleptic; administer amantadine or anticholinergics

Tardive syndromes
(Abnormal involuntary movements caused by exposure to neuroleptic dopamine-receptor blocking agents, persisting for at least one month after withdrawal of the inciting drug)

Classical tardive dyskinesia	Chronic, late, persistent	Repetitive, orobuccolingual chewing movements; tongue popping	Administer reserpine, tetrabenazine, clozapine
Tardive dystonia	Chronic, late, persistent	Sustained movements of neck, trunk, oral region, or face	Administer anticholinergics, reserpine, or tetrabenazine
Tardive akathisia	Chronic, late, persistent	Sensation of inner restlessness and intolerance of remaining still, with overt movements of restlessness, pacing, marching in place, fidgetiness	Administer reserpine, tetrabenazine, clozapine

Withdrawal-emergence syndrome

	Occurs following abrupt withdrawal from chronic neuroleptic therapy; usually occurs in children	Generalized choreic movements involving trunk, limbs, neck, and rarely, face	Spontaneous resolution; movements resolve immediately if neuroleptics are reinstated

Neuroleptic malignant syndrome

	Begins abruptly while patient is on therapeutic doses of neuroleptic	Fever, autonomic hyperactivity, muscle rigidity, and alteration of mental status	Discontinuation of neuroleptics; administer bromocriptine, dantrolene

Figure 9-77. Movement disorders induced by dopamine-receptor blocking agents. Dopamine-receptor blocking agents may cause a variety of acute, subacute, and chronic movement disorders. The acute disorders tend to resolve spontaneously and upon discontinuation of the offending agent. The tardive dyskinesia syndromes are late-appearing involuntary movements resulting from chronic administration of dopamine-receptor blocking agents. The tardive syndromes present a variety of movement disorder phenomena, and may persist indefinitely despite discontinuation of the medication.

Drugs That May Cause Tardive Syndromes

Indication	Drug class	Drug name	Trade name
Antipsychotics	Phenothiazine	Chlorpromazine	Thorazine (SmithKline Beecham, Philadelphia, PA)
		Trifluopromazine	Vesprin (Apothecon, New York, NY)
		Thioridazine	Mellaril (Sandoz, East Hanover, NJ)
		Mesoridazine	Serentil (Boehringer Ingelheim, Ridgefield, CT)
		Trifluoperazine	Stelazine (SmithKline Beecham, Philadelphia, PA),
		Perphenazine	Trilafon (Schering, Kenilworth, NJ), Triavil (Merck, West Point, PA)
		Fluphenazine	Prolixin (Apothecon, New York, NY), Permitil (Schering, Kenilworth, NJ)
		Pimozide	Orap (Lemmon, Sellersville, PA)
		Acetophenazine	Tindal (Schering, Kenilworth, NJ)
	Thioxanthene	Chlorprothixine	Taractan (Hoffmann-LaRoche, Nutley, NJ)
		Thiothixene	Navane (Roerig, New York, NY)
	Butyrophenone	Haloperidol	Haldol (McNeil, Fort Washington, PA)
		Droperidol	Inapsine, Innovar (Janssen, Titusville, NJ)
	Dibenzazepine	Loxapine	Loxitane (Lederle, Wayne, NJ), Daxolin (Miles, Elkhart, IN)
	Indolone	Molindone	Moban (DuPont Merck, Wilmington, DE), Lidone (Abbott, Abbott Park, IL)
	Pyrimidinone	Risperidone	Risperdal (Janssen, Titusville, NJ)
	Thienobenzodiazepine	Olanzapine	Zyprexa (Eli Lilly, Indianapolis, IN)
	Substituted benzamide	Tiapride	
		Sulpiride	
		Clebopride	
		Remoxipride	
Drugs used as antiemetics, cough suppressants, or as treatment for intractable hiccoughs	Phenothiazine Substituted benzamide	Prochlorperazine	Compazine (SmithKline Beecham, Philadelphia, PA)
		Promethazine	Phenergan (Wyeth-Ayerst, Philadelphia, PA)
		Chlorpromazine	Thorazine (SmithKline Beecham, Philadelphia, PA)
		Triethylperazine	Torecan (Roxane Laboratories, Columbus, OH)
		Triflupromazine	Vesprin (Apothecon, New York, NY)
		Metoclopramide	Reglan (A.H. Robins, Richmond, VA)
Antidepressants	Tricyclic	Amoxapine	Asendin (Lederle, Wayne, NJ), Triavil
Antihypertensives	Calcium channel blockers	Flunarizine	
		Cinnarizine	

Figure 9-78. Drugs that may cause tardive syndromes. Many different drugs used to treat a variety of psychiatric and medical conditions can induce tardive dyskinesias. All agents have in common the property of blocking brain dopamine receptors. Physicians prescribing these drugs have an obligation to explain to patients that the rare development of tardive syndromes may be permanent. Two antipsychotic drugs, clozapine (Clozaril) and quetiapine (Seroquel), are atypical antipsychotics and do not appear to cause tardive syndromes, and rarely drug-induced parkinsonism.

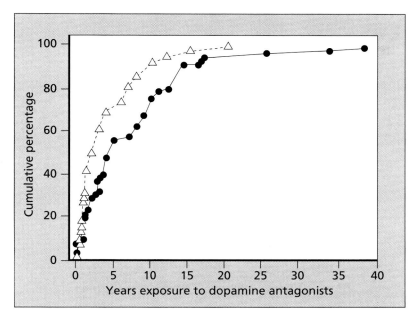

Figure 9-79. Relationship between exposure to neuroleptics and development of tardive dystonia. The cumulative percentage of patients with tardive dystonia is shown in relation to years of exposure to dopamine receptor antagonists in two different series of patients. The first series (*black circles*) comprises 67 patients followed at Columbia-Presbyterian Medical Center, and the second group (*open triangles*) consists of 43 patients reported in the literature before 1986. In both groups, cases of tardive dystonia developed shortly after exposure to neuroleptics, and no minimum safe duration of exposure was detected. (*Adapted from* Kang and colleagues [67].)

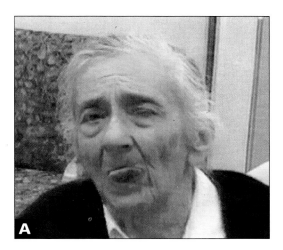
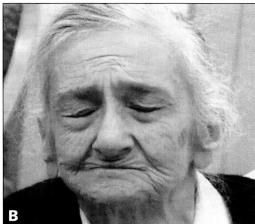

Figure 9-80. A patient with classical tardive dyskinesia of the oral-buccal-lingual type. **A,** Tongue popping movements. **B,** Other mouthing movements and eyelid closure.

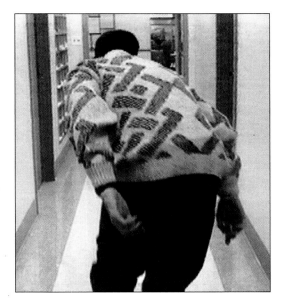

Figure 9-81. A patient with tardive dystonia showing flexion of his trunk as he walks. The elbows are extended and the wrists flexed. More common than trunk flexion in tardive dystonia is trunk extension with opisthotonus and retrocollis.

Peripheral and Miscellaneous Movement Disorders

Hemifacial Spasm

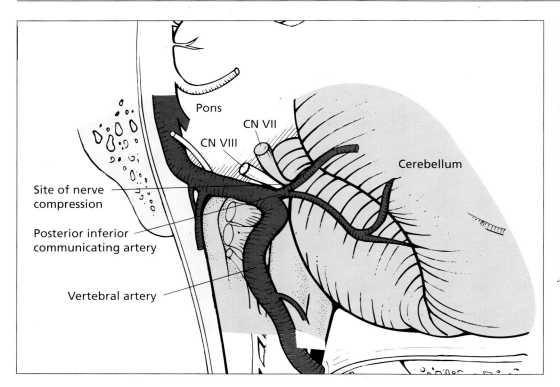

Pons

CN VII

CN VIII

Cerebellum

Site of nerve compression

Posterior inferior communicating artery

Vertebral artery

Figure 9-82. Compression of the facial nerve exit zone by the vertebral and posterior inferior cerebellar arteries in a patient with hemifacial spasm. Hemifacial spasm is a condition of recurrent unilateral contractions of the facial musculature innervated by CN VII. Hemifacial spasm was traditionally considered to be an idiopathic condition, but evidence from imaging studies and intraoperative visualization indicates that many, if not most, cases are associated with microvascular compression of the facial nerve. Rare causes of hemifacial spasm include posterior fossa tumors, aneurysms, arteriovenous malformations, arachnoid cysts, intrinsic glial tumors, brain stem infarction, and multiple sclerosis [68]. Hemifacial spasm can be treated with microvascular decompression of the nerve or with injections of botulinum toxin into the facial muscles. (*Adapted from* Jannetta [69].)

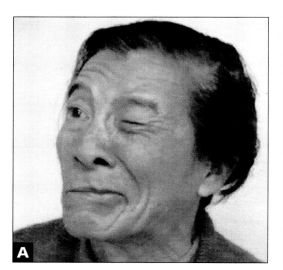

A

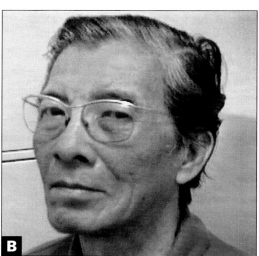

B

Figure 9-83. A patient with hemifacial spasm before (**A**) and after (**B**) being treated with injections of botulinum toxin.

Psychogenic Movement Disorders

A. Psychogenic Movement Disorders

Clinical features of psychogenic movement disorders

Abrupt onset, with clear inciting event

Multiple movement disorder manifestations

Variable and inconsistent motor manifestations, fluctuating within the same examination session

Motor manifestations that are incongruous with organic pathology

Movements increase or become more elaborate when examination focuses upon the affected body part

Movements diminish or resolve when not the clear focus of attention or inquiry

Movements diminish or resolve during tests requiring concentration or other tasks

Hyperekplexia, or excessive startle response

Movements respond to placebo or suggestion

Associated false or incongruous neurologic signs

Associated psychiatric features

Movement disorder resolves with psychotherapy, or when patient is unaware of being observed

Figure 9-84. Psychogenic movement disorders (**A–C**). Psychogenic movement disorders are abnormal movements that do not result from a known organic cause but are caused by psychiatric conditions. Most psychogenic movements can be categorized as tremor, chorea, dystonia, myoclonus, parkinsonism, or gait disturbance. Psychogenic movements that are generalized may overlap with the symptoms of epilepsy. The two most important clues suggesting a possible psychogenic cause are abnormal movements that are incongruous with typical organic disease and movements that are inconsistent or fluctuate during the examination. The importance of an accurate diagnosis cannot be overstated, and there is no substitute for a careful assessment by an experienced observer of movement disorders. The diagnosis is certain only when the movement disorder is

B. Psychogenic Movement Disorders

Features of psychogenic tremor

Tremor similar in all positions and at rest, posture-holding, and with action

Variability of examination: changes in frequency, distribution, direction, and amplitude

Spontaneous remission

Selective or intermittent disability

Entrainment of tremor by tests of coordination

C. Psychogenic Movement Disorders

Features of psychogenic dystonia

Onset of dystonia at rest

Onset in foot in adults

Specific incongruities: absence of dystonic tremor, absence of null point, absence of modifying sensory tricks

Spontaneous pain with passive movement

Contractures do not exclude diagnosis

Startle-induced elaboration of dystonic postures

Abrupt changes in dystonia

persistently relieved by psychotherapy. The psychiatric diagnoses in cases of psychogenic movement disorders include conversion disorder, somatization disorder, factitious disorder, and malingering. Effective treatment generally requires a combination of intensive psychotherapy, physical therapy, pharmacotherapy, and other rehabilitation techniques. (*Adapted from* Williams and colleagues [70].)

Paroxysmal Dyskinesias

Clinical Features of Paroxysmal Kinesigenic Dyskinesia, Nonkinesigenic Dyskinesia, and Exertional Dyskinesia

Feature	PKD	PNKD	PED
Male:female	4:1	1.4:1	1:1
Inheritance	AD	AD	AD
Genetic mapping	16p11.2–q12.1	Mount-Reback syndrome, 2q33–35 With diplopia and spasticity (CSE), chromosome 1p	?
Age at onset			
Range	<1–40	<1–30	2–30
Median	12	12	11.5
Mean	12	12	12
Attacks			
Duration	<5 min	2 min–4 h	5 min–2 h
Frequency	100/d–1/mo	3/d–2/y	1/d–2/mo
Trigger	Sudden movement, startle, hyperventilation	—	Prolonged exercise
Precipitant	Stress	Ethanol, stress, caffeine, fatigue	Stress
Movement pattern	Any combination of dystonic postures, chorea, athetosis, and ballism; unilateral or bilateral		
Treatment	Anticonvulsants	Clonazepam, benzodiazepines, acetazolamide, antimuscarinics	Acetazolamide, antimuscarinics, benzodiazepines

Figure 9-85. Clinical features of paroxysmal dyskinesias. The most common paroxysmal dyskinesias are paroxysmal kinesigenic dyskinesia (PKD) (induced by sudden movement or startle), paroxysmal nonkinesiogenic dyskinesia or the *Mount-Reback syndrome* (PNKD) (induced by fatigue, caffeine, or stress), and paroxysmal exertional dyskinesia (PED) (induced by prolonged exertion). Characteristically, attacks of PKD are very brief, usually lasting seconds, with many attacks per day. Attacks of PKND are usually long, lasting many minutes to hours, with attacks usually less than once a day. Attacks of PED usually last about half an hour. Paroxysmal dyskinesias can be secondary to cerebral injury, with multiple sclerosis the most common cause. Sporadic PNKD is often of psychogenic etiology [71]. AD—autosomal dominant.

Clinical and Genetic Features of Episodic Ataxias

Type	Age at onset, y	Clinical	Acetazolamide response	Precipitant	Frequency/ duration	Interictal	Gene
Myokymia, neuromyotonia (EA-1)	2–15	Aura of weightlessness or weakness, then ataxia, dysarthria, tremor, facial twitching	In some kindreds; anticonvulsants may help	Startle, movement, exercise, excitement, fatigue	Up to 15/d; usually one or less per day; seconds to minutes, usually 2–10 min	Myokymia, shortened Achilles tendon; PKD	12p13, K+ channel, different point mutations in KCNA1
Vestibular (EA-2)	0–40, usually 5–15	Ataxia, vertigo, nystagmus, dysarthria, headache, ptosis, ocular palsy, vermis atrophy	Very effective	Stress, alcohol, fatigue, exercise, caffeine	Daily to q 2 mo; usually hours; 5 min to weeks	Nystagmus, mild ataxia, less common; dysarthria and progressive cerebellar	19p13, Ca+ channel, CACNL1A4 familial hemiplegic migraine?
Ocular	20–50	Ataxia, diplopia, vertigo, nausea	No response	Sudden change in head position	Daily to year; minutes to hours	Symptoms gradually become constant	Unknown

Figure 9-86. Clinical and genetic features of episodic ataxias. The episodic ataxias are rare familial conditions, of which two (EA-1 and EA-2) have now been identified with mutations of genes for the potassium and calcium channels, respectively. EA-2 is effectively treated with acetazolamide. PKD—paroxysmal kinesigenic dyskinesia.

References

1. Hughes AJ, Daniel SE, Kilford L, Lees AJ: Accuracy of clinical diagnosis of idiopathic Parkinson's disease: a clinico-pathological study of 100 cases. *J Neurol Neurosurg Psychiat* 1992, 55:181–184.

2. Wichmann T, DeLong MR: Pathophysiology of parkinsonian motor abnormalities. *Adv Neurol* 1993, 60:53–61.

3. Duvoisin RC, Eldridge R, Williams A, *et al.*: Twin study of Parkinson disease. *Neurology* 1981, 31:77–80.

4. Chase, TN, Mouradian MM, Engber TM: Motor response complications and the function of striatal efferent systems. *Neurology* 1993, 43(suppl 6):S23–S27.

5. Mouradian MM, Juncos JL, Fabbrini G, *et al.*: Motor fluctuations in Parkinson's disease: central pathophysiological mechanisms, part II. *Ann Neurol* 1988, 24:372–378.

6. Laitinen LV, Bergenheim AT, Hariz MI: Leksell's posteroventral pallidotomy in the treatment of Parkinson's disease. *J Neurosurg* 1992, 76:53–61.

7. Limousin P, Krack P, Pollak P, *et al.*: Electrical stimulation of the subthalamic nucleus in advanced Parkinson's disease. *N Engl J Med* 1998, 339:1105–1111.

8. Steele RC, Richardson JC, Olszewski J: Progressive supranuclear palsy: a heterogeneous degeneration involving the brain stem, basal ganglia and cerebellum with vertical gaze and pseudobulbar palsy, nuchal dystonia and dementia. *Arch Neurol* 1964, 10:333–359.

9. Lepore FE, Duvoisin RC: "Apraxia" of eyelid opening: an involuntary levator inhibition. *Neurology* 1985, 35:423–427.

10. Lantos PL: The Neuropathology of Progressive Supranuclear Palsy. In *Progressive Supranuclear Palsy: Diagnosis, Pathology and Therapy.* Edited by Tolosa E, Duvoisin R, Cruz-Sanchez FF. New York: Springer-Verlag, Wein; 1994:137–152.

11. Brooks DJ: PET Studies in Progressive Supranuclear Palsy. In *Progressive Supranuclear Palsy: Diagnosis, Pathology, and Therapy.* Edited by Toloso E, Duvoisin R, Cruz-Sanchez FF. New York: Springer-Verlag; 1994:119–132.

12. Graham JG, Oppenheimer DR: Orthostatic hypotension and nicotinic sensitivity in a case of multiple system atrophy. *J Neurol Neurosurg Psychiatry* 1969, 32:28–34.

13. Lantos PL, Papp MI: Cellular pathology of multiple system atrophy: a review. *J Neurol Neurosurg Psychiatry* 1994, 57:129–133.

14. Gilman S, Koeppe RA, Junck L, *et al.*: Patterns of cerebral glucose metabolism detected with positron emission tomography differ in multiple system atrophy and olivopontocerebellar atrophy. *Ann Neurol* 1994, 36:166–175.

15. Rutledge JN, Schallert T, Hall S: Magnetic resonance imaging in parkinsonisms. *Adv Neurol* 1993, 60:529–534.

16. Rebeiz JJ, Kolodny EH, Richardson EP Jr: Corticodentatonigral degeneration with neuronal achromasia. *Arch Neurol* 1968, 18:20–33.

17. Uchihara T, Mitani K, Mori H, *et al.*: Abnormal cytoskeletal pathology peculiar to corticobasal degeneration is different from that of Alzheimer's disease or progressive supranuclear palsy. *Acta Neuropathol* 1994, 88:379–383.

18. Klawans HL: Hemiparkinsonism as a late complication of hemiatrophy: a new syndrome. *Neurology* 1981, 31:625–628.

19. Perry RH, Irving D, Blessed G, *et al.*: Senile dementia of Lewy body type. *J Neurol Sci* 1990, 95:119–139.

20. Hakim S, Adams RD: The special clinical problem of symptomatic hydrocephalus with normal cerebrospinal fluid pressure: observations on cerebrospinal fluid hydrodynamics. *J Neurol Sci* 1965, 2:307–327.

21. Greene PE, Kang UJ, Fahn S: Spread of symptoms in idiopathic torsion dystonia. *Mov Disord* 1995, 10:143–152.

22. Kramer PL, Heiman GA, Gasser T, *et al.*: The DYT1 gene on 9q34 is responsible for most cases of early limb-onset idiopathic torsion dystonia in non-Jews. *Am J Hum Genet* 1994, 55:468–475.

23. Rothwell JC, Obeso JA, Day BL, Marsden CD: Pathophysiology of dystonias. In *Motor Control Mechanisms in Health and Disease.* Edited by Desmedt JE. New York: Raven Press; 1983:851–863.

24. Marsden, CD, Obeso JA, Zarranz JJ, Lang AE: The anatomical basis of symptomatic hemidystonia. *Brain* 1985, 108:461–483.

25. Zilber N, Korcyn AD, Kahana E, *et al.*: Inheritance of idiopathic torsion dystonia among Jews. *J Med Genet* 1984, 21:13–26.

26. Waddy HM, Fletcher NA, Harding AE, Marsden CD: A genetic study of idiopathic focal dystonias. *Ann Neurol* 1991, 29:320–324.

27. Bressman SB, deLeon D, Brin MF, *et al.*: Idiopathic dystonia among Ashkenazi Jews: evidence for autosomal dominant inheritance. *Ann Neurol* 1989, 26:612–620.

28. Bressman SB, Sabatti C, Raymond D, *et al.*: The DYT1 phenotype and guidelines for diagnostic tsting. *Neurology* 2000, 54:1746–1752.

29. Holmgren G, Ozelius L, Forsgren L, *et al*: Adult-onset idiopathic torsion dystonia is excluded from the DYT1 region (9q34) in a Swedish family. *J Neurol Neurosurg Psychiatry* 1995, 59:178–181.

30. Bressman SB, Hunt AL, Heiman GA, *et al.*: Exclusion of the DYT1 locus in a non-Jewish family with early-onset dystonia. *Mov Disord* 1994, 9:626–632.

31. Leube B, Rudnicki D, Ratzlaff T, *et al.*: Idiopathic torsion dystonia: assignment of a gene to chromosome 18p in a German family with adult onset, autosomal dominant inheritance and purely focal distribution. *Hum Mol Genet* 1996, 5:1673–1677.

32. Ichinose H, Ohye T, Takahashi E, *et al*: Hereditary progressive dystonia with marked diurnal fluctuation caused by mutations in the GTP cyclohydrolase I gene. *Nat Genet* 1994, 8:229–235.

33. Nygaard TG, Waran SP, Levine RA, *et al.*: Dopa-responsive dystonia simulating cerebral palsy. *Pediat Neurol* 1994, 11:236–240.

34. Bull PD, Thomas GR, Rommens JM, *et al.*: The Wilson disease gene is a putative copper transporting P-type ATPase similar to the Menkes gene [published erratum appears in *Nat Genet* 1994, 6(2):214]. *Nat Genet* 1993, 5:327–237.

35. Tanzi RE, Petrukhin K, Chernov I, *et al.*: The Wilson disease gene is a copper transporting ATPase with homology to the Menkes disease gene. *Nat Gen* 1993, 5:344–350.

36. Thomas GR, Forbes JR, Roberts EA, *et al.*: The Wilson disease gene: spectrum of mutations and their consequences. *Nat Genet* 1995, 9:210–217.

37. Wiebers DO, Hollenhorst RW, Goldstein NP: The ophthalmologic manifestations of Wilson's disease. *Mayo Clin Proc* 1977, 52:409–416.

38. Higgins JJ, Patterson MC, Papadopoulos NM, *et al.*: Hypoprebetalipoproteinemia, acanthocytosis, retinitis-pigmentosa, and pallidal degeneration (HARP syndrome). *Neurology* 1992, 42:194–198.

39. Sethi KD, Adams RJ, Loring DW, Gammal TE: Hallervorden-Spatz syndrome: clinical and magnetic resonance imaging correlations. *Ann Neurol* 1988, 24:692–694.

40. Feinberg TE, Cianci CD, Morrow JS, *et al.*: Diagnostic tests for choreoacanthocytosis. *Neurology* 1991, 41:1000–1006.

41. Rubio JP, Danek A, Stone C, *et al.*: Chorea-acanthocytosis: genetic linkage to chromosome 9q21. *Am J Hum Genet* 1997; 61:899–908.

42. Witt TN, Danek A, Hein MU, *et al.*: McLeod syndrome: a distinct form of neuroacanthocytosis. *J Neurol* 1992, 239:302–306.

43. Orrell RW, Amrolia PJ, Heald A, *et al.*: Acanthocytosis, retinitis pigmentosa, and pallidal degeneration: a report of three patients, including the second reported case with hypoprebetalipoproteinemia (HARP syndrome). *Neurology* 1995, 45:487–491.

44. Huntington's Disease Collaborative Research Group: A novel gene containing a trinucleotide repeat that is expanded and unstable on Huntington's disease chromosomes. *Cell* 1993, 72:971–983.

45. Albin RL, Tagle DA: Genetics and molecular biology of Huntington's disease. *Trends Neurosci* 1995, 18:11–14.

46. Kremer B, Goldberg P, Andrew SE, *et al.*: A worldwide study of the Huntington's disease mutation—the sensitivity and specificity of measuring CAG repeats. *N Engl J Med* 1994, 330:1401–1406.

47. Bressman SB, Risch NJ: Genetics of Movement Disorders: Dystonia, Dopa-responsive Dystonia and Huntington's Disease. In *Movement and Allied Disorders in Childhood.* Edited by Robertson MM, Eapen V. London: John Wiley and Sons; 1995:327–356.

48. Myers RH, MacDonald ME, Koroshetew J, *et al.*: De novo expansion of a (CAG)n repeat in sporadic Huntington's disease. *Nat Genet* 1993, 5:168–173.

49. Martin WRW, Calne DB: Imaging Techniques and Movement Disorders. In *Movement Disorders.* Edited by Marsden CD, Fahn S. Boston: Butterworth; 1987: 14–16.

50. Harris GJ, Pearlson GD, Peyser CE, *et al.*: Putamen volume reduction on magnetic resonance imaging exceeds caudate changes in mild Huntington's disease. *Ann Neurol* 1992, 31:69–75.

51. DeLong MR: Primate models of movement disorders of basal ganglia origin. *Trends Neurosci* 1990, 13:281–285.

52. Pauls DL, Raymond CL, Stevenson JM, Leckman JF: A family study of Gilles de la Tourette syndrome. *Am J Human Genet* 1991, 43: 154–163.

53. Singer HS, Hahn IH, Krowiak E, *et al*.: Tourette's syndrome: a neurochemical analysis of postmortem cortical brain tissue. *Ann Neurol* 1990, 27:443–446.

54. Obeso JA, Rothwell JC, Marsden CD: The neurophysiology of Tourette syndrome. *Adv Neurol* 1982, 35:105–114.

55. Elble RJ: Mechanisms of Physiological Tremor and Relationship to Essential Tremor. In *Handbook of Tremor Disorders.* Edited by Findley LJ, Koller WC. New York: Marcel Dekker; 1995.

56. Vitek JL, Wichmann T, DeLong MR: Current Concepts of Basal Ganglia Neurophysiology Relative to Tremorgenesis. In *Handbook of Tremor Disorders.* Edited by Findley LJ, Koller WC. New York: Marcel Dekker; 1995:37–50.

57. Louis ED, Ford B, Lee H, *et al*.: Diagnostic criteria for essential tremor: a population perspective. *Arch Neurol* 1998, 55:222–227.

58. Caparros-Lefebvre D, Ruchoux MM, Blond S, *et al*.: Long-term thalamic stimulation in Parkinson's disease. *Neurology* 1994, 44:1856–1860.

59. Bogousslavsky J, Maeder P, Regli F, Meuli R: Pure midbrain infarction: clinical syndromes, MRI, and etiologic patterns. *Neurology* 1994, 44:2032–2040.

60. Wall M: Brainstem Syndromes. In *Neurology in Clinical Practice.* Bradley WG, Daroff RB, Fenichel GM, Marsden CD. Boston: Butterworth-Heinemann; 1991:347–362.

61. Weiner WJ, Lang AE: *Movement Disorders: A Comprehensive Survey.* Mount Kisco, NY: Futura; 1989:457–530.

62. Carpenter MB: *Core Text of Neuroanatomy*, edn 3. Baltimore: Williams & Wilkins; 1985.

63. Shibasaki H, Kuriowa Y: Electroencephalographic correlates of myoclonus. *Electroencephalog Clin Neurophysiol* 1975, 39:455–463.

64. Shibasaki H, Yamashita Y, Kuriowa Y: Electroencephalographic studies of myoclonus; myoclonus-related cortical spikes and high amplitude somatosensory evoked potentials. *Brain* 1978, 101:447–460.

65. Shibasaki H, Yamashita Y, Tobimatsu S, Neshige R: Electroencephalographic correlates of myoclonus. In *Adv Neurol* 1986, 43:357–372.

66. Young RH, Shahani BT: Asterixis: one type of negative myoclonus. *Adv Neurol* 1986, 43:137–156.

67. Kang UJ, Burke RE, Fahn S: Natural history and treatment of tardive dystonia. *Mov Disord* 1986, 1:193–208.

68. Barker FG, Jannetta PJ, Bissonette DJ, *et al*.: Microvascular compression for hemifacial spasm. *J Neurosurg* 1995, 82:201–210.

69. Jannetta PJ: Cranial Rhizotomies. In *Neurological Surgery.* Edited by Youmans JR. vol 6, edn 3. Philadelphia: WB Saunders; 1990, 4169–4182.

70. Williams DT, Ford B, Fahn S: Phenomenology and psychopathology related to psychogenic movement disorders. *Adv Neurol* 1995, 65:231–257.

71. Fahn S: Paroxysmal Dyskinesias. In *Movement Disorders III.* Edited by Marsden CD, Fahn S. Oxford: Butterworth-Heinemann; 1994:310-345.

10

The Epilepsies

Paul C. Van Ness

EPILEPSY is a common and disabling neurologic disorder that can be especially gratifying to treat. Successful treatment depends on proper classification of seizure type and epilepsy syndrome followed by the selection of an appropriate antiepileptic drug at an appropriate dosage. Patients with epilepsy frequently receive inadequate care for their condition because of misdiagnosis, inappropriate treatment, complicated drug regimens, and inappropriate use of diagnostic testing. Attitudes among physicians that occasional seizures are tolerable and indicate good control need to be altered, because virtually all epileptologists agree that the only acceptable outcome should be freedom from seizures and the disabilities associated with them.

For the majority of patients, seizure control is associated with and usually essential for a good psychosocial outcome, including full and meaningful employment and driving privileges. Being that epilepsy is often a chronic, lifelong condition, most neurologists develop a long-term relationship with their patients.

Epilepsies are classified into two major categories, partial (localization related) and generalized. Partial epilepsies are usually related to structural lesions, either macroscopic or microscopic, whereas generalized epilepsies often are genetic or secondary to diffuse, but nonspecific, brain insults. The clinical features and etiologies are quite diverse, and the classification system may change as new epilepsy syndromes are characterized.

Most epilepsies and seizure disorders can be diagnosed from a history and physical examination, with imaging and neurophysiologic tests as a supplement to the evaluation. Important points to consider when taking a patient's history are the number of seizure types, age at seizure onset, and a description of the attack from the patient and a reliable observer. The physician should inquire about an aura or prodrome, ictal behavior and impairment of consciousness, seizure evolution, and postictal deficits. Patterns of occurrence, precipitating factors, seizure frequency, and changes with maturation are important as well.

Patients may have tried a variety of medications, so the history should include information about the drug sequence, duration of therapy, effectiveness, toxicity, dosages, and levels. Monotherapy or polypharmacy trials may have been used, and failure of a drug may be related more to drug interactions than other factors.

Etiologies of the epilepsies are more easily determined, and the history should look for causative factors in the birth and development of the patient. Head trauma, febrile convulsions, central nervous system (CNS) infections, drug or toxin exposure, other CNS insults, and systemic illnesses may all be important. A family history can be difficult to obtain because epilepsy is often hidden from relatives. With the expanding list of genetic epilepsies, obtaining a detailed family history is critical.

A psychosocial history may reveal psychiatric difficulties, educational disabilities, unemployment or underemployment, unsafe driving practices, and other safety issues whether or not seizures are controlled. Many patients with intractable epilepsy are disabled and may require assistance with insurance or government benefits.

The exam should include a search for neurocutaneous syndromes, dysmorphic features, scalp scars, and signs of systemic disease in addition to a detailed neurologic exam to demonstrate a specific neurologic dysfunction of lesions. Often there are no neurologic abnormalities, but subtle features can include slight body size asymmetry, pathologic left handedness, subtle facial asymmetry, and mirror movements or impairment of fine motor skills.

Seizure observation by video or direct observation is extremely helpful and is occasionally possible in the office. When a seizure is witnessed it is helpful to note ictal and postictal behavior, transient postictal neurologic deficits, and amnesia or other cognitive alteration. Various ictal behaviors have localizing value. Adversive head turning before a secondarily generalized tonic-clonic seizure is contralateral to the focus [1,2]. Dystonic posturing of an upper extremity is almost always contralateral to the focus [3]. Ictal speech suggests nondominant hemisphere localization [2,4–9], whereas ictal vomiting suggests right temporal localization [10,11]. Ictal fear suggests amygdalar localization [12,13]. Postictal findings may also localize or lateralize, eg, aphasia suggests a dominant hemisphere focus, whereas Todd's paresis is contralateral to focus and postictal sensory losses are all contralateral to the ictal focus. The postictal deficits usually are typical to the region in which the seizure began and are motor sensory or cognitive.

This chapter conveys the highlights of seizure and epilepsy diagnosis and treatment as well as an understanding of the etiologies that underlie the majority of epileptic disorders.

Classification of Seizures and Epilepsy

Seizure Classification

Simple partial seizures

With motor signs	With autonomic symptoms or signs
Focal motor without march	Epigastric sensation
Focal motor with march (Jacksonian)	Pallor
Versive	Sweating
Postural	Flushing
Phonatory (vocalization or speech arrest)	Piloerection
With somatosensory or special sensory symptoms	Pupillary dilation
(simple hallucinations)	Cardiac arrhythmia
Somatosensory	With psychic symptoms (rare without impairment of consciousness)
Visual	Dysphasic
Auditory	Dysmnesic (eg, déjà-vu)
Olfactory	Cognitive (eg, dreamy states, distortion of time sense)
Gustatory	Affective (fear, anger, etc.)
Vertiginous	Illusions (eg, macropsia)
	Structured hallucinations (eg, music, scenes)

Complex partial seizures

Simple partial onset followed by impairment of consciousness	With impairment of consciousness at onset
With simple partial features only prior to impaired consciousness	Impairment of consciousness only
With automatisms	With automatisms

Partial seizures evolving to secondarily generalized tonic-clonic convulsions

Simple partial seizures to generalized tonic-clonic convulsions
Complex partial seizures to generalized tonic-clonic convulsions
Simple partial seizures to complex partial seizures to generalized tonic-clonic convulsions

Figure 10-1. Seizure classification. Seizures and epilepsy are not synonymous. Seizures are clinical manifestations of a paroxysmal, abnormal, excessive or hypersynchronous, usually self-limited, cerebral cortical neuronal discharge. Epilepsy is a chronic neurologic condition that is characterized by recurrent epileptic seizures, which are unprovoked by any known proximate insult [14,15]. Based on epidemiologic studies in Rochester Minnesota, Hauser estimated that about 10% of the population have a seizure by age 74; 3% develop epilepsy, a condition with recurring epileptic seizures; and 4.1% have unprovoked seizures [16]. Most seizures and epilepsies develop in the very young and very old, because a variety of disorders damage or affect the brain in these age groups [17].

To properly classify the type of epilepsy the patient has, it is usually necessary to understand what type of seizures occur. Seizures are divided into partial (focal, localized) seizures and generalized seizures. Simple partial seizures are seizures in which consciousness is not lost. Simple partial seizures may have motor signs, sensory signs, autonomic symptoms or signs, and even psychic or cognitive effects, depending in which region of the brain they start.

Complex partial seizures are partial seizures that involve alteration of consciousness. Consciousness is a very difficult term to define and some patients are quite reactive and may even be able to speak during the seizure, but they are amnestic for everything that happens. Therefore, most epileptologists define loss of consciousness as a lack of memory for the event, confusion, or disorientation.

Seizures can evolve to secondarily generalized tonic-clonic seizures. It is important to note the initial focal findings to properly classify these patients and differentiate them from patients with generalized seizures only. (*Adapted from* Commission on Classification and Terminology of the International League Against Epilepsy [18].)

Classification of Generalized Seizures (Convulsive or Nonconvulsive)

Absence seizures (signs alone or a combination)
  Impairment of consciousness only
  With mild clonic components
  With atonic components
  With tonic components
  With automatisms
  With autonomic components
Atypical absence
  Changes in tone that are more pronounced than
    typical absence
  Onset or cessation that is not abrupt
Myoclonic seizures
  Myoclonic jerks (single or multiple)
Clonic seizures
Tonic seizures
Tonic-clonic seizures
Atonic seizures (astatic)
Repeated epileptic seizures occuring under a variety of
  circumstances
  Fortuitous attacks
  Cyclic attacks (menstrual, sleep-wake cycle)
  Attacks provoked by nonsensory factors such as fatigue,
    alcohol, emotion, etc.
  Attacks provoked by sensory factors such as reflex seizures
Status epilepticus
  Convulsive
  Nonconvulsive

Figure 10-2. Classification of generalized seizures. Classification of generalized seizures is based primarily on clinical signs. Absence seizures typically begin with a stare and may contain other motor manifestations if they are long lasting. A typical absence seizure is difficult to differentiate from complex partial seizures, particularly if automatisms occur, so an electroencephalogram (EEG) is very useful in separating these two entities. Myoclonic seizures are important to recognize because of the long treatment implications. Many patients remember myoclonic jerks before their generalized seizure and these movements should not be mistaken for a focal ictal onset. Myoclonic jerks can be single or multiple and can be seen in idiopathic epilepsies such as juvenile myoclonic epilepsy or in symptomatic generalized epilepsies such as the progressive myoclonus epilepsies. Clonic seizure semiology can be difficult to differentiate from myoclonic jerks, but usually involves loss of consciousness and often precedes a generalized convulsion, whereas myoclonic jerks may not be associated with alteration of consciousness in all cases. Tonic seizures consist of stiffening of the extremities and trunk. These patients tend to fall and injure themselves and thus are often misdiagnosed with atonic seizures in which muscle tone is lost. Electromyogram monitoring or videotaping during EEG is helpful in differentiating these entities. Tonic-clonic seizures represent the endpoint of a variety of initial seizure types, and seizures that are generalized from onset can be tonic-clonic with the initial phase as a tonic event.

Provoked seizures are not generally considered diagnostic of epilepsy unless unprovoked attacks occur. Often treatment is aimed at elimination of the provocative factors. Status epilepticus is a condition characterized by repetitive seizures, or continuous seizures lasting 30 minutes. Most physicians treat the patient before the situation reaches this point to avoid progression to classical status. Status epilepticus is classified into two categories, convulsive and nonconvulsive. Any seizure type can occur repetitively and can constitute status epilepticus.

Idiopathic Localization-Related Epilepsies and Syndromes With Age-Related Onset

Benign childhood epilepsy with centro-temporal spike
Childhood epilepsy with occipital paroxysms
Autosomal dominant nocturnal frontal lobe epilepsy
Familial temporal lobe epilepsy
Primary reading epilepsy

Figure 10-3. Idiopathic localization-related epilepsies and syndromes with age-related onset. It is very likely that more of these epilepsies will be described over time since the genetic disorders are only now being discovered. Idiopathic epilepsies in general have no brain abnormality grossly, and are typically associated with normal intelligence and normal electroencephalogram (EEG) backgrounds. Most idiopathic epilepsies are generalized epilepsies, and these focal epilepsies are exceptions. Autosomal dominant nocturnal frontal lobe epilepsy [19] is a recent example of a genetic partial epilepsy that is easily treated with carbamazepine. The genetic defect involves a subunit of the nicotinic acetylcholine receptor. Familial temporal lobe epilepsy has not been as well characterized [20]. (*Adapted from* Commission on Classification and Terminology of the International League Against Epilepsy [21].)

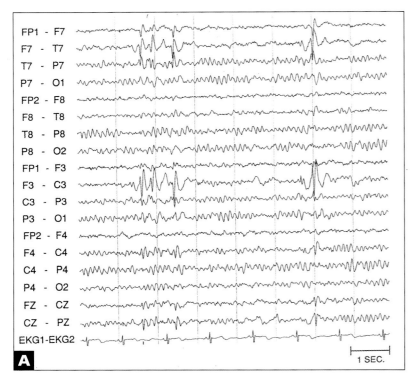

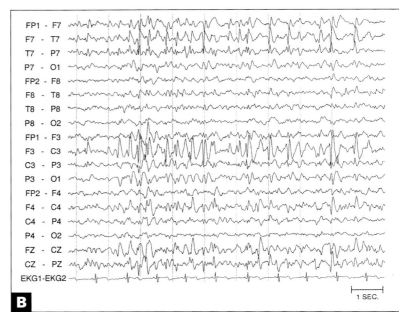

Figure 10-4. Benign rolandic epilepsy. Electroencephalograms (EEGs) from a 9-year-old boy with a history of nocturnal generalized tonic-clonic seizures that responded well to antiepileptic drugs. **A,** EEG from the awake background with several sharp waves in the left centrotemporal region. This distribution is typical for benign rolandic epilepsy, but it is not diagnostic for rolandic epilepsy, since other entities such as structural lesions can present with similar spiking. If the clinical history is appropriate, however, the best clinical correlation of these waveforms would be rolandic epilepsy. **B,** There is significant activation of the EEG spiking in sleep. The discharges are often quite continuous. The patients are usually asymptomatic at this time. This fascinating disorder may have a genetic component, and is almost always resolved by the age of 16. If seizures occur they can include simple partial motor seizures of the lower face and generalized tonic-clonic seizures [22–30].

Figure 10-5. Symptomatic localization-related epilepsies and syndromes. Symptomatic epilepsies are those that are due to underlying localized central nervous system (CNS) disorder. When the insult is localized to a specific brain region, seizures often occur with typical behaviors for that area. Thus, these epilepsies are classified according to lobe. Most localization epilepsies originate in the temporal lobe, with a frontal lobe source being slightly less common. Parietal and occipital lobe epilepsies are rare and may be underdiagnosed because some patients cannot recall an aura that would assist localization, so that all witnesses describe is a complex partial or secondarily generalized seizure.

Symptomatic Localization-Related Epilepsies and Syndromes

Frontal lobe epilepsies
  Supplementary motor
  Cingulate
  Anterior frontopolar region
  Orbitofrontal
  Dorsolateral
  Opercular
  Epilepsies of the motor cortex
    Lower prerolandic
    Rolandic
    Paracentral lobule
Kojewnikow's syndrome
  Rasmussen's syndrome
  Variable lesion of motor cortex with late myoclonus
    (epilepsia partialis continua)
Temporal lobe epilepsies
  Hippocampal epilepsy
  Amygdalar
  Lateral temporal
  Opercular (insular)
Parietal lobe epilepsies
  Anterior
  Posterior
Occipital lobe epilepsies
  Supracalcarine
  Infracalcarine

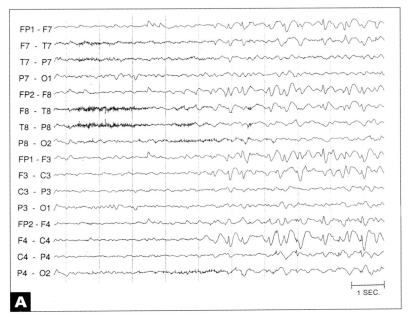

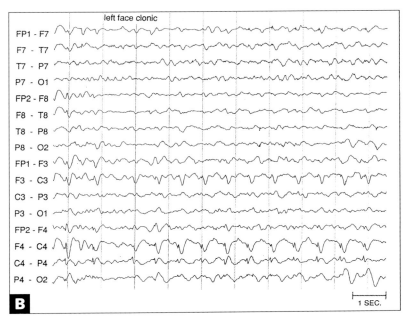

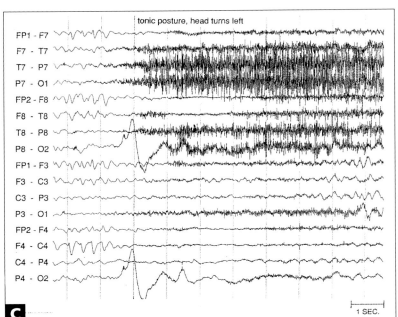

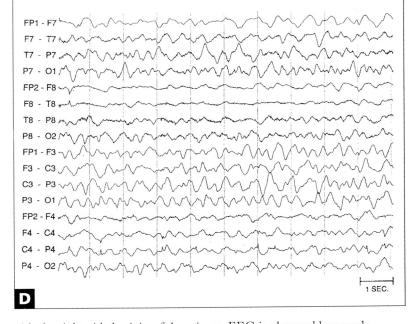

Figure 10-6. Electroencephalograms (EEGs) showing right frontal lobe seizures in a 7-year-old girl with a severe right frontal cortical dysplasia. **A,** The EEG onset is rather difficult to localize, though in the C4 electrode there is more prominent spiking. **B,** The spiking develops in a more rhythmical pattern and was associated clinically with left facial clonic activity. This is a highly reliable feature of a right hemisphere seizure involving the motor strip at the time those symptoms occurred. **C,** The patient suddenly developed tonic posturing and head version to the left side, again fitting with the right-sided origin of the seizure. EEG is obscured by muscle artifact at that point and the seizure did secondarily generalize. **D,** However, after the seizure had ended, significant postictal slowing is noted over the left side and amplitude attenuation is seen over the right hemisphere, with some persistent spiking at the C4 electrode. Postictal slowing is not always reliable for localization but certainly provides convincing evidence a seizure occurred and may agree occasionally with the localization of this seizure focus [31].

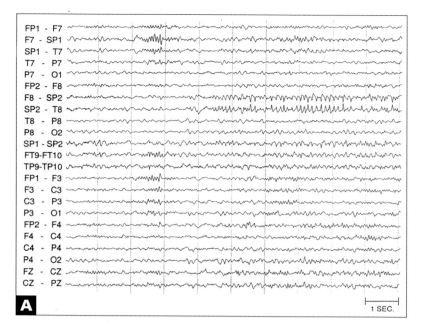

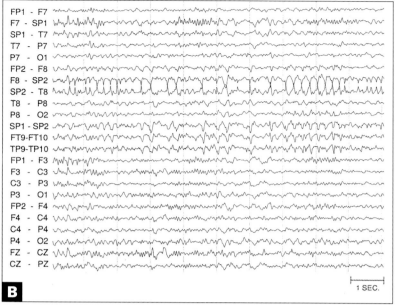

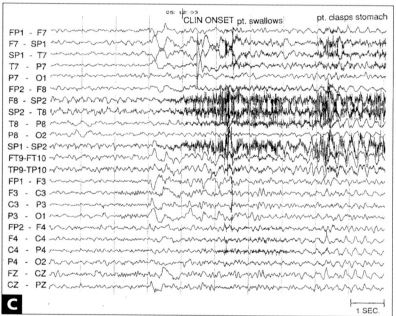

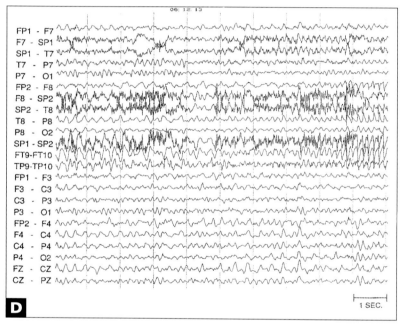

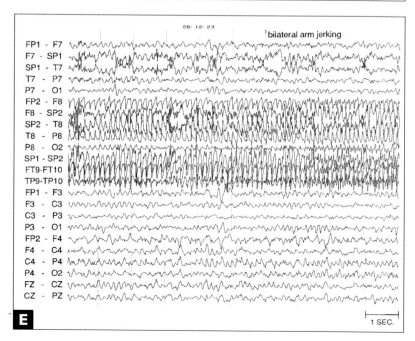

Figure 10-7. Sequence of electroencephalograms (EEGs) showing 10-second pages during a right temporal lobe partial seizure. This EEG pattern is the best localized scalp pattern that can be seen and is highly predictive of localization of the epileptogenic zone on the EEG [32]. **A**, Midway on the EEG there is a buildup of repetitive 7 to 8 Hz sharp activity limited to the right sphenoidal electrode. **B**, This pattern evolves by slowing, but becomes higher in amplitude as the seizure spreads to other brain regions. The patient is asymptomatic at this time. **C**, The clinical onset is marked when the patient begins to swallow and grasp his stomach, a typical aura for temporal lobe epilepsy. The EEG artifact does somewhat interfere with the viewing of the ictal patterns. **D**, There is more diffuse slowing at this point in time, but the seizure continues to evolve into a more well-defined, sustained rhythmic theta pattern. **E**, Again, there is phase reversing at the right sphenoidal electrode. These seizures can last several minutes and may not always progress to a more severe seizure type.

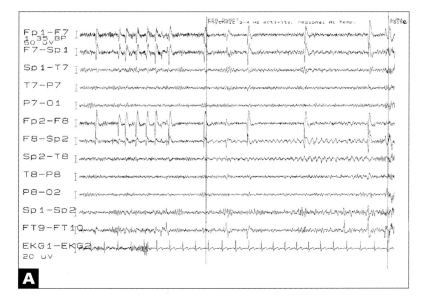

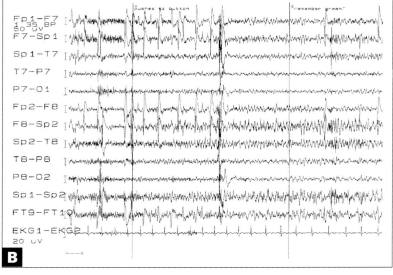

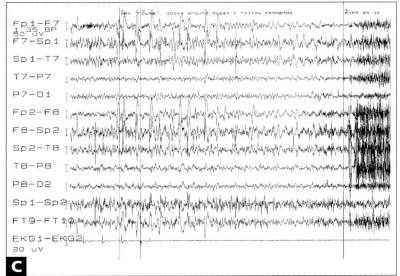

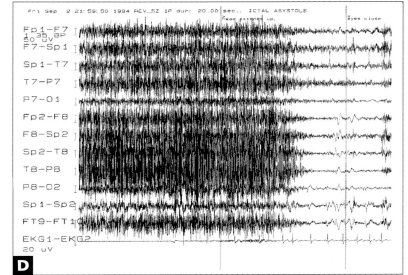

Figure 10-8. A patient with right temporal lobe epilepsy developed asystole during a complex partial seizure. This rare and potentially life-threatening complication has sometimes been referred to as a form of temporal lobe syncope [33–36]. Fortunately, the patient survived this attack. Two asystolic events were recorded during her evaluation. **A,** Electroencephalogram (EEG) showing the ictal onset over the right sphenoidal electrode at SP2 with rhythmic activity. **B,** Bradycardia appears at the end of the EEG as the EEG pattern develops. **C,** Asystole occurs. Clinically, without a video recording, it is difficult to appreciate the patient's behavior, but she suddenly became limp and developed tonic posturing and a few clonic jerks late in the seizure, suggesting a convulsive syncope. **D,** The cardiac rhythm returned and convulsive movements stopped. This patient was given a cardiac pacemaker to prevent sudden death because her seizures were uncontrolled.

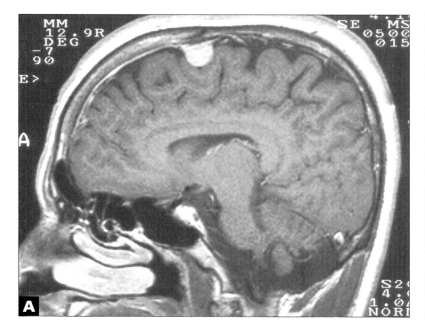

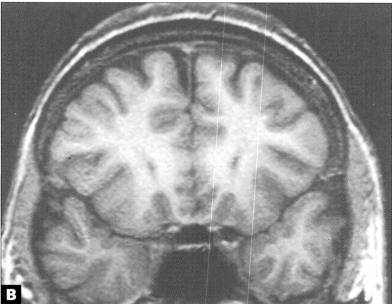

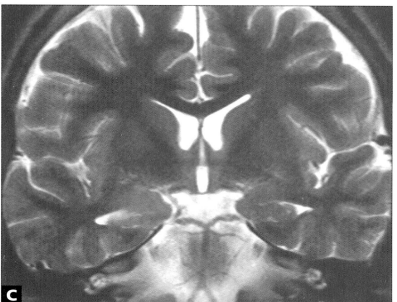

Figure 10-9. Magnetic resonance imaging (MRI) scans of a 20-year-old man with a history of febrile seizures as an infant, a latent period, and recurrence of seizures as a 17-year-old. The patient's seizures have been medically refractory. These scans demonstrate the complexities of evaluating patients for epilepsy surgery. **A,** A midline parasagittal meningioma that is visible slightly to the right side; however, after video electroencephalogram (EEG) monitoring it was clear that the patient had right temporal epilepsy based on the EEG seizure patterns and the clinical semiology of the seizure. Other MRI techniques in these series of pictures demonstrate right mesial temporal sclerosis. **B,** A more anterior coronal T1-weighted MRI view showing the distortion of the gray-white boundaries in the right anterior temporal lobe when compared to the left side. **C,** A more posterior coronal T2-weighted MRI view demonstrating marked hippocampal atrophy on the right side compared to the left. The undulations of the dentate gyrus can be appreciated in these 2-mm thick sections. MRI has become an essential tool in the evaluation of epilepsy [37–48].

Idiopathic Generalized Epilepsies and Syndromes With Age-Related Onset, Listed in Order of Age

Benign neonatal familial convulsions
Benign neonatal convulsions
Benign myoclonic epilepsy in infancy
Childhood absence epilepsy (pyknolepsy)
Juvenile absence epilepsy
Juvenile myoclonic epilepsy
Epilepsy with generalized tonic-clonic seizures on awakening
Other generalized idiopathic epilepsies not defined above
Epilepsies with seizures precipitated by specific modes of activation (most reflex epilepsies)

Figure 10-10. Idiopathic generalized epilepsies and syndromes with age-related onset, listed in order of age. Idiopathic generalized epilepsies are disorders that are presumably of genetic origin for most patients. Each syndrome has its characteristic age of seizure onset and prognosis. For example, benign neonatal familial convulsions resolve in the neonatal period. Childhood absence epilepsy often resolves in adolescence, whereas juvenile absence epilepsy carries a poorer long-term prognosis [49,50]. Juvenile myoclonic epilepsy is a lifelong condition and requires lifelong treatment [51].

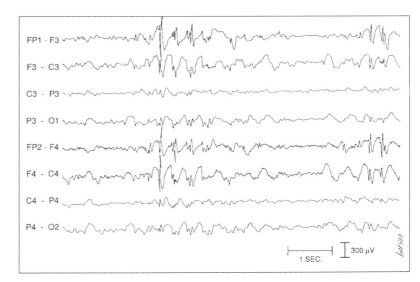

Figure 10-11. Electroencephalogram (EEG) showing a high amplitude 3-Hz generalized maximum bifrontal interictal spike wave complex in an 11-year-old patient with juvenile absence epilepsy. The spiking is often enhanced by hyperventilation or photic stimulation. Longer bursts of 3-Hz spike wave complexes may be associated with absence seizures.

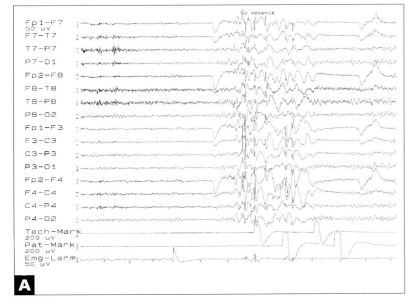

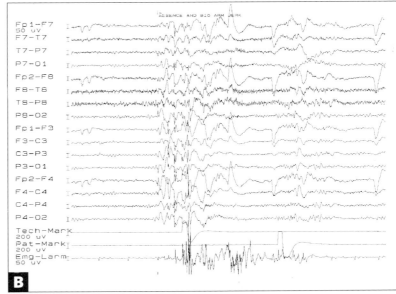

Figure 10-12. Electroencephalograms (EEGs) showing myoclonic jerk in a patient with myoclonic epilepsy. **A,** Ten seconds of EEG in a 14-year-old patient with recent onset of early morning myoclonic and tonic-clonic seizures. The bottom channels of the EEG tracing depict a clicking device that the technologist sounds during interesting EEG segments. The patient is then supposed to respond with a click at the same time, using her own handheld clicker. The bottom channel contains an electromyogram (EMG) monitor of the left arm. This EEG shows no alteration of consciousness or delay in response time with the 2- to 3-second bursts of generalized 4 to 5 Hz spike wave complexes.

B, The same patient has a myoclonic jerk in the arms associated with the electrographic spike and wave discharges. There is also a long delay before she is able to respond to the clicking noise, suggesting that consciousness may have been briefly altered, or perhaps the jerking interfered with the response.

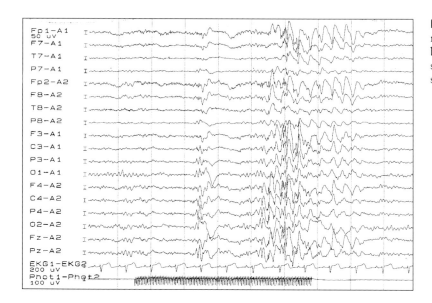

Figure 10-13. Electroencephalogram from a 13-year-old girl with juvenile myoclonic epilepsy who had a photoparoxysmal response that was sustained beyond the time of the flashing lights. The bottom channel of the recording shows the photic stimulation frequency. The vertical bars represent one-second intervals.

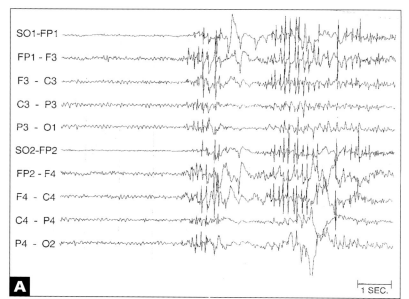

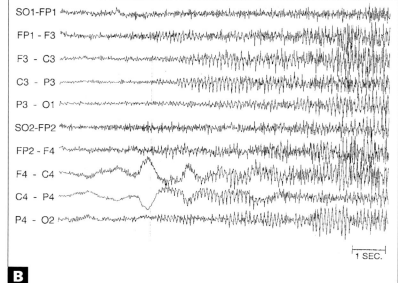

Figure 10-14. Electroencephalograms (EEGs) showing myoclonic jerks and a tonic-clonic seizure in a 35-year-old patient. **A,** Myoclonic jerks. **B,** A tonic-clonic seizure. The EEG rhythm evolves from motion artifact to a low voltage fast activity, building up to rapid generalized spike-wave discharges. Patients with myoclonic jerks followed by tonic-clonic seizures often have juvenile myoclonic epilepsy. This hereditary disorder is almost always successfully treated with divalproex sodium.

Cryptogenic or Symptomatic Epilepsies, in Order of Age of Appearance

Cryptogenic epilepsies
  West syndrome
  Lennox-Gastaut syndrome
  Epilepsy with myoclonic-astatic seizures
  Epilepsy with myoclonic absences
Symptomatic generalized epilepsies and syndromes
  Nonspecific etiology
    Early myoclonic encephalopathy
    Early infantile epileptic encephalopathy with burst
      suppression EEG
    Other symptomatic generalized epilepsies not defined above

Symptomatic generalized epilepsies and syndromes (*continued*)
  Specific syndromes
    Malformations
    Proven or suspected inborn error of metabolism
Epilepsies and syndromes undetermined—focal or generalized
  With both generalized and focal seizures
    Neonatal seizures
    Severe myoclonic epilepsy in infancy
    Epilepsy with continuous spike waves during slow wave sleep
    Acquired epileptic aphasia (Landau-Kleffner syndrome)
    Other undetermined epilepsies not defined above

(*Table continued on next page*)

Figure 10-15. Cryptogenic or symptomatic epilepsies, in order of age of appearances. Symptomatic generalized epilepsies are the most disabling forms of epilepsy. Patients are usually mentally retarded, have multiple seizure types, and are frequently medically intractable. In infants, infantile

(*Continued on next page*)

Cryptogenic or Symptomatic Epilepsies, in Order of Age of Appearance (*continued*)

Without unequivocal generalized or focal features
Special syndromes—situation-related seizures
  Febrile convulsions
  Isolated seizures or isolated status epilepticus
  Seizures occurring only when there is an acute metabolic or toxic event involving, *eg*, alcohol, drugs, eclampsia, nonketotic hyperglycemia

Figure 10-15. (*Continued*) spasms and hypsarrhythmia on electroencephalogram (EEG) are commonly followed by development of the Lennox-Gastaut syndrome with an EEG pattern of slow spike-wave complexes [52]. Occasionally, independent multifocal spike discharges are seen in EEGs [53], and all patterns can develop over time in an individual, with slow spike-wave complexes usually as the most stable pattern [54]. A variety of disorders that affect the nervous system can produce epilepsy as part of the symptom complex, but unlike the idiopathic epilepsies in which epilepsy is the primary neurologic symptom, mental retardation and other neurologic disability often are the major problems, and the epilepsy is only part of the illness.

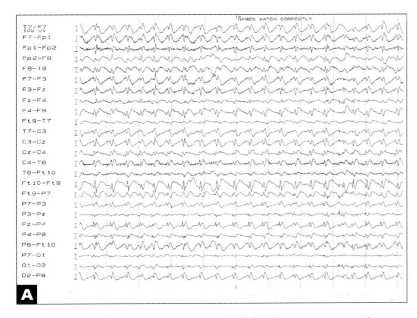

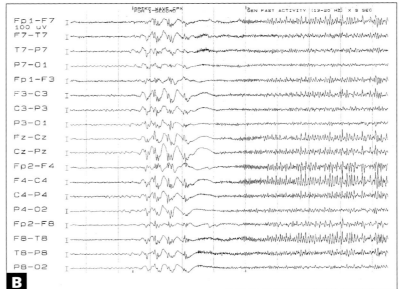

Figure 10-16. Electroencephalograms (EEGs) from a patient with Lennox-Gastaut syndrome. **A**, EEG showing slow spike-wave complexes typical of the Lennox-Gastaut syndrome. While the EEG is severely abnormal in these patients they are fully conscious and able to talk. **B**, The same patient with a seizure has the first 2 seconds of nonepileptiform EEG followed by bursts of generalized spike and wave complexes that evolve to low voltage fast activity and a tonic seizure. This is one of the seizure types that is typical of the Lennox-Gastaut syndrome, which often includes generalized tonic-clonic seizures, atypical absences, and even partial seizures.

Epidemiology of Epilepsy

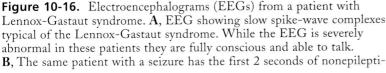

Incidences of Uncontrolled Epilepsy

Previously diagnosed patients

Ages, y	% With intractable seizures
0–14	28.1
15–64	51.9
65+	36.6

Newly diagnosed patients

Ages, y	% With intractable seizures 1–7 years after onset
0–15	24.2
15–64	24.3
65+	26.7

Figure 10-17. Incidences of uncontrolled epilepsy. Of all patients with epilepsy, 54% experience initial or delayed seizure control while 46% remain intractable, with at least occasional seizures. Incidences of uncontrolled epilepsy in previously diagnosed patients versus those in newly diagnosed patients are categorized by age [55]. As of 1995, there were 2.3 million patients in the United States diagnosed with epilepsy. Although epilepsy may begin in childhood, most people with epilepsy are of working age. The majority (62%) are between the ages of 15 and 64; 24% are age 65 or older; and 14% are under 14 years of age. Most patients (42%) newly diagnosed with epilepsy are between the ages of 15 and 64; 33% are age 65 or older; and 25% are under 14 years of age. A minority (24%) of these patients are refractory to treatment; 76% achieve seizure control.

The annual direct medical cost of epilepsy in the United States is $12.5 billion (includes medical costs but not long-term care costs or lost wages). Lifetime costs for 181,000 new cases each year is $11.1 billion. The average direct medical cost for 6 years is $6,429. Cost for the elderly is highest at $10,612; this figure does not include expenses for the 253,000 patients living in nursing homes. Men who continue to have seizures reduce their lifetime wages by 35% or $317,000, while women reduce their lifetime wages by 25% or $140,000. Even if seizures become controlled, lifetime lost wages are estimated at $59,000 for women and $210,000 for men. The lower figure for women reflects lower wage norms for women [55].

Causes of Epilepsy

Syndromes and Conditions That May Cause Epilepsy

Perinatal insults
  Perinatal asphyxia
Migrational disturbances
  Lissencephaly
  Bilateral perisylvian syndrome
  Cortical dysplasia
  Microdysgenesis in primary generalized epilepsies [77,78]
  Heterotopia
    Nodular [66]
    Microscopic
Hamartoma
Other malformations
Sturge Weber syndrome

Figure 10-18. Developmental or perinatal conditions that may cause epilepsy. In recent years it has been clear that a variety of migrational disturbances underlie many devastating childhood epilepsies [56]. Severe migrational disturbances such as lissencephaly and cortical dysphasia may be responsible for a third to half of all childhood epilepsy syndromes. It is unclear whether these represent a specific disease entity or rather a general response to an insult at a certain stage of neurologic development. Most likely, both occur with regard to cortical dysplasia. The bilateral perisylvian syndrome may represent an intrauterine vascular event. Some of the migrational and lamination disturbances are not visible on magnetic resonance imaging scan, particularly when subtle, and these entities can be very focal and produce focal seizures, or very widespread and produce generalized seizures and epilepsies.

Febrile convulsions may be benign or have been associated with the later development of chronic epilepsy, usually associated with mesial temporal sclerosis [39,57] particularly if prolonged [58]. A familial association exists [59]. Between 2% to 4% of children have a febrile convulsion [60].

Genetic Localization-related Epilepsies

Syndrome (nomenclature)	Gene locus	Gene product
AD nocturnal frontal lobe epilepsy (ADNFLE type 1): ENFL1 (75% penetrant)	20q13.2–q13.3 [61]	Alpha-4 subunit of the nicotinic acetylcholine receptor CHRNA4 [62]
AD nocturnal frontal lobe epilepsy (ADNFLE type 2): ENFL2	15q24 [63]	?
AD partial epilepsy with variable foci	22q11–q12 [64,65]	?
AD rolandic epilepsy with speech dyspraxia	? Possible triplet repeat [66]	?
Familial temporal lobe epilepsy (autosomal dominant, 60% penetrant)	? [67], 10q [68]	?
Benign occipital epilepsy (BOE)	? [69]	?
Benign rolandic epilepsy	?	?
Periventricular nodular heterotopia	Xq28 [70]	Filamin-1 [71]

Figure 10-19. Etiologies of genetic localization-related and generalized epilepsies. As of October 2000, McKusick [100] listed 194 genetic disorders with epilepsy as part of the syndrome. Genetic epilepsies are growing in number and many more entities await discovery. Most genetic epilepsies are known from the study of a few informative families and linkage analysis. Only a few gene products are known, such as the t-RNA lysine

Table continued on opposite page

Genetic Generalized Epilepsies

Syndrome (nomenclature)	Gene locus	Gene product
Benign familial neonatal convulsions (EBN1)	20q13.2–13.3 [72,73]	Potassium voltage-gated channel (KCNQ2)
Benign familial neonatal convulsions (EBN2)	8q24 [74,75]	KCNQ3
Benign familial infantile convulsions (BFIC) (onset 3–12 months, AD)	19q [76]	?
Familial infantile convulsions with paroxysmal choreoathetosis (ICCA syndrome)	16p12–q12 [77,78]	?
Febrile convulsions (FEB1) (AD)	8q13–21 [79]	?
Febrile convulsions (FEB2) (AD)	19p13.3 [80]	?
Febrile convulsions (FEB3) (AD)	2q23–24 [81]	?
Febrile convulsions (FEB4)	5q14–q15 [82]	?
Generalized epilepsy with febrile seizures plus (GEFS+)	19q13 [83] SCN1 gene	Sodium channel, voltage-gated, type I, alpha polypeptide
Generalized epilepsy with febrile seizures plus, type 2 (GEFSP2)	2q24	SCN1A gene
Childhood absence epilepsy	Possible 1p	?
Juvenile absence epilepsy (ECA1)	8q24 [84]	?
Juvenile myoclonic epilepsy, 1 (EJM1)	6p11 [85,86]	?
Juvenile myoclonic epilepsy, 2 (EJM2)	15q14 [87]	Possibly alpha-7 subunit of nAChR (CHRNA7)
Epilepsy with generalized tonic clonic seizures on awakening	6p	?
Lafora's disease (EPM2A)	6q24 [88,89]	Laforin
Epilepsy, progressive, with mental retardation (EPMR) (Northern Epilepsy syndrome)	8p [90]	?
Unverricht-Lundborg disease (baltic myoclonic epilepsy) (EPM1)	21q22.3 [91,92,93]	Cystatin B [94]
Benign adult familial myoclonic epilepsy (BAFME)	8q23.3–q24.11 [95]	?
Myoclonic epilepsy with ragged red fibers (MERRF)	Mitochondrial DNA	t-RNA lysine [96,97]
Angelman syndrome (AS)	15q11–q13 [98]	UBE3A [99]

Figure 10-19. *(continued)* defect in myoclonic with ragged red fibers (MERRF) [96,97]. This is an area of intense research interest because understanding the genetics of epilepsies may lead to effective and disease-specific therapies. AD—autosomal dominant.

Cortical Dysplasia

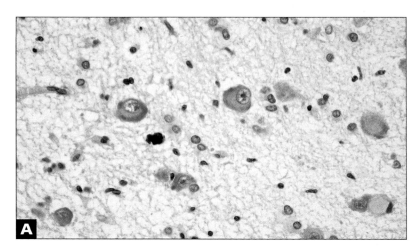

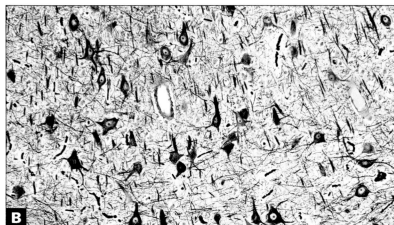

Figure 10-20. Histologic slides showing cortical dysplasia. Cortical dysplasia is a disorder that arises during neuronal migration. The cortex, which consists of disorganized and sometimes bizarrely shaped neural elements, is highly epileptogenic. Electroencephalographic activity is very epileptiform compared with other structural lesions [101,102]. When dysplasia is severe, seizures often are extremely severe and have an early age of onset. They can lead to progressive neurologic deterioration, which can be slowed with successful surgical intervention [103]. Cortical dysplasia can also be extremely focal, present in just one gyrus, and cause epilepsy later in life in an otherwise normal individual. **A,** Unlike heterotopic neurons in the white matter, which consist of more normal appearing neurons, dysplastic neurons are often enlarged as balloon cells as the giant neurons scatter in the cortical mantle. Balloon cells are seen in the most severe form of cortical dysplasia, whereas in milder forms the findings may be more subtle and neuroimaging studies may be normal [38,104,105]. **B,** Bielschowsky's stain highlights the cytoskeletal elements that demonstrate the bizarrely shaped neurons oriented in various directions, which suggest the chaotic abnormalities of the cortical architecture and synaptic connections. (*Courtesy of* H. Vinters, UCLA School of Medicine, Department of Neuropathology, Los Angeles, CA.)

Nodular Heterotopia

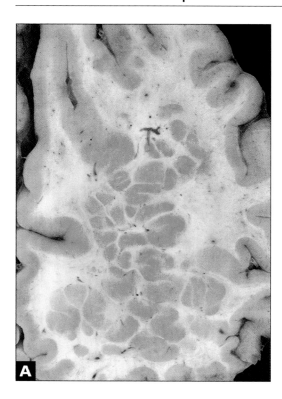

Figure 10-21. Nodular heterotopia. **A,** Pathologic specimen of a brain demonstrating severe neuronal heterotopia within the white matter. Heterotopic neurons most likely originate during neuronal migration when masses of neurons from the germinal matrix migrate to assume their position in the cortex. Recently this disorder has been found to be an X-linked genetic disorder expressed in women and lethal to male fetuses as exemplified by a high rate of miscarriage [70,106–108]. Some patients have normal intelligence and mild epilepsy.

(*Continued on next page*)

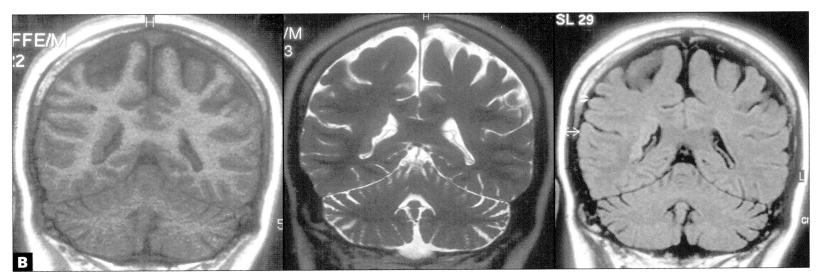

Figure 10-21. (*Continued*) **B**, Magnetic resonancing imaging scan showing predominantly right-sided trigonal nodular heterotopia with T1, T2, and FLAIR (fluid-attenuated inversion recovery) image sequences. This is a 27-year-old woman diagnosed with epilepsy at age 16 with complex partial and occasional secondarily generalized tonic-clonic seizures. She was born 6 weeks premature and had no other epilepsy risk factors. There is no family history of females with epilepsy or excessive miscarriages of male offspring. Interictal electroencephalogram (EEG) showed right temporal spikes and sharp waves; ictal EEG showed a posterior temporal ictal onset at the P8 and TP10 electrodes. (Panel A *courtesy of* H. Vinters, UCLA School of Medicine, Department of Neuropathology, Los Angeles, CA.)

Middle Cranial Meningocele

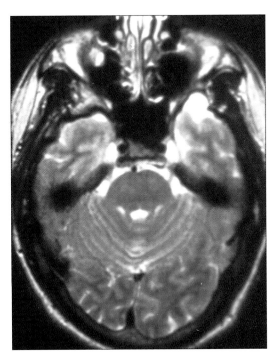

Figure 10-22.
Magnetic resonance imaging scan showing a bony defect in the floor of the middle cranial fossa in a patient with a middle cranial fossa meningocele. The meningocele in this 41-year-old patient was most likely a congenital abnormality. He did not develop epilepsy until he was 31 years old, and his seizures consist of an aura of déjà vu and only rarely have led to alteration of consciousness.

Tumors Causing Epilepsy

Low grade neoplasms
  Ganglioglioma
  Dysembryoplastic neuroepithelial tumor (DNT)
  Low grade astrocytoma
Malignant neoplasms
  Anaplastic astrocytoma
  Glioblastoma
  Oligodendroglioma
  Metastatic neoplasms

Figure 10-23. Tumors causing epilepsy. Tumors are a major cause of epilepsy in adults. Low grade tumors, such as gangliogliomas, have a tendency to present as chronic epilepsy because they are not often seen on computed tomography scans. Neuroimaging studies should be done in patients who have not had such studies in recent years, particularly if they have focal epilepsy that has been difficult to control. Low grade neoplasms are treatable with surgical resection in many cases and may not require radiation or chemotherapy. Malignant neoplasms, on the other hand, may often present with recent seizures that are not difficult to control, but the main clinical issue is mass effect and the tumors' progression, thus these tumors often require a more aggressive approach.

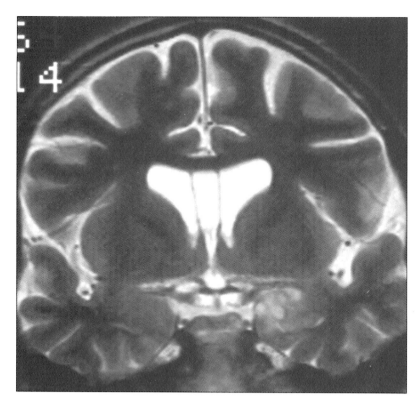

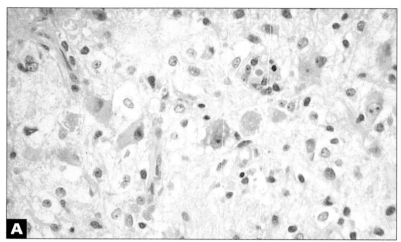

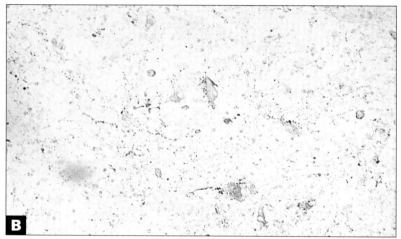

Figure 10-24. Magnetic resonance imaging (MRI) scan from a 35-year-old right-handed patient with a ganglioglioma of the left amygdala. He has had seizures since he was 14 years old. The seizures consist of an aura of déjà vu or a smell of butterscotch followed by speech arrest and, rarely, loss of consciousness. An electroencephalogram showed left temporal spikes in a left temporal ictal pattern. An MRI scan done 6 years earlier showed a similar lesion, although it was not recognized at the time. The lesion in the left amygdala does not enhance with gadolinium and represents a ganglioglioma. A dysembryoplastic neuroepithelial tumor would be another diagnostic consideration. These lesions tend to grow very slowly, if at all. The patient also has a cavum septum pellucidum.

Figure 10-25. Histologic slides showing a ganglioglioma. Gangliogliomas are a low-grade neoplasm with mixed neuronal and glial elements. These are a common cause of epileptic seizures, particularly when the seizures are chronic. Morris and colleagues have shown that seizures are the main presenting symptom [109]. With complete resection, prognosis is excellent for a seizure-free outcome [110,111]. **A, B,** The key features of ganglioglioma consist of neuronal elements in a more benign-appearing glial background [112]. Low-grade neoplasms are occasionally associated with cortical dysplasia, suggesting a developmental etiology [113,114]. (*Courtesy of* H. Vinters, UCLA School of Medicine, Department of Neuropathology, Los Angeles, CA.)

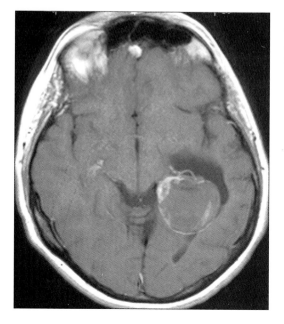

Figure 10-26. Magnetic resonance imaging (MRI) scan with gadolinium from a 40-year-old patient with an epidermoid tumor. She had two seizures in her life, at an interval of 16 years. The second seizure prompted the MRI scan. This lesion, an intraventricular epidermoid neoplasm, was resected and she has remained seizure free.

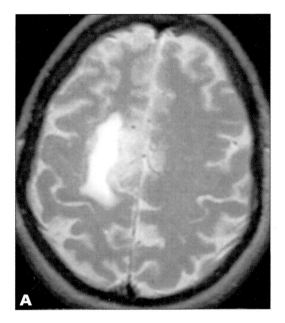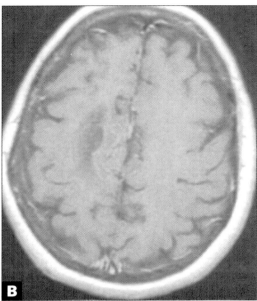

Figure 10-27. Tumoral epilepsy. Magnetic resonance imaging (MRI) scans showing an oligodendroglioma. **A,** MRI scan showing a large low-grade astrocytoma in the right premotor area in a 51-year-old woman with a nearly normal neurologic exam (except for left arm hyperreflexia) and a 9-year history of infrequent seizures. Frontal lobe tumors can get quite large without causing symptoms other than seizures. **B,** T1-weighted MRI scan of the right premotor area appears hypointense and there is some mass effect, but not as much as would be seen with more malignant neoplasms. The sulcus at the bottom of the lesion most likely represents the central sulcus. Preoperatively, the patient's seizures consisted of secondarily generalized tonic-clonic seizures. There has been no recurrence on MRI two and a half years after resection of the tumor. The patient remained seizure-free for one and a half years and then experienced several simple partial motor seizures of the left foot after attempted medication reduction.

Cerebrovascular Disease

Epilepsy Caused by Cerebrovascular Disease

Infarct
Hematoma
Vascular malformation
  Arteriovenous malformation
  Venous angioma
  Cavernous angioma
Vasculitis
Hypoperfusion

Figure 10-28. Epilepsy caused by cerebrovascular disease. Cerebrovascular disease is a common etiology of epilepsy, particularly in the elderly population, but in young individuals one should suspect an underlying vascular malformation. Many of these epilepsies are pharmacoresistant and would require surgical intervention for either seizures or management of the vascular malformation.

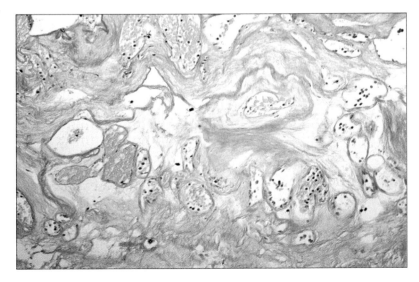

Figure 10-29. Cavernous angioma. Pathologic specimen showing cavernous angioma (magnification × 10). Cavernous angiomas are a common etiology for epilepsy and in some families are hereditary [115]. Approximately 50% of patients who have cavernous angiomas found on imaging studies initially present with epilepsy. According to Robinson and colleagues, the natural history of cavernous angiomas is fairly benign, with only a 0.7% per year incidence of hemorrhage, which is usually not severe enough to cause significant long-term neurologic disability, unless lesions are infratentorial [116,117]. Hemosiderin deposition around the cavernous angioma is an irritant that may provoke seizures [118]. In addition, there is occasionally a localized dysplasia around the cavernous angioma. These lesions can be multiple and, if seizures are intractable, it is sometimes difficult to determine which specific cavernous angioma is responsible for the epilepsy. When lesions are situated near the cerebral cortex they are more likely to be epileptogenic. (*Courtesy of* H. Vinters, UCLA School of Medicine, Department of Neuropathology, Los Angeles, CA.)

Infections and Inflammation

Epilepsy Caused by Infections and Inflammation

Meningitis
  Bacterial
  Fungal
  Mycobacteria
Encephalitis
  Herpes
  HIV
  Rasmussen's encephalitis
  Others
Parasitic
  Cysticercosis

Figure 10-30. Epilepsy caused by infections and inflammation. Infections are another common etiology of epilepsy. Interestingly, when children acquire meningitis or encephalitis before the age of 5 they often present with mesial temporal sclerosis later in life [119], whereas these infections in adults are often more devastating and present with neocortical seizures. One of the most common etiologies for epilepsy in the developing world is cysticercosis, particularly in Latin America [120]. It is derived from undercooked pork and poor sanitary practices.

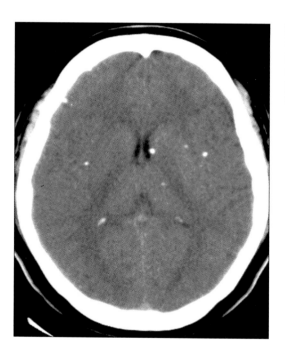

Figure 10-31. Computed tomography (CT) scan from a patient with cysticercosis, one of the most frequent causes of epilepsy worldwide. The patient is a 31-year-old woman, who is a native of Mexico and who has a history of seizures since she was 8 years old. They are complex partial seizures without an aura, which occasionally secondarily generalize. Calcifications can be seen throughout the brain parenchyma in multiple locations. Fortunately, the patient is on medications that have kept her free of seizures, as the number of lesions would make surgery difficult.

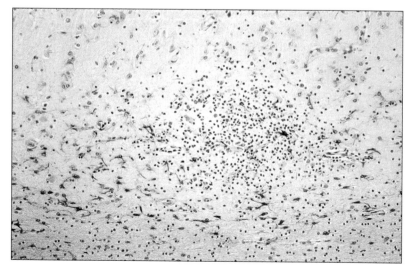

Figure 10-32. Histologic slide showing Rasmussen's encephalitis. Rasmussen's encephalitis is a poorly understood progressive form of epilepsy that results in progressive cortical atrophy and intractable seizures, often with simple partial motor seizures being the most common seizure type. Children are most often affected, but this syndrome can occur in adults. While an infectious agent is suspected in the pathogenesis of the inflammation, no specific virus has been consistently implicated [121,122]. Until lately, the treatment of this disorder included hemispherectomy [123–126]. Recently, the presence of anti-glutamate receptor subunit 3 (GluR3) antibodies in several patients with this disorder has suggested an autoimmune etiology [127–129]. Rasmussen's encephalitis demonstrates inflammatory cells within the cortical mantle (glial fibrillary acid protein [GFAP] stain, magnification ×10) [130]. (*Courtesy of* H. Vinters, UCLA School of Medicine, Department of Neuropathology, Los Angeles, CA.)

Head Trauma

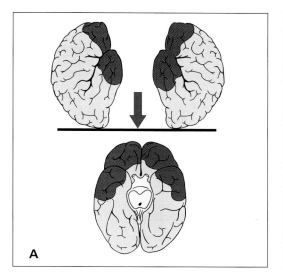

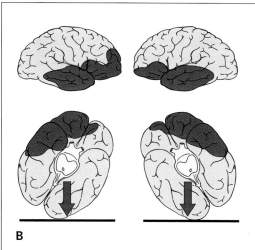

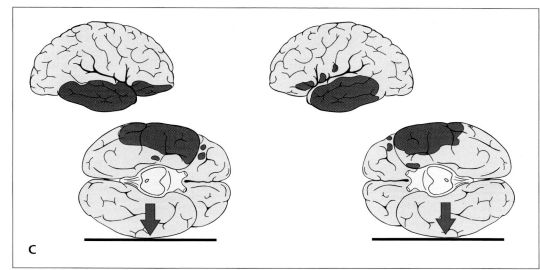

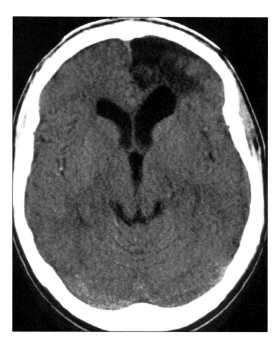

Figure 10-34. Computed tomography (CT) scan showing a large area of encephalomalacia in the left frontal lobe with dilation of the left frontal horn of the lateral ventricle. The CT scan is from a 21-year-old man who was in a motor vehicle accident at age 16. He suffered a right-sided skull fracture and early seizures and was in a coma for 3 weeks. He has simple partial adversive seizures that secondarily generalize but are well controlled with phenytoin and gabapentin.

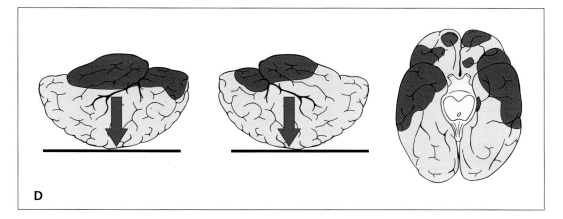

Figure 10-33. Epilepsy caused by head trauma. Head trauma is a frequent cause of epilepsy, but usually the injuries are quite severe, often involving penetration of the dura and intracranial bleeding [131]. Concussions are very common, and many patients recall having a head injury before seizures, although these are likely unrelated. Early seizures, occurring less than 1 week after trauma, confer a significant risk factor for chronic epilepsy to develop, probably within 1 to 4 years [132]. Late seizures, occurring 1 week after the trauma, are an ominous predictor of chronic epilepsy, with about half of the cases developing seizures within the first post-injury year. Electroencephalogram may not be a good predictor of late epilepsy after trauma [133]. Courville studied head trauma victims in a large series of autopsied cases to correlate contusion location and the direction of impact [134]. No matter what the direction of impact, the frontal and temporal lobes seem to bear the brunt of contusions, which may explain why posttraumatic epilepsy often involves the frontal or temporal lobes when there is closed head injury. **A,** Contusions of the temporal lobe from a posterior impact. **B,** Contusions of the temporal lobe from posterolateral impact. **C,** Contusions of the temporal lobe from lateral impact; **D,** Contusions of the temporal lobe from vertical impact.

Diagnosis of Epileptic Seizures

Differential Diagnosis of Non-epileptic Seizures

Syncope
Hyperventilation
Breath holding spell
Sleep disorder
  Narcolepsy/cataplexy
  Sleep apnea
  Parasomnia
Migraine
Cerebrovascular disease movement disorders
Transient global amnesia
Toxic/metabolic encephalopathy
Movement disorders
Vertigo
Psychiatric/behavioral
  Psychogenic seizures
    Conversion disorder
    Malingering
  Episodic lack of control
  Panic disorder
  Obsessive-compulsive behavior
  Stereotypy
  Dissociative states
    Psychogenic fugue
    Multiple personality
    Psychogenic amnesia
    Depersonalization disorder
  Normal daydreaming

Figure 10-35. Differential diagnosis of non-epileptic seizures. A wide variety of disorders can mimic epilepsy and be misdiagnosed as epileptic seizures. These include syncope, hyperventilation, breath holding spells, and sleep disorders. Certainly vascular disease movement disorders, vertigo, and migraine are also considerations in the differential diagnosis. Usually electroencephalogram and a good clinical history are able to separate the nonepileptic events from the epileptic. Psychogenic seizures are particularly disturbing aspects that neurologists encounter frequently. Patients who are susceptible to psychogenic seizures usually have a history of physical or sexual abuse, and the most common etiology is conversion disorder, however, malingering and other dissociative states may also be present.

Laboratory Investigation of Seizures

Blood work
Routine EEG
  Timing
  Activation procedures
    Photic, hyperventilation, sleep
Sleep deprived EEG
Video-EEG monitoring
Cognitive testing
Neuroimaging structure and function
  MRI, CT
  PET, SPECT
  MR Spectroscopy, functional MRI
  Angiography, MR angiography
  MEG

Figure 10-36. Laboratory investigation of seizures. A variety of tests have been used to determine the causes of seizures or epilepsy, as treatment may be needed for an underlying disorder. Blood chemistries and other blood work occasionally identify an underlying metabolic disturbance responsible for seizures. Electroencephalogram (EEG) is the single most useful test, but it is best if recording is done during a seizure or just after it, when spiking is more prevalent. Before specific epileptiform discharges can be identified, several EEGs are often necessary, including an EEG done during sleep or after sleep deprivation. When the diagnosis is unclear, video-EEG is the best way to confirm a diagnosis of epilepsy or nonepileptic seizures. Cognitive testing is useful in patients with complaints of memory problems or who display psychiatric symptoms or signs, because depression is common in epilepsy and cognitive training or psychiatric intervention may help minimize disability. Neuroimaging is as important as EEG in the diagnosis of epilepsy etiology. Computed tomography (CT) scan is rarely useful and even if an abnormality is detected, magnetic resonance imaging (MRI) almost always shows it better. MRI is the procedure of choice, and epilepsy protocols exist to look for hippocampal sclerosis and migrational disturbances, which are common causes of partial epilepsy. The remaining tests listed here are not routine, but in select cases they may be helpful in planning epilepsy surgery. Magnetic resonance (MR) spectroscopy, functional MRI, and magnetoencephalography (MEG) currently are under investigation for their usefulness as neuroimaging tools for localization of the epileptogenic zone. PET—positron emission tomography; SPECT—single photon emission computed tomography.

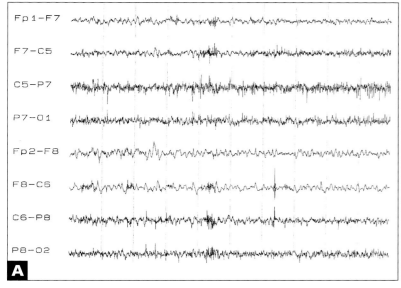 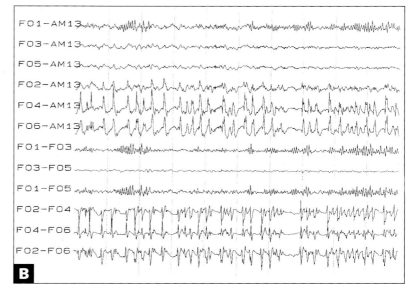

Figure 10-37. Electroencephalograms (EEGs) in a patient with temporal lobe epilepsy experiencing an aura. **A,** Scalp EEG showing an ongoing seizure, but changes are minimal, if any, and certainly no recognizable seizure pattern is present. **B,** However, with foramen ovale (FO in montage) electrodes one can clearly see a right-sided ictal pattern. FO electrode contacts that are evenly numbered are adjacent to the right mesial temporal lobe and odd numbered contacts are left sided. The AM13 electrode was a left lateral temporal depth electrode contact used as a reference for this particular recording. This proves that patients may have seizures without scalp EEG changes. This is a particular problem with simple partial non-motor seizures because only 15% have scalp EEG changes, whereas if motor activity was seen during the simple partial seizure, 33% of seizures had EEG changes [135]. Use of additional scalp electrodes may increase the yield of scalp EEG [136].

Treatment of Epilepsy

Drugs

Drugs Used in the Treatment of Epilepsy

Drugs for partial epilepsies		Drugs for generalized epilepsies	
First line	Second line	For absence seizures only	Second line
Phenytoin	Lamotrigine	Ethosuximide	Primidone
Carbamazepine	Topiramate	For all generalized seizures	Phenobarbital
Oxcarbazepine	Tiagabine	First line	Clonazepam
Gabapentin	Zonisamide	Divalproex sodium or	Felbamate
Levetiracetam	Felbamate	valproic acid	Possible
Divalproex sodium or	Primidone	Lamotrigine	Levetiracetam
valproic acid	Phenobarbital	Topiramate	Zonisamide
	Benzodiazepines		

Figure 10-38. Drugs used in the treatment of epilepsy. The goals of epilepsy treatment include freedom from seizures without side effects, maximal quality of life, minimal disability, simple monotherapy regimens, and the use of antiepileptic drugs without drug interactions. If seizures are provoked, it is reasonable to eliminate the provocative factors and expect a good outcome without treatment. If seizures are unprovoked and it is a first seizure, it still may not be necessary to treat, because many patients have a single seizure in their lifetime, and it may not be possible to identify the provocative factors [137,138]. However, if the history is highly suggestive of focal onset, the neuroimaging studies are abnormal, the neurologic exam is abnormal, and the electroencephalogram (EEG) shows epileptiform abnormalities indicating a high risk of seizure recurrence, it would be reasonable to begin treatment after a single seizure. A good example of this would be a patient with a brain tumor, stroke, or other obvious structural lesion; the EEG may show slowing or spiking and the clinical exam fits with the neuroimaging studies. These patients may be harmed by additional seizures while they are acutely ill, and it is rea-sonable to treat them to prevent further seizures. If more than one unprovoked seizure occurs, the patient has epilepsy, and by classifying the seizure and epilepsy type, an appropriate antiepileptic drug (AED) can be chosen. Most patients should begin treatment with first-line antiepileptic drugs. Drugs are considered first line owing to their ease of use or low toxicity or second line owing to their slow titration to effective dose, higher risk for toxicity, or need for more intensive laboratory monitoring. With numerous new antiepileptic drugs available in recent years, and no comparative studies to decide the appropriate order of medication trials, the designation of drugs as first line or second line is an approximation and will likely change as new data become available. Individual patient characteristics will influence dose, timing, compliance, need for polypharmacy, and the type of formulation (tablet, liquid, capsule). Individual pharmacokinetic variables can increase or decrease the daily dosage necessary. Patient compliance is improved if the physician allows the patient to choose the formulation of the drug.

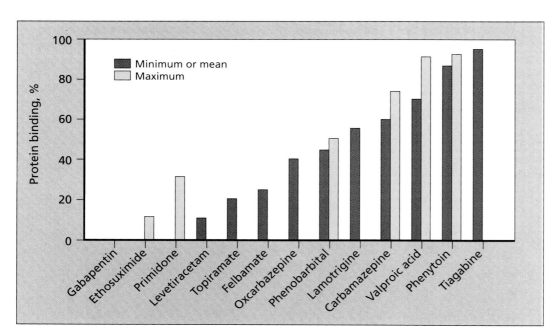

Figure 10-39. Antiepileptic drug protein binding. After absorption, drugs may bind to plasma proteins, usually albumin. The unbound portion, or free level, is what enters the brain and is pharmacologically active. Drugs that have minimal protein binding will not have clinically relevant changes in brain levels of the drug in the presence of other highly protein-bound drugs or disease states that alter protein binding, such as uremia. In uremia, free phenytoin levels can approach 30% of the total level and cause toxicity despite the "normal" total phenytoin level. Thus, adjustment of the total level is necessary to maintain an appropriate brain level of phenytoin. The disadvantage of no protein binding is that the drug is more completely removed in hemodialysis. A drug like gabapentin must be dosed after each dialysis to make up for what has been removed.

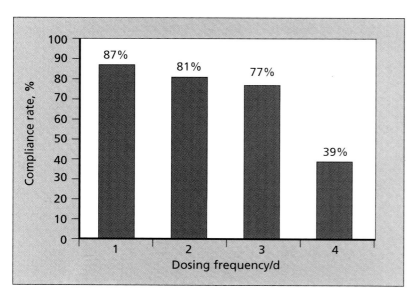

Figure 10-40. Compliance and dosing schedules. Besides using an ineffective antiepileptic drug, noncompliance is another major reason for uncontrolled seizures. A study investigating dosing frequency and compliance using standard pill bottles with microprocessors in the caps recorded every bottle opening as a presumptive dose. The results indicated that a regimen of a drug given four times a day was not possible for the majority of patients [139]. Simple drug regimens work best and the newer antiepileptic drugs, with the exception of gabapentin, have been approved for dosing twice a day. Physicians, nurses, pharmacists, and family can work together to improve medication compliance. Patient education, written instructions, monitoring of antiepileptic drug levels, and communication by phone, e-mail, and clinic visits will all enhance medication compliance.

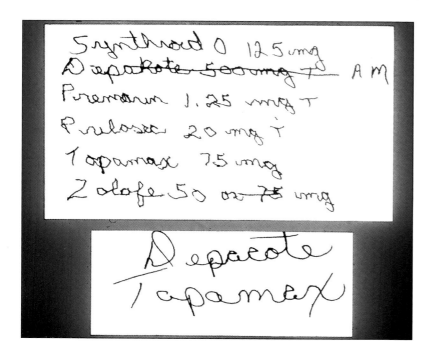

Figure 10-41. Tremor with divalproex sodium (VPA) illustrated by handwriting sample from a 50-year-old woman with partial epilepsy. Initially seen when taking VPA and topiramate, she complained of tremor so severe that her handwriting deteriorated (*top*). Two months later, after VPA was tapered, she returned much improved and was able to write more clearly (*bottom*).

Antiepileptic Drug Toxicity

Dose-related effects	Idiosyncratic reactions
Sedation	Allergy
Impaired cognition	Rash
Ataxia	Stevens-Johnson syndrome
Nystagmus	Drug-induced lupus
Tremor	Hematologic
Long-term effects	Aplastic anemia platelet dysfunction
Osteoporosis	Hepatitis
Cerebellar atrophy	Teratogenic
Nephrolithiasis	
Neuropathy	**Drug interactions**

Figure 10-42. Antiepileptic drug toxicity. Patients should be educated about the major categories of antiepileptic drug toxicity common to many first- and second-line agents. Specific drugs or clinical situations may require additional warnings, *eg*, aplastic anemia with felbamate or the high risk of hepatotoxicity with valproic acid in infants. Depending on the medication, antiepileptic drug failure due to toxicity occurs in 5% to 50% of patients. Dose-related effects are managed by dose reduction, change in dosing schedule, or both. Long-term effects necessitate periodic clinic visits with appropriate examination. Idiosyncratic reactions vary by drug and are customarily evaluated by routine hematology or blood chemistry monitoring. Often, severe idiosyncratic reactions are first noticed by the patient, prompting an unscheduled clinic visit.

Surgery

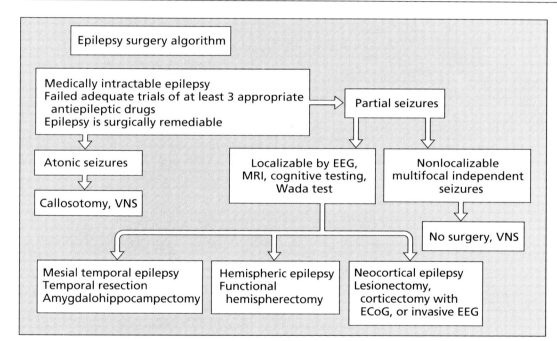

Figure 10-43. Algorithm for determining the need for epilepsy surgery. When seizures are refractory to medical management the patient should be evaluated at an epilepsy center for possible epilepsy surgery [140]. It usually takes no more than 2 years to determine whether a patient is medically intractable, after the failure of three appropriate antiepileptic drugs given at adequate doses for an adequate period of time with adequate compliance. There are a variety of surgical procedures available [141,142]. The most common surgical procedure is the anterior temporal lobectomy for medial temporal lobe epilepsy, which has a success rate of about 70% to 80% of patients remaining seizure free. Ideal patients have intractable complex partial seizures, and their neuroimaging studies such as magnetic resonance imaging (MRI), positron emission test scan, ictal single photon emission computed tomography (SPECT) study, cognitive testing, and the Wada test show concordant information for localization. The usual pathology is hippocampal sclerosis, particularly with early insults such as complicated febrile convulsions. Epilepsy surgery can be done in other brain regions, and the patients with the best outcomes usually have obvious structural lesions that can be completely resected without inducing a neurologic deficit. It is important to include the entire epileptogenic zone if it extends beyond the lesion itself. This is more of a problem with lesions such as cortical dysplasia with its indistinct boundaries than with extremely focal lesions such as a cavernous angioma. A vagus nerve stimulator (VNS) is another option for patients with refractory epilepsy previously not considered surgically remediable [143]. Although approved in the United States for localization-related epilepsies only, some physicians are trying the device for treatment of generalized epilepsies.

Some young patients with symptomatic generalized epilepsy or Lennox-Gastaut syndrome who have frequent atonic seizures leading to falls and serious injuries are candidates for corpus callosotomy. While this procedure does not eliminate all seizures in all patients, it may improve safety and quality of life for the patient and caregivers [144–151]. ECoG—echocardiogram; EEG—electroencephalogram.

Treatment of Status Epilepticus

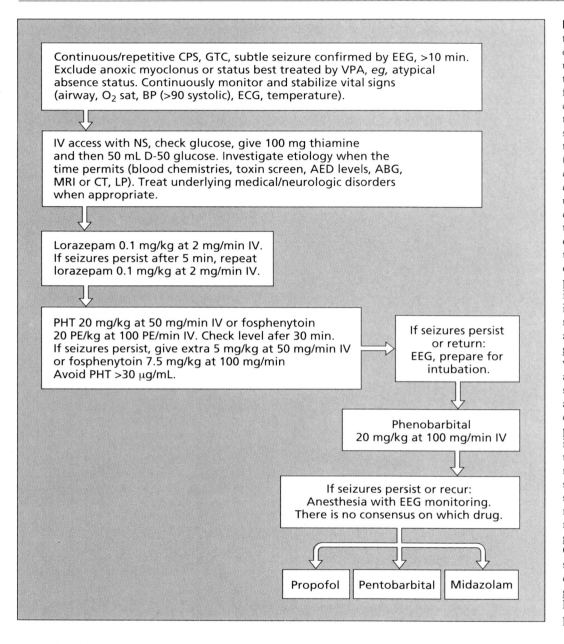

Continuous/repetitive CPS, GTC, subtle seizure confirmed by EEG, >10 min. Exclude anoxic myoclonus or status best treated by VPA, *eg*, atypical absence status. Continuously monitor and stabilize vital signs (airway, O₂ sat, BP (>90 systolic), ECG, temperature).

IV access with NS, check glucose, give 100 mg thiamine and then 50 mL D-50 glucose. Investigate etiology when the time permits (blood chemistries, toxin screen, AED levels, ABG, MRI or CT, LP). Treat underlying medical/neurologic disorders when appropriate.

Lorazepam 0.1 mg/kg at 2 mg/min IV. If seizures persist after 5 min, repeat lorazepam 0.1 mg/kg at 2 mg/min IV.

PHT 20 mg/kg at 50 mg/min IV or fosphenytoin 20 PE/kg at 100 PE/min IV. Check level afer 30 min. If seizures persist, give extra 5 mg/kg at 50 mg/min IV or fosphenytoin 7.5 mg/kg at 100 mg/min Avoid PHT >30 µg/mL.

If seizures persist or return: EEG, prepare for intubation.

Phenobarbital 20 mg/kg at 100 mg/min IV

If seizures persist or recur: Anesthesia with EEG monitoring. There is no consensus on which drug.

Propofol | Pentobarbital | Midazolam

Figure 10-44. Protocol for treatment of status epilepticus in adults. Status epilepticus is defined as continuous or frequent seizures without recovery for 30 minutes. Most physicians do not wait 30 minutes to begin treatment; the goal of therapy is first to prevent status from developing and then to treat it aggressively if it does occur. This is one method of treating status epilepticus in adults. It is important that other types of status, such as absence status, be excluded because they are treated differently, for example with valproic acid (VPA). The key to successfully treating status epilepticus is to recognize the disorder and begin treatment quickly. While one must always keep in mind the underlying etiology, the patient must not be sent off for computed tomography scans or other diagnostic tests if they are actively convulsing, because brain damage can occur if the seizures last 30 minutes or longer. This protocol is somewhat modified from the recommendations of the Epilepsy Foundation of America [152] and each physician may develop his or her own method of treating status. Fosphenytoin will probably become the intravenous treatment of choice within a short time to replace phenytoin (PHT). The drug is currently dosed as phenytoin equivalents rather than milligram per kilogram, but it is much more expensive. The main controversy with status epilepticus is what to do if a benzodiazepine followed by fosphenytoin fails to stop the seizures. Phenobarbital is the next logical choice, although one could advocate the use of anesthesia more quickly with short-acting drugs such as pentobarbital, propofol, or midazolam. There is no consensus regarding the third or fourth agent in refractory status epilepticus. It is clear that an electroencephalogram will help manage these cases because many patients stop having seizures clinically yet continue to have electrographic seizures. When a patient does not awaken after treatment of convulsive status epilepticus one should suspect nonconvulsive status (NS) [153]. ABG—arterial blood gas; AED—antiepileptic drug; BP—blood pressure; CBC—complete blood count; CPS—complete partial seizure; CT—computed tomography; ECG—electrocardiogram; EEG—electroencephalogram; GTC—generalized tonic-clonic seizure; IV—intravenous; LP—lumbar puncture; PE—PHT equivalent (1.5 mg fosphenytoin is equivalent to 1.0 mg PHT).

Sudden Unexplained Death

Sudden Unexplained Death in Epilepsy

Study	Population	SUDEP incidence
Nashef *et al.* [135]	Adult outpatients, tertiary referral center	1/200
Nashef *et al.* [136]	Residential school	1/295
Klenerman *et al.* [137]	Severe epilepsy, institutionalized	1/480
Timmings [133]	Epilepsy unit population	1/500
Tennis *et al.* [132]	Saskatchewan Canada outpatients using AEDs	1/740–1/1852

Figure 10-45. Sudden unexplained death in epilepsy (SUDEP). Sudden death in epilepsy patients is a major concern, with a lifetime risk of 10% [154]. These risks exceed the risk of epilepsy surgery and are a major justification for early surgical intervention in medically intractable patients. Cardiac arrhythmia [155] and respiratory compromise [154] are postulated causes. Other risk factors include uncontrolled seizures, in children [154]; noncompliance [154]; living alone or unsupervised; male sex [156]; being age 20 to 40 years [157,158]; tonic-clonic seizures [157]; polypharmacy [156]; and alcohol abuse [158]. Physicians should strive to reduce the risk factors in epilepsy patients wherever possible, particularly with drug compliance and education about safety and substance abuse. AED—antiepileptic drugs.

References

1. Salanova V, Morris HH, Van Ness P, *et al.*: Frontal lobe seizures: electroclinical syndromes. *Epilepsia* 1995, 36:16–24.

2. Chee MW, Kotagal P, Van Ness PC, *et al.*: Lateralizing signs in intractable partial epilepsy: blinded multiple-observer analysis. *Neurology* 1993, 43:2519–2525.

3. Newton MR, Berkovic SF, Austin MC, *et al.*: Dystonia, clinical lateralization, and regional blood flow changes in temporal lobe seizures. *Neurology* 1992, 42:371–372.

4. Yen DJ, Su MS, Yiu CH, *et al.*: Ictal speech manifestations in temporal lobe epilepsy: a video-EEG study. *Epilepsia* 1996, 37:45–49.

5. Abou-Khalil B, Welch L, Blumenkopf B, *et al.*: Global aphasia with seizure onset in the dominant basal temporal region. *Epilepsia* 1994, 35:1079–1084.

6. Devinsky O, Kelley K, Yacubian EM, *et al.*: Postictal behavior. A clinical and subdural electroencephalographic study. *Arch Neurol* 1994, 51:254–259.

7. Fakhoury T, Abou-Khalil B, Peguero E: Differentiating clinical features of right and left temporal lobe seizures. *Epilepsia* 1994, 35:1038–1044.

8. Koerner M, Laxer KD: Ictal speech, postictal language dysfunction, and seizure lateralization. *Neurology* 1988, 38:634–636.

9. Gabr M, Luders H, Dinner D, *et al.*: Speech manifestations in lateralization of temporal lobe seizures. *Ann Neurol* 1989, 25:82–87.

10. Kotagal P, Luders HO, Williams G, *et al.*: Psychomotor seizures of temporal lobe onset: analysis of symptom clusters and sequences. *Epilepsy Res* 1995, 20:49–67.

11. Devinsky O, Frasca J, Pacia SV, *et al.*: Ictus emeticus: further evidence of non-dominant temporal involvement. *Neurology* 1995, 45:1158–1160.

12. Cendes F, Andermann F, Gloor P, *et al.*: Relationship between atrophy of the amygdala and ictal fear in temporal lobe epilepsy. *Brain* 1994, 117:739–746.

13. Manford M, Fish DR, Shorvon SD: An analysis of clinical seizure patterns and their localizing value in frontal and temporal lobe epilepsies. *Brain* 1996, 119:17–40.

14. Hauser W, Hesdorffer D: *Epilepsy Frequency, Causes and Consequences.* New York: Demos; 1990.

15. Engel J Jr: *Seizures and Epilepsy.* Philadelphia: FA Davis, 1989.

16. Hauser WA, Annegers JF, Rocca WA: Descriptive epidemiology of epilepsy: contributions of population-based studies from Rochester, Minnesota. *Mayo Clin Proc* 1996, 71:576–586.

17. Camfield CS, Camfield PR, Gordon K, *et al.*: Incidence of epilepsy in childhood and adolescence: a population-based study in Nova Scotia from 1977 to 1985. *Epilepsia* 1996, 37:19–23.

18. Commission on Classification and Terminology of the International League Against Epilepsy. Proposal for revised clinical and electroencephalographic classification of epileptic seizures. *Epilepsia* 1981, 22:489–501.

19. Scheffer IE, Bhatia KP, Lopes-Cendes I, *et al.*: Autosomal dominant nocturnal frontal lobe epilepsy. A distinctive clinical disorder. *Brain* 1995, 118:61–73.

20. Berkovic S, McIntosh A, Howell R, Hopper J: Familial temporal lobe epilepsy: a benign, unrecognized and common disorder. *Epilepsia* 1994, (suppl 8)35:109.

21. Commission on Classification and Terminology of the International League Against Epilepsy. Proposal for revised classification of epilepsies and epileptic syndromes. *Epilepsia* 1989, 30:389–399.

22. Wirrell EC, Camfield PR, Gordon KE, *et al.*: Benign rolandic epilepsy: atypical features are very common. *J Child Neurol* 1995, 10:455–458.

23. Legarda S, Jayakar P: Electroclinical significance of rolandic spikes and dipoles in neurodevelopmentally normal children. *Electroencephalogr Clin Neurophysiol* 1995, 95:257–259.

24. Legarda S, Jayakar P, Duchowny M, *et al.*: Benign rolandic epilepsy: high central and low central subgroups. *Epilepsia* 1994, 35:1125–1129.

25. Loiseau P, Duche B: Benign rolandic epilepsy. *Adv Neurol* 1992, 57:411–417.

26. Loiseau P, Duche B, Cohadon S: The prognosis of benign localized epilepsy in early childhood. *Epilepsy Res* (suppl) 1992, 6:75–81.

27. Holmes GL: Benign focal epilepsies of childhood. *Epilepsia* 1993, 34:S49–S61.

28. Holmes GL: Rolandic epilepsy: clinical and electroencephalographic features. *Epilepsy Res* (suppl) 1992, 6:29–43.

29. Loiseau P, Duche B, Cordova S, *et al.*: Prognosis of benign childhood epilepsy with centrotemporal spikes: a follow-up study of 168 patients. *Epilepsia* 1988, 29:229–235.

30. Doose H: Symptomatology in children with focal sharp waves of genetic origin. *Eur J Pediatr* 1989, 149:210–205.

31. Kaibara M, Blume WT: The postictal electroencephalogram. *Electroencephalogr Clin Neurophysiol* 1988, 70:99–104.

32. Risinger MW, Engel J Jr, Van Ness PC, *et al.*: Ictal localization of temporal lobe seizures with scalp/sphenoidal recordings. *Neurology* 1989, 39:1288–1293.

33. Constantin L, Martins JB, Fincham RW, Dagli RD: Bradycardia and syncope as manifestations of partial epilepsy. *J Am Coll Cardiol* 1990, 15:900–905.

34. Joske DJ, Davis MJ: Sino-atrial arrest due to temporal lobe epilepsy. *Aust N Z J Med* 1991, 21:62–64.

35. Nashef L, Walker F, Allen P, *et al.*: Apnoea and bradycardia during epileptic seizures: relation to sudden death in epilepsy. *J Neurol Neurosurg Psychiatry* 1996, 60:297–300.

36. Li LM, Roche J, Sander JW: Ictal ECG changes in temporal lobe epilepsy. *Arquivos de Neuro-Psiquiatria* 1995, 53:619–624.

37. Spencer SS, McCarthy G, Spencer DD: Diagnosis of medial temporal lobe seizure onset: relative specificity and sensitivity of quantitative MRI. *Neurology* 1993, 43:2117–2124.

38. Raymond AA, Fish DR, Sisodiya SM, *et al.*: Abnormalities of gyration, heterotopias, tuberous sclerosis, focal cortical dysplasia, microdysgenesis, dysembryoplastic neuroepithelial tumour and dysgenesis of the archicortex in epilepsy. Clinical, EEG and neuroimaging features in 100 adult patients. *Brain* 1995, 118:629–660.

39. Cendes F, Andermann F, Dubeau F, *et al.*: Early childhood prolonged febrile convulsions, atrophy and sclerosis of mesial structures, and temporal lobe epilepsy: an MRI volumetric study. *Neurology* 1993, 43:1083–1087.

40. Benbadis SR, So NK, Antar MA, *et al.*: The value of PET scan (and MRI and Wada test) in patients with bitemporal epileptiform abnormalities. *Arch Neurol* 1995, 52:1062–1068.

41. Cascino GD: Structural neuroimaging in partial epilepsy. Magnetic resonance imaging. *Neurosurg Clin N Am* 1995, 6:455–464.

42. Lorenzo NY, Parisi JE, Cascino GD, *et al.*: Intractable frontal lobe epilepsy: pathological and MRI features. *Epilepsy Res* 1995, 20:171–178.

43. Kuzniecky RI, Burgard S, Bilir E, *et al.*: Qualitative MRI segmentation in mesial temporal sclerosis: clinical correlations. *Epilepsia* 1996, 37:433–439.

44. Kuzniecky RI: Neuroimaging in pediatric epilepsy. *Epilepsia* 1996, 37:S10–S21.

45. Jack CR Jr: MRI-based hippocampal volume measurements in epilepsy. *Epilepsia* 1994, 35:S21–S29.

46. Cascino GD, Jack CR Jr, Parisi JE, *et al.*: MRI in the presurgical evaluation of patients with frontal lobe epilepsy and children with temporal lobe epilepsy: pathologic correlation and prognostic importance. *Epilepsy Res* 1992, 11:51–59.

47. Cendes F, Leproux F, Melanson D, *et al.*: MRI of amygdala and hippocampus in temporal lobe epilepsy. *J Comput Assist Tomogr* 1993, 17:206–210.

48. Cendes F, Andermann F, Dubeau F, *et al.*: Early childhood prolonged febrile convulsions, atrophy and sclerosis of mesial structures, and temporal lobe epilepsy: an MRI volumetric study. *Neurology* 1993, 43:1083–1087.

49. Loiseau P, Duche B, Pedespan JM: Absence epilepsies. *Epilepsia* 1995, 36:1182–1186.

50. Olsson I, Hagberg G: Epidemiology of absence epilepsy. III. Clinical aspects. *Acta Paediatr Scand* 1991, 80:1066–1072.

51. Porter RJ: The absence epilepsies. *Epilepsia* 1993, 34:S42–S48.

52. Hrachovy RA, Frost JD Jr: Infantile spasms. *Pediatr Clin North Am* 1989, 36:311–329.

53. Markand ON: Slow spike-wave activity in EEG and associated clinical features: often called 'Lennox' or "Lennox-Gastaut" syndrome. *Neurology* 1977, 27:746–757.

54. Kotagal P: Multifocal independent Spike syndrome: relationship to hypsarrhythmia and the slow spike-wave (Lennox-Gastaut) syndrome. *Clin Electroencephalogr* 1995, 26:23–29.

55. Begley CE, Famulari M, Annegers JF, *et al.*: The cost of epilepsy in the United States: an estimate from population-based clinical and survey data. *Epilepsia* 2000, 41:342–351.

56. Meencke HJ, Veith G: Migration disturbances in epilepsy. *Epilepsy Res* (suppl) 1992, 9:31–39 (discussion 39–40).

57. Abou-Khalil B, Andermann E, Andermann F, *et al.*: Temporal lobe epilepsy after prolonged febrile convulsions: excellent outcome after surgical treatment. *Epilepsia* 1993, 34:878–883.

58. Maher J, McLachlan RS: Febrile convulsions. Is seizure duration the most important predictor of temporal lobe epilepsy? *Brain* 1995, 118:1521–1528.

59. Rich SS, Annegers JF, Hauser WA, Anderson VE: Complex segregation analysis of febrile convulsions. *Am J Hum Genet* 1987, 41:249–257.

60. Hauser WA: The prevalence and incidence of convulsive disorders in children. *Epilepsia* 1994, 35:S1–S6.

61. Phillips HA, Scheffer IE, Berkovic SF, *et al.*: Localization of a gene for autosomal dominant nocturnal frontal lobe epilepsy to chromosome 20q 13.2 [letter] [see comments]. *Nat Genet* 1995, 10:117–118.

62. Steinlein OK: Neuronal nicotinic receptors in human epilepsy. *Eur J Pharmacol* 2000, 393:243–247.

63. Phillips HA, Scheffer IE, Crossland KM, *et al.*: Autosomal dominant nocturnal frontal-lobe epilepsy: genetic heterogeneity and evidence for a second locus at 15q24. *Am J Hum Genet* 1998, 63:1108–1116.

64. Scheffer I, Phillips H, Mulley J, *et al.*: Autosomal dominant partial epilepsy with variable foci is not allelic to autosomal dominant nocturnal frontal lobe epilepsy. *Epilepsia* (suppl 3) 1995, 36:S28.

65. Xiong L, Labuda M, Li DS, *et al.*: Mapping of a gene determining familial partial epilepsy with variable foci to chromosome 22q11-q12. *Am J Hum Genet* 1999, 65:1698–1710.

66. Scheffer IE, Jones L, Pozzebon M, *et al.*: Autosomal dominant rolandic epilepsy and speech dyspraxia: a new syndrome with anticipation. *Ann Neurol* 1995, 38:633–642.

67. Berkovic S, McIntosh A, Howell R, Hopper J: Familial temporal lobe epilepsy: a benign, unrecognized and common disorder. *Epilepsia* 1994, (suppl 8)35:109.

68. Ottman R, Risch N, Hauser WA, *et al.*: Localization of a gene for partial epilepsy to chromosome 10q [see comments]. *Nat Genet* 1995, 10:56–60.

69. Kuzniecky R, Rosenblatt B: Benign occipital epilepsy: a family study. *Epilepsia* 1987, 28:346–350.

70. Eksioglu YZ, Scheffer IE, Cardenas P, *et al.*: Periventricular heterotopia: an X-linked dominant epilepsy locus causing aberrant cerebral cortical development. *Neuron* 1996, 16:77–87.

71. Fox JW, Lamperti ED, Eksioglu YZ, *et al.*: Mutations in filamin 1 prevent migration of cerebral cortical neurons in human periventricular heterotopia. *Neuron* 1998, 21:1315–1325.

72. Leppert M, Anderson VE, Quattlebaum T, *et al.*: Benign familial neonatal convulsions linked to genetic markers on chromosome 20. *Nature* 1989, 337:647–648.

73. Singh NA, Charlier C, Stauffer D, *et al.*: A novel potassium channel gene, KCNQ2, is mutated in an inherited epilepsy of newborns. *Nat Genet* 1998, 18:25–29.

74. Lewis TB, Leach RJ, Warck K, *et al.*: Genetic heterogeneity in benign familial neonatal convulsions: identification of a new locus on chromosome 8q. *Am J Human Genet* 53:670–675.

75. Charlier C, Singh NA, Ryan SG, *et al.*: A pore mutation in a novel KQT-like potassium channel gene in an idiopathic epilepsy family. *Nat Genet* 1998, 18:53–55.

76. Guipponi M, Rivier F, Vigevano F, *et al.*: Linkage mapping of benign familial infantile convulsions (BFIC) to chromosome 19q. *Hum Mol Genet* 1997, 6:473–477.

77. Szepetowski P, Rochette J, Berquin P, *et al.*: Familial infantile convulsions and paroxysmal choreoathetosis: a new neurological syndrome linked to the pericentromeric region of human chromosome 16. *Am J Hum Genet* 1997, 61:889–898.

78. Lee WL, Tay A, Ong HT, *et al.*: Association of infantile convulsions with paroxysmal dyskinesias (ICCA syndrome): confirmation of linkage to human chromosome 16p12-q12 in a Chinese family. *Hum Genet* 1998, 103:608–612.

79. Wallace R, Berkovic S, Howell R, *et al.*: *J Med Genet* 1996, 33:308–312.

80. Johnson EW, Dubovsky J, Rich SS, *et al.*: Evidence for a novel gene for familial febrile convulsions, FEB2, linked to chromosome 19p in an extended family from the Midwest. *Hum Mol Genet* 1998, 7:63–67.

81. Peiffer A, Thompson J, Charlier C, *et al.*: A locus for febrile seizures (FEB3) maps to chromosome 2q23-24. *Ann Neurol* 1999, 46:671–678.

82. Nakayama J, Hamano K, Iwasaki N, *et al.*: Significant evidence for linkage of febrile seizures to chromosome 5q14-q15. *Hum Mol Genet* 2000, 9:87–91.

83. Wallace RH, Wang DW, Singh R, *et al.*: Febrile seizures and generalized epilepsy associated with a mutation in the Na(+)-channel beta-1 subunit gene SCN1B. *Nat Genet* 1998, 19:366–370.

84. Fong GCY, Shah PU, Gee MN, *et al.*: Childhood absence epilepsy with tonic-clonic seizures and electroencephalogram 3–4-Hz spike and multispike-slow wave complexes: linkage to chromosome 8q24. *Am J Hum Genet* 1998, 63:1117–1129.

85. Greenberg DA, Delgado-Escueta AV, Widelitz H, *et al.*: Juvenile myoclonic epilepsy (JME) may be linked to the BF and HLA loci on human chromosome 6. *Am J Med Genet* 1988, 31:185–192.

86. Liu AW, Delgado-Escueta AV, Serratosa JM, *et al.*: Juvenile myoclonic epilepsy locus in chromosome 6p21.2-p11: linkage to convulsions and electroencephalography trait. *Am J Hum Genet* 1995, 57:368–381.

87. Elmslie FV, Rees M, Williamson MP, *et al.*: Genetic mapping of a major susceptibility locus for juvenile myoclonic epilepsy on chromosome 15q. *Hum Mol Genet* 1997, 6:1329–1334.

88. Serratosa JM, Delgado-Escueta AV, Posada I, *et al.*: The gene for progressive myoclonus epilepsy of the Lafora type maps to chromosome 6q. *Hum Mol Genet* 1995, 4:1657–1663.

89. Minassian BA, Ianzano L, Meloche M, *et al.*: Mutation spectrum and predicted function of laforin in Lafora's progressive myoclonus epilepsy. *Neurology* 2000, 55:341–346.

90. Tahvanainen E, Ranta S, Hirvasniemi A, *et al.*: The gene for a recessively inherited human childhood progressive epilepsy with mental retardation maps to the distal short arm of chromosome 8. *Proc Natl Acad Sci U S A* 1994, 91:7267–7270.

91. Lehesjoki AE, Koskiniemi M, Norio R, *et al.*: Localization of the EPM1 gene for progressive myoclonus epilepsy on chromosome 21: linkage disequilibrium allows high resolution mapping. *Hum Mol Genet* 1993, 2:1229–1234.

92. Lehesjoki AE, Eldridge R, Eldridge J, *et al.*: Progressive myoclonus epilepsy of Unverricht-Lundborg type: a clinical and molecular genetic study of a family from the United States with four affected sibs. *Neurology* 1993, 43:2384–2386.

93. Alakurtti K, Virtaneva K, Joensuu T, *et al.*: Characterization of the cystatin B gene promoter harboring the dodecamer repeat expanded in progressive myoclonus epilepsy, EPM1. *Gene* 2000, 242:65–73.

94. Pennacchio LA, Lehesjoki AE, Stone NE, *et al.*: Mutations in the gene encoding cystatin B in progressive myoclonus epilepsy (EPM1) [see comments]. *Science* 1996, 271:1731–1734.

95. Mikami M, Yasuda T, Terao A, *et al.*: Localization of a gene for benign adult familial myoclonic epilepsy to chromosome 8q23.3-q24.1. *Am J Hum Genet* 1999, 65:745–751.

96. Chomyn A, Lai ST, Shakeley R, *et al.*: Platelet-mediated transformation of mtDNA-less human cells: analysis of phenotypic variability among clones from normal individuals—and complementation behavior of the tRNALys mutation causing myoclonic epilepsy and ragged red fibers. *Am J Hum Genet* 1994, 54:966–974.

97. Shoffner JM, Wallace DC: Mitochondrial genetics: principles and practice. *Am J Hum Genet* 1992, 51:1179–1186.

98. Minassian BA, DeLorey TM, Olsen RW, *et al.*: Angelman syndrome: correlations between epilepsy phenotypes and genotypes. *Ann Neurol* 1998, 43:485–493.

99. Matsuura T, Sutcliffe JS, Fang P, *et al.*: De novo truncating mutations in E6-AP ubiquitin-protein ligase gene (UBE3A) in Angelman syndrome. *Nat Genet* 1997, 15:74–77.

100. McKusick VA, ed. *Online Mendelian Inheritance in Man.* Bethesda, MD: National Center for Biotechnology Information, National Library of Medicine; 2000. Available at: http://www.ncbi.nlm.nih.gov/omim/. Accessed October, 2000.

101. Gambardella A, Palmini A, Andermann F, *et al.*: Usefulness of focal rhythmic discharges on scalp EEG of patients with focal cortical dysplasia and intractable epilepsy. *Electroencephalogr Clin Neurophysiol* 1996, 98:243–249.

102. Roper SN, Gilmore RL, Houser CR: Experimentally induced disorders of neuronal migration produce an increased propensity for electrographic seizures in rats. *Epilepsy Res* 1995, 21:205–219.

103. Wyllie E: Surgery for catastrophic localization-related epilepsy in infants. *Epilepsia* 1996, 37:S22–S25.

104. Mischel PS, Nguyen LP, Vinters HV: Cerebral cortical dysplasia associated with pediatric epilepsy. Review of neuropathologic features and proposal for a grading system. *J Neuropathol Exp Neurol* 1995, 54:137–153.

105. Prayson RA, Estes ML: Cortical dysplasia: a histopathologic study of 52 cases of partial lobectomy in patients with epilepsy. *Hum Pathol* 1995, 26:493–500.

106. Dubeau F, Tampieri D, Lee N, *et al.*: Periventricular and subcortical nodular heterotopia. A study of 33 patients. *Brain* 1995, 118:1273–1287.

107. Huttenlocher PR, Taravath S, Mojtahedi S: Periventricular heterotopia and epilepsy. *Neurology* 1994, 44:51–55.

108. Kamuro K, Tenokuchi Y: Familial periventricular nodular heterotopia. *Brain Dev* 1993, 15:237–241.

109. Morris HH, Estes ML, Gilmore R, *et al.*: Chronic intractable epilepsy as the only symptom of primary brain tumor. *Epilepsia* 1993, 34:1038–1043.

110. Pilcher WH, Silbergeld DL, Berger MS, Ojemann GA: Intraoperative electrocorticography during tumor resection: impact on seizure outcome in patients with gangliogliomas. *J Neurosurg* 1993, 78:891–902.

111. Packer RJ, Sutton LN, Patel KM, *et al.*: Seizure control following tumor surgery for childhood cortical low-grade gliomas. *J Neurosurg* 1994, 80:998–1003.

112. Wolf HK, Muller MB, Spanle M, *et al.*: Ganglioglioma: a detailed histopathological and immunohistochemical analysis of 61 cases. *Acta Neuropathol* 1994, 88:166–173.

113. Prayson RA, Estes ML, Morris HH: Coexistence of neoplasia and cortical dysplasia in patients presenting with seizures. *Epilepsia* 1993, 34:609–615.

114. Becker LE: Central neuronal tumors in childhood: relationship to dysplasia. *J Neurooncol* 1995, 24:13–19.

115. Gunel M, Awad IA, Anson J, Lifton RP: Mapping a gene causing cerebral cavernous malformation to 7q11.2-q21. *Proc Natl Acad Sci U S A* 1995, 92:6620–6624.

116. Robinson JR, Awad IA, Little JR: Natural history of the cavernous angioma. *J Neurosurg* 1991, 75:709–714.

117. Robinson JR Jr, Awad IA, Magdinec M, Paranandi L: Factors predisposing to clinical disability in patients with cavernous malformations of the brain. *Neurosurgery* 1993, 32:730–735 (discussion 735–736).

118. Kraemer DL, Awad IA: Vascular malformations and epilepsy: clinical considerations and basic mechanisms. *Epilepsia* 1994, 35:S30–S43.

119. Cendes F, Cook MJ, Watson C, *et al.*: Frequency and characteristics of dual pathology in patients with lesional epilepsy. *Neurology* 1995, 45:2058–2064.

120. Garcia HH, Gilman R, Martinez M, *et al.*: Cysticercosis as a major cause of epilepsy in Peru. The Cysticercosis Working Group in Peru (CWG) [see comments]. *Lancet* 1993, 341:197–200.

121. Jay V, Becker LE, Otsubo H, *et al.*: Chronic encephalitis and epilepsy (Rasmussen's encephalitis): detection of cytomegalovirus and herpes simplex virus 1 by the polymerase chain reaction and in situ hybridization. *Neurology* 1995, 45:108–117.

122. Atkins MR, Terrell W, Hulette CM: Rasmussen's syndrome: a study of potential viral etiology. *Clin Neuropathol* 1995, 14:7–12.

123. Honavar M, Janota I, Polkey CE: Rasmussen's encephalitis in surgery for epilepsy. *Dev Med Child Neurol* 1992, 34:3–14.

124. Villemure JG, Rasmussen T: Functional hemispherectomy in children. *Neuropediatrics* 1993, 24:53–55.

125. Oguni H, Andermann F, Rasmussen TB: The syndrome of chronic encephalitis and epilepsy. A study based on the MNI series of 48 cases. *Adv Neurol* 1992, 57:419–433.

126. McLachlan RS, Girvin JP, Blume WT, Reichman H: Rasmussen's chronic encephalitis in adults. *Arch Neurol* 1993, 50:269–274.

127. Twyman RE, Gahring LC, Spiess J, Rogers SW: Glutamate receptor antibodies activate a subset of receptors and reveal an agonist binding site. *Neuron* 1995, 14:755–762.

128. Andrews PI, Dichter MA, Berkovic SF, *et al.*: Plasmapheresis in Rasmussen's encephalitis [see comments]. *Neurology* 1996, 46:242–246.

129. Rogers SW, Andrews PI, Gahring LC, *et al.*: Autoantibodies to glutamate receptor GluR3 in Rasmussen's encephalitis. *Science* 1994, 265:648–651.

130. Farrell MA, Droogan O, Secor DL, *et al.*: Chronic encephalitis associated with epilepsy: immunohistochemical and ultrastructural studies. *Acta Neuropathol* 1995, 89:313–321.

131. Jennett B: Epilepsy and acute traumatic intracranial haematoma. *J Neurol Neurosurg Psychiatry* 1975, 38:378–381.

132. Jennett B: Early traumatic epilepsy. Incidence and significance after nonmissile injuries. *Arch Neurol* 1974, 30:394–398.

133. Jennett B, Van De Sande J: EEG prediction of post-traumatic epilepsy. *Epilepsia* 1975, 16:251–256.

134. Courville CB: Traumatic Lesions of the Temporal Lobe as the Essential Cause of Psychomotor Epilepsy. In *Temporal Lobe Epilepsy*. Edited by Baldwin M, Bailey P. Springfield, IL: Charles C. Thomas; 1958:220–239.

135. Devinsky O, Kelley K, Porter RJ, Theodore WH: Clinical and electroencephalographic features of simple partial seizures. *Neurology* 1988, 38:1347–1352.

136. Bare MA, Burnstine TH, Fisher RS, Lesser RP: Electroencephalographic changes during simple partial seizures. *Epilepsia* 1994, 35:715–720.

137. Hauser WA, Anderson VE, Loewenson RB, McRoberts SM: Seizure recurrence after a first unprovoked seizure. *N Engl J Med* 1982, 307:522–528.

138. Hart RG, Easton JD: Seizure recurrence after a first, unprovoked seizure. *Arch Neurol* 1986, 43:1289–1290.

139. Cramer JA, Mattson RH, Prevey ML, et al.: How often is medication taken as prescribed? A novel assessment technique. *JAMA* 1989, 261:3273–3277.

140. Engel J Jr: Epilepsy surgery. *Curr Opin Neurol* 1994, 7:140–147.

141. Luders HO: *Epilepsy Surgery*. New York: Raven Press, 1992.

142. Engel J Jr: *Surgical Treatment of the Epilepsies*, edn 2. New York: Raven Press, 1993.

143. Handforth A, DeGiorgio CM, Schachter SC, et al.: Vagus nerve stimulation therapy for partial-onset seizures: a randomized active-control trial. *Neurology* 1998, 51:48–55.

144. Cendes F, Ragazzo PC, da Costa V, Martins LF: Corpus callosotomy in treatment of medically resistant epilepsy: preliminary results in a pediatric population. *Epilepsia* 1993, 34:910–917.

145. Fiol ME, Gates JR, Mireles R, *et al.*: Value of intraoperative EEG changes during corpus callosotomy in predicting surgical results. *Epilepsia* 1993, 34:74–78.

146. Landy HJ, Curless RG, Ramsay RE, *et al.*: Corpus callosotomy for seizures associated with band heterotopia. *Epilepsia* 1993, 34:79–83.

147. Madsen JR, Carmant L, Holmes GL, Black PM: Corpus callosotomy in children. *Neurosurg Clin N Am* 1995, 6:541–548.

148. Mamelak AN, Barbaro NM, Walker JA, Laxer KD: Corpus callosotomy: a quantitative study of the extent of resection, seizure control, and neuropsychological outcome [see comments]. *J Neurosurg* 1993, 79:688–695.

149. Pallini R, Aglioti S, Tassinari G, *et al.*: Callosotomy for intractable epilepsy from bihemispheric cortical dysplasias. *Acta Neurochir* 1995, 132:79–86.

150. Reutens DC, Bye AM, Hopkins IJ, *et al.*: Corpus callosotomy for intractable epilepsy: seizure outcome and prognostic factors. *Epilepsia* 1993, 34:904–909.

151. Spencer SS, Spencer DD, Sass K, *et al.*: Anterior, total, and two-stage corpus callosum section: differential and incremental seizure responses. *Epilepsia* 1993, 34:561–567.

152. Working Group on Status Epilepticus: Treatment of convulsive status epilepticus. Recommendations of the Epilepsy Foundation of America's Working Group on Status Epilepticus [see comments]. *JAMA* 1993, 270:854–859.

153. Treiman DM: Electroclinical features of status epilepticus. *J Clin Neurophysiol* 1995, 12:343–362.

154. Earnest MP, Thomas GE, Eden RA, Hossack KF: The sudden unexplained death syndrome in epilepsy: demographic, clinical, and postmortem features. *Epilepsia* 1992, 33:310–316.

155. Dasheiff RM, Dickinson LJ: Sudden unexpected death of epileptic patient due to cardiac arrhythmia after seizure. *Arch Neurol* 1986, 43:194–196.

156. Tennis P, Cole TB, Annegers JF, *et al.*: Cohort study of incidence of sudden unexplained death in persons with seizure disorder treated with antiepileptic drugs in Saskatchewan, Canada. *Epilepsia* 1995, 36:29–36.

157. Timmings PL: Sudden unexpected death in epilepsy: a local audit. *Seizure* 1993, 2:287–290.

158. Leestma JE, Walczak T, Hughes JR, *et al.*: A prospective study on sudden unexpected death in epilepsy. *Ann Neurol* 1989, 26:195–203.

11

Neuromuscular Disease

David Pleasure • Shawn Bird • Steven Scherer
John Sladky • Donald Schotland

THIS chapter illustrates diseases that involve the peripheral nervous system and skeletal muscle. In such diseases, the history and physical examination frequently provide sufficient data to arrive at the correct diagnosis. For example, autonomic dysfunction, distal limb weakness, hyporeflexia, and sensory loss in an adult with long-standing diabetes mellitus are probably due to diabetic neuropathy, and fluctuating weakness of bulbar and ocular muscles without sensory or reflex alterations strongly suggests myasthenia gravis. The clinical diagnosis can often be validated by specific immunochemical, biochemical, or molecular blood tests (Fig. 11-1).

Electromyography (EMG) and nerve conduction velocity studies are extensions of the neurologic examination. They are minimally invasive, permit rapid sampling of many nerves and skeletal muscles, and often allow unequivocal localization of a disease process to motor neurons, axons, the myelin sheath, the neuromuscular junction, or skeletal muscle. By combining the results of these electrical studies with the medical, social, and family histories and the neurologic examination, flow charts can be devised to guide the clinician to a definitive diagnosis and management scheme (Fig. 11-2).

In some instances, the history, neurologic examination, electrophysiologic studies, and analysis of biologic fluids are not sufficient to arrive at the definitive diagnosis, and biopsy of skeletal muscle or peripheral nerve is required. These biopsy studies are usually done under local anesthesia. In general, the optimal site for biopsy is a muscle that is mildly weakened by the disease process. This avoids the difficulty in interpreting end-stage muscle, in which myofibers may be almost completely replaced by fibrous tissue and fat. Biopsy of a skeletal muscle that was recently examined by EMG should be avoided because needle penetrations can cause microfoci of inflammation and muscle fiber necrosis, complicating interpretation of the histology.

Nerve biopsy is used less frequently than skeletal muscle biopsy. Sensory nerve biopsy often results in a patch of permanent cutaneous numbness, sometimes leads to a painful neuroma, and may be nondiagnostic in motor-denervating disorders. Nerve biopsy, however, is valuable in diagnosing familial and acquired amyloid neuropathy as well as vasculitic processes that preferentially involve the peripheral nervous system (*eg*, periarteritis nodosa). In some instances, information useful in diagnosing or quantifying the severity of neuropathy can be obtained by examination of sensory nerve twigs in cutaneous biopsies [1].

The next section of this chapter depicts aspects of the electrophysiologic examination, including EMG, motor nerve conduction studies, F waves and H reflexes, and repetitive stimulation studies of the function of neuromuscular junctions. This discussion is followed by illustrations of skeletal muscle and peripheral nerve biopsy findings in various myopathic and denervating diseases.

Diagnostic Studies

Diagnostic Immunologic, Biochemical, and Molecular Blood Studies in Neuromuscular Diseases

Figure 11-1. Examples of immunologic, biochemical, and molecular blood studies that provide specific diagnostic information in neuromuscular diseases. ALS—amyotrophic lateral sclerosis; HNPP—hereditary neuropathy with predisposition to pressure palsies; MAG—myelin-associated glycoprotein; PCR—polymerase chain reaction; SMN—survival motor neuron; SOD—superoxide dismutase.

Lyme Western and PCR	Lyme neuritis
Anti-Hu titer	Paraneoplastic sensory neuropathy
Cryoglobulins	Cryoglobulinemic neuropathy
anti-MAG titer	MAG paraproteinemic sensory neuropathy
Phytanic acid	Refsum's disease
Long-chain fatty acids	Adrenoleukodystrophy
Arylsulfatase	Metachromatic leukodystrophy

Leukocyte DNA analysis for:

Chromosome 17 duplication	Charcot-Marie-Tooth disease type 1A
Chromosome 17 deletion	HNPP (tomaculous neuropathy)
Transthyretin mutations	Familial amyloid neuropathy
Connexin 32 mutations	Charcot-Marie-Tooth disease type 1X
SOD mutations	Familial ALS
SMN mutations	Familial spinal muscular atrophy
Androgen receptor triplet repeat	Bulbospinal motor neuron disease

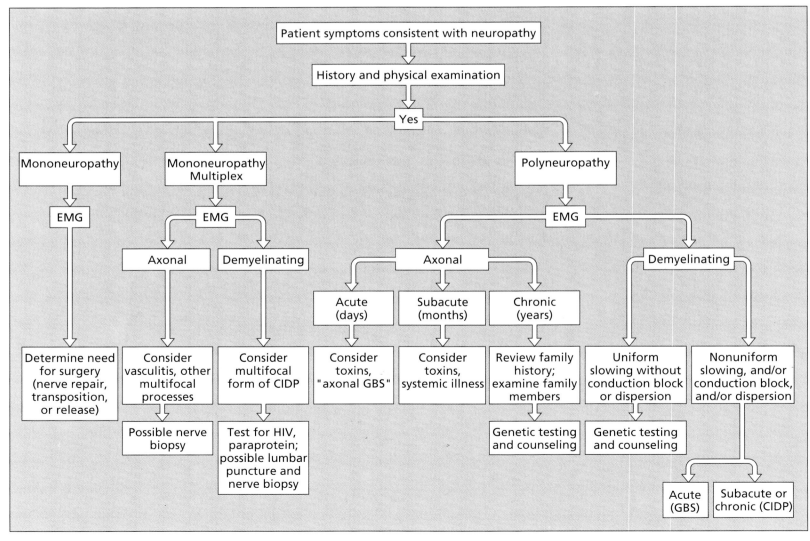

Figure 11-2. Evaluation of patients with neuropathy. CIDP—chronic inflammatory demyelinating polyneuropathy; EMG—electromyogram; GBS—Guillain-Barré syndrome. (*Adapted from* Asbury [2]).

Electrophysiologic Studies

Electromyography

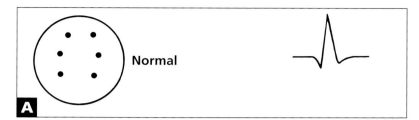

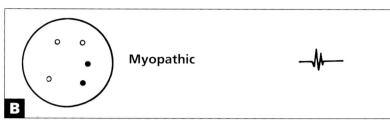

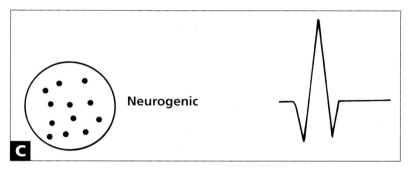

Figure 11-3. The motor unit and its relation to motor unit potential. The motor unit territory (*left*) is schematized by the large circle, which represents the recording area of the needle electromyogram (EMG) electrode. The small dark circles represent individual muscle fibers of one motor unit (the motor neuron and all the muscle fibers it innervates) in that recording area. In a needle EMG recording area, there are at least several overlapping motor units (not shown). The EMG needle records the nearly synchronous muscle fiber action potentials from all the muscle fibers in the recording area. This summated waveform is the motor unit potential (MUP). Thus, the MUP is longer, larger, and more complex than the action potential of a single muscle fiber. The morphology (amplitude, duration, and number of phases) of the MUP is determined by the number and distribution of muscle fibers of the motor unit in that recording area. Normally, (**A**) the amplitude is determined by the few fibers closest to the needle, and the duration by the number and location of more distant fibers. In myopathic disorders (**B**), there is loss of muscle fibers in the motor unit (*small open circles*), so that the recorded MUP is both smaller in amplitude and shorter in duration than normal. In neurogenic disorders (**C**), there is a loss of motor axons to other motor units in that recording area. Collateral sprouting from surviving axons innervates some of those muscle fibers, shown as an increased number of dark circles. There are more muscle fibers close to the needle, and they are more widely distributed, resulting in a larger and longer MUP. The extra components of the MUP may result in greater complexity of the waveform, producing a polyphasic appearance (greater than four phases).

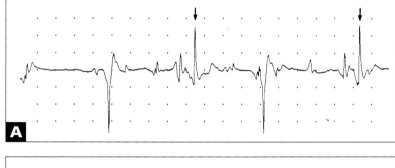

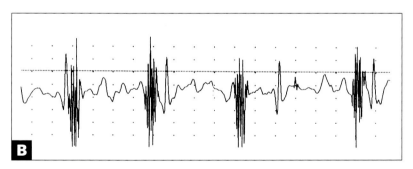

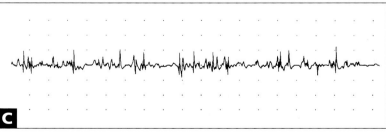

Figure 11-4. Needle electromyogram recording of the morphology and recruitment of motor unit potentials. **A**, Normal motor unit potential (MUP) morphology and recruitment. To characterize MUP morphology, MUPs are examined at a level of contractile force that results in the appearance of only a few MUPs in each area of muscle studied. MUP morphology (amplitude and duration) depends on a number of physiologic variables (*eg*, specific muscle, age of the subject) as well as on technical factors (type of needle used, location of needle in the muscle). Normal MUP duration ranges between 5 and 15 ms, and amplitude ranges between 200 and 2000 μV. Usually, only a small proportion of MUPs examined are polyphasic (more than four phases). In addition to MUP morphology, MUP recruitment is also examined. Recruitment is the manner in which MUPs increase their firing rates and new MUPs begin to fire as the muscle contraction is increased in a graded fashion. In normal muscle, recruitment of new units occurs as relatively low effort, with only a modest increase in firing rates of those MUPs already recruited. The usual MUP firing rate in normal muscle is no greater than 10 to 15 Hz. A normal MUP (*arrow*) is shown firing at 10 Hz. **B**, Neurogenic MUP morphology and recruitment. In neurogenic disorders, the MUP morphology is larger and longer and includes a greater number of polyphasic MUPs. In this example, a long polyphasic MUP is recruited in a neurogenic fashion, at a firing rate of greater than 20 Hz, with only mild muscle contraction. **C**, Myopathic MUP morphology and recruitment. In myopathic disorders, and in skeletal muscle–wasting disorders such as Cushing's syndrome, the MUPs are smaller, shorter, and often polyphasic. The MUPs shown here are all less than 200 μV in amplitude and shorter than 5 ms in duration. In addition, recruitment is abnormal, with numerous MUPs recruited at a very low contractile force (sensitivity = 200 μV/div; sweep speed = 10 ms/div).

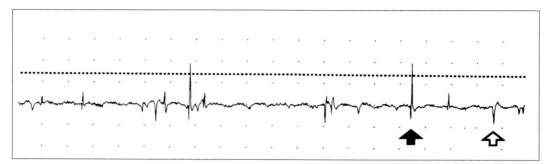

Figure 11-5. Fibrillation potentials and positive sharp waves. Fibrillation potentials and positive sharp waves are the action potentials of single muscle fibers that spontaneously discharge in the absence of innervation. The potentials typically fire at a constant rate, most often at 1 to 15 Hz. Fibrillation potentials (*closed arrow*) are biphasic or triphasic spikes (initial phase is electropositive or downward) and are usually 20 to 200 μV in amplitude. Positive sharp waves (*open arrow*) are biphasic potentials with an initial positivity followed by a long negative phase. These potentials are also individual muscle action potentials, like fibrillations, but are recorded with the needle electromyogram electrode from an injured portion of a muscle fiber (occasionally, this injury is caused by the needle itself). Thus, positive sharp waves have the same significance as fibrillation potentials. Both of these potentials are seen in disorders that cause loss of muscle fiber innervation. Neurogenic disorders produce denervated muscle fibers because of the loss of motor axons. However, fibrillations may also be seen in myopathic disorders and after muscle trauma. This is because each muscle fiber is innervated only at the motor endpoint region, and myopathy can cause segmental fiber necrosis, with the generation of one or more denervated segments of that myofiber. These surviving, denervated segments may generate fibrillation potentials or positive sharp waves.

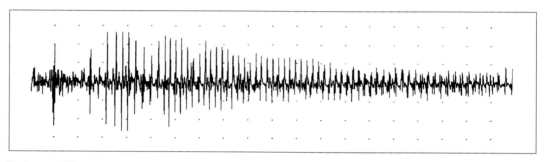

Figure 11-6. Myotonic discharges. These repetitive discharges are seen after needle movement or with muscle percussion. They are defined by the characteristic waxing and waning of the amplitude and frequency of the potentials within the discharge. This variability within the discharge produces an easily identifiable sound due to the corresponding change in patch, often described as a dive-bomber. These discharges vary in frequency from 40 to 100 Hz. Myotonic discharges can occur with or without clinical myotonia and are commonly seen in myotonic dystrophy, myotonia congenita, and paramyotonia; in association with the myopathy of acid maltase deficiency; and in some forms of hyperkalemic periodic paralysis (sensitivity = 100 μV/div; sweep speed = 100 ms/div).

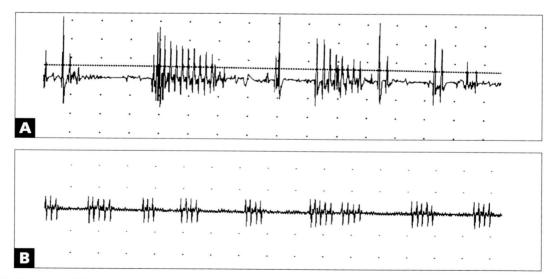

Figure 11-7. Myokymic discharges. These spontaneous electrical discharges are groups of normal-appearing motor unit potentials that fire with a fixed pattern and rhythm. They are also referred to as *grouped discharges* or *grouped fasciculations*. Variations can occur in both the frequency of discharges and the frequency of motor unit potentials within the discharge. The discharges are associated with clinical myokymia (quivering movements of the muscle). They are sometimes seen in the facial muscles in multiple sclerosis, brain stem neoplasm, or facial palsy. In the limbs, they are commonly seen after radiation-induced plexopathy, and occasionally with chronic nerve root or nerve compression (*eg*, in carpal tunnel syndrome). **A,** Two bursts of 8 to 12 potentials firing at 100 Hz (sensitivity = 500 μV/div; sweep speed = 50 ms/div). **B,** Multiple bursts of 3 to 5 small potentials firing at 30 to 40 Hz (sensitivity = 50 μV/div; sweep speed = 100 ms/div). Bursts repeat at intervals of about 0.1 to 0.3 seconds.

Nerve Conduction Studies

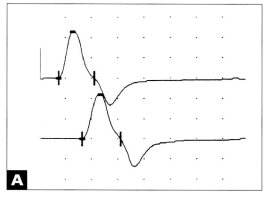 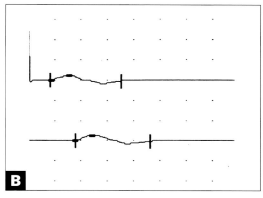 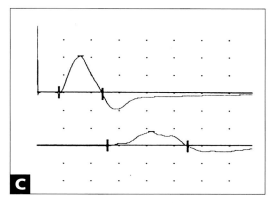

Figure 11-8. Motor nerve conduction studies: normal, axonal loss, and conduction block. **A,** A normal compound muscle action potential (CMAP) is obtained by stimulating the ulnar nerve at the wrist (*upper trace*) or at the elbow (*lower trace*), recording with surface electrodes over the abductor digiti minimi muscle. The amplitude is measured from the baseline to the negative peak (upward by convention and, in this example, 11.6 mV). The conduction velocity is calculated using the distance measured between the two sites of stimulation and the time difference of the onset of the two responses (in this example, 288 mm/4.5 ms = 62.2 m/s). Note that the amplitude of the response is about the same with distal (wrist) and proximal (elbow) stimulation. **B,** Ulnar motor response in a patient with significant axonal loss (due, for example, to motor neuron disease, axonal neuropathy, or nerve trauma). The amplitude of the CMAP is reduced to 1.2 mV (normal is greater than 4 mV). The velocity is mildly reduced, to 46 m/s. The amplitude of the distal CMAP is the same as the proximal response, although both are reduced. The hallmark of axonal loss in motor conduction studies is a reduced CMAP amplitude proximally and distally, reflecting the loss of axons along the length of the nerve. The conduction velocity may be mildly reduced, owing to loss of the fastest conducting motor fibers, but does not fall below 70% of the lower limit of normal values for that nerve. **C,** Ulnar motor response from a patient with chronic inflammatory demyelinating polyneuropathy. The CMAP with distal stimulation is normal. With proximal stimulation, however, the CMAP amplitude is only 40% of that of the distal CMAP, and the duration of the negative peak is greatly increased. This reflects conduction block and temporal dispersion between the proximal and distal sites, a physiologic hallmark of focal segmental demyelination. The conduction velocity is 30 m/s (normal is greater than 49 m/s), which is slower than can be produced by axonal loss alone, and is characteristic of demyelination.

Conduction velocity slowing to the degree illustrated here is typical in immune-mediated demyelinative neuropathies (*eg*, chronic inflammatory demyelinating polyneuropathy, Guillain-Barré syndrome) and in genetic disorders of peripheral nervous system myelin (*eg*, Charcot-Marie-Tooth disease types 1A and 1X). In Dejerine-Sottas syndrome, nerve conduction velocities are often below 10 m/s. Two other features that may be observed with demyelination are prolonged distal latency (Fig. 11-9) and conduction block (Fig. 11-10).

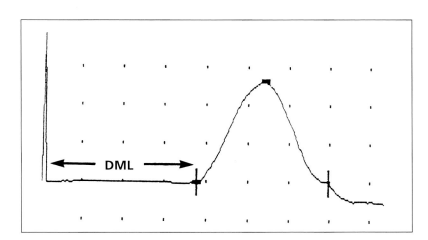

Figure 11-9. Prolonged distal motor latency in a patient with carpal tunnel syndrome. A compound motor action potential is obtained with stimulation of the median nerve at the wrist and surface electrode recording over the abductor pollicis brevis muscle. The distal motor latency (DML) is the time delay from the stimulus artifact (*far left*) to the onset of the response. This is a reflection of the conduction time in the distal motor nerve (and neuromuscular transmission). It is frequently prolonged in distal compressive neuropathies (*eg*, carpal tunnel syndrome, tarsal tunnel syndrome) and with distal demyelination (*eg*, Guillain-Barré syndrome). In this example, the DML is prolonged at 7.5 ms (normal is less than 4.6 ms; sensitivity = 2 mV/div; sweep speed = 2 ms/div).

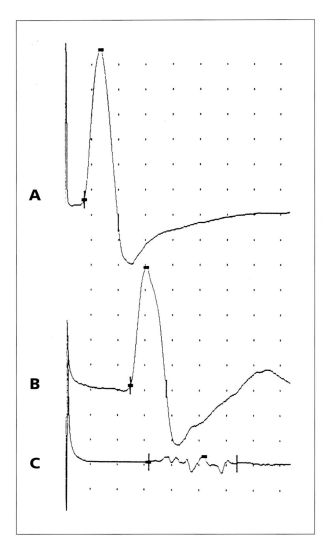

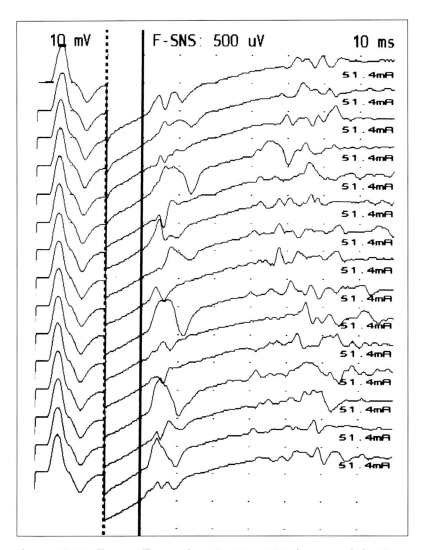

Figure 11-10. Acute conduction block in a patient with acute compressive neuropathy. This peroneal motor conduction study was performed in a man who had a foot drop after prolonged unconsciousness, during which there was compression of the lateral aspect of the knee against a hard surface. Responses from the extensor digitorum brevis muscle were obtained 2 weeks later with stimulation at the ankle (**A**), below the fibular head (**B**), and above the fibular head (**C**). The preserved compound motor action potential amplitudes distal (*A* and *B*) to the site of nerve compression at the fibular head demonstrate minimal axonal loss. The markedly reduced amplitude proximal (*C*) to the site of the lesion reflects block of conduction through that segment. This focal conduction block (or neurapraxia) is due to changes in the myelin architecture as a result of the compression injury. This patient completely recovered within 4 weeks, as expected, with conduction block (sensitivity = 200 μV/div; sweep speed = 5 ms/div.)

Figure 11-11. F waves. F waves (*to right of the solid line*) are recorded with supramaximal stimulation of the ulnar nerve at the wrist and surface recording electrodes over the abductor digiti minimi muscle (sensitivity = 500 μV/div; sweep speed = 10 ms/div). The F wave is the surface recorded response of a late motor unit discharge due to the antidromic activation and "backfiring" of a motor neuron. Note that the F wave has a smaller amplitude (1% to 5%) than the M wave (the compound muscle action potential; shown on the left; sensitivity = 10 mV/div). F waves also vary in latency (minimum latency is 29.6 ms; *marked by solid bar*) and morphology, owing to the discharge of different motor neurons with each trial. The latency reflects the time from the stimulus that it takes the action potential to reach the motor neuron antidromically and then travel orthodromically back down the motor axon to the muscle. As a result, it involves conduction through the proximal portions of the motor axon not directly accessible by other means. F waves are often absent, or the latency is markedly delayed, in disorders that produce demyelination in proximal motor axons, such as the Guillain-Barré syndrome or chronic inflammatory demyelinating polyneuropathy.

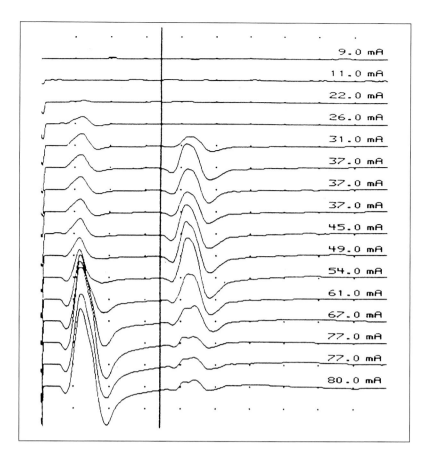

	9.0 mA
	11.0 mA
	22.0 mA
	26.0 mA
	31.0 mA
	37.0 mA
	37.0 mA
	37.0 mA
	45.0 mA
	49.0 mA
	54.0 mA
	61.0 mA
	67.0 mA
	77.0 mA
	77.0 mA
	80.0 mA

Figure 11-12. H reflex. The H reflex or H waves are recorded with surface electrodes over the soleus muscle and are elicited by electrical stimulation of the posterior tibial nerve in the popliteal fossa. The H reflex is the electrical equivalent of the ankle jerk reflex but is provoked by electrical stimulation of afferents in the mixed nerve rather than mechanical stretch. The H wave is shown on the right, with a latency of 34.2 ms (*dark bar*). The M wave (or direct compound muscle action potential) from the soleus is shown on the left. The H-reflex latency does not vary from trial to trial, unlike F waves. In addition, the H wave appears maximally at lower stimulus strengths and is abolished or reduced with intensity sufficient to elicit a maximal M wave. The H reflex is lost, or the latency is prolonged, in processes that affect the first sacral nerve root, such as radiculopathy or proximal demyelination (sensitivity = 5 mV/div; sweep speed = 10 ms/div).

Repetitive Stimulation Studies of Neuromuscular Junctions

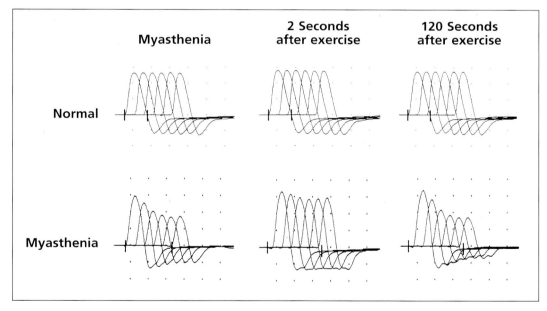

Figure 11-13. Repetitive stimulation studies in healthy patients and in those with myasthenia gravis. Defective transmission at neuromuscular junctions can be caused either by impaired release of acetylcholine-containing vesicles from the motor terminal (Lambert-Eaton myasthenic syndrome and botulism) or by a reduction in the capacity of postsynaptic skeletal muscle receptors to respond to acetylcholine (myasthenia gravis). These neuromuscular junction abnormalities can be diagnosed by repetitive stimulation studies. In the upper three tracings, responses are shown in a normal individual before exercise, immediately after exercise, and 120 seconds after exercise. Exercise is maximal voluntary contraction of the muscle under study for 30 to 60 seconds. The successive compound motor action potentials (CMAPs) are displayed after six supramaximal stimuli at 2 Hz (cycles/second). Note that the amplitude and configuration of the CMAP does not change in each series. In the lower left tracing, a decrementing response is shown at rest with stimulation at 3 Hz in a patient with myasthenia gravis. A decrement, reflecting abnormal neuromuscular transmission of any cause, is best seen with low rates of stimulation (2 to 5 Hz). A decrementing response is a reproducible decline in the CMAP amplitude (or area) with repetitive stimulation. In this example, there is a 38% decrement in the rested muscle. Immediately after maximal exercise, there is brief improvement in neuromuscular transmission, termed *postexercise facilitation*. This is reflected in a smaller decrement (in this example, of 13%). For several minutes after maximal exercise, there is a larger decrementing response than is seen in the rested muscle, termed *postexercise depression* or *exhaustion*. The decrement in this example is 48% when tested 120 seconds after exercise. These abnormalities with low rates of stimulation are seen in disorders that produce abnormal neuromuscular transmission, including myasthenia gravis, Lambert-Eaton syndrome, and botulism (sensitivity = 5 mV/div; sweep speed = 5 ms/div).

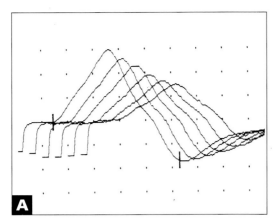 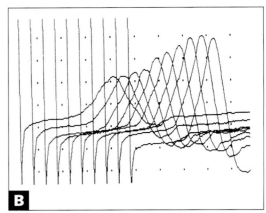

Figure 11-14. Repetitive stimulation studies in Lambert-Eaton myasthenic syndrome and botulism. **A,** A decrementing response is seen at low rates of stimulation (2 Hz), as in myasthenia gravis. **B,** An incrementing response, where the compound motor action potential amplitude (or area) increases after successive stimuli, is seen at high rates of stimulation (20 to 50 Hz). A three-fold increment is shown in this example at 20 Hz. This incrementing response seen at high rates of stimulation is characteristic of presynaptic disorders of neuromuscular transmission (Lambert-Eaton myasthenic syndrome and botu- lism) and is not seen in healthy patients or patients with myasthenia gravis (sensitivity = 200 µV/div; sweep speed = 2 ms/div).

The Lambert-Eaton syndrome is most frequently seen in patients with lung carcinoma. It is caused by autoantibodies recognizing calcium channels involved in the release of acetylcholine-containing vesicles from motor nerve ter- minals [3]. Botulism in adults is most often due to ingestion of foods containing the toxin and occasionally is caused by infection of a wound. In infants, botulism is most often due to *Clostridium botulinum* colonization of the gut [4].

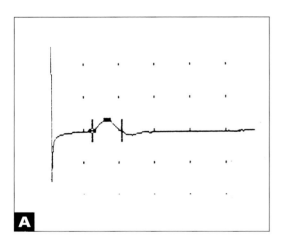 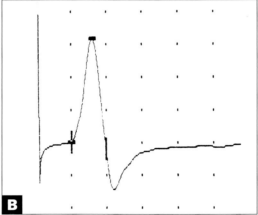

Figure 11-15. Postexercise increment in Lambert-Eaton myasthenic syndrome. **A,** The compound motor action potential (CMAP) ampli- tude is characteristically reduced in all rested limb muscles in Lambert-Eaton myasthenic syndrome (LEMS). In this example, the peroneal motor response amplitude is 0.35 mV (normal is greater than 1 mV). **B,** An incrementing response is seen after brief maximal exercise (10 to 15 seconds) in patients with LEMS, but not in healthy or myas- thenic patients. In this example, the increment is almost 10-fold, with a CMAP of 3.2 mV after exercise. This method is preferable for the diagnosis of LEMS in cooperative patients because high-fre- quency stimulation (Fig. 11-14) is uncomfortable (sensitivity = 1 mV/div; sweep speed = 5 ms/div).

Biopsy Studies of Skeletal Muscle and Peripheral Nerve

Myopathic Disorders

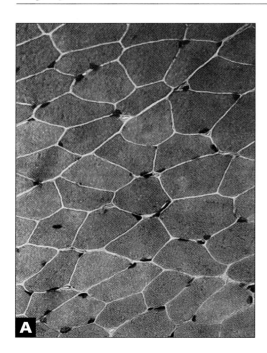 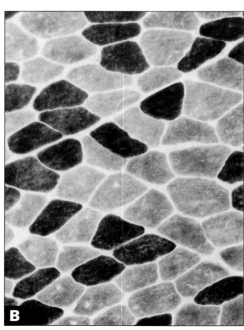

Figure 11-16. Normal skeletal muscle. **A,** Frozen cross-section of a limb skeletal muscle stained with hematoxylin-eosin (H-E). Note the polygonal configu- ration and normal variability in myofiber diameter. Most nuclei lie at the myofiber periphery in mature skeletal muscle (a color illustration of a normal skeletal muscle cross-section stained with H-E is shown in Fig. 11-18B). **B,** Frozen cross-section that has been histo- chemically stained by the ATPase (pH 9.4) procedure to show the normal bimodal distribution of type I (pale) and type II (dark) myofibers. Although individ- ual motor units (Fig. 11-3) contain only a single fiber type, the territories of individual motor units overlap in normal skeletal muscle, producing this montage of myofiber types. Motor unit overlap may be lost in the skeletal muscles of patients with anterior horn cell dis- ease or chronic motor neuropathy.

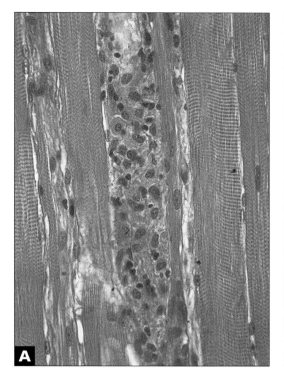

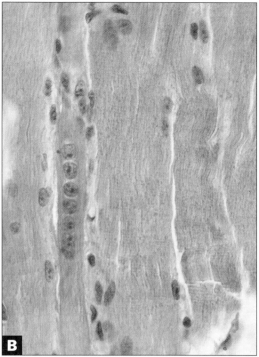

Figure 11-17. Myonecrosis and muscle regeneration. The presence of necrotic and regenerating myofibers in a skeletal muscle biopsy specimen strongly suggests a myopathic disorder. The loss of plasma membrane integrity during myonecrosis is responsible for the elevation in serum creatine kinase. If many myofibers simultaneously undergo myonecrosis, as may occur, for example, with massive muscle trauma or in patients with myophosphorylase deficiency, sufficient myoglobin may be released to cause acute renal failure. **A,** Myonecrosis. In this longitudinal section of skeletal muscle, one necrotic myofiber contains a large collection of phagocytic mononuclear cells, whereas adjacent myofibers appear normal. **B,** Regeneration. A small-caliber regenerating myofiber is seen in this longitudinal section of skeletal muscle. The hallmark of regeneration is the appearance of a string of large, centrally located nuclei with prominent nucleoli within a myofiber.

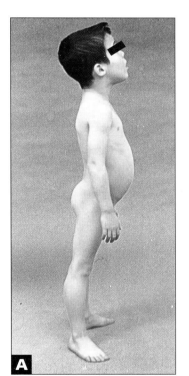

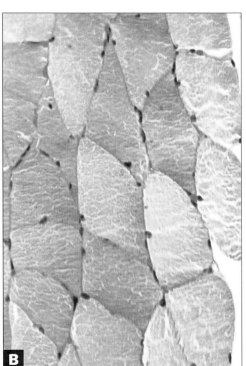

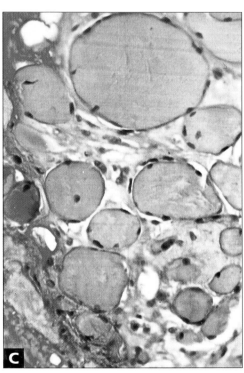

Figure 11-18. Duchenne dystrophy. Duchenne dystrophy is an X-linked progressive myopathy of childhood caused by mutations of the dystrophin gene. **A,** Lateral photograph of a boy with Duchenne dystrophy. Note the lumbar lordosis and enlarged calves. **B,** Cross-section of a normal skeletal muscle biopsy specimen, stained with hematoxylin and eosin (H&E). There is a similarity between muscle fibers in diameter, the presence of nuclei at the periphery of the fibers, and the lack of endomysial fibrosis. **C,** Cross-section of a skeletal muscle biopsy specimen from a child with Duchenne dystrophy, stained with H&E. There is a variation in fiber size, the presence of central nuclei, and the increased amounts of endomysial fibrous tissue and fat. **D,** Girls with one mutant and one normal copy of the dystrophin gene sometimes have symptoms, including elevated serum creatine kinase levels and mild weakness. This section, prepared from a skeletal muscle biopsy from a female Duchenne carrier, was immunostained with an antibody to dystrophin, then studied by indirect immunofluorescence using a rhodamine-conjugated second antibody. Most myofibers show some dystrophin staining, although some fibers (especially smaller-diameter fibers) are nearly devoid of staining. In addition, the staining pattern is nonuniform along the sacrolemmal membrane in some fibers. These features indicate the presence of a reduced quantity of the normal dystrophin molecule in this patient and are typical of heterozygous, female Duchenne carriers. Dystrophin, the skeletal muscle protein mutated in Duchenne dystrophy, appears to have primarily a structural function [5]. Mutations of other dystrophin-associated skeletal muscle structural proteins have also been found to cause muscular dystrophy phenotypes [6].

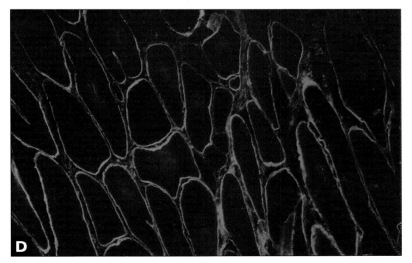

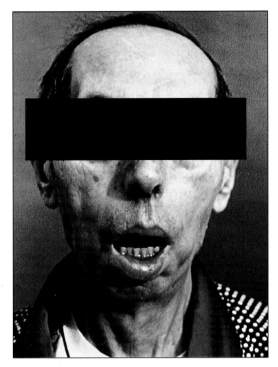

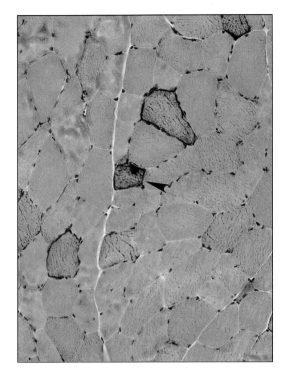

Figure 11-19. A patient with myotonic dystrophy who has the typical symptoms of muscle wasting, ptosis, and frontal balding. Myotonic dystrophy is a relatively common form of muscular dystrophy. It can present in children and adults and is inherited as an autosomal dominant trait. The characteristic myotonic discharges are illustrated in Figure 11-6 and correlate with clinical myotonia. Weakness is also a feature of myotonic dystrophy and often affects distal as well as proximal muscles. Other features common in adults with myotonic dystrophy include cataracts, testicular atrophy, and an organic mental syndrome. Skeletal muscle biopsy usually shows nonspecific myopathic changes. Affected family members demonstrate a triplet repeat (CTG) expansion in the 3′ untranslated region of the myotonic dystrophy gene, and, as in other triplet repeat–associated neural degenerative disorders (*eg*, X-linked spinal and bulbar muscular atrophy, Huntington's disease, Machado-Joseph disease, and fragile X syndrome), clinical severity tends to be worse in the affected children of an adult with myotonic dystrophy [7,8].

Figure 11-20. Low-power light microscopic view of a trichrome-stained frozen cross-section of skeletal muscle demonstrating myofibers with increased intramyofibrillar network and, in the center of the field, a fiber with dense, purple-staining subsarcolemmal material (*arrowhead*). These features correspond to accumulations of cytoskeletally normal or abnormal mitochondria in the subsarcolemmal region, which evolve over time in some patients with defects in mitochondrial oxidative phosphorylation. These "ragged red fibers" are unusual in children and rare in infants and toddlers. Mitochondrial myopathies are maternally inherited. Skeletal muscle weakness, correlated with the presence of ragged red skeletal muscle fibers, may occur in conjunction with central nervous system stroke-like episodes (the mitochondrial myopathy, encephalopathy, lactic acidosis, and stroke-like [MELAS] syndrome) or with progressive external ophthalmoplegia [9].

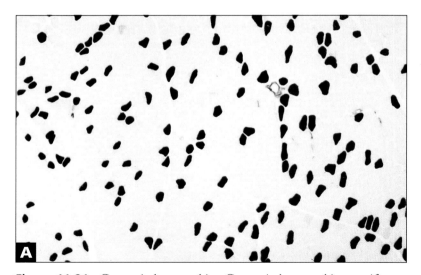

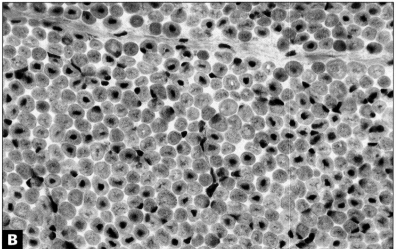

Figure 11-21. Congenital myopathies. Congenital myopathies manifest in early childhood with diffuse weakness and sometimes with congenital joint contractures (arthrogryposis). Mutations responsible for some of the familial forms of congenital myopathy (nemaline myopathy and central core myopathy) have recently been elucidated [10–12]. **A,** Congenital myopathy with fiber-type disproportion. This ATPase stained (pH 9.4) frozen muscle cross-section demonstrates an abnormal distribution of type I (pale-staining) and type II (dark-staining) myofibers. In normal muscle, these two fiber types are represented roughly equally, depending on the muscle sampled. In this muscle, there is type I predominance, with excessive variability of myofibrillary caliber predominantly affecting type I fibers. This finding is not specific, and congenital fiber-type disproportion can be a feature of otherwise nonspecific congenital myopathies. **B,** Congenital myopathy with central nuclei. This hematoxylin-eosin–stained frozen skeletal muscle cross-section demonstrates a marked increase in centrally located nuclei within small myofibers. Where the nucleus is not in the plane of section, a central "hole" represents absence of myofibrillar apparatus adjacent to the central nucleus. These disorders are almost certainly polygenic and have been termed *centronuclear myopathy* or *myotubular myopathy*.

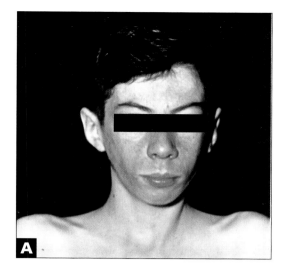

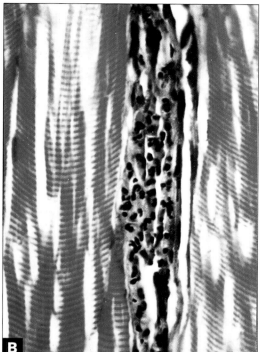

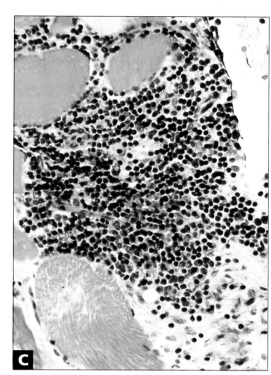

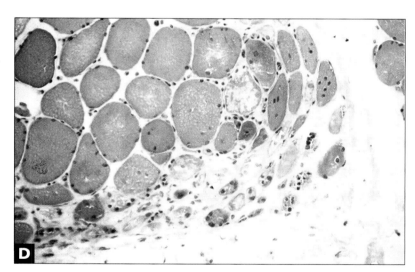

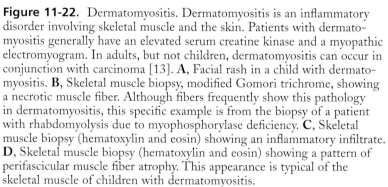

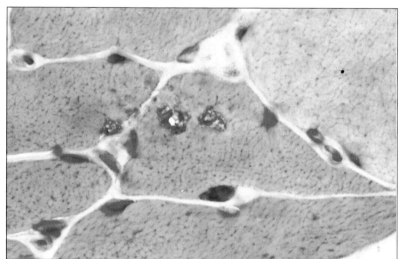

Figure 11-22. Dermatomyositis. Dermatomyositis is an inflammatory disorder involving skeletal muscle and the skin. Patients with dermatomyositis generally have an elevated serum creatine kinase and a myopathic electromyogram. In adults, but not children, dermatomyositis can occur in conjunction with carcinoma [13]. **A,** Facial rash in a child with dermatomyositis. **B,** Skeletal muscle biopsy, modified Gomori trichrome, showing a necrotic muscle fiber. Although fibers frequently show this pathology in dermatomyositis, this specific example is from the biopsy of a patient with rhabdomyolysis due to myophosphorylase deficiency. **C,** Skeletal muscle biopsy (hematoxylin and eosin) showing an inflammatory infiltrate. **D,** Skeletal muscle biopsy (hematoxylin and eosin) showing a pattern of perifascicular muscle fiber atrophy. This appearance is typical of the skeletal muscle of children with dermatomyositis.

Figure 11-23. Skeletal muscle biopsy from a patient with inclusion body myositis (hematoxylin and eosin) showing a rimmed vacuole. Inclusion body myositis can be either sporadic or familial. The inclusion bodies contain paired helical filaments and beta-amyloid precursor proteins [14].

Denervating Disorders

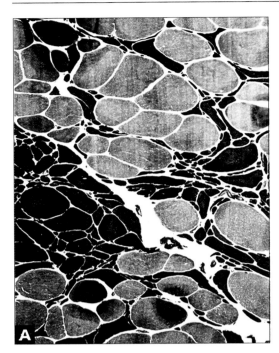 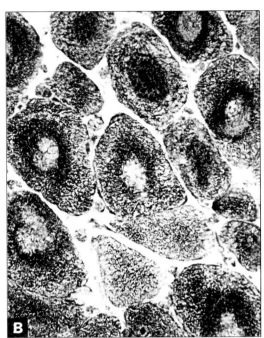

Figure 11-24. Neurogenic changes in skeletal muscle. Exciting progress has been made in determining the genetic mechanisms responsible for inherited denervating disorders. Transthyretin mutations are responsible for the many familial cases of amyloid neuropathy. Prognosis in these patients is improved by liver transplantation [15]. Point mutations and duplications or deletions of chromosomal segments that alter the structure or rate of synthesis of myelin proteins cause demyelinative neuropathies [16]. A triplet repeat expansion in the androgen receptor and mutations in the *SMN* or superoxide dismutase genes each result in progressive loss of spinal cord motor neurons [17–19]. As the fund of molecular information about these familial denervating diseases continues to increase, the need for biopsy of neural tissue to establish the diagnosis will continue to fall. We still have much to learn about the pathophysiology of denervating diseases by biopsy. Furthermore, biopsy is likely to continue to have an important role in the diagnosis of acquired denervating diseases. Loss of innervation causes skeletal muscle fibers to become small and angular. Muscle fiber–type grouping occurs after chronic denervation and compensatory extension of the territory of individual motor neurons by collateral sprouting. When all myofibers in a particular region are innervated by a single motor neuron, they share similar physiologic and histochemical characteristics, and this phenomenon of fiber-type grouping ensues. Target fibers may also be seen with skeletal muscle reinnervation but are a nonspecific finding. **A,** Skeletal muscle biopsy cross-section, ATPase (pH 9.4) histochemical reaction, showing small, angular muscle fibers, mostly type II (dark), and type grouping. **B,** Skeletal muscle biopsy cross-section, NADH tetrazolium reductase histochemistry, showing target fibers. The designation of target fiber requires the identification of three distinct zones within the myofiber. With the NADH stain, the central "bull's eye" is pale, reflecting an absence of mitochondrial membranes, surrounded by a dense ring and then by normal-staining peripheral sarcoplasm.

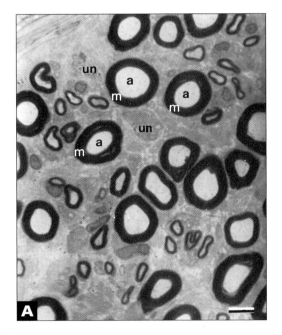 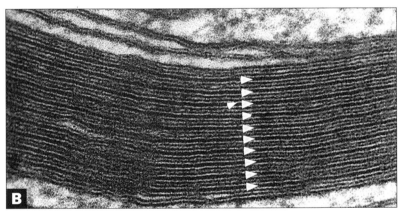

Figure 11-25. Myelin sheaths. **A,** Transverse section of a sural nerve from a 27-year-old man. Each myelin sheath (m) surrounds a single axon (a) and forms about 40% of the total diameter of the myelinated fiber. Unmyelinated axons (un) and their associated Schwann cells lie in the interstices between the myelinated axons. **B,** Electron micrograph showing that compact myelin is composed of alternating layers of major dense lines (*arrowheads*) and interperiod lines, which are double because they are the two apposed Schwann cell membranes. In glutaraldehyde-fixed samples such as this one, the distance between the major dense lines is about 15 nm [20]. (Scale bar: A, 10 μm.)

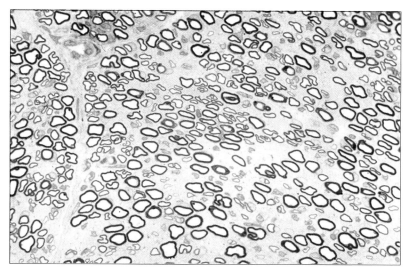

Figure 11-26. Sural nerve biopsy from a normal 2-month-old infant. Note the variability in axon caliber, the relatively small myelin sheath thickness to axonal diameter ratio, and the variability in myelin thickness to axonal diameter ratio. Compare this with the morphology of an adult nerve (Fig. 11-25A). Studies of nerve conduction velocity and amplitude (Figs. 11-8–11-12) permit the distinction of neuropathies affecting primarily axons (often with secondary demyelination caused by degeneration of myelinated axons) from neuropathies affecting primarily Schwann cells and the myelin sheath, causing segmental demyelination with relative sparing of axons.

Figure 11-27. Wallerian degeneration caused by vasculitis. Many types of systemic vasculitis affect the epineurial blood vessels that supply peripheral nerves, typically causing mononeuropathy multiplex owing to nerve ischemia. **A**, **B**, Transverse and longitudinal sections of a sural nerve from a patient who had an acute, severe neuropathy caused by Churg-Strauss syndrome. The axons have already degenerated, and myelin sheaths have begun to segment into myelin ovoids (o), some of which have been further broken down into smaller fragments (f) and lipid droplets (ld) by Schwann cells and macrophages (m). **C**, Mononuclear cells surrounding and infiltrating epineurial blood vessels (v) in a sural nerve biopsy specimen from a patient who had cryoglobulinemia stemming from a hepatitis C infection [21]. **D**, Epineurial arteriole from a patient with periarteritis nodosa. The media and elastic lamina (*arrows*) are disrupted by infiltrating mononuclear cells. (Scale bars: A, B, D, 10 μm; C, 50 μm.)

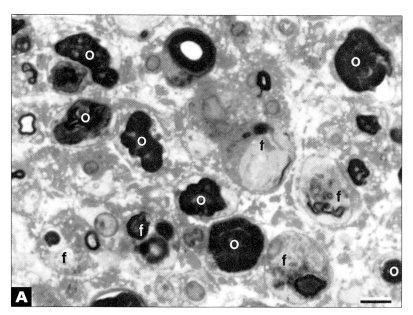

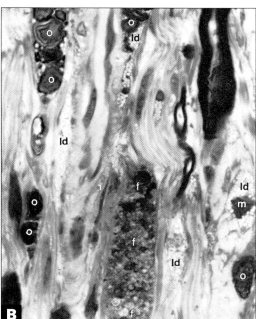

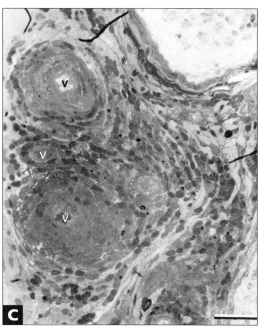

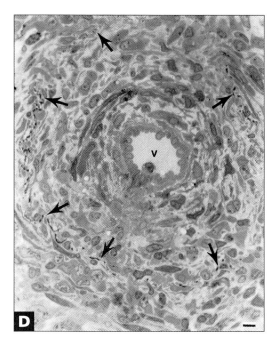

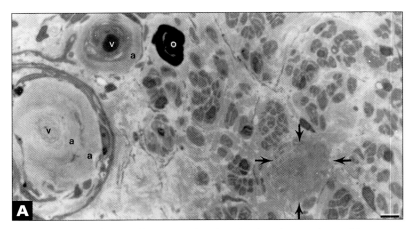

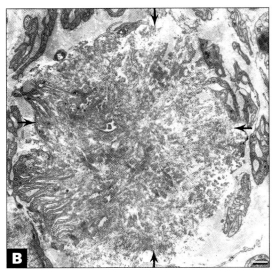

Figure 11-28. Amyloid neuropathy. Amyloid is the product of incompletely degraded proteins and can be caused by inherited transthyretin mutations or occur in conjunction with paraproteinemia [15,22]. **A,** Sural nerve biopsy from a patient who had a paraprotein [22] in which both myelinated and unmyelinated axons are lost in amyloid neuropathy. One degenerating myelin sheath is indicated (o). The amyloid (a) accumulates around endoneurial blood vessels (v) and also in the endoneurium (*arrows*). **B,** Electron micrograph of an endoneurial amyloid deposit (*arrows*), which is surrounded by denervated Schwann cells that have

lost their axons. (Scale bars: A, 10 µm; B, 1 µm.) The electron microscopic appearance of peripheral nervous system myelin is illustrated in Figure 11-25.

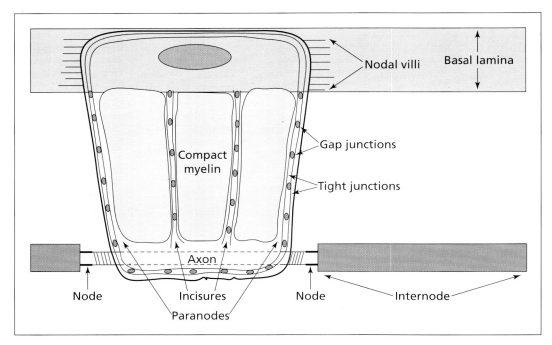

Figure 11-29. Schematic view of a myelinating Schwann cell. A myelinating Schwann cell has been unrolled, revealing the regions that form compact myelin, incisures, and paranodes. Two rows of tight junctions are depicted as continuous lines; these form a circumferential belt and are also found in the incisures [23]. Gap junctions are depicted as ovals; these are found between the rows of tight junctions. The abaxonal portion of the myelinating Schwann cell apposes the basal lamina, whereas the adaxonal portion apposes the axon. Peripheral nervous system myelin contains characteristic lipids and proteins that play roles in inherited and acquired demyelinative neuropathies. For example, mutations of lysosomal enzymes that diminish the capacity to degrade myelin galactocerebroside and sulfatide cause Krabbe's disease (globoid cell leukodystrophy) and metachromatic leukodystrophy (sulfatide lipidosis), respectively. Some of the proteins associated with peripheral nervous system myelin are depicted in Figure 11-30.

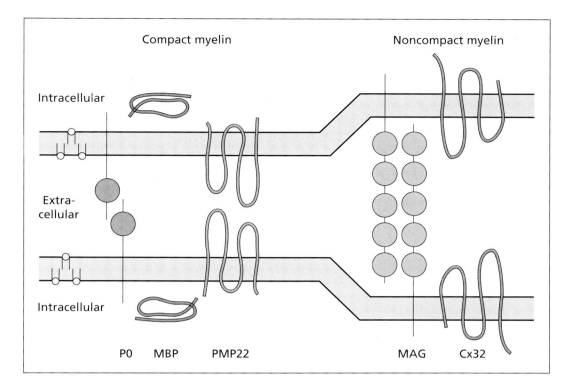

Figure 11-30. Schematic view of the major myelin-related proteins of the myelin sheath. In the peripheral nervous system, compact myelin contains protein zero (P0), peripheral myelin protein 22 kD (PMP22), myelin basic protein (MBP), and myelin P2 basic protein (not shown). The noncompact myelin of the paranodes and incisures contains myelin-associated glycoprotein (MAG) and connexin 32 (Cx32). P0 and MAG have extracellular immunoglobulin-like domains (circles) and PMP22 and Cx32 have four transmembrane domains. These myelin proteins play prominent roles in acquired and inherited demyelinative neuropathies. For example, patients (generally adult men) who express monoclonal autoantibodies against MAG may develop a demyelinative neuropathy affecting selectively large myelinated afferent fibers and causing sensory ataxia [24]. The roles of these Schwann cell proteins in inherited neuropathies are outlined in Figure 11-31.

Figure 11-31. The relation between inherited demyelinating neuropathies and mutations in myelin-related genes. CMT—Charcot-Marie-Tooth disease; Cx32—connexin 32; DSD—Duchenne dystrophy; HNPP—hereditary neuropathy with predisposition to pressure palsies; P0—protein zero; PMP22—peripheral myelin protein 22 kD.

The Relation Between Inherited Demyelinating Neuropathies and Mutations in Myelin-Related Genes

Disease	Genes affected	How genes are affected
CMT1A	PMP22	Duplication of one PMP22 gene; occasionally missense mutations
CMT1B	P0	Missense mutations
CMTX	Cx32	Missense mutations, nonsense mutations, small deletions, premature terminations
DSD	P0, PMP22	New dominant, gain-of-function PMP22
		Po missense mutations; duplication of PMP22 genes
HNPP	PMP22	Deletion of one PMP22 gene; loss of (nonsense) point mutations

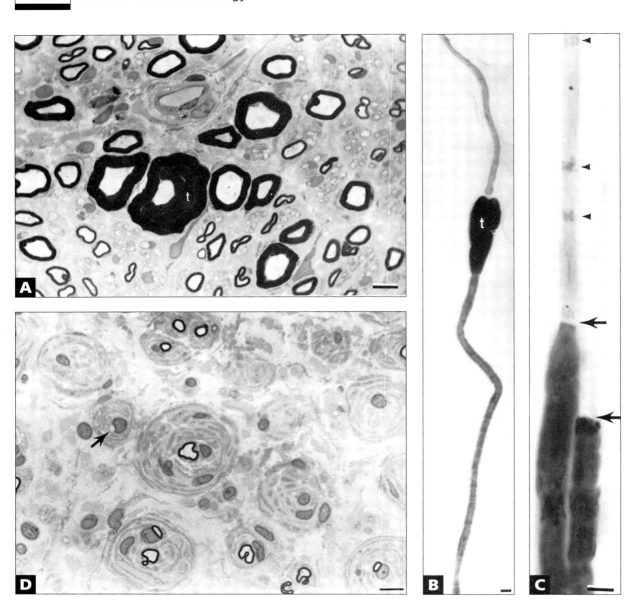

Figure 11-32. Nerve biopsies in patients with hereditary neuropathy with predisposition to palsies (HNPP) and chronic inflammatory demyelinating polyneuropathy (CIDP). HNPP is an inherited demyelinating neuropathy with conspicuous, focal thickening of the myelin sheaths, called *tomaculi*. **A,** Transverse section of a sural nerve showing a tomacula (*t*). **B,** Teased fiber from a sural nerve showing a tomacula (*t*). **C,** A pair of teased myelinated fibers from a patient with CIDP. The thickness of the myelin sheath changes abruptly at the nodes (*arrows*). The fiber on the left has a thin myelin sheath, as evidenced by the presence of incisures (*arrowheads*); whereas the fiber on the right appears to be demyelinated. **D,** Transverse section of a sural nerve from a patient who had CIDP, showing well-developed onion bulbs, which develop after repeated episodes of demyelination and remyelination. One of the axons at the center of an onion bulb is demyelinated (*arrow*), and the rest of the axons have abnormally thin myelin sheaths. (Scale bars: 10 μm.)

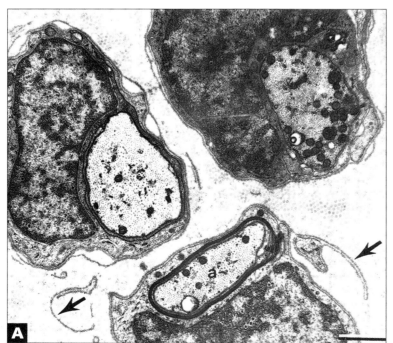

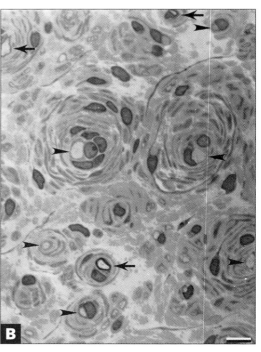

Figure 11-33. Nerve biopsies in congenital hypomyelinating neuropathy, Dejerine-Sottas syndrome and Charcot-Marie-Tooth disease (CMT) type 1. **A,** Electron micrograph of a sural nerve biopsy taken from an infant with congenital hypomyelinating neuropathy. An abnormally thin myelin sheath surrounds one axon (a); the other two axons are demyelinated. Excessive basal laminae are present (*arrows*), but not onion bulbs. **B,** Transverse section of a sural nerve from a 16-year-old girl with Dejerine-Sottas syndrome. Only three axons in this field are myelinated (*arrows*), and even these myelin sheaths are abnormally thin; other axons of comparable size are demyelinated (*arrowheads*). (*Continued on next page*)

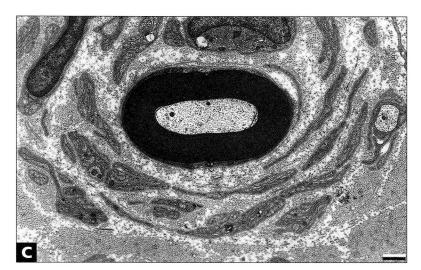

Figure 11-33. (*Continued*) Onion bulbs are conspicuous. The electron micrograph in **C** is from a sural nerve biopsy of a 59-year-old woman who has the demyelinating form of CMT disease. It shows that onions bulbs are composed of Schwann cell processes that are circumferentially disposed around an axon, which in this example is well myelinated. (Scale bars: A, C, 1 μm; B, 10 μm.)

References

1. Hermann DN, Griffin JW, Hauer P, *et al.*: Epidermal nerve fiber density and sural nerve morphometry in peripheral neuropathies. *Neurology* 1999, 53:1634–1640.

2. Asbury AK, Gilliatt RW: The Clinical Approach to Neuropathy. In *Peripheral Nerve Disorders*. Edited by Asbury AK, Gilliatt RW. London: Butterworths; 1994:1–20.

3. Lennon VA, Kryzer TJ, Griesmann GE, *et al.*: Calcium channel antibodies in the Lambert-Eaton syndrome and other paraneoplastic syndromes. *N Engl J Med* 1995, 332:1467–1474.

4. Chaudhry V, Crawford TO: Stimulation single-fiber EMG in infant botulism. *Muscle Nerve* 1999, 22:1698–1703.

5. Pasternak C, Wong S, Elson EL: Mechanical function of dystrophin in muscle cells. *J Cell Biol* 1995, 128:355–361.

6. Chan YM, Bonnemann CG, Lidov HGM, Kunkel LM: Molecular organization of sarcoglycan complex in mouse myotubes in culture. *J Cell Biol* 1998, 143:2033–2044.

7. Mahadevan M, Tsilfidis C, Sabourin L, *et al.*: Myotonic dystrophy mutation: an unstable CTG repeat in the 3′ untranslated region of the gene. *Science* 1992, 255:1253–1255.

8. Lieberman AP, Fischbeck KH: Triplet repeat expansion in neuromuscular disease. *Muscle Nerve* 2000, 23:843–850.

9. DiMauro S, Bonilla E, Davidson M, *et al.*: Mitochondria in neuromuscular disorders. *Biochim Biophys Acta* 1998, 1366:199–210.

10. Laing NG, Wilton SD, Akkari PA, *et al.*: A mutation in the alpha tropomyosin gene TPM3 associated with autosomal dominant nemaline myopathy. *Nature Genet* 1995, 9:75–79.

11. Johnston JJ, Kelley RI, Crawford TO, *et al.*: A novel nemaline myopathy in the Amish caused by a mutation in troponin TL. *Am J Hum Genet* 2000, 67:814–821.

12. McCarthy TV, Quane KA, Lynch PJ: Ryanodine receptor mutations in malignant hyperthermia and central core disease. *Hum Mutat* 2000, 15:410–417.

13. Sigurgeirsson B, Lindelof B, Edhag O, Allander E: Risk of cancer in patients with dermatomyositis or polymyositis: a population-based study. *N Engl J Med* 1992, 326:363–367.

14. Askanas V, Engel WK: Sporadic inclusion-body myositis and hereditary inclusion-body myopathies: current concepts of diagnosis and pathogenesis. *Curr Opin Rheumatol* 1998, 10:530–542.

15. Adams D, Samuel D, Goulon-Goeau C, *et al.*: The course and prognostic factors of familial amyloid polyneuropathy after liver transplantation. *Brain* 2000, 123:1495–1504.

16. Keller MP, Chance PF: Inherited neuropathies: from gene to disease. *Brain Pathol* 1999, 9:327–341.

17. La Spada AR, Roling DB, Harding AE, *et al.*: Meiotic stability and genotype-phenotype correlation of the trinucleotide repeat in X-linked spinal and bulbar muscular atrophy. *Nature Genet* 1992, 2:301–304.

18. Pellizzoni L, Charroux B, Dreyfuss G: SMN mutants of spinal muscular atrophy patients are defective in binding to snRNP proteins. *Proc Natl Acad Sci USA* 1999, 96:11167–111672.

19. Gurney ME, Liu R, Althaus JS, *et al.*: Mutant CuZn superoxide dismutase in motor neuron disease. *J Inherit Metab Dis* 1998; 21:587–597.

20. Peters A, Palay SL, Webster H deF: *The Fine Structure of the Nervous System*. New York: Oxford University Press; 1994.

21. Khella SL, Frost S, Hermann GA, *et al.*: Hepatitis C infection, cryoglobulinemia, and vasculitic neuropathy. Treatment with interferon alpha: case report and literature review. *Neurology* 1995, 45:407–411.

22. Rajkumar SV, Gertz MA, Kyle RA: Prognosis of patients with primary systemic amyloidosis who present with dominant neuropathy. *Am J Med* 1998, 104:232–237.

23. Arroyo EJ, Scherer SS: On the molecular architecture of myelinated fibers. *Histochem Cell Biol* 2000, 113:1–18.

24. Nobile-Orazio E, Meucci N, Baldini L, *et al.*: Long-term prognosis of neuropathy associated with anti-MAG IgM M-proteins and its relationship to immune therapies. *Brain* 2000, 123:710–717.

12

Infectious Diseases of the Nervous System

Burk Jubelt • Stacie Ropka

I N this chapter infectious diseases of the nervous system are discussed. These include bacterial, viral, fungal, spirochetal, and parasitic infections.

Although the central nervous system (CNS) is protected from bacterial invasion by the intact blood-brain barrier (BBB), bacterial invasion is enhanced by the special surface properties of bacteria as well as host immune deficiencies. Similar to any type of infection of the nervous system, bacteria may involve any of the nervous system compartments: the epidural space (epidural abscess); the dura (pachymeningitis); the subdural space (subdural empyema); the leptomeninges and the subarachnoid space containing cerebrospinal fluid (meningitis or leptomeningitis); and the brain parenchyma (brain abscess). The clinical manifestations, pathogenesis, pathology, etiology, epidemiology, diagnosis, differential diagnosis, and treatment of these syndromes are presented.

The list of viruses capable of causing neurologic disease is extensive. Most viral infections of the nervous system represent unusual complications of common systemic infections. After replication in extraneural tissue, viruses reach the CNS by the blood stream or spread along nerve fibers. Although rabies and poliomyelitis have been known since antiquity, only in the early part of the twentieth century were they demonstrated to be caused by "filterable agents" (viruses). In the 1930s, arboviruses were isolated from the brains of patients dying of encephalitides (Eastern and Western equine, St. Louis, and Japanese encephalitis), and lymphocytic choriomeningitis virus was isolated from the spinal fluid of patients with aseptic meningitis, being the first virus demonstrated to cause this syndrome. The coxsackie- and echoviruses were isolated and recognized to cause viral meningitis in the 1950s. The 1960s and 1970s were the decades during which slow virus infections were recognized, with conventional viruses and atypical agents (prions) isolated from chronic neurologic diseases. The 1980s ushered in the identification of the retroviruses with the AIDS epidemic and tropical spastic paraparesis. In the late 1990s, West Nile virus began to cause disease in North America. We have yet to discover what other viruses are unrecognized as causes of unusual neurologic diseases.

The last 30 years have seen a steady increase in the frequency of fungal infections of the CNS, primarily due to the increased use of immunosuppressive drugs and the AIDS epidemic. Most fungal infections are caused by opportunistic organisms except those caused by the pathogenic fungi (histoplasmosis, blastomycosis, coccidioidomycosis, and paracoccidioidomycosis). In most fungal infections, spread to the CNS occurs after obvious extraneural primary infection of the lungs, skin, and hair, the main exception being cryptococcosis.

The spirochetal diseases that involve the nervous system include syphilis, Lyme disease, and leptospirosis. Syphilis and Lyme disease regularly cause both meningeal and parenchymal disease; humans are the only host in syphilis and an important dead-end host in Lyme disease. Both of these diseases can be chronic and are relatively common; they are discussed in detail. Leptospirosis, in contrast, is a disease of both wild and domestic animals with humans being incidental hosts. Human infection occurs through contact with infected animal tissue or urine or from exposure to contaminated ground water, soil, or vegetation. Leptospirosis is a self-limited illness that primarily manifests as aseptic meningitis. Rarely, encephalitis, myelitis, optic neuritis, and peripheral neuropathy have been reported. Penicillin or tetracycline as an alternative therapy is the antibiotic of choice; fewer than 100 cases of leptospirosis are reported per year.

Parasitic infections can be divided into two major categories: protozoan and helminthic (worms). Helminths include nematodes (roundworms), trematodes (flukes), and cestodes (tapeworms). Parasitic diseases occur worldwide but are most common in tropical and underdeveloped areas of the world, where poverty and poor housing conditions contribute to their pathogenesis and spread. Tropical climates are also ideal for the vectors that spread these infections. In these areas, parasitic infections are the most common infectious disease, and they exact a heavy toll on the human population.

Bacterial Infections

Acute Bacterial Meningitis

Clinical Manifestations of Acute Bacterial Meningitis by Age Group

Age group	Symptoms	Signs
Infants (≤2 years)	Irritability	Fever
	Poor feeding	Lethargy
	Vomiting	Stupor, coma
	Unconsciousness	Bulging fontanel
	Respiratory symptoms	Seizures
	Apnea	Petechial or purpuric rash
Children and adults	Headache	Fever
	Neck stiffness or pain	Nuchal rigidity
	Unconsciousness	Lethargy, confusion, stupor, coma
	Nausea and vomiting	Seizures
	Photophobia	Focal neurologic deficits, including cranial nerve palsies
	Respiratory symptoms	Ataxia (in children)
		Petechial or purpuric rash

Figure 12-1. Clinical manifestations of acute bacterial meningitis by age group. The symptoms and signs of bacterial meningitis in infants are nonspecific and typical of a severe systemic infection including sepsis. In children and adults, the classic signs of meningeal irritation are nuchal rigidity, Kernig's sign, and Brudzinski's sign. Nuchal rigidity is present when the patient has resistance to passive flexion of the neck. Kernig's sign is elicited by flexing the thigh and knee while the patient is in the supine position; in the presence of meningeal inflammation, there is resistance to passive extension of the leg at the knee with the thigh flexed. Brudzinski's sign is positive when passive flexion of the neck causes flexion of the hips and knees. Neurologic complications are frequently associated with bacterial meningitis. *Seizures* occur in 40% of cases. Generalized seizures usually occur early due to fever, metabolic derangements, or toxic factors (*eg*, alcohol withdrawal); focal seizures are more likely to occur after 4 to 10 days and are caused by arterial thrombosis, cortical vein thrombosis, or abscess formation. *Cranial nerve (CN) palsies*, especially of CN III, VI, VII, and VIII, are due to purulent exudates in the arachnoid sheaths of the specific cranial nerve. Sensorineural hearing loss is a major complication in infants and children, occurring in 30% of cases. *Cerebral edema and increased intracranial pressure* may be due to noncommunicating hydrocephalus caused by basilar exudates, or to exudates in the Virchow-Robin spaces invading the parenchyma. *Focal cerebral signs* are most likely to occur at the end of the first week of infection but may occur later as well; they are due to arterial thrombosis causing infarction, cortical vein thrombosis with secondary hemorrhagic infarction, or abscess formation.

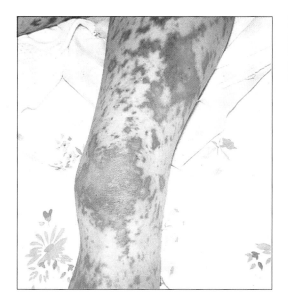

Figure 12-2. Meningococcal rash. Meningococcus is the only bacterium that frequently causes a rash, which is probably the most important clue to the diagnosis of meningococcal meningitis (Fig. 12-13). It usually begins as a diffuse erythematous maculopapular rash. As the rash evolves, petechiae and purpura appear primarily on the trunk and lower extremities. (*From* Roos and colleagues [1]; with permission.)

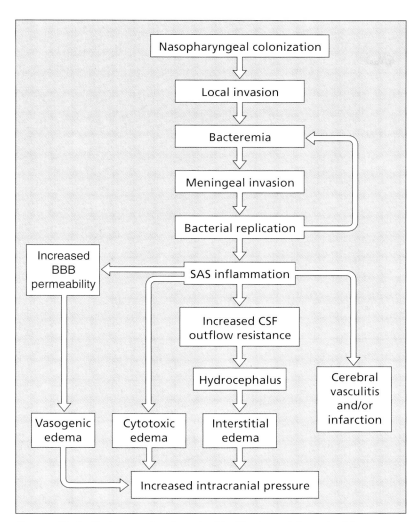

Figure 12-3. Pathogenesis of meningitis. For bacterial meningitis to occur, the host usually acquires a new organism by colonization of the nasopharynx. This may lead to direct seeding of cerebral spinal fluid (CSF) spaces, but more likely causes local spread to the sinuses or the lungs (pneumonia) or bacteremia, which then results in meningeal invasion. BBB—blood-brain barrier; SAS—subarachnoid space. (*Adapted from* Roos and colleagues [1].)

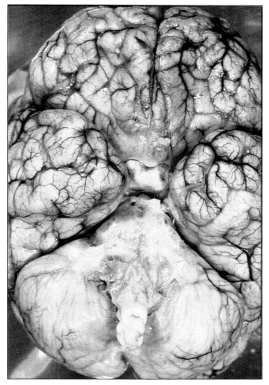

Figure 12-4.
Purulent exudate of bacterial meningitis at the base of the brain. The neurologic complications of cranial nerve palsies and increased intracranial pressure are often caused by inflammation of the base of the brain. The increased intracranial pressure occurs because cerebrospinal fluid pathways are blocked, resulting in obstructive hydrocephalus. (*From* Roos and colleague [2]; with permission.)

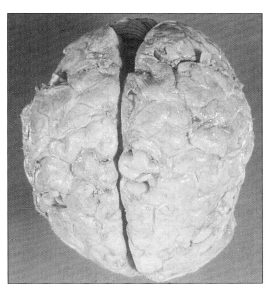

Figure 12-5. Purulent exudate of leptomeningitis (inflammation of pia and arachnoid spaces) over the convexities of the cerebral cortex. This may result in the additional complications of arterial or venous thrombosis with infarction and hemorrhage, both of which may lead to focal neurologic defects. Initially exudates over the convexity appear yellow, but later turn gray as they become thicker. (*From* Kaplan [3]; with permission.)

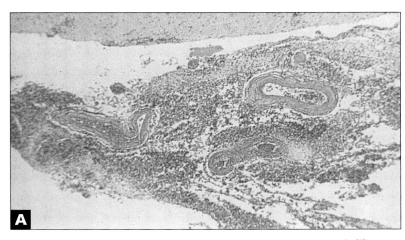

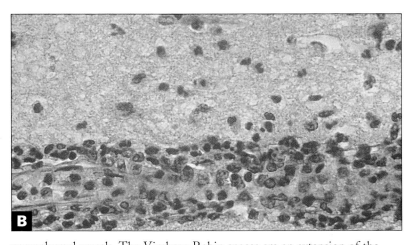

Figure 12-6. Microscopic examination in bacterial meningitis. **A,** The meninges are thickened by both polymorphonuclear (PMNs) and mononuclear inflammatory cells. Thickening of blood vessels may eventually lead to thrombotic occlusion, cerebral infarcts, and focal neurologic deficits. **B,** Inflammatory cells in the Virchow-Robin spaces around penetrating parenchymal vessels. The Virchow-Robin spaces are an extension of the subarachnoid space. Occasionally, inflammation may extend into the perivascular parenchyma, as shown here. (Panel A *from* Kaplan [3]; with permission; Panel B *from* Wilson [4]; with permission.)

Predisposing Factors in 404 Single Episodes of Bacterial Meningitis

Factor	Community-acquired, % (n = 253)	Nosocomial, % (n = 151)
Acute otitis media	19	1
Chronic otitis media	7	0
Sinusitis	12	4
Pneumonia	15	8
Endocarditis	7	1
Head injury*		
Recent	5	13
Remote	4	0
Recent neurosurgery*	0	68
Neurosurgical device†	1	32
Altered immune state	19	31
Diabetes mellitus	10	6
Alcoholism	18	5
Cerebrospinal fluid leak	8	13
None of the 13 factors	25	8

*Recent denotes head injury or neurosurgery within 1 month of the onset of meningitis; remote, more than 1 month before the onset of meningitis.

†Neurosurgical devices included ventriculostomy, ventriculoperitoneal or ventriculoatrial shunt, lumbar epidural catheter, lumboperitoneal catheter, and dorsal-column stimulator.

Figure 12-7. Predisposing factors in bacterial meningitis. Predisposing factors for community-acquired meningitis are somewhat different than those seen in nosocomial infections. Predisposing factors for nosocomial infections are primarily caused by openings into the central nervous system. (*Adapted from* Durand and colleagues [5].)

Percentage of Causative Organisms in Single Episodes of Meningitis, 1962 Through 1988*

Nosocomial organism	Community-acquired, % (n = 253)	Nosocomial, % (n = 151)
Streptococcus pneumoniae	38	5
Gram-negative bacilli†	4	38
Neisseria meningitidis	14	1
Streptococci‡	7	9
Enterococcus	0	3
Staphylococcus aureus	5	9
Listeria monocytogenes	11	3
Haemophilus influenzae	4	4
Mixed bacterial species	2	7
Coagulase-negative staphylococci	0	9
Other§	2	3
Culture negative	13	11

*Percentages do not always total 100 because of rounding.

†In community-acquired meningitis, the causative organisms were Escherichia coli (4 episodes), and species of Klebsiella (3), Enterobacter (1), and Proteus (1); in nosocomial meningitis, E. coli (17), Klebsiella (13), Pseudomonas (6), Acinetobacter (6), Enterobacter (5), Serratia (5), Citrobacter (2), Proteus (1), "coliform" bacteria (1), and "nonenteric gram-negative rods" (1).

‡In community-acquired meningitis, the causative organisms were group A (4 episodes), group B (1), nonenterococcal group D (3), group D, not further identified (1), other groups (5), and non-hemolytic, nongrouped (3); in nosocomial meningitis, the causative organisms were group B (4), nonenterococcal group D (3), other groups (2), α-hemolytic, nongrouped (3), and nonhemolytic, nongrouped (1).

§In community-acquired meningitis, the causative organisms were anaerobes (3 episodes) and diphtheroids (1); in nosocomial meningitis, the causative organisms were micrococci (2), Neisseria species (1), propionibacteria (1), and diphtheroids (1).

Figure 12-8. Causative organisms of bacterial meningitis. The causative organisms are somewhat different for community-acquired as opposed to nosocomial meningitis. (*Adapted from* Durand and colleagues [5].)

Causative Organisms of Bacterial Meningitis (Percentage of Cases by Age)

Organism	<1 mo	1–23 mo	2–29 y	30–59 y	≥60 y
Haemophilus influenzae	0	0.7	5.4	12.1	2.5
Neisseria meningitidis	0	30.8	59.8	18.2	3.6
Streptococcus pneumoniae	8.7	45.2	27.2	60.6	68.6
Streptococci group B	69.5	19.2	5.4	3	3.6
Listeria monocytogenes	21.8	0	2.2	0.1	21.7

Figure 12-9. Causative organisms of bacterial meningitis by age-related relative frequency. *Haemophilus influenzae* type b was the leading cause of meningitis until widespread use of vaccine. Now *H. influenzae* is not a significant cause of bacterial meningitis in the vaccinated population [6]. Meningococcal meningitis caused by *Neisseria meningitidis* affects mostly children and young adults. As of 1995, *N. meningitidi* had replaced *H. influenzae* as the leading cause of bacterial meningitis in these age groups in the United States [7]. Congenital terminal complement deficiencies (C5-C8) predispose to meningococcemia. Pneumococcal meningitis caused by *Streptococcus pneumoniae* is the most common cause of bacterial meningitis in adults. Predisposing factors include pneumonia, otitis media, sinusitis, head trauma, CSF leaks, sickle cell disease, splenectomy, diabetes and alcoholism. (*Adapted from* Schuchat and colleagues [8].)

Causative Organisms of Recurrent Meningitis*

Organism	Community-acquired (*n* = 38)	Nosocomial, % (*n* = 41)
Streptococcus pneumoniae	13 (34)	1 (2)
Gram-negative bacilli[†]	0	19 (46)
Neisseria meningitidis	3 (8)	0
Streptococci[‡]	4 (11)	1 (2)
Staphylococcus aureus	1 (3)	6 (15)
Haemophilus influenzae	4 (11)	0
Mixed bacterial species	0	2 (5)
Coagulase-negative staphylococci	0	3 (7)
Other[§]	2 (5)	1 (2)
Culture negative	11 (29)	8 (20)

Both initial and recurrent episodes in the 17 patients who had more than one episode of community-acquired meningitis and the 19 patients who had more than one episode of nosocomial meningitis are included. Not included are five patients, each of whom had one episode of community-acquired meningitis and one episode of nosocomial meningitis. The community-acquired episodes in these patients were caused by group A streptococcus (1), N. meningitidis (1), and Staph. aureus (1); two episodes were culture-negative. The nosocomial episodes were caused by Staph. aureus (2), klebsiella (1), and Strep. pneumoniae (1); one episode was culture-negative. Percentages do not total 100 because of rounding.

†*The causative organisms were as follows:* Pseudomonas *(5 episodes),* Klebsiella *(4),* Enterobacter *(3),* Acinetobacter *(2),* Serratia *(1),* Escherichia coli *(1),* Proteus *(1),* Citrobacter *(1), and "gram-negative rods" (1).*

‡*In community-acquired meningitis:* α-hemolytic, nongrouped *(3 episodes), and group D, not further identified (1); in nosocomial meningitis: nonhemolytic (1).*

§*In community-acquired meningitis: anaerobes (1 episode) and* Campylobacter fetus *(1); in nosocomial meningitis:* Propionibacterium acnes *(1).*

Figure 12-10. Causative organisms of recurrent meningitis. *Streptococcus pneumoniae* is the most frequent cause of community-acquired recurrent meningitis. Gram–negative bacilli are the most frequent causes for nosocomial infections. The most frequent risk factors are head trauma, neurosurgical procedures, and cerebrospinal fluid leaks. Other risk factors include immunodeficiencies, immunosuppressant therapy, splenectomy, and parameningeal infection (*eg*, sinusitis, otitis media). (*Adapted from* Durand and colleagues [5].)

Initial Cerebrospinal Fluid Values in 493 Episodes of Bacterial Meningitis*

Variable	Community-acquired, % (*n* = 296)	Nosocomial, % (*n* = 197)
Opening pressure (mm of water)		
0–139	9	23
140–299	52	52
300–399	20	11
≥400	19	15
White-cell count per mm³[†]		
0–99	10 (13)	17 (19)
100–4999	61 (59)	65 (62)
5000–9999	15 (15)	11 (12)
≥10,000	13 (13)	7 (8)
Percent neutrophils		
0–19	2	2
20–79	19	31
≥80	79	66
Total protein (mg/dL)		
0–45	4	6
46–199	40	42
≥200	56	52
Glucose <40 mg/dL	50	45
Positive Gram stain	60	46
Culture positive	73	83

The values shown are percentages of all the episodes in which the results of a given study were reported on initial examination of cerebrospinal fluid. Of the 296 community-acquired episodes, opening pressure was reported in 205, the white-cell count in 286, percent neutrophils in 271, protein level in 263, glucose level in 269, results of Gram's staining in 272, and culture results in 289. Of the 197 nosocomial episodes, opening pressure was reported in 102, white-cell count in 167, percent neutrophils in 163, protein level in 159, glucose level in 164, results of Gram's staining in 126, and culture results in 180. Percentages do not always total 100 because of rounding.

†*Because the data for pleocytosis may be biased by our criteria for culture-negative episodes, the percentages of culture-positive episodes alone are given in parentheses.*

Figure 12-11. Cerebrospinal fluid (CSF) abnormalities in acute bacterial meningitis. The characteristic CSF picture in acute bacterial meningitis usually includes an increased opening pressure (greater than 200 mm H_2O); an increased white cell count with a predominance of polymorphonuclear leukocytes (PMNs) or neutrophils; a decreased glucose level (less than 40 mg/dL) or decreased CSF to serum glucose ratio (less than 0.3); and an increased protein level (greater than 45 mg/dL). Turbid CSF seen on visual inspection suggests more than 400 white cells per mm³. (*Adapted from* Durand and colleagues [5].)

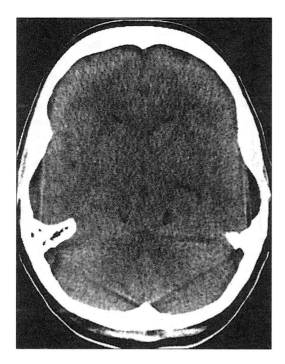

Figure 12-12. Computed tomography (CT) scan done as part of a diagnostic work-up for acute bacterial meningitis. Diagnostic studies include blood cultures (three sets) and cerebrospinal fluid (CSF) analysis. In addition to routine CSF studies, specialized immunochemical tests should be performed in patients who have been partially treated, even with oral antibiotics. These special tests include latex agglutination, counterimmunoelectrophoresis, *limulus* amoebocyte lysate and coagglutination. If the patient shows signs suggestive of increased intracranial pressure (impaired mental status, focal neurologic signs, papilledema, dilated nonreactive pupil, cranial nerve VI palsy), then a brain CT scan should be performed before lumbar puncture (LP). The CT scan may show diffuse cerebral edema (as here) or a focal lesion, which are contraindications to LP. (*From* Roos and colleague [1]; with permission.)

Differential Diagnosis of Bacterial Meningitis

Differential diagnosis	Diagnostic test
Viral meningitis	CSF
Viral encephalitis	CSF, EEG, MRI
Tuberculous meningitis	CSF
Fungal meningitis	CSF
Brain abscess	CT
Subdural empyema	CT
Rocky Mountain spotted fever	Rash biopsy with FA staining of specimen
Bacterial endocarditis	Cardiac murmur
Subarachnoid hemorrhage	CSF
Neoplastic meningitis	CSF

Figure 12-13. Differential diagnosis of acute bacterial meningitis. Viral meningitis is a diagnostic consideration of very early bacterial meningitis. In viral meningitis, fever is not as prominent, and cerebrospinal fluid (CSF) studies usually reveal normal glucose levels and mononuclear pleocytosis, although polymorphonuclear neutrophils (PMNs) may be seen in the first 12 to 24 hours. In viral encephalitis, the CSF analysis is similar to that of viral meningitis, but mental status is altered. Tuberculous (TB) meningitis may be subacute or have a rapid downhill course, but mononuclear cells are present in the CSF and usually the glucose level is low. Fungal meningitis has a more chronic course. CSF studies reveal a mononuclear pleocytosis and low glucose. Brain abscess and subdural empyema usually present with focal abnormalities on examination, increased intracranial pressure, and a CSF pleocytosis with normal glucose. Rocky Mountain spotted fever may clinically resemble bacterial meningitis, with patients exhibiting fever, headache, altered mental status, and a petechial rash. The rash is usually different than that seen in meningococcemia (Fig. 12-2), beginning on wrists and ankles, then spreading to the body and face; the mucous membranes are not involved. The CSF is usually normal, and a history of tick bite is elicited in 80% of patients. Bacterial endocarditis causes a new heart murmur, petechial lesions of the nailbeds, mucous membranes, and extremities, and hematuria, as well as altered mental status. Subarachnoid hemorrhage presents with sudden, excruciating headache, meningismus, fever at times, usually a normal mental status (unless intracerebral bleeding occurred), and CSF xanthochromia with a large number of red blood cells. Neoplastic meningitis (meningeal carcinomatosis) often causes cranial nerve palsies, mononuclear cells in the CSF, and low glucose levels; the cytologic appearance is diagnostic. A diffuse erythematous maculopapular rash is present in over 50% of patients with meningococcemia. This presents as petechiae and purpura on the trunk and lower extremities (Fig. 12-2). The petechiae may appear on mucous membranes and conjunctivae but never in the nailbeds. Other organisms that cause meningitis less frequently cause similar rashes (*Staphylococcus aureus*, *Acinetobacter* species, *Streptococcus pneumoniae*, and *Haemophilus influenzae*). The rash of staphylococcal endocarditis involves the nailbeds in addition to the mucous membranes and the extremities. Echovirus type 9 infections often also cause a petechial or purpuric rash. CT—computed tomography; EEG—electroencephalogram; FA—fluorescent antibody; MRI—magnetic resonance imaging.

Differential Diagnosis in Acute Bacterial Meningitis Based Upon Typical Cerebrospinal Abnormalities

Type of infection	Predominant cells (per mm³)	Glucose (mg/dL)	Stain for organisms	Diagnosis
Bacterial meningitis	PMNs	Very low (0–10)	Gram stain	Culture, CIE, LA, LAL, CoA
Tuberculous meningitis	Monos	Low to very low (10–20)	Ziehl-Neilson	Culture
Viral meningitis	Monos	Normal	—	Culture
Fungal meningitis	Monos	Low (15–30)	Cryptococcus—India ink stain	Culture; various Ab & Ag tests
Parameningeal (serous) meningitis	Subacute and chronic—monos (usual picture); acute—PMNs (uncommon)	Normal	—	CT, MRI; myelogram
Neoplastic meningitis	Monos	Low or normal (30–50)	—	Cytologic studies

Figure 12-14. Differential diagnosis of cerebrospinal fluid (CSF) abnormalities in acute bacterial meningitis. Rarely in bacterial meningitis monocytes may predominate in the CSF (Listeria monocytogenes and especially Brucellosis). In viral meningitis, polymorphonuclear (PMNs) leukocytes may appear in the first 12 to 24 hours, and then there is a shift to mononuclear cells. Most parameningeal foci of infection (*eg*, brain abscess, epidural abscess) cause a subacute to chronic condition of mononuclear cells in the CSF. Subdural empyema, however, may cause an acute parameningeal CSF appearance of a large number of PMNs. Ab—antibody; Ag—antigen; CIE—counter immunoelectrophoresis; CoA—coagglutination; CT—computed tomography; LA—latex agglutination; LAL—limulus amoebocyte lysate; Monos—mononuclear leukocytes; MRI—magnetic resonance imaging; PMNs—polymorphonuclear leukocytes.

Empiric Antimicrobial Therapy for Bacterial Meningitis

	Antimicrobial agent
Neonates	Ampicillin plus cefotaxime
Infants and children	Cefotaxime or ceftriaxone
Adults (15–50 y)	Third-generation cephalosporin or penicillin G
Older adults	Third-generation cephalosporin (ceftriaxone or ceftazidime) plus ampicillin
Neurosurgical procedure	Third-generation cephalosporin (ceftazidime) plus aminoglycoside plus vancomycin
Immunocompromised state	Ampicillin plus third-generation cephalosporin
Neutropenic state	Ceftazidime plus ampicillin

Figure 12-15. Empiric antimicrobial therapy for acute bacterial meningitis. Empiric antibiotic therapy must be given before the causative organism can be definitively identified. The choice of the empiric agent depends on the patient's age and associated conditions (such as neurosurgical procedure, immunodeficiency), with modifications based on a positive Gram stain. To achieve adequate antibiotic levels in the cerebrospinal fluid, antibiotics should be given intravenously. (*Adapted from* Roos and colleague [2].)

Antibiotic Therapy for Acute Bacterial Meningitis

Organism	Antibiotics*
Haemophilus influenzae	Third-generation cephalosporin, ampicillin (if sensitive), chloramphenicol[†]
Streptococcus pneumoniae	Penicillin G, third-generation cephalosporin Chloramphenicol[†]
Reduced penicillin-sensitive	Third-generation cephalosporin
Penicillin-resistant	Third-generation cephalosporin plus vancomycin or rifampin
Neisseria meningitidis	Penicillin G, chloramphenicol[†]
Streptococcus agalactiae	Penicillin G or ampicillin
Listeria monocytogenes	Ampicillin (plus aminoglycoside) or trimethoprim-sulfamethoxazole
Enterobacteriaceae	Third-generation cephalosporin with or without aminoglycoside
Pseudomonas aeruginosa	Ceftazidime plus aminoglycoside or fluoroquinolone (*eg* ciprofloxacin)
Staphylococcus aureus	Nafcillin

*Third-generation cephalosporins: cefotaxime, ceftriaxone, ceftizoxime.

[†]For penicillin-allergic patients.

Figure 12-16. Specific antibiotic therapy for acute bacterial meningitis. Once the causative organism is cultured and sensitivities determined, therapy should be adjusted to be as narrow as possible. The duration of treatment is somewhat empiric with the following general recommendations: *Neisseria meningitidis*, 7 days; *Haemophilus influenzae*, 7 to 10 days; *Streptococcus pneumoniae*, 10 to 14 days; gram-negative bacilli, 21 days. (*Adapted from* Täuber and colleagues [9]; Klugman and Madhi [10].)

Adjunctive Therapy and Supportive Care for Bacterial Meningitis

Adjunctive dexamethasone—0.15 mg/kg every 6 hours
 for 4 days, for children only
Supportive care
 Fluid and electrolyte balance—monitor for syndrome of
 inappropriate antidiuretic hormone
 Maintenance of normal systemic blood pressure because of
 loss of autoregulation
 Intracranial pressure (ICP) monitoring for critically ill
 patients
 Treatment for increased ICP
 Elevate head of bed to 30°
 Hyperventilation to $PaCO_2$ to 27–30 mm Hg
 Hyperosmolar agents—mannitol, glycerol
 Glucocorticoids—dexamethasone
 Monitor and treat obstructive hydrocephalus
 Seizure control—lorazepam, phenytoin, phenobarbital

Figure 12-17. Adjunctive therapy and supportive care of acute bacterial meningitis. Several studies have demonstrated that dexamethasone decreases sensorineural hearing loss and improves neurologic outcome in children older than 2 months of age [11]. The dexamethasone should be started shortly before giving the first dose of antibiotics because the drug inhibits the production of inflammatory cytokines. The role of dexamethasone in the treatment of adults has not been clarified. $PaCO_2$—arterial carbon dioxide pressure.

Mortality Rates of Treated Cases of Bacterial Meningitis

Organism	Number of episodes	Case fatality rate (%)	
		Meningitis-related	Total
Streptococcus pneumoniae	120	25	28
Gram-negative bacilli	86	23	36
Neisseria meningitidis	40	10	10
Streptococci	36	17	25
Enterococcus	4	25	50
Staphylococcus aureus	36	28	39
Listeria monocytogenes	34	21	32
Haemophilus influenzae	19	11	11
Mixed bacterial species	18	39	44
Coagulase-negative staphylococci	16	0	0
Other*	12	0	8
Culture negative	72	7	10
All causes	493	19	25
1962–1970	172	21	24
1971–1979	186	18	26
1980–1988	135	17	24

*Other organisms were as follows: anaerobes (4 episodes), propionibacteria (2),
diphtheroids (2), micrococci (2), Neisseria species (1), and Campylobacter fetus (1).*

Figure 12-18. Mortality rates of treated cases of acute bacterial meningitis. The mortality rate for treated cases of acute bacterial meningitis remains significant because of the numerous potential complications (increased intracranial pressure, hydrocephalus, focal neurologic deficits, seizures, brain abscess, subdural empyema, sepsis). Factors associated with significantly higher overall mortality rates were age of 60 years or older, obtundation on admission, and seizures occurring within 24 hours of admission. (*Adapted from* Durand and colleagues [5].)

Vaccination for Acute Bacterial Meningitis

Hib vaccine recommendations	Indicators for meningococcal and pneumococcal vaccines
Vaccinate all infants at 2, 4, and 6 months of age	Meningococcal quadrivalent vaccine
Unvaccinated infants 7–11 months of age receive two doses 2 months apart	Vaccination during epidemic outbreaks due to represented serogroup
Unvaccinated children 12–14 months of age receive one dose plus booster at 15 months	Travel to hyperepidemic areas
Unvaccinated children 15–60 months of age receive one dose	High-risk immunodeficient groups
Children older than 5 years are vaccinated if increased disease risk (asplenia, sickle cell disease, immunodeficiency, or immunosuppression)	Terminal coagulant deficiency
	Properdin deficiency
	Pneumococcal vaccine
Children with history of invasive Hib disease or vaccinated at greater than 2 years with polyribosylribitol phosphate vaccine do not need revaccination	Elderly over 65 years of age
	Those with chronic cardiorespiratory conditions
	Chronic alcoholics
	Those with asplenic states, multiple myelemia, Wiskott-Aldrich syndrome
	Human immunodeficiency virus infection
	Those with diabetes mellitis or significant hepatitic or renal disease

Figure 12-19. Vaccination for acute bacterial meningitis. Vaccines are now available for *Hemophilus influenzae* type b (Hib), *Neisseria meningitides*, and *Streptococcus pneumoniae*. The routine use of Hib vaccine has greatly decreased the incidence of meningitis due to this agent [12]. Meningococcal and pneumococcal vaccines are used for specific circumstances or "at risk" populations. Meningococcal vaccine is available for serogroups A, C, Y, and W135 (quadrivalent vaccine), but the response is poor in young children, and there is no vaccine for serogroup B, which is responsible for over 50% of infections in the United States [13]. Pneumococcal vaccine is indicated for high-risk groups older than 2 years of age. It is recommended that close household, day care center, and medical personnel contacts for meningococcal and *H. influenzae* meningitis be treated prophylactically with rifampin.

Chronic Bacterial Meningitis

Differential Diagnosis of Chronic Meningitis

Infectious causes	Noninfectious causes
Bacterial infections	Neoplasm
Tuberculosis	Sarcoidosis
Spirochetal (syphilis, Lyme disease, *Leptospira* infection)	Vasculitis
Agents that form sinus tracts (*Actinomyces, Arachnia, Nocardia*)	Primary central nervous system angiitis
Brucellosis	Systemic: giant cell arteritis, systemic lupus erythematosus, Sjögren's syndrome, rheumatoid arthritis, lymphomatoid granulomatosis, polyarteritis nodosa, Wegener's granulomatosis)
Listeria monocytogenes (rare cause)	
Fungal infections	
Common (*Candida, Coccidioides, Cryptococcus, Histoplasma*)	
Uncommon (*Aspergillus, Blastomyces, Dematiaceous paracoccidioides, Pseudoallescheria, Sporothrix, Mucormycetes*)	
Parasitic diseases	Behçet's disease
Cysticercosis	Chemical meningitis
Granulomatous amebic meningoencephalitis (acanthamoeba)	Endogenous
Eosinophilic meningitis (angiostrongylus)	Exogenous
Toxoplasmosis	Chronic benign lymphocytic meningitis
Coenurus cerebralis	Idiopathic hypertrophic pachymeningitis
Viral infections	Vogt-Koyanagi-Harada disease
Retrovirus (HIV-1, HTLV-1)	
Enterovirus (in hypogammaglobulinemia)	
Parameningeal infections (epidural abscess, subdural empyema, brain abscess)	

Figure 12-20. Differential diagnosis of chronic meningitis. Chronic meningitis accounts for about 10% of all meningitis cases. Clinical features include a subacute to chronic onset of various combinations of fever, headache, and stiff neck, often with signs of encephalitis (parenchymal involvement), mental status changes, seizures, and focal deficits. Therefore, chronic meningitis is often referred to as a meningoencephalitis. The cerebrospinal fluid (CSF) is abnormal with a pleocytosis (usually mononuclear), elevated protein levels, and a moderately decreased glucose level (see Fig. 12-14 for comparison). Some require that these manifestations persist for 4 weeks as a criterion for the diagnosis of chronic meningitis; however, the differential diagnosis is usually considered before this period on the basis of the suggestive CSF profile. The differential diagnosis is quite extensive and includes both infectious and noninfectious causes. The most common infectious causes of chronic meningitis are tuberculosis, cryptococcosis and toxoplasmosis; the common noninfectious causes are neoplasms and vasculitis. HTLV—human T-cell lymphotropic virus. (*Adapted from* Roos and colleague [2].)

Historical and Clinical Clues to Diagnosis of Chronic Meningitis

History	Examination
Exposure history	**Dermatologic lesions**
To patient with tuberculosis (TB)	Erythema chronicum migraines (ECM)—Lyme disease
Ingestion of unpasteurized milk or dairy products (brucellosis)	Depigmentation of skin (vitiligo) and hair (poliosis)—VKH
To farm animals or swimming in farm ponds (leptospirosis)	Macular hyperpigmented lesions of trunk, palms, and soles—secondary syphilis
To deer ticks (Lyme disease)	Subcutaneous nodules, abscesses, draining sinuses—fungal infections, especially blastomycosis, mucormycosis, aspergillosis
Swimming in warm fresh water ponds (acanthamebiasis)	
Sexual transmission (syphilis, retroviruses)	**Ophthalmologic disease**
Intravenous drug use (retroviruses)	Uveitis—sarcoidosis, Behçet's syndrome, VKH
Travel and geographic history	Choroidal tubercles—TB, sarcoidosis
Mexico and Latin America (cysticercosis)	**Organ disease**
Southeast Asia and Pacific (angiostrongylosis)	Primary disease—sarcoidosis, TB, histoplasmosis, aspergillosis, blastomycosis
US Northeast, North Central (Lyme disease)	
US Midwest (histoplasmosis, blastomycosis)	Enlarged liver—potential biopsy sites for TB, histoplasmosis
US Southwest (coccidiomycosis)	Muscle nodules—biopsy site for sarcoidosis, vasculitis
US Southeast (acanthamebiasis)	Adenopathy—biopsy site for TB, systemic fungi
History of extraneural or systemic disease	**Neurologic features**
Pulmonary disease (TB, histoplasmosis, sarcoidosis)	Cranial nerve involvement—sarcoidosis, Lyme disease
Polyarthritis (Lyme disease, Behçet's syndrome, systemic lupus erythematosus, rheumatoid arthritis)	**Focal lesions**
	Abscess—TB, fungal meningitis, toxoplasmosis
Uveitis (sarcoidosis, Behçet's syndrome, Vogt-Koyanagi-Harada [VKH], leptospirosis)	Strokes—TB, aspergillosis, mucormycosis, vasculitis
	Hydrocephalus—TB, fungal meningitis, especially cryptococcosis, cystinosis
Skin lesions (syphilis, Lyme disease, VKH)	
Prior diagnosed disease (diabetes, malignancy, TB, syphilis, AIDS)	Peripheral neuropathy—Lyme disease, sarcoidosis, brucellosis, vasculitis
History of immunodeficiency	Multiple levels—carcinomatous meningitis
Congenital	
Agammaglobulinemia (enteroviruses)	
Acquired	
AIDS (toxoplasmosis, cryptococcosis, syphilis, etc.)	
Organ transplant immunosuppression (toxoplasmosis, listeriosis, candidiasis, nocardiosis, aspergillosis)	
Chronic steroid use (TB, cryptococcosis, candidiasis)	
Malignancy and chemotherapy (TB, cryptococcosis, listeriosis)	

Figure 12-21. Historical and examination clues to chronic meningitis. Exploring the history may reveal clues to an etiologic diagnosis, although unfortunately such a clue is not found in most cases, which does not exclude any of the possible diagnoses. The history can be explored in four major areas: exposure history; travel and geographic history; extraneural or systemic diseases; and immunologic deficiency. The physical examination of patients with chronic meningitis is directed at finding extraneural signs that provide clues to the central nervous system disease, identifying potential sites for biopsy, and documenting the exact location and extent of neurologic involvement. For example, skin and eye involvement support specific diagnoses, and skin, adenopathy, and organomegaly indicate potential biopsy sites. (*Adapted from* Roos and colleague [2].)

Laboratory Tests in Chronic Meningitis

Blood tests: CBC, serum chemistry
    studies, ANA, ANCA, ESR,
    VDRL, ACE
Cultures of draining skin lesions, sinuses,
    nodes, blood, sputum, urine, CSF
  Multiple sites
  Multiple times (≥3)
Skin testing
  Intermediate PPD
  Anergy battery
Antibody studies
  Paired serum and CSF samples

CSF studies (x 3 if needed)
  Cells, protein, glucose, antigen assays
    (fungus only), antibody assays,
    culture, cytologic analyses (Gram
    stain, India ink preparations,
    acid-fast stains)
Imaging
  Chest radiography
  Contrast-enhanced MRI preferred
    over CT
  Angiography
Biopsy
  Extraneural
  Meningeal/cerebral

Figure 12-22. Laboratory tests in chronic meningitis. A complete blood count (CBC) may reveal bone marrow disease (tuberculosis [TB], vasculitis, neoplasms). Abnormal results of serum chemistry tests may include a low sodium level (syndrome of inappropriate antidiuretic hormone [SIADH] from TB); a high sodium level from diabetes insipidus (sarcoid); high levels of calcium and angiotensin-converting enzyme (ACE) (sarcoid); elevated liver function tests (TB, sarcoid, histoplasmosis); and positive antinuclear antibodies (ANA) and antineutrophil cytoplasmic antibodies (ANCA) (systemic vasculitis). Cerebrospinal fluid (CSF) examination is the most important test for the diagnosis of chronic meningitis. If several lumbar CSF studies have negative results, then cisternal or lateral cervical CSF studies are needed, because basilar meningitis commonly occurs with chronic meningeal processes. A ventricular tap for CSF may ultimately be necessary. Chest radiographs are needed to determine the presence of TB, sarcoid, histoplasmosis, or tumor. Brain imaging studies should be performed before a spinal tap to exclude focal brain lesions (abscess or stroke) and hydrocephalus. Enhancements help to localize abscesses as well as reveal chronic meningeal inflammation. Magnetic resonance imaging (MRI) is needed for spinal disease. Angiography may be useful for diagnosing systemic or central nervous system vasculitis. If these tests are not diagnostic, then biopsies may be required, especially if the patient continues to deteriorate. CT—computed tomography; ESR—erythrocyte sedimentation rate; PPD—purified protein derivative; VDRL—Veneral Disease Research Laboratory test.

CSF Finding in Diagnosis of Chronic Meningitis

Type of pleocytosis	Differential diagnosis
Mononuclear cells with low glucose levels	Noninfectious meningitis (usually <50 cells/mL) Neoplastic meningitis Sarcoid Tuberculous meningitis Fungal meningitis Syphilis Lyme disease Cysticercosis Toxoplasmosis
Mononuclear cells with normal glucose levels	Neoplastic meningitis Sarcoid Lyme disease Vasculitis Parameningeal infection Chronic benign lymphocytic meningitis Chemical meningitis
Neutrophilic predominance	Bacterial infection (*Actinomyces, Brucella, Nocardia,* early TB) Fungal infection (*Aspergillus, Blastomyces, Candida, Coccidioides, Histoplasma, Pseudoallescheria, Mucomycetes*) Noninfectious meningitis (chemical, vasculitis)
Eosinophilic predominance	Parasitic infection (*Angiostrongylus,* cysticercus, *Gnathostoma*) Bacterial infection (*Coccidioides*) Noninfectious meningitis (vasculitis, chemical) Neoplastic meningitis (lymphomatous, Hodgkin's disease)

Figure 12-23. Cerebrospinal fluid (CSF) finding in differential diagnosis of chronic meningitis. In the CSF, the cellular infiltrate is mononuclear for most causes of chronic meningitis. The glucose is low or normal. However, there are a few chronic infections that predominately have a neutrophilic response, which is the type of response usually seen in acute infections. Also, a few organisms elicit allergic eosinophilic responses.

Central Nervous System Tuberculosis

Clinical Staging of Tuberculous Meningitis

Stage I (early)	Nonspecific symptoms and signs
	No clouding of consciousness
	No neurologic deficits
Stage II (intermediate)	Lethargy or alteration in behavior
	Meningeal irritation
	Minor neurologic deficits (cranial nerve palsies)
Stage III (advanced)	Abnormal movements
	Convulsions
	Stupor or coma
	Severe neurologic deficits (pareses)

Figure 12-24. Clinical staging of tuberculous meningitis. Because the clinical picture of meningitis due to tuberculosis (TB) varies, especially by age at onset, a clinical staging system was introduced 50 years ago. Stage I patients have only a nonspecific prodrome without neurologic manifestations, which includes headache, malaise, and low-grade fever. This stage usually lasts up to 2 weeks. Stage II is often referred to as the meningitic phase, as symptoms and signs of meningitis occur along with cranial nerve palsies. Behavior alteration and lethargy may be seen. This stage progresses over days to weeks to stage III (advanced), in which seizures, stupor or coma, focal neurologic signs, and decorticate or decerebrate posturing occur. Without treatment, the course proceeds steadily downhill to death in 6 to 12 weeks. Disease progression tends to occur faster in adults. Rarely, other forms of tuberculous meningitis may be seen. It can present acutely, similar to acute bacterial meningitis, with a more rapid course. Infrequently, it has a more chronic course, with slowly developing hydrocephalus, similar to fungal meningitis. A stroke syndrome has also been associated with tuberculous meningitis. (*Adapted from* Zuger and colleague [14].)

Symptoms and Signs of Tuberculous Meningitis at Presentation

Manifestations	Children, %	Adults, %
Symptoms		
Headache	20–50	50–60
Nausea/vomiting	50–75	8–40
Apathy/behavioral changes	30–70	30–70
Seizures	10–20	0–13
Prior history of tuberculosis	55	8–12
Signs		
Fever	50–100	60–100
Meningismus	70–100	60–70
Cranial nerve palsy	15–30	15–40
Coma	30–45	20–30
Purified protein derivative-positive	85–90	40–65

Figure 12-25. Symptoms and signs of tuberculous meningitis at presentation. The clinical presentation in children is somewhat different than that seen in adults. Nausea and vomiting as well as behavioral changes are more common in children, whereas headache is clearly more common in adults. Children also frequently complain of abdominal pain and constipation. In both groups, seizures increase in frequency with disease progression. On examination, fever and meningismus are the most common signs in both age groups, although the frequency varies greatly. Cranial nerve palsies are present in some patients at presentation but eventually occur in about half of all cases. The sixth cranial nerve is involved most commonly, followed by the third, fourth, and seventh cranial nerves. Examination of the optic fundus may reveal tubercles in a small percentage of patients. Funduscopic examination may also reveal papilledema due to increased intracranial pressure from hydrocephalus. Hydrocephalus correlates well with the duration of disease and eventually occurs in most cases.

Additional manifestations of central nervous system tuberculosis include the following. Caseating granulomas of epithelioid cells and macrophages containing mycobacteria may occur in the brain as single or multiple focal lesions. Infrequently, caseating necrosis occurs, forming a *tuberculous (cold) abscess*. Both lesions often occur without meningitis. Most often, the initial presentation of tuberculoma and abscess is similar to that of a brain tumor, with headaches from increased intracranial pressure, seizures, focal deficits, and altered mental status. Less frequently, seizure or focal deficits may be the first manifestations. The most common form of *tuberculosis of the spine* is epidural compression of the thoracic cord from vertebral and disc destruction by caseating granulomas (tuberculous osteomyelitis). Less frequently the lumbar or cervical spine may be affected. The clinical manifestations are those of chronic epidural cord compression with back pain increased with weight bearing; percussion tenderness over the spine; a spastic paraparesis, often with a sensory level; and bowel and bladder dysfunction. Localized and severe percussion spine tenderness with painful limitation of spinal motility is referred to as a "spinal gibbus." *Tuberculous meningomyelitis* is the rare occurrence of infection of the spinal leptomeninges without spine involvement; it has also been referred to as spinal meningitis, spinal arachnoiditis, and spinal radiculomyelitis. Thick exudates and tubercles encase the nerve roots and spinal cord. This process presents as subacute to chronic radiculomyelitis or as cauda equina syndrome. It appears mainly in highly endemic areas but has been reported in AIDS patients in the United States. Intramedullary tuberculomas are rare and have clinical presentations similar to other spinal cord tumors. (*Adapted from* Zuger and colleague [14].)

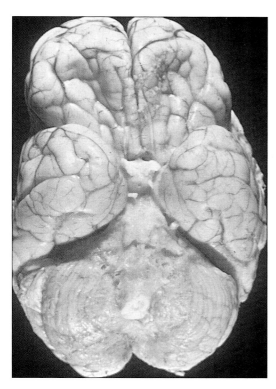

Figure 12-26. Tuberculous basilar meningitis. The tubercle bacillus enters the human host through inhalation. Airborne droplets reach the alveoli and multiply there or in alveolar and circulating macrophages. During this 2 to 4 week stage of infection, hematogenous dissemination occurs, and delayed secondary hematogenous dissemination may also occur. During dissemination, tubercles form in multiple organs, including the brain. Eventually tubercles rupture into the subarachnoid space or ventricular system to cause meningitis. The initial pathologic event after tubercle rupture is the formation of a thick exudate in the subarachnoid space. This exudate initially begins at the base of the brain, where it is especially thick, and envelops cranial nerves, causing cranial nerve palsies. (*From* Wilson [4]; with permission.)

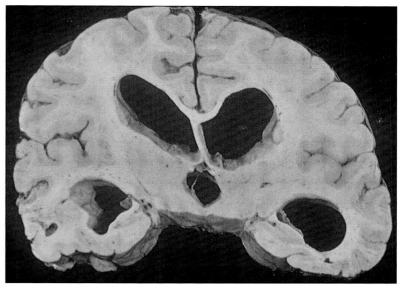

Figure 12-27. Tuberculous hydrocephalus. With the thick basilar exudate of tuberculous meningitis, often the foramina of Luschka and Magendie become obstructed. Obstruction may also occur at the level of the aqueduct, causing noncommunicating hydrocephalus, increased intracranial pressure, and papilledema. Communicating hydrocephalus caused by blockage of the basilar cisterns, interfering with the resorption of cerebrospinal fluid, may also occur. Either type of hydrocephalus may result in brain atrophy. (*From* Wilson [4]; with permission.)

Prevalence of CNS Tuberculosis in AIDS Patients

Location	Year	Cases of active TB/cases of AIDS	Cases of TB with CNS disease
Florida	1984	27/45 (60%)	2 of 27 (7%)
New Jersey	1986	52/420 (12%)	10 of 52 (19%)
New York City	1986	24/280 (9%)	1 of 24 (4%)
San Francisco	1987	35/1705 (2%)	2 of 35 (6%)
Barcelona, Spain	1988	Not available	5 of 65 (8%)

Figure 12-28. Prevalence of tuberculosis (TB) of the central nervous system (CNS) in AIDS patients. In the first half of the twentieth century, autopsy studies revealed that 5% to 10% of patients with TB had CNS involvement. TB in AIDS patients is thought to occur because of reactivation; most cases are pulmonary, but the incidence of extrapulmonary disease is much greater than that of the general population. Rates of tuberculin purified protein derivative (PPD) reactivity are lower than those in the general population, ranging from 33% to 50% as compared to 50% to 90%. The incidence of CNS involvement is similar to that of the general population. (*Adapted from* Zuger and colleague [14].)

Chemotherapeutic Options for Tuberculous Meningitis in Adults*

Drug	Dose	Frequency	Duration
Low probability of drug resistance			
Alternative regimen I			
Isoniazid	300 mg	Daily	6 mo†
Rifampin	600 mg	Daily	6 mo†
Pyrazinamide	15–30 mg/kg	Daily	2 mo
Alternative regimen II			
Isoniazid	300 mg	Daily	9 mo
Rifampin	600 mg	Daily	9 mo
Pyrazinamide	15–30 mg/kg	Daily	2 mo
Ethambutol	25 mg/kg	Daily	2 mo
High probability of drug resistance			
Isoniazid	300 mg	Daily	12–18 mo
Rifampin	600 mg	Daily	12–18 mo
Pyrazinamide	15–30 mg/kg	Daily	9–18 mo
+			
Streptomycin	1 g	Daily	2 mo
or			
Ethambutol	25 mg/kg	Daily	2 mo
± Ethionamide	15 mg/kg	Daily	2–18 mo

In cases of documented drug resistance, chemotherapy must be tailored to demonstrated sensitivities.

†Duration should be 10 months for children.

Figure 12-29. Chemotherapeutic options for tuberculous meningitis in adults. The usefulness of these regimens has been extrapolated from the treatment of other forms of tuberculosis (TB). Because of the rarity of tuberculous meningitis in developed countries, questions related to the optimal regimen, doses, routes of administration, and length of treatment have not been clarified. The number of drugs used depends on the probability of drug resistance. Most drug-resistant cases in the United States occur in AIDS patients and prisoners. Antituberculous chemotherapy must be initiated as soon as tuberculous meningitis is suspected based upon the cerebrospinal fluid (CSF) formula. Delays in treatment due to waiting for positive results from smears or cultures usually result in increased mortality and morbidity. (*Adapted from* Zuger and colleague [14].)

Results of Treatment of Tuberculous Meningitis with Corticosteroids

Stage of disease	Steroids		No steroids	
	Patients, *n*	TB deaths, %	Patients, *n*	TB deaths, %
I	33	0	22	0
II	206	5	61	12
III	100	30	23	61
Totals	339	12	106	20

Figure 12-30. Treatment of tuberculous meningitis with corticosteroids. The role of corticosteroids in the treatment of tuberculous meningitis is controversial but the weight of evidence favors their use in stage II (intermediate) and stage III (advanced or late) disease. Suggested regimens have included prednisone (adults: 60 to 80 mg for 1 to 2 weeks, then taper off over 4 to 6 weeks) and dexamethasone (adults: 16 mg/d for 3 weeks then taper off over 3 weeks; children: 0.3 mg/kg/d for 3 weeks and taper off over 3 weeks). Other adjunctive therapy includes ventricular drainage for hydrocephalus. Tuberculomas presenting with swelling and edema should also be treated with steroids, in which case surgical removal is required infrequently. TB—tuberculosis. (*Adapted from* Shaw and colleagues [15].)

Mortality Rates for Tuberculous Meningitis

	Percentage
Age	
<5 y	20
5–50 y	8
>50 y	60
Duration of symptoms	
0–2 mo	9
>2 mo	80
Stage	
Stage I	0
Stage II	10
Stage III	45

Figure 12-31. Mortality and morbidity rates of tuberculous meningitis. Mortality and morbidity rates depend upon several factors, including the patient's age, the duration of symptoms, and the stage of the disease. (*Adapted from* Kennedy and colleague [16].)

Intracranial Epidural Abscess

Clinical Manifestations and Pathogenesis of Intracranial Epidural Abscess

Clinical manifestations	Sources of infection
Early	Extension of contiguous infections
Fever	Paranasal sinusitis
Symptoms related to the source of infection	Orbital cellulitis
Sinusitis, otitis, etc.	Otitis
Headache	Mastoiditis
Localized skull tenderness from osteomyelitis	Cranial defects
Scalp and face cellulitis from osteomyelitis	Skull fracture
Cranial nerve palsies—rare	Neurosurgical procedures
Late	
Seizures	
Focal neurologic deficits	
Meningismis	
Nausea and vomiting from increased ICP	
Papilledema from increased ICP	
Altered mental status from increased ICP	
Cranial nerve palsies—rare	

Figure 12-32. Clinical manifestations and pathogenesis of intracranial epidural abscess. An intracranial epidural abscess is a localized area of infection between the skull and dura caused by the spread of infection from contiguous locations, such as the paranasal sinuses, the ear, and the orbit or because of skull defects. Because the abscess grows by pushing the dura away from the skull, the process is slow and the lesion well-circumscribed. Osteomyelitis of the skull may accompany the process, causing swelling and edema of the scalp and face, and skull tenderness. Because the abscess grows slowly, seizures, focal neurologic deficits, and an altered level of consciousness with increased intracranial pressure (ICP) occur late in the course. Cranial nerve palsies are uncommon, but may occur from increased ICP or when the abscess involves sites in which cranial nerves penetrate the dura. Infection of the apex of the petrous temporal bone may involve cranial nerves V and VI, causing facial pain, sensory loss, and lateral rectus palsy ("Gradenigo's syndrome"). Complications from the spread of infection include dural sinus or cortical vein thrombosis with infarction, subdural empyema, meningitis, and brain abscess.

Organisms Commonly Causing Intracranial Epidural Abscess (by Location of Primary Infection)

Paranasal sinuses
  Hemolytic streptococci
  Microaerophilic streptococci
  Gram-negative aerobes
  Bacteroides or other anaerobes
  Rhinocerebral mucormycosis (in diabetic or immunosuppressed patients)
Otitis media
  Streptococcus pneumoniae
  Haemophilus influenzae
  Hemolytic streptococci
  Gram-negative aerobes
  Bacteroides or other anaerobes
Cranial trauma or surgery
  Staphylococci
  Streptococcal pneumonia

Figure 12-33. Etiology of intracranial epidural abscess. The responsible organisms are those commonly associated with the primary infectious process. Cranial epidural abscess is rare in young children, occurring mainly in adolescents and adults. The exact incidence of intracranial abscess is not known, but it is less common than subdural empyema and brain abscess.

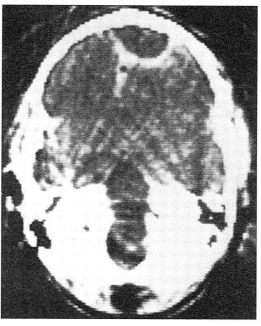

Figure 12-34. Computed tomography (CT) scan of an epidural abscess revealing a lesion that is well-localized, extracerebral, hypodense, and lenticularly shaped, with a nonenhancing hyperdense medial capsule. Diagnosis of intracranial epidural abscess is made by CT or magnetic resonance imaging (MRI). Even if the initial CT is not diagnostic, contrast-enhanced MRI scanning should clarify the diagnosis. The cerebrospinal fluid (CSF) usually reveals a picture of a chronic parameningeal focus with mononuclear pleocytosis, normal glucose levels, and sterile cultures. Differential diagnoses include epidural tumor, epidural hematoma, subdural hemorrhage, subdural empyema, dural sinus or cortical vein thrombosis, and less frequently, brain abscess or brain tumor. (*From* Weisberg and colleagues [17]; with permission.)

Treatment of Intracranial Epidural Abscess

Empiric antibiotic therapy
  Paranasal sinus or otitis source of infection
    Ceftriaxone plus metronidazole
  Cranial trauma or surgery
    Vancomycin plus ceftazidime
Surgical drainage and decompression
  Gram stain and culture for bacteria and fungi
  Craniectomy for osteomyelitis
  Dural débridement; excision and grafting not usually
    required
  Closure of any communication between sinus cavity and
    epidural space to prevent reaccumulation
Institute specific antibiotic therapy based on culture results

Figure 12-35. Treatment of intracranial epidural abscess. Therapy for intracranial epidural abscess consists of antibiotic therapy combined with neurosurgical drainage and decompression. The prognosis for these epidural infections is excellent, with no mortality in recent series, probably because the process is usually subacute to chronic and computed tomography and magnetic resonance imaging are excellent diagnostic tools.

Spinal Epidural Abscess

Clinical Stages of Progression of Spinal Epidural Abscess

Stage I	Severe localized back pain	
	Exquisite spinal percussion tenderness	
	Paraspinal muscle spasm	
Stage II	Nerve root irritation with radiating pain and paresthesia (radiculopathy)	
	Focal weakness or reflex changes	
Stage III	Spinal cord compression, with	
	Progressive weakness	
	Sensory loss	
	Bowel and bladder dysfunction	
Stage IV	Complete paralysis	
	Sensation is impaired below sensory level at or near the cord segment of the lesion	

Figure 12-36. Clinical manifestations of spinal epidural abscess by stages of progression. The epidural space in the spinal cord is a true space, unlike the potential epidural intracranial space. In the spinal cord, the dura and arachnoid are closely approximated, so that the subdural space is only a potential space, and spinal subdural empyema or abscess is rare; spinal epidural abscess is much more common. Spinal epidural abscess is an emergency because spinal cord compression and paraplegia are possible complications. It can be acute (symptoms are present less than 2 weeks) or chronic (symptoms are present for more than 2 weeks); the acute form is more common. Four stages of progression of spinal epidural abscess have been recognized. The acute form presents as an acute cord compression. Progression from stages I to II and from stages II to III usually takes 1 to 4 days each. Once stage III is reached, complete paralysis may occur in hours. In the acute form fever, malaise, and a "flu-like" prodrome may occur. The chronic form presents as an expanding tumor, usually without fever or other prodromal symptoms.

A. Pathogenesis and Pathophysiology of Spinal Epidural Abscess: Location of Spinal Epidural Abscess

Location	Patients, *n* (%)
Cervical	20 (14)
Thoracic	71 (51)
Lumbar	48 (35)
	Total: 139 (100)
Anterior	28 (21)
Posterior	105 (79)
	Total: 133 (100)

Figure 12-37. Pathogenesis and pathophysiology of spinal epidural abscess. **A,** Locations of spinal epidural abscess. Spinal epidural abscesses tend to occur most frequently in the thoracic and lumbar levels, posterior to the cord where the epidural space is largest and contains more epidural fat. **B,** Source of infection of spinal epidural abscess. Hematogenous or metastatic seeding is the most common source of infection, occurring from cutaneous, respiratory, abdominal, pelvic, urinary, cardiac, and dental sites of infection as well as from intravenous drug use. Hematogenous seeding is most likely to occur in the thoracic area owing to the end-anastomotic blood supply in this area. Contiguous sources of infection include vertebral body osteomyelitis and retroperitoneal and perinephric infections. Trauma and surgery (back surgery, epidural catheterization for anesthesia and pain control, dorsal column stimulators, lumbar puncture) play a lesser role.

(Continued on next page)

B. Pathogenesis and Pathophysiology of Spinal Epidural Abscess: Source of Infection of Spinal Epidural Abscess

Source	Percentage of patients*
Hematogenous seeding	43
Skin and soft tissues	20
Abdomen and pelvis	7
Respiratory system	6
Intravenous drug use	5
Urinary tract	2
Cardiac system	2
Dental infection	1
Contiguous location	27
Vertebral osteomyelitis	8
Retroperitoneal or retromediastinal infection	7
Perinephric or psoas abscess	8
Decubitis ulcers	4
Surgery and trauma	5
No source identified	25
Total	100%

Estimates compiled from various series.

Figure 12-37. (*Continued*) Medical conditions associated with spinal epidural abscess include diabetes, malignancy, cirrhosis, renal failure, and alcoholism. The most common etiologic agent is *Staphylococcus aureus*, although gram-negative aerobic bacilli (especially *Escherichia coli* and *Pseudomonas* species) have accounted for an increasing percentage of cases. In addition, tuberculosis has accounted for up to 25% of cases in recent series. (*Adapted from* Danner and colleague [18].)

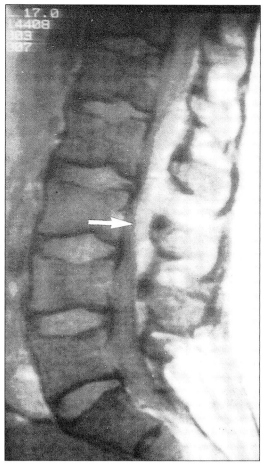

Figure 12-38. Contrast-enhanced T1-weighted magnetic resonance image (MRI) done as part of a diagnostic work-up for spinal epidural abscess. This scan reveals an epidural mass (*arrow*) extending from the lower part of the L1 vertebral body to the upper part of the L4 vertebral body. Patients with acute spinal epidural abscess have a high peripheral leukocytic count from 12,000 to 15,000 cells per mm^3. If the process is chronic, the peripheral leukocyte count may be normal. Cerebrospinal fluid (CSF) examination is consistent with parameningeal infection, with an elevated cell count, elevated protein level, normal glucose level, and negative cultures. When the process is acute, usually polymorphonuclear leukocytes predominate, with up to 100 to 200 cells per mm^3; in chronic cases, mononuclear cells predominate, usually with fewer than 50 cells per mm^3. CSF cultures are negative unless the organism has spread to the CSF and subsequently caused meningitis. Blood cultures are positive 60% to 70% of the time. The definitive diagnostic studies, however, are computed tomography myelograms and MRI scans, with MRI the study of choice. MRI scans directly visualize the extent of the abscess and should include T1-weighted images before and after contrast enhancement and a T2-weighted image. (*From* Gelfand and colleagues [19]; with permission.)

Intracranial Subdural Empyema

Clinical Manifestations of Subdural Empyema

Signs/symptoms	Patients, *n**	Percentage
Fever	420	77
Headache	467	74
Hemiparesis	389	71
Altered consciousness	544	69
Nuchal rigidity	385	63
Seizures	576	48
Papilledema	238	33
Altered speech	364	22
Other focal deficits	265	45

Total number of patients assessed for the specific manifestation.

Figure 12-39. Clinical manifestations of intracranial subdural empyema. Subdural empyema is a fulminant, purulent infection that spreads over the cerebral hemispheres in the existing subdural space. It is usually confined to one side of the brain by the anatomic barriers of the falx and tentorium. Undiagnosed and untreated, subdural empyema is rapidly fatal and therefore is a neurologic emergency. Usually patients have a nonspecific prodrome for several days to a week and then become acutely ill. After head trauma or surgery, the presentation may be milder and more subacute. The presenting manifestations usually include fever, headache, hemiparesis, nuchal rigidity, and seizures. As the process continues, increased intracranial pressure causes papilledema and alteration of consciousness. At the end of the first week and into the second, cortical vein thrombosis begins to occur, causing infarcts and additional focal deficits. (*Adapted from* Helfgott and colleagues [20].)

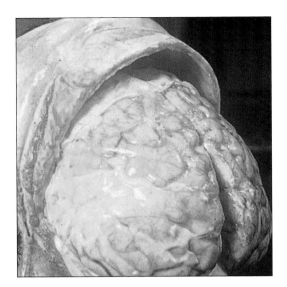

Figure 12-40. Pathologic specimen showing acute subdural empyema with large amounts of exudate overlying parts of the left cerebral hemisphere. The exudate is usually grey or yellowish. The histologic findings in subdural empyema are typical of acute inflammatory processes: the exudate is composed primarily of polymorphonuclear leukocytes, although a few lymphocytes and plasma cells may be present. (*From* Wilson [4]; with permission.)

Etiology of Adult Subdural Empyema

Organism	Incidence* (%)
Streptococci	
Aerobic†	32
Anaerobic	16
Staphylococci	
Coagulase-positive	11
Coagulase-negative	5
Aerobic gram-negative bacilli‡	8
Other anaerobes	5
Sterile	34

*200 evaluated cases, total greater than 100% because of multiple isolates from single cases.

†Includes α-hemolytic, β-hemolytic, and nonhemolytic.

‡Mostly enteric bacilli.

Figure 12-41. Predisposing causes, pathogenesis, and etiology of subdural empyema. The vast majority of cases of subdural empyema occur in males (about 75%). It has been suggested that this is related to the growth of the frontal sinuses in boys during puberty. The most common predisposing cause of subdural empyema is sinusitis (54%). After infection has started in the sinuses, the middle ear, or other areas of the head, it spreads to the subdural space by means of venous drainage. Emissary veins connect the large veins of the scalp and face with the dural venous sinuses, and because the veins of the head and brain are valveless, retrograde spread of thrombophlebitis into the dural and cortical veins from infected venous sinuses may occur. The frontal sinus is probably the single most predisposing site of infection; the incidence of subdural empyema following frontal sinusitis is 1% to 2%. Another predisposing cause of subdural empyema is infection and trauma of the head (about 13%). This is followed by otogenic infections (otitis, mastoiditis—about 13%), which may also spread to the subdural space by erosion of bone. Otogenic infections usually cause a posterior fossa (infratentorial) subdural empyema; about 10% of all cases are infratentorial. A minor predisposing cause of subdural empyema is hematogenous spread (about 3%). Most cases of subdural empyema occur during the second decade of life (about 40%), followed by the third (about 15%), first (about 11%), fourth (about 10%), and fifth (about 9%) decades. Streptococci and staphylococci are the most common causative organisms. Sinus and ear infections usually result in streptococcal subdural empyema, while head trauma or surgery usually results in a staphylococcal subdural empyema. Meningitis is an important predisposing condition in infants but not in adults. (*Adapted from* Helfgott and colleagues [20].)

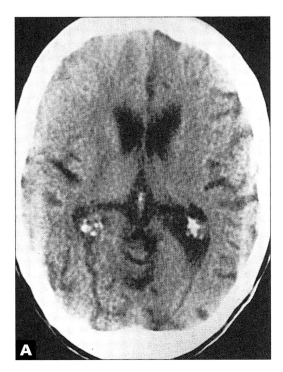

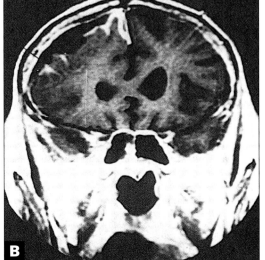

Figure 12-42. Computed tomography (CT) scan with contrast and a magnetic resonance imaging (MRI) scan of subdural empyema done as part of a diagnostic work-up. **A**, CT scan reveals effaced sulci over the right hemisphere, with only minimal mass effect. **B**, However, MRI scanning with contrast reveals the large subdural empyema with mass effect.

Computed tomography with contrast and MRI scans are the diagnostic studies of choice for subdural empyema. Routine blood tests may reveal an elevated leukocyte count, especially in acute subdural empyema. Lumbar puncture is usually contraindicated because of focal deficits, increased intracranial pressure, and abnormalities on CT or MRI scans. When lumbar puncture is performed, the picture is one of parameningeal inflammatory response with an increased cell count; about 15% of cases have more than 1000 cells per mm³. The response is acute with greater than 50% polymorphonuclear leukocytes in about 70% of cases. The glucose level is usually normal and cultures are usually negative (in greater than 90% of cases). The differential diagnosis includes epidural abscess, brain abscess, intracerebral thrombophlebitis, subdural hematoma, meningoencephalitis, pyogenic meningitis (especially after infarction has occurred), herpes simplex encephalitis, cysticercosis, and cerebral neoplasm. (*From* Greenlee [21]; with permission.)

Brain Abscess

Clinical Manifestations of Brain Abscess

Manifestation	Percent (approximations)
Headache	75
Fever	50
Nausea/vomiting	50
Focal neurologic deficits	50
Altered mental status	50
Seizures	30
Signs of systemic infection	30
Nuchal rigidity	25
Papilledema	25

Figure 12-43. Clinical manifestations of brain abscess. The clinical manifestations of brain abscess depend upon the location of the lesion, whether the lesion is single (75% of cases) or multiple, and the duration of the process (fulminant or indolent, hours to several months—average 10 to 13 days). In most cases, the manifestations are those of an expanding intracerebral mass with few signs of infection. The headache may be focal, from a mass lesion, or diffuse, suggesting increased intracranial pressure. Focal neurologic deficits and seizures are usually caused by the mass itself, while nausea or vomiting, papilledema, and altered mental status are due to increased intracranial pressure. Focal deficits include hemiparesis, hemianopsia, hemisensory loss, and aphasia. About 25% of abscesses involve the posterior fossa, primarily the cerebellum.

Brain Abscess: Predisposing Conditions, Site of Abscess, and Microbiology

Predisposing conditions	Site of abscess	Usual isolate(s) from abscess
Contiguous site of primary infection		
Otitis media and mastoiditis	Temporal lobe or cerebellar hemisphere	Streptococci (anaerobic or aerobic), *Bacteroides fragilis*, Enterobacteriaceae
Frontoethmoidal sinusitis	Frontal lobe	Predominantly streptococci, *Bacteroides*, Enterobacteriaceae, *Staphylococcus aureus*, and *Haemophilus* species
Sphenoidal sinusitis	Frontal or temporal lobe	Same as in frontoethmoidal sinusitis
Dental sepsis	Frontal lobe	Mixed *Fusobacterium*, *Bacteroides*, and *Streptococcus* species
Penetrating cranial trauma or postsurgical infection	Related to wound	*S. aureus*, streptococci, Enterobacteriaceae, *Clostridium* species
Distant site of primary infection		
Congenital heart disease	Multiple abscess cavities; middle cerebral artery distribution common but may occur at any site	Viridans, anaerobic, and microaerophilic streptococci; *Haemophilus* species
Lung abscess, empyema, bronchiectases	Same as in congenital heart disease	*Fusobacterium*, *Actinomyces*, *Bacteroides*, streptococci, *Nocardia asteroides*
Bacterial endocarditis	Same as in congenital heart disease	*S. aureus*, streptococci
Compromised host (immunosuppressive therapy or malignancy)	Same as in congenital heart disease	*Toxoplasma*, fungi, Enterobacteriaceae, *Nocardia*

Figure 12-44. Predisposing conditions, site of abscess, and microbiology in brain abscess. Brain abscesses are usually associated with a contiguous site of infection, head trauma or surgery, and hematogenous spread from distant sites of infection. A contiguous site of infection usually accounts for about 40% to 50% of the cases; hematogenous spread, for about 25% to 35%; head trauma or surgery, for about 10%; and there is no obvious predisposing factor in about 15%. Unlike other age groups, brain abscess complicates meningitis in neonates. The predisposing condition plays a definite role regarding the site of the abscess in the brain and which organisms cause the abscess. (*Adapted from* Wispelwey and colleagues [22].)

A. Brain Abscess in the Immunologically Uncompromised Host

Etiologic organisms	Isolation frequency (%)
Staphylococcus aureus	10–15
Enterobacteriaceae	23–33
Streptococcus pneumoniae	<1
Haemophilus influenzae	<1
Streptococci (S. *intermedius* group, including S. *anginosus*	60–70
Bacteroides and *Prevotella* species	20–40
Fungi	10–15
Protozoa, helminths*	<1

Heavily dependent on geographic locale.

Figure 12-45. Microbiologic etiology of brain abscess. **A,** In the immunologically uncompromised host. In the preantibiotic era, *Staphylococcus aureus*, streptococci, and coliform bacteria were the common isolates from brain

B. Brain Abscess in the Immunologically Compromised Host

Abnormal cell-mediated immunity	Neutropenia or neutrophil defects
Toxoplasma gondii	Aerobic gram-negative bacteria
Nocardia asteroides	*Aspergillus* species
Cryptococcus neoformans	Zygomycetes
Listeria monocytogenes	*Candida* species
Mycobacterium species	

abscess. In the last 20 years, however, anaerobes (streptococci intermedius group, *Bacteroides* species) are probably the most common cause. **B,** In the immunologically compromised host. Patients with AIDS, underlying malignancy, or those treated with immunosuppressive agents are at an increased risk for developing brain abscess. Fungi and parasites are also important diagnostic considerations in these patients. Neutropenia and neutrophilic defects are most often due to chemotherapy. (Panel A *adapted from* Wispelwey and colleague [23]; Panel B *adapted from* Wispelwey and colleagues [22].)

A. Differential Diagnosis of Brain Abscess in the Immunologically Uncompromised Host

Subdural empyema
Pyogenic meningitis
Viral encephalitis (esp. herpes simplex)
Cysticercosis
Cerebral infarction
Mycotic aneurysms
Epidural abscess
Cerebral neoplasms

Hemorrhagic leukoencephalitis
Echinococcosis
Cryptococcosis
Central nervous system vasculitis
Chronic subdural hematoma
Intracerebral thrombophlebitis

Figure 12-46. Differential diagnosis of brain abscess. **A,** The differential diagnosis in the immunologically uncompromised host includes entities causing focal neurologic deficits, which are usually seen early in the course, and diffuse entities, which are seen later in the course of brain abscess.

B. Differential Diagnosis of Brain Abscesses in Patient With AIDS

Toxoplasmosis
Primary central nervous system lymphoma
Mycobacterium tuberculosis
Mycobacterium avium-intracellulare
Progressive multifocal leukoencephalopathy

Cryptococcus neoformans
Candida species
Listeria monocytogenes
Nocardia asteroides
Salmonella group B
Aspergillus species

B, In AIDS patients, focal neurologic infections and processes of diverse and unusual etiologies have been recognized. The most common cause of focal neurologic lesions is toxoplasmosis, followed by lymphoma. (Panel A *adapted from* Wispelwey [24]; Panel B *adapted from* Wispelwey and colleagues [22].)

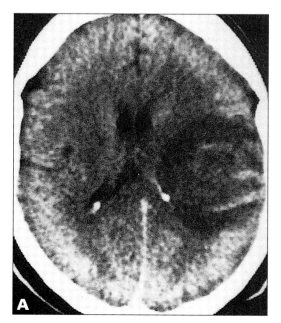

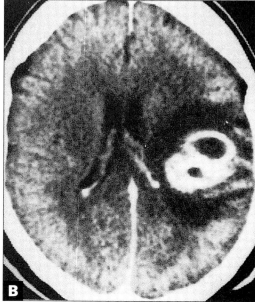

Figure 12-47. Computed tomography (CT) imaging studies for brain abscess. Routine laboratory studies are usually not helpful; they may show peripheral leukocytosis and increased erythrocyte sedimentation rate, but these findings are nonspecific. In addition to complete blood count, chest radiograph, electrocardiogram, and echocardiogram as needed, blood cultures should also be obtained. Lumbar puncture may reveal a parameningeal response, but the procedure is usually contraindicated until an imaging study of the brain has been performed. CT plain imaging and with contrast should be performed. Magnetic resonance imaging (MRI) is even more sensitive, and reveals abscess or cerebritis at earlier stages of development than CT. **A,** Plain axial CT reveals mass effect in the left hemisphere with effacement of the sylvian fissure and the ipsilateral ventricle. **B,** With contrast, CT reveals a multiloculated ring enhanced lesion. The surrounding area of decreased attenuation represents cerebral edema. (Panel A *from* Wispelwey and colleagues [22]; with permission; Panel B *from* Falcone and colleagues [25]; with permission.)

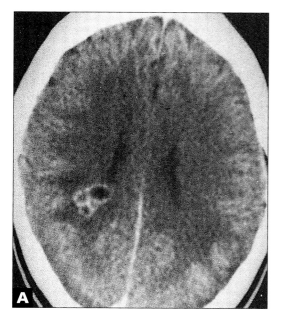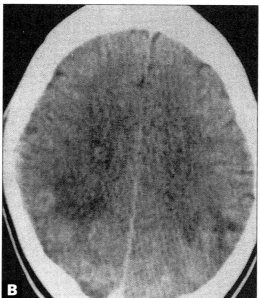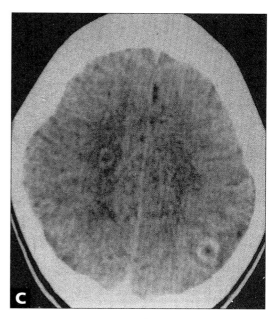

Figure 12-48. Computed tomography (CT) images of multiple brain abscesses. Hematogenous spread of septic emboli may cause multiple cerebral abscesses. In this case, the abscesses are due to *Staphylococcus aureus* septicemia. Periventricular (**A**) centrum semiovale (**B**) and gray-white matter junction (**C**) abscesses are seen. (*From* Wispelwey and colleagues [23]; with permission.)

Viral Infections

Viral Infections of the Nervous System

RNA viruses	Representative viruses responsible for neurologic disease
Enterovirus (Picornavirus)	Poliovirus
	Coxsackievirus
	Echovirus
	Enterovirus 70 and 71
	Hepatitis A
Togavirus: alphavirus (arbovirus)	Equine encephalitis (Eastern, Western, Venezuela)
Flavivirus (arbovirus)	St. Louis encephalitis
	West Nile encephalitis
	Japanese encephalitis
Bunyavirus (arbovirus)	Tick-borne encephalitis
Reovirus: coltivirus (arbovirus)	California encephalitis
Togavirus: rubivirus	Colorado tick fever
Orthomyxovirus	Rubella
Paramyxovirus	Influenza
	Measles and subacute sclerosing panencephalitis
Arenavirus	Mumps
Rhabdovirus	Lymphocytic choriomeningitis
Retrovirus	Rabies
	HIV, AIDS
DNA viruses	Human T-cell lymphotropic virus (HTLV)
Herpesviruses	
	Herpes simplex (HSV)
	Varicella-zoster (VZV)
	Cytomegalovirus (CMV)
Papovavirus	Epstein-Barr (EBV) (infectious mononucleosis)
Poxvirus	Progressive multifocal leukoencephalopathy (PML)
Adenovirus	Vaccinia
	Adenovirus serotypes

Figure 12-49. Viral infections of the nervous system. The numerous viruses causing nervous system infections can be classified according to virus characteristics and the type of disease produced. Viruses are classified according to their nucleic acid type, sensitivity to lipid solvents (enveloped vs nonenveloped), and by their size. The infections produced may be either acute or chronic. In temperate zones of the northern hemisphere some of the viruses causing meningitis and encephalitis have a distinct seasonal activity. This is especially true for the enteroviruses and the mosquito-borne and tick-borne arboviruses that have peak epidemic activity in the spring and summer. Mumps is more often seen in late winter or spring and lymphocytic choriomeningitis in the fall and winter. Herpes viruses are endemic and cause disease in any season. (*Adapted from* Jubelt and colleague [26].)

Acute Viral Infections

Relative Frequency of Meningitis and Encephalitis of Known Viral Etiology

Viral agent	Viral meningitis, 1976*, patients, n (%)	Viral encephalitis, 1976[†], [‡], patients, n (%)	Viral encephalitis, 1981[‡], [§], patients, n (%)
Enteroviruses	324 (83)	13 (2)	82 (23)
Mumps	28 (7)	71 (10)	7 (2)
Arboviruses	6 (2)	424 (60)	107 (30)
Herpes simplex	15 (4)	69 (10)	97 (27)
Measles	3 (1)	44 (6)	1 (0.3)
Varicella	5 (1)	58 (8)	30 (8)

Data from Centers for Disease Control and Prevention: Aseptic Meningitis Surveillance, Annual Summary 1976. Issued January 1979. There were 2534 cases of indeterminate etiology.

[†]*Data from Centers for Disease Control and Prevention: MMWR - Annual Summary 1977, 26(53):13, 1978. There were 1121 cases of indeterminate etiology.*

[‡]*Includes both primary and postinfectious encephalitis. Almost all cases caused by measles and varicella are postinfectious.*

[§]*There were 1121 cases of indeterminate etiology.*

Figure 12-50. Acute viral syndromes of the central nervous system (CNS). Acute viral infections of the CNS may cause three syndromes: viral (aseptic) meningitis, encephalitis, and myelitis. Acute viral meningitis is a self-limited illness, accompanied by fever, headache, photophobia, and nuchal rigidity.

Encephalitis implies involvement of the brain parenchyma, causing alteration of consciousness, seizures, and focal neurologic deficits. When both meningeal and encephalitic signs are present on examination, the term *meningoencephalitis* is sometimes used in the diagnosis. Viral myelitis is an infection of the spinal cord. The myelitis is most often considered a demyelinating white matter syndrome (transverse myelitis), but spinal motor neurons (poliomyelitis, paralytic disease), sensory neurons, and autonomic neurons (bladder paralysis) may be affected. If encephalitis and myelitis occur together, the term *encephalomyelitis* is used. The cerebrospinal fluid (CSF) formula in all these viral syndromes is similar, usually showing mononuclear pleocytosis of 50 to 500 cells per mm^3, normal glucose level, and elevated protein level and pressure. A clinical continuum exists between viral meningitis and encephalitis, as the same spectrum of viruses cause both syndromes, although some viruses more often cause meningitis and others, encephalitis. The role of mumps virus in the etiology of these syndromes has decreased greatly since the 1970s because of vaccination programs. (*Adapted from* Centers for Disease Control and Prevention [27].)

Virologic and Serologic Studies for Acute CNS Viral Syndromes

Agent	Specimens for virus detection	Serologic studies
Enteroviruses		
Polio	Throat washing, stool, and CSF (culture and PCR)	Acute/convalescent sera
Coxsackie		
Echovirus		
Lymphocytic chorio-meningitis virus	Blood, CSF	Acute/convalescent sera
Mumps	Saliva, throat washing, CSF, urine	Acute/convalescent sera
Measles	Throat washing, urine, conjunctival secretions	Acute/convalescent sera IgM ELISA of serum
Arboviruses	Blood, CSF	IgM antibody ELISA of CSF or serum Acute/convalescent sera
Herpesviruses		
Herpes simplex (HSV)		
Type 1	Brain biopsy, PCR of CSF	CSF antibody detection after day 10 Acute/convalescent sera (±)
Type 2	CSF, genital and vesicle fluid, blood	Acute/convalescent sera
Varicella-zoster	Vesicle fluid, CSF	Acute/convalescent sera
Cytomegalovirus	Urine, saliva, blood (circulating leukocytes), CSF PCR amplification	Acute/convalescent sera
Epstein-Barr virus	Rarely cultured	Acute sera for antibody profile
Rabies	Saliva, CSF, neck skin biopsy, brain biopsy	Serum after day 15
Adenovirus	Nasal or conjunctival swab, urine, stool	Acute/convalescent sera
Influenza	Throat washing	Acute/convalescent sera

Figure 12-51. Specific virologic and serologic studies for the diagnosis of acute central nervous system (CNS) viral syndromes. Viruses may be isolated from extraneural sites. For most infections, except reactivated infections such as with herpes simplex virus type 1 (HSV-1) or herpes zoster, extraneural isolation is usually diagnostic. Obviously if virus can be isolated from the cerebrospinal fluid (CSF), that is preferred. Detection of virus-specific nucleic acid by polymerase chain reaction (PCR) is readily available for enteroviruses and some herpesviruses [28]. Serologic studies require a fourfold increase between the acute and convalescent specimen to be considered positive. Acute phase sera should be obtained immediately or as soon as infection is suspected. If the acute phase sera is not obtained until the end of the first week of the disease, the chances of seeing a fourfold rise drops to 50%. Most viral infections of the CNS result in the *intrathecal* synthesis of specific antibody. When analyzing CSF antibody synthesis one looks for an increased CSF to serum antibody ratio. Therefore, paired CSF and serum samples are required. A correction should also be used for blood brain barrier breakdown, which results in serum to CSF antibody leakage. This can be done by using CSF to serum albumin or other viral antibody ratios. Unfortunately, most antibody studies are not positive until at least 1 week after the onset of infection. ELISA—enzyme-linked immunosorbent assay. (*Adapted from* Jubelt [29].)

Viral Meningitis

Clinical Manifestations of Acute Viral Meningitis

Systemic manifestations	Central nervous system manifestations
Fever	Headache, usually frontal or retro-orbital
Malaise	Nuchal rigidity
Anorexia	Photophobia
Myalgia	Lethargy
Nausea and vomiting	
Agent-specific pharyngitis, URI, abdominal pain, diarrhea	

Figure 12-52. Clinical manifestations of acute viral meningitis. Acute viral meningitis is sometimes referred to as "aseptic" meningitis, but the terms are not synonymous, because agents other than viruses also cause aseptic meningitis, for example, parameningeal infection, autoimmune disease, vasculitis, and chemicals. Acute viral meningitis usually begins abruptly with a combination of central nervous system signs of nuchal rigidity, headache, and occasionally lethargy along with systemic manifestations. If the alteration in the level of consciousness is more pronounced than lethargy, another diagnosis should be considered. The cerebrospinal fluid (CSF) profile is that of all viral syndromes, with lymphocytic pleocytosis, mildly elevated protein levels, and a normal glucose level. Because the intensity of the inflammatory response in the CSF is low (usually 0 to 500 cells per mm³), nuchal rigidity is usually the only sign of meningeal irritation, and Kernig's and Brudzinski's signs are often absent. In a few cases, however, marked pleocytosis may be seen (greater than 1000 cells per mm³), often accompanied by Kernig's and Brudzinski's signs. The meningitis is self-limited, resolving usually in 1 week. URI—upper respiratory infection.

Differential Diagnosis of Acute Viral Meningitis

Bacterial meningitis
  Early (0–24 h)
  Also listeriosis, mycoplasmosis, brucellosis
Tuberculous meningitis
Fungal meningitis
Spirochetal meningitis: syphilis, Lyme disease, leptospirosis
Parasitic meningitis
Parameningeal infections
Neoplastic meningitis

Autoimmune and inflammatory diseases; lupus, sarcoid, vasculitis
Drug reactions: nonsteroidal anti-inflammatory agents, sulfamethizole, trimethoprim, trimethoprim-sulfamethoxazole, isoniazid, carbamazepine, azathioprine, intravenous immune globulin, intravenous monoclonal OKT3
Chemical meningitis: intrathecal drugs, central nervous system tumors, myelography, isotope cisternography

Figure 12-53. Differential diagnosis of acute viral meningitis. It is important to exclude nonviral causes of meningitis that may require specific therapy or more emergent therapy. During the first 24 hours of viral meningitis polymorphonuclear leukocytes may appear in the cerebrospinal fluid sample, similar to bacterial meningitis. In partially treated bacterial meningitis, the glucose level may be normal. Usually in tuberculous, fungal, spirochetal, and parasitic meningitis, the glucose level is depressed. Cytologic examination should differentiate neoplastic meningitis, whereas serologic studies help exclude autoimmune disease. Imaging studies usually detect parameningeal foci.

Neurologic Syndromes Associated with Enteroviruses

Syndrome	Virus type
Aseptic meningitis	Polioviruses 1–3 Coxsackieviruses A1–11, 14, 16–18, 22, 24 Coxsackieviruses B1–6 Echoviruses 1–7, 9, 11–25, 27, 30–33
Encephalitis	Enterovirus 71 Polioviruses 1–3 Coxsackieviruses A2, 4–9 Coxsackieviruses B1–6 Echoviruses 2–4, 6, 7, 9, 11, 14, 17–19, 25 Enterovirus 71 Enterovirus 72 (hepatitis A virus)
Paralytic disease	Poliovirus 1–3 Coxsackieviruses A2–4, 6–11, 14, 16, 21 Coxsackieviruses B1–6 Echoviruses 1–4, 6, 7, 9, 11, 13, 14, 16, 18–20, 30, 31 Enteroviruses 70, 71

(Table continued on next page)

Figure 12-54. Neurologic syndromes associated with enteroviruses. In addition to aseptic meningitis, several other syndromes have been associated with enteroviruses. Encephalitis is the second most common syndrome caused by enteroviruses, and in some years, enteroviruses account for a fourth of all cases of encephalitis of known etiology. The encephalitis is usually mild, with obtundation, coma (rarely), isolated seizures, behavior changes, and mild focal defects (rarely severe). The prognosis is excellent with resolution in 3 to 4 weeks, although concentration and intellectual abilities may not resolve for 3 to 6 months. The exceptions to this good prognosis are the fulminant encephalitis seen with group B coxsackievirus systemic neonatal infections, and the chronic encephalitis that appears with chronic persistent infection in agammaglobulinemic patients.

(Continued on next page)

Neurologic Syndromes Associated with Enteroviruses (*continued*)

Syndrome	Virus type
Acute cerebellar ataxia	Polioviruses 1, 3 Coxsackieviruses A2, 4, 7, 9, B1–6 Echoviruses 6, 9 Enterovirus 71
Isolated cranial nerve palsies, especially facial	Poliovirus 1–3 Coxsackieviruses A10, B5 Echoviruses 4 Enteroviruses 70
Chronic infections	Polioviruses 1–3 (vaccine-like strains) Coxsackieviruses A15, B3 Echoviruses 2, 3, 5, 7, 9, 11, 15, 17–19, 22, 24, 25, 27, 29, 30, 33

Figure 12-54. (*Continued*) Paralytic disease is discussed in the section on myelitis and related infections (Figures 12-75–12-77). Acute cerebellar ataxia and isolated cranial nerve palsies are infrequent and have a good prognosis. Chronic (persistent) enterovirus infections are caused mainly by echoviruses and a vaccine strain of polioviruses in agammaglobulinemic children. The echoviruses cause chronic encephalitis that progresses over several years, possibly accompanied by dermatomyositis. Polioviruses cause chronic encephalitis, but because of ensuing paralysis the course usually lasts only months to a year. The prognosis is poor despite the intrathecal administration of specific antibody, which may result in temporary remissions but usually not clearance of virus from the central nervous system. (*Adapted from* Jubelt and colleague [30].)

Herpes Simplex Virus Type 2

Pathogenesis of Herpes Simplex Type 2 Infections

	Adolescents and adults	Newborns	Immunocompromised host
Transmission	Venereal	In utero or at delivery	Venereal
Primary infection	Genital herpes; aseptic meningitis	Disseminated infection with hepatic and adrenal necrosis and encephalitis	Genital herpes Cutaneous herpes Disseminated infection with encephalitis
Latency	Sacral dorsal root ganglia	Unknown, usually fatal	Same as adolescent and adults
Recurrence	Genital herpes Cutaneous herpes Aseptic meningitis Radiculitis	—	Same as adolescent and adults if patient survives

Figure 12-55. Pathogenesis of herpes simplex type 2 (HSV-2) meningitis. HSV-2 is spread primarily by venereal contact. Most primary infections occur between the ages of 14 and 35 years, and most often manifest as genital infections of the penis in men and of the vulva, perineum, buttocks, cervix, and vagina in women. Approximately 25% of those infected by venereal transmission develop aseptic meningitis as part of the primary infection. Primary infection of a fetus can occur in utero or during delivery through an infected birth canal, which may result in severe and often fatal disseminated infection with encephalitis of the neonate. A similar disseminated infection may occur in the immunocompromised host after venereal transmission. Because the sacral ganglia receive sensory fibers from the external genitalia, the virus is transported axonally to the ganglia, where it becomes latent; the virus later reactivates and causes recurrent disease. Recurrent disease usually is limited to the genitalia, but aseptic meningitis and radiculitis may occur. Radiculitis is manifested by dysesthesia, which is often painful, may be burning or lancinating in character, and may cause sciatica. Sacral radiculitis may also result in bladder and bowel dysfunction, such as retention or incontinence.

Acyclovir Treatment of Herpes Simplex Type 2 Infections

Type of infection	Recommended treatment
Primary infection	
Genital lesions	Oral acyclovir, 200 mg daily 5x for 10 d
Aseptic meningitis	None or oral acyclovir (but not studied)
Disseminated infection with or without encephalitis	IV acyclovir, 10 mg/kg q8h for 21 d
Recurrent infection	
Immunocompetent host	
Infrequent	No treatment
Frequent	Oral acyclovir for suppression for up to 1 y, 200 mg tid or qid
Immunocompromised host	
Localized infection	Oral or IV acyclovir
Disseminated infection	IV acyclovir
Preventative	Oral acyclovir, 200 to 400 mg 2x to 5x per day

Figure 12-56. Treatment of herpes simplex type 2 infections. Acyclovir is the major drug in use today for treating herpes simplex infections. It is available in three formulations: intravenous (IV), oral, and topical (5% ointment). For the primary genital infection, oral acyclovir is indicated. Treatment for aseptic meningitis has not been studied, but it is a self-limited disease. Intravenous acyclovir is needed for disseminated infection with or without encephalitis. Frequent recurrences are usually treated, in the immunocompetent host, with 1 year of oral acyclovir for suppression. The immunocompromised host requires treatment for each recurrence and probably continuous oral treatment for suppression as a preventative measure.

Viral Encephalitis

Clinical Manifestations of Acute Viral Encephalitis

Acute febrile illness of abrupt onset

Systemic manifestations—malaise, anorexia, myalgias, pharyngitis, upper respiratory infection, abdominal pain, pain, nausea and vomiting, diarrhea

Meningeal irritation—headache, photophobia, nuchal rigidity

Parenchymal (brain) dysfunction

Altered level of consciousness

Lethargy to coma

Confusion, disorientation

Delirium

Mental changes—personality and behavioral changes, including agitation, hallucinations, and psychosis

Seizures—focal or generalized

Extensor plantar responses and hyperreflexia

Focal deficits—less frequent

Aphasia

Ataxia

Hemiparesis

Tremor

Cranial nerve palsies

Figure 12-57. Clinical manifestations of acute viral encephalitis. The term *encephalitis* implies involvement of the brain parenchyma. Often the meningeal manifestations seen in acute viral meningitis are also present in addition to the signs of brain dysfunction (meningoencephalitis). The signs of brain dysfunction may be focal or diffuse; these may manifest as mental status changes, seizures (in greater than 50% of cases), or hard focal signs. All types of focal deficits have been reported. Viral encephalitis can be divided into primary and secondary types. In primary encephalitis, there is viral invasion and infection of the brain parenchyma, usually of the gray matter. Secondary encephalitis is postinfectious encephalitis (or encephalomyelitis) in which an immune-mediated attack against myelin and white matter apparently occurs. Despite the different locations (gray vs white matter) of these pathologic insults, one cannot distinguish between the two based on the clinical symptoms and signs. The cerebrospinal fluid profile is similar to that of any acute viral syndrome, with lymphocytic pleocytosis (usually 5 to 500 cells per mm^3), normal glucose levels, increased protein levels, and increased pressure.

Differential Diagnosis of Acute Viral Encephalitis

Bacterial infections
  Parameningeal—epidural abscess, subdural empyema,
    brain abscess
  Tuberculous meningitis—late with parenchymal involvement
  Bacterial endocarditis
  Rocky Mountain spotted fever
  Brucellosis
  Mycoplasma pneumonia
  Legionella pneumonia

Fungal infections
  Fungal abscess
  Fungal meningitis—late with parenchymal involvement

Parasitic infections
  Toxoplasmosis
  Amebic meningoencephalitis
  Cysticercosis
  Malaria
  Trichinellosis
  Trypanosomiasis

Spirochete infections
  Lyme disease
  Leptospirosis

Noninfectious causes
  Encephalopathy—toxins, drugs, metabolic disorders
  Autoimmune and inflammatory causes—collagen vascular
    disease, vasculitis, sarcoid

Neoplasia
  Primary brain tumors
  Metastatic brain lesions

Figure 12-58. Differential diagnosis of acute viral encephalitis. A wide variety of diseases that affect the brain parenchyma can simulate acute viral encephalitis. The differential diagnoses includes both infectious and noninfectious diseases.

A. Geographic Distribution of the Major Viral Encephalitides

Virus	Geographic distribution
Japanese encephalitis	Eastern Asia, India
St. Louis encephalitis	US, Caribbean
California group encephalitis	North America
Eastern equine encephalitis	US Atlantic and Gulf coasts, Caribbean, South America
Western equine encephalitis	Western US and Canada, Central and South America
Venezuelan equine encephalitis	Texas, Florida, Central and South America
West Nile encephalitis	Africa, Middle East, eastern Europe, northeast US
Murray Valley encephalitis	Australia, New Guinea
Rocio	Brazil
Tick-borne encephalitis complex	Worldwide
Lymphocytic choriomeningitis	Americas, Europe, Africa
Mumps	Worldwide
Measles	Worldwide
Rabies	Worldwide (except UK and Japan)
Herpes simplex encephalitis	Worldwide
Epstein-Barr encephalitis	Worldwide
Varicella-zoster encephalitis	Worldwide
HIV	Worldwide

B. Most Causes of Viral Encephalitides in the United States

Virus	Geographic distribution
Herpes simplex	Nationwide
Mumps	Nationwide
St. Louis	Nationwide (esp. south and central)
California/La Crosse	Central and eastern US
Western equine	Western US
Eastern equine	Atlantic and Gulf coasts
West Nile encephalitis	Northeast US
Colorado tick fever	Western US
Venezuelan equine	Texas and Florida
Rabies	Nationwide

Figure 12-59. Geographic distribution of major causes of encephalitides. The arboviruses (insect-borne) have distinct geographic locations throughout the world. Other viruses may occur in seasonal, epidemic, or endemic fashion depending on the geographic location. Therefore, the travel history may be very important for making the diagnosis. **A,** Major causes of viral encephalitides worldwide. **B,** Major causes of viral encephalitides in the United States. (*Adapted from* Hanley and colleagues [31]; Miller and colleagues [32].)

Herpes Simplex Type 1 Encephalitis

Clinical Manifestations of Herpes Simplex Encephalitis at Presentation

	NIAID Collaborative Study*	Swedish Study†
Symptoms		
Altered consciousness	97% (109/112)	100% (53/53)
Fever	90% (101/112)	100% (53/53)
Headache	81% (89/110)	74% (39/53)
Seizures	67% (73/109)	
Vomiting	46% (51/111)	38% (20/53)
Hemiparesis	33% (33/100)	
Memory Loss	24% (14/59)	
Signs		
Fever	92% (101/110)	
Personality alteration (confusion, disorientation)	85% (69/81)	57% (30/53)
Dysphasia	76% (58/76)	36% (19/53)
Autonomic dysfunction	60% (53/88)	
Ataxia	40% (22/55)	
Hemiparesis	38% (41/107)	40% (21/33)
Seizures	38% (43/112)	62% (33/53)
Focal	(28/43)	
Generalized	(10/43)	
Both	(5/43)	
Cranial nerve deficits	32% (34/105)	
Papilledema	14% (16/111)	

*Adapted from *Whitley and colleagues [33].*

†Adapted from *Skoldenberg and colleagues [34].*

Figure 12-60. Clinical manifestations of herpes simplex type 1 (HSV-1) encephalitis. HSV-1 causes a focal encephalitis involving the medial temporal and orbitofrontal lobes. However, at presentation, when the diagnosis needs to be made for institution of therapy, hard focal signs are present only in the minority of patients. The most common manifestations at presentation (alteration in consciousness and personality changes including bizarre behavior and hallucinations) are not very localizing and can be seen in diffuse processes. Localization of the lesion depends upon diagnostic tests. The numbers in parentheses are absolute numbers that represent the number of patients presenting with symptoms or signs divided by the total number of points for which they were asked or for which they looked. NIAID—National Institute of Allergy and Infectious Diseases.

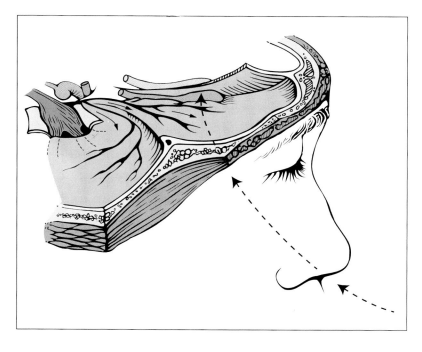

Figure 12-61. Pathogenesis of herpes simplex virus (HSV) encephalitis. Anatomical pathways may explain the localization of herpes simplex virus type 1 (HSV-1) encephalitis to the orbitofrontal and medial temporal lobes. Direct infections via the olfactory bulb could cause orbital-frontal infection with secondary spread to the temporal lobe. Recurrent sensory branches from the trigeminal ganglia project to the basilar dura of the anterior and middle cranial fossa. This may explain temporal lobe localization of HSV encephalitis when the virus reactivates in the trigeminal ganglia. Based upon serologic studies, about 30% of HSV encephalitis is due to direct invasion and 70% from reactivation. (*Adapted from* Johnson [35].)

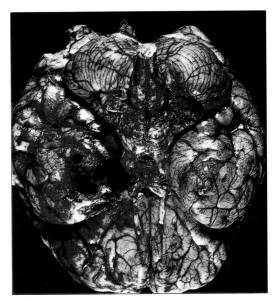

Figure 12-62. Gross anatomy of the brain in herpes simplex virus encephalitis. There is a hemorrhagic necrotic lesion of the left medial temporal lobe. As in this case, subarachnoid hemorrhage is frequent and results in the large number of erythrocytes often found in the cerebrospinal fluid. (*From* Hirano and colleagues [36]; with permission.)

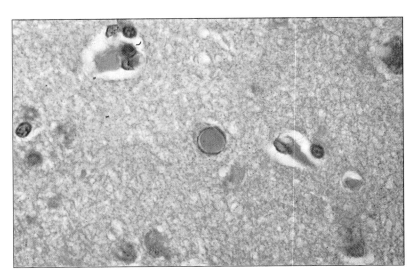

Figure 12-63. Histologic slide showing microscopic anatomy of herpes simplex virus (HSV) encephalitis (hematoxylin-eosin stain). Shown is a type A intranuclear inclusion body within the nucleus of a small nerve cell. These eosinophilic inclusion bodies may be seen in other herpes virus infections and subacute measles encephalitis. This section was taken from the temporal lobe cortex of a person with HSV encephalitis. The nuclear chromatin is marginated. These inclusion bodies can also be seen in glia and are a helpful diagnostic sign. (*From* Wilson [4]; with permission.)

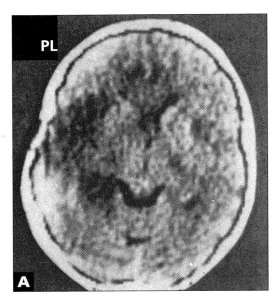
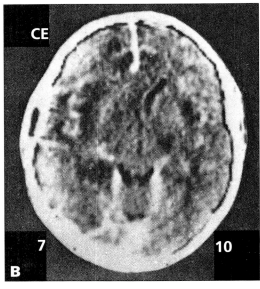

Figure 12-64. Computed tomography (CT) scans of herpes simplex virus (HSV) encephalitis. The initial diagnostic test should be a brain CT scan to exclude other lesions and to check for mass effect. Usually the CT scan does not become positive until the end of the first week of infection. If there is mass effect, treatment should commence with mannitol or steroids and acyclovir. Diagnosis can then be confirmed by magnetic resonance imaging (MRI) scanning. If the CT is normal or there is no mass effect, lumbar puncture should be performed. Within the first day or two of onset, 5% to 10% of cerebrospinal fluid (CSF) examinations are normal, but usually there is a lymphocytic pleocytosis, normal glucose, elevated protein, and pressure similar to other central nervous system viral infections. However, in HSV encephalitis there may be significant necrosis, hemorrhage, and erythrocytes in the CSF. The use of polymerase chain reaction (PCR) for amplification of HSV DNA from the CSF is still experimental but eventually will provide a rapid and sensitive method of diagnosis. If the CSF is abnormal, MRI scanning should be performed, and acyclovir should be started if the MRI is consistent with herpes encephalitis. The electroencephalogram (EEG) can also be a useful test as it may reveal temporal lobe foci earlier than CT scanning. If the diagnosis is not confirmed from the MRI and EEG, then a brain biopsy may be needed. **A,** CT scan on day 10 revealing low density lesion in the right temporal and deep frontal lobes. **B,** The corresponding enhanced CT scan reveals gyral enhancement in the sylvian fissure and insular regions, which are greater on the right. (*From* Davis and colleagues [37]; with permission.)

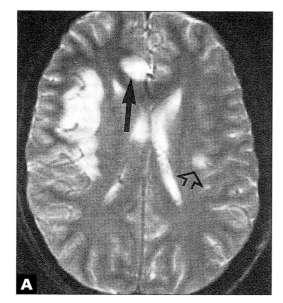

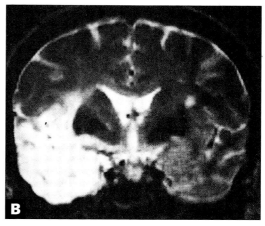

Figure 12-65. Magnetic resonance imaging (MRI) scans used in the diagnosis of herpes simplex virus (HSV). MRI has become the diagnostic test of choice for HSV encephalitis. MRI will usually reveal a hyperintense lesion with T2 weighting due to inflammation and edema within a day or two of onset, even when the computed tomography scan is normal. Lesions may not only be seen in the temporal lobe but also in the orbital frontal lobes and insular cortex. **A**, T2-weighted axial MRI shows high signal intensity in the right insular cortex, medial right frontal cortex (*solid arrow*), and left insular cortex (*open arrow*). **B**, T2-weighted coronal image shows increased signal in the left temporal lobe and beginning involvement of the right side. Coronal images are the most useful for seeing the lesion. (Panel A *from* Runge [38]; with permission; Panel B *from* Schroth and colleagues [39]; with permission.)

Arbovirus Encephalitis

Major Arboviral Encephalitides

Mosquito-borne viruses	Location	Tick-borne viruses	Location
Togaviridae (alphaviruses)		Flaviviridae (flaviruses)	
Eastern equine encephalitis	US Atlantic and Gulf coasts, Caribbean	Tick-borne complex	
		Far Eastern	Eastern Russia
Venezuelan equine encephalitis	Texas, Florida, Central and South America	Central European	Eastern Europe, Scandinavia, France, Switzerland
Western equine encephalitis	Western US and Canada, Central and South America	Russian spring-summer	Eastern Europe, Asia
		Kyasanur Forest disease complex	India
Flaviviridae (flaviruses)		Negishi	Japan
St. Louis encephalitis	US, Caribbean	Powassan	Northcentral US, eastern Canada
Japanese encephalitis	Eastern Asia, India	Louping ill	Great Britain
Murray Valley encephalitis	Australia, New Guinea	Reoviridae (coltivirus)	
Rocio	Brazil	Colorado tick fever	US and Canadian Rocky Mountains
West Nile	Africa, Middle East, eastern Europe, notheast US		
Ilheus	Central and South America		
Bunyaviridae (bunyaviruses)			
California encephalitis group			
California	Western US		
La Crosse	Central and eastern US		
Tahyna (phlebovirus)	Central and southern Europe		
Rift Valley fever	East and South Africa		

Figure 12-66. Major arbovirus encephalitides in the world. The term *arbovirus* is no longer used as official viral nomenclature. However, it is still useful to designate all the anthropod-borne viruses. There are about 20 arboviruses worldwide that primarily cause encephalitis. Many other arboviruses cause systemic febrile illnesses or hemorrhagic fevers (eg, yellow fever virus) but only infrequently, encephalitis. Arboviruses are usually geographically localized and seasonally restricted. (*Adapted from* Hanley and colleagues [31]; Miller and colleagues [32].)

Rabies

Clinical Manifestations of Rabies

Finding	%
Fever	73
Dysphagia	58
Altered mental state	55
Pain, paresthesia referable to site of exposure	45
Excitement, agitation	45
Paralysis, weakness	26
Hydrophobia	21
Hypersalivation	16
Nausea, vomiting	18.6
Malaise	16.3
Dyspnea	14.0
Headache	14.0
Convulsions, spasms	9.1
Coma	4.5
Miscellaneous (lethargy, dysuria, anorexia, hydrophobia)	16.3
No history of rabies exposure	16

Figure 12-67. Clinical manifestations of rabies, frequency during the course of the disease. At onset, about half of the patients have pain or paresthesia at the exposure site. Other initial manifestations include fever, malaise, anorexia, and drowsiness. (*Adapted from* Robinson [40].)

Clinical Progression of Rabies

Stage	Duration	Clinical association
Incubation period	30–90 days: ~ 50% of cases <30 days: ~ 25% >90 days to 1 year: ~ 20% >1 year: ~ 5%	No clinical findings
Prodrome and early clinical symptoms	2–10 days	Paresthesia and/or pain at site of bite Fever, malaise Anorexia, nausea, vomiting Headache
Acute neurologic disease	2–7 days	"Furious rabies" (80% of cases) Hallucinations, bizarre behavior, anxiety, agitation, biting Hydrophobia Autonomic dysfunction "Paralytic rabies" (20% of cases) Flaccid paralysis Paresis and plegias Ascending paralysis
Coma	0–14 days	SIADH Diabetes insipidus Multiorgan failure Respiratory or cardiac failure
Death (common) (rare)	Variable	—
Recovery (rare)	Variable	Severe sequelae

Figure 12-68. Clinical progression of rabies. The clinical course of rabies consists of five stages. The prolonged incubation period lasts more than 90 days in 25% and more than 1 year in 5% of cases. After the initial manifestations with lethargy, a state of excitability ensues, when external stimuli may cause focal or generalized convulsions. Spasmodic contractions of the larynx and pharynx are precipitated by any attempt to drink or eat, thus the term *hydrophobia*. During this stage the temperature may reach 105° to 107° F. This hyperexcitability stage passes into the comatose stage, with generalized paralysis. Occasionally, the disease begins as "dumb rabies," in which flaccid paralysis of one or more limbs occurs rather than a hyperexcitable period. Death is usually caused by respiratory paralysis followed by cardiovascular collapse. SIADH—syndrome of inappropriate secretion of antidiuretic hormone. (*Adapted from* Whitley and colleague [41].)

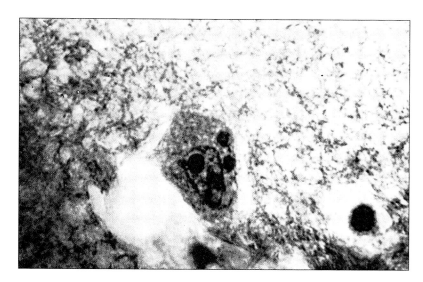

Figure 12-69. Negri body, a cytoplasmic eosinophilic inclusion with central basophilic granules, which is pathognomic of rabies. Unfortunately, these inclusions are present in only 70% to 80% of cases, and might not be seen. The inclusions contain rabies virus antigens. Negri bodies are only found in neurons, most commonly the hippocampal pyramidal cells and cerebellar Purkinje cells, but they may occur in other cortical neurons and other regions of the central nervous system. Perivascular inflammation is mild to minimal, perhaps because rabies virus is transported axonally and transynaptically, with little extracellular virus extension. A microglial rod cell response usually occurs, as do diffuse degenerative changes of neurons. (*From* Jubelt and colleague [26]; with permission.)

Diagnostic Tests for Rabies

No preclinical diagnostic tests
Cerebropspinal fluid—standard viral syndrome
  Lymphocytic pleocytosis
  Increased pressure
  Increased protein level
  Normal glucose level
Neck skin biopsy for fluorescent antibody test
  Need 6–8 mm full-thickness specimen
  Posterior aspects of neck just above hairline
  First week of illness 50% positive, greater thereafter
Corneal impression test—less sensitive, less specific than neck skin biopsy
Rabies antibody in serum and CSF—high CSF titers seen only in clinical disease
Culture of rabies virus from saliva, urine sediment, CSF and brain tissue (brain biopsy)

Figure 12-70. Diagnostic tests for rabies. Rabies cannot be diagnosed before the onset of clinical disease. Biopsy of neck skin for fluorescent staining and the cerebrospinal fluid (CSF) antibody response (which is not present until at least the second week) are the most useful diagnostic tests, except for biopsy of the brain. The differential diagnosis includes all causes of encephalitis, both primary and postinfectious. In Australia, the closely related Lyssavirus has caused several cases of fatal encephalitis clinically similar to rabies [42]. Treatable causes such as herpes simplex virus encephalitis are especially important to exclude. Muscular rigidity due to tetanus is also an important differential consideration. Hydrophobia is virtually diagnostic of rabies. In countries where rabies is common, rabies psychosis or hysteria may be seen in those exposed to possibly rabid animals. Paralytic disease caused by poliomyelitis, other enterovirus infections, paralytic zoster, transverse myelitis, and Guillain-Barré syndrome must be excluded.

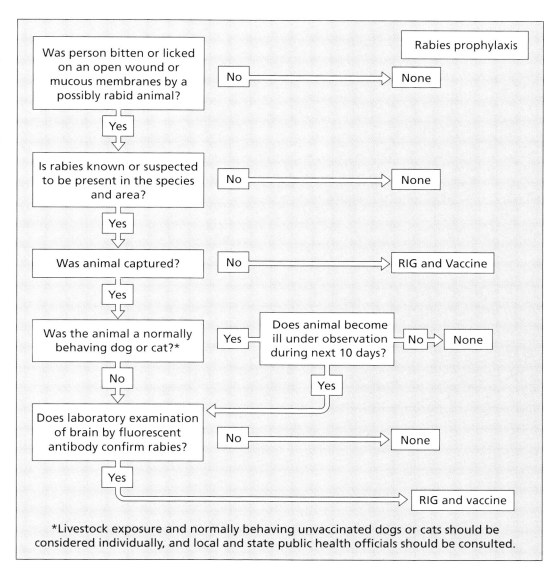

*Livestock exposure and normally behaving unvaccinated dogs or cats should be considered individually, and local and state public health officials should be consulted.

Figure 12-71. Rabies postexposure prophylaxis algorithm. Over 1 million people in the United States are bitten by animals each year; thus, for each of these bites, a decision must be made about instituting postexposure prophylaxis. Worldwide, dog bites are the main cause of rabies. Fortunately, because of the domestic animal rabies control programs instituted in the 1950s, the chances of getting rabies from a dog in the United States is minimal. RIG—rabies immune globulin. (*Adapted from* Corey [43].)

Postexposure Rabies Prophylaxis Regimen in the United States

	Rabies-naïve patients	Previously immunized patients
Local wound care and passive immunization with rabies antiserum	Cleanse wound with soap and water HRIG, up to 20 U/kg, with as much as possible by local infiltration into wound; any remaining HRIG given intramuscularly in gluteus or thigh	Cleanse wound with soap and water. Administration of HRIG is contraindicated
Active immunization with rabies vaccine	Rabies vaccine, 1-mL dose intramuscularly in deltoid or thigh, X 5 doses (given on days 0, 3, 7, 14, and 28)	Rabies vaccine, 1-mL dose intramuscularly in deltoid or thigh, X 2 doses (given on days 0 and 3)

Figure 12-72. Postexposure rabies prophylaxis regimen. There is no specific treatment for rabies once the clinical disease begins; maximum supportive care in an intensive care unit is the patient's only hope for survival. For individuals at high risk (rabies laboratory workers, some veterinarians, animal control and wildlife workers in endemic areas, and spelunkers and travelers to highly endemic areas in which exposure could occur), pre-exposure prophylaxis should be used. Postexposure prophylaxis includes local wound care, passive immunization with rabies antiserum, and active immunization with rabies vaccine. Both the antiserum and the vaccine should be started immediately. To avoid the formation of antigen-antibody complexes, vaccine and antisera should not be given in the same inoculation or even inoculated into the same geographic site. If human rabies immune globulin (HRIG) is not available, equine antirabies serum (ARS) can be used, but serum sickness may result. Human diploid cell vaccine (HDCV) and rabies vaccine absorbed are equally effective and both safe; severe reactions are rare. There have been three cases of recovery from rabies; these patients were treated ineffectively with pre-exposure or postexposure prophylaxis with the older nonhuman rabies animal vaccines before the onset of clinical disease. Rabies postexposure prophylaxis with HRIG and HDCV (or rabies vaccine) has been 100% effective in the United States. Case reports of failure from outside the United States may relate to the use of inappropriate inoculation sites and failure to treat the wound adequately. (*Adapted from* Dreesen and colleagues [44].)

Postinfectious Encephalitis

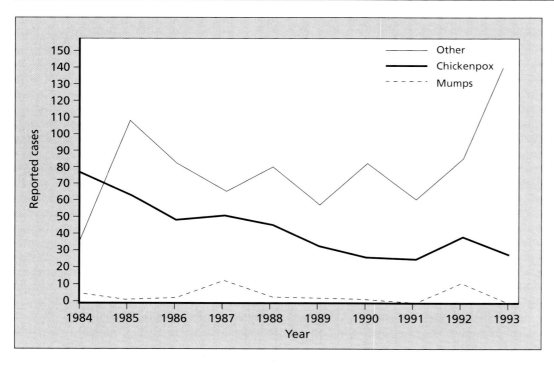

Figure 12-73. Incidence of postinfectious encephalitis (PIE) in the United States from 1984 to 1993. PIE is secondary encephalitis in which an immune-mediated attack appears to be mounted against central myelin. At times the spinal cord is also involved, causing encephalo-myelitis. Presumably virus does not need to invade the central nervous system to cause the syndrome, as the immune system can become sensitized to myelin peripherally by sequence homology between viral proteins and myelin proteins. The common causes of postinfectious encephalitis are chickenpox (varicella), mumps, and nonspecific upper respiratory infections. Usually this syndrome begins 3 days to 3 weeks after onset of the preceding infection. PIE occurs in cerebral and cerebellar forms. Clinically the cerebral form looks like primary encephalitis (Fig. 12-57). The acute cerebellar ataxic form is the type most often caused by chickenpox and has a good prognosis. Between 100 to 200 cases are reported annually in the United States. (*Adapted from* Centers for Disease Control and Prevention [45].)

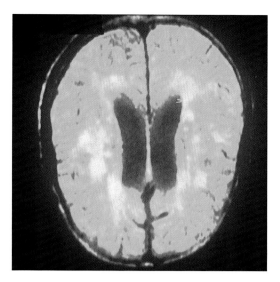

Figure 12-74. Proton-density magnetic resonance imaging (MRI) scan showing demyelination in postinfectious encephalitis (PIE) that occurred 2 weeks after a nonspecific upper respiratory infection. The best diagnostic test for PIE is MRI, which demonstrates white matter disease. Whether the form is cerebral or cerebellar, the cerebrospinal fluid (CSF) profile is similar to that of other acute viral syndromes, with lymphocytic pleocytosis, normal glucose level, elevated protein level, and pressure. One CSF test that may be helpful is the myelin basic protein (MBP) level, which is usually elevated; unfortunately, in most places, it takes 1 to 2 weeks to receive results. Treatment should be started once the diagnosis is made based upon the clinical presentation, including causative disease, a CSF picture consistent with encephalitis, and a positive MRI scan. Treatment consists of high-dose intravenous steroids (1.0 g methylprednisolone daily for 7 to 10 days) that will stop perivascular demyelination.

Poliomyelitis, Myelitis, and Radiculitis

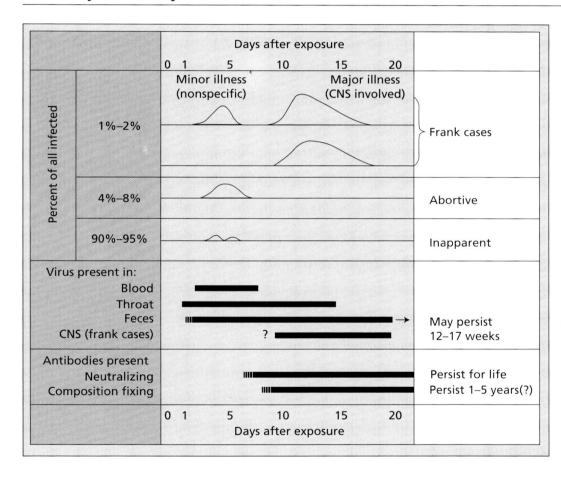

Figure 12-75. Correlation of clinical forms of poliomyelitis with the time of viral replication and antibody production. The term *poliomyelitis* is from the Greek words for gray marrow ("polio") and spinal cord ("myelitis"): "the gray marrow of the spinal cord." Sometimes the term *anterior* is added as a reminder that it is the anterior rather than the posterior horns that are inflamed in poliomyelitis. Only about 1% to 2% of those infected with the virus develop paralysis (major illness) with or without the nonspecific, systemic, febrile minor illness. Paralysis is usually asymmetric and flaccid, and can occur in all four extremities, as well as in the brain stem, causing bulbar polio with cranial nerve palsies, respiratory insufficiency, dysphagia, and coma. The use of oral polio vaccine has eradicated poliomyelitis caused by wild type virus in the United States and other developed countries. However, poliomyelitis is still a significant problem in underdeveloped areas. CNS—central nervous system. (*Adapted from* Horstmann [46].)

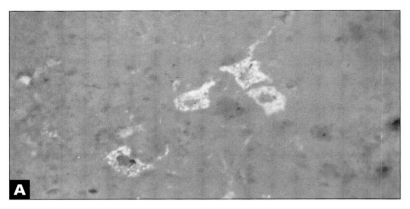 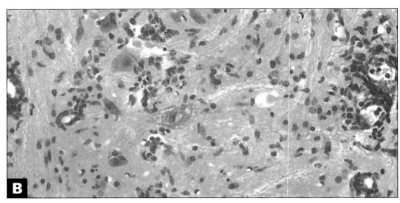

Figure 12-76. Histology slides showing pathogenesis and pathology of poliomyelitis. The paralysis in poliomyelitis is caused by poliovirus infecting the large anterior horn motor neurons. With destruction of these motor neurons, an intense inflammatory response ensues. **A**, Fluorescent antibody staining of type 2 poliovirus antigen in large anterior horn cells of the lumbar spinal cord in a mouse model of human poliomyelitis. Immunofluorescence in the cytoplasm and processes of these cells is prominent. Poliovirus is an RNA virus that replicates in the cytoplasm; therefore there is no immunofluorescence in the nucleus. Adjacent to the infected cells are dark unstained, uninfected neurons. **B**, Cervical cord showing poliomyelitis due to intracerebral injection of Lansing type 2 poliovirus in a mouse model of human poliomyelitis. Anterior horn cells show various stages of neuronal degeneration. The inflammatory response consists of perivascular mononuclear cell cuffing, parenchymal mononuclear and microglial cell infiltrates and neuronophagia. (*From* Jubelt and colleagues [47]; with permission.)

Differential Diagnosis of Poliomyelitis

Non-polio enteroviruses (EV)
  Coxsackieviruses—rare, mild paralysis
  Echoviruses—rare, mild paralysis
  EV 70—severe paralysis in Asia, Africa, Europe; no paralysis in the New World
  EV 71—severe paralysis in Eastern Europe; rare mild paralysis in the New World
Rabies virus—paralytic or "dumb" rabies
Herpes zoster—"zoster paresis"
Guillain-Barré syndrome—usually symmetric
Botulism—symmetric
Acute toxic neuropathies—symmetric with stocking/glove sensory loss
Acute intermittent porphyria—symmetric paralysis, psychiatric symptoms, delirium, abdominal pain, seizures
Acute transverse myelitis—usually symmetric with sensory level and bowel and bladder involvement
Cord compression from epidural abscess—same as transverse myelitis, also localized back percussion tenderness

Figure 12-77. Differential diagnosis of poliomyelitis. The diagnosis of poliomyelitis is based upon the clinical paralysis, the cerebrospinal fluid profile picture of an acute viral syndrome, isolation of virus from the throat or stool, and a fourfold rise in the serum antibody level. The differential diagnosis includes other causes of acute lower motor neuron flaccid paralysis. Paralysis is usually asymmetric, without bladder or sensory involvement. Bladder and sensory involvement, however, resulting in a picture of transverse myelitis, has been caused by poliovirus, thus expanding the differential diagnosis to this entity. The only specific treatment for poliomyelitis is prevention with poliovirus vaccine. Both the live attenuated oral vaccine (Sabin type) and the inactive injectable vaccine (Salk type) are used throughout the world. Treatment of the acute disease is supportive.

Acute Transverse Myelitis

Viruses Causing Acute Transverse Myelitis*

Common	Uncommon	Rare
Herpes simplex virus type 2	Mumps	Poliovirus
	Influenza	Coxsackievirus
Cytomegalovirus	Rubella	Echovirus
Varicella-zoster virus		Rabies
Epstein-Barr virus		Hepatitis A and B
		Measles

Viruses causing encephalomyelitis, in which myelitis occurs only with encephalitis, are not listed.

Figure 12-78. Viruses causing acute transverse myelitis. The syndrome of "acute transverse myelitis" consists of acute flaccid paralysis with hypoflexia (later may develop spasticity with hyperreflexia), sensory loss usually with a sensory level, and bowel and bladder involvement. The paralysis is symmetric and thus different from the usual asymmetric paralysis seen in poliomyelitis. In addition to viruses, this clinical syndrome may be caused by cord compression from epidural abscess or epidural tumor that hemorrhages; intraspinal abscess or intraspinal hemorrhaging tumor; spinal cord infarct; vasculitis (*eg*, systemic lupus erythematosus) causing infarction; postinfectious immune-mediated myelitis; multiple sclerosis; and remote effects of cancer.

Cytomegalovirus Polyradiculitis

Cytomegalovirus Neurologic Infections

Disease and features	Host and frequency

Cytomegalic inclusion body disease
  Encephalitis
    Microencephaly
    Seizures
    Mental retardation
    Periventricular calcifications
  Disseminated disease
	Neonate, congenital
	  disease—rare

Encephalitis/ventriculitis
  Subacute course: (1–3 mo)
  Progressive mental status changes
  Disseminated disease in the immuno-compromised
    patient
  MRI—periventricular hyperintensities, meningeal
    enhancement
	Immunocompromised
	  patient (described
	  primarily in AIDS
	  patients)—uncommon
	Immunocompetent
	  patient—rare

Polyradiculitis/polyradiculomyelitis
  Pain and paresthesia in legs and perineum
  Sacral hypesthesia
  Urinary retention
  Subacute ascending hypotonic paraparesis
  Eventually ascends to cause myelitis
  CSF—pleocytosis (PMNs > lymphocytes), low
    glucose level, high protein level, CMV positive
    by culture or PCR
  Usually disseminated disease
  MRI—lumbosacral leptomeningeal enhancement
	Immunocompromised
	  patient (described only in
	  AIDS patients)—common

Multifocal neuropathy
  Markedly asymmetric
  Numbness, painful paresthesia for months, followed
    by sensorimotor neuropathy
  Usually disseminated disease
  CMV positive in CSF by culture or PCR
	Immunocompromised
	  patient (described only
	  in AIDS)—uncommon

Figure 12-79. Cytomegalovirus (CMV) neurologic infections. Prior to the occurrence of the AIDS epidemic in the United States, CMV was known primarily for causing cytomegalic inclusion body disease, an infrequent congenital disease of newborns. Cases of CMV encephalitis have been recognized rarely in immunocompetent individuals. CMV ventriculitis and encephalitis occur most often as an opportunistic infection in AIDS patients. The most common syndrome caused by CMV today, however, is the CMV polyradiculitis (polyradiculopathy)/polyradiculomyelitis (polyradiculomyelopathy). This syndrome occurs relatively late in the course of AIDS when the CD4$^+$ T lymphocyte count is usually less than 100. Less frequent and also late in the course of AIDS is CMV multifocal neuropathy. Ganciclovir and foscarnet have been reported to be beneficial in some postnatally acquired infections [48]. CSF—cerebrospinal fluid; MRI—magnetic resonance imaging; PCR—polymerase chain reaction; PMNs—polymorphonuclear leukocytes.

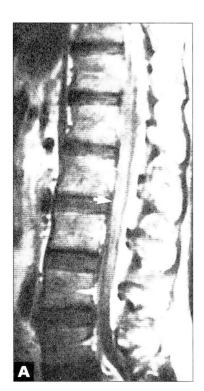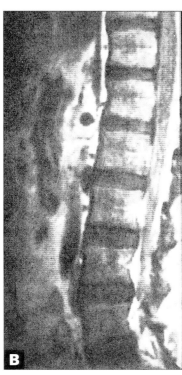

Figure 12-80. Enhanced T1-weighted sagittal magnetic resonance image of nerve roots from L1 to L4 and the cauda equina region (*arrows*) in a patient with cytomegalovirus polyradiculitis/polyradiculomyelitis (**A, B**). In the right half of the picture, the pial lining of the sac is also enhanced (*small arrows*). Usually these lesions are visible only with enhancement. (*From* Talpes and colleagues [49]; with permission.)

Herpes Zoster

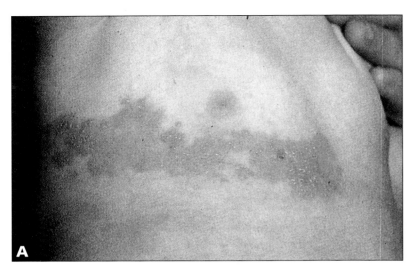

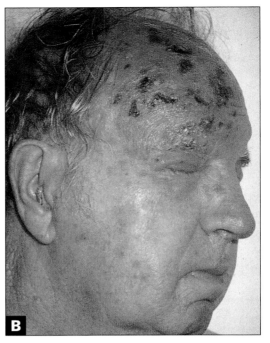

Figure 12-81. Herpes zoster. Herpes zoster is a distinctive syndrome caused by the varicella-zoster virus (VZV), which also causes chickenpox (varicella). The chickenpox virus travels from the skin up the sensory nerves to become latent in the dorsal root ganglia. Later in life, the virus reactivates, replicates in the ganglia, and travels down the nerve to the skin to cause a dermatomal vesicular eruption. The incidence of zoster increases with age and is more common in those with compromised cellular immunity. Typically, patients experience dermatomal paresthesia or dysesthesias (itching, burning pain, tingling) for 1 to 2 days, after which the vesicular eruption occurs. Most patients have hypalgesia and hypesthesia in the affected dermatome. **A**, Herpes zoster in a thoracic dermatome. **B**, Herpes zoster ophthalmicus. Herpes zoster of the ophthalmic division of the trigeminal nerve. (Panel A *from* Murray and colleagues [50]; with permission; Panel B *from* Rosencrance [51]; with permission.)

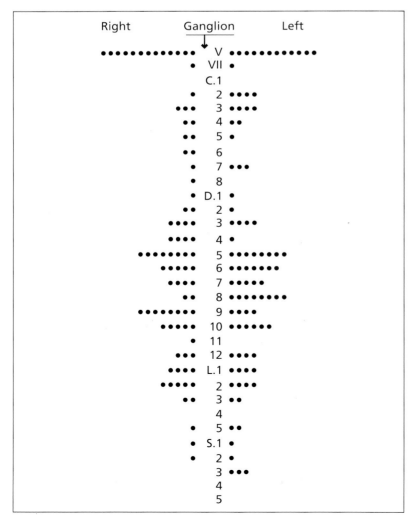

Figure 12-82. Segmental distribution of herpes zoster. Most cases occur in the thoracic nerves, the lumbar nerves, and the ophthalmic divisions of the trigeminal nerve (ophthalmic zoster). Approximately 40% to 50% of patients younger than 50 years of age develop postherpetic neuralgia (PHN), which is pain persisting for more than 6 weeks after the rash clears. The pain can be severe. PHN can be helped with amitriptyline and carbamazepine; local application of capsaicin may also help. For patients over 50 years of age, the use of oral acyclovir seems prudent in the hope of preventing PHN. Complications of herpes zoster include zoster paresis, myelitis, encephalitis, disseminated disease, and infection of the eye. Secondary to ophthalmic zoster (Fig. 12-81B) are keratitis, conjunctivitis, ocular muscle palsies, ptosis, mydriasis, contralateral hemiplegia due to viral spread to the ipsilateral carotid or middle cerebral artery, and the Ramsay Hunt syndrome (geniculate zoster, herpes zoster oticus) with facial palsy, loss of taste, and vesicles in the external auditory meatus. Intravenous acyclovir is indicated for disseminated zoster and probably for most of these complications, although controlled studies of its use for complications have not been reported. (*Adapted from* Hope-Simpson [52].)

Slow or Chronic Viral Infections

Slow Viral Infections of the Central Nervous System

Conventional viruses
  Retroviruses
    AIDS
    HTLV-1-associated myelopathy/tropical spastic
      paraparesis (HAM/TSP)
  Progressive multifocal leukoencephalopathy (PML)
  Subacute sclerosing panencephalitis (SSPE)
  Subacute measles encephalitis (SME)
  Progressive rubella panencephalitis (PRP)
  Enteroviruses—polio-, echoviruses
  Other—cytomegalovirus (CMV), adenovirus

Prion diseases (spongiform encephalopathy agents)
  Kuru
  Creutzfeldt-Jakob disease
  Gerstmann-Straussler syndrome (GSS)
  Fatal familial insomnia (FFI)

Figure 12-83. Slow viral infections of the central nervous system (CNS). Slow or chronic viral infections that result in chronic neurologic disease are caused by conventional viruses. Prion agents (unconventional transmissible spongiform encephalopathy agents) are not true viruses and are reviewed in the next section. The conventional viruses are true viruses with RNA or DNA genetic material and a recognizable structure on electron microscopy. Slow infections to be reviewed in detail are caused by retroviruses (acquired immunodeficiency syndrome, HTLV-1-associated myelopathy/tropical spastic paraparesis), papovaviruses (progressive multifocal leukoencephalopathy), and measles virus (subacute sclerosing panencephalitis [SSPE]).

Subacute measles encephalitis (SME) has also been referred to as "immunosuppressive measles encephalitis" and "measles inclusion body encephalitis" because of the large number of Cowdry Type A intranuclear inclusions present. SME occurs most often in children immunosuppressed with chemotherapy for lymphoma or leukemia. A few cases have occurred in adults. The incubation period is less than 6 months from the time of measles exposure. Clinical manifestations are seizures, hemiparesis, retinitis, and cortical blindness followed by coma and death in weeks to months. There is no treatment. The cerebrospinal fluid (CSF) is usually normal except for increased measles antibody titers. The electroencephalogram (EEG) may reveal focal slowing but no periodic complexes. Because of the immunosuppressed state, a large load of virus appears to reach the CNS.

Progressive rubella panencephalitis (PRP) was recognized as a distinct disease entity in 1974, at which time only several dozen cases had been reported. The disease develops during adolescence, usually in patients having stigmata of congenital rubella. Clinically the disease resembles SSPE in onset with dementia. Myoclonus and seizures are less prominent than in SSPE, but cerebellar ataxia is more prominent. The course is protracted over 8 to 10 years to death. There is no treatment. High levels of rubella antibody appear in the serum and CSF. Both CSF protein and IgG are increased, oligoclonal bands are present, and some patients have CSF pleocytosis (10 to 40 monocytes/mm^3). The EEG reveals diffuse slowing (rarely periodicity). Persistent infection is believed to cause the formation of immune complexes that are deposited in vessel walls, causing vasculitis.

Persistent enterovirus infections in agammaglobulinemic children have been caused by both attenuated polioviruses (vaccine strains) and echoviruses. The illness caused by polioviruses consists of a course of 2 to 3 months with both diffuse encephalitis and lower motor neuron paralysis. In the echovirus infections, the course may last months to several years with just encephalitis. About half the patients, however, have a polymyositis-like syndrome from echoviral infection of muscles. These patients may have remissions with intrathecal administration of antibodies, although as yet there are no definite cures. As previously noted (Fig. 12-79), cytomegalovirus (CMV) can cause subacute to chronic infections in AIDS patients, as can adenovirus, but less frequently.

Acquired Immunodeficiency Syndrome (AIDS)

Neurologic Syndromes in Patients With HIV Infection

Syndrome	HIV related	Opportunistic process
Leptomeningeal disease	Acute aseptic meningitis Chronic meningitis	Other viruses: HSV, VZV, EBV, CMV, hepatitis B Fungal: primarily cryptococcus* Bacterial: syphilis, mycobacteria*, listeriosis, pyogenic bacteria Lymphomatosis meningitis

Cerebral syndromes	Acute HIV encephalopathy*
	Chronic HIV-encephalopathy/
	  encephalitis
	  (AIDS dementia complex)
		Toxoplasmosis*
		CMV encephalitis*
		HSV encephalitis
		PML*
		Abscesses; bacterial, fungal
		Diffuse atypical mycobacterium*
		Primary central nervous system lymphoma*
		Metastatic lymphoma*, Kaposi's sarcoma*

(Table continued on next page)

*AIDS indicator diseases.

Figure 12-84. Major neurologic syndromes in patients with HIV infection. The various neurologic syndromes occurring in HIV-infected patients are caused by the direct effects of HIV or opportunistic processes. CMV—cytomegalovirus; EBV—Epstein-Barr virus;

HAM/TSP—HTLV-1-associated myelopathy and tropical spastic paraparesis; HSV—herpes simplex virus; PML—progressive multifocal leukoencephalopathy; VZV—varicella-zoster virus.

(Continued on next page)

Neurologic Syndromes in Patients With HIV Infection (*continued*)

Syndrome	HIV related	Opportunistic process
Spinal cord syndromes	HIV vacuolar myelopathy Anterior horn cell disease	Viral myelitis: HSV, VZV, CMV CMV anterior horn cell disease? HAM/TSP
Cranial neuropathies	Immune-complex retinopathy Others secondary to meningitis	CMV, toxoplasmosis, and candida retinitis Others secondary to meningitis
Peripheral neuropathies	Predominantly sensory polyneuropathy Acute and chronic inflammatory demyelinating polyneuropathies (AIDP, CIDP) Mononeuritis multiplex	CMV polyradiculitis CMV mononeuritis multiplex
Muscle disease	HIV myopathy	Toxoplasma myositis

Figure 12-84. (*Continued*)

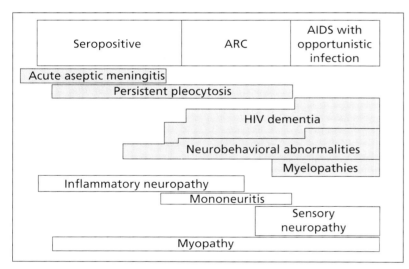

Figure 12-85. Timing and relative frequency of neurologic complications due to the direct effects of HIV infection. Diseases that affect the central nervous system (CNS) are shaded, whereas those affecting the peripheral nervous system (PNS) are not. The relative frequency of each complication is indicated by the height of each box. No clinical or cerebrospinal fluid (CSF) features distinguish HIV acute aseptic meningitis from other viral meningitides, but the HIV p24 core protein and HIV antibody are often found in the CSF. The chronic persistent pleocytosis is more often asymptomatic than symptomatic. As noted in Figure 12-84, both acute and chronic demyelinating polyneuropathies (AIDP, CIDP) may occur, which are clinically similar to non-HIV AIDP (Guillain-Barré syndrome) and CIDP. Usually, however, a CSF pleocytosis appears rather than the typical albumino-cytologic dissociation. Treatment is plasmapheresis or intravenous administration of immunoglobulins.

As the HIV infection progresses, patients become symptomatic with neurobehavioral abnormalities and dementia (HIV encephalopathy), also referred to as the AIDS dementia complex. At approximately the same time, a mononeuritis multiplex may occur, which is thought to be due to ischemic injury. It must be distinguished from cytomegalovirus (CMV) mononeuritis multiplex.

Late in the course of infection when patients have met the criteria for the diagnosis of AIDS (less than 200 CD4+ T lymphocytes or the occurrence of indicator diseases), opportunistic infections are more likely to occur, but HIV also causes several syndromes. One is the chronic vacuolar myelopathy that results in corticospinal tract and posterior column sensory signs (vibration and position sense loss). It needs to be distinguished from secondary HTLV-1-associated myelopathy and tropical spastic paraparesis (HAM/TSP). Other viral myelitides are too acute (herpes simplex virus, varicella-zoster virus) or subacute (CMV) to fit the picture. Also, distal, primarily sensory polyneuropathy may occur, which is the most common neuropathy to appear late in the disease, occurring in about a third of AIDS patients. The neuropathy is painful and there is loss of pain sensation, temperature sensation, light touch, and reflexes. CMV polyradiculitis is the primary differential diagnosis. An HIV myopathy may also be seen but is infrequent; a myopathy secondary to zidovudine therapy is more likely. ARC—AIDS-related complex. (*Adapted from* Johnson and colleagues [53].)

Figure 12-86. Clinical features of HIV encephalopathy (AIDS-dementia complex). **A,** In the early manifestation of AIDS dementia, HIV encephalopathy presents as a subcortical white matter disconnection syndrome with psychomotor slowing and impaired concentration. Gait ataxia is also a common early sign.
(*Continued on next page*)

A. Early Manifestations of the AIDS Dementia Complex

Symptoms	Signs
Cognition	Mental status
Impaired concentration	Psychomotor slowing
Forgetfulness	Impaired serial 7s or reversals
Mental slowing	Organic psychosis
Motor	Neurologic examination
Unsteady gait	Impaired rapid movements (limbs, eyes)
Leg weakness	Hyperreflexia
Loss of coordination, impaired handwriting	Release reflexes (snout, glabellar, grasp)
Tremor	Gait ataxia (impaired tandem gait, rapid turns)
Behavior	Tremor (postural)
Apathy, withdrawal, personality change	Leg weakness
Agitation, confusion, hallucinations	

B. Late Manifestations of the AIDS Dementia Complex

Mental status	Neurologic signs
Global dementia	Weakness (legs, arms)
Psychomotor slowing: verbal responses delayed, near or absolute mutism, vacant stare	Ataxia
	Pyramidal tract signs: spasticity, hyperreflexia, extensor plantar responses
Unawareness of illness, disinhibition	Bladder and bowel incontinence
Confusion, disorientation	Myoclonus
Organic psychosis	

Figure 12-86. (*Continued*)
B, In the late manifestations, AIDS dementia becomes global and psychomotor slowing severe. Patients often do not speak spontaneously and exhibit a delayed response to questions. (*Adapted from* Price and colleagues [54].)

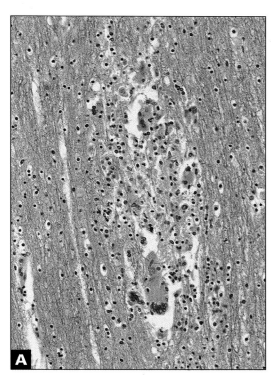
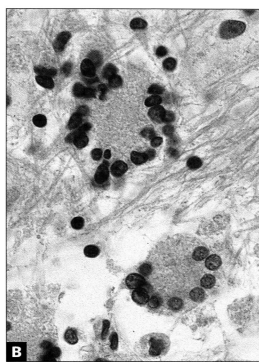
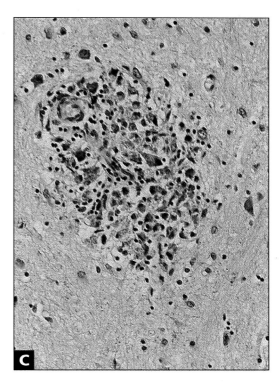

Figure 12-87. Pathology of HIV encephalopathy. The hallmarks of HIV encephalopathy are the multinucleated giant cells and microglial nodules. These cells appear throughout the cortex and white matter and are infected with HIV. HIV antigen is also found in glia and endothelial cells, but not neurons. Therefore, neuronal dysfunction is not the result of viral replication, and has not been clarified. **A,** Focal area of inflammation with a multinucleated giant cell and tissue disruption in HIV encephalopathy. Lesions are usually composed of macrophages and microglia. **B,** Multinucleated giant cells of macrophage origin. These cells appear to be the result of syncytial fusion of HIV-infected macrophages and microglia. **C,** Microglial nodule composed of macrophages and microglia. (*From* Hanley and colleagues; with permission [31].)

Differential Diagnosis of HIV Encephalopathy and Common Complications of AIDS

| Disorder | Approximate incidence (%) | Clinical manifestations | | | Neuroimaging findings | | |
		Onset	Alertness	Features	Lesions, *n*	Type of lesions	Location of lesions
AIDS dementia (HIV) encephalopathy	67	Weeks to months	Preserved	Personality change, unsteady gait, seizures, dementia	None, multiple, or diffuse	Increased MRI T2 signal, no enhancement or mass effect	White matter, basal ganglia
Cerebral toxoplasmosis	15	Days	Reduced	Fever, headaches, focal deficits, seizures	Multiple	Multiple, low-density ring-enhancing lesions on CT and T1-weighted MRI; spherical, increased T2-weighted MRI signal; mass effect	Cortex, basal ganglia
Cryptococcal meningitis	~ 9	Weeks	Variable	Fever, headaches, nausea and vomiting, confusion	None, hydrocephalus	—	—
Progressive multifocal leukoencephalopathy	4	Weeks	Preserved	Multiple focal deficits, late dementia	Multiple	Multiple, diffuse nonenhancing; no mass effect	White matter, adjacent to cortex
Primary central nervous system lymphoma	1	Days to weeks	Variable	Headache, focal deficits, seizures	One or few	Single > multiple; diffuse > ring enhancement; mass effect	Periventricular, white matter

Figure 12-88. Differential diagnosis of HIV encephalopathy and common complications of AIDS. By the end of October 1995, just over 500,000 cumulative cases of AIDS had been reported to the Centers for Disease Control and Prevention (CDC) from the United States and its territories. Of these cases 62% of patients had died. The World Health Organization estimates that there are 4.5 million cases worldwide. It is estimated that about two thirds of AIDS patients develop HIV encephalopathy. The figure lists the common complications of AIDS. Obviously less frequent complications such as bacterial brain abscesses (less than 1%), tuberculous meningitis with hydrocephalus and infection (1%), and other encephalitides (herpes simplex virus, varicella-zoster virus, and cytomegalovirus) may be part of the differential diagnosis at times. CT—computed tomography; MRI—magnetic resonance imaging. (*Adapted from* Price and colleagues [54]; Fauci and colleague [55].)

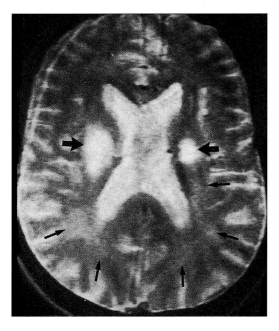

Figure 12-89. T2-weighted magnetic resonance imaging (MRI) scan showing bilateral diffuse (*small arrows*) and patchy white matter lesions (*large arrows*) in the brain of an AIDS patient. Computed tomography scans of HIV encephalopathy are nonspecific and only reveal diffuse atrophy with diffuse cortical atrophy and enlarged ventricles. T1-weighted MRI scans will also reveal diffuse atrophy. On T2-weighted MRI scans, in addition to atrophy, increased signal in the white matter is seen in 25% to 30% of AIDS patients. These changes may be diffuse or may be focal, patchy, or punctate. (*From* Olsen and colleagues [56]; with permission.)

Approved Anti-HIV Agents—2000

Agent	Mechanism of action	Limiting side effects	Indication
Zidovudine (ZDV) (Retrovir, Glaxo Wellcome, Research Triangle Park, NC)	nRTI	Anemia Neutropenia Myopathy Hepatitis (hepatic steatosis with lactic acidosis)	Initial therapy when <500 CD4+ T cells/µl
Didanosine (DDI) (Videx, Bristol-Myers Squib, Princeton, NJ)	nRTI	Painful sensory neuropathy Pancreatitis	Progressive disease while on ZDV, as monotherapy or with ZDV
Zalcitabine (ddC) (Hivid, Roche Laboratories, Nutley, NJ)	nRTI	Same as DDI	Only in combination with ZDV
Stavudine (d4T) (Zerit, Bristol-Myers Squib, Princeton, NJ)	nRTI	Painful sensory neuropathy Hepatitis (hepatic steatosis with lactic acidosis)	Intolerance or failure of ZDV or DDI
Lamivudine (3TC) (Epivir, Glaxo Wellcome, Research Triangle Park, NC)	nRTI	Nausea, vomiting, diarrhea Leukopenia/anemia Painful sensory neuropathy	Failure or intolerance of other drugs
Abacavir (Ziagan, Glaxo Wellcome, Research Triangle Park, NC)	nRTI	Hypersensitivity reactions	Initial regimens, naïve patients
ZDV + 3TC (Combivir, Glaxo Wellcome, Research Triangle Park, NC)	nRTI	See ZDV and 3TC above	Reduces "pill burden overload" in combination therapy
Saquinavir (Inverase, Fortovase, Glaxo Wellcome, Research Triangle Park, NC)	PI	Diarrhea Abdominal pain	Combination therapy
Ritonavir (Norvir, Abbott, North Chicago, IL)	PI	Diarrhea, nausea, vomiting	Combination therapy
Indinavir (Crixivan, Merck & Co., West Point, PA)	PI	Same as Ritonavir Hyperbilirubinemia Nephrolithiasis	Combination therapy
Nelfinavir (Viracept, Agouron, La Jolla, CA)	PI	Diarrhea	Combination therapy
Amprenavir (Agenerase, Glaxo Wellcome, Research Triangle Park, NC)	PI	Nausea, vomiting, diarrhea Rash including Stevens-Johnson Perioral paresthesias	Combination therapy
Nevirapine (Viramune, Roxane, Columbus, OH)	NNRTI	Hepatitis Rash	Combination therapy
Delaviradine (Pharmacia & Upjohn, Kalamazoo, MI)	NNRTI	Rash	Combination therapy
Efavirenz (Sustiva, DuPont Pharmaceuticals, Wilmington, DE)	NNRTI	Hepatitis Encephalopathy Transient 25% Limiting 3% Rash	Combination therapy

Figure 12-90. Treatment of HIV encephalopathy and other syndromes caused by the direct effects of HIV infection. Specific antiretroviral agents can be used for all syndromes caused directly by HIV. Symptomatic treatment such as antidepressants or antipsychotics for HIV encephalopathy may be useful. For the painful sensory neuropathy, analgesics, antidepressants (especially tricyclics), anticonvulsants (carbamazepine, phenytoin), and topical capsaicin ointment may be helpful. Specific agents for the treatment of HIV infections include nucleoside reverse transcriptase inhibitors (nRTI), protease inhibitors (PI), and nonnucleoside reverse transcriptase inhibitors (NNRTI). Therapy is recommended for all patients with symptomatic established HIV infection. Combination therapy is used but definitive data regarding the superiority of one regimen over another is not yet available. Initial regimens of two nRTIs plus a PI (or two PIs) or two nRTIs plus a NNRTI is recommended [57]. Both CD4+ cell and HIV RNA levels are used to decide when to start and change therapy [57]. Triple combination therapies with RTIs and PIs have been referred to as highly active antiretroviral therapy (HAART) [58]. When prescribing anti-HIV therapy, it is important to know the interactions between these agents as well as the interactions between these agents and other medication classes (antihistamines, antifungals, antimycobacterials, oral contraceptives, cytochrome P450 metabolized drugs, benzodiazepines, antibiotics, methadone, anticonvulsants, antiarrhythmics, calcium channel blockers, and ergot alkaloids).

HTLV-1 Associated Myelopathy and Tropical Spastic Paraparesis

Neurologic Signs of HAM/TSP

Abnormal signs	Affected, %
Corticospinal signs	
Legs	
Spasticity	100
Weakness	90–100
Arms	
Spasticity	60–90
Weakness	20–50
Increased jaw jerk	30–70
Bladder dysfunction	70–90
Impaired position, vibration sense	10–60
Root or cord sensation	20–65
Optic atrophy	2–20
Cerebellar signs	3–10

Figure 12-91. Neurologic signs of HTLV-1 associated myelopathy and tropical spastic paraparesis (HAM/TSP). HAM/TSP is characterized by a chronic progressive spastic paraparesis, usually with a neurogenic bladder. Patients may have paresthesia and pain in the legs. Both posterior column and spinothalamic sensory loss have been seen but usually in a minority of cases. Infrequently, cranial nerve (CN) signs are seen, with optic atrophy the most common. Other CN signs include nystagmus, diplopia, deafness, and facial paresis. Antibodies to HTLV-1 have been found in 80% to 100% of cases, and HTLV-1 has been isolated from the cerebrospinal fluid (CSF). The pathogenesis appears more likely to be an immune-mediated process, as cytotoxic-T lymphocytes rather than HTLV-1 viral titer levels are related to the demyelinating lesions. Pathologic changes include inflammation of the leptomeninges, perivascular cuffing, and inflammation of the cord parenchyma. Symmetrical demyelination of the corticospinal tracts occurs, and to a lesser degree and frequency, demyelination of the posterior columns and spinothalamic and spinocerebellar tracts.

Most cases of HAM/TSP occur in warm areas along the equator, where the virus is endemic. Isolated cases have occurred in more northern and southern latitudes, including northern areas of the United States. The disease usually begins in the third or fourth decade and women are more commonly affected, with a female to male ratio of about 2 to 1. The virus appears to be transmitted by vertical transmission from the mother to the fetus, sexual contact, intravenous drug use, and blood transfusions. For cases reported from the United States, except for the endemic area of South Florida, 20% to 25% of the time the mode of transmission cannot be determined. (*Adapted from* Rodgers-Johnson and colleagues [59].)

Differential Diagnosis of HAM/TSP

Cervical or thoracic cord compression
  Chiari malformations
  Foramen magnum tumors
  Cervical spondylosis
  Cervical and thoracic herniated discs
  Arteriovenous malformations

Motor neuron disease or related
    syndromes
  Amyotrophic lateral sclerosis
  Primary lateral sclerosis
  Hereditary spastic paraplegia

Inflammatory disorders
  Multiple sclerosis
  Systemic lupus erythematosus
  Sarcoid

Infectious diseases
  HIV myelopathy
  Bacterial disease
    Syphilis
    Tuberculosis (cord tuberculoma,
      compression)

  Parasites
    Schistosomiasis
    Strongyloidosis

Nutritional disorders
  Combined systems disease (B$_{12}$ deficiency)
  Vitamin E (tocopherol) deficiency
  Lathyrisin

Neoplastic disease
  Extramedullary (metastatic) or
    intramedullary tumors (primary or
    metastatic)
  Paraneoplastic myelopathy

Other disorders
  Adrenoleukodystrophy
  Hepatic myelopathy

Figure 12-92. Differential diagnosis of HTLV-1 associated myelopathy and tropical spastic paraparesis (HAM/TSP). The differential diagnosis of HAM/TSP is that of a chronic spastic progressive paraparesis. The diagnosis can be made by analysis of the cerebrospinal fluid (CSF). Less than half of patients have mild pleocytosis, while more than half have an elevated protein level. Specific CSF tests include the presence of HTLV-1 antibody and HTLV-1 oligoclonal bands, virus isolation from the CSF, and the detection of the HTLV-1 genome using polymerase chain reaction amplification. Magnetic resonance imaging (MRI) may reveal nonspecific demyelination in the spinal cord and brain. For treatment, prednisone and danazol have been reported to be beneficial but have not been tested in a controlled fashion. In a recent double-blind, controlled study, however, two thirds of the patients reported a benefit from 3.0 million units per day of interferon-α. (*Adapted from* Izumo and colleagues [60].)

Progressive Multifocal Leukoencephalopathy

Clinical Manifestations of Progressive Multifocal Leukoencephalopathy

Multifocal symptoms and signs
  Hemiparesis
  Hemianopsia
  Hemisensory deficit
  Aphasia
  Ataxia
  Dysarthria
Late mental status changes
  Personality changes
  Dementia

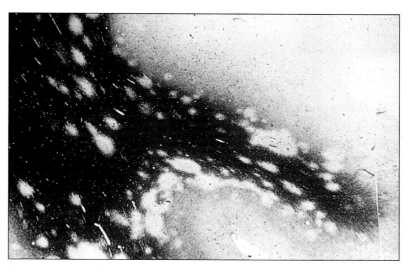

Figure 12-93. Clinical manifestations of progressive multifocal leuko-encephalopathy (PML). PML is caused by the opportunistic JC papova-virus. Multiple areas of demyelination occur, leading to the accumulation of different focal deficits (multifocal). When the lesions become extensive throughout the white matter, mental status changes ensue. The disease progresses to death in months. There is no specific treatment.

Figure 12-94. Photomicrograph showing the multiple pale areas of demyelination that are usually well-circumscribed in progressive multifocal leukoencephalopathy (PML). These areas contain macrophages and virally infected astrocytes and oligodendroglia (lower power, myelin stain). The opportunistic JC papovavirus infects oligodendroglia of immunocompromised patients. This results in multiple areas of demyelination, which are greater in the cerebral white matter than the brain stem and cerebellum. Hyperplasia of astrocytes also occurs, and eosinophilic intranuclear inclusions are visible in enlarged oligodendroglia nuclei. (*Courtesy of* Richard Johnson, MD, Johns Hopkins Medical School, Baltimore, MD.)

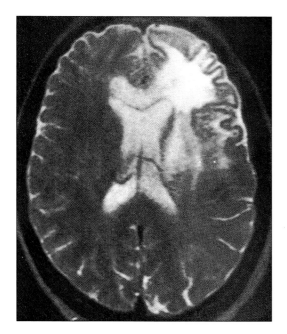

Figure 12-95. T2-weighted axial magnetic resonance imaging (MRI) scan, with increased signal intensity in the left frontal lobe and corona radiata with extension across the midline in a patient with progressive multifocal leukoencephalopathy (PML). As is characteristic, the subcortical U-fibers are involved. No specific findings occur in the cerebrospinal fluid (CSF), which is normal. The electroencephalographic (EEG) changes are nonspecific. Serologic testing is not helpful, as most adults already have antibody to JC virus. Amplification of JC viral DNA from the CSF has been reported on an experimental basis. Computed tomography (CT) scans reveal low-density nonenhancing lesions. MRI scans reveal increased signal intensity of T2-weighted images; enhancement is minimal in 10% to 15% of cases. Biopsy of the brain is necessary for a definitive diagnosis. In patients with AIDS, however, the disease is usually well-recognized and diagnosed based upon the clinical features and CT and MRI scanning. There is no specific treatment. A good outcome was reported in one patient with underlying sarcoid who was treated with cytarabine and interferon α, but other progressive multifocal leuko-encephalopathy (PML) cases treated with this regimen have shown no response. (*From* Whiteman and colleagues [61]; with permission.)

Subacute Sclerosing Panencephalitis

Clinical Stages of Subacute Sclerosing Panencephalitis (SSPE)

Stage I: Cerebral signs (mental, behavioral)

Irritability
Affectionate displays
Lethargy
Forgetfulness
Indifference
Withdrawal
Drooling
Regressive speech
Slurred speech

Stage II: Convulsive, motor signs

Myoclonus of head, limbs, trunk
Incoordination of trunk, limbs
Dyskinesia—choreoathetoid postures, movements, tremors

Stage III: Coma, opisthotonus

No responsiveness to any stimulus
Extensor hypertonus
Decerebrate rigidity
Irregular, stertorous respiration

Stage IV: Mutism, loss of cerebral cortex function, myoclonus

Pathologic laughter, crying
Wandering of eyes
Flexion of upper and lower limbs
Hypotonia
Turning of head to one side
Occasional limb myoclonus
Startling by noise

Figure 12-96. Clinical stages of subacute sclerosing panencephalitis (SSPE). SSPE has become a rare disease in the United States, with fewer than 10 cases per year, since the introduction of measles vaccine. Most patients had their measles infection prior to the age of 2 years, followed by a latent period before the onset of disease, which occurs between the ages of 5 to 15 years in 85% of patients. The disease usually begins with poor school performance, personality changes and then dementia (forgetfulness, regressive speech), which is referred to as stage I. Myoclonus, seizures, and movement disorders occur in stage II. Eventually the comatose and akinetic mutism stages ensue. Death usually occurs in 1 to 3 years, but has ranged from several months to 15 years.

SSPE apparently is caused by the lack of production of the measles virus M protein, which is needed by the virus to bud out of the cell and spread efficiently to the next cell. This results in a cell-associated infection. The measles virus can spread only by cell fusion, which is slow and inefficient. Diagnosis is made from clinical manifestations and the characteristic laboratory abnormalities. One of the most characteristic laboratory tests is the electroencephalogram, which reveals periodic patterns of bursts occurring every 5 to 7 seconds followed by periods of background attenuation (burst-suppression). The cerebrospinal fluid (CSF) gamma globulin and measles antibody titers are usually elevated. Computed tomography (CT) and magnetic resonance imaging (MRI) performed late in the course reveal diffuse atrophy of the cortex and white matter, with *ex vacuo* ventricular enlargement. MRI usually reveals multifocal white matter lesions. Although there is no specific treatment, intrathecal administration of interferon α has resulted in good remissions. (*Adapted from* Ohya and colleagues [62].)

The Prion Diseases

Prion Diseases of Humans and Animals

Disease	Host
Scrapie	Sheep, goats
Transmissible mink encephalopathy (TME)	Mink
Chronic wasting disease	Mule deer, elk
Bovine spongiform encephalopathy (BSE)	Cattle
Feline spongiform encephalopathy (FSE)	Cats
Kuru	Humans
Creutzfeldt-Jakob disease (CJD)	Humans
New variant CJD (nvCJD)	Humans
Gerstmann-Straussler syndrome (GSS)	Humans
Fatal familial insomnia (FFI)	Humans

Figure 12-97. Prion diseases of humans and animals. The prion diseases have also been referred to as transmissible spongiform encephalopathy agents. The first of these diseases, scrapie, was recognized to be transmissible in sheep in the 1930s. The latest epidemic of BSE in Britain, referred to by the lay public as "mad cow disease," is believed to have been transmitted to humans via the ingestion of contaminated beef resulting in a progressive dementia that has been named *new variant CJD* (nvCJD). The disease caused by nvCJD occurs in younger people and disease progression is slower [62]. *Kuru* is of historical interest because it was the first human prion disease to be recognized as transmissible. It occurs in the Fore Indians of New Guinea beginning with gait, trunk, and limb ataxia and involuntary movements (myoclonus, chorea, tremor) followed by dementia at a later date. Because it is transmitted primarily through cannibalistic rituals, which are now restricted, kuru is rare.

Characteristics of Prion Diseases and Agents

Prolonged incubation period of months to years

Progressive course of weeks to months to death

No host immune response (except astrocytosis)

Pathologic lesions confined to the central nervous system

Similar histopathology

No specific treatment

Causative agents (prions) have specific properties:

  No detectable nucleic acid

  Resistant to alcohol, formalin, heat, ultraviolet (UV)
  irradiation, nucleases*

  Susceptible to proteolytic enzymes, denaturing agents,
  organic solvents†

  Sterilized by:

    Steam autoclaving 1 hour at 132° C

    Immersion in 1N NaOH for 1 hour at room temperature

Agents that hydrolyze or modify nucleic acids.

†*Agents that digest, denature, or modify proteins.*

Figure 12-98. Characteristics of the prion diseases and agents. One of the important characteristics of these agents is that they do not contain detectable nucleic acids (DNA, RNA) but do contain a protein, the prion protein (PrP), that must be transmitted for disease to occur. This finding led to the "prion" terminology, which was derived from "protein" and "infectious." There is no specific treatment for the various prion diseases. However, the agent (prions) can be disinfected with various sterilization procedures.

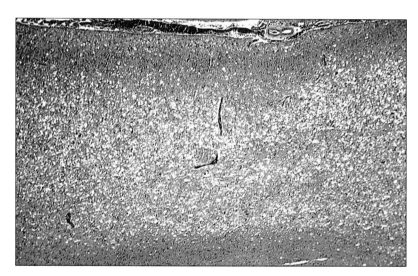

Figure 12-99. Low power view of hematoxylin-eosin stain, spongiform change confined to the cerebral cortex with sparing of the white matter. Other gray matter areas such as the basal ganglia, thalamus, and cerebellum may also be involved. Spongiform change can also be due to the development of vacuoles in the neurons more than in the astrocytes. This would result in an overall loss of neurons. As previously noted, the prion protein (PrP) is associated with the transmission of disease. It is a hydrophobic protein with a molecular weight of 27-30 kD, referred to as PrPSc 27-30. Scrapie (Sc) is the prototype prion disease that has been analyzed in these studies. PrPSc 27-30 is the protease-resistant component of a larger protein, PrPSc 33-35. Subsequently, it was found that uninfected brains also contained a similar protein, PrPC 33-35, which in humans has its gene (*PRNP*) on the short arm of chromosome 20. PrPC 33-35 is fully degraded but PrPSc 33-35 is only degraded to PrPSc 27-30, which collapses to produce amyloid deposition. On electron micrographs "prion rods" (or "scrapie associated fibrils") may be seen. PrPC is found on the cell surface and has two transmembrane domains, while PrPSc accumulates within cells and extracellularly. The role of PrPC is unknown. These findings have lead to the hypothesis that in infected animals, PrPC undergoes post-translational modification being converted to the PrPSc isoform. This post-translational modification would be the explanation for the *sporadic* prion diseases (Creutzfeldt-Jakob disease [CJD]). Prion disease can also be *infectious* (Kuru, accidental CJD), or *genetic* (familial CJD, Gerstmann-Straussler syndrome, Fatal Familial Insomnia). Kuru is infectious and is transmitted most often during cannibalistic rituals. CJD has been transmitted by surgical instruments, stereotactic electroencephalogram needles, growth hormone preparations, dura matter grafts, and corneal transplants. In the genetic cases there are mutations in the *PRNP* gene. How the agent actually replicates in the sporadic and infectious cases is unclear. Pathologic changes are similar in all prion diseases with varying degrees of each feature. These features include spongiform change, astrocytosis, and deposition of amyloid or kuru plaques. (*From* Hirano and colleagues [36]; with permission.)

Creutzfeldt-Jakob Disease

Clinical Characteristics of 232 Experimentally Transmitted Cases of Sporadic Creutzfeldt-Jakob Disease

Symptoms/Signs	Patients with symptoms or signs, %		
	At onset	On first exam	During course
Mental deterioration	69	85	100
Memory loss	48	66	100
Behavioral abnormalities	29	40	57
Higher cortical functions	16	36	73
Cerebellar	33	56	71
Visual/oculomotor	19	32	42
Vertigo/dizziness	13	15	19
Headache	11	11	18
Sensory	6	7	11
Involuntary movements	4	18	91
Myoclonus	1	9	78
Other (including tremor)	3	12	36
Pyramidal	2	15	62
Extrapyramidal	0.5	9	56
Lower motor neuron	0.5	3	12
Seizures	0	2	19
Pseudobulbar	0.5	1	7
Periodic electroencephalogram*	0	0	60
Triphasic 1 cycle/sec	0	0	48
Burst suppression	0	0	14

*The figures shown are much lower than those in published small series of repeatedly studied patients.

Figure 12-100. Clinical and epidemiologic features of Creutzfeldt-Jakob disease (CJD). Usually there is a gradual onset of dementia in middle or late life. Prodromal symptoms may include anxiety, dizziness, blurred vision, unusual behavior, poor judgment, and fatigue. In addition to dementia, cerebellar signs often occur early and involuntary movements (especially myoclonus) and corticospinal tract and extrapyramidal signs eventually become prominent. So-called variant types, for example, lower motor neuron type and occipital type, have been categorized when these features are prominent early in the course. The incidence of CJD is 1 case per 1 million people per year and is the same throughout the world except for a few areas of high incidence (Libya, North Africa, Slovakia). CJD is not contagious but is transmissible, and general trauma, head and neck trauma, and head and neck surgery predispose a patient to the disease. Five percent to 15% of cases are familial, with an autosomal dominant pattern of inheritance. Mutations have been found in the *PRNP* gene in some of these familial cases and most often occur at codons 178 and 200. In a recent series the range for the age of onset was 16 to 82 years but only one patient was younger than 30 years old and four were younger than 40 years old. The mean duration of disease was 8 months; 80% to 90% die in 1 year. As previously noted, CJD is not contagious but the mode of transmission is unknown. The agent is not found in saliva or stool and only very rarely in urine. Therefore, it does not seem necessary to isolate patients. Because the agent is present in internal organs, blood and cerebrospinal fluid serum hepatitis precautions should be taken. (*Adapted from* Brown and colleagues [64].)

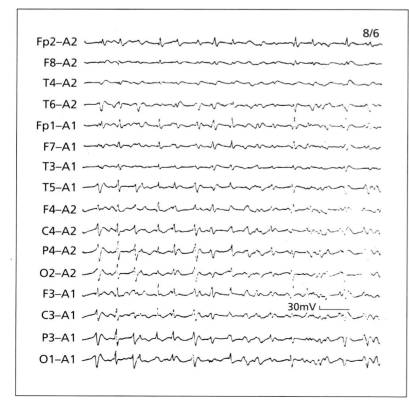

Figure 12-101. Diagnostic studies and diagnosis of Creutzfeldt-Jakob disease (CJD). Routine blood studies are normal. The cerebrospinal fluid (CSF) is also usually normal although the protein may be increased. Two dimensional isoelectric focusing of CSF proteins have revealed two abnormal protein species (designated 130 and 131), which may be relatively specific for CJD, but additional testing is needed to clarify specificity and sensitivity. Computed tomography and magnetic resonance imaging may show nonspecific atrophy. The electroencephalogram (EEG) is the diagnostic test of choice. Various series report 60% to 95% of patients will have periodic complexes occurring on the average of one per second (range 0.5 to 2.5 seconds). Serial EEG may be needed to detect the periodicity, as it is usually absent at onset and early in the course and may also be absent late in the course. Diagnosis can also be made from brain biopsy but usually is not required. This electroencephalogram from a 65-year-old man with Creutzfeldt-Jakob disease shows periodic spikes or sharp waves every 0.7 seconds. (*Adapted from* Jubelt and colleague [26].)

Clinical Features in New Variant Creutzfeldt-Jakob Disease

Symptoms/Signs	Patients with symptoms or signs, % (*n* = 35)	
	At onset	During course
Psychiatric	63	97
Sensory symptoms	20	68
Limb pain	11	37
Ataxia	8	100
Forgetfulness	17	83
Involuntary movements	6	94
Dystonia	6	34
Chorea	0	57
Myoclonus	0	71
Upgaze paresis	0	40
Dementia	0	100
Akinetic	0	57

Figure 12-102. Clinical features of new variant CJD (nvCJD). nvCJD occurs at a younger age than classic CJD, with 89% dying before the age of 40. The duration of nvCJD is also longer, with a median duration of illness of 14 months as compared to 9 to 11 months for classic CJD. nvCJD usually begins with psychiatric symptoms and painful sensory symptoms rather than memory loss. Similar to classic CJD, dementia, ataxia, and involuntary movements eventually occur (see Fig. 12-100). Another unusual feature of nvCJD is that the typical periodic triphasic complexes seen on electroencephalograms from classsic CJD patients have not been reported. (*Adapted from* Will and colleagues [65].)

Gerstmann-Sträussler-Schenker Syndrome

Characteristics of Gerstmann-Sträussler-Schenker Syndrome

Familial autosomal dominant disease—*PRNP* gene mutations, most frequently at codons 102, 117, 198

Age of onset—midlife

Clinical signs

Early—cerebellar ataxia with gait ataxia

Later—limb ataxia, dysarthria, nystagmus, dementia, parkinsonism, deafness, blindness, gaze palsies

Eventually—corticospinal tract signs

Course—lengthy, 2 to 10 years

Treatment—supportive

Figure 12-103. Characteristics of Gerstmann-Sträussler-Schenker syndrome (GSS). GSS is an autosomal dominant familial disease. Clinically, patients appear to have spinocerebellar degeneration or olivopontocerebellar degeneration with cerebellar ataxia, which is the first most severe manifestation of the disease. Myoclonus is much less common. Eventually dementia and parkinsonism develop in most patients. The electroencephalogram does not usually show periodicity.

Fatal Familial Insomnia

Clinical Features of Fatal Familial Insomnia

Case	Sex	Age of onset (years)	Course (months)	Insomnia	Dysautonomia	Ataxia	Myoclonus	Seizures	EEG
IV-20	F	48	7	+	+	+	+	—	—
IV-21*	M	52	9	+++[†]	+++	+	+	—	—
IV-34	F	45	7	+++	+(?)	+++	+	?	—
IV-37*	M	61	18	+++	+(?)	++	+	—	—
IV-75	M	54	18	++	++	++	+	—	—
IV-92	M	45	7	++	+++	?	+	—	+[§]
V-58*	F	35	25	+[†]	+++	+++	+++	+[‡]	

Clinically examined and longitudinally observed.

[†]*Polygraphically proven.*

[‡]*Grand mal type.*

[§]*Periodic spike activity.*

+ *Minimal.*

++ *Mild.*

+++ *Severe.*

Figure 12-104. Clinical features of fatal familial insomnia (FFI). FFI is a rapidly progressive autosomal dominant disease of middle or late life. Mutation at codon 178 of the *PRNP* gene has been demonstrated. This change is similar to that reported for some cases of familial Creutzfeldt-Jakob disease, but the clinical picture is much different. FFI is characterized primarily by insomnia, dysautonomia, and ataxia. Dementia and a periodic electroencephalogram (EEG) are uncommon. The course progresses to death in a half to 2 years. (*Adapted from* Manetto and colleagues [66].)

Mutations in the Prion Protein Gene Associated with Familial Prion Diseases*

Codon no.	Normal amino acid	Mutant amino acid	Familial prion disease
51–91	5 octarepeats	Additional 2–9 octarepeats	CJD
178	Asp	Asn	CJD
180	Val	Ile	CJD
200	Glu	Lys	CJD
210	Val	Ile	CJD
232	Met	Arg	CJD
102	Pro	Leu	GSS
105	Pro	Leu	GSS
117	Ala	Val	GSS
145	Tyr	Stop	GSS
198	Phe	Ser	GSS
217	Glu	Arg	GSS
129	Val or Met	Val	178[ASN] CJD
		Met	178[ASN] FFI

Other mutations have been described but only in single cases.

Figure 12-105. Familial prion diseases. Prion disease can be genetic and include familial Creutzfeld-Jakob disease (CJD), Gerstmann-Sträussler-Schenker syndrome (GSS), and fatal familial insomnia (FFI). Specific mutations in the prion protein gene have been found to be associated with specific prion diseases. (*Adapted from* Jubelt [67]).

Fungal Infections

Spectrum of Involvement for Fungi That Can Infect the CNS*

Organisms	Incidence	Predilection to involve the CNS†	Chief pathologic manifestations		
			Meningitis	Abscess or inflammatory mass	Infarct
Cryptococcus	Common	++++	++++	+	+
Coccidioides	Common	+++	++++	+	+
Candida	Common	++	++	++	—
Aspergillus	Occasional	++	+	+++	++++
Zygomycetes‡	Occasional	++	+	+++	++++
Histoplasma	Occasional	+	+	+	+
Blastomyces	Occasional	+	+	+	—
Sporothrix	Occasional	+	+	—	—
Paracoccidioides	Rare	±	±	±	—
Dematiaceous fungi	Rare	+++	±	++++	—
Pseudallescheria	Rare	+	++	++	—

*Key: ++++, common; ±, rare; —, does not occur.

†Versus other body sites.

‡The class of Zygomycetes or Phycomycetes includes genera Rhizopus and Mucor.

Figure 12-106. Clinical syndromes and frequencies of fungal infections that can affect the central nervous system (CNS). The clinical syndromes caused by fungi invading the CNS can be divided into meningitis, abscess or inflammatory mass (granuloma formations), and arterial thrombosis causing infarction. Fungi exist in two forms: yeasts and molds. Yeasts are unicellular organisms that have a thick cell wall surrounded by a well-defined capsule (Fig. 12-110). Molds are composed of tubular filaments that sometimes have a branched form (hyphae). In the brain, dimorphic and fungal yeasts are more likely to cause meningitis, while molds are more likely to cause vasculitis with subsequent thrombosis and infarction. The major pathogenic molds are species of the genes *Aspergillus* and the class of Zygomycetes. (*Adapted from* Perfect and colleague [68].)

Factors Predisposing to Fungal CNS Infections

Predisposing factors	Typical organisms
Prematurity	*Candida*
Inherited immune defects CGD, SCID, etc.	*Candida, Cryptococcus, Aspergillus*
Acquired immune defects	
Corticosteroids	*Cryptococcus, Candida*
Cytotoxic agents	*Aspergillus, Candida*
HIV infection	*Cryptococcus, Histoplasma*
Alcoholism	*Sporothrix*
Hematologic malignances	*Candida, Aspergillus, Cryptococcus, Histoplasma*
Iron chelator therapy	
Deferoxamine	Zygomycetes
Intravenous drug abuse	Zygomycetes, *Candida*
Diabetic ketoacidosis	Zygomycetes, *Candida*
Trauma, surgery, foreign body, near-drowning	*Candida, Pseudallescheria,* dematiaceous fungi

Figure 12-107. Predisposing factors to fungal infections of the central nervous system (CNS). As previously noted, most fungal infections are opportunistic. Specific factors predispose to specific fungal infections. CGD—chronic granulomatous disease; SCID—severe combined immune deficiency. (*Adapted from* Tunkel and colleague [69]; Gozdasoglu and colleagues [70].)

Fungal Meningitis

Signs and Symptoms of Fungal Meningitis

Fungal organism	Fever (>101°F)	Headache	Stiff neck	Change in mentation	Focal signs	Visual disturbance
Blastomyces	+	+++	+++	+	++	+
Candida	+++	+++	++	+	+	+
Coccidioides	+	+++	+	++	++	++
Cryptococcus	+	+++	+++	+	+	+++
Histoplasma	++	+	++	+	+	+
Sporothrix	+	++	++	++	+	?

Key: +, rare; ++, occasionally to moderately frequently; +++, usually.

Figure 12-108. Signs and symptoms of fungal meningitis. The symptoms and signs of fungal meningitis, one of the many causes of chronic meningitis, vary somewhat depending on the specific organism. (*Adapted from* Tucker and colleague [71].)

Cryptococcal Meningitis

A. Clinical Presentation in Non-AIDS and AIDS Patients

Clinical presentation	Non-AIDS (%)	AIDS (%)
Headache	87	81
Fever	60	88
Nausea, vomiting, malaise	53	38
Mental status changes	52	19
Meningeal signs	50	31
Visual changes, photophobia	33	19
Seizures	15	8
No symptoms or signs	10	12

B. Laboratory Studies in Non-AIDS and AIDS Patients

Laboratory findings	Non-AIDS (%)	AIDS (%)
Positive blood culture	—	30–63
Positive serum cryptococcal antigen	66	99
CSF opening pressure >200 mm H_2O	72	62
CSF glucose <2.2 mmol/L (40 mg/dL)	73	33
CSF protein >0.45 g/L (45 mg/dL)	89	58
CSF leukocytes >20 × 10^6/L	70	23
Positive CSF India ink preparation	60	74
Positive CSF culture	96	95
Positive CSF cryptococcal antigen	86	91–100

Figure 12-109. Clinical presentations (**A**) and laboratory studies (**B**) of cryptococcal meningitis. Cryptococcus is the most frequent cause of fungal meningitis in both non-AIDS and AIDS patients. It is a chronic meningitis, but in AIDS patients it may progress even more slowly and present only with fever and headache instead of the usual manifestations of meningeal signs, mental status changes, and cranial nerve palsies.

The usual cerebrospinal fluid profile (CSF) in cryptococcal meningitis, as well as most causes of fungal meningitis is that of mononuclear (lymphocytic) pleocytosis, a low glucose level, and an elevated protein level. AIDS patients, however, often do not fit this typical CSF picture. Most striking is the fact that 65% of AIDS patients have a normal CSF cell count of fewer than 5 cells/mm^3. Diagnosis is confirmed by positive CSF culture result or a positive CSF cryptococcal antigen test. (*Adapted from* Tunkel and colleague [72].)

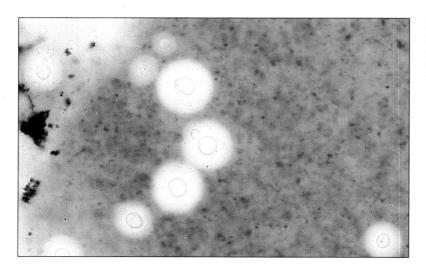

Figure 12-110. An India ink preparation used in the diagnosis of cryptococcal meningitis that demonstrates the prominent capsule of *Cryptococcus neoformans.* The India ink test is positive 50% to 60% of the time, and slightly more frequently in patients with AIDS (Fig. 12-109B). (*From* Tunkel and colleague [69]; with permission.)

Coccidioidal Meningitis

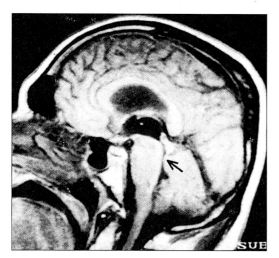

Figure 12-111. Magnetic resonance image showing enlargement of the third ventricle and the patent aqueduct (*arrow*), which are consistent findings with a communicating hydrocephalus. The diagnosis of coccidioidal meningitis depends on the recognition of the clinical picture of fungal meningitis and the extraneural manifestations of pulmonary and skin involvement. Positive cerebrospinal fluid (CSF) culture and antibody assays are required as the definitive criteria. Hydrocephalus is a common complication of coccidioidal meningitis and may be communicating or noncommunicating.

The clinical features of "cocci" meningitis are similar to those of cryptococcal meningitis except that changes in the patient's mental state are more likely to occur because of the earlier development of hydrocephalus. Other manifestations include fever, headache, and meningismus. Coccidioides is a common cause of fungal meningitis in areas where it is endemic. Fortunately, it is endemic only in the San Joaquin Valley and the desert areas of Central California. (*From* Galgiani [73]; with permission.)

Extraneural Manifestations of Fungi That Cause Meningitis

	Clinical manifestations			
Species	Respiratory tract	Skin/membranes	Hair	Bone/joints
Coccidioides	+++	++	—	+
Candida	+	+++	++	+
Histoplasma	++	+	—	—
Blastomyces	+++	+++	+	+
Sporothrix	+	++	—	++

Key: +, low frequency; ++, moderate frequency; +++, high frequency.

Figure 12-112. Extraneural clinical manifestations of fungal meningitides. Unlike cryptococcosis, other fungi that cause meningitis have extraneural clinical manifestations that may be diagnostically valuable. These extraneural infections usually involve the respiratory tract, the skin, and hair. Clinical respiratory manifestations may be upper respiratory infection or pneumonia; the chest radiogram is often abnormal.

CSF Tests for Fungal Meningitis

Species	Positive culture results	CSF serologic tests
Blastomyces dermatitidis	Rare	Ab
Candida spp.	50%	Ab/Ag
Coccidioides immitis	25%–45%	Ab
Cryptococcus neoformans	75%–80%	Ag
Dematiaceous fungi	Rare	None
Histoplasma capsulatum	50%	Ab
Paracoccidioides brasiliensis	Rare	Ab
Sporothrix schenckii	Rare	Ab

Figure 12-113. Cerebral spinal fluid (CSF) diagnostic tests for fungal meningitis. Other than extraneural manifestations, the main diagnostic studies are those performed on the CSF. Most patients with fungal meningitis have mononuclear pleocytosis, low glucose levels, and a high protein level similar to that seen in cryptococcal meningitis (Fig. 12-109). Conclusive proof of diagnosis relies on culture and antigen (Ag) and antibody (Ab) tests. Unfortunately, CSF cultures often are not positive, but the likelihood of a positive result increases by culturing a large volume of CSF (15 to 30 mL). Computed tomography or magnetic resonance imaging scans usually reveal at least some degree of hydrocephalus. Less frequently, single or multiple enhancing parenchymal lesions (abscesses) may be seen. (*Adapted from* Perfect and colleague [68].)

Differential Diagnosis of Fungal Meningitis Syndrome

Infectious	Noninfectious
Bacterial	Neoplasm
Tuberculosis	Sarcoidosis
Spirochetal (Lyme disease, syphilis, *Leptospira*)	Vasculitis
Agents that cause sinus tracts (*Actinomyces, Arachnia, Nocardia*)	Primary central nervous system angiitis
Brucellosis	Systemic (giant cell arteritis, systemic lupus erythematosus, Sjögren's syndrome, rheumatoid arthritis, lymphomatoid granulomatosis, polyarteritis nodosa, Wegener's granulomatosis)
Listeria monocytogenes	
Fungal	
Common (*Candida, Coccidioides, Cryptococcus, Histoplasma*)	
Uncommon (*Aspergillus, Blastomyces, Dematiaceous fungi, Paracoccidioides, Pseudoallescheria, Sporothrix, Mucormycetes*)	Behçet's disease
Parasitic	Chemical meningitis
Cysticercosis	Endogenous
Granulomatous amebic meningoencephalitis (acanthamoebiasis)	Exogenous
Eosinophilic meningitis (angiostrongyloidiasis)	Chronic benign lymphocytic meningitis
Toxoplasmosis	Idiopathic hypertrophic pachymeningitis
Coenurus cerebralis	Vogt-Koyanagi-Harada disease
Viral	
Retrovirus (HIV-1, human T-cell lymphotropic virus [HTLV-1])	
Enterovirus (in hypogammaglobulinemia)	
Parameningeal infections—epidural abscess, subdural empyema, brain abscess	

Figure 12-114. Differential diagnosis of fungal meningitis syndrome. Fungal meningitis is a subacute to chronic process with a course lasting over weeks to months, and the differential diagnosis of chronic meningitis is extensive. (*Adapted from* Perfect and colleague [68].)

Primary Antifungal Therapy for Fungal Meningitides

Blastomyces dermatitidis	Amphotericin B
Candida spp.	Amphotericin B/Flucytosine
Coccidioides immitis	First: Fluconazole
	Second: Amphotericin B (intrathecal)
Cryptococcus neoformans	Amphotericin B/Flucytosine
	Fluconazole for suppression in AIDS patients
Dematiaceous fungi	Surgery
Histoplasma capsulatum	Amphotericin B
Paracoccidioides brasiliensis	Intraconazole/Amphotericin B
Sporothrix schenckii	Amphotericin B

Figure 12-115. Treatment of fungal meningitis. Amphotericin B has been the main drug used for treatment of fungal meningitis for over 30 years. It remains the agent of choice alone or in combination with other treatment for most species. (*Adapted from* Perfect and colleague [68]; Davis [74].)

Fungal Abscess and Infarction

Etiology of CNS Fungal Abscess

Species	Distribution of cases (%)	Years of survey	Reference*
Total cases, 39		1964–1973	(8)
Candida spp.	49		
Crytococcus n.	23		
Mucormycoses	13		
Aspergillus spp.	5		
Histoplasmosis	5		
Total cases, 11		1955–1971	(9)
Aspergillus spp.	64		
Mucormycoses	27		
Candida spp.	9		
Total cases, 61†		1956–1985	(11)
Candida spp.	44		
Aspergillus spp.	28		
Cryptococcus n.	23		
Mucormycoses	3		
Histoplasmosis	2		
Total cases, 57‡		1984–1992	(12)
Aspergillus spp.	58		
Candida spp.	33		
Mucormycoses	5		

*References from Sepkowitz and colleague [61].

†Includes meningitis plus abscess cases.

‡Bone marrow transplant recipients.

Figure 12-116. Etiology of fungal abscess of the central nervous system (CNS). Over the last 30 years fungal abscess has become more frequent due to the use of broad-spectrum antibiotics and immunosuppressive agents as well as the AIDS epidemic. Treatment may require agents to decrease intracranial pressure (mannitol, corticosteroids), surgical decompression, and antifungal chemotherapy agents (Fig. 12-115). (*Adapted from* Sepkowitz and colleague [75].)

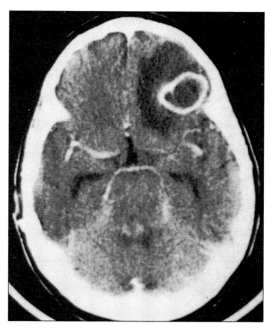

Figure 12-117. Contrast-enhanced computed tomography (CT) scan that shows an aspergilloma in a 9-year-old boy with glioblastoma multiforme. For focal central nervous system fungal infections, CT or magnetic resonance imaging are the diagnostic tests of choice. The cerebrospinal fluid analysis may be contraindicated because of increased intracranial pressure with a focal lesion. Culture specimens must be obtained at the time of surgical drainage and decompression. (*From* Sepkowitz and colleague [75]; with permission.)

Pathogenic Molds in the Central Nervous System

	Aspergillus species	Mucorales	*Pseudallescheria boydii*
Patients at risk	Hematologic neoplasm Neutropenia on broad-spectrum antibiotics Corticosteroids Organ transplants Intravenous drug use Liver disease Postcraniotomy	Diabetes with ketoacidosis (>70%) Hematologic neoplasm Neutropenia on broad-spectrum antibiotics Renal transplant Intravenous drug use Desfuroxamine Acidosis	Near-drowning Intravenous drug use Neutropenia on broad-spectrum antibiotics Hematologic malignancy
Pathogenesis	Hematogeneous Direct extension, including rhinocerebral (rare)	Rhinocerebral Hematogenous	Hematogenous Direct extension Traumatic implantation
Microscopic appearance	Septate hyphae Acute branching	Nonseptate hyphae Broad right-angle branching	Narrow septate hyphae with rare branching
Culture from CSF	Rare	Never	Occasional
Treatment	Surgery Amphotericin B ± Rifampin ? ± Fluconazole ? Itraconazole	Surgery Amphotericin B	Surgery Miconazole ? Fluconazole ? Itraconazole (Amphotericin B-resistant)

Figure 12-118. Pathogenic molds in the central nervous system. Molds may cause disease by direct extension, including rhinocerebral disease, and by invading blood vessels causing infarctions. It is rarely possible to culture these organisms from the cerebrospinal fluid (CSF) sample, but CSF antigen and antibody assays are available for *Aspergillus* sp., as is a CSF antibody assay for Zygomycetes genera (Mucorales or *Mucor*). There are no CSF antigen or antibody tests for *Pseudallescheria boydii*. Aggressive treatment with surgery to remove necrotic tissue and anti-fungal chemotherapy are needed to cure these infections. (*Adapted from* Sepkowitz and colleague [75].)

Spirochete Infections

Neurosyphilis

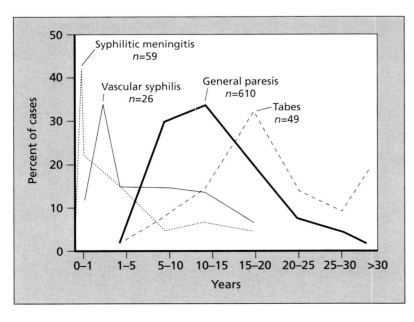

Figure 12-119. Time course for the appearance of neurosyphilic manifestations. Starting with the onset of the primary syphilitic infection of skin chancre, usually on the penis or perineum, the development of neurosyphilic syndromes over three decades is shown. Syphilitic meningitis occurs with either secondary or tertiary syphilis. All other syndromes of neurosyphilis occur during the tertiary stage. All forms of syphilis of the central nervous system ultimately result from active meningeal inflammation. When the meningeal inflammation extends to the cerebral blood vessels, cerebrovascular neurosyphilis results, usually within 5 years after the primary infection. The parenchymal forms of neurosyphilis—general paresis (dementia) and tabes dorsalis—occur after 5 years. Although each syndrome has a predictable time course, appearances often overlap and several syndromes may occur at the same time. (*Adapted from* Simon [76].)

Classification of Neurosyphilis

Type	Clinical symptoms	Pathologic	CSF leukocyte (cells/mm^3)	Brain CT or MRI
Asymptomatic	No symptoms; CSF abnormal	Various. Chiefly leptomeningitis; arteritis or encephalitis may be present	<5 >5	Normal Meningeal enhancement
Meningeal and vascular Cerebral meningeal Diffuse (syphilitic meningitis)	Increased intracranial pressure; cranial nerve palsies	Leptomeningitis with hydrocephalus; degeneration of cranial nerves; arteritis	5 or more	Meningeal enhancement
Focal (gumma)	Increased intracranial pressure; focal cerebral symptoms and signs of slow onset	Granuloma formation (gumma)	Any	Mass lesion
Cerebrovascular	Focal cerebral symptoms and signs of sudden onset	Endarteritis with infarcts	Any	Subcortical or cortical infarct
Spinal meningeal and vascular	Paresthesia, weakness, atrophy, and sensory loss in limbs and trunk	Admixture of endarteritis and meningeal infiltration and thickening with degeneration of nerve roots and substance of the cord—myelomalacia	Any	NA
Parenchymatous Tabetic	Pain, paresthesia, crises, ataxia, impairment of pupillary reflexes, loss of tendon reflexes, impaired proprioceptive sensation, and trophic changes	Leptomeningitis and degenerative changes in posterior roots, dorsal funiculi, and brain stem	Any	NA
Paretic	Personality changes, convulsions, and dementia	Meningoencephalitis	Any	Optic atrophy
Optic atrophy	Loss of vision, pallor of optic discs	Leptomeningitis and atrophy of optic nerves	Any	NA

Figure 12-120. Classification of neurosyphilis. Neurosyphilis encompasses several different syndromes because the causative organism, *Treponema pallidum*, is able to infect the meninges, the blood vessels, and the brain and spinal cord parenchyma. Asymptomatic neurosyphilis is diagnosed by positive serologic findings in both the blood and the cerebrospinal fluid (CSF). CSF pleocytosis with mononuclear cells could allow diagnosis of asymptomatic syphilitic meningitis. CT—computed tomography; MRI—magnetic resonance imaging. NA—not applicable. (*Adapted from* Rowland [77].)

Cranial Nerve Palsies in Syphilitic Meningitis*

Cranial nerves	Percent of abnormalities
I	2
II	27
III	24
IV	2
V	12
VI	22
VII	41
VIII	42
IX–X	6
XI	1
XII	4

354 cranial nerve palsies in 195 patients.

Figure 12-121. Cranial nerve palsies in syphilitic meningitis. Symptomatic meningeal syphilis usually occurs during the first 2 years after the primary infection. In approximately 10% of cases, syphilitic meningitis occurs with the rash of secondary syphilis, but most cases occur during the tertiary stage. Patients present with headache, meningismus, and malaise. They may or may not have a low-grade fever. Lymphocytic pleocytosis of up to several hundred cells occurs; the cerebrospinal fluid (CSF) glucose level is reduced, but usually is greater than 25 mg/dL; CSF protein level is increased and may exceed 100 mg/dL; and the CSF pressure may be elevated. This syndrome is diagnosed with positive blood and CSF serologic tests (serologic tests for syphilis: Veneral Disease Research Laboratories [VDRL], rapid plasma reagin [RPR]). The syndrome may resolve on its own or complications may ensue. Because the meningitis is most concentrated at the base, cranial nerve palsies are often seen, sometimes bilaterally but usually asymmetrically. Obstruction of CSF pathways may result in subacute to chronic hydrocephalus. (*Adapted from* Merrit and colleagues [78].)

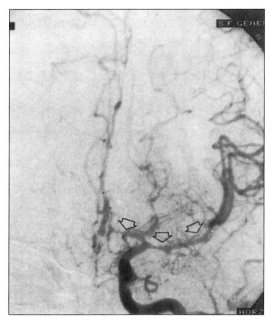

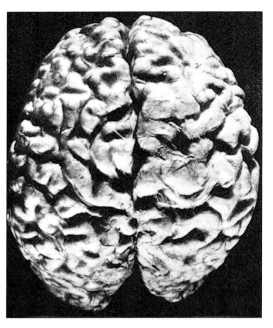

Figure 12-122. Anteroposterior view, left carotid angiogram, of a 26-year-old man with meningovascular syphilis, showing constriction (*arrows*) of the anterior and middle segments of the middle cerebral artery. Cerebrovascular syphilis occurs when the inflammation in the subarachnoid space compromises arteries traversing this space. Vasculitis of middle-sized vessels occurs, resulting in ischemia. The middle cerebral artery is affected most often, but any cerebral or spinal vessel may be involved. Stroke syndromes occurring in neurosyphilis are no different than those seen from other causes; focal clinical manifestations are determined by which vessel is involved. The patients exhibit risk factors for venereal disease and are usually younger than those with athrosclerotic infarction. Differentiation depends upon the blood and cerebrospinal fluid serologic results. Computed tomographic or magnetic resonance imaging scans of the brain reveal cortical or subcortical infarction. If the meningeal inflammation is intense enough, a prodrome of headache and personality change may precede the stroke by weeks (meningovascular syphilis). Penicillin effectively cures the infection, preventing further infarctions. (*From* Simon and colleague [79].)

Figure 12-123. Pathologic specimen from a brain with paretic neurosyphilis. Paretic neurosyphilis has also been referred to as general paresis of the insane, syphilitic meningoencephalitis, dementia paralytica, and syphilitic dementia. Symptoms usually begin 5 to 15 years after the primary infection, with a range of 3 to 30 years. Paretic neurosyphilis was common in the pre-antibiotic era but is now infrequent. The symptoms and signs of general paresis are similar to any organic brain syndrome. Progressive dementia with personality changes is the most common feature. Behavioral changes with psychosis and grandiose delusional states are unusual. Seizures also are seen. Masked facies, tremors of the face, tongue, lips, and extremities, dysarthria and hyperactive reflexes may also occur. Pathologically there is chronic meningoencephalitis with cortical atrophy, enlarged ventricles, thickened meninges, and granular ependymitis. Microscopic lesions include mononuclear inflammatory cells, a prominent microglial rod cell response, and the presence of the organisms. Diagnosis depends upon cerebrospinal fluid (CSF) abnormalities and serologic results. Usually patients are younger (less than 50 years of age) than those with other causes of dementia. Penicillin is an effective therapy and usually arrests the progression of the dementia but will not reverse the existing damage. (*From* Merrit and colleagues [78]; with permission.)

A. Symptoms and Signs of Tabetic Neurosyphilis (Analysis of 150 Cases)

Symptoms	%	Signs	%
Lancinating pain	75	Abnormal pupils	94
Ataxia	42	Argyll-Robertson	48
Bladder disturbance	33	Other abnormalities	46
Paresthesia	24	Absent reflexes	
Gastric or visceral crises	18	Ankle jerks	94
Optic atrophy	16	Knee jerks	81
Rectal incontinence	14	Biceps and triceps	11
Deafness	7	Romberg sign	55
Impotence	4	Impaired sensations	
		Vibratory sense	52
		Position sense	45
		Touch and pain	13
		Ocular palsy	10
		Charcot joints	7

Figure 12-124. Symptoms and signs of tabetic neurosyphilis. Tabetic neurosyphilis is also referred to as tabes dorsalis because of the degeneration of the posterior columns. Tabes usually begins 10 to 20 years after the primary infection, but some cases have had onset after 30 years (range 5 to 50 years). **A,** The most common and classic symptoms of tabes are the lancinating or lightning-like pains, ataxia, and bladder dysfunction. Prominent signs include abnormal pupils including Argyll Robertson pupils, absent reflexes in the lower extremities, loss of posterior column sensations, Romberg sign, and gait ataxia. As the disease progresses, bladder dysfunction and the sensory gait ataxia usually become the most disabling problems. Loss of deep pain sensation may occur with Abadie's sign (loss or delayed recognition of pain when the Achilles tendon is squeezed). Charcot's joints and distal extremity ulcerations may be seen.

(Continued on next page)

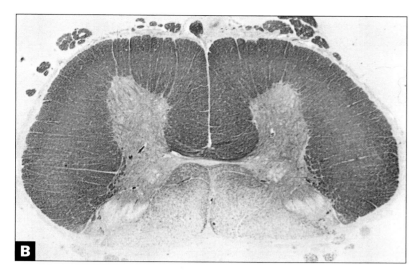

Figure 12-124. (*Continued*) **B**, Pathologically, degeneration of the posterior columns and dorsal roots occurs. Diagnosis is relatively easy because of the classic clinical manifestations, with positive serologic results, at least in the blood samples. The disease may arrest spontaneously or may be arrested with antibiotic treatment. The latter is more likely to occur when there are signs of active inflammation in the cerebrospinal fluid (CSF). Even after treatment, and even when there is no active CSF inflammation (as regards CSF pleocytosis), many of the manifestations may continue to progress. The pathogenesis of tabes is not understood. In contrast to paretic cortical lesions, spirochetes are not found in the affected areas of the spinal cord, which may explain why antibiotic therapy may not stop progression. (Panel A *adapted from* Merrit and colleagues [78]; Panel B *from* Wilson [4]; with permission.)

Frequency of Different Forms of Symptomatic Neurosyphilis*

| | Preantibiotic era | | | Antibiotic era | | AIDS era | |
| | | | | | | HIV (-) | HIV (+) or AIDS |
	1	2	3	4	5	6	7
Tabetic	45	48	45	15	11	5	0
Paretic	17	18	8	12	4	9	4
Taboparetic	4	7	9	23	23	—	—
Vascular	15	19	9	19	61	41	38
Meningeal	8	8	19	23	0	23	46
Optic neuritis	4	—	—	—	—	14	42
Spinal cord	4	—	10	8	—	—	—

*Numbers are a percentage of cases.

1 Merritt, Adams, Solomon, 1946 (457 patients).

2 Kierland et al., 1942 (2019 patients).

3 Wolters, 1987 (518 patients, 1930–1940).

4 Wolters, 1987 (121 patients, 1970–1984).

5 Burke, Schaberg, 1985 (26 patients).

6, 7 Katz et al., 1993.

Figure 12-125. Frequency of different forms of symptomatic neurosyphilis. Following the introduction of penicillin, the frequency of neurosyphilis per hospital admission fell from 5.9 per 100,000 population in 1942 to 0.1 per 100,000 in 1965. Beginning in the 1980s and coincident with the AIDS epidemic, this trend has been reversed. The incidence of neurosyphilis is unknown, but the incidence of primary and secondary syphilis has risen from 13.7 per 100,000 population in 1981 to a peak of 20.1 per 100,000 in 1990. Since then the incidence has dropped significantly, perhaps because of better surveillance and education. The overall frequency of neurosyphilis in HIV-positive and AIDS patients is estimated to be 2%. Also during the 1980s and 1990s, a shift has occurred toward meningeal and vascular forms of neurosyphilis and a decline in the parenchymal forms. This may be related to cerebrospinal fluid abnormalities of neurosyphilis in HIV-infected patients, which are more intense than those of non–HIV-infected patients. As the mean leukocyte count increases, the mean protein level becomes higher and the mean glucose level becomes lower [80]. In addition, this shift may be an artifact of closer follow-up studies and earlier diagnoses of other diseases of AIDS patients. (*Adapted from* Rowland [76].)

CSF Findings in Neurosyphilis by Clinical Syndrome (Subtype)

Neurosyphilic syndrome	OP mm H$_2$O	Leukocyte level (per mm^3)	Glucose level (mg/dL)	Protein level (mg/dL)	VDRL Blood	VDRL CSF
Meningitic	210–400* (<200->400)	100–500[†] (<10–2000)	20–40 (<20->80)	45–200 (<45–400)	1:64	1:4
Cerebrovascular	<200 (>200–250)	10–100 (<10->100)	Normal to mildly decreased	100–200 (15–260)	1:512	1:16
Paretic	<200 (<200–300)	10–100 (<10->100	Normal to mildly decreased	45–100 (29–500)	1:128	1:8
Tabetic	<200 (<200–300)	Active 5–50 (5–165) Inactive 0–5	Normal	45–100 (14–250)	Active 1:15 Inactive 1:16	1:28 1:2

Numbers without parentheses are the common range. Numbers in parentheses are the overall range.

[†]*CSF pleocytosis is usually 80% to 100% lymphocytic mononuclear.*

Figure 12-126. Abnormalities of cerebrospinal fluid (CSF) in neurosyphilis. The diagnosis of active neurosyphilis is based upon a compatible clinical syndrome, an inflammatory CSF profile, and reactive serologic tests in the blood (treponemal antibody test) and CSF (nontreponemal test). CSF pleocytosis (primarily lymphocytic) is the best measure of disease activity. The number of cells varies with each clinical subtype, being maximal in the earlier acute-like stage of syphilitic meningitis. The glucose level is usually low in syphilitic meningitis and is more likely to be normal for other subtypes. CSF protein levels are usually elevated for all subtypes. The CSF gamma globulin level may be increased and oligoclonal bands may be present. OP—opening pressure, VDRL—Venereal Disease Research Laboratory. (*Adapted from* Simon and colleague [79].)

Serologic Tests Used in the Diagnosis of Neurosyphilis

Test	Abnormality required for diagnosis	False/positive tests
FTA-ABS or MHA-TP	+ in blood required - excludes diagnosis	Rare Other spirochete diseases Autoimmune diseases, especially systemic lupus erythematosus (SLE)

VDRL	+ in CSF required for diagnosis - in CSF inactive or no neurosyphilis	Contamination of CSF by blood
		CSF paraprotein
		Very high CSF protein level
		Autoimmune disease (such as SLE)
		Strong immunologic stimulus
		  Acute bacterial or viral infections
		  Early HIV infection
		  Vaccination
		Central nervous system neoplasia
		Drug addiction
		Pregnancy
		Chronic liver disease

Figure 12-127. Serologic tests used in the diagnosis of neurosyphilis. Diagnosis of neurosyphilis depends on a compatible clinical syndrome, an inflammatory cerebrospinal fluid (CSF) profile, and reactive serologic tests. The treponemal antibody tests are the fluorescent treponemal antibody-absorption (FTA-ABS) test and the microhemagglutination test for *Treponema pallidum* (MHA-TP). Positive blood FTA-ABS and MHA-TP are diagnostic for syphilis, as they are highly specific and remain positive for years. If these tests are negative, the diagnosis of neurosyphilis is essentially excluded; they are not useful, however, for following disease activity because they do not revert with successful treatment. These treponemal antibody tests are not useful for CSF analysis. The serologic diagnosis of neurosyphilis requires a positive blood serologic result and a reactive CSF serologic test for syphilis (STS). The two STS tests used currently are the Venereal Disease Research Laboratory (VDRL) test and the rapid plasma reagin (RPR) test. The RPR test cannot be used on the CSF. The CSF VDRL test can be used to follow disease activity after treatment but is not as reliable as the CSF pleocytosis.

Treatment Regimens for Neurosyphilis

Established

Aqueous crystalline penicillin G, 12 to 24 million U IV daily (divided doses q4h) for 10–14 d

Approved

Aqueous procaine penicillin G, 2.4 million U IM daily, plus probenecid 500 mg po qid for 10–14 d

Under study

Ceftriaxone 1 g IV q12h

Alternate drug regimens for penicillin-allergic patients

Desensitize to penicillin (preferred alternative)

Tetracycline hydrochloride 500 mg po qid for 30 d

Doxycycline 200 mg po bid for 21 d

Erythromycin 500 mg po qid for 30 d

Chloramphenicol 1 g IV qid for 14 d

Ceftriaxone 1 g q12h (under study)

Recommended treatment regimens for syphilis in HIV-coinfected patients

No change in therapy for early syphilis (CSF examination may be a useful guide to adequate treatment)

Benzathine penicillin should not be used

Examine CSF before and following treatment as a treatment guide

Aqueous crystalline penicillin G IV, 12–24 million U daily (2–4 million U q4h)

Aqueous or procaine penicillin G, 2.4 million U IM daily plus probenecid 500 mg po qid

Figure 12-128. Treatment regimens for neurosyphilis. The cerebrospinal fluid (CSF) inflammatory process (increased cell count) is the best indicator of disease activity and should be monitored for successful treatment. Normalization of CSF pleocytosis and protein level is the ultimate goal of treatment. The CSF Venereal Disease Research Laboratory test titer should also be followed, but it is not as sensitive to treatment as the CSF pleocytosis. Penicillin remains the drug of choice with the regimens shown here. Benzathine penicillin G does not produce adequate levels in the CSF for treatment. After treatment, the clinical examination should stabilize and the blood serologic test levels should decline. The CSF is examined at 6 and 12 months after treatment. At 6 months, the cell count should be normal and protein level falling; by 12 months, both are usually normal. If cells are still present at 6 or 12 months, retreatment is required. If the protein level is still elevated at 12 months, the CSF should be reexamined in 2 years. Retreatment is required if there has been clinical progression or the CSF is still abnormal. The same treatment regimen is recommended for HIV-coinfected patients as for non-HIV patients. IV—intravenous; IM—intramuscular; po—per os (by mouth). (*Adapted from* Simon and colleague [79].)

Lyme Disease

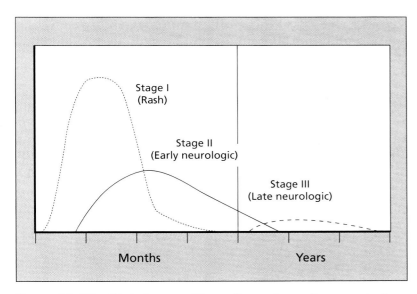

Figure 12-129. Clinical stages of Lyme disease. Lyme disease results from infection by the spirochete *Borrelia burgdoferi*, which is transmitted by ticks. Lyme disease may develop into a chronic persistent infection in a fashion somewhat similar to syphilis. For this reason, Lyme disease has been divided into stages. The nervous system is involved clinically in 10% to 15% of patients. Stage I, the acute stage, is characterized by a rash—erythema chronicum migrans (ECM)—which is an erythematous ring that develops around the tick bite site about 8 to 9 (range 3 to 32) days after exposure.

Smaller secondary (migratory) rings may occur later. Neurologic manifestations may occur in stage I concurrently with ECM, but they are more frequent in stage II. Stage II, the subacute stage, is characterized by prominent cardiac and neurologic manifestations. This stage usually begins several months after the bite and the onset of ECM. Stage III, the chronic stage, is characterized by chronic arthritis. Neurologic manifestations also occur in stage III but they are less prominent than those of stage II. Stage III usually begins about 1 year after onset.

In the acute stage I, a systemic flu-like syndrome with fever, chills, and malaise may occur. Neurologic manifestations include headache and neck stiffness but normal cerebrospinal fluid (CSF) parameters. Stage II is also referred to as the "early neurologic stage" because dissemination of the organism to the central nervous system begins. During this stage, aseptic meningitis with complications of cranial nerve palsies, especially facial (Bell's palsy), and radiculoneuritis are most prominent. The facial or Bell's palsy is usually bilateral. The radiculoneuritis may take the form of a Guillain-Barré-like syndrome, but the CSF shows pleocytosis; sometimes the radiculoneuritis is focal. Occasionally, mild meningoencephalitis along with irritability, emotional lability, decreased concentration and memory, and sleep abnormalities may occur.

Stage III or the chronic stage is also referred to as the "late neurologic stage." This stage is characterized by chronic or late persistent infection of the nervous system. Syndromes included in this stage are encephalopathy, encephalomyelopathy, and polyneuropathy. The encephalopathy is characterized by memory and other cognitive dysfunction. The encephalomyelopathic signs are combined with progressive long tract signs and optic nerve involvement. White matter lesions may be visible on magnetic resonance imaging of the brain. The late polyneuropathy is primarily sensory. (*Adapted from* Davis [81].)

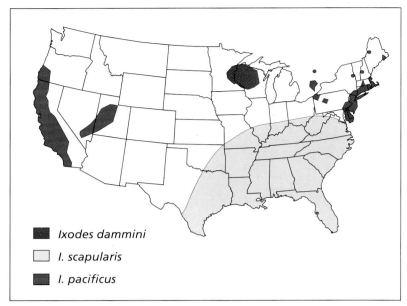

Ixodes dammini

I. scapularis

I. pacificus

Figure 12-130. Epidemiology of Lyme disease. Lyme disease accounts for about 90% of the vector-borne infections in the United States. In 2000, nearly 20,000 cases were reported to the Centers for Disease Control and Prevention. *Borrelia burgdorferi*, the spirochete that causes Lyme disease, is transmitted by *Ixodes* species (hard body) ticks. Up to 50% of human infections are asymptomatic. The infection rate of different *Ixodes* species carrying the spirochete depends on the species. *I. dammini* (deer tick) is the principal vector in the Northeast (30% to 60% infection rate) and the Midwest (10% to 15% infection rate). *I. pacificanus* (Western black-legged tick) is the vector in the West (1% to 5% infection rate). In the southeastern United States, *I. scapularis* is the vector but its infection rate is much lower even than that of *I. pacificanus*. The various infection rates of the different *Ixodes* species explains why 10 states account for almost 90% of the cases: New York (40%), followed by Connecticut, New Jersey, Pennsylvania, Rhode Island, Massachusetts, Maryland, Wisconsin, Minnesota, and California. In the figure, the circles with center dots indicate collection sites outside the main range of *I. dammini*. (*Adapted from* Anderson [82].)

CSF Analysis in Lyme Disease Encephalomyelitis

Test	CSF findings
Opening pressure*	Normal
Total leukocytes/mm^3	166 (15–700)†
Percent lymphocytes	93 (40–100)
Glucose (mg/dL)‡	49 (33–61)
Protein (mg/dL)	79 (8–400)
IgG/albumin ratio (*n* = 20)	0.18 (0.9–0.44)
Oligoclonal bands (*n* = 4)	Present
Myelin basic protein (*n* = 5)	Absent
VDRL (*n* = 20)	Negative

*n = 38, except where noted.
†Median (range).
‡Serum glucose = 95 (87–113).

Figure 12-131. Cerebrospinal fluid (CSF) analysis in Lyme disease encephalomyelitis. CSF is usually abnormal in central nervous system Lyme disease and generally normal in peripheral nervous system (PNS) syndromes unless there is radicular involvement. CSF analysis is usually abnormal and has a higher diagnostic yield than electroencephalography (usually normal or nonspecific) or magnetic resonance imaging (25% have small cerebral white matter lesions). CSF analysis also offers the opportunity to test for the intrathecal production of *Borrelia burgdorferi* antibodies. VDRL—Venereal Disease Research Laboratory. (*Adapted from* Pachner and colleague [83].)

Causes of False-Positive and False-Negative Lyme Serologic Tests

False-positive
  Cross-reactive spirochetal infection (*eg*, mouth treponemes, syphilis, leptospirosis, relapsing fever)
  Severe bacterial infections
  Hypergammaglobulinemia
  Epstein-Barr virus
  Autoimmune disorders with high autoantibody titers
  Human immunodeficiency virus infection
  Unreliable assay
False-Negative
  Too early in the infection
  Early antibiotics with blunted humoral response
  Unreliable assay

Figure 12-132. Causes of false-positive and false-negative Lyme disease serologic tests. Serum antibodies, when present, prove exposure to the agent but cannot be used to determine when the infection occurred. Most antibody assays are now performed by an enzyme-linked immunosorbent assay (ELISA) technique. Western blots should be used on a restricted basis to pursue suspected false-positive ELISA results. The demonstration of elevated *Borrelia burgdorferi* antibodies in the cerebrospinal fluid is essentially diagnostic. About 95% of Lyme disease patients are seropositive, but false-positive and false-negative test results may occur. (*Adapted from* Coyle [84].)

Neurologic Conditions in Which Lyme Disease Should Be Considered

Central Nervous System	Peripheral Nervous System
Acute aseptic meningitis	Cranial neuritis (Bell's palsy)
Chronic lymphocytic meningitis	Mononeuritis simplex or multiplex
Acute meningoencephalitis	Radiculoneuritis
Acute focal encephalitis	Plexitis
Brain stem encephalitis	Distal axonal neuropathy
Progressive encephalomyelitis	Demyelinating neuropathy
Cerebral demyelination, including multiple sclerosis	Carpal tunnel syndrome
Cerebral vasculitis	Focal myositis
Dementia	
Transverse myelitis	

Figure 12-133. Differential diagnosis of Lyme disease. The combination of meningitis, neuritis, and radiculitis without fever is highly suggestive of Lyme disease. If a history of tick exposure or erythema chronicum migrans is obtained, the diagnosis can be made with confidence. Because of the involvement of both the peripheral and the central nervous systems, the differential diagnosis is varied and extensive. (*Adapted from* Reik [85].)

Antibiotic Therapy for Neurologic Symptoms of Lyme Disease

Manifestations	Treatment
ECM and systemic symptoms	
Adults	Amoxicillin, 500 mg po tid for 14–28 d (plus probenecid, 500 mg po tid)*
	Doxycycline, 100 mg po bid for 14–28 d
	Cefuroxime axetil, 500 mg po bid for 14–28 d†
Children (≤8 y)	Amoxicillin, 25–50 mg/kg po daily in 3 divided doses for 14–28 d
	Erythromycin, 30 mg/kg po daily in 4 divided doses for 14–28 d
	Cefuroxime axetil, 250 mg po bid for 14–28 d†
Early neurologic involvement	
Facial palsy alone	Oral antibiotics as for ECM -
All others	
Adults	Ceftriaxone, 2 g IV daily for 14–28 d
	Cefotaxime, 2 g IV tid for 14–28 d
	Penicillin G, 20–24 million U IV daily for 10–14 days
	Doxycycline, 100 mg po bid for 14–28 d
Children	Ceftriaxone, 75–100 mg/kg IV daily for 14–28 d
	Penicillin G, 300,000 U/kg IV daily for 10–14 d
Late neurologic involvement	
Adults	Penicillin, ceftriaxone, or cefotaxime IV as for early involvement
	Doxycycline, 100–200 mg po bid for 30 d
Children	Penicillin or ceftriaxone IV as for early involvement

* Optional

† Alternative

Figure 12-134. Antibiotic therapy for neurologic syndromes of Lyme disease. The antibiotic therapy for neurologic syndromes depends on the specific stage of Lyme disease. Ceftriaxone IV is now usually considered the drug of choice for stages II (early neurologic stage) or III (late neurologic stage). Most symptoms resolve with antibiotic treatment, but motor signs may last for 7 to 8 weeks. The duration of therapy has never been clarified. A postinfectious syndrome with symptoms of fatigue, headache, and muscle and joint pain may last for months to several years. ECM—erythema chronic migrans; IV—intravenous; po—per os (by mouth). (*Adapted from* Reik [86].)

Parasitic Infections

Major Protozoan and Helminthic Infections of the Central Nervous System

Protozoan	Nematodes (roundworms)	Trematodes (flukes)
Toxoplasmosis	Trichinosis	Schistosomiasis
Cerebral malaria	Eosinophilic meningoencephalitis	Paragonimiasis
Trypanosomiasis	*Angiostrongylus cantonensis*	Cestodes (tapeworms)
Amebic meningo-encephalitis	*Gnathostoma spinigerum*	Cysticercosis
	Strongyloidiasis	Hydatid disease (*Echinococcus*)
	Toxocariasis (visceral larva migrans)	
	Human filariases	
	Onchocerciasis (river blindness)	
	Dracunculiasis	

Figure 12-135. Major protozoan and helminthic infections of the central nervous system. Toxoplasmosis is the most important protozoan infection in developed countries, where it occurs in immunosuppressed individuals. Worldwide malaria is the most important protozoan infection. Cysticercosis is probably the most important helminthic infection causing central nervous system disease. (*Adapted from* Coda [87].)

Protozoa

Protozoan Infections of the Nervous System

Disease/parasite	Geographic distribution	Risk factors	Neurologic disease
Toxoplasmosis			
Toxoplasma gondii	Worldwide	Perinatal infection, immunosuppression	Diffuse, focal, or multifocal encephalitis, chorioretinitis
Malaria			
Plasmodium falciparum	Tropics and subtropics	Mosquitoes	Acute encephalopathy
Trypanosomiasis			
African			
Trypanosoma gambiense	Tropical West African forest	Tsetse flies	Chronic encephalitis
T. rhodesiense	East equatorial Africa		Subacute meningoencephalitis
South American			
T. cruzi	Mexico to South America	Reduviid bugs	Acute meningoencephalitis (rare)
			Chronic parasympathetic denervation of gastrointestinal tract
Amebiasis			
Entamoeba histolytica	Worldwide	Poor water and sewage, institutionalized persons, homosexuals	Brain abscess (rare)
Naegleria	Worldwide	Freshwater sports	Acute meningoencephalitis
Acanthamoeba	Worldwide	Immunosuppression	Subacute or chronic meningoencephalitis

Figure 12-136. Protozoan infections of the nervous system. Protozoa are small, single-cell organisms that cause diffuse more often than focal encephalitis of the nervous system. Protozoa do not cause allergic reactions and eosinophilia as do many of the helminthic infections. (*Adapted from* Johnson and colleagues [88].)

Toxoplasmosis

Clinical Manifestations of Toxoplasmosis

Congenital disease	%	Immunocompromised host	%
Retinochoroiditis	87	Altered mental status	75
Abnormal cerebrospinal fluid	55	Fever	10–72
Anemia	51	Seizures	33
Convulsions	50	Headache	56
Intracranial calcifications	50	Focal neurologic signs	60
Jaundice	29	Motor deficits	
Fever	25	Cranial nerve palsies	
Splenomegaly	21	Movement disorders	
Hepatomegaly	17	Dysmetria	
		Visual field loss	
		Aphasia	

Figure 12-137. Clinical manifestations of toxoplasmosis. Congenital toxoplasmosis is a systemic illness causing chorioretinitis, microencephaly, seizures, mental retardation (from encephalitis), and cerebral calcifications in newborns. Cases in immunocompromised patients are frequent, thus, toxoplasmosis is a common opportunistic infection in AIDS patients that usually occurs because of reactivation. (*Adapted from* Luft and colleague [89].)

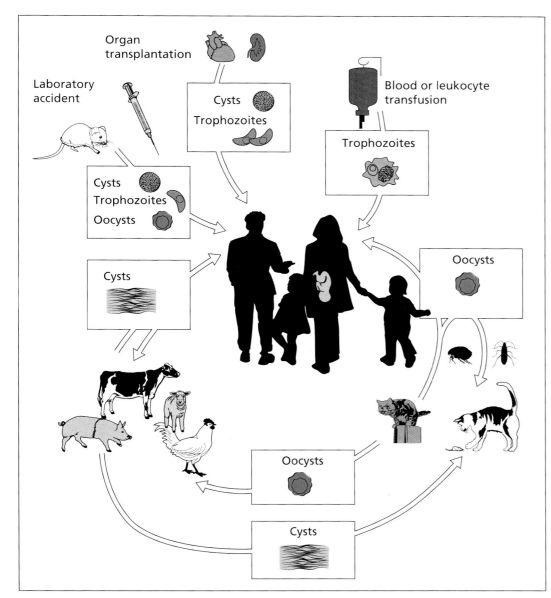

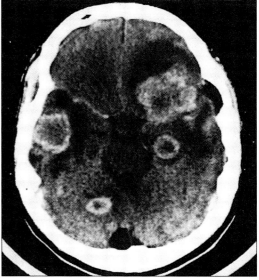

Figure 12-139. Enhanced T1-weighted magnetic resonance image (MRI) of toxoplasmosis in an AIDS patient showing multiple ring and nodular enhancing lesions. The complete blood count may reveal anemia, leukopenia, or leukocytosis in congenital toxoplasmosis. In most AIDS patients, disease is limited to the brain. The cerebrospinal fluid (CSF) is abnormal in about half the patients with congenital toxoplasmosis and in most patients with AIDS. Lymphocytic pleocytosis is usually mild but may be as high as several thousand cells/mm^3. The protein level is increased and the glucose level is usually normal or rarely mildly reduced. Isolation of the organism is difficult, as it requires inoculation of laboratory mice; therefore, a presumptive diagnosis can be made based on serologic tests in the appropriate clinical setting. The demonstration of IgM antibodies is most helpful for the diagnosis of congenital or acute acquired infection. In AIDS and other immunosuppressed patients, IgG, but not IgM, antibody is usually present. CSF antibodies may also be detected. Other than serologic testing, neuroimaging is the diagnostic study of choice. In congenital toxoplasmosis the skull radiograph may reveal multiple intracerebral calcifications. The enhanced computed tomography scan of toxoplasmosis in AIDS patients reveals multiple ring enhancing, hypodense lesions with surrounding edema as does the MRI scan shown here. (*From* Farrar and colleagues [91]; with permission.)

Figure 12-138. Transmission of toxoplasmosis. Most often *Toxoplasma gondii* infection occurs by eating undercooked meat or other foods contaminated with cat feces containing oocysts. Common-source outbreaks have occurred in families from contaminated food. Unpasteurized milk and water are also possible sources of infection. In addition to exposure to cats and eating undercooked meats, warm humid climates and poor sanitation correlate with a greater prevalence of infection. Primary infection in the immunocompetent host is usually asymptomatic. Rarely, symptomatic severe primary infection occurs. Usually tissue cysts persist and reactivation is prevented unless immunity wanes, as occurs in AIDS or other immunosuppressive events (such as therapy for cancer and transplantation). (*Adapted from* Berger [90].)

Guidelines for Treatment of Toxoplasma Encephalitis in AIDS

Drug	Dosage schedule
Standard regimens	
Pyrimethamine	Oral, 200 mg loading dose, then 50 to 75 mg daily
Folinic acid (leucovorin)	Oral, IV, or IM, 10–20 mg daily (up to 50 mg daily)
plus	
Sulfadiazine	Oral, 1–1.5 g q6h
or	
Clindamycin	Oral or IV, 600 mg q6h (up to IV 1200 mg q6h)
Possible alternative regimens	
Trimethoprim/sulfamethoxazole	Oral or IV 5 mg (trimethoprim component)/kg q6h
Pyrimethamine and folinic acid	As in standard regimens plus one of the following:
Clarithromycin	Oral, 1 g q12h
Azithromycin	Oral, 1200–1500 mg daily
Atovaquone	Oral, 750 mg q6h
Dapsone	Oral, 100 mg daily

Figure 12-140. Guidelines for treatment of toxoplasma encephalitis in AIDS. The prognosis is poor in the congenital form of toxoplasmosis, with death occurring within weeks of birth in more than 50% of cases. Mental retardation and other neurologic defects are common in survivors. The prognosis for reactivated infections in immunocompromised patients is also poor. In AIDS patients, empiric therapy is instituted when IgG antibody and characteristic computed tomography findings are found. Pyrimethamine and sulfadiazine are the agents of choice. IM—intramuscular; IV—intravenous. (*Adapted from* Beaman and colleagues [92].)

Cerebral Malaria

Clinical Manifestations of Cerebral Malaria

Common	Less common	Possible systemic manifestations
Headache, meningismus, photophobia	Monoparesis and hemiparesis	Hyperpyrexia
Seizures	Aphasia	Anemia
Behavioral and cognitive changes	Hemianopia	Hepatosplenomegaly
Delirium	Ataxia, tremor, myoclonus	Hypoglycemia
Coma	Cranial nerve palsies	Disseminated intravascular coagulation
	Papilledema	Pulmonary edema
	Blindness	Renal failure
	Deafness	Shock
	Spinal cord lesions	
	Polyneuritis	

Figure 12-141. Clinical manifestations of cerebral malaria. The symptoms and signs of cerebral malaria are primarily those of acute encephalopathy. These neurologic manifestations usually occur in the second or third week of infection. The disease occurs most often in infants, children, and nonimmune travelers to endemic areas. (*Adapted from* Berger [90].)

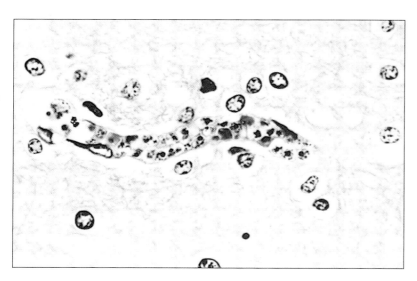

Figure 12-142. A brain capillary with parasitized erythrocytes in a patient with cerebral malaria. The neurologic manifestations are due to the congestion and obstruction of capillaries and venules with parasitized erythrocytes. Parasitized erythrocytes are less deformable than normal erythrocytes and more adherent to vascular endothelial cells. Thrombotic occlusions, microinfarctions, microhemorrhages, and cerebral edema result. Large infarctions and hemorrhage are unusual.

Malaria is the most common human parasitic disease in the world, with a prevalence of 250 to 300 million people and a yearly death rate of 1 to 2 million. The disease is endemic in tropical and subtropical areas of Asia, Africa, and Central and South America. Nervous system involvement occurs in about 2% of infected patients. Cerebral malaria is caused only by *Plasmodium falciparum*. (*From* Oo and colleagues [93]; with permission.)

Parenteral Antimalarial Therapy for Cerebral Malaria

	Type of dose	Dosage
Cinchona alkaloids*	IV	
Quinine dichloride	Loading	7 mg salt/kg over 30 min (infusion pump) followed immediately by 10 mg/kg over 4 h
		or
		20 mg salt/kg over 4 h
	Maintenance	10 mg/kg over 4 h repeated 8–12 h[†,‡]
	IM	
	Loading	20 mg salt/kg (dilute IV formulation to 60 mg/ml given by deep IM injection divided between both anterior thighs)
Quinidine gluconate	Maintenance	10 mg salt/kg 8–12 h[†,‡]
	IV	
	Loading	10 mg salt/kg infused over 1–2 h
		or
		20 mg salt/kg infused over 4 h
Artemisinin derivatives¶	Maintenance	0.02 mg salt/kg/min continuously for up to 72 h[†,‡,§]
Artesunate**		*or*
		10 mg salt/kg infused over 4 h q8–12 h[†,‡]
Artemether	Loading	2.4 mg/kg
	Maintenance	1.2 mg/kg daily for 6 d
	Loading	3.2 mg/kg
	Maintenance	1.6 mg/kg daily for 6 d

*Avoid loading dose if quinine, quinidine, or mefloquine was taken in previous 24 h.

†Change to oral quinine as soon as possible and complete 7 days' treatment.

‡Add tetracycline 1 g/d in 4 divided doses for 7 days in nonpregnant adults in some areas.

§Adjust rate of quinidine infusion to maintain blood level at 3–7 mg/L and prevent prolongation of QRS >50%, QTc >25% of pretreatment values.

¶Not marketed/licensed in many countries.

**Artesunate is reconstituted with bicarbonate solution immediately before use.

Figure 12-143.
Treatment of cerebral malaria. The diagnosis of cerebral malaria is made from the clinical presentation and by finding the organisms in the blood. The mortality rate for cerebral malaria is 15% to 40%, with the highest mortality rate in those patients with coma and seizures. Treatment has classically been with chloroquine, but chloroquine-resistant falciparum malaria requires treatment with quinine plus Fansidar. IM—intramuscular; IV—intravenous. (*Adapted from* Newtown and colleague [94].)

Trypanosomiasis

Comparison of West African and East African Trypanosomiasis

	West African (*T. gambiense*)	East African (*T. rhodesiense*)
Organism	*T. b. gambiense*	*T. b. rhodesiense*
Vectors	Tsetse flies (*palpalis* group)	Tsetse flies (*morsitans* group)
Primary reservoir	Humans	Antelope and cattle
Human illness	Chronic (late CNS disease)	Acute (early CNS disease)
Duration of illness	Months to years	<9 months
Lymphadenopathy	Prominent	Minimal
Parasitemia	Low	High
Diagnosis by rodent inoculation	No	Yes
Epidemiology	Rural populations	Tourists in game parks Workers in wild areas Rural populations

Figure 12-144. Comparison of West African and East African trypanosomiasis. There are two varieties of human trypanosomiasis, an African form (sleeping sickness) and a South American form (Chagas disease), which is caused by *Trypanosoma cruzi*. The African disease is of two types. The West African form is caused by *Trypanosoma brucei gambiense* and the East African variety by *T. brucei rhodesiense*. The East African disease is more acute, leading to death in weeks to months. CNS—central nervous system. (*Adapted from* Kirchhoff [95].)

Clinical Manifestations of African Trypanosomiasis

Stage I—febrile or hemolymphatic stage
  Remitting fever
  Circinate rash and pruritus
  Lymphadenitis
  Transient edema of face and hands
  Hepatosplenomegaly
  Headache
  Asthenia
  Arthralgia
  Myalgia
  Weight loss

Stage II—lethargic or meningo-
    encephalitic stage
  Headache
  Irritability
  Personality change with apathy
  Organic mental syndrome
  Insomnia or somnolence
  Tremor
  Ataxia
  Convulsions
  Paralysis
  Coma

Figure 12-145. Clinical manifestations of African trypanosomiasis. The signs and symptoms of West and East African trypanosomiasis are basically the same, except that the West African form has a more acute course of weeks to months while the East African form has a more chronic course of months to years. These diseases pass through two stages: stage I is the systemic illness, with organisms present in the blood; stage II is neurologic. The first stage usually passes imperceptibly into the second.

Clinical Manifestations of South American Trypanosomiasis

Acute stage
  Fever
  Conjunctivitis
  Palpebral and facial edema
  Lymphadenopathy
  Hepatosplenomegaly
  Acute encephalitis (rare)

Chronic stage
  Cardiac disease
  Gastrointestinal disease
  Mental alterations
  Convulsions
  Choreoathetosis
  Hemiplegia
  Ataxia
  Aphasia

Figure 12-146. Clinical manifestations of South American trypanosomiasis. The acute stage lasts about 1 month, during which trypanosomes are present in the blood. In the chronic stage, organ involvement including the nervous system occurs. This disease affects about 16 million people in Central and South America, primarily children living in rural areas. The disease is transmitted by the reduviid bug, which lives in the walls of houses. Death usually occurs within a few months or years.

Treatment of Human Trypanosomiasis

African trypanosomiasis
  Hemolymphatic (stage I)
    Suramin, 100–200 mg test dose IV, *then* 1 g IV on days 1, 3, 7, 14, 21
      or
    Eflornithine, 100 mg/kg qid × 14 days, *then* 300 mg/kg/d po × 3–4 wk
  CNS involvement (stage II)
    Eflornithine, 100 mg/kg qid × 14 days, *then* 300 mg/kg/d po × 3–4 wk
      or
    Melarsoprol, 2–3.6 mg/kg/d IV in 3 doses × 3 days, *then*, after 1 wk, 3.6 mg/kg/d IV in 3 doses × 3 days
    Repeat latter course after 10–21 days
American trypanosomiasis
  Nifurtimox, 8–10 mg/kg/d po in 4 doses × 90–120 days

Figure 12-147. Diagnosis and treatment of trypanosomiasis. Anemia occurs in all forms of trypanosomiasis. The erythrocyte sedimentation rate and serum IgM may be increased. The cerebrospinal fluid (CSF) has lymphocytic pleocytosis, normal glucose level, increased protein level, and increased IgG and IgM levels. The diagnosis is established by identifying the organism in the blood, CSF, or biopsied lymph nodes. Except for the chronic stage of American trypanosomiasis, chemotherapy is relatively effective. CNS—central nervous system; IV—intravenous; po—per os (by mouth). (*Adapted from* Berger [90].)

Amebic Meningoencephalitis

Species of Amebae Causing Amebic Meningoencephalitis

Taxonomy	Host	Pathogen	Disease
Order Amoebida			
Family Endamoebidae			
Entamoeba histolytica	Humans	Yes	Colitis, hepatic, lung, and brain abscess
Endolimax nana	Humans	No	None
Iodamoeba butschlii	Humans	No	None
Family Acanthamoebidae			
Acanthamoeba culbertsoni, A. polyphaga, A. castellani, A. astronyxis, A. palestinensis, A. rhysodes, others	Humans, mice	Yes	GAE, keratoconjunctivitis, skin lesions, mandibular bone graft infection
Order Schizopyrenida			
Family Vahlkampfidae			
Naegleria fowleri	Yes	Humans	PAM
N. australiensis	Yes	Mice	Experimental PAM
N. gruberi, N. lovaniensis	No	None known	None known
Vahlkampfia	Unproven	? Humans	? GAE or PAM
Order Leptomyxida			
Balamuthia mandrillaris	Yes	Humans, primates, sheep	GAE
Leptomyxa	No	?	?

Figure 12-148. Species of amebae causing amebic meningoencephalitis. The species primarily causing meningoencephalitis are the free-living amebae *Naegleria fowleri* and *Acanthamoeba* species. *Entamoeba histolytica* may rarely invade the brain and cause brain abscess. *Naegleria* causes acute primary amebic meningoencephalitis (PAM), whereas Acanthamoeba causes subacute or chronic PAM and granulomatous amebic encephalitis (GAE). The Leptomyxida *Balamuthia mandrillaris* has also caused GAE. These infections occur worldwide. Most cases in the United States occur in the Southeast. (*Adapted from* Durack [96].)

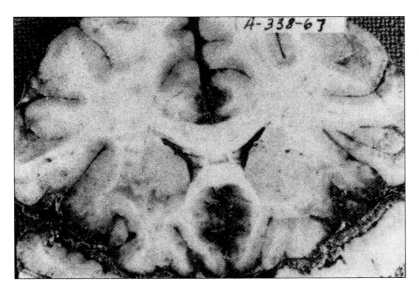

Figure 12-149. Acute primary amebic meningoencephalitis (PAM), with the most severe lesions in the basal meninges and adjacent cortex. *Acanthamoeba* causes subacute or chronic PAM, including granulomatous amebic encephalitis (GAE), usually as an opportunistic infection in immunosuppressed patients. The respiratory tract is probably the portal of entry, resulting in systemic infection with seeding of the brain through hematogenous spread. GAE may ensue with multiple focal areas (cortical, subcortical white matter, and basal ganglia) of infection.

Naegleria infections usually occur in children and young adults who have been swimming in fresh water lakes and ponds, although inhalation of dust-borne cysts occurs in arid regions. The organism does not cause a systemic infection but invades the brain through olfactory nerves. (*From* Durack [96]; with permission.)

Clinical Manifestations of Primary Amebic Meningoencephalitis

Acute	Subacute or chronic, including granulomatous
Abrupt onset	Insidious onset
Fever	Chronic fever
Headache	Headache
Nuchal rigidity	Gradual onset of focal signs:
Vomiting	Aphasia
Lethargy	Focal seizures
Disorientation	Hemiparesis
Seizures	Ataxia
Increased intracranial pressure	Altered mentation
Coma	Systemic manifestations:
	Skin lesions
	Corneal ulcers
	Uveitis
	Pneumonitis

Figure 12-150. Clinical manifestations of primary amebic meningoencephalitis (PAM). Acute PAM caused by *Naegleria* presents as acute meningoencephalitis after an incubation period of several days to a week. The cerebrospinal fluid (CSF) profile is similar to that of acute bacterial meningitis, with several hundred to thousand leukocytes, primarily polymorphonuclear leukocytes, and a low glucose level. Amebae may be seen on wet preparations or with Wright or Giemsa stains. The organisms can be cultured on special media or isolated by mouse inoculation. A serologic test is available at the Centers for Disease Control and Prevention. The disease is rapidly fatal. Amphotericin B is the drug of choice. Subacute or chronic PAM (including granulomatous amebic encephalitis) presents more gradually, similar to a brain abscess or tumor. The CSF pleocytosis is more often lymphocytic, with a normal or only slightly decreased glucose level. Amebae can be found in the CSF only occasionally. Neuroimaging reveals focal lesions; biopsy is usually required for diagnosis. This disease is usually fatal. *In vitro* the organism is usually sensitive to pentamidine, ketoconazole, and flucytosine.

Helminthic Infections

Nematode (Roundworm) Infections of the Nervous System

Disease/parasite	Geographic distribution	Risk factors	Neurologic disease
Trichinella spiralis	Worldwide	Eating rare pork or bear meat	Acute meningoencephalitis myositis
Angiostrongylus cantonensis	Southeast Asia, Oceania	Eating freshwater snails, crabs, and raw vegetables	Acute eosinophilic meningitis
Gnathostoma	Japan, Thailand, Phillippines, Taiwan	Eating raw fish or meat	Hemorrhages, infarcts (rare)
Strongyloides	Tropics	Penetration of skin or gut by filariform; dissemination with immunosuppression	Meningitis (rare), paralytic ileus due to autonomic involvement
Toxocara	Worldwide	Children with pica, contamination with dog or cat feces	Small granulomas (rare), ocular granuloma
Filaria loa loa	Tropical Africa	Bites by deer flies, horseflies	Acute cerebral edema, subacute encephalitis (rare)
Onchocerca volvulus	Equatorial Africa, Latin America	Black flies	Chorioretinal lesions

Figure 12-151. Nematode (roundworm) infections of the nervous system. These infections are no longer common in the United States or other developed countries. *Trichinosis* was common in the United States during the first half of the twentieth century but is now almost nonexistent because of improved sanitation and public health measures. *Angiostrongylus* causes eosinophilic meningitis with headache, paresthesia, and a mean cerebro-spinal fluid leukocyte count of 500 to 600 cells/mm^3, of which the mean eosinophil count is approximately 50%. Most patients recover in 1 to 2 weeks. Additional causes of eosinophilic meningitis include other helminths, coccidioidomycosis, foreign bodies, drug allergies, and neoplasia. The other roundworm infections less frequently involve the nervous system. (*Adapted from* Johnson and colleague [97].)

Trematode (Fluke) Infections of the Nervous System

Disease/parasite	Geographic distribution	Risk factors	Neurologic disease
Schistosomiasis			
Schistosoma japonicum	Far East	Walking or swimming in infested waters (snails)	Cerebral granulomas
S. mansoni	South America, Caribbean, Africa		Myelitis (rare)
S. hematobium	Africa, Middle East		Myelitis (rare)
Paragonimus sp.	Asia, Central Africa, Central and South America	Eating infected freshwater crabs and crayfish	Cerebral granulomas

Figure 12-152. Trematode (fluke) infections of the nervous system. Many species of trematodes can infect humans, although schistosomiasis and paragonimiasis are the most common. With the exception of some schistosomes, most trematodes have wild or domestic animals as definitive hosts, with humans infected accidentally. Eosinophilia is common during acute trematode infections. *Paragonimus* are lung flukes, the lungs being the final habitat. Acute purulent (meningoencephalitic) forms, chronic granulomatous (tumorous) forms, and late inactive forms are seen. In the acute meningoencephalitic form, there is fever, headache, seizures, hemiparesis and other focal deficits, and confusion. The cerebrospinal fluid (CSF) pleocytosis consists of polymorphonuclear leukocytes (PMN) in the acute form and lymphocytes in the chronic form. Eosinophils occasionally appear in the cerebrospinal fluid. Serologic tests are generally available. Diagnosis is confirmed by finding ova in the stool or sputum or by biopsy. Computerized tomography may reveal "soap bubble" calcifications. The acute form has a 10% mortality rate; the chronic form is benign. The acute form is treated with praziquantel or bithionol; the chronic form, with surgery. (*Adapted from* Johnson and colleague [88].)

Species of *Schistosoma* That Infect Humans

Species infecting humans	Intermediate hosts		Final habitat
	Primary	Secondary	
S. haematobium	Snails	None	Vesical plexus
S. japonicum	Snails	None	Superior mesenteric veins
S. mansoni	Snails	None	Inferior mesenteric veins
S. mekongi	Snails	None	Mesenteric veins
S. intercalatum	Snails	None	Mesenteric veins

Figure 12-153. Species of *Schistosoma* that infect humans. Five species of this trematode infect over 200 million people in the world. It is estimated that over 400,000 cases exist in the United States, primarily in immigrants from infected areas (Puerto Rico, Brazil, Philippines, Middle East).

Fortunately, the organism cannot be transmitted in this country because of the absence of the appropriate male intermediate host. *Schistosoma* are blood flukes; their final habitat are veins or venous plexi. The predilection for a specific region of the central nervous system (CNS) appears to relate to the location of the adult worms when ova are released. *S. japonicum* resides in the superior mesenteric veins; it infects the CNS in about 3% of cases. The small eggs of this organism are able to reach the brain; ectopic worms have been found in cerebral veins. *S. mansoni* and *S. haematobium*, residing in the inferior mesenteric veins and vesical plexus respectively, have larger eggs that most commonly affect the spinal cord. This CNS involvement occurs less frequently than that seen with *S. japonicum*. Neurologic disease has not been well characterized for *S. mekongi* and *S. intercalatum*. (*Adapted from* Mahmoud [98].)

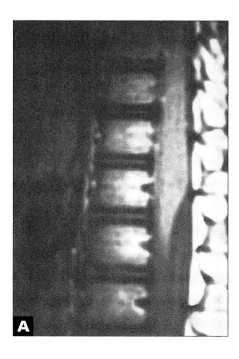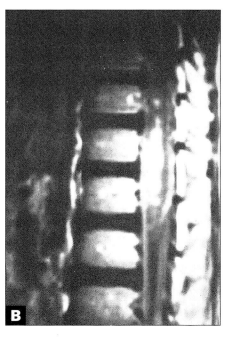

Figure 12-154. T1-weighted magnetic resonance image (MRI) showing sagittal view of a spinal cord in a case of *Schistosoma mansoni*. **A**, Precontrast MRI scan showing increased anteroposterior diameter of the spinal cord at T11–T12. **B**, Postcontrast MRI scan showing enhancement of the schistosomal lesion. Cerebral schistosomiasis may be acute or chronic. The acute form presents as fulminating meningoencephalitis with fever, headache, confusion, lethargy, seizures, focal deficits, and coma. The presentation of the chronic cerebral form is similar to a tumor, with focal deficits, seizures, increased intracranial pressure, and papilledema. The spinal cord disease is almost always acute, presenting as incomplete transverse myelitis. There is a peripheral leukocytosis with eosinophilia except in the chronic cerebral form. The cerebrospinal fluid shows slight to moderate pleocytosis, sometimes with eosinophilia. Cerebral lesions may be seen with computed tomography or MRI; spinal lesions, with MRI or myelography. Diagnosis can be made by finding ova in the stool or urine, by using serologic tests, and rectal mucosal biopsy. Treatment includes the use of praziquantel, corticosteroids for edema, anticonvulsants for seizure, and often decompressive laminectomy for a spinal block. (*From* Selwa and colleagues [99]; with permission.)

Cestode (Tapeworm) Infections of the Nervous System

Disease/parasite	Geographic distribution	Risk factors	Neurologic disease
Cysticercosis			
Taenia solium	Central and South America, Asia, Africa, East Europe	Ingestion of eggs in human fecal contamination	Small cysts or basilar arachnoiditis with hydrocephalus; ocular lesions
Hydatid disease			
Echinococcus granulosus	Worldwide	Ingestion of eggs in canine fecal contamination	Large cysts
Coenurosis			
Multiceps multiceps	Europe, Americas	Ingestion of eggs in carnivore fecal contamination	Budding cysts (rare)

Figure 12-155. Cestode infections of the nervous system. Cestode, or human tapeworm, infections can be divided into two groups. In the first, humans are the definitive host and the adult worms (*Taenia saginata* and others) live in the gastrointestinal tract and the central nervous system (CNS) is not involved. In the second group, humans are the intermediate host and the larvae spread to the tissues, including the CNS (echinococcosis, coenurosis, and others less common). In *Taenia solium*, the pork tapeworm infection, humans may be either the definitive host (*T. solium*) or the intermediate host (cysticercosis).

Ingestion of undercooked pork containing the encysted larvae (*Cysticercus cellulosae*; tissue larval stage) results in infection of the human intestine by the adult tapeworm (definitive host). There are usually no symptoms at this stage. The terminal gravid proglottids of the worm are excreted in the feces with thousands of ova. These ova contaminate the environment, where they are ingested by pigs or humans (intermediate hosts). The shells of these eggs are digested by gastric juices, liberating the embryos (oncospheres), which penetrate the intestinal wall, migrate to tissues, and become encysted (cysticerci). In humans they primarily localize to the brain and CNS. Cysticercosis is clearly the most important cestode infection of humans. Coenurosis is the rare larval-disease caused by the dog tapeworm, *Taenia (Multiceps) multiceps*. (*Adapted from* Johnson and colleague [88].)

Clinical Manifestations of Neurocysticercosis

Symptoms and signs	Approximate frequency, %
Headache	23–98
Seizures	37–92
Papilledema	48–84
Meningeal signs	29–33
Nausea/vomiting	74–80
Altered mental status	9–47
Dementia	1–6
Psychosis	1–17
Focal sensory or motor deficits	3–36
Cranial nerve palsies	1–36
Altered vision	5–34
Ataxia	5–24
Spinal cord compression	<1

Figure 12-156. Clinical manifestations of neurocysticercosis. The manifestations of neurocysticercosis depend on the location of the lesions. The clinical disease can be divided into four types based upon the anatomic location of infection: parenchymal, subarachnoid (meningitic), intraventricular, and spinal. In the parenchymal form, the manifestations are related to the location of the cysts. Focal seizures and focal neurologic deficits are seen in the parenchymal form. The meningitic form results in headache, nuchal rigidity, and communicating hydrocephalus. Intraventricular disease may result in obstructive hydrocephalus. Spinal disease may result in arachnoiditis and subarachnoid block. (*Adapted from* Cameron and colleague [100].)

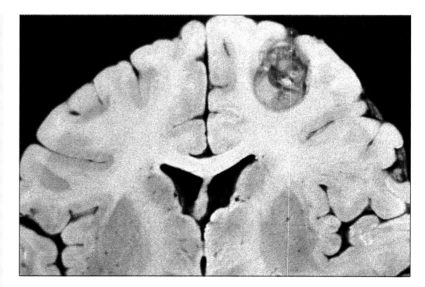

Figure 12-157. Pathologic sample showing the parenchymal cysticerci that are typically found at gray-white matter junctions. The encysted larvae (cysticerci) are fluid-filled cysts that may be deposited in parenchymal cerebrospinal fluid (CSF) spaces, where they may displace or compress tissue or block CSF pathways. (*From* Berger [90]; with permission.)

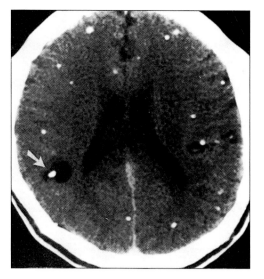

Figure 12-158. Noncontrast computed tomography (CT) scan showing numerous calcified (inactive) cysticerci and an active cyst with scolex (*arrow*) with contrast ring enhancement of active cysts in a patient with neurocysticercosis. The diagnosis of cysticercosis should be considered in patients who reside in endemic areas (Fig. 12-155) and have seizures, meningitis, or papilledema (increased intracranial pressure). CT and magnetic resonance imaging (MRI) are especially useful, as they may demonstrate live parenchymal cysts with enhancement (diffuse or ring pattern), calcified dead cysts, hydrocephalus, and intraventricular and subarachnoid cysts with enhancement. Usually the cerebrospinal fluid (CSF) shows mild pleocytosis, but may be normal or show severe pleocytosis due to meningitis when subarachnoid or intraventricular cysts die. There may be up to several thousand leukocytes (usually mononuclear), a low glucose level, and an elevated protein level. CSF and serum antibody tests are usually positive (80% to 98% sensitivity depending on the test). (*From* Cameron and colleague [100]; with permission.)

Treatment of Neurocysticercosis

Medical therapy
  Praziquantel   50 mg/kg/d in 3 doses × 15 d
  Albendazole   15 mg/kg/d in 3 doses × 8 d
  Plus adjunctive corticosteroids
    or
Surgical excision

Figure 12-159. Treatment of neurocysticercosis. For symptomatic patients, both praziquantel and albendazole are effective. Because dying cysticerci provoke a severe inflammatory reaction with edema, corticosteroids should be used concomitantly. Seizures can usually be controlled with anticonvulsants, but if intractable, surgical removal of cysts may be required. Ventricular shunting is usually adequate for hydrocephalus. Symptomatic ocular and spinal lesions usually require surgical excision. (*Adapted from* Berger [90].)

Clinical Manifestations of CNS Echinococcosis

Headache
Increased intracranial pressure
  Nausea and vomiting
  Papilledema
Seizures
Focal neurologic signs
  Hemiparesis
  Hemisensory loss
  Aphasia
  Ataxia
Cranial nerve palsies
Spinal cord compression

Figure 12-160. Clinical manifestations of central nervous system (CNS) echinococcosis (hydatid disease, hydatid cysts). Echinococciasis is the tissue infection caused by the larvae of a dog tapeworm. Most cases are caused by *Echinococcus granulosus*, but a few have been caused by *E. multilocularis*, *E. vogeli*, and *E. oligarthrus*. The disease primarily occurs in sheep-herding regions of Africa, South America, Eastern Europe, the former Soviet Union, and the Mediterranean. Sheep and cattle are the usual intermediate hosts. In the brain, the disease presents as a slowly expanding mass lesion.

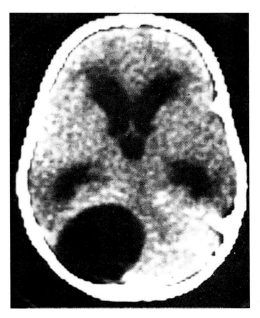

Figure 12-161. Computed tomography (CT) scan of a patient with a hydatid cyst of the brain. CT and magnetic resonance imaging (MRI) scans localize the lesions, which are usually single, nonenhancing, and have the density of cerebrospinal fluid. Needle biopsy is usually precluded because of severe allergic reactions, including anaphylaxis, caused by cyst rupture. Additional cysts may be found in the lungs and liver. The enzyme-linked immunosorbent assay antibody test has a 95% sensitivity. Surgical removal of cysts is the preferred treatment. Drug treatment with albendazole may decrease the size of the cysts, but it should be started before surgery to prevent allergic reactions and secondary hydatidosis at the time of surgery. (*From* Abbassioun and colleagues [101]; with permission.)

References

1. Roos KL, Tunkel AR, Scheld WM: Acute Bacterial Meningitis in Children and Adults. In *Infections of the Central Nervous System*, edn 2. Edited by Scheld WM, Whitley RJ, Durack PT. Philadelphia: Lippincott-Raven; 1997:335–401.

2. Roos KL, Bonnin JM: Acute bacterial meningitides. In *Atlas of Infectious Diseases: Central Nervous System and Eye Infections*, vol 3. Edited by Mandell GL, Bleck TP. Philadelphia: Current Medicine; 1995:1.2–1.25.

3. Kaplan MH: Part 1: Bacterial and Viral Causes. In *Meningitis and CNS Infection*. Garden Grove, CA: Medcom; 1979: Slide 2.

4. Wilson N: Infections of the Nervous System. In *Neuropathology: An Illustrated Course*. Edited by Duffy PE. Philadelphia: FA Davis; 1977: Slide 12.

5. Durand ML, Calderwood SB, Weber DJ, *et al.*: Acute bacterial meningitis in adults: a review of 493 episodes. *N Engl J Med* 1993, 328:21–28.

6. Gold R: Epidemiology of bacterial meningitis. *Infect Dis Clin North Am* 1999, 13:515–525.

7. Rosenstein NE, Perkins BA: Update on Haemophilus influenzae serotype b and meningococcal vaccines. *Pediatr Clin North Am* 2000, 47:337–352.

8. Schuchat A, Robinson K, Wenger JD, *et al.*: Bacterial meningitis in the United States in 1995. *N Engl J Med* 1997, 14:970–976.

9. Täuber MG, Turren JH, Sande MA: Bacterial Meningitis. In *Current Therapy in Neurologic Disease*, edn 4. Edited by Johnson RT, Griffin JW. St. Louis: Mosby–Year Book; 1993:109–113.

10. Klugman KP, Madhi SA: Emergence of drug resistance. Impact on bacterial Meningitis. *Infect Dis Clin North Am* 1999, 13:637–647.

11. Schaad UB, Lips U, Gnehm HE, *et al.*: Dexamethasone therapy for bacterial meningitis in children. Swiss Meningitis Study Group. *Lancet* 1993, 342:457–461.

12. Centers for Disease Control and Prevention: Standards for pediatric immunization practices. *MMWR* 1993, 42(RR-5):1.

13. Centers for Disease Control and Prevention: Prevention and control of meningococcal disease. Recommendations of the Advisory Committee on Immunization Practices (ACIP). *MMWR* 2000, 49(RR-7):1–10.

14. Zuger A, Lowy FD: Tuberculosis of the Central Nervous System. In *Infections of the Central Nervous System*, edn 2. Edited by Scheld WM, Whitley RJ, Durack DT. Philadelphia: Lippincott-Raven; 1997:417–443.

15. Shaw PP, Wang SM, Tung SG, *et al.*: Clinical analysis of 445 adult cases of tuberculous meningitis. *Chinese J Tuberc Respir Dis* 1984, 3:131–132.

16. Kennedy DH, Fallon RJ: Tuberculous meningitis. *JAMA* 1979, 241:264–268.

17. Weisberg L, Nice C, Katz M: Infectious Inflammatory Conditions. In *Cerebral Computed Tomography, A Text Atlas*, edn 2. Philadelphia: WB Saunders; 1984:229–248.

18. Danner RL, Hartman BJ: Update of spinal epidural abscess: 35 cases and review of the literature. *Rev Infect Dis* 1987, 9:265–274.

19. Gelfand MS, Bakhtian BJ, Simmons BP: Spinal sepsis due to *Streptococcus milleri*: two cases and review. *Rev Infect Dis* 1991, 13:559–563.

20. Helfgott DC, Weingarten K, Hartman BJ: Subdural Empyema. In *Infections of the Central Nervous System*, edn 2. Edited by Scheld WM, Whitley RJ, Durack DT. Philadelphia: Lippincott-Raven; 1997:495–505.

21. Greenlee JE: Subdural empyema. In *Principles and Practice of Infectious Diseases*, edn 4. Edited by Mandell GL, Bennet JE, Dolin R. New York: Churchill Livingstone; 1995:900–903.

22. Wispelwey B, Dacey RG Jr, Scheld WM: Brain Abscess. In *Infections of the Central Nervous System*, edn 2. Edited by Scheld WM, Whitley RJ, Durack DT. Philadelphia: Lippincott-Raven; 1997:463–493.

23. Wispelwey B, Scheld WM: Brain Abscess. In *Principles and Practice of Infectious Diseases*, edn 4. Edited by Mandell GL, Douglas RG Jr, Bennett JE. New York: Churchill Livingstone; 1995:889–891.

24. Wispelwey B: Brain Abscess. In *Atlas of Infectious Diseases: Central Nervous System and Eye Infections*, vol. III. Edited by Mandell GL, Bleck TP. Philadelphia: Current Medicine; 1995:4.2–4.14.

25. Falcone S, Post MJ: Encephalitis, cerebritis, and brain abscess: pathophysiology and imaging findings. *Neuroimaging Clin North Am* 2000, 10:333–353.

26. Jubelt B, Miller JR: Viral Infections. In *Merritt's Textbook of Neurology*, edn 9. Edited by Rowland LP. Philadelphia: Williams & Wilkins; 1995:142–179.

27. Centers for Disease Control and Prevention: Annual summary 1981: reported morbidity and mortality in the United States. *MMWR* 1982, 30(54).

28. Read SJ, Kurtz JB: Laboratory diagnosis of common viral infections of the central nervous system by using a single multiplex PCR screening assay. *J Clin Microbiol* 1999, 37:1352–1355.

29. Jubelt B: The Diagnosis of Viral Meningitis and Encephalitis. In *Neurology and Neurosurgery Update Series*, vol 2, no 30. Edited by Scheinberg P, Davidoff RA, Arnason BGW. Princeton NJ: Education Center; 1981.

30. Jubelt B, Lipton HL: Enterovirus Infections. In *Handbook of Clinical Neurology*, vol 12. Edited by Vinken PJ, Bruyn GW, Klawans HL. Amsterdam: Elsevier Science Publishing; 1989:326.

31. Hanley DF, Glass JD, McArthur JC, Johnson RT: Viral Encephalitis and Related Conditions. In *Atlas of Infectious Diseases: Central Nervous System and Eye Infections*. Edited by Mandell GL, Bleck TB. Philadelphia: Current Medicine; 1995:3.2–3.40.

32. Miller BR, Masci RS, Godsey MS, *et al.*: First field evidence for natural vertical transmission of West Nile virus in Culex univittatus complex mosquitoes from Rift Valley province, Kenya. *Am J Trop Med Hyg* 2000, 62:240–246.

33. Whitley RJ, Alford CA, Hirsch MS, *et al.*: Vidarabine versus acyclovir therapy in herpes simplex encephalitis. *N Engl J Med* 1986, 314:144–149.

34. Skoldenberg B, Forsgren M, Alestig K, *et al.*: Acyclovir versus vidarabine in herpes simplex encephalitis. Randomised multicenter study in consecutive Swedish patients. *Lancet* 1984, 2:707–711.

35. Johnson RT: In *Viral Infections of the Nervous System*. New York: Raven Press; 1984:129–157.

36. Hirano A, Iwato M, Kato T, *et al.*: In *Color Atlas of Pathology of the Nervous System*, edn 2. Edited by Hirano A. Tokyo: Igaku-Shoin, 1988:231.

37. Davis JM, Davis KR, Kleinman GM, *et al.*: Computed tomography of herpes simplex encephalitis with clinicopathological correlation. *Radiology* 1978, 129:409–417.

38. Runge VM: Skull and Its Contents. In *Magnetic Resonance Imaging of the Brain*. Philadelphia: JB Lippincott; 1994:180.

39. Schroth G, Gawehn J, Thron A, Vollbracht A, Voight K: Early diagnosis of herpes simplex encephalitis by MRI. *Neurology* 1987, 37:179–183.

40. Robinson P: Rabies. In *Infectious Diseases*. Edited by Gorbach SL, Bartlett JG, Blacklow NR. Philadelphia: WB Saunders; 1992:1269–1277.

41. Whitley RJ, Middlebrook M: Rabies. In *Infections of the Central Nervous System*, edn 2. Edited by Scheld WM, Whitley RJ, Durack DT. Philadelphia: Lippincott-Raven; 1997:181–198.

42. Hanna JN, Carney IK, Smith GA, *et al.*: Australian bat lyssavirus infection: a second human case, with a long incubation period. *Med J Aust* 2000, 172:597–599.

43. Corey L: Rabies, Rhabdoviruses, and Marburg-like Agents. In *Harrison's Principles of Internal Medicine*, edn 13. Edited by Isselbacher KJ, Braunwald E, Wilson JD. New York: McGraw Hill; 1994:834.

44. Dreesen DW, Hanlon CA: Current recommendations for the prophylaxis and treatment of rabies. *Drugs* 1998, 56:801–809.

45. Centers for Disease Control and Prevention: Summary of notifiable disease, United States, 1993. *MMWR* 1993, 42(53):27.

46. Horstmann DM: Epidemiology of poliomyelitis and allied diseases—1963. *Yale J Biol Med* 1964, 36:5–26.

47. Jubelt B, Gallez-Hawkins G, Narayan O, Johnson RT: Pathogenesis of human poliovirus infection in mice. I. Clinical and pathological studies. *J Neuropathol Exp Neurol* 1980, 39:138–148.

48. Anders HJ, Goebel FD: Cytomegalovirus polyradiculopathy in patients with AIDS. *Clin Infect Dis* 1998, 27:345–352.

49. Talpes D, Tien RD, Hesselink JR: Magnetic resonance imaging of AIDS-related polyradiculopathy. *Neurology* 1991, 41:1995–1997.

50. Murray RP, Kobayashi GS, Pfaller MA, Rosenthal KD: Picorna viruses. In *Medical Microbiology*, edn 2.; St. Louis: Mosby; 1994:583.

51. Rosencrance G: Images in clinical medicine. Herpes zoster. *N Engl J Med* 1994, 330:906.

52. Hope-Simpson R: The nature of herpes zoster: a long-term study and a new hypothesis. *Proc Roy Soc Med* 1965, 58:1–12.

53. Johnson RT, McArthur JC, Narayan O: The neurobiology of HIV infections. *FASEB J* 1988, 2:2970–2981.

54. Price RW, Brew BJ, Roke M: Central and Peripheral Nervous System Complications of HIV-1 Infections and AIDS. In *AIDS: Etiology, Diagnosis, Treatment, and Prevention*. Edited by DeVita VT, Hellman S, Rosenberg SA. Philadelphia: JB Lippincott; 1992:237–254.

55. Fauci AS, Lane HC: Human Immunity Deficiency Virus (HIV) Disease: AIDS and Related Disorders. In *Harrison's Principles of Internal Medicine*, edn 13. Edited by Isselbacher KJ, Braunwald E, Wilson JD, *et al.* New York: McGraw-Hill; 1994:1590.

56. Olsen WL, Longo FM, Mills CM, Norman D: White matter disease in AIDS: findings at MR imaging. *Radiology* 1988, 169:445–448.

57. Carpenter CCJ, Cooper DA, Fischl MA, *et al.*: Antiretroviral therapy in adults: updated recommendations of the International AIDS Society–USA Panel. *JAMA* 2000, 283:381–390.

58. Blankson J, Siliciano RF: Interleukin 2 treatment for HIV infection. *JAMA* 2000, 284:236–238.

59. Rodgers-Johnson PEB, Ono SG, Asher DM, Gibbs CL: Tropical Spastic Paraparesis and HTLV-1 Myelopathy: Clinical Features and Pathogenesis. In *Immunologic Mechanisms in Neurologic and Psychiatric Disease*. Edited by Waksman BD. New York: Raven Press; 1990.

60. Izumo S, Goto MD, Itoyama MD, *et al.*: Interferon-alpha is effective in HTLV-1-associated myelopathy: a multicenter, randomized, double blind, controlled trial. *Neurology* 1996, 46:1016–1021.

61. Whiteman ML, Post MJ, Berger JK, *et al.*: Progressive multifocal leukoencephalopathy in 47 HIV-seropositive patients: neuroimaging with clinical and pathologic correlation. *Radiology* 1993, 187:233–240.

62. Ohya T, Martinez AJ, Jabbour JT, *et al.*: Subacute sclerosing panencephalitis. Correlation of clinical, neurophysiologic and neuropathologic findings. *Neurology* 1974, 24:211–218.

63. Weihl CC, Roos RP: Creutzfeldt-Jakob disease, new variant Creutzfeldt-Jakob disease, and bovine spongiform encephalopathy. *Neurol Clin* 1999, 17:835–859.

64. Brown P, Gibbs CJ Jr, Rodgers-Johnson P, *et al.*: Human spongiform encephalopathy: the NIH series of 300 cases of experimentally transmitted disease. *Ann Neurol* 1994, 35:513–529.

65. Will RG, Zeidler M, Stewart GE, *et al.*: Diagnosis of new variant Creutzfeldt-Jakob disease. *Ann Neurol* 2000, 47:575–582.

66. Manetto V, Medori R, Cortelli P, *et al.*: Fatal familial insomnia: clinical and pathologic study of five new cases. *Neurology* 1992, 42:312–319.

67. Jubelt B: Prion diseases. In *Merritt's Textbook of Neurology*, edn 10. Edited by Rowland LP. Philadelphia: Lippincott Williams & Wilkins; 2000:206–211.

68. Perfect JR, Durack DT: Fungal Meningitis. In *Infections of the Central Nervous System*, edn 2. Edited by Whitley RJ, Durack DT. Philadelphia: Lippincott-Raven; 1997:721–739.

69. Tunkel AR, Crous SE: Subacute and chronic meningitides. In *Atlas of Infectious Diseases: Central Nervous System and Eye Infections*, vol 3. Edited by Mandell GL, Bleck TP. Philadelphia: Current Medicine; 1995:2.13.

70. Gozdasoglu S, Ertem M, Buyukkececi Z, *et al.*: Fungal colonization and infection in children with acute leukemia and lymphoma during induction therapy. *Med Ped Oncol* 1999, 32:344–348.

71. Tucker T, Ellner JJ: Chronic Meningitis. In *Infections of the Central Nervous System*. Edited by Scheld WM, Whitley RJ, Durack DT. New York: Raven Press; 1991:703–728.

72. Tunkel AR, Scheld WM: Central Nervous System Infections in the Compromised Host. In *Clinical Approach to Infection in the Compromised Host*, edn 3. Edited by Rubin RH, Young LS. New York: Plenum; 1994:187.

73. Galgiani JN: Coccidioidomycosis. *West J Med* 1993, 159:153–171.

74. Davis LE: Fungal infections of the central nervous system. *Neurol Clin* 1999, 17:761–781.

75. Sepkowitz K, Armstrong D: Space-occupying Fungal Lesions. In *Infections of the Central Nervous System*, edn 2. Edited by Scheld WM, Whitley RJ, Durack DT. Philadelphia: Lippincott-Raven Publishing; 1997:741–762.

76. Simon RP: Neurosyphilis. *Arch Neurol* 1995, 42:606–613.

77. Rowland LP: Spirochete Infections: Neurosyphilis. In *Merritt's Textbook of Neurology*, edn 9. Edited by Rowland LP. Baltimore: Williams & Wilkins; 1995:200–208.

78. Merrit HH, Adams RD, Solomon HC: In *Neurosyphilis*. New York: Oxford University Press; 1946:24–67.

79. Simon R, Bayne L: Neurosyphilis. In *Infectious Diseases of the Central Nervous System*. Edited by Tyler KL, Martin JB. Philadelphia: FA Davis; 1993:237–255.

80. Katz DA, Berger JR, Duncan RC: Neurosyphilis. A comparative study of the effects of infection with human immunodeficiency virus. *Arch Neurol* 1993, 50:243–249.

81. Davis E: Spirochetal Disease. In *Diseases of the Nervous System: Clinical Neurobiology*, edn 2. Edited by Asbury AK, McKhann GM, McDonald WI. Philadelphia: WB Saunders; 1992:1359–1370.

82. Anderson JF: Epizootiology of *Borrelia* in *Ixodes* tick vectors and reservoir hosts. *Rev Infect Dis* 1989, 11(suppl 6):S1451–S1459.

83. Pachner AR, Steere AC: The triad of neurologic manifestations of Lyme disease, meningitis, cranial neuritis and radiculoneuritis. *Neurology* 1985, 35:47–53.

84. Coyle PK: Lyme Disease. In *Current Diagnosis in Neurology*. Edited by Feldman E. St. Louis: CV Mosby; 1994:113.

85. Reik L Jr: Lyme Disease. In *Infections of the Central Nervous System*, edn 2. Edited by Scheld WM, Whitley RJ, Durack DT. Philadelphia: Lippincott-Raven; 1997:685–718.

86. Reik L Jr.: Lyme Disease. In *Infections Diseases of the Central Nervous System*, edn 2. Edited by Scheld WM, Whitley RJ, Durack DT. Philadelphia: Lippincott-Raven; 1996:685–718.

87. Coda GC: Protozoan and Helminthic Infections. In *Infections of the Central Nervous System*. Edited by Lambert HP. Philadelphia: BC Decker; 1991:264–282.

88. Johnson RT, Warren KS: Parasitic Infections. In *Diseases of the Nervous System: Clinical Neurobiology*, edn 2. Edited by Asbury AK, McKhann GM, McDonald WI. Philadelphia: WB Saunders; 1992:1350–1358.

89. Luft BJ, Remington JS: Toxoplasmosis of the Central Nervous System. In *Current Topics in Infectious Diseases*, vol 6. Edited by Remington SJ, Swartz MN. New York: McGraw-Hill; 1985:315–358.

90. Berger JR: Parasitic diseases of the Nervous System. In *Atlas of Infectious Diseases: Central Nervous System and Eye Infections*. Edited by Mandell GL, Bleck TP. Philadelphia: Current Medicine; 1995:5.4–5.25.

91. Farrar WE, Wood MJ, Innes JA, Tubbs H: *Infectious Diseases: Text and Color Atlas*, edn 2. London: Gower Medical Publishers; 1992:3.30

92. Beaman MH, McCabe RE, Wong S-Y, Remington JS: *Toxoplasma gondii*. In *Principles and Practice of Infectious Diseases*, edn 4. Edited by Mandell GL, Bennett JE, Dolin R. New York: Churchill Livingstone; 1995:2455–2475.

93. Oo MM, Aikawa M, Than T, *et al.*: Human cerebral malaria: a pathological study. *J Neuropathol Exp Neurol* 1987, 46:223–231.

94. Newton CRJC, Warrell DA: Neurological manifestations of falciparum malaria. *Ann Neurol* 1998, 43:696–702.

95. Kirchhoff LV: Agents of African Trypanosomiasis (Sleeping Sickness). In *Principles and Practice of Infectious Diseases*, edn 4. Edited by Mandell GL, Bennett JE, Dolin R. New York: Churchill Livingstone; 1995:2450–2455.

96. Durack DT: Amebic Infections. In *Infections of the Central Nervous System*, edn 2. Edited by Scheld WM, Whitley RJ, Durack DT. Philadelphia: Lippincott-Raven; 1997:831–844.

97. Johnson RT, Warren KS: Parasitic Infections. In *Diseases of the Nervous System: Clinical Neurobiology*, edn 2. Edited by Asbury AK, McKhann GM, McDonald WI. Philadelphia: WB Saunders; 1992:1350–1358.

98. Mahmoud AAF: Trematodes (Schistosomiasis) and Other Flukes. In *Principles and Practices of Infectious Diseases*, edn 4. Edited by Mandell GL, Bennett JE, Dolin R. New York: Churchill Livingstone; 1995:2538–2544.

99. Selwa LM, Brumberg JA, Mandell SH, Garofalo EA: Spinal cord schistosomiasis: a pediatric case mimicking intrinsic cord neoplasm. *Neurology* 1991, 41:755–757.

100. Cameron ML, Durack DT: Helminthic infections. In *Infections of the Central Nervous System*, edn 2. Edited by Scheld WM, Whitley RJ, Durack DT. New York: Raven Press; 1997:845–878.

101. Abbassioun K, Rahmat H, Ameli NO, Tafazoli M: Computerized tomography in hydatid cyst of the brain. *J Neurosurg* 1978, 49:408–411.

13

Neuroimmunology

Michael R. Swenson

THE immune system is that collection of tissues and organs devoted to the defense of self, an action usually directed against infectious pathogens—parasites, fungi, viruses, and bacteria. Antigens are the distinguishing characteristics of pathogens, usually foreign molecules, used by the immune system as a target for identification of an invader and for direction of attack.

The immune system can be functionally divided into two subsystems: innate immunity and adaptive immunity. The innate immune system is nondiscriminating, reacting to antigen at first encounter and mounting a first line of defense. Skin, membranes, mucus, cilia, and soluble factors such as complement are components of the innate system. The phagocytes are its cellular elements. They scavenge for invaders and act as antigen-presenting cells.

The adaptive immune system is the standing army of immunity. Its forces divide into lymphocytes, which engage in the operations of command and control, and the antibodies, which perform the basic work of the immune system. The lymphocytes identify distinguishing components of the antigen, develop a response specific to the pathogen, mobilize and direct forces, and remember and anticipate recurrent antigenic challenges. T lymphocytes occur in two major types: CD8 cells and CD4 cells. CD8 lymphocytes recognize antigenic fragments (epitopes) complexed with major histocompatibility (MHC) class I and expressed from within other cells. Virally infected cells express MHC class I, calling in the CD8 lymphocyte for killing the infected cell. CD4 cells become actively involved in activation and control of the immune response, reacting to MHC class II–epitope complexes expressed on the surfaces of antigen-presenting scavenger cells.

The antigen-presenting cell serves a reconnaissance function, capturing invaders and bringing in antigen fragments for recognition and initiation of action by the CD4 lymphocytes. Activated CD4 cells release cytokines to stimulate B cells; activated B cells proliferate and differentiate to become plasma cells; plasma cells manufacture and secrete antibodies, which are the soluble form of the B-cell receptor.

Antibodies in the immune system take the form of immunoglobulin molecules. Antibodies recognize intact antigen. They can bind and directly neutralize antigen, or they can opsonize antigen for phagocytosis. Antibodies also may act by sensitizing target cells to initiate the inflammatory response or by activating complement to mediate cell lysis.

Anatomy and Function of the Immune System

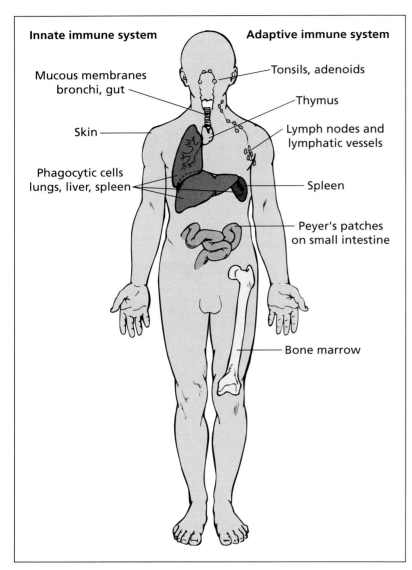

Figure 13-1. Gross anatomy of the immune system. Immune reactions to infection must occur at widely scattered sites, so the lymph nodes, spleen, adenoids, tonsils, and other lymphoid tissues of the immune system are diffusely arranged. T cells originate in the thymus and B cells in the bone marrow. Once matured, T cells and B cells migrate to lymph organs, where they process antigen, reacting to nonself components. The thymus, a bilobed lymphoid organ in the anterior mediastinum, is the proving ground for maturing T cells. Self-tolerance is learned by maturing T cells in the thymus. T cells, B cells, and immunoglobulins are the reactive components for adaptive immunity. They are capable of specific antigen recognition followed by activation and proliferation of the components needed to mount an attack on invaders. The adaptive immune system also has memory, reacting more quickly and more forcefully with repeated antigenic challenge. The innate immune system, acting nonselectively and without memory, is composed of skin, mucous membranes, and phagocytic cells. These components react to any antigen. Phagocytes, however, participate in adaptive immunity by presenting antigen to lymphocytes.

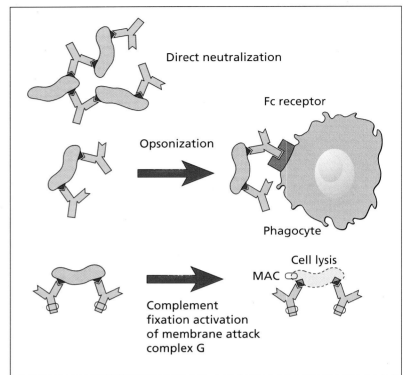

Figure 13-2. Mechanisms of antibody function. Antibodies, through their Fab regions, bind to antigen, either free in solution or on cell surfaces. Antibody can directly neutralize antigen, but more commonly it acts by cross-linking antigen to host cells of the immune system that have surface receptors for the Fc portion. Some antigen–antibody complexes activate the classic complement cascade, resulting in, among other actions, the formation of membrane attack complex (MAC) that destroys cell membrane and lyses cells.

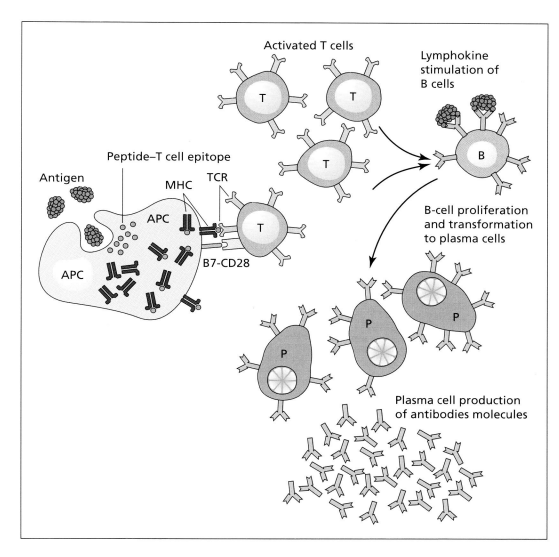

Figure 13-3. Lymphocyte activation and antibody production. Antigen-presenting cells (APCs) are found in many organs, including lymph nodes, thymus, spleen, liver, lung, and gut. APCs perform reconnaissance activity, scavenging for antigens. Antigen is phagocytosed and broken into short (10 to 20 amino acid) peptide fragments. These peptides are used by the immune system as the distinguishing and identifying characteristic of the antigen, called the *T-cell epitope*, for T-cell signaling. The peptides are complexed with major histocompatibility complex (MHC) class II and expressed on the APC surface. The APC seeks out and docks on a helper T cell bearing a compatible receptor, the T-cell receptor (TCR). The "handshake" between APC and T cell—MHC–peptide–TCR—is called the trimolecular complex (TMC). The TMC stimulates the T cell when appropriate co-stimulatory signals are present (*eg*, B7-CD28). The stimulated T cells proliferate and secrete cytokines called *interleukins* (*eg*, IL-2, IL-4). These cytokines activate other lymphocytes, including B lymphocytes, for antibody production.

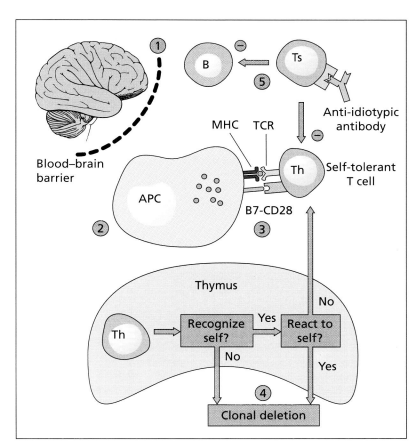

Figure 13-4. Mechanisms of self-tolerance. In dedication to the defense of self, the immune system has been required to define self—a definition that occurs at the cellular and molecular levels. Tolerance relies on the talent of self-recognition that B cells and T cells probably acquire during maturation. Lymphocytes unable to recognize self or lacking the willingness to tolerate self are deleted or rendered anergic by mechanisms still not fully understood. These mechanisms are sequestration, lack of antigen presentation, clonal energy, clonal deletion, and suppressor cells.

In *sequestration* (1) some tissue proteins (*eg*, myelin basic protein, lens of the eye) are anatomically isolated from exposure to lymphocytes; anatomic barriers (*eg*, the blood–brain barrier) preclude contact with helper T cells. The development of T-cell tolerance is also blocked, so a later breakdown of sequestration can lead to lymphocyte activation and the development of autoimmune disease.

In *lack of antigen presentation* (2) some tissues contain cells lacking the capability of antigen presenting cells (APC)—cells unable to express major histocompatibility complex (MHC). Neurons, for example, cannot express MHC.

In *clonal anergy* (3) T-cell activation requires a secondary co-stimulatory signal received by the CD28 complex. If a T cell confronts an antigen on a cell that lacks a functional B7 protein, the T cell becomes inactivated or tolerant.

In *clonal deletion* (4), during maturation, T cells must demonstrate recognition of self and tolerance of self. This takes place in the thymus (Th). T-cell lines failing to pass these tests are deleted or inactivated.

Suppressor cells (5) (T_S) and other cells have been proposed to induce self-tolerance. For development of tolerance, T_S cells may be activated by binding to anti-idiotypic antibodies. TCR—T-cell receptor.

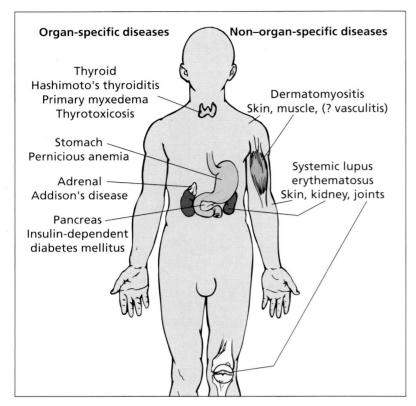

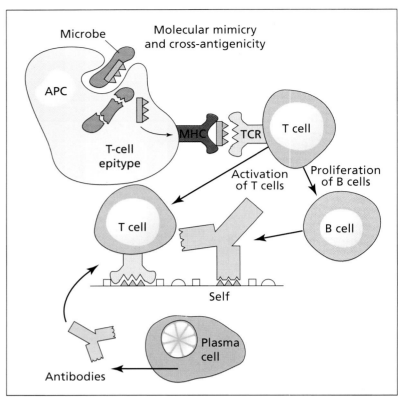

Figure 13-5. Types of autoimmunity. Autoimmunity occurs when the protective mechanisms of self-tolerance fail or are bypassed; pathologic reactions against self-antigens may result. Anti-self antibodies and self-reacting cells disrupt tissues and cause organ damage, or autoimmune disease. The spectrum of autoimmune disease spans two major categories. In *organ specific disorders*, typified by thyroiditis and myasthenia gravis, attack is directed against a single antigen in a single organ or tissue. *Non–organ-specific diseases* target widespread self-antigens such as nucleic acids in systemic lupus erythematosus. Organ damage is widely disseminated owing to the ubiquitous distribution of the antigen, and immune complex deposition may cause remote systemic injury. The organ-specific diseases occur together with greater than expected likelihood. For example, 5% to 10% of patients with myasthenia gravis also have antibody-mediated thyroid disease [1]. Disease clustering also occurs at the other end of the spectrum, with frequent overlap between, for example, dermatomyositis and other rheumatologic syndromes [2].

Figure 13-6. Mechanisms of autoimmunity. The causes of a breakdown of self-tolerance are not fully understood, but proposed mechanisms include the following: 1) In *molecular mimicry*, cell surface antigens of some microbial pathogens resemble self-proteins. Presumably, the forces of evolution have selected those pathogens that are cloaked in such a camouflage. When the immune system recognizes these pathogens, self-proteins are attacked by "friendly fire"—a case of mistaken identity. The connection between strep throat and rheumatic heart diseases is one of the simplest examples of such cross-antigenicity. 2) Activation of tolerant T cells may be due to a bypass of the normal controls of autoreactivity. Self-antigens may, for example, lose their tolerated status when bound to drugs (*eg*, procainamide). 3) Cells of self-tissue may be induced to express major histocompatibility complex when stimulated with γ-interferon. 4) Excessive cytokine release during infections or inflammations may awaken self-tolerant T cells, a theory in line with flare-ups of autoimmune disease observed after viral infections [3]. APC—antigen-presenting cell; MHC—major histocompatibility complex; TCR—T-cell receptor.

Multiple Sclerosis

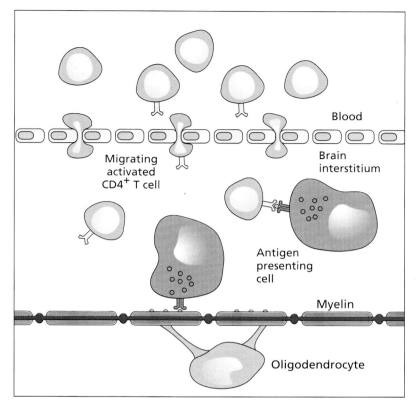

Figure 13-7. Pathogenesis of multiple sclerosis (MS). MS, a potentially disabling inflammatory central nervous system disease, affects about 250,000 Americans, mostly young adults, often during the most productive years of life. A strong regional variation of prevalence, demonstrating a steep gradient from south to north, suggests an environmental exposure, perhaps a childhood virus with re-exposure to a secondary factor during adulthood, that triggers a complex autoimmune response. Inflammatory lesions aggregate around venules, mostly in white-matter regions, suggesting that the blood–brain barrier is breached and that serum antimyelin factors gain access to antigenic targets on myelin sheaths. Disruption of motor and sensory transmission in heavily myelinated pathways of the brain, brain stem, cerebellum, and spinal cord cause a diverse spectrum of neurologic symptoms and disabilities. The widely scattered regions of injury, combined with an unpredictable relapsing and remitting time course, make accurate diagnosis a challenge, especially in the early years of the disease.

Presumably, activated helper T cells (CD4+) induced by some systemic factor breach the blood–brain barrier into the central nervous system and demonstrate specificity for peptide subunits of myelin. Secretion of γ-interferon leads to release of tumor necrosis factor and other cytokines that damage myelin and contribute to myelin phagocytosis.

Gadolinium-enhanced magnetic resonance image scanning of brain, cerebellum, brain stem, and spinal cord allows detection of MS lesions with remarkable sensitivity. The diagnosis of MS, once reliant on a demonstration of a typical clinical pattern of attacks (disseminated in time and space), is made much easier by these techniques.

Revolutionary discoveries in the treatment of MS are just breaking. The two available β-interferons and copolymer 1 have each been shown to reduce annual attack rates by about 30%. Corticosteroids, methotrexate, cytoxan, and other general immunosuppressant methods are still under study with some encouraging results. Antigen-specific therapies, or "silver bullet" methods, rely on recognition of antigenic peptides (epitopes) or their specific lymphocyte receptors. Once identified, methods are envisioned that would interfere with cellular signaling and enable an intervention that would inhibit the immune response to the specific target antigens in MS. Because these antigens are still unknown, these methods remain investigational but are the source of much hope.

Autoreactive T cells in the circulation, stimulated by some environmental challenge, breach the blood–brain barrier and migrate into the central nervous system, accompanied by other recruited lymphocytes. Macrophages and microglial cells are activated directly and by cytokine release. Self-reactivity against some lamellar component may result in myelin attack and destruction.

The regulatory effects of cytokines play a significant role in the development of experimental allergic encephalitis and, presumably, MS. Putative cytokines involved in the process include γ-interleukins, interferon, and tumor necrosis factor. Subsets of these substances engage in a complex interplay of cell signaling that leads to directed attack and myelin damage [4].

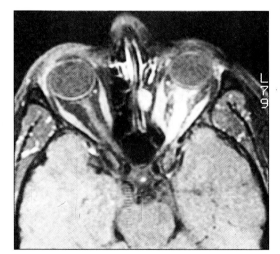

Figure 13-8. Magnetic resonance image showing optic neuritis in a patient with multiple sclerosis (MS). Optic neuritis, internuclear ophthalmoplegia, and various patterns of nystagmus are the most common ophthalmologic declarations of MS. Optic neuritis causes relatively acute impairment of vision, progressing over hours to days, reaching a nadir in about 1 week. During the acute phase, orbital pain, brow pain, and pain with eye movement occur. Depression of vision affects the whole field of one eye, sometimes both [5]. The disc is spared with retrobulbar neuritis: "The patient sees nothing—neither does the doctor." Optic neuritis is the presenting feature in 25% of MS cases and occurs at some stage of the illness in 73%. Conversely, 50% to 75% of patients with isolated optic neuritis later develop definite MS within 12 to 15 years [6]. Bilateral optic neuritis, occurring acutely in the company of transverse myelitis, is termed *neuromyelitis optica* or *Devic's disease*. This form of MS attack occurs most often in young people and carries a poorer prognosis [7].

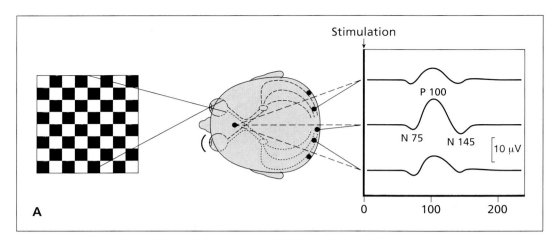

Figure 13-9. Central scotoma and pattern-reversal visual-evoked potentials in optic neuritis. **A,B,** Optic neuritis typically causes a central or centrocecal scotoma, usually involving the central 20°. Diminished acuity, color desaturation, and reduced contrast sensitivity are detectable. Pattern-reversal visual-evoked potentials show delayed latency and reduced amplitude with stimulation of the affected eye. Abnormal visual-evoked potentials are nonspecific, but are useful in detecting asymptomatic lesions of the optic nerve. Abnormal visual-evoked potentials may be detected in up to 20% of patients with definite multiple sclerosis who do not provide a history of optic neuritis.

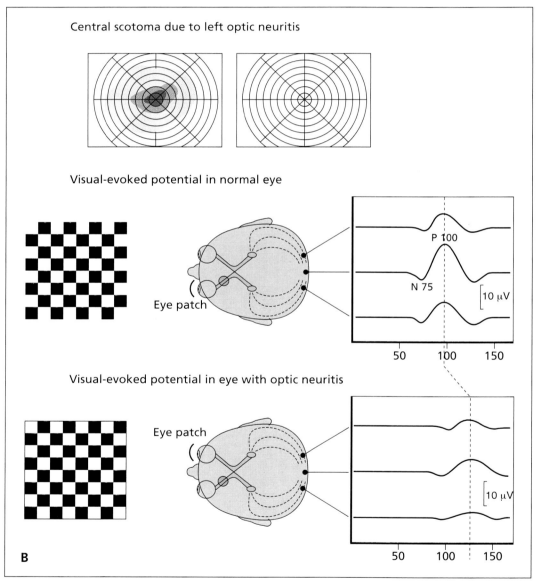

Cerebrospinal Fluid Abnormalities in Multiple Sclerosis

Quantitation of IgG synthesis rate
IgG index
$(IgG_{CSF}/IgG_{serum})/(alb_{CSF}/alb_{serum})$
Cerebrospinal fluid electrophoresis demonstrating
  oligoclonal bands
Myelin basic protein
Leukocyte count

Figure 13-10. Cerebrospinal fluid (CSF) abnormalities in the diagnosis of multiple sclerosis (MS). Clinical criteria for the diagnosis of MS typically include objective neurologic signs of central nervous system dysfunction at two distinct sites on two or more occasions in a patient between the ages of 10 and 50 years. The diagnosis should be made in the absence of other neurologic disease. Magnetic resonance imaging has greatly enhanced the diagnostic yield and is required in most suspected cases. Spinal fluid testing is still a useful adjunctive test and is an important supporting laboratory test in Poser's criteria [8].

About 70% of patients with clinically confirmed MS have an elevated intrathecal rate of immunoglobulin synthesis. This can be determined directly, or it can be expressed as an index that allows compensation for the serum levels and ratios of IgG to albumin [alb]. IgG indices of greater than 0.7 are abnormal, and ratios greater than 1.7 indicate a high probability of MS [9].

Agarose gel electrophoresis of CSF demonstrates migration of γ-globulins in discrete populations—the so-called oligoclonal bands. Oligoclonal band patterns appear early in MS patients and tend to remain constant during the course of the disease. They are not abolished by treatment. Other inflammatory diseases, including subacute sclerosing panencephalitis, aseptic meningitis, Guillain-Barré syndrome, and other encephalitides, may also generate bands. The presence of oligoclonal bands in patients with early or isolated attacks suggests a higher risk of subsequent progression [10]. High-resolution techniques and isoelectric focusing techniques add sensitivity to the determination of oligoclonal bands. Immunofixation techniques, though not widely available, can be used to make the test very specific.

High levels of myelin basic protein are seen in the spinal fluid during acute attacks; levels tend to be lower in progressive disease and revert to normal during remissions. The test is not widely available.

Leukocytes are often found during acute attacks, reflecting the inflammatory nature of MS. Cell counts are usually less than 50/mm³, but in rapidly progressive cases or more severe attacks, the count can exceed 100. Lymphocytes are predominant, usually T cells.

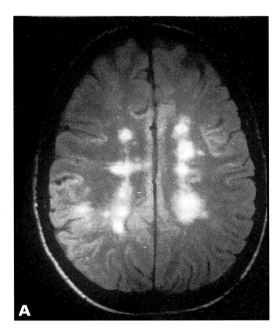
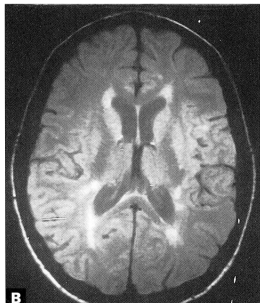

Figure 13-11. Periventricular plaques. The utility of magnetic resonance imaging (MRI) is seen most dramatically in images of the brain of patients with multiple sclerosis (MS). The periventricular white matter is typically involved, demonstrating multiple lesions with characteristically prominent T1 prolongation (**A**) and high T2-weighted signal density (**B**). Elliptical lesions deep in the white matter directed toward the ventricular margin appear in the corona radiata and tend to point toward the ventricular margin—a morphology known as *Dawson's finger* [11]. Subependymal lesions may be nodular or confluent. Subcortical–cortical junction lesions and callosal lesions distinguish MS from vascular diseases. Brain MRI is abnormal in more than 95% of patients with MS [12].

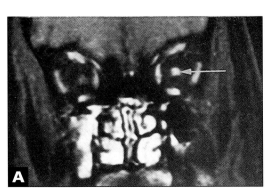
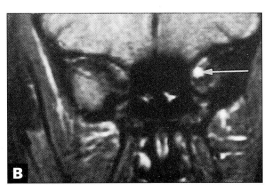

Figure 13-12. Magnetic resonance imaging (MRI) scans showing multiple sclerosis (MS) of the optic nerve, brain stem, and spinal cord. **A,B,** Accurate visualization of the intraorbital portion of the optic nerve (*arrows*) can demonstrate unilateral optic neuritis. Fat-saturation sequences enhance the signal contrast between optic nerve and orbital fat. (*Continued on next page*)

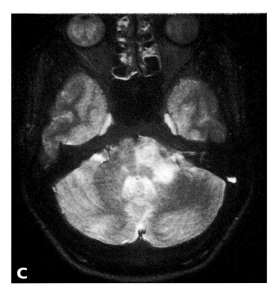
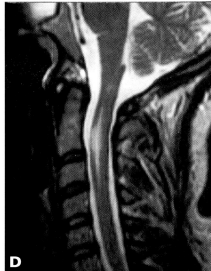
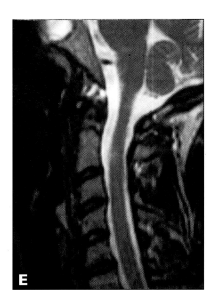

Figure 13-12. (*Continued*) **C**, Focal brain stem and cerebellar peduncular foci, especially the middle cerebellar peduncle (brachium pontis), are common sites of involvement in MS. These lesions are usually symptomatic in the acute phase, often correlating with internuclear ophthalmoplegia or other brain stem signs. Comi and colleagues [13] found brain stem lesions by MRI scanning of 50 patients with clinical signs of brain stem involvement. Seventy-four percent of these lesions correlated with clinical findings.

D,E, Transverse myelitis may involve thoracic or cervical segments and may overlap in appearance with spinal astrocytoma, even with contrast-enhanced techniques. McDonald and Miller [14] identified 139 lesions in 74% of 59 patients, more commonly in the cervical segments. Spinal cord atrophy, found in 40%, correlated more with clinical disability than did discrete cord lesions. Curiously, the burden of plaque detectable by MRI typically goes far beyond the clinical signs and symptoms. The burden of dis-

ease increases about 10% per year [15,16], and a high rate of MRI activity correlates with poor prognosis [17].

Although the MRI findings should not stand alone to establish a diagnosis of MS, cases of a single clinical attack may be considered as clinically probable MS if new lesions can be shown to develop on serial scans.

Fazekas' criteria specify the finding of a periventricular lesion, an infratentorial lesion, and a lesion 6 mm or greater in diameter. These criteria are 89% specific for the diagnosis of MS [18].

Filippi and colleagues [19] studied 100 patients with multiple sclerosis who had undergone neuropsychologic testing to evaluate cognitive impairment. Atrophy of the corpus callosum and dilation of the ventricles correlated significantly with lower mean scores on neuropsychologic testing. Widening of the cortical sulci and higher lesion scores correlated inversely with performance intelligence quotient (IQ) and total IQ, suggesting that MRI pathology correlates with cognitive dysfunction in patients with MS.

Current Therapies for Multiple Sclerosis

FDA-approved therapies:
Interferon β-1b (Betaseron, Berlex Laboratories, Richmond, CA)
  Approved for relapsing or remitting MS
  Results in a 30% reduction in attack rate [20]
  Results in an 80% reduction in plaque burden seen on MRI scans
  Minimal side effects [21]
    Injection site irritation
    Flu-like symptoms
  Long-term benefits unclear
  Every-other-day dosing
Interferon β-1a (Avonex, Biogen, Inc., Cambridge, MA)
  Reported effective and safe in relapsing and remitting MS
  About a 30% reduction in attack rate [22]
  Slower rate of progression of disability
  Minimal side effects
    Flu-like symptoms
  Weekly dosing
Glatiramer (previously copolymer-1, Copaxone, Teva Pharmaceuticals)
Results in a 29% reduction in annual relapse rate
  Significant improvement or stabilization of disability scores

Daily injections but few side effects and minimal site reaction
Mitoxantrone (Novantrone, Immunex, Olney, MD)
Results in a 60+% reduction in annual relapse rate
Results in a 1 point deterioration in Expanded Disability Status Score reduced by half
Reduced rate of new lesion formation seen on MRI scans
IV infusion every 3 months
Cumulative cardiotoxicity limits the duration of treatment
Non-FDA approved therapies:
Corticosteroids
  May lengthen the intervals between attacks [23]
  Commonly used for treatment of acute attacks, but proof of effect still lacking
  Numerous side effects with chronic use
Cyclophosphamide
  Monthly pulse therapy useful in younger patients [24]
  Canadian Cooperative Study Group found disappointing results [25]
Methotrexate
  Demonstrated effect in patients with chronic progressive MS [26]

2-Chlorodeoxyadenosine (Leustatin, Ortho Biotech, Inc., Raritan, NJ)
  Induces lymphocyte apoptosis
  Clinical and MRI scan improvement in chronic–progressive MS [27]
Isoprinosine [28]
Total lymphoid irradiation [29–31]
Intravenous immunoglobulin
  Reduced exacerbation rate and slow disease progression
  Very small clinical trials [32]
Plasmapheresis
  Minimal clinical trial evidence
  Dramatic improvement reported but remains unsubstantiated [33]
Antigen-specific therapies
  T-cell tolerogens
  B-cell tolerogens
  Monoclonal antibodies
Symptomatic treatment
  Antispasticity therapy
  4-Aminopyridine (4-AP); 3,4-diaminopyridine (3,4 DAP)
  Rehabilitative techniques

Figure 13-13. Current therapies for multiple sclerosis (MS). The approvals of β-interferons [34], glatiramer [35], and now mitoxantrone [36] for clinical use signal the beginning of a new era in therapy for MS. The challenge is in deciding which treatments, single drugs, or combinations are the most efficacious. MRI—magnetic resonance imaging.

Antibody-Associated Central Nervous System Disorders

Paraneoplastic Syndromes

Central Nervous System Paraneoplastic Syndromes

Syndrome	Putative antigen	Associated antibody
Paraneoplastic cerebellar degeneration	Ovarian or breast cancer	Anti-Yo, type 1, PCA-1, APCA
Paraneoplastic encephalomyelitis or limbic encephalitis	Small cell lung cancer	Anti-Hu, type IIa, ANNA-1
Paraneoplastic sensory ganglioneuritis	Small cell lung cancer	Anti-Hu
Opsoclonus	Neuroblastoma, retinoblastoma, or breast cancer	Anti-Ri, type IIb, ANNA-2
Paraneoplastic retinal degeneration	Small cell lung cancer	Antiretinal antibody

Figure 13-14. Central nervous system (CNS) paraneoplastic syndromes. Cerebellar degeneration is the most familiar paraneoplastic syndrome. This syndrome manifests with pancerebellar dysfunction, including oculomotor nystagmus, dysarthria, and wide-based ataxic gait. Anti-Yo antibody is directed against Purkinje cells. Less commonly, anti-Hu antibody or an atypical antibody is found. Seventy-seven percent of patients with paraneoplastic encephalomyelitis or limbic encephalitis have an underlying small cell lung cancer [37]. Symptoms reflect the region of involvement: lower-extremity weakness with myelitis, bulbar palsy with brain stem encephalitis, and memory loss and cognitive impairment with limbic encephalitis. Paraneoplastic sensory ganglioneuritis is a frequent accompaniment. The correlation is high with anti-Hu antibody. Anti-Hu cross-reacts with neuronal protein components in the CNS and the dorsal root ganglia. As with other paraneoplastic syndromes, symptoms may precede detection of tumor by many months.

The opsoclonus syndromes are rare paraneoplastic disorders characterized by rapid arrhythmic conjugate square wave gaze jerks, often accompanied by myoclonic jerks of appendicular musculature. Ataxia, dysarthria, myoclonus, vertigo, and encephalopathy are other signs associated with this relapsing and remitting syndrome, usually related to the antineuronal antibody of type II (anti-Ri or type IIb).

Rasmussen's encephalitis, Bickerstaff's encephalitis, and stiff-man syndrome are other inflammatory CNS disorders with reported antibody association.

Paraneoplastic retinal degeneration causes painless visual loss, most commonly in association with small cell lung cancer [38]. Autoreactive antigens against retinal cell components have been found, most frequently identified with photoreceptor cells. Immunosuppressive agents may be helpful [39]. ANNA—antineuronal nuclear antibody; APCA—anti-Purkinje cell antibody; PCA—Purkinje cell antibody.

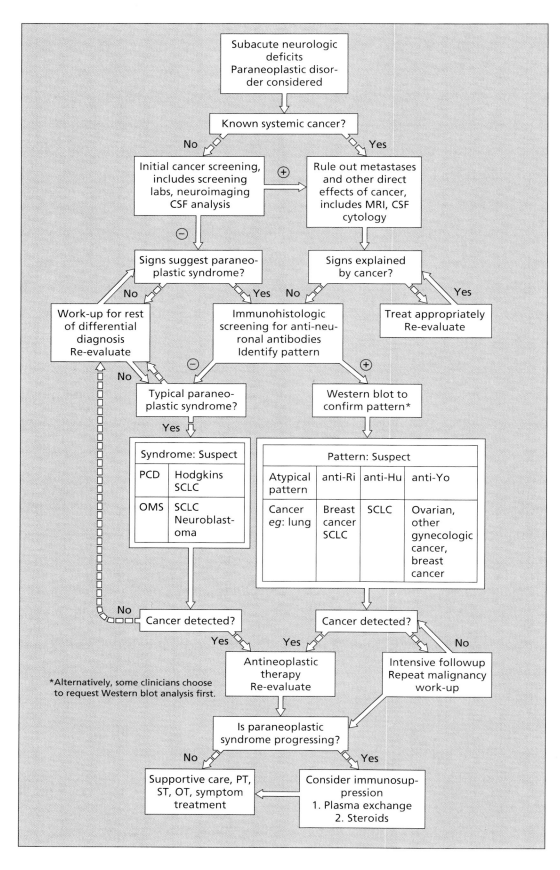

Figure 13-15. Algorithm for the evaluation of central nervous system (CNS) paraneoplastic syndromes. Detection of antibodies associated with disorders of the central nervous system has led to the discovery that these diseases are often acquired through association with tumors and viruses. Some antibody tests are now used as diagnostic markers in the clinic. The mediation of these diseases by antibody suggests opportunities for treatment by a variety of immunosuppressant methods.

The paraneoplastic syndromes occur rarely in patients with known cancer but may be the heralding symptom and may be the most disabling and potentially treatable aspect of the disorder (about half of patients develop neurologic symptoms preceding the diagnosis of systemic cancer).

Paraneoplastic syndromes often occur when the causative cancer is relatively small, opening greater opportunity for effective treatment. The paraneoplastic syndromes are also important to consider because they frequently cause symptoms that are mistaken for metastatic disease or for the adverse effects of chemotherapy or malnutrition.

The theory that these disorders are autoimmune in pathogenesis implies that tumor antigens or viral antigens cross-react with antigenically similar molecular

(Continued on next page)

Figure 13-15. (*Continued*) components of neurons or other CNS structures. The role of antineuronal antibodies (Hu, Ri, Yo) is still debated. Antibody titer may be high in the presence of minimal disease and present in the absence of disease [40], and paraneoplastic syndromes may occur without measurable antibody titer. Stated more simply, antibody testing is neither specific nor sensitive for the presence of paraneoplastic disease. The evidence for cross-antigenicity between tumor (or virus) in target neurons is still compelling, both clinically and in the laboratory.

Treatment of paraneoplastic CNS disorders relies on an aggressive search for underlying malignancy to interrupt tumor progression early. Tumor removal may also cure or ease the treatment of paraneoplastic syndromes. Because anti-body-mediated attack against tumor may be part of an antineoplastic defense, immunosuppressant therapy before tumor removal might accelerate tumor growth and disinhibit metastases formation. Many of these syndromes occur even in the absence of tumor or may continue after tumor removal, so immunosuppressant techniques or plasma exchange may be warranted [41]. Brashear [42] recommends concurrent plasmapheresis with high-dose steroids after clinical response and antibody titer determination. CSF—cerebrospinal fluid; MRI—magnetic resonance imaging; OMS—opsoclonus myoclonus syndrome; OT—occupational therapy; PCD—paraneoplastic cerebellar degeneration; PT—physical therapy; SCLC—small cell lung cancer; ST—speech therapy. (*Adapted from* Brashear [42].)

Viral Syndromes

Antibody-Associated Central Nervous System Viral Syndromes

Syndrome	Putative antigen	Associated antibody
Stiff-man syndrome (Moersch-Woltman syndrome)	Unknown	Anti-GAD
Rasmussen's encephalitis	Possibly cytomegalovirus or herpes simplex virus	Possibly GluR3
Bickerstaff's encephalitis	Possibly cytomegalovirus	Possibly anti-GQ1b
Possibly amyotrophic lateral sclerosis	Unknown	Possibly anti-VGCC

Figure 13-16. Antibody-associated central nervous system viral syndromes. Stiff-man syndrome (SMS) is a rare disorder characterized by rigidity and continuous electromyographic motor activity affecting axial musculature. Paroxysmal autonomic dysfunction has been reported to cause sudden death. The painful axial stiffening is often triggered by startling noises, touch, emotion, or attempted voluntary movements. The frequent association with insulin-dependent diabetes and autoimmune thyroid disorders, identification of associated antibodies to glutamic acid decarboxylase (anti-GAD), and reports of successful reversal with immunosuppressant methods all suggest an immune-mediated cause of SMS [43,44].

Reportedly, SMS is caused by an antibody-mediated attack against inhibitory glutamatergic inhibitory interneurons. Rare cases have been associated with breast cancer [45]. Treatment of idiopathic cases has been successful with plasmapheresis, corticosteroids, and intravenous immunoglobulin.

A chronic inflammatory encephalopathy, often unilateral and associated with hemiparesis and intractable focal epilepsy, is known as Rasmussen's encephalitis [46]. Children and young teens are affected. Viral associations (herpes simplex virus types 1 and 2, cytomegalovirus) and detection of serum antibody to glutamate receptor 3 (GluR3) indicate an autoimmune cause [47]. Antiviral agents and immunosuppressants have been tried with some success. Bickerstaff's encephalitis is a similar inflammatory disease of the brain stem, also associated with cytomegalovirus and with detectable amounts of anti-GQ1b antibody.

Sporadic amyotrophic lateral sclerosis (ALS) has been mimicked in guinea pig models of autoimmune motor neuron disease. Clinical observations suggest an autoimmune-mediated cause of ALS based on the following evidence: 1) 3% to 5% of patients have other autoimmune disorders (*eg*, thyroid disease); 2) immunoglobulin monoclonal spikes occur with three to five times the prevalence in ALS; 3) immune complex deposition can be seen at the neuromuscular junction and in kidneys; and 4) paraproteinemias are more common. Smith and colleagues [46] have shown increased intracellular Ca^{2+} concentrations and postulate immune-mediated disruption of voltage-gated calcium-channel (VGCC) function, perhaps leading to apoptotic motor neuron cell death. Attempts to treat ALS with immunosuppressant medication, however, have been futile.

Autoimmune Peripheral Nervous System

Inflammatory Demyelinating Nerve Disease

Syndrome	Putative antigen	Associated antibody
Acute inflammatory demyelinating polyradiculoneuropathy (Guillain-Barré syndrome)	*Campylobacter jejuni* viruses	Possibly anti-GM$_1$
Chronic inflammatory demyelinating polyradiculoneuropathy	Unknown	Possibly cell mediated
Neuropathies in diabetes mellitus	Unknown	Unknown
Vasculitic neuropathies	Unknown	Unknown

Figure 13-17. Inflammatory demyelinating nerve disease. The inflammatory demyelinating polyradiculopathies occur in acute, chronic, and chronic relapsing forms (AIDP, CIDP, CRIP). AIDP leads to arreflexic weakness. Respiratory failure occurs in 20% of cases and leaves 15% of patients with significant neurologic residual impairments. Because conventional immunosuppressant methods (*eg*, corticosteroids) have failed to show benefit, positive therapeutic trials of plasmapheresis and intravenous immunoglobulin (IVIg) have been greeted eagerly. The large studies of plasmapheresis for AIDP, reported in the early 1980s, showed an impact on respirator time and time to independent ambulation, cutting each about in half when treatment was given during the first weeks of the disease. IVIg has also been proved beneficial.

CIDP is a different syndrome, evolving insidiously over weeks or months and progressing slowly. Weakness is usually symmetric, involving proximal and distal muscles. Reflexes are lost or depressed. Respiratory failure is rare. Nerve conduction studies show reduced velocities and scattered regions of conduction block [48]. A wide array of treatment options are available for CIDP, including corticosteroids, azathioprine, and cyclosporine A. Plasma

exchange is also useful, but the benefits of therapy fade after 10 to 14 days, so maintenance with concomitant steroid therapy is required [49]. Chronic plasma exchange therapy has obvious drawbacks in terms of expense, vascular access, and complications.

Dyck and colleagues [50] have shown that weekly IVIg is equal in effect to plasma exchange and may be the preferable therapy in terms of availability and lower rate of complications.

Krendel and colleagues [51] reported successful treatment of neuropathies in some diabetic patients using immunosuppressant methods (IVIg, prednisone, cyclophosphamide, pheresis, or azathioprine) alone or in various combinations. Diabetic patients with CIDP-like illness were insulin dependent only, suggesting a common underlying immunopathogenesis.

Vasculitic neuropathies manifest as mononeuritis multiplex or polyneuropathy with equal likelihood, either as part of a systemic vasculitis or in isolation, without other organ involvement [52,53]. Circulating immune complex deposits, inflammation, and cell-mediated mechanisms of injury to nerve have been postulated.

Acute Inflammatory Demyelinating Polyneuropathy

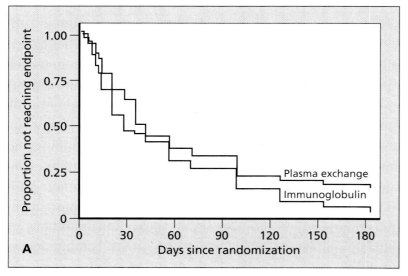
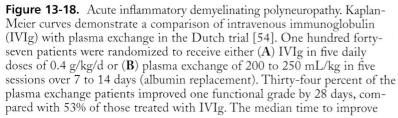
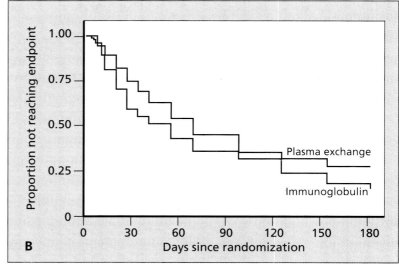

Figure 13-18. Acute inflammatory demyelinating polyneuropathy. Kaplan-Meier curves demonstrate a comparison of intravenous immunoglobulin (IVIg) with plasma exchange in the Dutch trial [54]. One hundred forty-seven patients were randomized to receive either (**A**) IVIg in five daily doses of 0.4 g/kg/d or (**B**) plasma exchange of 200 to 250 mL/kg in five sessions over 7 to 14 days (albumin replacement). Thirty-four percent of the plasma exchange patients improved one functional grade by 28 days, compared with 53% of those treated with IVIg. The median time to improve

one grade was 41 days with plasma exchange but only 27 days with IVIg therapy. Other measures included a shorter hospital stay by 14 days, shorter intubation time by 7 days, greater safety and fewer complications in the IVIg group. Relapse rates were higher with IVIg treatment. Nonetheless, the wide availability of IVIg and the ease of administration have made this technique a welcome therapeutic option, especially in smaller hospitals and in outlying areas where plasma exchange is unavailable. (*Adapted from* Parry [48].)

Inflammatory Demyelinating Polyradiculoneuropathy

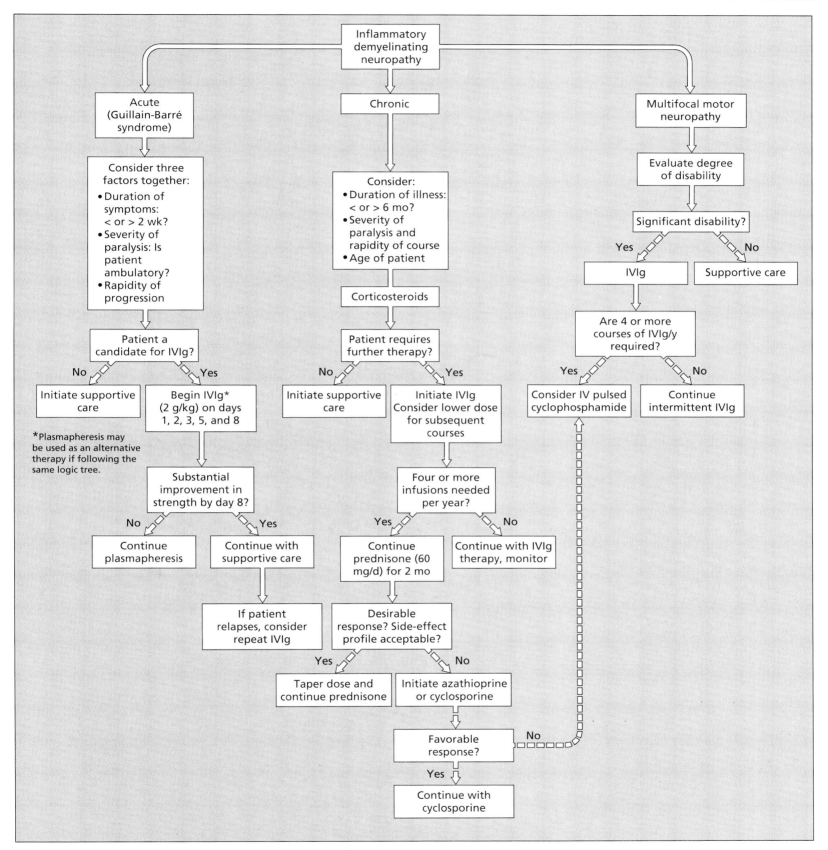

Figure 13-19. Suggested clinical algorithm for treatment of inflammatory demyelinating polyradiculoneuropathy [48]. This algorithm favors early use of intravenous immunoglobulin (IVIg). In centers where plasma exchange is easily available, either option could be exercised. (*Adapted from* Parry [48].)

Other Antibody-Mediated Disorders

Other Antibody-Mediated Disorders

Syndrome	Putative antigen	Associated antibody
Multifocal motor neuropathy	Unknown	Anti-GM$_1$
Anti-MAG–associated neuropathy	Unknown	Anti-MAG
Isaac's syndrome (acquired neuromyotonia)	Unknown	Nerve K$^+$ channels

Figure 13-20. Other antibody-mediated disorders. Autoimmunity to gangliosides (glycoproteins and glycolipid components of cell membranes) may underlie two or more peripheral neuropathies. In multifocal motor neuropathy (MMN), a focal or multifocal, predominantly distal motor impairment develops in a step-wise or gradually progressive fashion with minimal sensory expression. Nerve conduction testing reveals localizable regions of conduction block when involved sites are accessible; conduction block may be too proximal or too distal to detect. High antibody titers to GM$_1$ ganglioside are seen in about half of these patients. Recovery may be dramatic, even in chronic cases [55].

Sensorimotor neuropathy associated with a monoclonal paraprotein is recognized. Antibodies against myelin-associated glycoprotein (MAG) are thought to account for a monoclonal spike and are considered the causative agent targeting myelin and leading to demyelination of motor and sensory nerve fibers. Plasma exchange, steroids, cyclophosphamide, and intravenous immunoglobulin have been tried with variable success. Parry and Swenson [56] favor plasmapheresis followed by cyclophosphamide and chlorambucil.

Acquired myotonia, known as Isaacs' syndrome, is characterized by muscle activity causing visible myokymia. This excessive muscle activity is of peripheral nerve origin. Electromyographically, bursts of multiple, single-unit discharges occur in high frequency. Transfer of disease to mice by injection with affected patients' immunoglobulin suggests an autoimmune cause. Antibodies to peripheral nerve potassium channels may be the pathophysiologic explanation. Treatment with plasma exchange has been of benefit in a few patients [57,58]. Occurrence of Isaacs' syndrome with chronic inflammatory demyelinating polyradiculopathy, with other neuropathies, and in association with malignancies has been reported [59].

Glycoconjugates

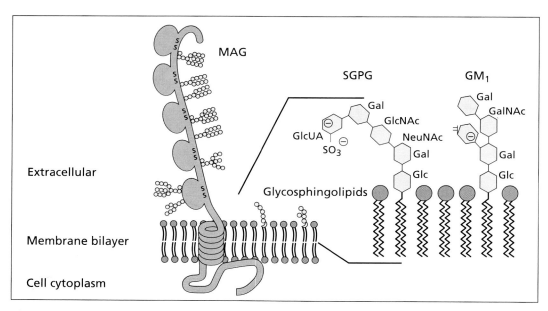

Figure 13-21. Cell surface glycoconjugates implicated as potential target antigens in immune-mediated neuropathy. Glycolipids, glycoproteins, and proteoglycans contain complex oligosaccharide moieties exposed on the outside of cell membranes. These cell surface glycoconjugates are exposed to become foci of an immune attack and have been implicated as potential target antigens in immune-mediated neuropathy. The myelin-associated glycoprotein (MAG) may be involved in myelin layer adhesion or in the interaction between Schwann cells and the axolemma.

Sulfate-3-glucuronyl paragloboside (SGPG) is a glycolipid that shares structural features with MAG and that is implicated in neuronal function. SGPG may also be antigenic.

GM$_1$ is presumably the antigen attacked in multifocal motor neuropathy as well as in some forms of Guillain-Barré syndrome. Labeled anti-GM$_1$ antibodies have been shown to bind preferentially to the nodes of Ranvier, perhaps blocking sodium-channel function. This would also explain the rapid reversibility of multifocal motor neuropathy with immunotherapeutic methods [60,61]. Gal—galactose; GalNAc—N-acetylgalactosamine; Glc—glucose; GlcNAc—N-acetylglucosamine; GlcUA—glucuronic acid; NeuNAc—N-acetylneuraminic acid (sialic acid). (*Adapted from* Quarles [61]; *courtesy of* Richard H. Quarles, PhD, National Institute of Neurological Disorders and Stroke.)

Neuromuscular Junction

Neuromuscular Junction

Syndrome	Putative antigen	Associated antibody
Myasthenia gravis	Possibly thymus	Anti-AChR
Lambert-Eaton myasthenic syndrome	Small cell lung cancer	Anti-VGCC

Figure 13-22. Neuromuscular junction. Few neurologic studies have yielded so clear a connection of pathophysiology with disease as have the disorders of the neuromuscular junction, especially myasthenia gravis and Lambert-Eaton myasthenic syndrome (LEMS). The acetylcholine receptor (AChR) is attacked by autoantibody, uncoupling the activation of muscle fibers from incoming nerve impulses. Painless fatigability and weakness of skeletal musculature, the identifying symptoms of myasthenia gravis, result. Sensation, autonomic function, reflexes, and cognitive powers remain intact—myasthenia gravis specifically affects only skeletal muscle [62].

Anti–acetylcholine receptor antibodies (anti-AChR-Ab) are of IgG subtype, mostly binding to the main immunogenic region of the AChR α-subunit, causing cross-linking of adjacent receptors, accelerated receptor turnover, and complement-mediated injury to the postsynaptic junction. Cross-antigenicity with thymic components, with or without thymoma, presumably plays a role in the disease development and explains the improvement seen in some patients after thymus removal. Diagnosis relies on antibody serology, repetitive nerve stimulation studies, and single-fiber electromyography. Careful and cautious management is mandated by the clinical instability and potential for rapid deterioration of respiratory power in patients with generalized disease. Anticholinesterase medication (*eg*, pyridostigmine) is the mainstay of therapy, with additional use of prednisone, azathioprine, cyclosporine, plasma exchange, and intravenous immunoglobulin, depending on severity and degree of disability [63].

LEMS differs from myasthenia gravis in that patients usually have more constant degrees of weakness, accompanied by autonomic features such as dry mouth, impotence, and constipation. Proximal muscle weakness may be reversed by brief exercise. Antibodies to presynaptic voltage-gated calcium channels, also of IgG subtype, impair calcium influx during nerve terminal depolarization, inhibiting release of acetylcholine [64,65].

Most patients with LEMS have an underlying small cell lung cancer, but cases accompanying autoimmune disease are not uncommon. Diagnosis relies on recognition of the clinical syndrome and demonstration of marked enhancement of compound motor action potential amplitude (greater than 200%) after brief exercise. Treatment is directed at the underlying lung cancer or immunosuppressant medication in non-neoplastic cases. Immunosuppression should be used cautiously if an underlying cancer cannot be excluded because suppression of tumor growth by LEMS antibody could be reversed, creating a potential for rapid tumor growth. Pyridostigmine is useful in some cases [66]. VGCC—voltage-gated Ca^{2+} channel.

Myasthenia Gravis

Clinical Groups in Myasthenia Gravis

	Early onset (55%)	Thymoma (10%)	Late onset (20%)	Seronegativity (15%)
Weakness	Generalized	Generalized	Generalized or ocular	Ocular or generalized
Age at onset	<40 years of age	Any	>40 years of age	Any
Sex incidence	M < F	M = F	M > F	M > F
Anti-acetylcholine receptors	High	Intermediate	Low	Absent
Thymus	Hyperplasia	Thymoma	Normal	Normal
HLA associations (whites)	B8, DR3		B7, DR2	

Figure 13-23. Clinical groups in myasthenia gravis. Patients with myasthenia gravis can be categorized into four groups relating to age of onset, presence of thymoma, and presence or absence of antibody. Myasthenia gravis has been called a disease of young women and old men, but cases with thymoma occur at any age without gender predilection. Seronegative patients are more commonly mildly affected, but generalized and severe weakness can occur in the absence of detectable antibodies. Passive transfer of disease to mice suggests that the antibody in these cases is simply not detectable by current methods [67,68]. HLA—human lymphocyte antigen. (*Adapted from* Newsom-Davis [69].)

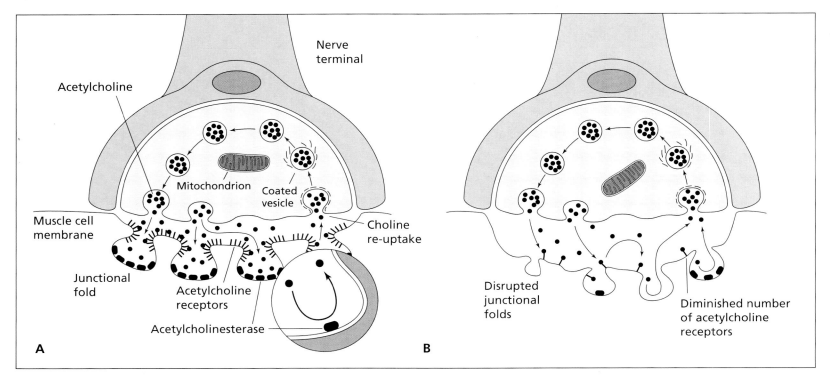

Figure 13-24. Neuromuscular junction in myasthenia gravis. **A**, The normal neuromuscular junction releases acetylcholine from presynaptic vesicles that bind to acetycholine receptors (AChR) at the apices of postsynaptic junctional folds. Bound AChRs allow sodium influx, which causes depolarization of post-synaptic membranes. Acetycholine (ACh) is degraded by acetylcholinesterase, located deep within the postsynaptic crypts. **B**, AChR-Abs bind to AChR, causing: accelerated endocytosis and degradation of receptors, blockade of acetylcholine binding sites, and complement-mediated damage to the post-synaptic membrane. The density of AChR is reduced, and the remaining receptors are blockaded by the presence of bound antibody. Postsynaptic junctional folds are flattened, damaged, and disorganized by this complement-mediated attack. The reduced population of receptor disallows sufficient membrane depolarization to originate a propagating muscle membrane action potential. (*Adapted from* Lindstrom [68].)

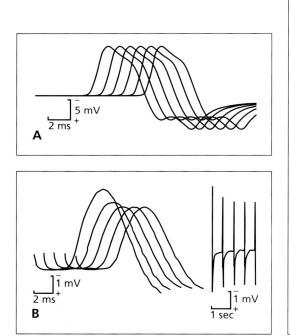

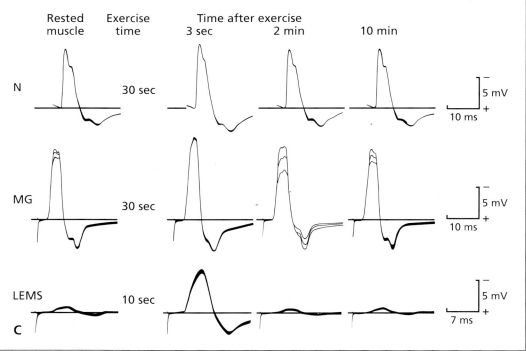

Figure 13-25. Neurophysiologic testing in myasthenia gravis. **A**, Repetitive nerve conduction testing in a normal subject demonstrates a constant compound motor action potential (CMAP) amplitude with repetitive nerve stimulation at slow and rapid rates. **B**, In a patient with symptomatic myasthenia gravis, the amplitude of the compound motor action potential decrements at low rates of 2 to 5 Hz, showing greatest change between the first and second responses. This decrement may correct with administration of intravenous edrophonium (Tensilon, Hoffmann-LaRoche, Nutley, NJ), a short-acting acetylcholinesterase inhibitor. **C**, Comparison of repetitive nerve stimulation in normal (N) subjects, myasthenia gravis (MG) patients, and Lambert-Eaton myasthenic syndrome (LEMS) patients. The decrementing seen in symptomatic MG can be repaired by 30 seconds of exercise, but increasing decrementation then occurs after about 2 minutes. In LEMS, the initial CMAP is of very low amplitude, increasing by greater than 200% after brief, 10-second exercise. After a few minutes, the amplitude again is low.

(*Continued on next page*)

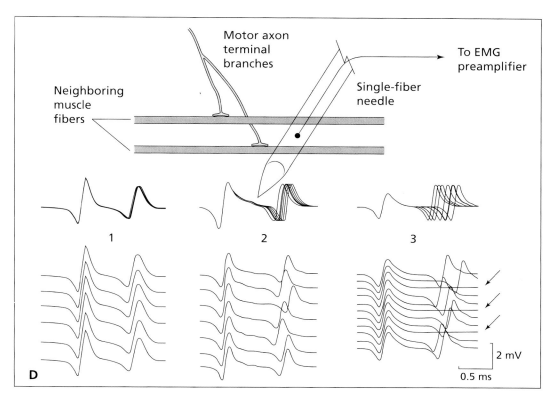

Figure 13-25. (*Continued*) **D,** Use of a special single fiber needle allows the recording of action potentials from individual muscle fibers. Triggering on one muscle cell action potential, the potential from a neighboring fiber of the same motor unit is also captured and appears time-locked with the first as a pair on the oscilloscope. (1) The first potential is held steady on the screen by the instrument; the second fires with variable timing, a phenomenon called *jitter*. The jitter is increased in myasthenia gravis, (2) and blocking of the second potential occurs when the neuromuscular junction fails (3) (*arrows*). EMG—electromyograph. (*Adapted from* Muscle & Nerve [70].)

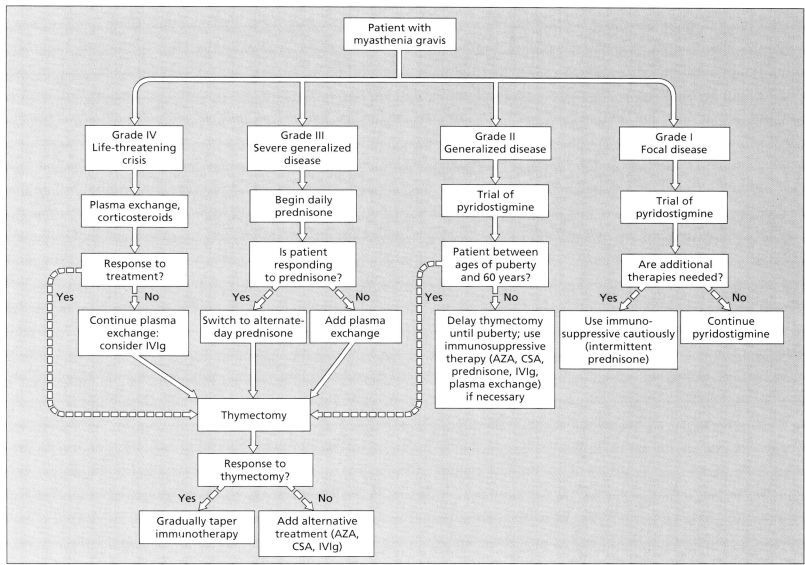

Figure 13-26. Clinical algorithm for the treatment of myasthenia gravis. Treatment strategies in myasthenia gravis include the use of pharmacologic agents directed at the function of the neuromuscular junction; immunosuppressant and immunomodulating techniques; surgical thymectomy. AZA—azathioprine; CSA—cyclosporine; IVIg—intravenous immunoglobulin. (*Adapted from* Mendell [71].)

Lambert-Eaton Syndrome

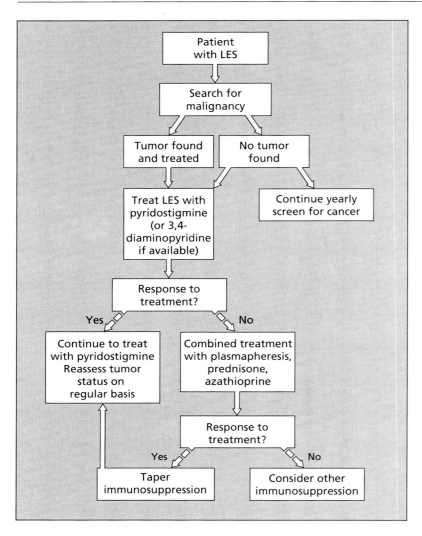

Figure 13-27. Clinical algorithm for the treatment of Lambert-Eaton syndrome (LES). The management of Lambert-Eaton syndrome assumes the presence of an underlying malignancy, although 30% of patients may have no tumor found. Pharmacologic treatment is a second step. Immunosuppressive treatment should only be used when tumor is absent. (*Adapted from* Mendell [71].)

Inflammatory Myopathies

Diagnostic Criteria for Inflammatory Myopathies

Criterion	Polymyositis		Dermatomyositis		Inclusion body myositis
	Definite	Probable*	Definite	Mild or Early	Definite
Muscle strength	Myopathic muscle weakness[†]	Myopathic muscle weakness[†]	Myopathic muscle weakness[†]	Seemingly normal strength[‡]	Myopathic muscle weakness with early involvement of distal muscles[†]
Electromyographic findings	Myopathic	Myopathic	Myopathic	Myopathic or nonspecific	Myopathic with mixed potentials
Muscle enzymes	Elevated (up to 50-fold)	Elevated (up to 50-fold)	Elevated (up to 50-fold) or normal	Elevated (up to 10-fold) or normal	Elevated (up to 10-fold) or normal
Muscle biopsy findings	Diagnostic for this type of inflammatory myopathy	Nonspecific myopathy without signs of primary inflammation	Diagnostic	Nonspecific or diagnostic	Diagnostic
Rash or calcinosis	Absent	Absent	Present	Present	Absent

An adequate trial of prednisone or other immunosuppressive drugs is warranted in probable cases. If, in retrospect, the disease is unresponsive to therapy, another muscle biopsy should be considered to exclude other diseases or possible evolution to inclusion body myositis.

[†]*Myopathic muscle weakness, affecting proximal muscles more than distal ones and sparing eye and facial muscles, is characterized by a subacute onset (weeks to months) and rapid progression in patients who have no family history of neuromuscular disease, no endocrinopathy, no exposure to myotoxic drugs or toxins, and no biochemical muscle disease (excluded on the basis of muscle biopsy findings).*

[‡]*Although strength is seemingly normal, patients often have new onset of easy fatigue, myalgia, and reduced endurance. Careful muscle testing may reveal mild muscle weakness.*

Figure 13-28. Diagnostic criteria for inflammatory myopathy. The autoimmune nature of acquired inflammatory muscle disease is generally accepted, and both cellular and humeral factors are involved. Cellular attack directed against muscle fiber components mediates the muscle invasion and phagocytosis that are seen in polymyositis (PM) [24,72]. Dermatomyositis (DM), by contrast, appears to be mediated by an autoantibody or immune complex response directed against a component of the vascular endothelium. Damage to muscle and other tissues results from disruption of endothelial cells and capillaries, a theory in line with the appearance of perifascicular atrophy in muscle biopsy.

The skin manifestations of DM set it apart. Psoriatic rash over the knuckles (Gottron's sign), forehead and malar rash, periorbital discoloration, nail signs, and subcutaneous calcifications are distinctive, but these may be noticed only in retrospect after biopsy diagnosis. Proximal painless muscle weakness in PM is unaccompanied by other unique clinical features, so diagnosis relies on biopsy and the exclusion of other causes of muscle inflammation. Inclusion body myositis (IBM) is clinically and histologically distinct from PM and DM. The inflammatory myopathy in IBM may only be a secondary response to some underlying myopathic process [2,73].

Later age of onset and mixed proximal and distal weakness characterize IBM. Finger flexors and ankle dorsiflexors are characteristically involved.

The muscle biopsy in IBM shows rimmed vacuoles within muscle fibers accompanied by endomysial inflammation [74].

No proof of therapeutic efficacy has been achieved in PM, DM, or IBM for any pharmacologic or procedural method. Prednisone is first line for PM and DM, but refractory cases call for the use of methotrexate, azathioprine, cyclophosphamide, irradiation (lymphoid or total body), plasmapheresis, and high dose intravenous immunoglobulin. Objective clinical measures such as an expanded Medical Research Council scale, and not creatine kinase levels, should be used to drive the therapeutic decision-making process.

The diagnosis of inflammatory myopathy relies on 1) demonstration of muscle weakness, usually proximal, in the absence of severe sensory loss; 2) elevated muscle enzymes; 3) electromyography demonstrating brief, small, polyphasic motor units in association with fibrillations, positive waves, and complex repetitive discharges; 4) muscle biopsy with characteristic features. Dermatomyositis shows accompanying features of rash and calcinosis. Distal weakness and mixed features on electromyography typify IBM. Care should be taken to exclude infectious processes, toxic myopathies, and other systemic diseases when making these diagnoses. (*Adapted from* Dalakas [75].)

Age Group Affected by and Conditions or Factors Associated With Inflammatory Myopathies

Characteristic	Dermatomyositis	Polymyositis	Inclusion body myositis
Age at onset of disease	Adulthood and childhood	>18 years of age	>50 years of age
Associated condition or factor			
Connective tissue diseases	Yes, with scleroderma and mixed connective tissue disease	Yes	Yes, in up to 15% of cases
Overlap syndrome	Yes, with scleroderma and mixed connective tissue disease	No	No
Systemic autoimmune diseases*	Infrequently	Frequently	Infrequently
Malignant conditions	Probably	No	No
Viruses	Unproved	Yes, with HIV, HTLV-1; possibly other viral or postviral conditions	Unproved
Parasites and bacteria	No	Yes†	No
Drug-induced myotoxicity‡	Yes	Yes	No
Familial association	No	No	Yes, in some cases

The most commonly associated systemic autoimmune diseases are Crohn's disease, vasculitis, sarcoidosis, primary biliary cirrhosis, adult celiac disease, chronic graft-versus-host disease, discoid lupus, ankylosing spondylitis, Behçet's syndrome, myasthenia gravis, acne fulminans, dermatitis herpetiformis, psoriasis, Hashimoto's disease, granulomatous diseases, agammaglobulinemia, monoclonal gammopathy, hypereosinophilic syndrome, Lyme disease, Kawasaki disease, autoimmune thrombocytopenia, hypergammaglobulinemic purpura, hereditary complement deficiency, and IgA deficiency.

†*Includes parasitic (protozoa, cestodes, and nematodes), tropical, and bacterial myositis.*

‡*Drugs include penicillamine (for dermatomyositis and polymyositis), zidovudine (for polymyositis), and contaminated tryptophan (for a dermatomyositis-like illness). Other myotoxic drugs may cause myopathy but not inflammatory myopathy.*

Figure 13-29. Age group affected by and conditions or factors associated with inflammatory myopathies. HTLV—human T-cell lymphotropic virus. (*Adapted from* Dalakas [75].)

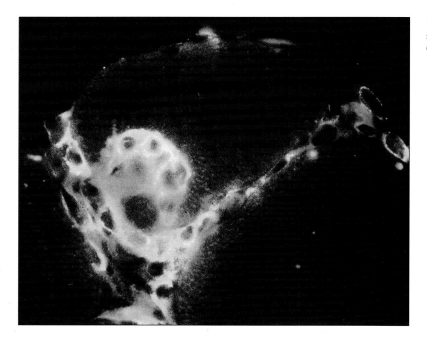

Figure 13-30. Micrograph showing non-necrotic muscle fibers surrounded and invaded by mononuclear cells in polymyositis. (*From* [76]; *courtesy of* Andrew G. Engel, MD, Mayo Clinic, Rochester, MN.)

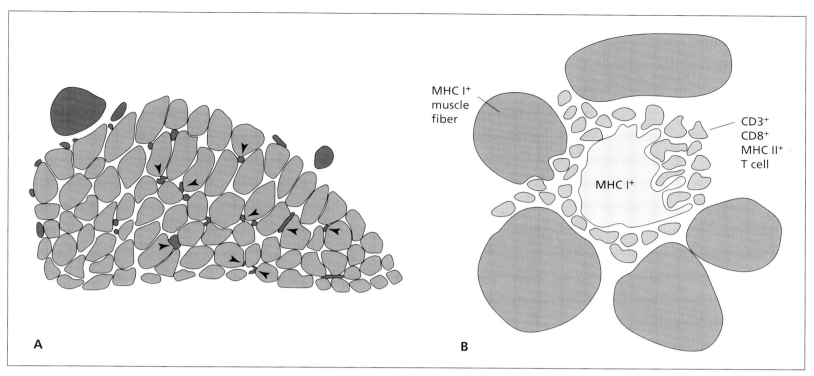

Figure 13-31. Representation of the typical histologic changes observed in inflammatory myopathies. **A**, Dermatomyositis. Muscle fibers are shown in tan, blood vessels in red. Note atrophic fibers at the lower edge of the fascicle (perifascicular atrophy). Clusters of capillaries and venules stain positively for complement membrane attack complex (MAC), and MAC-positive vessels are marked with black arrowheads. The capillary density is significantly reduced. **B**, Polymyositis or inclusion body myositis. T cells surround and focally invade a non-necrotic muscle fiber. All invaded muscle fibers, and some that are noninvaded, show surface reactivity for major histocompatibility complex class 1 (MHC 1). (*Adapted from* Hohlfeld [77].)

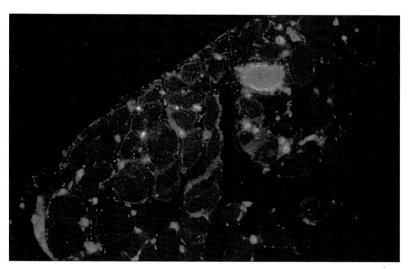

Figure 13-32. Micrograph showing immunolocalization of complement membrane attack complex (MAC) with red rhodamine fluorescence in a patient with dermatomyositis. Numerous capillaries are immunoreactive for MAC. The large MAC-positive profile at the upper right is a necrotic muscle fiber. Complement activation and MAC deposition occur nonspecifically when a muscle fiber undergoes necrosis from any cause. (*From* Hohlfeld [78]; *courtesy of* Andrew G. Engel, MD, Mayo Clinic, Rochester, MN.)

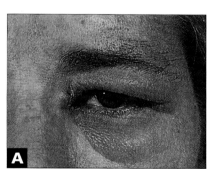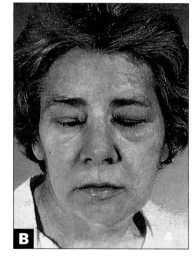

Figure 13-33. Blue-purple discoloration, the heliotrope rash, appearing on the upper eyelids and in the periorbital region in a patient with inflammatory myopathy (**A**). The forehead and malar areas are affected by a nonraised red rash (**B**). (*From* Griggs and colleagues [79]; with permission.)

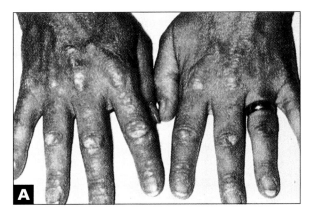
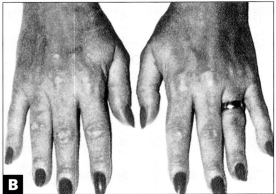

Figure 13-34. Gottron's sign in dermatomyositis, which is seen in some patients with inflammatory myopathies. **A,** A raised, violaceous, scaly eruption with a psoriatic appearance overlies the extensor surfaces of the knuckles. Similar lesions appear over the extensor surfaces of the elbows and other joints. **B,** The same patient after treatment with intravenous immune globulin. (*From* Dalakas and colleagues [80]; with permission.)

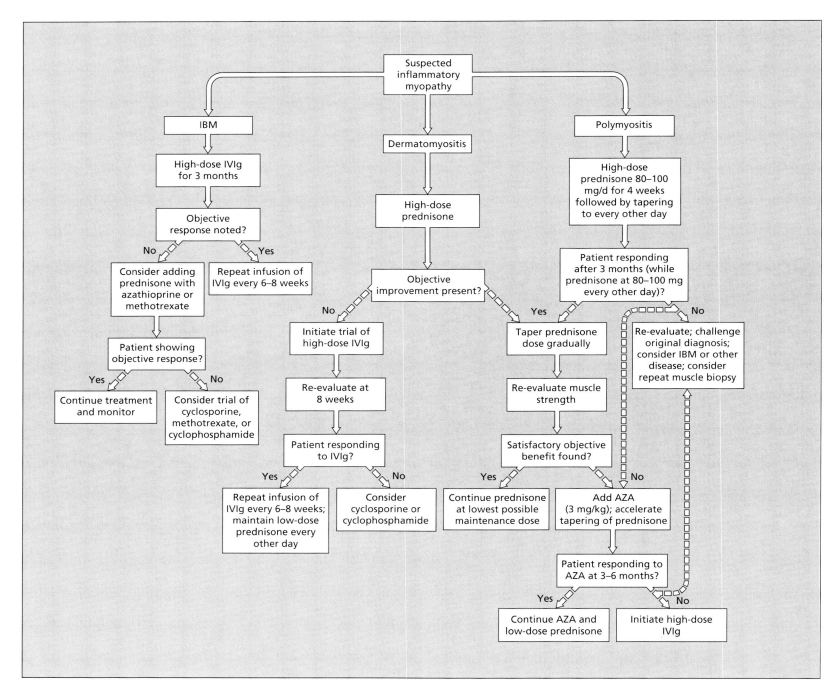

Figure 13-35. Clinical algorithm for the treatment of inflammatory myopathies. AZA—azathioprine; IBM—inclusion body myositis; IVIg—intravenous immunoglobulin. (*Adapted from* Dalakas [75].)

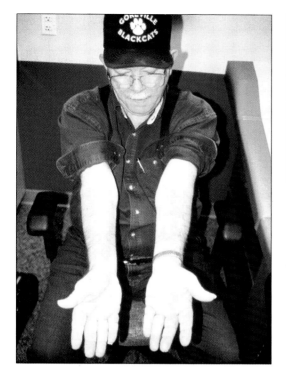

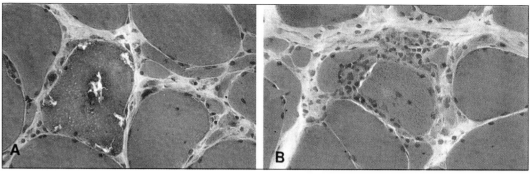

Figure 13-37. A, B, Modified trichrome stain showing intracytoplasmic vacuoles rimmed by dark-staining granules. Eosinophilic inclusion bodies lie adjacent to the vacuoles. Endomysial inflammatory infiltration and muscle cell phagocytosis leads to necrosis. Small, angulated fibers occur in groups and may indicate a component effect of denervation [84]. Amyloid filaments have been demonstrated [85] and type II adenovirus has been isolated from muscle biopsy [86]. (*From* Griggs and colleagues [87]; with permission.)

Figure 13-36. Signs and symptoms of inclusion body myositis (IBM). The signs and symptoms of IBM are typified in this patient, a 66-year-old man with weakness of the quadriceps muscles, bilateral foot-drop, and severe loss of grip strength, progressing over nine years [81]. This shows the characteristic scooped-out appearance of the volar forearms due to marked atrophy of the deep finger flexors. Dysphagia may be the first symptom of IBM [82] or may develop and worsen as the disease slowly progresses. The creatine phosphokinase may be only mildly elevated, so a misdiagnosis of motor neuron disease often occurs. Treatment for IBM is usually disappointing, although intravenous immunoglobulin has benefited a few cases [83].

References

1. Genkins G, Kornfeld P, Papatestas AE, *et al.*: Clinical experience in more than 2,000 patients with myasthenia gravis. *Ann NY Acad Sci* 1987, 505:500–513.

2. Dalakas MC: Polymyositis, dermatomyositis, and inclusion body myositis. *N Engl J Med* 1991, 325(21):1487–1498.

3. Sibley WA, Bamford CR, Clark K: Triggering Factors in Multiple Sclerosis. In *Diagnosis of Multiple Sclerosis*. Edited by Poser CM, Paty DW, Scheinberg L. New York: Thieme-Stratton; 1984:14.

4. Constantinescu CS, Cohen JA: Regulatory-cytokine therapy for autoimmune diseases: Implications for multiple sclerosis. *Multiple Sclerosis: Clinical Issues* 1994, 1(3):6–9.

5. Glaser JS: Topical Diagnosis: Prechiasmal Visual Pathways. In *Neuroophthalmology*, edn 2. Edited by Glaser JS. Philadelphia: JB Lippincott; 1990:123–128.

6. Francis DA, Compston DA, Batchelor JR, *et al.*: A reassessment of the risk of MS developing in patients with optic neuritis after extended follow-up. *J Neurol Neurosurg Psychiatry* 1987, 50(6):758–765.

7. Leys D, Petit H, Block AM, *et al.*: Neuromyelitis optica (Devic's disease): four cases. *Rev Neurol* (Paris) 1987, 143:722.

8. Poser CM, Paty DW, Scheinberg L, *et al.*: New diagnostic criteria for multiple sclerosis: guidelines for research protocols. *Ann Neurol* 1983, 13:227–231.

9. Ohman S, Ernerudh J, Forsberg P, *et al.*: Comparison of seven formulae and isoelectric focusing for determining of intrathecally producing IgG in neurological diseases. *Ann Clin Biochem* 1992, 29:405–410.

10. Stendahl Brodin L, Link H: Optic neuritis: oligoclonal bands increase the risk of multiple sclerosis. *Acta Neurol Scand* 1983, 67:301–304.

11. Yock DH: White Matter Disorders. In *Magnetic Resonance Imaging of CNS Disease*, Chap. 7. St. Louis: Mosby–Year Book; 1995.

12. Thorp JW, Miller DH: MRI: its application and impact. *Internat MS J* 1994, 1(1):7–15.

13. Comi G, Filippi M, Martinelli V, *et al.*: Brain stem magnetic resonance imaging and evoked potential studies of symptomatic multiple sclerosis patients. *Eur Neurol* 1993, 33:232–237.

14. McDonald WI, Miller DH: Spinal cord MRI using multi-array coils and fast spin echo. II. Findings in multiple sclerosis. *Neurology* 1993, 43:2632–2637.

15. Kastrukoff LF, Oger JJ, Hashimoto SA, *et al.*: Systemic lymphoblastoid interferon therapy in chronic progressive multiple sclerosis. I. Clinical and MRI evaluation. *Neurology* 1990, 40:479–486.

16. Koopmans RA, Li DKB, Zhao GJ, *et al.*: MRI assessment of cyclosporine therapy of MS in a multi-center trial. *Neurology* 1992, 42(suppl 3):210.

17. Thompson AJ, Miller D, Youl B, *et al.*: Serial gadolinium-enhanced MRI in relapsing/remitting multiple sclerosis of varying disease duration. *Neurology* 1992, 42:60–63.

18. Offenbacher H, Fazekas F, Schmidt R, *et al.*: Assessment of MRI criteria for a diagnosis of MS. *Neurology* 1993, 43:905–909.

19. Filippi M, Martinelli V, Sirabian G, *et al.*: Brain magnetic resonance imaging correlates of cognitive impairment in multiple sclerosis. *J Neurol Sci* 1993, 115(suppl):S66–S73.

20. IFNB Multiple Sclerosis Study Group: Interferon β-1b is effective in relapsing-remitting multiple sclerosis. I. Clinical results of a multicenter, randomized, double-blind, placebo controlled trial. *Neurology* 1993, 43(4):655–661.

21. Paty DW, Li DKB, UBC MS/MRI Study Group, IFNB Multiple Sclerosis Study Group: Interferon β-1b is effective in relapsing-remitting multiple sclerosis. II. MRI analysis results of a multicenter, randomized, double-blind, placebo controlled trial. *Neurology* 1993, 43(4):662–667.

22. Wolinsky JS: Copolymer 1: A most reasonable alternative therapy for early relapsing-remitting multiple sclerosis with mild disability. *Neurology* 1995, 45(7):1245–1247.

23. Beck RW, Cleary PA, Anderson MM, *et al.*: A randomized controlled trial of corticosteroids in the treatment of acute optic neuritis. *N Engl J Med* 1992, 326(9):581–588.

24. Weiner HL, Mackin GA, Orav EJ, *et al.*: Intermittent cyclophosphamide pulse therapy in progressive multiple sclerosis: final report of the Northeast Cooperative Multiple Sclerosis Treatment Group. *Neurology* 1993, 43(5):910–918.

25. Canadian Cooperative Multiple Sclerosis Study Group: The Canadian Cooperative Trial of cyclophosphamide and plasma exchange in progressive multiple sclerosis. *Lancet* 1991, 337:441—446.

26. Goodkin DE, Rudick RA, Medendorp SV, *et al.*: Low dose oral weekly methotrexate (MTX) significantly reduces the frequency of progression of impairment in patients with chronic progressive multiple sclerosis (CPMS). *Neurology* 1994, 44:A357.

27. Sipe JC, Romine JS, Koziol JA, *et al.*: Cladribine in treatment of chronic progressive multiple sclerosis. *Lancet* 1994, 344(8914):9–13.

28. Milligan NM, Miller DH, Compston DAS: A placebo-controlled trial of isoprinosine in patients with multiple sclerosis. *J Neurol Neurosurg Psychiatry* 1994, 57(2):164–168.

29. Wiles CM, Omar L, Swan AV, *et al.*: Total lymphoid irradiation in multiple sclerosis. *J Neurol Neurosurg Psychiatry* 1994, 57(2):154–163.

30. Miller A, Lider O, Roberts AB, *et al.*: Suppressor T cells generated by oral tolerization to myelin basic proteins suppress both *in vitro* and *in vivo* immune responses by the release of transforming growth factor after antigen specific triggering. *Proc Nat Acad Sci* 1992, 89:421.

31. Weiner HL, Mackin GE, Matsui M, *et al.*: Double-blind pilot trial of oral tolerization with myelin antigens in multiple sclerosis. *Science* 1993, 259(5099):1321–1324.

32. Achiron A, Pras E, Gilad R, *et al.*: Open controlled therapeutic trial of intravenous immunoglobulin in relapsing-remitting multiple sclerosis. *Arch Neurol* 1992, 49(12):1233–1236.

33. Rodriguez M, Karnes WE, Bartleson JD, *et al.*: Plasmapheresis in acute episodes of fulminant CNS inflammatory demyelination. *Neurology* 1993, 43(6):1100–1104.

34. IFNB Multiple Sclerosis Study Group and the University of British Columbia MS/MRI Analysis Group. Interferon β-1b in the treatment of multiple sclerosis: final outcome of the randomized controlled trial. *Neurology* 1995, 45:1277–1285.

35. Johnson KP, Brooks BR, Cohen JA, *et al.*, and the Copolymer 1 Multiple Sclerosis Study Group: Copolymer 1 reduces relapse rate and improves disability in relapsing-remitting multiple sclerosis: results of a phase III multicenter, double-blind, placebo controlled trial. *Neurology* 1995, 45:1268–1276.

36. Noseworthy JH, Hopkins MB, Vandervoort MK, *et al.*: An open trial evaluation of mitoxantrone in the treatment of progressive MS. *Neurology* 1993, 43(7):1401–1406.

37. Graus F, Dalmau JO: Management of paraneoplastic neurological syndromes. In *Neurological Complications of Cancer*. Edited by Wiley RO. New York: Marcel Dekker; 1995:167–198.

38. Posner JB: Paraneoplastic syndromes. In *Neurological Complications of Cancer*. Edited by Posner JB. Philadelphia: FA Davis; 1995:353–384.

39. Jacobson DM, Thirkill CL, Tipping SJ: A clinical triad to diagnose paraneoplastic retinopathy. *Ann Neurol* 1990, 28(2):162–167.

40. Dropcho EJ: Autoimmune central nervous system paraneoplastic disorders: Mechanisms, diagnosis and therapeutic options. *Ann Neurol* 1995, 37(suppl 1):S102–S113.

41. Greenlees J, Brashear HR: Remote effects of carcinoma. In *Current Therapy in Neurologic Disease*. Edited by Johnson RT, Griffin JW. St. Louis: Mosby–Year Book; 1995:167–198.

42. Brashear HR: Antibody testing: Finding the inside track to early diagnosis of CNS paraneoplastic syndromes. *Adv Neuroimmunol* 1995, 2(3):3–11.

43. Meinck HM, Ricker K, Hulser PJ, *et al.*: Stiff-man's syndrome: neurophysiological findings in 8 patients. *J Neurol* 1995, 242(3):134–142.

44. Meinck H, Ricker K, Hulser PJ, *et al.*: Stiff-man's syndrome: clinical and laboratory findings in 8 patients. *J Neurol* 1994, 241(3):157–166.

45. Folli F, Solimena M, Cofiell R, *et al.*: Autoantibodies to a 128-kd synaptic protein in 3 women with stiff-man syndrome and breast cancer. *N Engl J Med* 1993, 328(8):546–551.

46. Smith RG, Engelhardt JI, Tajti J, *et al.*: Experimental immune-mediated motor neuron diseases: models for human ALS. *Brain Res Bull* 1993, 30:373–380.

47. Rogers SW, Andrews PI, Gahring LC, *et al.*: Autoantibodies to glutamate receptor 3 in Rasmussen's encephalitis. *Science* 1994, 265:648–651.

48. Parry GJ: Inflammatory demyelinating polyneuropathies: new perspectives in treatment. *Adv Neuroimmunol* 1994, 1(1):9–15.

49. Dyck PJ, Daube J, O'Brien P, *et al.*: Plasma exchange in chronic inflammatory demyelinating polyradiculoneuropathy. *N Engl J Med* 1986, 314:461–465.

50. Dyck PJ, Litchy WJ, Kratz KM, *et al.*: A plasma exchange versus immune globulin infusion trial in chronic inflammatory demyelinating polyradiculoneuropathy. *Ann Neurol* 1994, 36(6):838–845.

51. Krendel DA, Successful treatment of neuropathies in patients with diabetes mellitus. *Arch Neurol* 1995, 52:1053–1061.

52. Kissel JT, Mendel JR: Vasculitic neuropathy. *Neurol Clin* 1992, 10:761–781.

53. Olney RK: Neuropathies in connective tissue disease. *Muscle Nerve* 1992, 15:531–542.

54. van der Meche FGA, Schmitz PIM, and the Dutch Guillain-Barré Study Group: A randomized trial comparing intravenous immune globulin and plasma exchange in Guillain-Barré syndrome. *N Engl J Med* 1992, 326(17):1123–1129.

55. Hayes MT: Analyzing new strategies to diagnose and treat autoimmune neuropathies. *Adv Neuroimmunol* 1995, 2(2):10–17.

56. Parry G, Swenson MR: When is antibody testing useful and what therapy is effective in immune-mediated neuropathies? *Adv Neuroimmunol* 1995, 2(2):18–22.

57. Odabasi Z, Joy JL, Claussen GC, *et al.*: Isaacs' syndrome associated with chronic inflammatory demyelinating polyneuropathy. *Muscle Nerve* 1996, 19:210–215.

58. Newsom-Davis J, Mills KR: Immunological associations of acquired neuromyotonia (Isaacs' syndrome): report of five cases and literature review. *Brain* 1993, 116 (part III):453–469.

59. Sinha S, Newsom-Davis J, Mills K, *et al.*: Autoimmune aetiology for acquired neuromyotonia (Isaacs' syndrome). *Lancet* 1991, 338(8759):75–77.

60. Quarles RH, Colman DR, Salzer JL, *et al.*: Myelin associated glycoprotein: structure-function relationships and involvement in neurological diseases. In *Myelin: Biology and Chemistry*. Edited by Martenson RE. Boca Raton, FL: CRC Press; 1992:413–448.

61. Quarles RH: Antibody mediated neuropathies exploring the pathogenic mechanisms. *Adv Neuroimmunol* 1995, 2(2):3–9.

62. Drachman DB: Myasthenia gravis. *N Engl J Med* 1994, 330:1797–1810.

63. Grob D, Arsura EL, Brunner NG, Namba T: The course of myasthenia gravis and therapies affecting outcome. *Ann NY Acad Sci* 1987, 505:472–479.

64. Engel AG: Review of evidence for loss of motor nerve terminal calcium channels in Lambert-Eaton myasthenic syndrome. *Ann NY Acad Sci* 1991, 635:246–258.

65. O'Neill JH, Murray NM, Newsom-Davis J: The Lambert-Eaton myasthenic syndrome: A review of 50 cases. *Brain* 1988, 111:577–596.

66. Chalk CH, Murray NM, Newsom-Davis J: Response of the Lambert-Eaton myasthenic syndrome to treatment of associated small cell lung carcinoma. *Neurology* 1990, 40:1552–1556.

67. Soliven BC, Lange DJ, Penn AS, *et al.*: Seronegative myasthenia gravis. *Neurology* 1988, 38:514–517.

68. Lindstrom JM: Pathophysiology of myasthenia gravis: the mechanisms behind the disease. *Adv Neuroimmunol* 1994, 1(2):3–8.

69. Newsom-Davis J: Myasthenia gravis: The Lambert-Eaton myasthenic syndrome and acquired myotonia. In *Diagnostic and Therapeutic Approaches to Myasthenia Gravis. Proceedings of the Annual Meeting of the Myasthenia Gravis Foundation of America*, Salt Lake City, Utah, April 28, 1995.

70. Section II: Illustrations of selected waveforms. *Muscle & Nerve* 1987, 10(8S):G24–G52.

71. Mendell J: Neuromuscular junction disorders: A guide to diagnosis and treatment. *Adv Neuroimmunol* 1994, 1(2):9–16.

72. Hohlfeld R, Engel AG, Kunio I, *et al.*: Polymyositis mediated by T cell lymphocytes that express the gamma delta receptor. *N Engl J Med* 1991, 324:877–881.

73. Barohn RJ, Amato AA, Sahenk Z, *et al.*: Inclusion body myositis: explanation for poor response to immunosuppressive therapy. *Neurology* 1995, 45:1302–1304.

74. Lotz BP, Engel AG, Nishino H, *et al.*: Inclusion body myositis. *Brain* 1989, 112:727–742.

75. Dalakas MC: Polymyositis, dermatomyositis, and inclusion-body myositis. *N Engl J Med* 1991, 325:1487–1498.

76. Cover photo from *Adv Neuroimmunol* 1995, 2(1).

77. Hohlfeld R, Engel AG, Kunio I, *et al.*: The immunobiology of muscle. *Immunol Today* 1994, 15:269–274.

78. Hohlfeld R: New concepts in the immunobiology of inflammatory myopathy. *Adv Neuroimmunol* 1995, 2(1):4–8.

79. Griggs R, Mendell J, Miller R: Inflammatory Myopathy. In *Evaluation and Treatment of Myopathy*. Philadelphia: FA Davis; 1995.

80. Dalakas MC, Illa I, Dambrosia JM, *et al.*: A controlled trial of high-dose intravenous immune globulin infusions as treatment for dermatomyositis. *N Engl J Med* 1993, 329(27):1993–1999.

81. Shaibani A, Harati Y: Idiopathic inflammatory myopathies: polymyositis, dermatomyositis, inclusion body myositis. In *Neuro-Immunology for the Clinician*. Edited by Rolak LA, Harati Y. Boston: Butterworth-Heinemann; 1997:301–316.

82. Riminton DS, Chambers ST, Darkin PJ, *et al.*: Inclusion body myositis presenting solely as dysphagia. *Neurology* 1993, 43:1241.

83. Dalakas MC, Dambrosia JM, Sekul EA, *et al.*: Inclusion body myositis: the efficacy of high-dose intravenous immunoglobulin (IVIg) in patients with inclusion body myositis. *Neurology* 1995, 45(suppl 4):A208.

84. Pruitt JN, Showalter CJ, Engel AG, *et al.*: Sporadic inclusion body myositis. Counts of different types of abnormal fibers. *Ann Neurol* 1996, 39:139.

85. Mendell JR, Sahenk Z, Gales T, Paul L: Amyloid filaments in inclusion body myositis. Novel findings provide insight into nature of filaments. *Arch Neurol* 1991, 48:1229–1234.

86. Mikol J, Felten-Papaiconomou A, Ferchal F, *et al.*: Inclusion-body myositis: clinicopathological studies and isolation of an adenovirus type 2 from muscle biopsy specimen. *Ann Neurol* 1982, 11:576–581.

87. Griggs RC, Mendell JR, Miller RG: *Evaluation and Treatment of Myopathies*. Philadelphia: FA Davis; 1995:172.

14

Neurotoxic Disorders

Bruce G. Gold • Jerome V. Schnell
Peter S. Spencer

THE nervous system is commonly impacted by chemicals found in nature, elaborated by organisms, or synthesized by chemists. The peculiar architecture of neural cells, their high-energy demands, and the mandate for electrochemical communication combine to place the nervous system at high risk for chemical perturbation. This inherent vulnerability is exploited by natural agents, synthetic chemicals, medications, and recreational substances designed or used to target the nervous system as well as by a host of other substances that are occasionally encountered in the environment. The neurotoxic actions of chemicals are expressed in a wide range of neurologic phenomena, some of which are associated with purely functional changes, others with structural damage, and still others with both. Many chemicals cause effects that appear and disappear rapidly; others produce effects that evolve over days or weeks and regress over months or years. Diagnosis is heavily dependent on the history and characteristic clinical phenomenology. Specific treatment other than termination of exposure is rare. Although clinical improvement is the rule, neurotoxic disorders leave scars or disappear without a trace.

Hundreds of substances are known to have neurotoxic potential. Neurologic illness is associated with certain gases, liquids, minerals, bacteria, fungi, plants, and primitive, intermediate, and higher members of the animal kingdom. Zootoxins often have high toxic potency and discrete biologic actions; they are among the best understood from the mechanistic standpoint. Many other, less potent, naturally occurring chemicals precipitate neurologic illness after repeated exposure to relatively large doses. Among the most common causes of functional or structural neurotoxicity are drugs used for their therapeutic or euphoric properties. Overt neurologic illness associated with chemicals in the workplace has become less common.

Tracking the probable cause of neurotoxic illness requires precise identification of exposure. Cause and effect are best shown by demonstrating under controlled conditions that the neurologic disorder is induced in a suitable mammal after comparable exposure to the suspect agent. Neurotoxic chemicals identified in this manner often become useful experimental tools to probe the structure of receptors or the vulnerability of neural cells, or to reproduce models of neurodegenerative and other disorders. These approaches will contribute to an understanding of the role of environmental chemicals in conditions that are currently idiopathic.

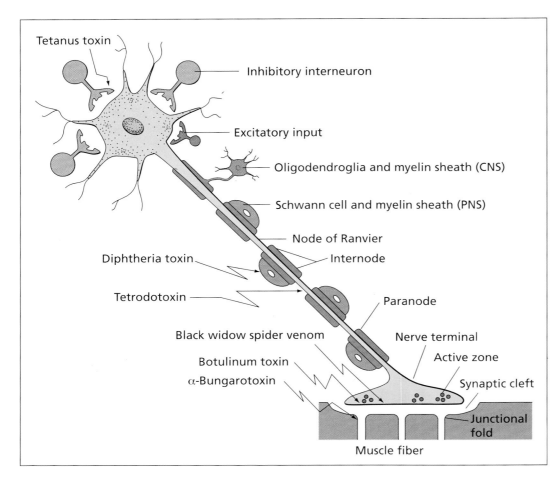

Figure 14-1. Subcellular targets of selected neurotoxins. A motor neuron showing normal anatomic landmarks on the right, and the sites of action of several biologic toxins on the left. The cell body, containing the nucleus, nucleolus, and Nissl substance, receives inhibitory and excitatory synaptic inputs. The intraspinal axon is ensheathed by processes derived from oligodendroglia, while the axons in the roots and the peripheral nerves have myelin sheaths maintained by Schwann cells. The nerve terminal occupies a depression on the muscle surface with presynaptic active zones opposite the receptor-rich convexities (junctional folds) of the postsynaptic (muscle) membrane. Tetanus toxin is taken up at nerve terminals and carried by retrograde axonal transport to the cell body from which it passes transsynaptically to bind to, and block, axosomatic inhibitory (glycinergic) synaptic inputs. Diphtheria toxin binds to Schwann cells and arrests protein synthesis. Tetrodotoxin (found in puffer and porcupine fish) blocks sodium channels at the nodes of Ranvier. Black widow spider venom causes massive release of transmitter by promoting fusion of synaptic vesicles at sites outside the active zones. Botulinum toxin impairs release of acetylcholine by interfering with exocytosis at active zones. α-Bungarotoxin (found in the venom of the snake *Bungarus multicinctus*) blocks transmission by binding to the acetylcholine receptor. CNS—central nervous system; PNS—peripheral nervous system. (*Adapted from* Price and colleague [1].)

Sources of Human Toxicants

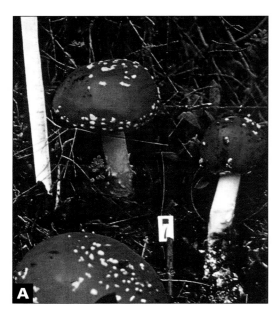

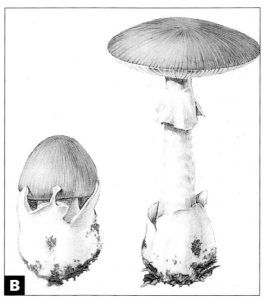

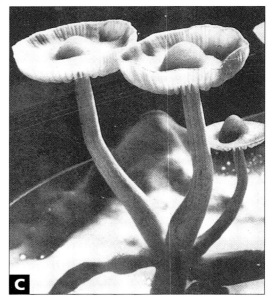

Figure 14-2. Mushroom neurotoxins. Two examples of highly toxic *Amanita* mushrooms. **A**, *Amanita muscaria*, found in temperate climates, contains the neurotoxins ibotenic acid, muscimol (which has lysergic acid diethylamide–like actions), and muscazone. Eating this mushroom results in a myriad of dose-related central nervous system effects, including dizziness, ataxia, euphoria, hallucinations, delirium, and, occasionally, convulsions. **B**, *Amanita phalloides*, one of the most toxic of all mushrooms and responsible for 95% of mushroom-related deaths, contains two classes of toxins: the amatoxins and the phallotoxins. Consumption results in the development of vomiting and diarrhea attributable to the phallotoxins and, after several days, the development of liver and kidney dysfunction. Intracranial hemorrhage may also occur. Although these toxins may have no direct neurotoxic effect, CNS dysfunction may result both from intracranial hemorrhage and hepatic encephalopathy. **C**, *Psilocybe mexicana* is a psychotropic species ("magic mushroom of Mexico") that contains the potent hallucinogen psilocybin and its dephosphorylated analog, psilocin. Euphoria results from small (milligrams) doses; higher doses induce hallucinations and visual alterations. Convulsions and death follow massive overdose. (Panels A and C *from* Toro-González and colleagues [2]; with permission; Panel B P. van der Maaden *from* Vinken and colleague [3]; with permission.)

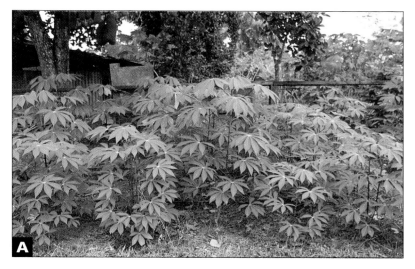

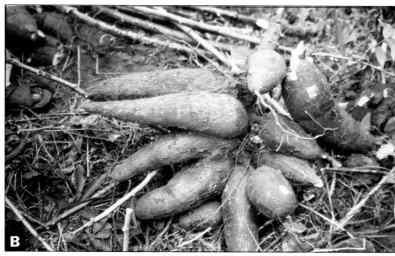

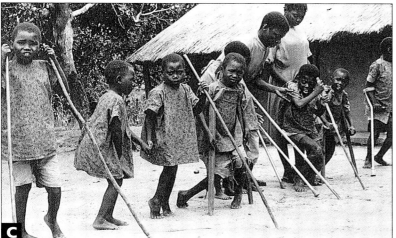

Figure 14-3. Cassava neurotoxicity. Eaten by more than 500 million people, the cassava plant is an important source of nutrition throughout the world. Both the leaves (**A**) and roots (**B**) are eaten, the latter after crushing, pounding, washing, and drying to remove toxic components. Tapioca is derived from cassava, and cassava plant materials are also used increasingly in processed food. The plant harbors cyanogenic glucosides, which liberate cyanide on consumption. Outbreaks of neurologic disease always occur in the setting of protein malnutrition in subjects (**C**) from communities dependent on cassava for their diet. If malnourished people fail to sufficiently process the roots, a variety of neurologic symptoms (notably headache) can follow. The onset of neurologic disease is subacute and featured by leg weakness and pyramidal signs. Spastic paraparesis may be accompanied by largely reversible visual difficulties and sensory neural dysfunction. Subjects subsisting on incompletely detoxified cassava may develop a slowly evolving central and peripheral nervous system disorder (tropical ataxia myeloneuropathy). (*From* Rosling [4]; with permission.)

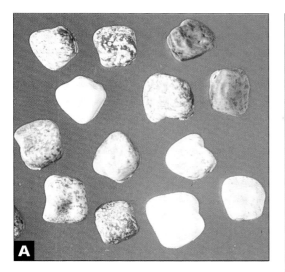

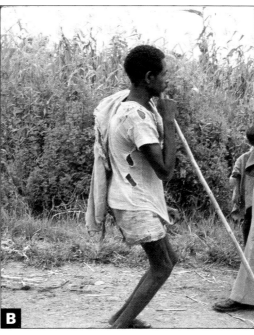

Figure 14-4. Lathyrism. *Lathyrus sativus* (grass pea, chickling pea) is a hardy legume resistant to both drought and flood, and is eaten in parts of Africa (Ethiopia), the Indian subcontinent, and China. International trade of this potentially neurotoxic legume may be increasing. **A,** The seed of the grass pea is a source of protein for food but also harbors a potent excitatory amino acid, β-*N*-oxalylamino-L-alanine (BOAA). BOAA is the culpable agent of human lathyrism, a form of irreversible spastic paraparesis clinically comparable to the cassava-related disease. **B,** Irreversible spastic paraparesis (lathyrism) is triggered by prolonged, heavy dietary reliance on the grass pea. Onset is usually subacute, with symptoms of heaviness and weakness in the legs, with sparing of the arms. Subjects develop increased muscle tone and walk with a scissoring gait on the balls of their feet. Degrees of spasticity increase with continued grass pea consumption. Most patients are mildly affected ("no-stick" cases), some use one stick as an ambulatory aid (as seen here), and severely affected patients employ a pair of crutches or are forced to move around on their rumps ("crawler stage"). Signs are consistent with disease of upper motor neurons, with evidence of pyramidal dysfunction. Strength is retained in the upper extremities, and mentation remains clear. (Panel A *courtesy of* Clayton C. Campbell, PhD, Morden, Manitoba, Canada.)

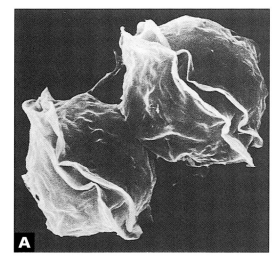

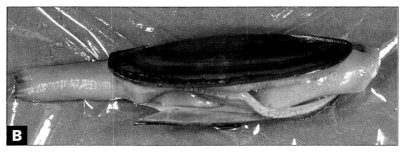

Figure 14-5. Dinoflagellate neurotoxins. Electron scanning micrograph (**A**) of *Gonyaulax catenella* isolated from a red tide sample showing a dorsal view of a two-celled chain. This dinoflagellate produces saxitoxin, which blocks sodium channels in nerve membranes and initially causes distal-extremity and circumoral paresthesias. This is followed by dizziness, ataxia, hypotonia, and death. Saxitoxin accumulates in shellfish that feed on the dinoflagellate, including the Alaska butter clam, mussels, the bay scallop *Argopecten irradians,* and the razor clam (**B**). Dinoflagellates of *Pseudonitzcshia americana* have been implicated in an acute neurologic disease featured by short-term memory loss and neuromuscular weakness. Domoic acid, the suspect neurotoxic agent, is a potent glutamate analog found in razor clams, anchovies, mussels, and crabs harvested from the entire length of the US West Coast. (Panel A *from* Halstead [5]; with permission; photograph by A.R. Loeblich III and L.A. Loeblich *courtesy of* World-Life Research Institute, Colton, CA; Panel B *courtesy of* John C. Wekell, PhD, Northwest Fisheries Science Center of Seattle, WA.)

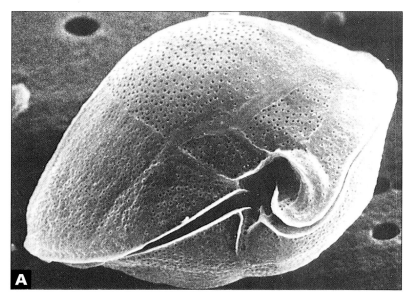

Figure 14-6. Dinoflagellate neurotoxins (ciguatoxins). Ciguatera toxins are manifold and include two major types: ciguatoxin and maitotoxin. Ciguatoxin acts selectively on voltage-dependent sodium channels of nerve and muscle cells and at synaptic terminals. Maitotoxin acts to increase calcium permeability through voltage-sensitive channels. Humans consuming tropical reef or in-shore fish containing ciguatoxin develop diarrhea, nausea, and vomiting. Paresthesia is a prominent symptom, a presentation that assists in the differential diagnosis from other fish poisons or gastroenteritis. Other neurologic symptoms include ataxia, auditory hallucinations, dizziness, extreme fatigue, headaches, muscular numbness, myalgia, pruritus, sweating with chilling, transient blurred vision or blindness, and vertigo. The neurologic signs may persist for months or even years. Ciguatoxicosis is seen in tropical and subtropical regions. **A**, This dinoflagellate (*Gambierdiscus toxicus*) is one of possibly several organisms responsible for ciguatera fish poisoning. **B**, Diagram depicting the origin of ciguatera fish poisoning and the ways in which it is contracted by humans. Both the fish that feed on the algae and the larger predators that eat the toxic bottom-feeding fish can be poisonous to humans. (Panel A *from* Halstead [5]; with permission; photograph by D.R. Tindall and G. Morey-Gaines, *courtesy of* World-Life Research Institute, Colton, CA; Panel B *adapted from* Anon [6].)

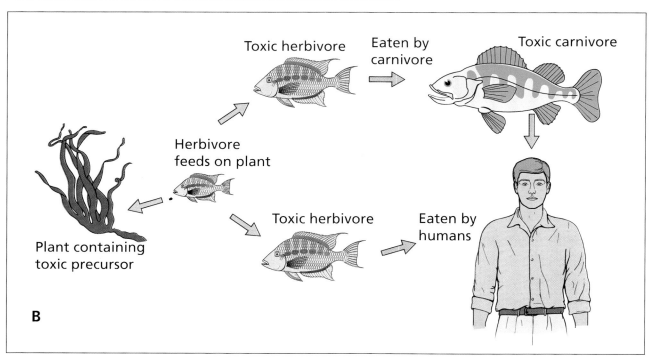

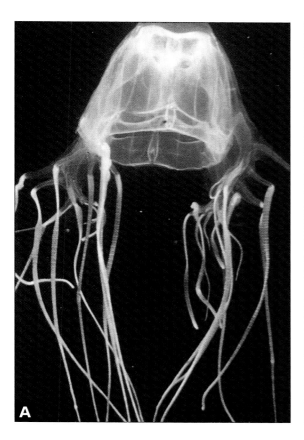
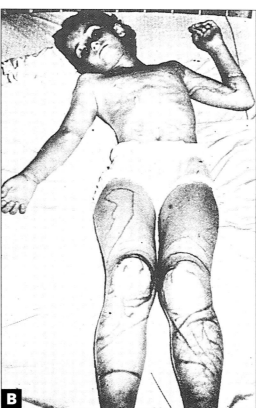

Figure 14-7. Coelenterate neurotoxicity. **A**, *Chironex fleckeri*, the lethal box jelly, likely accounts for most of the fatalities that occur in northern Australian waters. This is probably the most dangerous venomous marine animal known. It may cause death within a period of seconds to several minutes. Stings are extremely painful and may cause vesication and skin necrosis in survivors. Muscle spasms, dyspnea, prostration, and pulmonary edema occur. Cardiovascular effects include hypertension followed by hypotension, and cardiac arrhythmias. Stringent protective measures in the form of adequate diving clothing (*eg*, neoprene-coated nylon) must be worn to avoid contact with the tentacles. All exposed portions of the body must be covered. **B**, Child stung in north Queensland by *Chironex fleckeri*. The extensive weals cause severe pain and other neurotoxic and dermatonecrotic effects. (Panel A *from* Halstead [5]; with permission; photograph by K. Gillett, *courtesy of* World-Life Research Institute, Colton, CA; Panel B *from* Vinken and colleague [7]; with permission.)

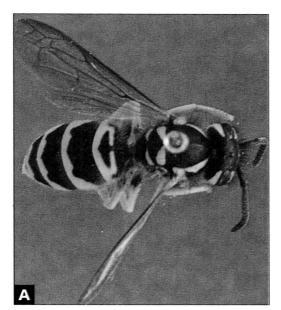
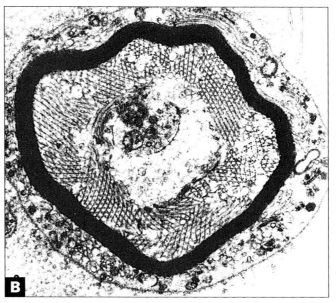

Figure 14-8. Insect envenomation. **A**, The yellow jacket (*Vespula* spp.) elaborates a toxin containing a range of pharmacologically active substances, including histamine, serotonin, polyamine, cinene, and catecholamines. A sting most commonly results in a mild local reaction accompanied by pain, urticaria, erythema, and swelling locally. **B**, Peripheral nerve. A honeycombed pattern involving the inner circumference of the myelin sheath is seen surrounding a shrunken, degenerated axon. The Schwann cell cytoplasm also shows degenerated organelles and irregularly shaped vesicles. Anaphylaxis with bronchial spasm may precipitate neurologic complications associated with hypoxia. It can manifest as changes in consciousness and as occasional, nonfocal seizures. Intracerebral hemorrhage and edema are seen on occasion. Delayed neurologic effects are uncommon but may include a progressive radiculomyelopathy associated with patchy demyelination of thoracic and lumbar roots and corresponding areas of the spinal cord. Application of the toxin to the sciatic nerve of a rat results in selective changes of the myelin sheath. True allergy to the venom can result in serious and occasionally fatal complications. (Panel A *from* Anon [8]; Panel B *from* Saida and colleagues [9]; with permission.)

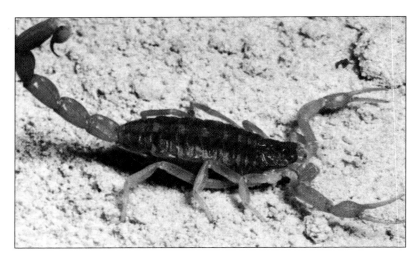

Figure 14-9. Scorpion envenomation. Scorpions secrete a complex mixture of substances, including an array of proteins with neuropharmacologic and enzymatic activity. The venom is delivered from a tail stinger. The sting of most scorpions is associated with dysesthesia, localized swelling, and ecchymosis without necrosis. However, certain species (*eg, Centruroides* spp.) can cause major neurologic manifestations associated with release of acetylcholine at neuromuscular junctions and cholinergic endings. Some venoms contain components that alter the permeability of sodium channels. Autonomic manifestations include dilated pupils, profuse sweating, salivation, vomiting, incontinence of urine and feces, and priapism. Abnormal eye movements, fasciculations, opisthotonus, jerking of limbs, and hemiballismus may occur. Dyspnea, respiratory arrest, and cardiac arrest may develop as early as 1 hour or up to several days after envenomation. Antivenin is available for *Centruroides* envenomation, and atropine counters the parasympathomimetic effects of the venom. (*From* Anon [8].)

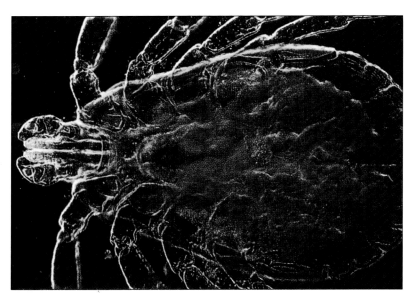

Figure 14-10. Tick neurotoxicity. *Dermancentor andersoni* is the tick most frequently implicated in the northwest United States with human neurologic illness. Other neurologically affected hosts are deer, llama, and sheep. Tick infestation precedes symptoms by several days. Anorexia, diarrhea, and irritability are noted first and are followed by weakness and atonia. Removal of the tick at this stage prevents the onset of true paralysis. Retained mouth parts should be excised and a thorough search instituted for other ticks. Improvement commences immediately and is often complete by 48 hours. Most cases of tick bite occur in the months of April to June, particularly in the northwest United States. Weakness usually begins about 5 days after attachment of the tick and is preceded by fatigue, irritability, and distal paresthesias. Flaccid weakness begins in the legs and ascends to the torso, arms, and face and may involve the bulbar and respiratory muscles. The paralysis may develop rapidly and resembles the Guillian-Barré syndrome. Diplopia and pupillary dilatation are common. Sensory deficits are absent. Death follows involvement of respiratory centers. (*From* Villee and colleagues [10]; with permission.)

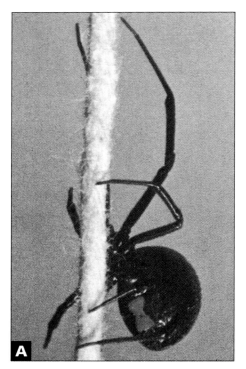

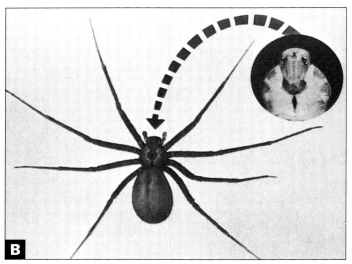

Figure 14-11. Poisonous arachnids. **A,** The black widow spider (*Latrodectus mactans*) elaborates a venom that can cause severe neurologic dysfunction. The venom (latrotoxin) promotes the release of acetylcholine at the neuromuscular junction and also indirectly releases catecholamines at adrenergic endings. The female (*shown here*) contains a red hourglass mark on the abdomen and is one of the most aggressive and most dangerous of the American spiders. The bite is accompanied by local sharp pain and followed by a generalized cramping sensation. Abdominal rigidity and trismus occur. Waves of excruciating pain cause the patient to scream and writhe. Headache, vomiting, and hypertension are common and are usually accompanied by paresthesias, fasciculation, tremor, and hyperreflexia. Convulsions are uncommon. **B,** The brown recluse spider (*Laxosceles reclusa*) causes a relatively painless bite followed by the development of a blue-gray macular halo around the puncture site; this is associated with local hemolysis and arterial spasm resulting in cyanosis. Systemic manifestations include urticaria, malaise, vomiting, headache, convulsions, hemolysis, delirium, shock, and coma. (Panels A, B *from* Anon [8].)

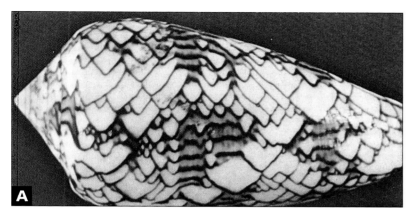

Figure 14-12. Mollusc envenomation. **A,** *Conus tulipa*, a cone snail, belongs to a family of predatory marine gastropods that have developed a salivary gland venom apparatus to assist them in the capture of prey. Humans stung by a cone snail experience a sharp burning or stinging sensation and slight numbness locally. Dysesthesias may spread rapidly and involve the entire body. In severe envenomation, limb paralysis, areflexia, and blurring of vision with diplopia may precede coma and respiratory failure. **B,** Neuromuscular junctions showing targets for the polypeptide toxins in *Conus* venoms. Calcium (Ca^{2+}) channels in the presynaptic terminus are targets for the ω-conotoxins; the acetylcholine receptor is a target for α-conotoxins, and voltage-activated sodium (Na^+) channels in muscle are targets for the μ-conotoxins. The left panel shows the neuromuscular junction in a quiescent state, the middle panel, in an activated state, and the right panel, how the different toxins found in *Conus geographus* venom block synaptic transmission even in the presence of a nerve impulse. K^+—Potassium. (Panel A *from* Toro-González and colleagues [2]; with permission; *courtesy of* Charles M. Poser, MD, Harvard Medical School; Panel B *adapted from* Tu [11].)

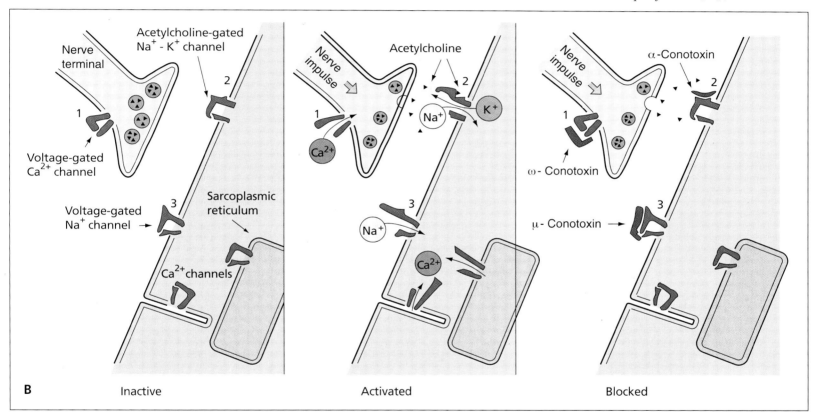

Figure 14-13. Wounding by a stingray. Stingrays are among the most important venomous fish. Rays are common in shallow coastal waters but are also found elsewhere. Stepping on a ray may result in the animal taking a defensive action, wielding its muscular tail and attached barb, which can cause extensive wounds. Local pain develops immediately, is intense, and may spread. Pain usually diminishes over a period of hours or days but may persist for more than 1 year. Other immediate symptoms include syncopy, nausea, anxiety, arrhythmia, muscle weakness, cramping and fasciculation, and respiratory distress. Stingray venoms have a direct action on cardiac muscle, depress respiration, and may provoke convulsions. (*Adapted from* Vinken and colleague [7].)

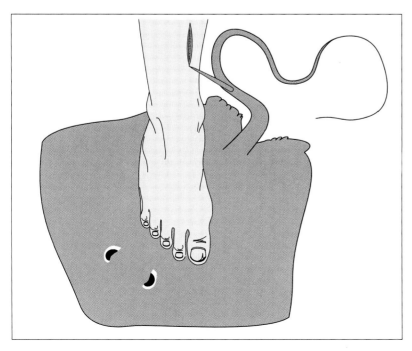

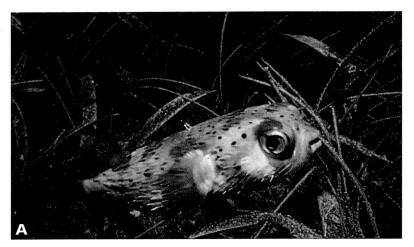
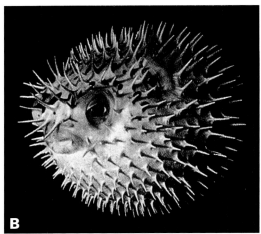

Figure 14-14. Fish that harbor neurotoxins. **A,** The porcupine fish (*Diodon hystrix*) is one of several fish species that harbor the sodium channel toxin tetrodotoxin, one of the most potent nonprotein poisons found in nature. Ingestion of the fish may result in a rapid onset of symptoms, including circumoral paresthesias, which rapidly progress to generalized paresthesias and lightheadedness. A wide variety of neurologic phenomena may follow. Incoordination and slurred speech may suggest drunkenness. Weakness and paralysis first develop in the upper extremities and subsequently in the lower extremities. Dyspnea and hypotension precede death. **B,** Tetrodotoxin is also present in the puffer fish, famous in Japanese culinary circles as the delicacy *fugu*. A satisfactory meal of *fugu* is accompanied by the development of mild paresthesias, flushing of the skin, and mood elevation. The toxin is concentrated in the liver, ovaries, intestines, and skin, but the flesh is easily contaminated when the fish is cleaned. (*From* Villee and colleagues [10]; with permission.)

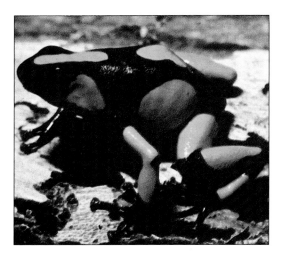

Figure 14-15. Poison-dart frog of the *Phyllobates* spp. These frogs are of little clinical concern but of interest experimentally and historically. Native people of South America and Africa have used the skin toxin (batrachotoxin) of these frogs to prepare poisonous darts that are used with a blowgun to kill animals. Batrachotoxin (a toxic steroidal compound) is one of the most toxic substances known. It acts on the nerve cell membrane, where it maintains sodium channels in the open state, causing persistent depolarization and paralysis. Its effect on sodium channels is therefore opposite to that of tetrodotoxin and saxitoxin, both of which can reverse depolarization caused by batrachotoxin. Inhalation of the skin secretion of *Phyllobates* spp. may result in dysesthesia of exposed areas such as the face. (*From* Toro-González and colleagues [2]; with permission.)

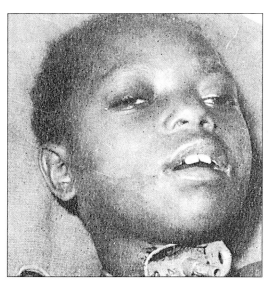

Figure 14-16. Snake envenomation. The South American rattlesnake (*Crotalus durissus terrificus*) is a member of the crotalid family of poisonous snakes. Other families include vipers, elapids, and colubrids. The active components of snake toxins form a complex array of neurotoxic agents active at presynaptic (β-toxin) and postsynaptic (α-neurotoxins, *eg*, α-bungarotoxin) sites. Venoms also contain cardiotoxins that cause hemolysis and cardiac arrest in addition to neuromuscular blockade. About 50,000 people are bitten annually by snakes in the United States. With crotalid snake bites, one or two fang marks are usually evident. Burning pain immediately follows the bite. Localized pitting edema may progress to involve the entire limb within hours. Neurologic signs are commonly minimal, but if paresthesias of the scalp, face, and lips are reported, or if a metallic taste occurs in the mouth, severe envenomation may have occurred. Shock, pulmonary edema, and renal failure may follow. Snake envenomation produces a syndrome resembling acute myasthenia. The victim, pictured 24 hours after a Papuan elapid bite, shows complete ptosis, external ophthalmoplegia, and paralysis of the jaw, tongue, and superficial muscles. A tracheostomy has been performed because respiratory paralysis may be fatal. (*From* Vinken and colleague [7]; with permission.)

Developmental Neurotoxicology and Teratology

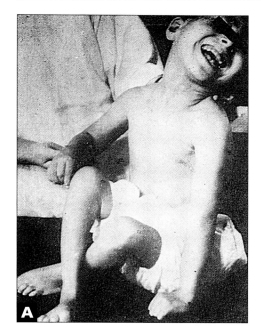

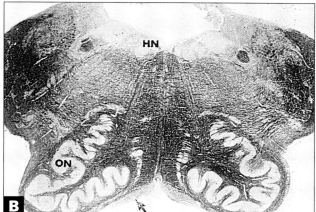

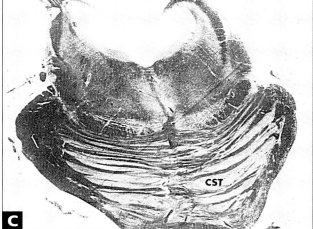

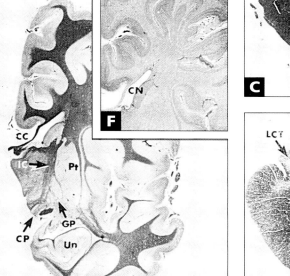

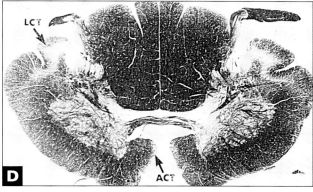

Figure 14-17. Minamata disease of prenatal origin associated with consumption of fish contaminated with organomercury compounds. **A**, Typical scissoring of the feet and contracture of upper limbs. **B**, Medulla oblongata. Conspicuous hypoplasia of both corticospinal tracts (CST) (magnification × 6.0, Woelcke myelin staining process); hypoglossal nucleus (HN), olivary nucleus (ON). **C**, Pons, similar to medulla oblongata; corticospinal tract (CST) (magnification × 4.2, Woelcke myelin staining process). **D**, Cervical cord. Severe symmetric hypoplasia of lateral corticospinal tract (LCT) and slight hypoplasia of anterior corticospinal tract (ACT) (magnification × 7.8, Woelcke myelin staining process). **E**, Frontal section of cerebral hemisphere through uncus (Un). Hypoplasia of cerebral white matter, particularly in corpus callosum (CC), cerebral peduncle (CP), ventral part of internal capsule (IC), globus pallidus (GP); putamen (Pt) (magnification × 1.1, Woelcke myelin staining method). **F**, Same section as in *E*. Well-developed cytoarchitecture in cortex, caudate nucleus (CN), and elsewhere (magnification × 1.1, thionin stain). (*From* Vinken and colleague [3]; with permission.)

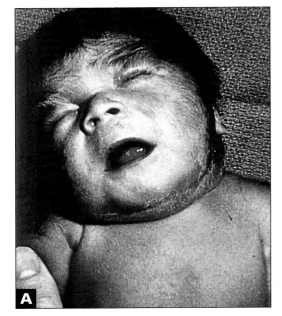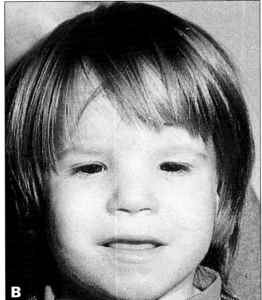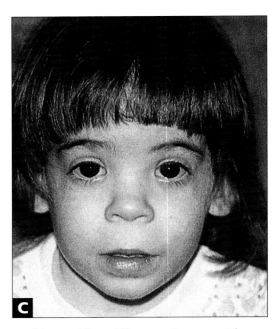

Figure 14-18. Fetal alcohol syndrome, the most commonly encountered of the many fetal drug syndromes. A newborn (**A**), toddler (**B**), and preschool child (**C**) with fetal alcohol syndrome. Even in subjects of different ages and races, palpebral fissures and perioral structures are consistently anomalous. The small nose and jaw and flat midface may improve with age. The brains of children with fetal alcohol syndrome have shown typical lesions of microcephaly and greatly reduced white matter. (*From* Clarren [12]; with permission.)

Adult Syndromes

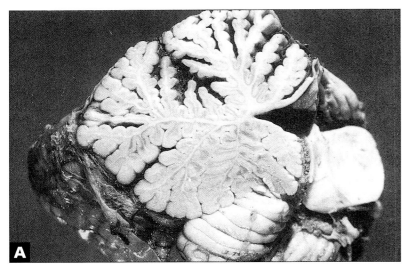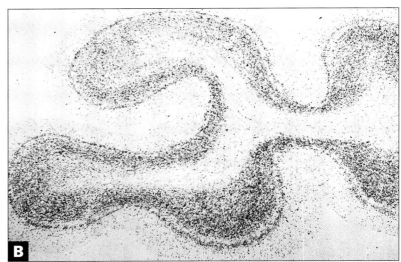

Figure 14-19. Chronic alcoholism. Cerebellar degeneration is seen in adults with impaired nutrition and a long history of excessive alcohol consumption. The cerebellar syndrome, which may be accompanied by peripheral neuropathy, sometimes appears abruptly but more commonly evolves over a period of several weeks or months, after which it remains unchanged for several years. **A**, Sagittal section through the middle of the vermis showing the typical atrophy of the anterosuperior lobules. **B**, Light microscopic section demonstrating severe involvement of the vermian cortex (cresyl violet stain). The molecular layer is narrow; Purkinje cells are absent, and the Bergmann glia are greatly increased; the granule cell layer is thinned. Gliosis of the molecular layer is apparent. Alcoholic women have a significantly smaller cross-sectional corpus callosum area than alcoholic men or control subjects of either gender. (Panel A *from* Victor and colleagues [13]; with permission; Panel B *from* Lieber [14]; with permission.)

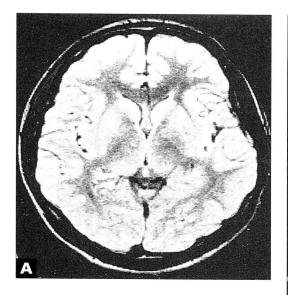
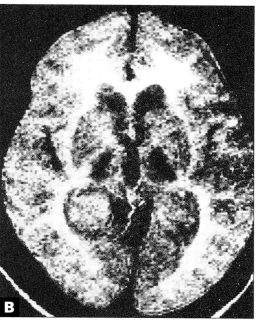

Figure 14-20. Toluene abuse. Many years of inhalation of high concentrations of toluene or toluene-containing mixtures for the purposes of inducing euphoria results in neurologic disease restricted to the central nervous system. Neurologic signs include cerebellar ataxia, dysarthria, nystagmus, incoordination, anosmia, ocular dysmetria, flutter opsoclonus, and cognitive impairment. Late weakness with or without spasticity may occur. **A,** Mildly T2-weighted magnetic resonance image spin-echo scans (TR = 2000 ms, TE = 30 ms) of the brain of a toluene abuser showing loss of normal gray and white differentiation and relatively hypointense posterior limbs of the internal capsule (*arrowheads*). Loss of volume and subtle periventricular hyperintensity are evident. **B,** T2-weighted spin-echo scan (TR = 2000 ms, TE = 60 ms) of a toluene abuser at the level of frontal horns of lateral ventricles. Severe, extensive hyperintensity of white matter is seen. Normal gray and white differentiation in nonhyperintense areas is lost. (*From* Rosenberg and colleagues [15]; with permission.)

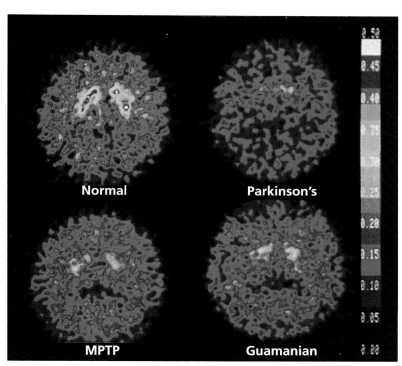
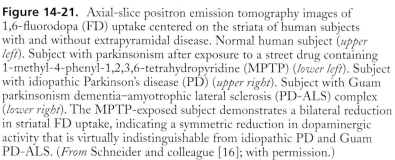

Figure 14-21. Axial-slice positron emission tomography images of 1,6-fluorodopa (FD) uptake centered on the striata of human subjects with and without extrapyramidal disease. Normal human subject (*upper left*). Subject with parkinsonism after exposure to a street drug containing 1-methyl-4-phenyl-1,2,3,6-tetrahydropyridine (MPTP) (*lower left*). Subject with idiopathic Parkinson's disease (PD) (*upper right*). Subject with Guam parkinsonism dementia–amyotrophic lateral sclerosis (PD-ALS) complex (*lower right*). The MPTP-exposed subject demonstrates a bilateral reduction in striatal FD uptake, indicating a symmetric reduction in dopaminergic activity that is virtually indistinguishable from idiopathic PD and Guam PD-ALS. (*From* Schneider and colleague [16]; with permission.)

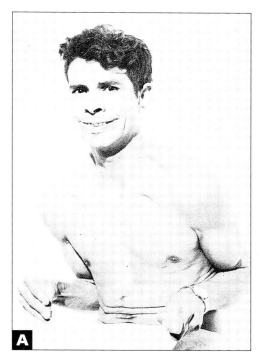
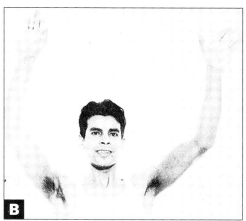

Figure 14-22. Chilean manganese ore miner with extrapyramidal dysfunction (manganism) featured by dystonic contraction of the face, neck, arms, and fingers. **A,** The patient before treatment. **B,** The patient after 4 months of daily levodopa treatment, showing normal facial expression and loss of dystonia. Psychomotor disturbances appear early in the disorder, with compulsive behavior and emotional instability. Generalized muscular weakness, with difficulty walking, impaired speech, and headaches, develops subsequently. Sialorrhea, clumsy movements, tremor, impotence, and sleep disorders may be present. Signs are dominated by disorders of gait, speech, and postural reflexes, with increased muscle tone and expressionless face. The major site of damage induced by manganese is the globus pallidus. Accordingly, subjects with manganism from the consumption of manganese-enriched plant products display intact striatal fluorodopa uptake by positron emission tomography [17], in contrast to the pronounced degeneration of the nigrostriatal pathway observed in Parkinson's disease (Fig. 14-21). (*From* Mena and colleagues [18]; with permission.)

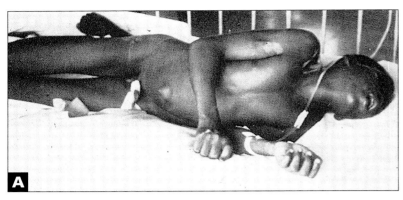

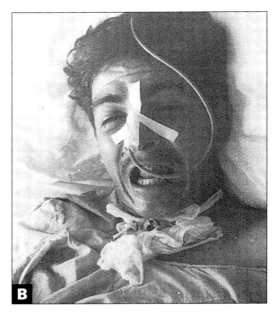

Figure 14-23. Tetanus. **A**, Tetanus in a Nigerian subject caused by tetanospasmin, a neurotoxic protein elaborated by the anerobe *Clostridium tetani*, which is found in soil, house dust, and as a contaminant of heroin. Tetanospasmin is composed of two components: a heavy and a light chain. Adults contract tetanospasmin when bacteria proliferate in deep wounds. The toxin gains access to axons within the region and is transported in a retrograde fashion to anterior horn cells, where it traverses the synaptic cleft and accumulates in the presynaptic terminals of spinal inhibitory neurons. Blockade of the inhibitory drive leads to uncontrolled activity of α and γ motoneurons, with consequent increased muscle tone and uncontrolled and simultaneous contraction of opposing muscle groups. A comparable chain of disinhibitory events of neurons in the intermediolateral column leads to dysautonomia. **B**, Clinical manifestations commence on average 2 weeks after injury. Muscle contraction is featured by stiff neck, trismus, dysphagia, painful spasms, apnea, opisthotonus, and risus sardonicus. Autonomic disorders include cardiac dysrhythmias, tachycardia, labile hypertension, hyperhidrosis, and fever. (Panel A *from* Spillane [19]; with permission; Panel B *from* Toro-González and colleagues [2]; with permission.)

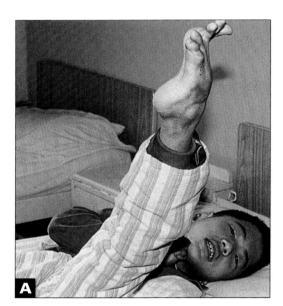

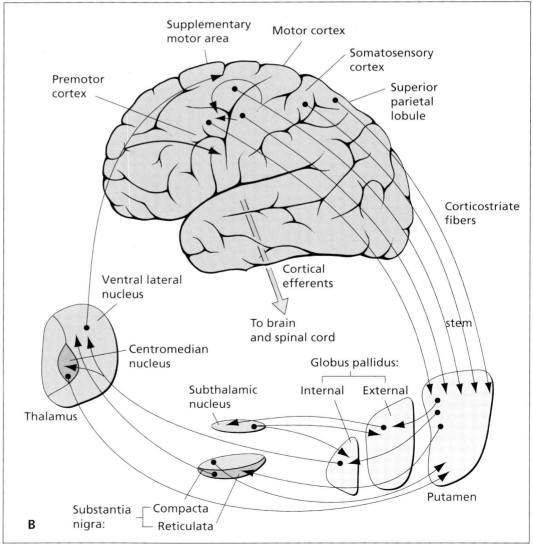

Figure 14-24. 3-Nitropropionic acid neurotoxicity (3-NPA). **A**, Young man with irreversible dystonia after acute poisoning with mildewed sugar cane containing the fungal toxin 3-NPA, an analog of succinic acid and a potent inhibitor of the mitochondrial enzyme succinic dehydrogenase (SDH). Illness is usually heralded by acute gastrointestinal distress, somnolence, convulsions, and coma. Extrapyramidal dysfunction usually appears weeks later in association with bilateral cavitation of the basal ganglia, notably the putamen. **B**, Studies of laboratory animals systemically intoxicated with 3-NPA demonstrate damage in the caudate putamen that is attenuated by transection of the glutamatergic corticostriate pathway before toxin administration. Neuronal lesions appear to result from glutamate excitotoxicity caused by reduced energy metabolism associated with SDH inhibition. (Panel B *adapted from* Kandel and colleagues [20].)

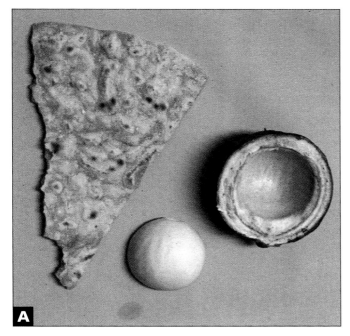
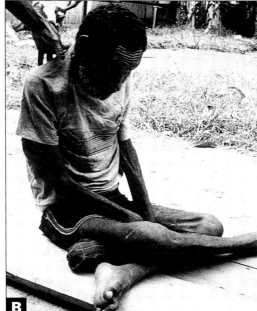
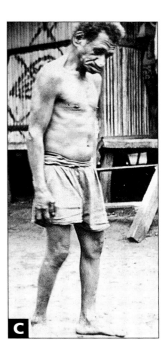

Figure 14-25. Cycad and Western Pacific neurodegenerative disease. Cycad (*Cycas* spp.) is a candidate environmental trigger for Western Pacific amyotrophic lateral sclerosis and parkinsonism dementia (ALS/PD) complex. Cycad seed is traditionally used for food and medicine on Guam by the indigenous people (Chamorro), who are at risk for ALS/PD. The incidence of ALS has declined steadily with the acculturation of the Chamorro people to Western ways. The inner part of the raw cycad seed, which induces neuromuscular disease in grazing animals, is traditionally used as a topical poultice for large open wounds on the extremities. For food preparation, seed is cut into pieces, soaked in water for several days to remove noxious elements, and dried for use as flour for various food products. **A,** Cycad flour used for tortillas prepared by Chamorro families contains residue of the principal cycad toxin (cycasin) [21], the concentration of which is strongly correlated with the historical incidence of motor neuron disease on Guam [22]. **B,** ALS and **C,** PD in male subjects indigenous to southwestern New Guinea (Irian Jaya, Indonesia), another high-incidence focus of Western Pacific ALS/PD. Epidemiologic links have been demonstrated between progressive motor neuron disease and the use of cycad seed to poultice wounds by the Auyu and Jaqai linguistic groups of this region of New Guinea.

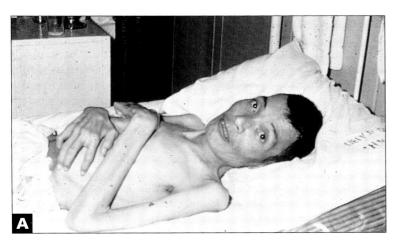

Figure 14-26. Spanish "toxic oil" syndrome. **A,** Patient with severe muscle wasting accompanied by muscle and skin fibrosis, prominent features of the Spanish toxic oil syndrome. Epidemiologic studies demonstrated that affected subjects consumed a rapeseed oil containing fatty acid anilides. Oil from France that had been deliberately adulterated with aniline to prevent food use was illegally intercepted in Spain, heated to remove the aniline, and sold in and around Madrid in 1981. (*Continued on next page*)

B. Clinical and Pathologic Findings of Five Cases of Toxic Oil Syndrome (TOS)

Case number	1	2	3	4	5
Autopsy, *n*	164	177	147	171	133
Age in years	17	10	18	24	32
Total course (weeks)	24	24	28	28	29
Clinical diagnosis	TOS	TOS	TOS	TOS	TOS
Clinical manifestations					
Central nervous system					
Consciousness	Clear	Clear	Clear	Clear	Clear
Motor	-	-	-	-	-
Sensory	-	-	-	-	-
Cranial nerves	nys	nys	nys	-	-
Peripheral nervous system					
Myalgias	+	+	+	+	-
Muscle weakness	+	+	+	+	+
Muscular atrophy	+	+	+	+	+
Areflexia	+	+	+	+	+
Distal sensory deficits	+	?	+	-	-
Respiratory insufficiency	+	+	+	+	+
Brain weight (g)	1280	1100	1310	1450	1430
Central chromatolysis					
Large cortical neurons	-	-	-	-	-
Locus coeruleus	+	+	+	+	+
Pontine nuclei	+	+	-	-	-
Median raphe nuclei	+	+	+	-	-
Descending trigeminal nuclei	-	+	-	+	+
Facial nerve nucleus	-	-	-	+	+
Vestibular nuclei	-	+	-	-	-
Medullary reticular substance	+	+	-	+	+
Cuneate nuclei	+	+	-	+	+
Anterior horn cells	+	+	+	+	+

Nys—occasional nystagmus.

Figure 14-26. (*Continued*) **B**, Clinical and pathologic findings in five cases are shown. In the late 1980s, a comparable syndrome impacted Americans using a synthetic tryptophan preparation. Both conditions were featured by early, prominent eosinophilia, myositis, and peripheral neuropathy. A complete animal model of these unusual conditions has yet to be developed. A direct toxic action of the culpable agents is unlikely. (*From* Tellez and colleagues [23]; with permission.)

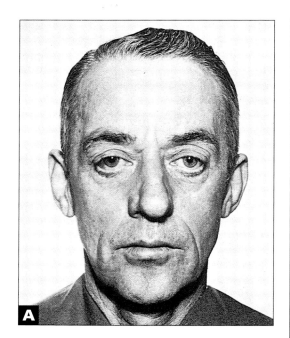

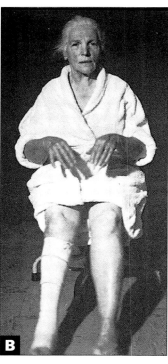

Figure 14-27. Drug-induced extrapyramidal dysfunction. **A**, A patient showing a staring, immobile, unblinking facial expression associated with phenothiazine toxicity. **B**, A patient with parkinsonism induced by promazine, 50 mg taken three times daily for 16 days. Coarse tremor and rigidity of the extremities appeared on the 10th day and disappeared within 3 days after withdrawing the drug. The blurred outlines of the hands and feet are the result of the tremor. (*Continued on next page*)

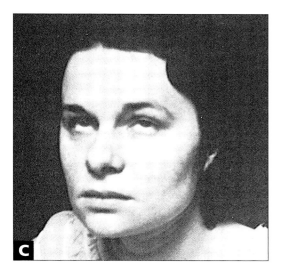

Figure 14-27. (*Continued*) **C**, A patient having an oculogyric crisis after intramuscular injection of perphenazine, 5 mg, during an episode of migraine. The following day, the subject felt dazed and experienced oculogyric crises, difficulty speaking, and stiffness of the hands and neck muscles. Symptoms subsided during the next 12 hours after intravenous injection of procyclidine, 10 mg. (*From* Spillane [24]; with permission.)

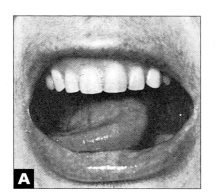
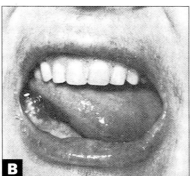
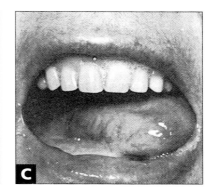
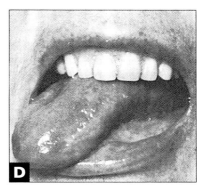
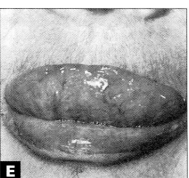
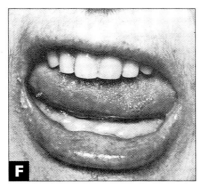

Figure 14-28. Drug-induced oral-buccal dyskinesia. **A–F**, The patient was suffering from agitated depression and was treated for 15 months with imipramine, 50 mg three times daily; trifluoperazine, 5 mg/d, and trihexyphenidyl (Benzhexol), 2 mg twice daily. The patient exhibited dysarthria, difficulty chewing, smacking of the lips, opening and closing of the mouth, and dyskinetic movements of the tongue. These photographs were taken 2 months after drug withdrawal. Twelve months later, the involuntary movements were still present but less marked. (*From* Spillane [24]; with permission.)

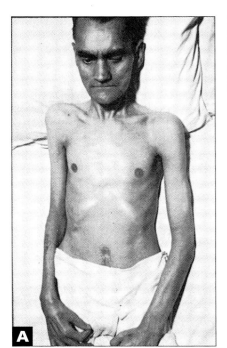
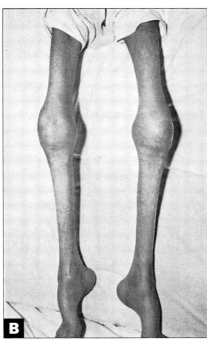

Figure 14-29. Neuropathy and convulsions. **A, B,** A patient with ankylosing spondylitis, arthritis, and pulmonary tuberculosis. Seizures resulted from cycloserine, and neuropathy followed isoniazid and phenylbutazone administration. (*Continued on next page*)

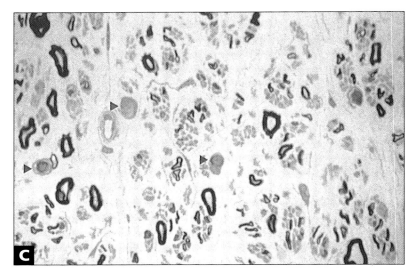

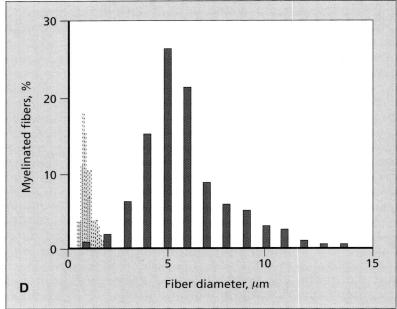

Figure 14-29. (*Continued*) **C**, Thalidomide neuropathy. A cross-section of the sural nerve showing marked depopulation of large myelinated fibers and signs of axon degeneration (*arrowheads*) (thionine-acridine orange stain, magnification × 40. Actual size: 370 for the image 13 × 9 cm). **D**, Abnormal distribution of myelinated fibers resulting from an absence of large-caliber axons (*solid bars*). The distribution of nonmyelinated fibers is unremarkable (*dotted bars*). (Panels A, B *from* Spillane [24]; with permission; Panel C *from* Chapon and colleagues [25]; with permission; Panel D *adapted from* Chapon and colleagues [25].)

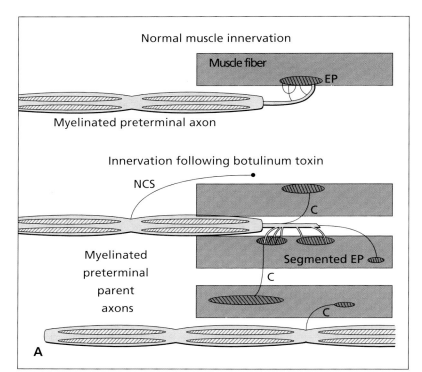

Figure 14-30. Effect of botulinum toxin. **A**, Patterns of innervation in orbicularis oculi before (*upper*) and after (*lower*) therapeutic treatment with botulinum toxin. In normal innervation (*upper*), the normal preterminal motor axon is unbranched after it leaves the intramuscular nerve. It is myelinated until immediately proximal to the muscle end plate (EP) region. The terminal axonal arborization branches over the muscle end plate. In reinnervation after botulinum toxin exposure (*lower*), motor axons develop noncollateral sprouts (NCS), which often run parallel to muscle fibers (top muscle fiber). NCS frequently end in a bulbous dilatation, considered the *terminus* of the sprout. These NCS originate from the preterminal axon; they can also originate from the terminal or ultraterminal regions of the axon. Axonal collaterals (C) extend toward end plates on

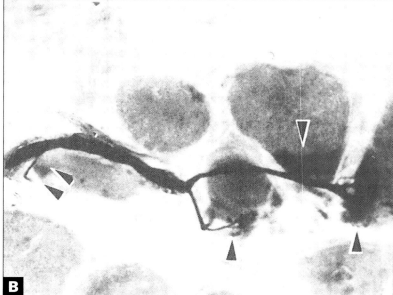

muscle fibers separate from the muscle fiber innervated by the parent axon. Collaterals arise from the unmyelinated terminal axon immediately proximal to the end plate (to the top muscle fiber), from the ultraterminal axonal arborization over the end plate (to the bottom muscle fiber), and from nodes of Ranvier of myelinated parent preterminal axons (from the lower preterminal axon to the bottom muscle fiber). End plates can appear segmented, with each segment innervated by an axonal process from the same motor axon (middle muscle fiber). More than one end plate can be present on a single muscle fiber, each innervated by axonal processes from different preterminal axons (bottom muscle fiber). **B**, Increased terminal innervation. A single myelinated preterminal axon innervates end plates on four muscle fibers, three through unmyelinated collaterals from the terminal axon (*single arrowheads*), the other through a more proximal collateral (*double arrowhead*) arising from a node of Ranvier (magnification × 450). (Panel A *adapted from* Alderson and colleagues [26]; Panel B *from* Alderson and colleagues [26]; with permission.)

Related Clinical Features

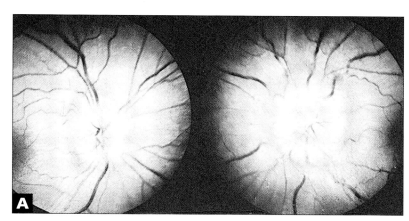
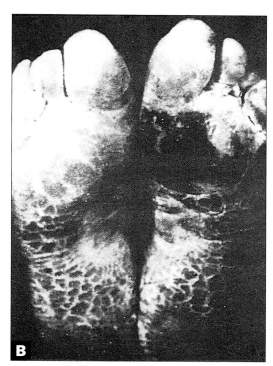
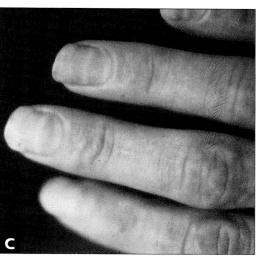
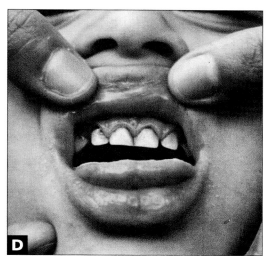
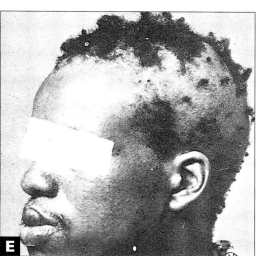
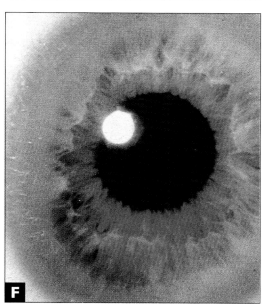

Figure 14-31. Signs of systemic intoxication. **A,** Bilateral papilledema in a subject with high blood, fat, and liver levels of chlordecone (Kepone), a cause of opsoclonus, tremor, anxiety, fatigue, and a sense of trembling (Kepone shakes), which was seen in workers producing this neurotoxic chlorinated insecticide. **B,** Severe hyperkeratosis in arsenic poisoning, a cause of sensorimotor peripheral neuropathy. **C,** Transverse striae (Mees' lines) on the fingernails of a subject intoxicated with arsenic. **D,** Linear black-green deposits (lead lines) on the gums in plumbism, a cause of encephalopathy in children and peripheral neuropathy (wrist drop) in metal workers. **E,** Scalp alopecia following thallotoxicosis, a cause of life-threatening cardiac dysfunction, alopecia, and painful distal sensory neuropathy. **F,** Copper deposition in the form of a golden-brown band in the peripheral area of Descemet's membrane (Kayser-Fleischer rings) in hepatolenticular degeneration (Wilson's disease), an inherited metabolic disorder of copper metabolism characterized by choreoathetosis, tremor, incoordination, dysphagia, rigidity, and personality changes. (Panel A *from* Sanborn and colleagues [27]; with permission; Panels B–D *from* Toro-González and colleagues [2]; with permission; *courtesy of* University Hospital San Juan de Bios, Bogota, Colombia; Panel E *from* Majoos and colleagues [28]; with permission; Panel F *from* Poirier [29]; with permission; *courtesy of* Howard M. Leibowitz, MD, Boston, MA.)

Neurotoxic Chemical-induced Animal Models of Human Neurodegenerative Disease

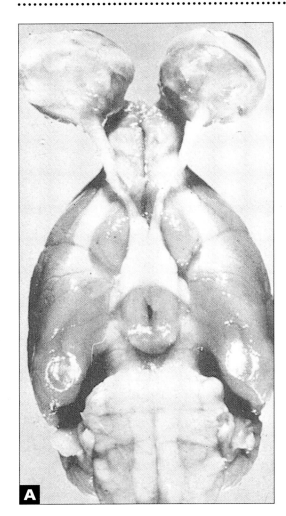

A

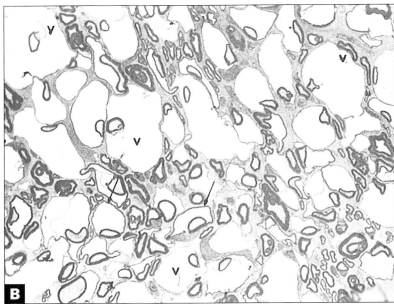

B

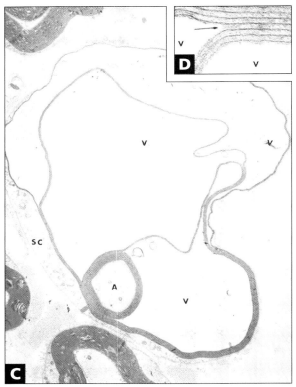

C

D

Figure 14-32.
Experimental toxic myelinopathy. A rodent model of hexachlorophene (HCP) neurotoxicity. In humans treated with this topical antimicrobial agent, toxicity is associated with convulsions, focal or generalized motor weakness, behavioral changes (withdrawal, irritability, or bizarre behavior), decreased levels of consciousness, coma, and death. Oral exposure is associated with systemic (hyperthermia, hypotension), gastrointestinal (diarrhea, vomiting), and neurologic findings. **A,** Brain of a young adult rat that received 900 ppm of HCP in the diet for 4 weeks. Note the enlargement of optic nerves and the chiasm (magnification × 3). **B,** Light micrograph of an epoxy cross-section of a sciatic nerve from an adult rat on 1000 ppm of HCP in the diet for 4 weeks showing large vacuoles (v) associated with myelinated axons (toluidine blue stain, magnification × 400.) **C,** Electron micrograph from same specimen as in *B*, showing large intramyelinic vacuoles (v). The axon (a) and corresponding Schwann cell cytoplasm (sc) lack pathologic changes (magnification × 6000). **D,** Higher magnification of *C*, showing intramyelinic vacuoles (v) produced from separation of myelin lamellae at intraperiod lines (*arrow*) (magnification × 175,000). (Panel A *from* Towfighi and colleagues [30]; with permission; Panel B *from* Towfighi [31]; with permission.)

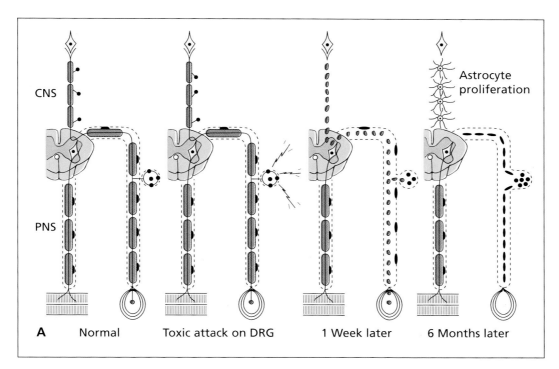

A   Normal   Toxic attack on DRG   1 Week later   6 Months later

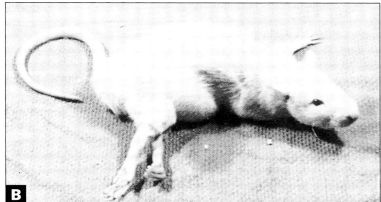

Figure 14-33. Experimental toxic sensory neuronopathy. **A,** Sequential events in a toxic sensory neuronopathy resulting from degeneration of dorsal root ganglion cells, a condition produced experimentally by intravenous doxorubicin therapy, mercury intoxication, or pyridoxine megavitaminosis. The jagged lines (*lightning bolts*) indicate that the toxin is directed at neurons in the dorsal root ganglion (DRG), where the blood–nerve barrier is normally absent. Degeneration of these cells is accompanied by fragmentation and phagocytosis of their peripherally and centrally directed axons. Denervated Schwann cell columns remain for some time; there is no axonal regeneration. **B,** Loss of proprioception in an animal treated intravenously with doxorubicin. The animal was placed in and retained the abnormal limb position. Neuropathologic examination displayed sensory neurons in lumbar dorsal root ganglia in various stages of degeneration. The animal was photographed 2 to 3 weeks after a single dose of 10 mg/kg doxorubicin was administered intravenously. CNS—central nervous system; PNS—peripheral nervous system. (Panel A *adapted from* Schaumburg and colleagues [32].)

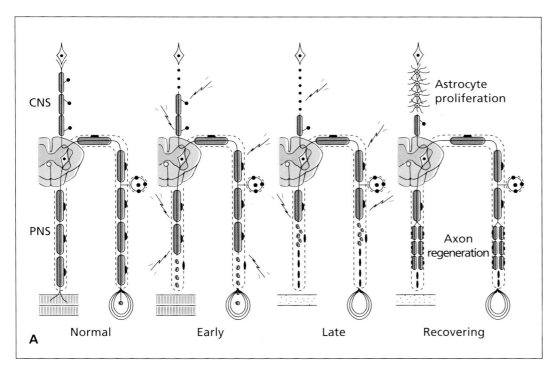

A   Normal   Early   Late   Recovering

Figure 14-34. Experimental toxic distal axonopathy. **A,** The sequential events in a central–peripheral distal axonopathy, the pattern of pathology associated with the majority of drug- and chemical-induced human and experimental symmetric peripheral neuropathies. Distal involvement of pyramidal and spinocerebellar tracts (not shown) may also occur. The jagged lines (*lightning bolts*) indicate that the toxin is acting at multiple sites along motor and sensory axons in the peripheral and central nervous systems. Axon degeneration has moved proximally ("dying-back") by the late stage. These pathologic changes are associated with a largely symmetric, stocking-and-glove pattern of sensory loss and motor weakness. Recovery of function is dependent on reinnervation and occurs in a proximal to distal manner. Recovery in the central nervous system is impeded by astroglial proliferation; failure to restore the integrity of pyramidal tracts is responsible for the appearance of mild spasticity in subjects in whom peripheral reinnervation has occurred. (*Continued on next page*)

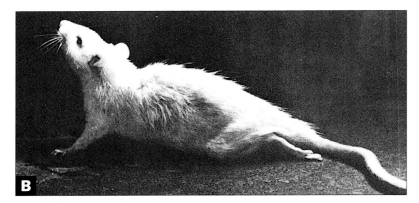

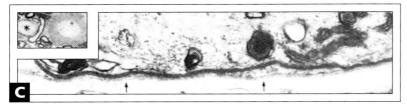

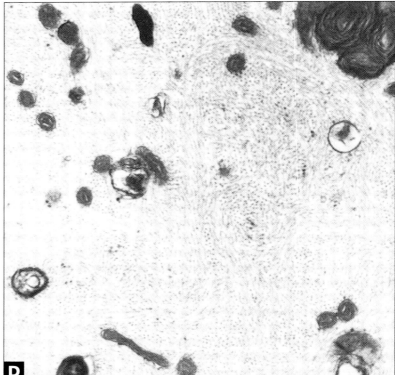

Figure 14-34. (*Continued*) **B**, Rat with symmetric hind-limb weakness and footdrop after 130 days of inhalation of continuous, controlled exposure to air containing 400 to 600 ppm of *n*-hexane, a solvent that generates the neurotoxic metabolite 2,5-hexanedione. Central–peripheral distal axonopathy is the underlying pathologic picture. Humans exposed to *n*-hexane in solvents used in the occupational environment or to induce euphoria have developed predominantly motor peripheral neuropathy. **C**, Electron micrographs of cross-sections of sensory nerve fibers in lumbar dorsal root ganglia of a 3-week-old rat given daily intraperitoneal injections of acrylamide (30 mg/kg) 6 days per week for 4 weeks, a substance used to form polymers employed in biochemical separations, grouting, and other jobs requiring a waterproof seal. Humans whose skin is exposed to acrylamide develop hyperhydrosis, palmar erythema, and a symmetric, sensorimotor neuropathy. In the upper portion of the micrography, the swelling is surrounded by a thin myelin sheath, Schwann cell cytoplasm, and basal lamina (*arrows*), confirming its axonal origin; abnor-

mal membranous organelles are present in the axoplasm. The inset (magnification × 475) is a light micrograph showing giant axonal swelling (*asterisks*) relative to the size of a neighboring neuronal perikaryon and other myelinated axons. Note that the swelling is surrounded by an attenuated myelin sheath (magnification x 18,800). **D**, Axoplasm is packed with neurofilaments and contains accumulations of membranous materials (magnification × 30,750). CNS—central nervous system; PNS—peripheral nervous system. (Panel A *adapted from* Schaumberg and colleagues [32]; with permission; Panel B *from* Schaumburg and colleague [33]; with permission; Panels C, D *from* Gold [34]; with permission.)

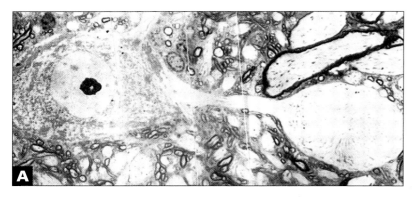

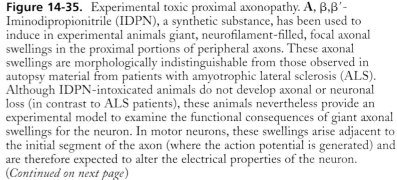

Figure 14-35. Experimental toxic proximal axonopathy. **A**, β,β′-Iminodipropionitrile (IDPN), a synthetic substance, has been used to induce in experimental animals giant, neurofilament-filled, focal axonal swellings in the proximal portions of peripheral axons. These axonal swellings are morphologically indistinguishable from those observed in autopsy material from patients with amyotrophic lateral sclerosis (ALS). Although IDPN-intoxicated animals do not develop axonal or neuronal loss (in contrast to ALS patients), these animals nevertheless provide an experimental model to examine the functional consequences of giant axonal swellings for the neuron. In motor neurons, these swellings arise adjacent to the initial segment of the axon (where the action potential is generated) and are therefore expected to alter the electrical properties of the neuron. (*Continued on next page*)

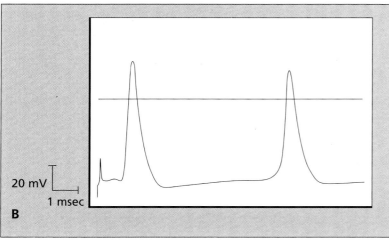

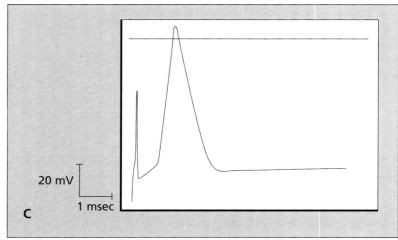

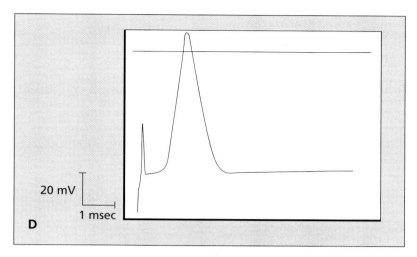

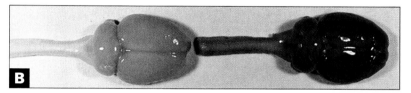

E. Comparison of Electrophysiologic Abnormalities in ALS and IDPN Neuropathy

ALS	IDPN neuropathy
Double motor unit discharges	Repetitive firing
Synchronous fasciculations and motor unit potentials	Crosstalk
Giant motor unit potentials	Crosstalk
	Increased excitability
	Decreased recurrent inhibition
Weakness	Conduction block

Figure 14-35. (*Continued*) **B, C, D,** Intracellular recordings from spinal cord motor neurons in IDPN-intoxicated cats reveal a number of significant electrophysiologic alterations. **E,** Comparable electrophysiologic alterations have been noted in ALS patients. Whether the proximal giant axonal swellings play a role in the development of the clinical hallmarks of the human disease is unknown. A single antidromic stimulus evokes two action potentials (*C*). Ephaptic interaction (electrical crosstalk) between motor neurons in a cat with IDPN neuropathy (*top* and *bottom* are the same cell, *D*). Independent antidromic stimulation of each half of the ventral root produces an action potential spike in the cell. Spikes are identical except for a small (150-s) increase in latency to spike in the top panel, as compared with the bottom panel. (Panels B–D *adapted from* Gold and colleague [35]; Panel E *adapted from* Gold [34].)

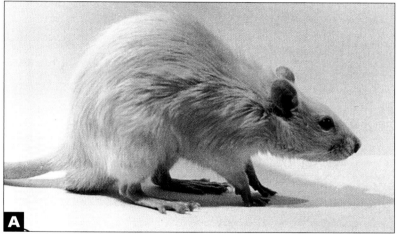

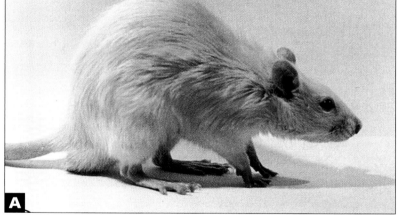

Figure 14-36. Experimental neuronopathy and vacuolar demyelination. **A,** Acetyl ethyl tetramethyl tetralin (AETT), formerly a widely used component of soaps, deodorants, and cosmetics, produced hyperirritability, arched back, and limb weakness in rats repeatedly exposed to the compound percutaneously or per os. Brain, spinal cord, and peripheral nerves were discolored blue, as was the skin of the face. Such changes were seen in animals treated with 25 to 50 mg/kg/d AETT for 2 to 3 weeks. The chromogenic and neurotoxic properties of AETT in rats appeared to be linked. Diethyl benzene and its derivatives are also chromogenic, and humans occupationally exposed to tetralin reportedly excrete green urine. The possibility of human neurologic disease from exposure to these compounds has not been assessed. **B,** Brains removed from normal (*left*) and AETT-treated (*right*) animals after systemic perfusion with buffered glutaraldehyde fixative. **C,** Neuropathology of rats treated with AETT. Hypoglossal neuron showing an accumulation of dense lipopigment. Arrows indicate cytosomes that display the histochemical, fluorescence, and ultrastructural features of ceroid lipopigment. The neuronal nucleus (n) is shown. **D,** Single teased peripheral nerve fiber displaying intact myelin (m) adjacent to an internode with multiple myelin bubbles (b) and a short length of demyelinated axons (d). **E,** Lumbar ventral root containing two cross-sectional fibers displaying prominent myelin bubbling (b). One vacuolated fiber contains an intramyelinic phagocyte (p). Bright-field micrographs; left and right are 1-μm epoxy sections stained with toluidine blue. (Scale bars: C—5 μm; D—10 μm; E—5 μm.) (Panels A, B *from* Spencer and colleagues [36]; with permission; Panels C–E *from* Spencer and colleagues [38]; with permission.)

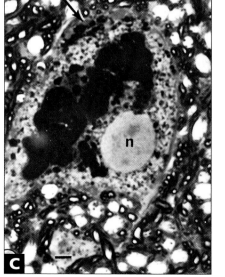

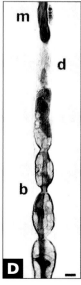

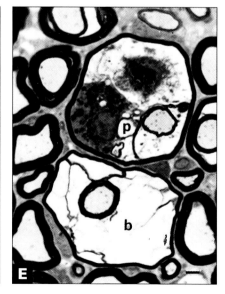

Acknowledgment

We thank Ms. Rhonda Marks for her assistance in preparing this manuscript.

References

1. Price DL, Griffin JW: Neurons and Ensheathing Cells as Targets of Disease Processes. In *Experimental and Clinical Neurotoxicology*. Edited by Spencer PS, Schaumburg HH. Baltimore: Williams & Wilkins; 1980:2–23.

2. Toro-González G, Román-Campos G, de Román LN: *Neurologia Tropical: Aspectos Neuropatologicos de la Medicina Tropical*. Bogota: Colombiana, Ltd.; 1983.

3. Vinken PJ, Bruyn GW: *Handbook of Clinical Neurology*, vol 36. *Intoxications of the Nervous System*, part I. Amsterdam: North-Holland Publishing; 1979.

4. Rosling H: *Cassava Toxicity and Food Security*, edn 2 Uppsala, Sweden: Tryck Kontact; 1988.

5. Halstead BW: *Poisonous and Venomous Marine Animals of the World*, edn 2. Princeton: Darwin Press; 1988.

6. Anon: *Toxic Fish and Mollusks*. Air Training Command of Maxwell Air Force Base, Alabama, Information Bulletin No. 12, US Government Printing Office, Washington, DC, Stock No. 008-070-00426-7, Class No. D301.38/8:12; June 1979.

7. Vinken PJ, Bruyn GW: *Handbook of Clinical Neurology*, vol 37. *Intoxications of the Nervous System*, part II. New York: North-Holland Publishing; 1979.

8. Anon: *Venomous Arthropod Handbook*. USAF School of Aerospace Medicine, Brooks Air Force Base, Texas 78235, US Government Printing Office, Washington, DC, Stock No. 008-070-00397-0, Catalog No. D 301.35: 161/43; 1977.

9. Saida K, Mendell JR, Sahenk Z: Peripheral nerve changes induced by local application of bee venom. *J Neuropathol Exp Neurol* 1977, 36:783–796.

10. Villee CA, Solomon EP, Martin CE, *et al.*: *Biology*, edn 2. Philadelphia: WB Saunders; 1989.

11. Tu AT: *Handbook of Natural Toxins*: vol 3. *Marine Toxins and Venoms*. New York: Marcel Dekker; 1988.

12. Clarren SK: Recognition of fetal alcohol syndrome. *JAMA* 1981, 245:2436–2439.

13. Victor M, Adams RD, Mancall EL: A restricted form of cerebellar cortical degeneration occurring in alcoholic patients. *AMA Arch Neurol* 1959, 1:579–688.

14. Lieber CS: *Medical and Nutritional Complications of Alcoholism*. New York: Plenum; 1992.

15. Rosenberg NL, Kleinschmidt-DeMasters BK, Davis KA, *et al.*: Toluene abuse causes diffuse central nervous system white matter changes. *Ann Neurol* 1988, 23:611–614.

16. Schneider JS, Gupta M: *Current Concepts in Parkinson's Disease Research*. Seattle: Hogrefe & Huber, 1993.

17. Calne DB, Chu NS, Huang C-C, *et al.*: Manganism and idiopathic parkinsonism: similarities and differences. *Neurology* 1994, 44:1583–1586.

18. Mena I, Court J, Fuenzalida S, *et al.*: Modification of chronic manganese poisoning: Treatment with L-dopa or 5-OH tryptophane. *N Engl J Med* 1970, 282:5–10.

19. Spillane JD: *Tropical Neurology*. London: Oxford University Press; 1973.

20. Kandel ER, Schwartz JH, Jessell TM: *Principles of Neural Science*, edn 3. Norwalk, CT: Appleton & Lange; 1991.

21. Kisby GE, Ellison M, Spencer PS: Content of the neurotoxins cycasin (methylazoxymethanol beta-D-glucoside) and BMAA (beta-N-methyl-L-alanine) in cycad flour prepared by Guam Chamorros. *Neurology* 1992, 42:1336–1340.

22. Zhang ZX, Anderson DW, Mantel N, Roman GC: Motor neuron disease on Guam: geographic and familial occurence 1956-85. *Acta Neurol Scand* 1996, 94:51–59.

23. Tellez I, Cabello A, Franch O, *et al.*: Chromatolytic changes in the central nervous system of patients with the toxic oil syndrome. *Acta Neuropathol (Berlin)* 1987, 74:354–361.

24. Spillane JD: *An Atlas of Clinical Neurology*. London: Oxford; 1968.

25. Chapon F, Lechevalier B, Da Silva DC, *et al.*: Neuropathies à la thalidomide. *Rev Neurol (Paris)* 1985, 141:719–728.

26. Alderson K, Holds JB, Anderson RL: Botulinum-induced alteration of nerve-muscle interactions in the human orbicularis oculi following treatment for blepharospasm. *Neurology* 1991, 41:1800–1805.

27. Sanborn GE, Selhorst JB, Calabrese VP, Taylor JR: Pseudomotor cerebri and insecticide intoxication. *Neurology* 1979, 29:1222–1227.

28. Majoos FL, Marais AD, Ames FR: Thallium poisoning. *S Afr Med J* 1983, 64:328–330.

29. Poirier RH: The Corneal Limbus. In *Corneal Disorders: Clinical Diagnosis and Management*. Edited by Leibowitz HM. Philadelphia: WB Saunders; 1984:185–211.

30. Towfighi J, Gonatas NK, McCree L: Hexachlorophene-induced changes in central and peripheral myelinated axons of developing and adult rats. *Lab Invest* 1975, 31:712–721.

31. Towfighi J, Gonatas NK, McCree L: Hexachlorophene neuropathy in rats. *Lab Invest* 1973, 29:428–436.

32. Schaumburg HH, Berger AR, Thomas PK: *Disorders of Peripheral Nerves*, edn 2. Philadelphia: FA Davis; 1992.

33. Schaumburg HH, Spencer PS: Degeneration in central and peripheral nervous systems produced by pure *n*-hexane: an experimental study. *Brain* 1976, 99:183–192.

34. Gold BG: The pathophysiology of proximal neurofilamentous giant axonal swellings: implications for the pathogenesis of amyotrophic lateral sclerosis. *Toxicology* 1987, 46:125–139.

35. Gold BG, Lowndes HE: Electrophysiological investigation of β,β′-iminodipropionitrile neuropathy: intracellular recordings in spinal cord. *Brain Res* 1984, 308:235–244.

36. Spencer PS, Sterman AB, Horoupian D, Bischoff M: Neurotoxic changes in rats exposed to the fragrance compound acetyl ethyl tetramethyl tetralin. *Neurotoxicology* 1979, 1:221–237.

37. Spencer PS, Sterman AB, Horoupian DS, Foulds MM: Neurotoxic fragrance produces ceroid and myelin disease. *Science* 1979, 204:633–635.

38. Spencer PS, Schaumberg HH, Ludolph AC: *Experimental and Clinical Neurotoxicology*, edn 2 New York: Oxford University Press; 2000.

15

Headache

Marc E. Lenaerts • James R. Couch, Jr

HEADACHE is one of the most common complaints of patients seeking medical attention. There are several important indications to warrant investigation of a headache: a patient's first or worst headache; a recent change in the patient's headache pattern; new neurologic findings; no response to treatment; and symptoms that do not correspond to a primary headache such as migraine, tension-type, or cluster [1].

The lifetime prevalence of headache in general is 93%; in women, it is 99% [2]. Migraine headache is reported by at least 12% of the population [3]. Episodic tension-type headache is much more frequent than migraine, at least 40%; however, it is rarely the object of medical attention [4]. Secondary headaches can be caused by tumors, trauma, vasculitis, infection, toxic exposure, or metabolic abnormalities.

Despite its frequency and frequent lack of specificity, a precisely described headache can be a critical clue to diagnosis and the source of a treatment from which the entire patient's well-being will benefit.

Classification and Diagnostic Criteria for Headache Disorders, Cranial Neuralgias, and Facial Pain

1 Migraine
1.1 Migraine without aura
1.2 Migraine with aura
1.3 Ophthalmoplegic migraine
1.4 Retinal migraine
1.5 Childhood periodic syndromes that may be precursor to or associated with migraine
1.6 Complications of migraine
1.7 Migrainous disorder not fulfilling above criteria
2 Tension-type headache
2.1 Episodic tension-type headache
2.2 Chronic tension-type headache
2.3 Tension-type headache not fulfilling above criteria
3 Cluster headache and chronic paroxysmal hemicrania
3.1 Cluster headache
3.2 Chronic paroxysmal hemicrania
3.3 Cluster headache-like disorder not fulfilling above criteria
4 Miscellaneous headaches unassociated with structural lesion
4.1 Idiopathic stabbing headache
4.2 External compression headache
4.3 Cold stimulus headache
4.4 Benign cough headache
4.5 Benign exertional headache
4.6 Headache associated with sexual activity
5 Headache associated with head trauma
5.1 Acute post-traumatic headache
5.2 Chronic post-traumatic headache
6 Headache associated with vascular disorder
6.1 Acute ischemic cerebrovascular disease
6.2 Intracranial hematoma
6.3 Subarachnoid hemorrhage
6.4 Unruptured vascular malformation
6.5 Arteritis
6.6 Carotid or vertebral artery pain
6.7 Venous thrombosis
6.8 Arterial hypertension
6.9 Headache associated with other vascular disorder
7 Headache associated with non-vascular intracranial disorder
7.1 High cerebrospinal fluid pressure
7.2 Low cerebrospinal fluid pressure
7.3 Intracranial infection
7.4 Intracranial sarcoidosis and other noninfectious inflammatory diseases
7.5 Headache associated with intrathecal injections

7.6 Intracranial neoplasm
7.7 Headache associated with other intracranial disorder
8 Headache associated with substances or their withdrawal
8.1 Headache induced by acute substance use or exposure
8.2 Headache induced by chronic substance use or exposure
8.3 Headache from substance withdrawal (acute use)
8.4 Headache from substance withdrawal (chronic use)
8.5 Headache associated with substances but with uncertain mechanism
9 Headache associated with noncephalic infection
9.1 Viral infection
9.2 Bacterial infection
9.3 Headache related to other infection
10 Headache associated with metabolic disorder
10.1 Hypoxia
10.2 Hypercapnia
10.3 Mixed hypoxia and hypercapnia
10.4 Hypoglycemia
10.5 Dialysis
10.6 Headache related to other metabolic abnormality
11 Headache or facial pain associated with disorder of cranium, neck, eyes, ears, nose, sinuses, teeth, mouth, or other facial or cranial structures
11.1 Cranial bone
11.2 Neck
11.3 Eyes
11.4 Ears
11.5 Nose and sinuses
11.6 Teeth, jaws, and related structures
11.7 Temporomandibular joint disease
12 Cranial neuralgias, nerve trunk pain, and deafferentation pain
12.1 Persistent pain of cranial origin
12.2 Trigeminal neuralgia
12.3 Glossopharyngeal neuralgia
12.4 Nervus intermedius neuralgia
12.5 Superior laryngeal neuralgia
12.6 Occipital neuralgia
12.7 Central causes of head and facial pain other than tic douloureux
12.8 Facial pain not fulfilling criteria in groups 11 or 12
13 Headache not classifiable

Figure 15-1. Classification and diagnostic criteria for headache disorders, cranial neuralgias, and facial pain. In 1988, a panel of international experts created a comprehensive classification of all headache types divided into 13 categories [5].

Primary Headaches

Migraine Headache

International Headache Society Criteria for the Migraine Syndrome

Migraine without aura

At least five attacks fulfilling the following three criteria

- Headache attacks lasting 4–72 hours
- Headache with at least two of the following characteristics
  - Unilateral location
  - Pulsating quality
  - Moderate or severe intensity
  - Aggravation by physical activity
- Patient experiences at least one of the following during headache
  - Nausea and/or vomiting
  - Photophobia and phonophobia

At least one of the following applies

Patient's history, physical, and neurologic examination do not suggest a disorder with secondary headache

Such a disorder is suggested but ruled out by appropriate investigations

Such a disorder is present but first incidence of migraine does not occur in close temporal relation with the disorder

Migraine with aura

At least two attacks fulfilling the following criterion

Headache has at least three of the following characteristics:

- One or more fully reversible aura symptom indicating focal cerebral, cortical, and/or brainstem dysfunction
- At least one aura symptom develops gradually over more than 4 minutes, or two or more symptoms occur in succession
- No individual aura symptom lasts more than 60 minutes.
- Headache follows aura with a free interval of less than 60 minutes (it can also begin before or simultaneously with the aura)

At least one of the following

- History and physical and neurologic examinations do not suggest a disorder with secondary headache
- Such a disorder is suggested but ruled out by appropriate investigations
- Such a disorder is present but migraine attacks do not occur for the first time in close temporal relation with the disorder.

Other migraine syndromes

Figure 15-2. International Headache Society (IHS) criteria for the migraine syndrome. In the IHS system, migraine is divided into migraine without aura, migraine with aura, and other migraine syndromes. All neurologic symptoms associated with migraine are termed *aura*, because of the presumption that the majority of neurologic phenomena occur immediately prior to a migraine headache. The IHS criteria are an extremely useful research tool, allowing studies on migraine to be done across cultural and language boundaries. Their specificity is high but, because patients who do not fit all the criteria can still have migraine, the sensitivity is lower.

Components of the Migraine Syndrome

Pain	Location: unilateral, bilateral, retro-orbital, occipital/suboccipital, parietal, or central facial
	Quality: throbbing, steady, aching, burning, boring, superficial, or deep
	Intensity: variable from mild to extremely severe and disabling
General irritability	Photophobia, phonophobia, osmophobia, kinesiophobia
Gastrointestinal symptoms	Anorexia, nausea, vomiting, diarrhea
Neurologic symptoms	Cortical symptoms
	Visual: spots, lines, grids, heat waves, fortification of spectra, lightning streak, "rope of light," "rockets" (can be positive with bright colors or lights or negative with black spots)
	Hemiparesis
	Hemisensory loss
	Aphasia (expressive or receptive), confusional states, transient global amnesia
	Brainstem symptoms
	Vertigo, loss of consciousness, forelimb weakness or numbness
Mood symptoms	Depression, euphoria, (hypo)mania, irritability, increased energy level

Figure 15-3. Components of the migraine syndrome. Migraine is very frequent; studies point to a previous underestimation although some experts believe the prevalence is increasing. Women share a higher burden, approximately 33% as opposed to 13% for men, especially during the reproductive years, mainly because of hormonal influences [6]. Patients usually begin the manifestations of migraine early in life [7]. The prevalence of migraine decreases from whites to blacks to Asians [8]. Fewer than a third of migraine patients report being very satisfied with their acute treatment [9]. Lost productivity secondary to migraine is approximately $13 million per year [10]. A high proportion of patients are not diagnosed, and many would benefit from therapeutic treatment. The burden on personal, familial, and professional life as well as on society as a whole is enormous [11].

Migraine, like the other primary headaches, is a syndrome and not a specific disease. It has a wide spectrum of manifestations, intensity, and symptoms [12]. Migraine also has comorbidities with other medical and psychiatric illnesses [13,14], and patients with migraine report a significantly worse quality of life than patients without migraine [11].

While migraine pain is classically described as throbbing, the pain can be steady, aching, or burning; the intensity of migraine pain is highly variable and can range from mild to extremely severe pain. The quality of migraine pain is also highly variable. There can be no pain at all, but other components of the migraine syndrome can be present. Symptoms of general irritability are an important part of the migraine syndrome. Photophobia, phonophobia, and aggravation by movement occur very commonly. Osmophobia is less common but still a major symptom for many migraine patients.

The gastrointestinal symptoms associated with migraine are the second most common cause of disability in migraine. There is a continuum from anorexia to vomiting. Nausea is present in 90% of migraine patients, and 60% of these patients experience vomiting. Diarrhea is seen in up to 25% of migraine patients. The intensity of these symptoms correlates with the head pain. There is comorbidity between migraine and irritable bowel syndrome, although this has not been studied in detail. The brainstem symptoms of vertigo, loss of consciousness, and forelimb numbness or weakness are less common. These features would typically occur with basilar artery migraine. The origin of the brainstem symptoms is unclear. The cortical symptoms are thought to relate to spreading depression occurring in the cortex, producing transient cortical dysfunction.

Mood changes, including increased energy and productiveness, euphoria, increased sex drive and appetite, irritability or depression, are often associated with migraine. While typically thought of as part of the prodrome, they can occur before, during, or after the headache.

Occurrence of Migraine-Associated Symptoms

	Whole, %	No VA,%	VA, %	5 min, %	1–4 min, %	<1 min, %	Multi R, %	LOV, %
Unilateral	52	51	55	59	46	38	63	42
Bilateral	25	27	24	26	21	29	19	35
Anorexia	23	24	22	22	25	19	20	27
Nausea	83	76	91	91	90	76	95	81
Vomiting	51	44	59	63	49	43	64	35
Diarrhea	27	22	33	32	40	19	33	15
Photophobia	86	78	94	94	98	90	94	81
Phonophobia	84	78	92	92	92	81	96	65
Osmophobia	35	26	45	44	48	38	48	19
Spots	20	0	40	37	48	43	43	0
Blurring	27	23	31	33	29	14	26	31
Loss of vision	9	0	12	14	11	5	12	100
Diplopia	4	3	6	5	11	10	3	0
Shapes/lights	31	0	62	64	59	52	62	0
Pressure	2	3	2	1	0	14	2	8
Giddiness	19	16	23	22	24	29	22	15
Vertigo	16	14	19	19	16	19	21	12
LOC	8	5	10	11	14	0	12	12
Presyncope	7	5	9	9	8	19	7	19
Steady pain	30	31	28	25	24	33	36	42
Throbbing pain	44	40	48	52	40	48	46	38
Tinnitus	14	11	17	20	10	10	18	12
Aphasia	13	9	17	14	27	24	14	4
Confusion	9	8	10	13	5	10	9	12
Dysphagia	1	1	1	1	2	5	0	4
HSL	19	13	24	28	30	14	19	31
HP	11	8	14	13	14	10	15	4
Bilateral weakness	2	1	3	2	6	0	1	4
BSL	2	2	3	3	3	0	2	4

Figure 15-4. Compilation of occurrence of migraine-associated symptoms. This compilation of clinical observations of 852 patients from the Oklahoma University Headache Clinic illustrates how symptoms correlate with the migraine syndrome [12]. Visual symptoms occurred during the aura period about 50% to 70% of the time but occurred during the headache and typically at the peak of the headache the remainder of the time. Approximately 10% of patients report having brief periods of visual symptoms occurring intermittently throughout the aura and the headache. Other neurologic symptoms tended to occur during the headache 80% to 90% of the time. Not reported in this study are acephalalgic migraine syndrome (aura in the absence of headache) and abdominal symptoms without headache in children (cyclic vomiting or abdominal cramps of childhood). BSL—bilateral sensory loss; BW—bilateral weakness; HP—hemiparesis; HSL—hemisensory loss; LOC—loss of consciousness; LOV—loss of vision; Multi R—multiple recurrence of visual phenomena; VA—visual aura.

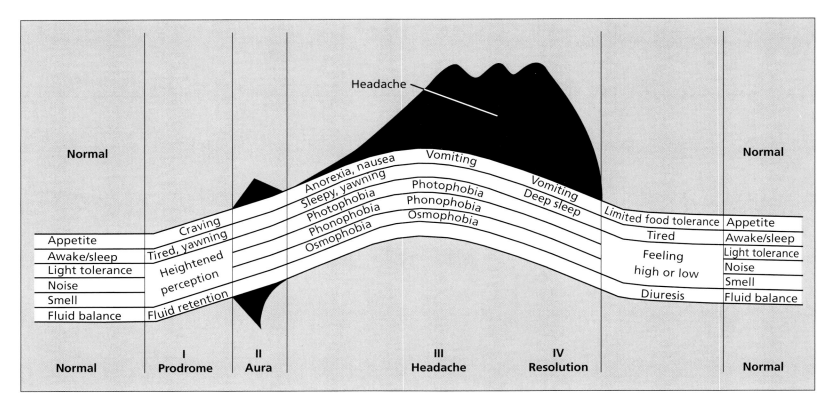

Figure 15-5. Four phases of classic migraine: prodrome, aura, headache, and resolution (postdrome). This model describes most migraine headaches and relates everything to the occurrence of pain. In the classic description, mood changes occur in the prodrome and postdrome.

Neurologic changes occur during the aura, and pain dominates the headache phase. Any of the components of migraine can occur at any time. (*Adapted from* Olesen and colleague [15].)

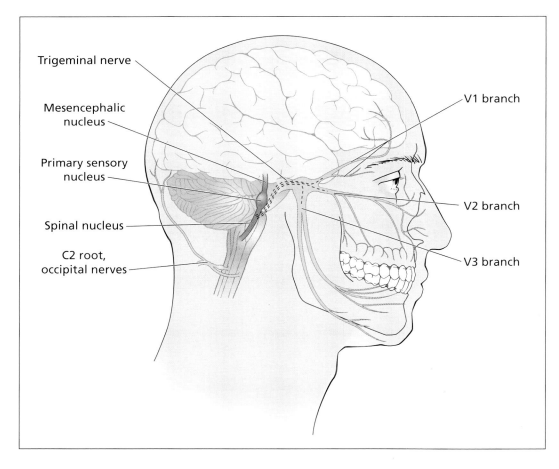

Figure 15-6. Head pain afferents. Referral of pain from the forehead to the upper neck and suboccipital region is common. As shown here, the trigeminal caudal nucleus divides into three branches: V1, extending into the orbit, cranium, meninges, and scalp; V2, extending into the nasal cavity, sinuses, and upper jaw; and V3, extending into the lower jaw and lower mouth structures. All pain messages converge toward the spinal nucleus, which converges with the C2 projection. This allows for referral of pain to the neck. The head pain can begin in the suboccipital region and refer to the distribution of the ophthalmic nerve. Complaints of neck pain in migraine commonly leads to the prescription of ineffective muscle relaxants. Typically, relief of the frontal headache will also relieve the suboccipital headache and neck pain, confirming the relationship described.

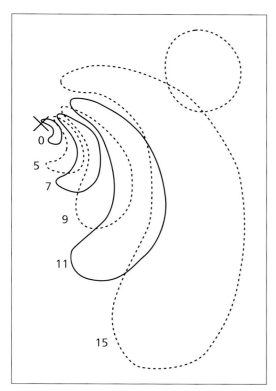

Figure 15-7. The aura. Visual aura experienced by Lashley illustrating the progression of the phenomenon in minutes across the visual cortex [15]. Fortification spectra can begin as a dot in the central vision and spread in a widening arch to the side. The dotted circle represents the blind spot; the point of visual fixation is marked by an X. There has been debate for decades between the vascular and neural origins of migraine. The vascular effect of ergotamine was known early in the last century and the vascular theory of migraine predominated for the next fifty years [16]. In 1944 Leão described the cortical spreading depression [17]. Because the progression of the visual symptoms and that of the cortical spreading depression was similar, it appeared that the latter could cause the former [18]. Any theory of migraine, however, must try to account for all of the symptoms. This has been and continues to be a problem. (*Adapted from* Olesen and colleague [15].)

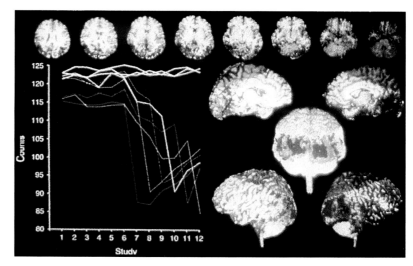

Figure 15-8. Spreading oligemia. Positron-emission tomography (PET) scan of a patient experiencing migraine aura. In 1984, Lauritzen and colleague described spreading oligemia in the occipital cortex of patients with migraine with aura [19]. Further studies demonstrated that oligemia spreads at a rate of 2 to 3 mm a minute across the cortex; this occurs irrespective of usual vascular distribution to the brain [20]. Also visible on magnetic resonance imaging [21], the aura is shown on this PET scan by decreased activity over time, area by area, in succession [22]. (*From* Woods and colleagues [22]; with permission.)

Figure 15-9. Temporal relationship between migraine symptoms and vascular tone. Although the aura is believed to occur during the hypoperfusion phase and the head pain during hyperperfusion, that is not always the case. CBF—cerebral blood flow. (*Adapted from* Olesen and colleagues [20].)

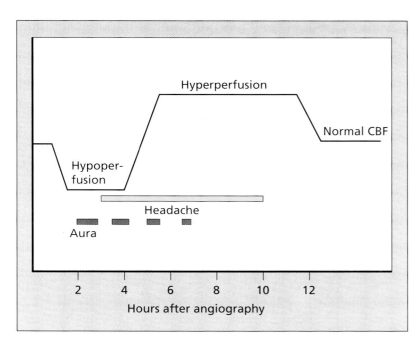

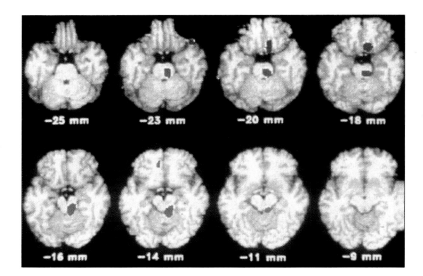

Figure 15-10. Migraine generator. The hypothesis that a center in the brainstem generates migraine symptoms has gained popularity. This positron-emission tomography scan demonstrates activation of an area at or near the periacqueductal gray matter [23]. The same concept is reflected in a study by Raskin of patients with cancer pain who had therapeutic stimulators placed in the periaqueductal gray matter; a subgroup of these patients developed typical migraine headaches [24]. (*From* Weiller and colleagues [23]; with permission.)

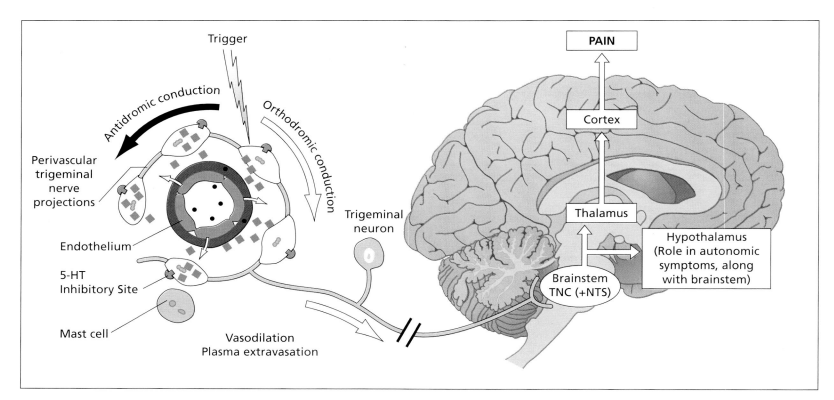

Figure 15-11. Trigeminovascular system. Trigeminal nerve antidromic activation triggers the release of neuropeptides (neuropeptide Y, calcitonin gene–related peptide, and substance P) (*orange squares*) which in turn induce vasodilation, blood-brain barrier disruption, local sterile neurogenic inflammation, and activation of the trigeminal nerve itself, with central transmission of pain afferent messages [25]. Such activation can be initiated by stress or food and possibly by cortical spreading depression. This has been extensively studied in animals, and there is evidence that it takes place in humans as well. Subsequently, Moskowitz and others showed that trigeminal nerve activation could spread orthodromically as well to the trigeminal caudal nucleus (TCN) [26]. Goadsby suggested that there was activation of the superior salivatory nucleus via the nucleus tractus solitarius (NTS) that in turn could be related to the gastrointestinal symptoms. Serotonergic agonists such as triptans act on the smooth muscle (vasoconstriction), the presynaptic boutons (decreased release of neuropeptides mentioned), and on the trigeminal afferents (central projection of pain). (*Adapted from* Moskowitz [26].)

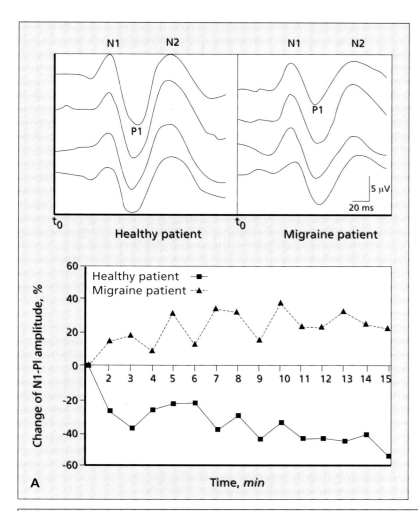

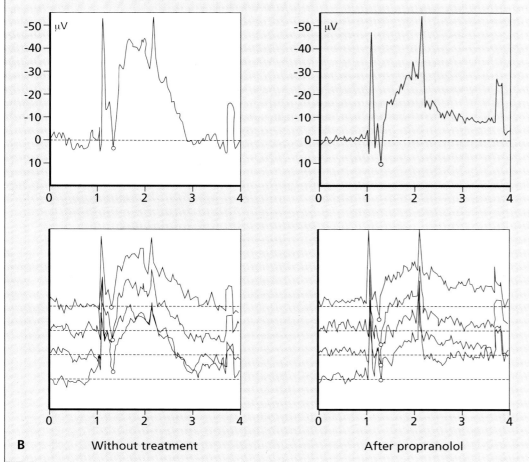

Figure 15-12. Cortical activity in migraine. Studies with evoked responses suggest that the brain of the migraine patient does not habituate to external stimuli as does that of the normal subject [28]. **A,** A study of visual evoked potentials in a patient with migraine compared with those in a healthy patient [29,30]. Not only do the responses not habituate over time, but there is an increase in amplitude. **B,** Contingent negative variation (CNV) in a 24-year-old patient with migraine without aura. An event-related cortical potential, CNV is dependent on norepinephrine and dopamine activity; CNV amplitude in migraine patients is high and there is no habituation [28]. CNV tends to normalize with prophylaxis using beta-blockers (propranolol), supposedly by correcting the excessive central catecholaminergic activity. The graphs on the left show CNV recording before treatment; those on the right show CNV recording in the same patient after a 3-month course of propranolol, 160 mg/d. Work with transcranial magnetic stimulation suggests that the occipital cortex in patients with migraine is hyperexcitable with a low threshold to transcranial magnetic stimulation [31]. A study of the genetics of migraine demonstrated a mutation in locus 12 of chromosome 19 in patients with familial hemiplegic migraine [32]. Ophoff and colleagues suggested that mutations in the alpha 1A subunit of the P-Q calcium channel gene (CACNL1A4) could alter cortical processing activity and can be related to the above observations [33]. There are also potential abnormalities in mitochondrial function as suggested by magnetic resonance spectroscopy by Barbiroli and colleagues [34] and Welch [35] and the efficacy of riboflavin in migraine prevention. (Panel A *adapted from* Schoenen and colleague [28]; Panel B *adapted from* Áfra and colleagues [29].)

Biochemistry of Migraine

Monoamines
  Serotonin (5-HT)
    Source: platelets and raphe nuclei
      Between attacks: decreased plasma 5-HT, increased plasma 5-HIAA
      During attacks: normal plasma 5-HT, decreased urine 5-HIAA [36,37]
    Source: turnover increased between and normalized during attacks [38]
    5-HT1B, 5-HT1D, ? 5-HT1F, 5-HT2, 5-HT3 are implicated [39–41]
  Dopamine
    Dopamine has been postulated to be associated with acceleration of migraine attack [42]
Neuroexcitatory amino acids
  Glu/Asp can trigger cortical spreading depression aura [43]
  NMDA modifies trigeminal reflex and pain transmission [44]
Magnesium
  Low level sensitizes NMDA receptors [38]
  In red blood cells and in brain during attack [45,46]
Estrogens
  Drop in level precipitates catamenial attacks [47]
  Can act via sympathetic system [48]

Figure 15-13. The biochemistry of migraine. The involvement of neurotransmitters in migraine, especially serotonin, has been the subject of many studies but the exact role played by each has yet to be integrated.

Considerations for Treatment of Migraine

Main categories of migraine treatment

Nonpharmacologic (biofeedback and/or relaxation)
Pharmacologic
Symptomatic (abortive)
Prophylactic

Components of treatment to consider

Headache frequency
Headache severity
Associated symptoms
Age
Comorbidity
Hormonal status/pregnancy
Psychologic status
Contraindications
Patient's functional status
Patient's preference
Triggers

Figure 15-14. Considerations for the treatment of migraine. These are general guidelines and each patient's situation must be considered individually. In general, patients who experience more than four moderate to severe headaches per month with a significant amount of disability are candidates for prophylactic therapy. If the patient has more than one type of headache, the patient must distinguish between more severe headaches that can require stronger medication and less severe headaches that can require a different approach. Symptomatic treatment of migraine does not merely consist of choosing a medication. The current tendency is to stratify therapy, beginning with the most efficient regimen, rather than using stepwise care in which patients are tried successively on medications from the least expensive and aspecific on up. Clinicians should begin with the simplest regimen possible, using enough nonhabituating medication to obtain relief. Patients should be followed up to determine if the medication regimen is achieving the desired effect.

Nonspecific and Semispecific Drug Therapies for Migraine

Non-specific	Usual dosage	Maximum dosage/d
NSAIDs		
Ibuprofen	400 mg–800 mg	3200 mg
Naproxen	250 mg–550 mg	1100 mg
Fenoprofen	300 mg–600 mg	2400 mg
Meclofenamate	100 mg	300 mg
Tolmetin	200 mg–400 mg	1800 mg
Aspirin	650 mg–1000 mg	4000 mg
Analgesics		
Acetaminophen	650 mg–1000 mg	4000 mg
Tramadol	50 mg	400 mg
Minor narcotics		
Codeine	30 mg–60 mg	360 mg
Hydrocodone	5 mg–75 mg	375 mg
Oxycodone	5 mg	30 mg
Semi-specific		
Isometheptene	65 mg	6 capsules/d
Butalbital	50 mg	200 mg–400 mg
Sodium valproate IV	500 mg	1500 mg

Figure 15-15. Nonspecific and semispecific drug therapies for migraine. Nonspecific therapies, such as nonsteroidal anti-inflammatory drugs (NSAIDs), analgesics, narcotics, and non-narcotics, relieve pain but do not attack the specific mechanism of migraine. For many patients with intermittent acute migraine, use of 800 mg ibuprofen, 500 mg naproxen, or another NSAID or acetaminophen can be sufficient. The addition of an antihistamine with antiemetic action (hydroxyzine 25 mg–50 mg) or dopamine antagonist (promethazine 25 mg–50 mg) can enhance the potential of this approach significantly. Codeine, oxycodone, and hydrocodone are effective for some patients but must be used carefully. If the patient requires more than 10 tablets per month, habituation should be suspected and alternative therapy sought. These minor narcotics can be used as individual agents or combined with an antihistamine or dopamine antagonist. Isometheptene or butalbital compounds are effective for some patients with migraine, but their mechanism of action is not fully elucidated. If the patient requires as many as 10 butalbital doses per month, habituation and rebound withdrawal headache should be considered and the use of butalbital discontinued. Slow intravenous (IV) injections of 500 mg sodium valproate have proven efficient in aborting a migraine attack [49].

A. Migraine Treatment: Triptans

Generic	Strength, mg	Max mg/24 h	1/2 life, h	T max, h	Efficacy,* %
First-generation triptans					
Sumatriptan PO	25, 50, 100	200	2.5	2	62/33
Sumatriptan NS	5, 20	40	2		64/31
Sumatriptan SC	6	12	2	12	80/40
Second-generation triptans					
Naratriptan	1, 2.5	5	6	1.5–3	58/27
Zolmitriptan	2.5, 5	10	3	2.5	67/33
Rizatriptan	5, 10	30	3	1.5	72/41

*Meta-analysis of patients at 2 hours: first number = improvement from moderate or severe headache to mild or none; second number = pain free.

Figure 15-16. Specific migraine treatment: first- and second-generation triptans. Triptans represent one of the most dramatic advances in migraine therapy of the last century. Since the development of sumatriptan newer triptans have been designed in an attempt to improve efficacy and decrease side effects. A main pharmacologic difference is their central nervous system penetration. They act on 5-HT1B/D receptors on meningeal and brain vessels, on presynaptic perivascular trigeminal nerve endings, and on the central projections of trigeminal fibers conveying pain [50–52]. Individual patient sensitivity to each triptan seems to vary. **A**, Dosing schedules for the first- and second-generation triptans. For most migraine patients, the triptans produce rapid and complete relief of the headache with relatively early return to functional status.

(*Continued on next page*)

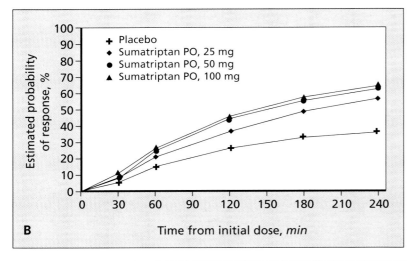

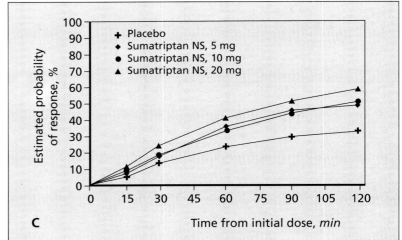

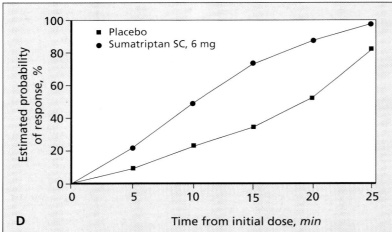

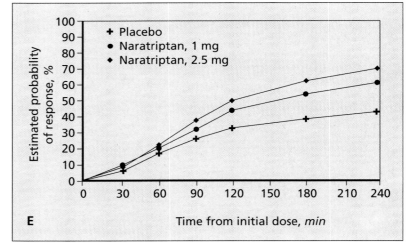

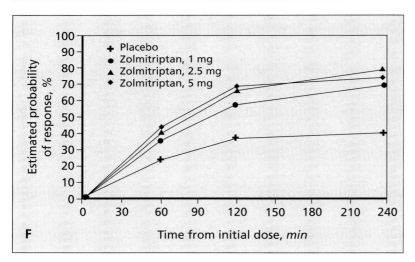

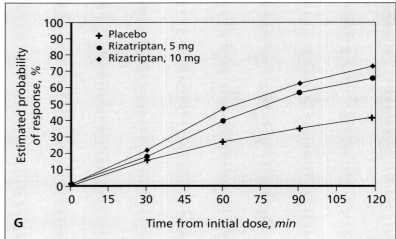

Figure 15-16. (*Continued*) **B**, Estimated probability of achieving initial headache response within 240 minutes with sumatriptan PO. **C**, Estimated probability of achieving initial headache response within 120 minutes with sumatriptan NS. **D**, Time to relief from time of injection with sumatriptan SC. **E**, Estimated probability of achieving initial headache response within 240 minutes with naratriptan. **F**, Estimated probability of achieving initial headache response within 240 minutes with zolmitriptan. **G**, Estimated probability of achieving initial headache response within 120 minutes with rizatriptan. In general, for uncomplicated intermittent migraine, 60% to 70% of patients will have good relief within 2 hours and more than 80% will have good relief within 4 hours [53–58]. Evidence suggests that even

milder migraine headaches can be effectively treated by a triptan [59,60]. Recurrence within 24 hours typically is 25% to 35%, but often recurrences are mild and will respond well to a second dose of triptan. In general, the triptans have onset of effect within 30 to 60 minutes, achieving peak effect at approximately 4 hours. About 50% of patients will maintain a response for 24 hours without recurrence or having to take supplementary medication. There do appear to be idiosyncratic differences between patients in response to the triptans. Patients who fail to respond to the one triptan can respond to one of the others. Consequently, it is worth trying all of the currently available triptans before assuming that the patient is "triptan-unresponsive." A simplistic approach to triptan usage is that patients can take a

(*Continued on next page*)

Figure 15-16. (*Continued*) dose of the medication and then repeat that dose once within 24 hours if necessary. For most of the triptans, repeating 2 doses within 24 hours is usually tolerated well. Of the available dose forms, most patients prefer tablets. Sumatriptan is available by both nasal spray and injection. The nasal spray at times produces an unpleasant taste for the patient and this can preclude usage. Patients with very rapidly progressing headache can prefer the subcutaneous injection to achieve relief as rapidly as possible. Between 30% and 40% of patients will have adverse events, typ-

ically mild but occasionally severe. Adverse events reported by more than 5% of patients include somnolence or fatigue, dizziness, paresthesia or sensation of chest/throat pressure, or nausea. These events tend to rarefy over time and are similar although more frequent or severe than those reported for dihydroergotamine. There is concern over the coronary arteries where ergots or triptans can produce up to a 20% constriction; however, this is not clinically significant in healthy individuals. Patients with coronary artery disease should not receive these drugs.

Therapy for Status Migrainosus

10 mg metoclopramide IV over 60 sec

Wait 5 min

0.5 mg DHE IV over 60 sec

Wait 5 min

Repeat 0.5 mg DHE IV over 60 sec; wait 5 min

Repeat above 5 steps every 8 h

Figure 15-17. Specific treatment for status migrainosus, a state marked by constantly recurring attacks of migraine: dihydroergotamine (DHE). Ergotamine is the oldest specific migraine abortive, but it has fallen into disuse since the advent of the triptans. Like the triptans, it has an effect on the serotonin 5HT1B and 5HT1D receptors, but is less specific and also binds to norepinephrine and dopamine. The usual dosage is 1 mg PO at the onset of the headache; the dosage can be repeated in 30 minutes and then hourly afterwards up to a maximum of 6 mg per day. DHE, a hydroxy derivative of ergotamine, can be given by intravenous injection (most effective), subcutaneous injection, or intramuscular injection and by nasal spray. Typically, a dose of 0.5 mg is given over 60 seconds and followed in 3 to 5 minutes by another 0.5 mg dose. Metoclopramide is given as a 10 mg injection over 60 seconds preceding the first dose of DHE by 3 to 5 minutes to decrease nausea, although it can also have intrinsic antimigraine action [61].

Migraine Prophylaxis

Generic	Efficacy*	Average dose/d	Frequent adverse effects	Remedy
Propranolol	51	80–180 mg	Sedation, hypotension, bradycardia	Check blood pressure
Amitriptyline	51	25–150 mg	Sedation, dry mouth, dizziness, constipation	
Valproate sodium	50	500–2000 mg	Nausea, alopecia, gastralgia, weight gain, liver toxicity	Check SGOT, SGPT
Verapamil	na	120–360 mg	Hypotension, dizziness	
Riboflavin	59	400 mg	None	
Gabapentin	na	600–2700 mg	Dizziness, drowsiness, nephrolithiasis	
Methysergide	50	3–6 mg	Retroperitoneal fibrosis, edema, fatigue	Maximum 6 months continuously

Efficacy expressed as percent of patients who had 50% or more improvement over baseline.

Figure 15-18. Migraine prophylaxis: most commonly used medications. Prophylaxis of migraine has to be individualized, and is typically given for a few months depending on the evolution of symptoms. Side effects must be carefully monitored since these are long-term treatments. Mechanisms of action vary [62]. Comorbidities must be kept in mind since often these agents can be therapeutic for other symptoms as

well [63,64]. Note that riboflavin appears to take 2 to 3 months to show results [65]. Other agents, such as metoprolol, are used but either they are not formally approved or definite proof of their efficacy is lacking. na—not available or not statistically significant; SGOT—serum glutamic-oxaloacetic transaminase; SGPT—serum glutamate pyruvate transaminase.

Tension-type Headache

International Headache Society Criteria for Tension-type Headache

At least 10 previous headache episodes fulfilling the following three criteria
  Headache from 30 min to 7 d
  At least two of the following pain characteristics
    Pressing/tightening quality
    Mild/moderate intensity
    Bilateral location
    No aggravation by physical activity
  Both of the following
    No nausea or vomiting
    Photophobia and phonophobia are absent, or at least not present together
At least one of the following
  History, physical, and neurologic examinations do not suggest a cause for a
  secondary headache
  If a cause for a secondary headache is suggested, it is ruled out by appropriate
  investigations
  If a cause for a secondary headache is present, it does not occur in close temporal
  relation to the present headache

Figure 15-19. International Headache Society criteria for tension-type headache. Subsequent classification distinguishes between episodic tension-type headache (fewer than 180 days/year with such headache) and chronic tension-type headache (more than 180 days/year with such headache). Tension-type headache is the most frequent headache type, experienced episodically by 40% of the population [4]. However, because patients are usually only mildly impaired, they rarely seek medical attention. Tension-type headache is somewhat difficult to define. There is no clearly distinctive positive feature for tension-type headache; most criteria are negative and tend to differentiate this headache type from migraine. A possible continuum has been suggested between tension-type headache and migraine [66]. It is likely that tension-type headache is a heterogeneous disorder. Episodic and chronic tension-type headache differ from a pathophysiologic standpoint and seem to respond differently to therapy.

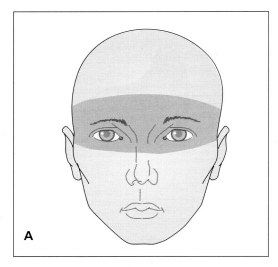 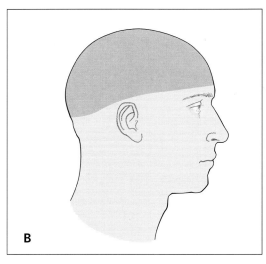

Figure 15-20. Clinical presentation. **A, B,** Pain distribution in tension-type headache is diffuse and bilateral in 90% of patients. It can sometimes predominate on one side; this is atypical, and the possibility of alternate diagnosis should be raised. The pain commonly varies in location. A band-like distribution is often reported. Patients typically describe a pressure sensation in the form of a helmet or a boring sensation. The intensity is mild or moderate, does not worsen with physical activities, and rarely interferes with the patient's routine. Nausea and vomiting are excluding factors, but anorexia can be present. Physical

examination typically reveals pericranial muscle tenderness; this is more prevalent during the headache phase. This finding defines the subclassification into tension-type headache associated with pericranial muscle disorder, which can be assessed by electromyography or algometer. Muscle contraction can in turn cause a reduction in the range of motion of the cervical spine, although there is no primary spine disorder. Pericranial tender and trigger points are best evaluated by a systematic methodology so as to allow the physician to better distinguish normal from abnormal. The presence of excessive muscle contraction in tension-type headache is clearly established. Its role in the pathogenesis of the pain remains difficult to establish. The pericranial pain threshold is decreased, at least in the chronic form of tension-type headache. Interestingly, a study of 30-minute–long teeth clenching established that headache was correlated with increased pericranial muscular tenderness [67]. Contrary to healthy patients, pericranial pain thresholds decrease with sustained contraction instead of increasing, pointing to a sensitization phenomenon.

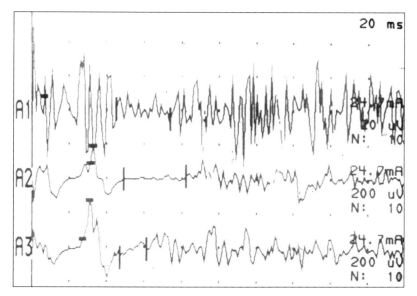

Figure 15-21. Electromyogram activity recorded with surface electrodes. A neurophysiologic tool has given insight into the role of brainstem and higher control centers in tension-type headache: the activity of jaw-closing muscles is normally inhibited by electrical stimulation at the lips. This is called the second exteroceptive silent period or ES-II. An electric stimulation at the lips during active jaw contraction normally provokes two phases of EMG activity interruption, ES-I and ES-II. This example is from a patient suffering from chronic tension-type headache; the ES-II period is between the two vertical markers, either reduced or inconsistent. This inhibition is reduced or abolished in chronic tension-type headache. This can in turn be modulated by central descending control.

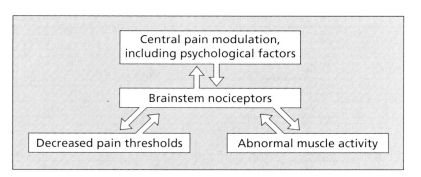

Figure 15-22. Pathophysiology of tension-type headache. An integrated approach to the mechanisms of tension-type headache was proposed by Schoenen and colleague [68].

Treatment of Tension-type Headache

NSAIDs (*eg*, naproxen sodium 500 mg PO QD-BID)
Other analgesics (*eg*, paracetamol 500–1000 mg PO BID–TID)
Tricyclic antidepressants (*eg*, amitriptyline 25-100 mg PO QD)
SSRIs (*eg*, fluoxetine 20 mg PO QD)
Nonpharmacologic treatments (*eg*, biofeedback, physical therapy, etc.)

Figure 15-23. Treatment of tension-type headache. Episodic tension-type headache seldom requires treatment. If necessary, nonsteroidal anti-inflammatory drugs (NSAIDs) or paracetamol can be used symptomatically. Chronic tension-type headache therapy will essentially be prophylactic. Tricyclic antidepressants are commonly used; the effective doses vary widely among individuals. Selective serotonin reuptake inhibitors (SSRIs) have generally failed to demonstrate efficacy. Non-pharmacologic treatments should be considered as well, and their efficacy is proven. These require experience and patients should be referred to a psychologist or a physical therapist with proficiency in the field. BID—twice a day; PO—by mouth; QD—each day; TID—three times a day.

Cluster Headache and Related Headaches

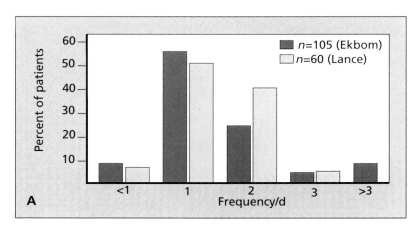

Figure 15-24. Characteristics of cluster headaches. **A**, A typical feature of cluster headache is its time course: "*clusters*" of frequently occurring headaches, especially at season changes, separated by several months or years without headache. There is a great deal of variation, however, and sometimes only a few weeks separate these periods. Cluster headaches can become chronic, in which case the episodes do not remit. There are also spontaneous complete remissions. The headaches often occur at the same time of the day for each patient, frequently evening or early morning. Patients occasionally have more than one attack a day.

(*Continued on next page*)

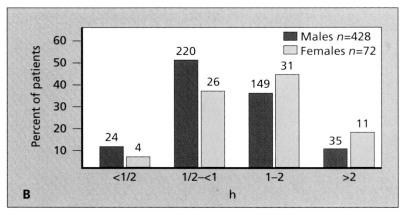

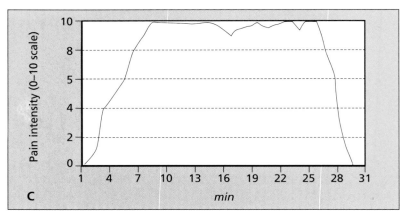

Figure 15-24. (*Continued*) **B,** Cluster headaches consist of the sudden onset of pain that lasts usually 30 to 60 minutes. **C,** The pain is very intense, often described as boring or sharp. The pain of cluster headache is periorbital and can extend into the jaw or toward the neck. Patients do not seek rest as with migraine but rather tend to pace the room. Ipsilateral autonomic symptoms accompany the pain: conjunctival injec-

tion, eyelid closure, and sometimes full Horner's syndrome, including facial flushing, lacrimation, rhinorrhea, and nasal obstruction. Exceptional cases of cluster headache with aura have been described. The attack can be triggered by alcohol or nitroglycerine but there are no physical triggers as in trigeminal neuralgia. (Panels A and B *adapted from* Lance and colleague [69].)

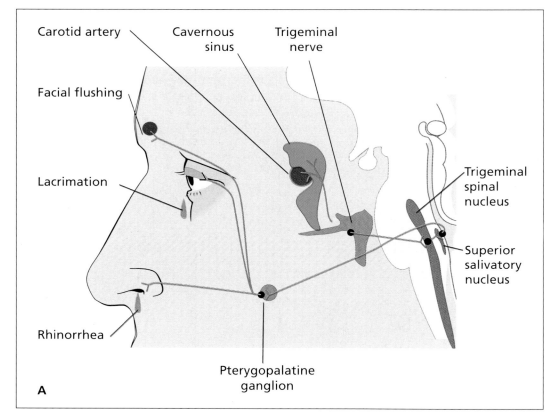

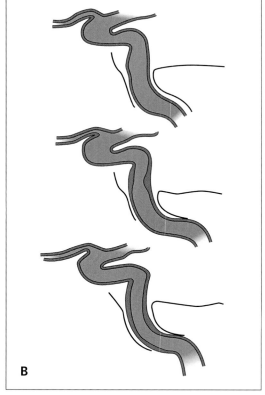

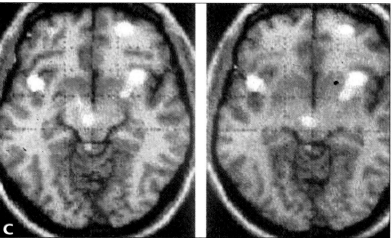

Figure 15-25. Anatomy of cluster headache. **A,** Dilated carotid artery and inflamed cavernous sinus activate the trigeminal nerve and pain ensues; projections from the trigeminal spinal nucleus to superior salivatory nucleus trigger autonomic symptoms via the pterygopalatine ganglion. **B,** Studies by Hardebo indicate cavernous sinus inflammation or blood flow obstruction [70]. The schematic illustrates the appearance of the carotid siphon before (*top*), during (*middle*), and near the end (*bottom*) of a cluster headache. Note the constrictions designated by thickened contours. The autonomic manifestations point to both a sympathetic inhibition and a parasympathetic activation. **C,** Positron-emission tomography/T1-weighted magnetic resonance coregistration imaging scans demonstrating activation of the hypothalamus, frontal cortex, and insulae seen in acute attacks of cluster headache. Significant activations are visible in the contralateral frontal cortex, bilateral insulae, and ipsilateral posterior hypothalamus. Serotonergic dysfunction has also been demonstrated [71]. (Panel B *adapted from* Hardebo [70]; Panel C *from* May and colleagues [71]; with permission.)

Drugs Used in the Treatment of Cluster Headache

Prophylactic

Steroids (prednisone 100 mg PO QD, tapered over a week; low dose may need to be maintained for a longer time)

Verapamil (240–720 mg PO QD)

Lithium (300–900 mg PO QD)

Methysergide (2–4 mg PO TID)

Valproate sodium (500 mg PO BID or TID, up to 2000 mg/day)

Ergotamine tartrate (1 mg PO QD or BID)

Symptomatic

Oxygen

Sumatriptan SC

Other triptans

DHE

Figure 15-26. Drugs used for cluster headache. Treatment of cluster headache can be either prophylactic or symptomatic. The acute and very intense nature of the headache render prevention difficult, hence the need to emphasize acute treatment. Prophylaxis must be given without delay for at least the presumed duration of the active period; combination therapy must be given in refractory cases. Steroids are the most effective treatment but it can be difficult to taper off after the headache is controlled. Verapamil is more effective for cluster headache than for migraine. Methysergide is effective in cluster headache but side effects limit its use. Several procedures have been found effective to control a cluster headache period: occipital nerve block, gasserian ganglion radiofrequency thermocoagulation, trigeminal nerve rhizotomy, and gamma knife radiosurgery. These procedures should only be considered after all attempts at pharmacologic treatment fail. Symptomatic treatment must be carefully chosen and adjusted until fast and adequate relief is obtained. The options are: oxygen by nasal cannula, 10 L/min for 10–15 minutes; sumatriptan 6 mg subcutaneously (SC) BID; or dihydroergotamine (DHE) 1 mg intravenously with or without pretreatment with a dopamine antagonist to counteract the adverse effects of DHE. Alternatively, intranasal DHE can be used, 1 mg TID. BID—twice a day; PO—by mouth; QD—each day; TID—three times a day.

Differential Diagnosis of Short-lasting Unilateral Headache

Headache type	Sex ratio	Duration	Frequency of attacks	Accompanying autonomic symptoms	Treatment
Cluster	Predominantly male	15–180 min	1–3/d	Prominent	Multiple
CPH	Predominantly female	min	Few to 100/d	Variable	Indomethacin (50–225 mg QD)
HC	Equal	Continuous, stabs (sec)	Constant, jabs many/d	Mild	Indomethacin (50–225 mg QD)
SUNCT	Predominantly male	sec–min	Few to 50/d	Variable	?
Idiopathic stabbing headache ("jabs and jolts")	Equal	sec	1 or several/d	None	Indomethacin?
Trigeminal neuralgia	Slightly predominantly female	sec		Few	Carbamazepine

Figure 15-27. Differential diagnosis of short-lasting unilateral headaches. These headaches share a paroxysmal course, are unilateral, and are often accompanied by local autonomic dysfunction. The underlying mechanisms for chronic paroxysmal hemicrania (CPH) and hemicrania continua (HC) are unknown. Short-lasting, unilateral, neuralgiform headache attacks with conjunctival injection and tearing (SUNCT) is rare; less than 50 cases have been described. Pathophysiology is unknown, but it has many similarities with cluster headache and it is frequently refractory to treatment. Idiopathic stabbing headache ("jabs and jolts") are very brief spells of lancinating pain that occur without a trigger and can be localized anywhere in the head and face. It tends to be more frequent in migraine patients. QD—each day.

Trigeminal Neuralgia

International Headache Society Criteria for Trigeminal Neuralgia

Paroxysmal attacks of facial or frontal pain lasting a few seconds to less than a minute

Pain has at least four of the following characteristics

Distribution along one or more divisions of the trigeminal nerve

Sudden, intense, sharp, superficial, stabbing, or burning character

Severe intensity

Precipitation by touching trigger areas or by daily activities such as eating, chewing, swallowing, talking, brushing teeth, etc.

No neurologic deficit

Triggers and attacks are stereotyped in a given individual

Exclusion of other causes of facial pain by history, physical examination, and ancillary investigations whenever necessary

Figure 15-28. International Headache Society criteria for trigeminal neuralgia. Also called tic douloureux, trigeminal neuralgia is the prototypic neuralgia, with lancinating pain that can be triggered, located in the strict distribution of a nerve. Patients complain of a severe, lightning-like pain in the distribution of V-2 and/or V-3, exceptionally V-1. Physical findings are observation of the trigger phenomenon, and a facial twitch during an attack. Autonomic dysfunction such as conjunctival injection and lacrimation can be present. There is no neurological deficit; if a sensory examination in the trigeminal nerve territory is abnormal, an underlying cause (secondary trigeminal neuralgia) should be sought. The underlying mechanism to this head pain is presumed to be recurrent action potentials in a demyelinated nerve, along with ephaptic transmission. The prevalence of this headache is about 0.1 to 0.2 per 100,000 people. It is twice as common in females and usually has begins in midadulthood [72].

Common Etiologies of Secondary Trigeminal Neuralgia

Inflammatory—immune
  Multiple sclerosis
  Sarcoidosis
  Lyme disease with trigeminal neuropathy
Vascular
  Pontine infarct
  Aneurysm
  Persistence of primitive trigeminal artery
  Pulsatile compression by superior cerebellar artery, more rarely the inferior
Neoplastic
  Pontine glioma
  Epidermoid
  Chordoma
  Lymphoma
Other
  Paraneoplastic?

Figure 15-29. Common etiologies of secondary trigeminal neuralgia. The distinction between primary and secondary trigeminal neuralgia must be addressed with every patient. Trigeminal neuralgia can be the heralding symptom of a lesion compressing or invading the trigeminal nerve or one of its nuclei. Treatment of trigeminal neuralgia is primarily prophylactic.

A. Prophylaxis and Treatment of Trigeminal Neuralgia

Prophylactic medications

Most effective
  Carbamazepine (100 mg PO BID, progressively increased to the maximum tolerated dose, usually 600–1200 mg QD)
  Baclofen (10–20 mg PO TID)
  Gabapentin (400–600 mg PO TID)
Less effective
  Phenytoin
  Clonazepam
  Amitriptyline
  Lamotrigine

Therapeutic procedures

Microvascular posterior fossa decompression (Jannetta procedure)
Alcohol injection of gasserian ganglion
Glycerol injection of gasserian ganglion
Percutaneous radiofrequency rhizotomy
Gamma-knife surgery

Figure 15-30. Prophylaxis and treatment options for trigeminal neuralgia. **A,** Drugs used in the prevention of trigeminal neuralgia, in descending order of efficacy, and therapeutic procedures. Carbamazepine remains the gold standard for trigeminal neuralgia, followed by baclofen and gabapentin. Phenytoin, clonazepam, amitriptyline, and lamotrigine can be useful in some patients, but they are generally less effective [73,74].

(*Continued on next page*)

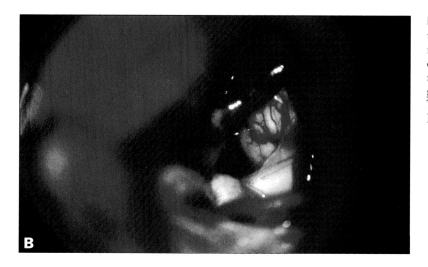

Figure 15-30. (*Continued*) **B,** The Janetta procedure. The most efficient therapeutic procedure is posterior fossa microvascular decompression, pioneered by Jannetta [75]. The procedure consists of separating the superior or anteroinferior cerebellar artery (pink) from the root of the trigeminal nerve (white) to reduce or eliminate the neurovascular conflict thought to generate the neuralgia. BID—twice a day; PO—by mouth; QD—each day; TID—three times a day. (*Courtesy of* PT Dang, MD, Department of Neurosurgery, Centre Hospitalier de Luxembourg, Luxembourg.)

Headache Due to Cerebrospinal Fluid Pressure Abnormalities

Etiologies of CSF Hypotension Headache

Spinal tap

Neurosurgical (cranial and/or spinal) procedures including shunt

Arnold-Chiari malformation

Traumatic root avulsion

Diabetes (insipidus or mellitus)

Rupture of arachnoid cyst

Dehydration

Sepsis

Figure 15-31. Etiology and diagnosis of cerebrospinal fluid (CSF) hypotension headache. Various causes, most frequently trauma, can provoke or exacerbate low-CSF pressure headache. The hallmark of CSF hypotension headache is its relation to position. It starts or worsens soon (less than 15 minutes per International Headache Society criteria) after the patient assumes orthostatic position and resolves or improves soon (less than 30 minutes) after the patient assumes recumbency. The pain, sharp or throbbing, varies from mild to intense and is classically distributed around the skull in a band-like fashion, although it can predominate in the neck or in the forehead. Variable features are cranial nerve dysfunction such as facial hypesthesia or paresthesia, diplopia, tinnitus, and rarely gastrointestinal discomfort. Physical examination can reveal neck stiffness, decreased blink reflex, or oculomotor paresis. Pathogenic mechanisms include a CSF leak, decreased production, or increased resorption. Traction on the meninges, veins, and venous sinuses ultimately causes pain. Diagnosis is based on the history and can be confirmed by a spinal tap measuring the CSF pressure in the resting decubitus position. More recently magnetic resonance imaging has demonstrated meningeal gadolinium enhancement. Isotope cisternography with spinal and cerebral images and iodine contrast computed tomography (CT) (CT myelogram) can help trace the site of a leak. They require a spinal puncture, however, potentially increasing the headache burden.

Determining and Nondetermining Factors in Post-spinal Tap Headache

Determining

Female sex, especially of child-bearing age

Small body-mass index

History of headaches before the spinal tap

Large needle size

Nondetermining

Needle type

Volume of cerebrospinal fluid collected

Post-procedure recumbency

Fluid intake after the procedure

Figure 15-32. Determining and nondetermining factors in post-spinal tap headache. Post-spinal tap headache occurs in about 15% of patients. The preventative effect of post-spinal tap decubitus has not been substantiated by controlled studies. Its therapeutic effect, on the other hand, is undisputed [76,77].

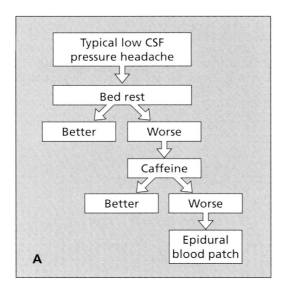

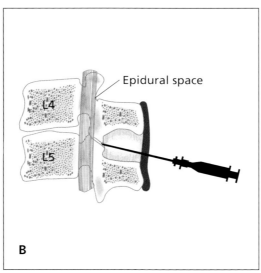

Figure 15-33. Treatment of cerebrospinal fluid (CSF) hypotension headache. **A,** Treatment consists of nonpharmacologic actions, medications, and procedures. Analgesics provide only marginal benefit. Caffeine can be taken orally but a large quantity is needed for this indication (at least 5 cups of strong coffee a day); subcutaneous or intravenous (IV) injections are more convenient. Caffeine benzoate 500 mg IV over 6 to 8 hours is recommended for venous vasoconstriction, and it can be repeated several times. **B,** Epidural blood patching is the ultimate treatment for refractory cases. In a trial, it did not prove useful as prophylaxis [78]. Ten to twenty ml of autologous blood are injected in the epidural space where the leak is, if known; the patient must rest for at least two hours to avoid breaking the clot, which would reduce the therapeutic benefit. The mechanism of action is a sealing effect, but there is also a pressure and volume effect by depressing the dura; this explains why the procedure also works in idiopathic cases where the site of the leak is unknown or no leak is present. In exceptional cases it can be repeated a second time if the first attempt has failed.

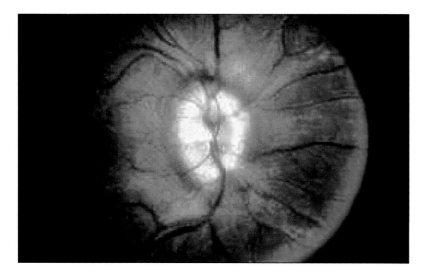

Treatment of Pseudotumor Cerebri

Weight loss
Removal of offending drug, if present
Acetazolamide
Other diuretics
Analgesics
Steroids
Octreotide?
Repeated spinal taps
Optic nerve fenestration
Ventriculoperitoneal shunt

Figure 15-34. Benign intracranial hypertension (BIH, or pseudotumor cerebri). Funduscopic view of patient with BIH, highlighting papilledema. The prevalence of BIH is about 1 per 100,000; however, it is 20 times more commonly seen in overweight women. Young adults are the most affected age group. The intracranial pressure is raised above 250 mm Hg, sometimes less, without apparent cause such as a tumor. The patient complains of headache and visual disturbances, frequently chronic. The head pain is aspecific: moderate or severe, throbbing or pressure-type, unilateral or bilateral, frontal and/or occipital. As in intracranial hypertension headache of other origins, it is worsened by recumbency. Patients complain of unilateral or bilateral visual blurring, nausea and vomiting, and papilledema. Other findings include reduction of visual fields concentrically or by cuts, blind spot enlargement, seventh nerve palsy, and stiff neck. Diagnosis is confirmed by measurement of cerebrospinal fluid (CSF) pressure by a spinal tap. Other causes of raised intracranial pressure must be ruled out, such as tumor or cerebral venous thrombosis. Pathophysiologic mechanisms include decreased resorption of CSF, vasomotor dysregulation, and, more recently suspected, excess growth hormone and decreased monoamine activity. The relation between the pressure and the pain is not direct. Vitamin A or D, tetracycline, retinoids and even steroids have been implicated in the etiology of this syndrome, even at therapeutic dosages.

Figure 15-35. Treatment of pseudotumor cerebri. Weight loss must be aggressively pursued. Whenever a causative agent such as a tetracycline is present, it must be removed. Symptomatic treatment includes medications to decrease cerebrospinal fluid production such as acetazolamide or other diuretics. Analgesics and steroids have been used. More recently, octreotide, a somatostatin analog, has been tried with success in an open study [79]. Repeated spinal taps are useful, and ultimately whenever full control is not obtained with these treatments, surgical shunting must be considered. Optic nerve fenestration should be considered whenever vision is impaired.

Cervical Spine and Headache

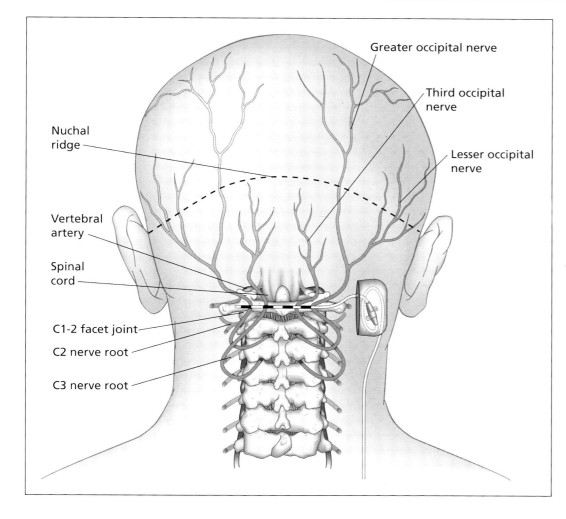

Greater occipital nerve

Third occipital nerve

Lesser occipital nerve

Nuchal ridge

Vertebral artery

Spinal cord

C1-2 facet joint

C2 nerve root

C3 nerve root

Figure 15-36. Occipital and C2 neuralgia. There is considerable overlap between occipital and C2 neuralgia, the difference being in the location of the underlying cause. Patients have a boring sensation in the occipital region radiating to the temporal and frontal areas punctuated by bouts of severe lancinating pain. In fewer than half the cases, hypertrophy of the zygapophyseal joint or atlanto-axial membrane or a local vascular malformation compressing the nerve can be demonstrated. Another site of compression is the nuchal ridge where the greater occipital nerve exits to the superficial subcutaneous tissues. Treatment consists of nerve blockade or rhizotomy of C2-3. More recently, electrical neurostimulators implanted in the suboccipital region have been tried and seem to offer relief [80]. (*Adapted from* Weiner [81].)

Diagnostic Criteria for Cervicogenic Headache

Major symptoms and signs
  Unilateral headache
  Neck involvement
    Pain precipitated by mechanical pressure to ipsilateral superior neck region or by awkward neck positioning
    Ipsilateral neck/shoulder/arm pain
    Reduced range of motion of cervical spine
Pain
  Of variable duration
  Moderate, usually nonthrobbing, starting in the neck and radiating forward
Other criteria
  Anesthetic blockade of the greater occipital nerve and/or C2 nerve root transiently relieve pain
  Female sex
  History of head/neck trauma

Figure 15-37. Diagnostic criteria for cervicogenic headache. In 1983 Sjaastad proposed the controversial concept of cervicogenic headache [82]. This array of symptoms is frequently encountered and can actually include some other more specific syndromes described earlier. The criteria do not stipulate a cause but rather a pattern of neck and head pain common to many neck disorders, including whiplash. Cervicogenic headache prompts radiographic, computed tomography, and/or magnetic resonance imaging focusing on the cervical spine; frequently, however, no abnormality is found. This headache often responds to nerve block with lidocaine and depot steroids in the greater occipital nerve or C2 area [83].

Secondary Headaches

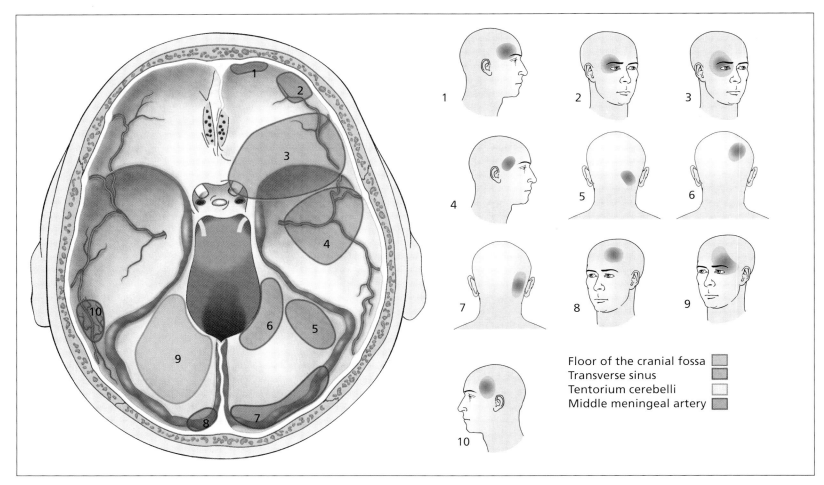

Figure 15-38. Pain-sensitive structures and their referred skin areas. The cutaneous projection of pain from intracranial structures can be extremely complex. Derived from stimulation of specific intracranial areas, this schematic highlights how unpredictable cutaneous projections can be. (*Adapted from* Dalessio [84].)

Floor of the cranial fossa
Transverse sinus
Tentorium cerebelli
Middle meningeal artery

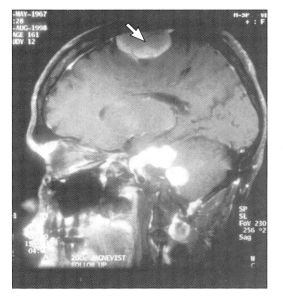

Figure 15-39. Neoplasm. Magnetic resonance imaging scan of a patient with neurofibromatosis type II. This patient presented with headache that fit all the International Headache Society criteria for migraine without aura except that it was secondary to the meningioma (*arrow*). The headache improved dramatically after removal of the tumor. Imaging was performed for this patient because of the high likelihood of finding an intracranial tumor.

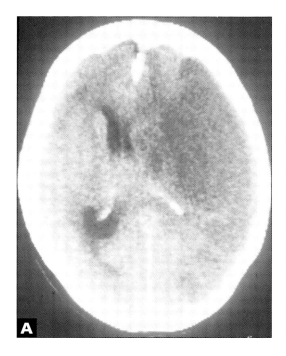
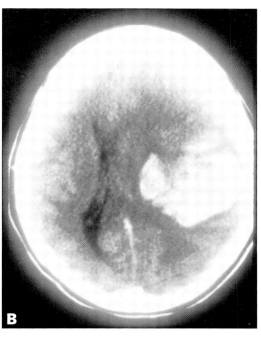

Figure 15-40. Cerebral herniation. **A,** Magnetic resonance imaging (MRI) scan showing herniation of brain tissue caused by an intracranial hemorrhage with underlying metastatic tumor, with definite midline shift (deviation of septum pellucidum and ventricles). **B,** MRI scan showing a massive subacute right middle cerebral infarct that developed enough edema to provoke herniation.

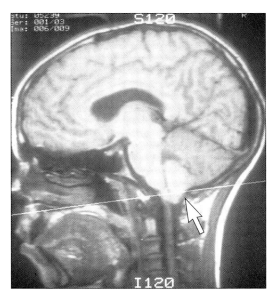

Figure 15-41. Arnold-Chiari malformation. The descent of cerebellar tonsils in the tight foramen magnum, the radiologic hallmark of this disease, is visible in this magnetic resonance imaging scan. *Arrow* marks the level of the foramen. Coughing, sneezing, or straining can suddenly push the cerebellar tonsils further into the foramen magnum, provoking headache at the base of the skull. Pressure on the posterior columns or their nuclei can cause numbness over the entire body.

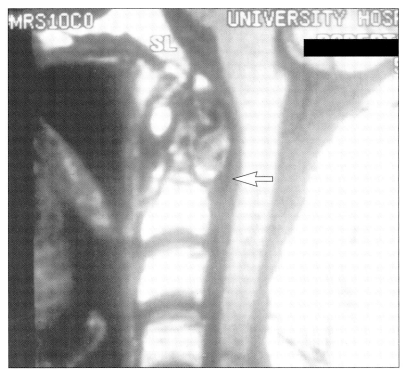

Figure 15-42. Traumatic headache. Magnetic resonance imaging scan of a patient with rheumatoid arthritis (RA) complaining of neck pain due to fracture of the odontoid of C2 (*arrow*), frequently observed in RA. Fractures of the skull or neck structures can produce pain from damage to periosteum or bone.

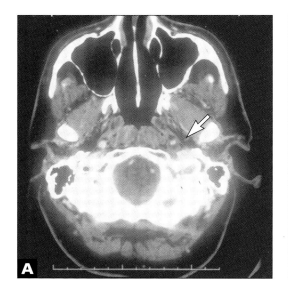 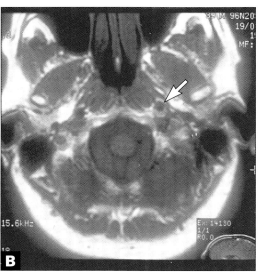

Figure 15-43. Carotid dissection. Spontaneous carotid dissection in a 40-year-old man who presented with two episodes of left frontal headache with no clinical abnormalities. **A,** Computed tomography revealed a defect in the lumen of the vessel on the left side, with a ring around it delineating the wall of the artery (*arrow*). **B,** Magnetic resonance (MR) imaging scan defined the lesion with a ring of hyperintensity around the lumen, itself defined by the classic dark round area corresponding to the flow void (*arrow*). MR angiography was of little help, barely showing an irregular lumen in the upper cervical portion of the carotid and in the intrapetrous carotid canal. The lesion was not visible on angiogram because of its subadventitial location. Carotid dissection commonly follows severe head or neck trauma, but sometimes occurs after only minor trauma or no trauma at all. Following three months' treatment with anticoagulant medication, this patient recovered completely.

Differential Diagnosis of Vascular Headache

Ischemic stroke
  Thrombotic
  Embolic
Vasculitis
  Arteritis
    Giant cell arteritis
      Temporal arteritis
      Takayasu's arteritis
    Polyarteritis nodosa
      Classic polyarteritis
      Allergic angiitis (Churg-Strauss syndrome)
      Systemic necrotizing vasculitis
    Isolated CNS angiitis
    Wegener's granulomatosis
    Hypersensitivity vasculitis
  Arteriolitis
    Systemic lupus erythematosus
    Behçet's disease
  Venous thrombosis
  Subarachnoid hemorrhage
  Intracerebral hemorrhage

Figure 15-44. Differential diagnosis of vascular headaches. The most common causes of vascular headaches are listed.

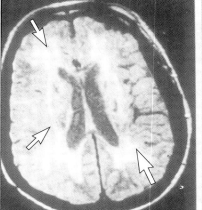 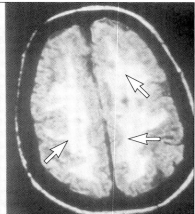

Figure 15-45. Cerebral autosomal dominant arteriopathy with subcortical infarcts and leukoencephalopathy (CADASIL). Magnetic resonance imaging scans demonstrating multiple subcortical infarcts (*arrows*). Patients with CADASIL typically present with migraine-type headaches; they also experience multiple subcortical strokes and often have encephalopathy. The disease is due to a mutation on chromosome 19, where the locus of familial hemiplegic migraine is also found [85]. (*From* Tournier-Lasserve [85]; with permission.)

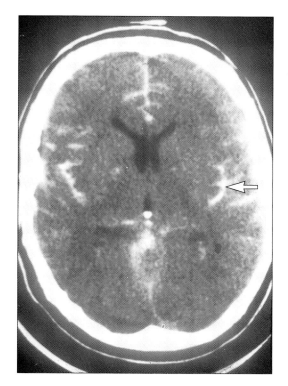

Figure 15-46. Subarachnoid hemorrhage (SAH). Computed tomography scan of a patient with SAH. Note that all the sulci are filled with blood (*arrow*). One of the most dramatic vascular causes of headache, SAH provokes a "thunderclap" headache [86]. The pain is sudden, severe, tends to migrate from head to neck, and frequently patients are obtunded and/or have a focal neurological deficit. When there is an aneurysm, there can be a first episode of headache (*sentinel headache*) that tends to resolve; this is probably due to a limited bleeding. However, it usually heralds a second episode, which is accompanied by massive bleeding. Note the absence of blood in ventricles.

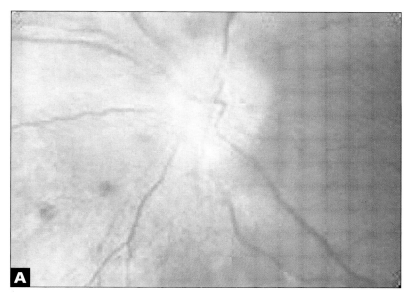

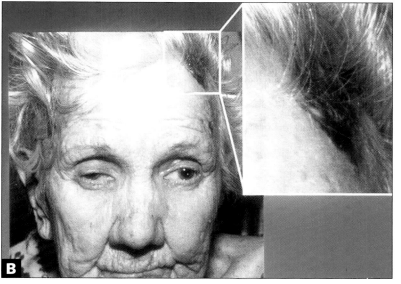

Figure 15-47. Giant cell arteritis. Also called temporal arteritis, this is the most common arteritis. Typically seen in patients over 50 years of age, this disease attacks the internal elastic membrane of extracranial arteries by the granulomatous process with giant cells. It involves midsize and large arteries but total occlusion is unusual. **A,** Fundoscopy demonstrating anterior ischemic optic neuropathy secondary to giant cell arteritis. Because it can become occluded rapidly, sudden onset of partial or complete blindness is possible. Rarely, intracranial arteries are involved, leading to hemispheric or brainstem stroke; other organs can be involved as well. Fever, malaise, weight loss, fatigue, and polymyalgia rheumatica are typical symptoms along with the headache. Diagnosis is suspected in the presence of a combination of the symptoms listed and an elevated erythrocyte sedimentation rate (ESR). Treatment consists of high-dose steroids, tapering to long-term maintenance, adjusted based on continued ESR monitoring. **B,** This patient suffered from headache, weight loss, anterior ischemic optic neuropathy, scalp necrosis, and multiple oculomotor nerve palsies. (*Courtesy of* Bradley K. Farris, MD, University of Oklahoma Health Sciences Center, Department of Ophthalmology, Oklahoma City, Oklahoma.)

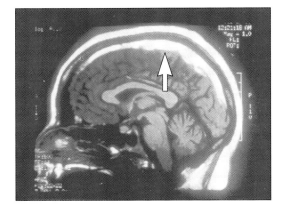
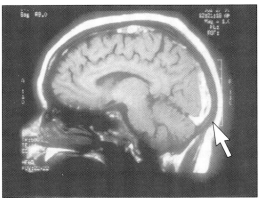
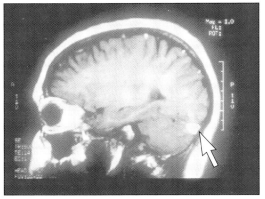
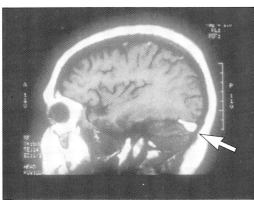

Figure 15-48. Intracranial venous thrombosis. Magnetic resonance (MR) imaging scans demonstrating the enhancement of the superior sagittal sinus (*arrows*), confirming intracranial venous thrombosis; alternatively, MR angiography can be diagnostic as well. Common in pregnancy, coagulopathies, dehydration, and Addison's disease, intracranial venous thrombosis can cause severe headaches as well as seizures and strokes.

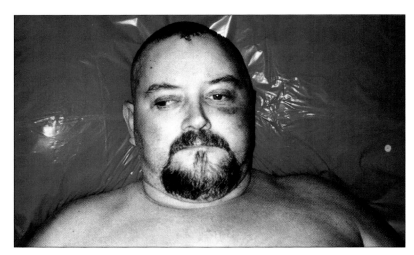

Figure 15-49. Tolosa-Hunt syndrome. This syndrome causes intense unilateral periorbital headaches accompanied by various cranial nerve palsies. This otherwise healthy patient developed a severe left periorbital headache with partial deficit of cranial nerves III and VI. A biopsy of the cavernous sinus confirmed the inflammatory nature of the disease; magnetic resonance imaging was normal. The patient improved dramatically on intravenous steroids.

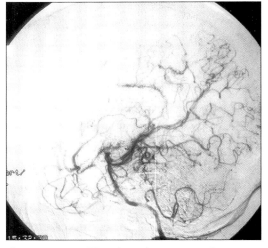

Figure 15-50. Vasculitis. Angiogram of a patient with systemic lupus erythematous who presented with headache. Note the irregular stenosis of mid-size arteries in the vertebral distribution. Angiitis can cause migraine-type headaches.

Differential Diagnosis of Infectious Headache

Intracerebral infections
  Acute infectious processes (bacterial or viral)
    Meningitis (*Neisseria, Streptococcus*)
    Parenchymal brain infections
      Encephalitis (herpes simplex)
      Abscess (*Staphylococcus*)
  Chronic infectious processes (bacterial, fungal, or viral)
    Meningitis (atypical tubercle bacillus, cryptococcus)
    Parenchymal
      Encephalitis (mucor mycosis, syphilis, HIV)
      Abscess (*Nocardia, Cryptococcus*)
  Infectious vasculitis
    Syphilis
Extracranial infections
  Infections of endothelial-lined cavities
  Infectious vasculitis
  Abscess

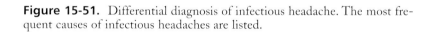

Figure 15-51. Differential diagnosis of infectious headache. The most frequent causes of infectious headaches are listed.

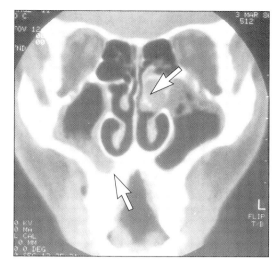

Figure 15-52. Sinusitis. Magnetic resonance imaging scan of a patient with bilateral (ethmoid and maxillary) sinusitis (*arrows*). Inflammation of the sinuses, mucous membranes of the nose, the middle ear cavity, and the mastoid air cells can produce significant pain that is often misdiagnosed as headache.

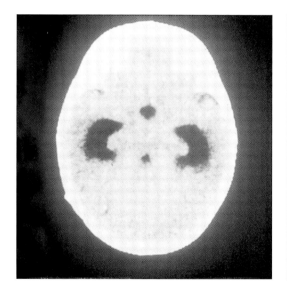
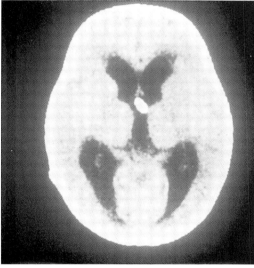

Figure 15-53. Tuberculous meningitis. Computed tomography scan of a patient with tuberculous meningitis; obstructive hydrocephalus was the ultimate cause of the patient's headache. Although this disease is typically revealed by cranial nerve palsies and other neurological deficits, and by systemic symptoms, occasionally headache can be the first complaint.

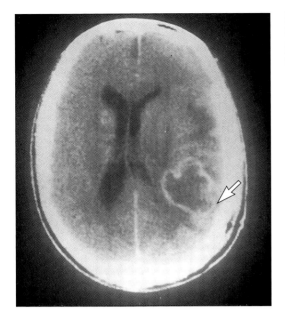

Figure 15-54. Toxoplasmosis. Magnetic resonance imaging scan of a patient with toxoplasmosis (*arrow*) initially revealed by a headache. Typically but not exclusively seen in immunosuppressed patients, toxoplasmosis can cause a headache due to intracranial hypertension, accompanied by cranial nerve palsies and blurred vision.

Differential Diagnosis of Toxic Headache

Toxic gases
  Suffocation or hypoxia (carbon monoxide, carbon dioxide, excess nitrogen)
  Direct toxic effect (sulfur-containing compounds, or gases from toxic compounds)
Organic solvents
Drugs (legitimate or illegal)
Exposure to heavy metals (lead, arsenic, mercury, bismuth)

Figure 15-55. Differential diagnosis of toxic headache. The most common toxic causes of headaches are listed.

Differential Diagnosis of Metabolic Headache

Major organ failure
  Hepatic failure
  Renal failure
  Pulmonary failure with carbon dioxide retention
Endocrinopathies
  Hyperthyroidism
  Hypothyroidism
  Hypoparathyroidism
  Addison's disease
  Cushing's disease
Conditions producing headache associated with vascular changes
  Fever
  Anemia
  Carbon dioxide retention with vasodilatation

Figure 15-56. Differential diagnosis of metabolic headache. The most frequent metabolic causes of headache are listed.

References

1. Couch JR: Headache to worry about. *Med Clin North Am* 1993, 77:141–167.

2. Rasmussen BK, Jensen R, Schroll M, Olesen J: Epidemiology of headache in a general population—a prevalence study. *J Clin Epidemiol* 1991, 44(11):1147–1157.

3. Lipton RB, Stewart WF: Migraine in the United States: a review of epidemiology and health care use. *Neurology* 1993, 43:S6–S10.

4. Schwartz BS, Stewart WF, Simon D, Lipton RB: Epidemiology of tension-type headache. *JAMA* 1998, 279(5):381–383.

5. Headache Classification Committee of the International Headache Society: Classification and diagnostic criteria for headache disorders, cranial neuralgias and facial pain. *Cephalalgia* 1988, 7:1–96.

6. Launer LJ, Terwindt GM, Ferrari MD: The prevalence and characteristics of migraine in a population-based cohort: the GEM study. *Neurology* 1999, 53(3):537–542.

7. Stewart WF, Linet MS, Celentano DD, *et al.*: Age- and sex-specific incidence rates of migraine with and without aura. *Am J Epidemiol* 1991, 134:1111–1120.

8. Stewart WF, Lipton RB, Liberman J: Variation in migraine prevalence by race. *Neurology* 1996, 47(1):52–59.

9. Lipton RB, Stewart WF: Acute migraine therapy. *Headache* 1999, 39:S20–S26.

10. Hu XH, Markson LE, Lipton RB, *et al.*: Burden of migraine in the United States: disability and economic costs. *Arch Intern Med* 1999, 159(8):813–818.

11. Terwindt GM, Ferrari MD, Tijhuis M, *et al.*: The impact of migraine on quality of life in the general population: the GEM study. *Neurology* 2000, 55:624–629.

12. Couch JR: Complexities of presentation and pathogenesis of migraine headache. In *Treating the Headache Patient*. Edited by Cady RK, Fox AW. New York: Marcel Dekker; 1995.

13. Lenaerts M: Migraine and epilepsy: comorbidity and temporal relationship. Paper presented at: Ninth Congress of the International Society; June 1999; Barcelona, Spain.

14. Merikangas KR, Merikangas JR, Angst J: Headache syndromes and psychiatric disorders: association and familial transmission. *J Psychiatr Res* 1993, 27:197–210.

15. Olesen J, Tfelt-Hansen P, Welch KMA: *The Headaches*. New York: Raven Press; 1993:256–266.

16. Lennox WG, Gibbs EL, Gibbs FA: Effect of ergotamine tartrate on the cerebral circulation of man. *J Pharmacol Exp Ther* 1935, 53:113.

17. Leão AAP: Spreading depression of activity in cerebral cortex. *J Neurophysiol* 1944, 7:359–390.

18. Lashley KS: Patterns of cerebral integration indicated by scotomas of migraine. *Arch Neurol Psychiat* 1941, 46:331.

19. Lauritzen M, Olesen J: Regional cerebral blood flow during migraine attacks by Xenon-133 inhalation and emission tomography. *Brain* 1984, 107:447–461.

20. Olesen J, Friberg L, Olsen TS, *et al.*: Timing and topography of cerebral blood flow, aura, and headache during migraine attacks. *Ann Neurol* 1990, 28:791–798.

21. Cutrer FM, Sorensen AG, Weisskoff RM, *et al.*: Perfusion-weighted imaging defects during spontaneous migrainous aura. *Ann Neurol* 1998, 43:25–31.

22. Woods RP, Iacoboni M, Mazziotta JC: Brief report: bilateral spreading cerebral hypoperfusion during spontaneous migraine headache. *N Engl J Med* 1994, 331:1689–1692.

23. Weiller C, May A, Limmroth V, *et al.*: Brain stem activation in spontaneous human migraine attacks. *Nat Med* 1995, 1:658–660.

24. Raskin NH, Hosobuchi Y, Lamb S: Headache may arise from perturbation of brain. *Headache* 1987, 27:416–420.

25. Goadsby PJ, Edvinsson L, Ekman R: Vasoactive peptide release in the extracerebral circulation of humans during migraine headache. *Ann Neurol* 1990, 28:183–187.

26. Moskowitz MA: Neurogenic versus vascular mechanisms of sumatriptan and ergot alkaloids in migraine. *Trends Pharmacol Sci* 1992, 13:307–311.

27. Goadsby PJ, Zagami AS, Lambert GA: Neural processing of craniovascular pain: a synthesis of the central structures involved in migraine. *Headache* 1991, 31:365–371.

28. Schoenen REF: Contingent negative variation: methods and potential interest in headache. *Cephalalgia* 1993, 13(1):28–32.

29. Áfra J, Cecchini AP, DePasqua V, *et al.*: Visual evoked potentials during long periods of pattern-reversal stimulation in migraine. *Brain* 1998, 121:233–241.

30. Wang W, Lenaerts M, Schoenen J: Reduced habituation of pattern-reversal visual evoked responses in migraine. Paper presented at: International Conference of the European Headache Federation; June 1994; Liege, Belgium.

31. Welch KMA, Cao Y, Aurora S, *et al.*: MRI of the occipital cortex, red nucleus, and substantia nigra during visual aura of migraine. *Neurology* 1998, 51:1465–1469.

32. Joutel A, Bousser MG, Biousse V, *et al.*: A gene for familial hemiplegic migraine maps to chromosome 19. *Nat Genet* 1993, 5:40–45.

33. Ophoff RA, Terwindt GM, Vergouwe MN, *et al.*: Familial hemiplegic migraine and episodic ataxia type-2 are caused by mutations in the Ca2+ channel gene CACNL1A4. *Cell* 1996, 87:543–552.

34. Barbiroli B, Montagna P, Cortelli P, *et al.*: Abnormal brain and muscle metabolism shown by 31P magnetic resonance spectroscopy in patients affected by migraine with aura. *Neurology* 1992, 42:1209–1214.

35. Welch KM, Levine SR, D'Andrea G, *et al.*: Preliminary observation on brain energy metabolism in migraine studied by in vivo phosphorus 31 NMR spectroscopy. *Neurology* 1989, 39:538–541.

36. Ferrari MD, Odink J, Tapparelli C, *et al.*: Serotonin metabolism in migraine. *Neurology* 1989, 39:1239–1242.

37. Humphrey PPA: 5-Hydroxytryptamine and the pathophysiology of migraine. *J Neurol* 1991, 238:S38–S44.

38. Ferrari MD: Systemic biochemistry. In *The Headaches*. Edited by Olesen J, Tfelt-Hansen P, Welch KMA. New York: Raven Press; 1993:179–183.

39. Parsons AA, Whalley ET: Characterization of the 5-HT receptor which mediates contraction of the human isolated basilar artery. *Cephalalgia* 1989, 9(S9):47–51.

40. Fozard JR, Kalkman HO: 5-HT in nervous system disease and migraine. *Curr Opin Neurol Neurosurg* 1992, 5(4):496–502.

41. Peroutka SJ: Antimigraine drug interactions with serotonin receptor subtypes in human brain. *Ann Neurol* 1988, 23(5):500–504.

42. Peroutka SJ: Dopamine and migraine. *Neurology* 1997, 49(3):650–656.

43. Goadsby PJ: The pathophysiology of primary headache. In *Headache in Clinical Practice*. Edited by Silberstein SD, Lipton RB, Goadsby PJ. Oxford: ISIS Medical Media; 1998.

44. Storer RJ, Goadsby PJ: Trigeminovascular nociceptive transmission involves N-methyl-D-aspartate and non-N-methyl-D-aspartate glutamate receptors. *Neuroscience* 1999, 90(4):1371–1376.

45. Schoenen J, Sianard-Gainko J, Lenaerts M: Blood magnesium levels in migraine. *Cephalalgia* 1991, 11:97–99.

46. Ramadan NM, Halvorson H, Vande-Linde A, *et al.* Low brain magnesium level in migraine. *Headache* 1989, 29(7):416–419.

47. Somerville BM: The role of estradiol withdrawal in the etiology of menstrual migraine. *Neurology* 1972, 22:355–365.

48. Welch KMA, Darnley D, Simkins RT: The role of estrogens in migraine: a review and hypothesis. *Cephalalgia* 1984, 4:227–236.

49. Mathew NT, Kailasam J, Meadors L, *et al.*: Intravenous valproate sodium (depacon) aborts migraine rapidly: a preliminary report. *Headache* 2000, 40(9):720–723.

50. Goadsby PJ, Hargreaves RJ: Mechanisms of action of serotonin 5-HT1B/D agonists: insights into migraine pathophysiology using rizatriptan. *Neurology* 2000, 55:S8–S14.

51. Goadsby PJ: The scientific basis of medication choice in symptomatic migraine treatment. *Can J Neurol Sci* 1999, 26:20–26.

52. Humphrey PP, Feniuk W: Mode of action of the anti-migraine drug sumatriptan. *Trends Pharmacol Sci* 1991, 12:444–446.

53. Silberstein SD: Rizatriptan versus usual care in long-term treatment of migraine. *Neurology* 2000, 55:S25–S28.

54. Solomon GD, Cady RK, Klapper JA, *et al.*: Clinical efficacy and tolerability of 2.5 mg zolmitriptan for the acute treatment of migraine. *Neurology* 1997, 49:1219–1225.

55. Nappi G, Sicuteri F, Byrne M, *et al.*: Oral sumatriptan compared with placebo in the acute treatment of migraine. *J Neurol* 1994, 241:138–144.

56. Sargent J, Kirchner J, Davis R, Kirkhart B: Oral sumatriptan is effective and well tolerated for the acute treatment of migraine: results of a multicenter study. *Neurology* 1995, 45:S10–S14.

57. Tfelt-Hansen P, Ryan RE Jr: Oral therapy for migraine: comparisons between rizatriptan and sumatriptan. A review of four randomized, double-blind clinical trials. *Neurology* 2000, 55:S19–S24.

58. The International 311C90 Long-term Study Group: The long-term tolerability and efficacy of oral zolmitriptan (Zomig, 311C90) in the acute treatment of migraine. An international study. *Headache* 1998, 38:173–183.

59. Cady RK, Lipton RB, Hall C, *et al.*: Treatment of mild headache in disabled migraine sufferers: results of the Spectrum Study. *Headache* 2000, 40(10):792–797.

60. Lipton RB, Stewart WF, Cady R, *et al.*: Sumatriptan for the range of headaches in migraine sufferers: results of the Spectrum Study. *Headache* 2000, 40(10):1–9.

61. Raskin NH: Repetitive intravenous dihydroergotamine as therapy for intractable migraine. *Neurology* 1986, 36(7): 995–997.

62. Goadsby PJ: How do the currently used prophylactic agents work in migraine? *Cephalalgia* 1997, 17:85–92.

63. Breslau N, Merikangas K, Bowden CL: Comorbidity of migraine and major affective disorders. *Neurology* 1994, 44:S17–S22.

64. Breslau N, Davis GC, Schultz LR, Peterson EL: Migraine and major depression: a longitudinal study. *Headache* 1994, 34:387–393.

65. Schoenen J, Jacquy J, Lenaerts M: Effectiveness of high-dose riboflavin in migraine prophylaxis. A randomized controlled trial. *Neurology* 1998, 50:466–470.

66. Silberstein SD, Silberstein MM: New concepts in the pathogenesis of headache: migraine versus tension-type headache. *Phys Assist* 1991, 9:67–81.

67. Jensen R, Olesen J: Initiating mechanisms of experimentally-induced tension-type headache. *Cephalalgia* 1996, 16:175.

68. Schoenen J, Sandor P: Headache. In *Textbook of Pain*, edn 4. Edited by Wall PD, Melzack R. New York: Churchill Livingstone; 1999.

69. Lance JW, Ekbom K: In *Cluster Headaches: Mechanism and Management*. Edited by Kudrow L. New York: Oxford University Press; 1980:27–28.

70. Hardebo JE: On pain mechanisms in cluster headache. *Headache* 1991, 31:91–106.

71. May A, Bahra A, Büchel, *et al.*: PET and MRA findings in cluster headache and MRA in experimental pain. *Neurology* 2000, 55:1328–1335.

72. Lenaerts M, Couch JR: Trigeminal neuralgia. *Emedicine* [serial online]. 2001. Available at: http://www.emedicine.com/oph/NEUROLOGIC_DISORDERS.htm. Accessed January 25, 2001.

73. Blom S: Trigeminal neuralgia: a treatment with a new anticonvulsant drug. *Lancet* 1962, 1:839–840.

74. Fromm GH, Terrence CF, Chattha AS: Baclofen in the treatment of trigeminal neuralgia: double-blind study and long-term follow-up. *Ann Neurol* 1984, 15(3):240–244.

75. McLaughlin MR, Jannetta PJ, Clyde BL, *et al.*: Microvascular decompression of cranial nerves: lessons learned after 4400 operations. *J Neurosurg* 1999, 90(1):1–8.

76. Evans RW, Armon C, Frohman EM, Goodin DS: Assessment: prevention of post-lumbar puncture headaches: report of the therapeutics and technology assessment subcommittee of the American Academy of Neurology. *Neurology* 2000, 55:909–914.

77. Lenaerts M, Pepin JL, Tombu S, Schoenen J: No significant effect of an "atraumatic" needle on the incidence of post-lumbar puncture headache or traumatic tap. *Cephalalgia* 1993, 13:296–297.

78. Williams E, Fawcett W, Jenkins G: Preventing headache after lumbar puncture. Optimism generally quoted for epidural blood patching is unwarranted. *BMJ* 1998, 317:1588–1589.

79. Panagopoulos G, Gotsi A, Piaditis G, *et al.*: Treatment of benign intracranial hypertension with octreotide [abstract]. *American Academy of Neurology.* 1998.

80. Lou L: Uncommon areas of electrical stimulation for pain relief. *Curr Rev Pain* 2000, 4(5):407–412.

81. Weiner RL: The future of peripheral nerve neurostimulation. *Neurol Res* 2000, 22:299–303.)

82. Sjaastad O, Saunte C, Hovdahl H, *et al.*: "Cervicogenic" headache: a hypothesis. *Cephalalgia* 1983, 3(4):249–256

83. Sjaastad O, Fredriksen TA, Pfaffenrath V: Cervicogenic headache: diagnostic criteria. *Headache* 1990, 30:725–726.

84. Dalessio JD: In *Wolff's Headache and Other Head Pain*, edn 3. Edited by Dalessio JD, Silberstein SD. New York: Oxford University Press; 1972:71.

85. Tournier-Lasserve E, Joutel A, Melki J, *et al.*: Cerebral autosomal dominant arteriopathy with subcortical infarcts and leukoencephalopathy maps to chromosome 19q12. *Nat Genet* 1993, 3:256–259.

86. Day JW, Raskin NH: Thunderclap headache: symptom of unruptured cerebral aneurysm. *Lancet* 1986, 2:1247–1248.

Index

N